Dedication

Dedicated to the memory of my parents, and to my sister, Connie.

CONTENTS

ACKNOWLEDGMENTS

I am indebted to the colleagues and clinicians who contributed chapters of outstanding quality to this textbook; their specialized interests provide unique perspectives on many aspects of women's health. I am also grateful to several friends, as well as some researchers whom I have never met; their willingness to read drafts of the original outline, guide decisions about topics for inclusion, and peer-review many chapters has greatly enhanced the value of the book. Special thanks to Dr. Sandro Galea for his support and that of the Department of Epidemiology at the Mailman School of Public Health.

During the book's gestation, women's health has received increased attention, often indicating the need for more gender-specific research to address the many unanswered questions raised by the authors in each chapter. Most epidemiology research relies on confidential questionnaire data collected from women and men; therefore, on behalf of all chapter authors, I express my gratitude to the vast number of people who have participated in the research referenced in this textbook and thank those who will be asked to contribute to future investigations.

The emotional support I received from my companion, Mario Fratti, my sister, Sally, and close friends, Danielle Maurice and Julie Olbert among many others, provided essential encouragement. I could not have functioned without the technical assistance provided by my sons, David and Daniel. I thank you all for your patience during this long and time-consuming project.

Ruby T. Senie

It is an honor to write a few words of introduction to this volume about the epidemiology of women's health. This book is a magisterial effort by Dr. Ruby Senie to bring together in one volume a vast body of literature about the morbidity and mortality that characterizes women's health at the beginning of the 21st century. The information gathered here is, of course, all available elsewhere, but is both made accessible and brought into sharp relief by its assembly in the same book.

This book starts with very helpful grounding chapters in the core concepts of epidemiology. This proves a valuable addition going forward, making the subsequent chapters accessible both to readers who are familiar and those who may be unfamiliar with epidemiologic terms. It then moves on to sections that cover health promotion, sexual health, sexually transmitted diseases, endocrine and autoimmune conditions, malignancies, chronic conditions, and aging. The book ends with two most interesting chapters about potential research directions in the field. The chapters, diverse and authored by a broad range of experts in the field, all well capture the state of the science in each particular area and contribute to a whole that is very much greater than the sum of the parts.

Many themes emerge from a reading of these chapters that are relevant not only to women's health but also to our understanding of the causes of morbidity and mortality more broadly. At the risk of minimizing the impact of other concepts covered in the book, I highlight here five themes that I thought emerged clearly from the book and that are at the conceptual core of the science summarized in this book.

First, it is clear from these chapters that events and exposures across the life course beginning in utero affect health conditions as women grow through adolescence into adulthood and senior ages. This argues very strongly for a life-course perspective on the production of health more broadly and for women's health in particular.

Second, foundational social factors inexorably shape the health of women, particularly those who live in poor urban communities and in rural settings. Of contemporary concern, the rapid democratization of health information is, in many ways, contributing to a widening in the health gap between women with and those without access to financial resources as the former fall farther and farther behind in access to health information and its attendant positive consequences.

Third, we have seen tremendous success in prevention, in delaying the onset of chronic disease both through health behavior modification (e.g., routine exercise, adequate nutrition, and avoidance of cigarette smoking) through minimizing adverse exposures. This has led to the now well-documented compression in morbidity in later life making an effort to focus on healthy aging and on finding dignified approaches to treatment in the later stages of life ever more important.

Fourth, even with success in prevention, emerging threats to women's health suggest that complacency in the area ill serves us. The epidemic of obesity especially among youth and young adults may, over the coming decades, undermine some of the progress that has lowered chronic disease rates. How to interrupt this growing problem has become the focus of much research as the proportion of the population classified as overweight and obese continues to go up, potentially increasing rates of hypertension, heart disease, and some cancers.

Fifth, the opportunities for innovative epidemiologic approaches to improve women's health in coming decades appear vast. The book includes chapters that highlight how research is addressing specific risks faced by women and their relatives whose genetic analyses indicate heightened susceptibility to psychological and physical conditions. It is not implausible that targeted health behavior changes and treatment options may contribute to optimizing prevention in the near future. Perhaps more exciting though, newer technologies and cells-to-society approaches to understanding the etiology of women's health stand to inspire new and as yet unknown approaches to population prevention that in the coming decades may very well have a deep and lasting impact on improving the health of women worldwide.

By pulling these chapters together in this book, Dr. Senie has succeeded, to my mind, on three very different fronts. First, this book serves to provide the reader who is unfamiliar with the topic a firm grounding in the science of women's health. Second, even in an age of widely available but fragmented information, the cataloging of knowledge in one place remains an indispensable service. The expert reader will find much use in the chapters as reference and I suspect that many will return to specific chapters many times over, finding much here that can usefully ground future writing in the area. Third, in painting a comprehensive picture, this book serves to jog the mind, to illustrate for us what we know and what we do not know in the field, sowing seeds of future inquiry.

Ultimately the task here is vast: mapping the epidemiology of the principal causes of morbidity and mortality faced by slightly more than half of the world's population. Within that vastness is the challenge for the field: posing questions that are focused, useful, and up to the challenge. Although many useful questions do indeed arise on a daily basis from a careful reading of the latest publications in the field, by connecting the scientific dots, our direct line to ever more specific inquiry runs the risk of losing sight of the big picture. Dr. Senie's book remedies that, giving us a big picture that stands to remind us of the even bigger questions and, it is hoped, nudges our science forward.

Sandro Galea, MD, DrPH
Gelman Professor and Chair
Department of Epidemiology
Mailman School of Public Health
Columbia University
New York, New York

Kimberly J. Alvarez, MPH
Department of Epidemiology
Mailman School of Public Health
Columbia University
New York, New York

Cornelia J. Baines, MD, MSc, FACE
Professor Emerita
Dalla Lana School of Public Health
University of Toronto
Toronto, Ontario, Canada

Grant T. Baldwin, PhD, MPH
National Center for Injury Prevention and Control
Centers for Disease Control and Prevention
Atlanta, Georgia

Michael F. Ballesteros, PhD
National Center for Injury Prevention and Control
Centers for Disease Control and Prevention
Atlanta, Georgia

Gloria L. A. Beckles, MD, MSc
Medical Epidemiologist
Centers for Disease Control and Prevention
Division of Diabetes Translation, NCCDPHP
Atlanta, Georgia

Wendy Chung, MD, PhD
Herbert Irving Assistant Professor of Pediatrics and Medicine
Departments of Pediatrics and Medicine
Director of Clinical Genetics
Columbia University
New York, New York

Leslie L. Davidson, MD, MSc
Professor of Epidemiology and Pediatrics
Mailman School of Public Health
Columbia University
New York, New York

Patrick Dawson, BA, MPH
Department of Epidemiology Alumnus
Mailman School of Public Health
Columbia University
New York, New York

Moise Desvarieux, MD, PhD
Associate Professor of Epidemiology
Mailman School of Public Health
Columbia University
New York, New York

Lois J. Eldred, PA-C, MPH, DrPH
Division of General Internal Medicine
Johns Hopkins University School of Medicine and
Bloomberg School of Public Health
Baltimore, Maryland

Susan E. Foster, MSW
Vice President and Director, Policy Research and Analysis
The National Center on Addiction and Substance Abuse
Columbia University (CASAColumbia)
New York, New York

Gina Gambone, MPH
Research Assistant
Heilbrunn Department of Population and Family Health
Mailman School of Public Health
Columbia University
New York, New York

Ellen M. Ginzler, MD, MPH
Distinguished Teaching Professor of Medicine
Division of Rheumatology
SUNY Downstate Medical Center
Brooklyn, New York

Cynthia Golembeski, MPH
Mailman School of Public Health Alumna
Columbia University
New York, New York

Mark W. Green, MD
Director of Pain and Headache Medicine
Professor of Neurology and Anesthesiology
Department of Neurology
Mount Sinai School of Medicine
New York, New York

Heidi Mochari Greenberger, PhD, MPH, RD
Post Doctoral Research Fellow
Preventive Cardiology Program
Columbia University Medical Center
New York, New York

Heather Greenlee, ND, PhD
Assistant Professor of Epidemiology and Medical Oncology (in
    Medicine)
Mailman School of Public Health
Columbia University
New York, New York

Judith S. Jacobson, DrPH, MBA
Associate Professor of Epidemiology
Mailman School of Public Health
Columbia University
New York, New York

Tamarra James-Todd, PhD, MPH
Research Fellow
Brigham and Women's Hospital
Harvard Medical School
Boston, Massachusetts

Sarah C. Janicki, MD, MPH
Assistant Professor
Gertrude H. Sergievsky Center
Department of Neurology
Columbia University
New York, New York

Leslie M. Kantor, MPH
Assistant Professor of Population and Family Health
Mailman School of Public Health
Columbia University
New York, New York

Wahida Karmally, DrPH, RD, CDE, CLS, FNLA
Associate Research Scientist Lecturer in Dentistry
Director of Nutrition
Irving Institute for Clinical and Translational Research
Columbia University Medical Center
New York, New York

Katherine M. Keyes, PhD
Assistant Professor of Epidemiology
Columbia University
New York, New York

Mary Kilty, MBA, MPH, MPhil
Department of Epidemiology
Mailman School of Public Health
Columbia University
New York, New York

Aimee Kroll-Desrosiers, MS
Biostatistician
University of Massachusetts Medical School
Department of Quantitative Health Sciences
Worcester, Massachusetts

Fredi Kronenberg, PhD
Consulting Professor
Department of Anesthesia, Stanford University College of
    Medicine
Michelle Clayman Institute for Gender Research
Stanford University
Stanford, California

Julie Ruckel Kumar, MPH
Clinical Research Manager
Department of Psychiatry and Behavioral Sciences
Memorial Sloan Kettering Cancer Center
New York, New York

Yuan-Chin Amy Lee, PhD
Visiting Instructor, Division of Public Health
Department of Family and Preventive Medicine
School of Medicine
University of Utah
Salt Lake City, Utah

Clara Li, MA
Neuropsychology Intern, Mt. Sinai Medical Center
Clinical Psychology Doctoral Student
Albert Einstein College of Medicine
Levittown, New York

Katherine M. Marconi, PhD, MS
Health Care Administration Program

University of Maryland University College
Adelphi, Maryland

Martha M. McKinney, PhD
Community Health Solutions
Asheville, North Carolina

Thelma J. Mielenz, PT, PhD, OCS
Assistant Professor of Epidemiology
Mailman School of Public Health
Columbia University
New York, New York

Stephen S. Morse, PhD
Professor of Epidemiology
Mailman School of Public Health
Columbia University
New York, New York

Jeri W. Nieves, PhD
Associate Professor of Epidemiology
Mailman School of Public Health
Columbia University
Clinical Research Center
Helen Hayes Hospital
West Haverstraw, New York

Rita K. Noonan, PhD
National Center for Injury Prevention and Control
Centers for Disease Control and Prevention
Atlanta, Georgia

Michelle D. Owens-Gary, PhD
Behavioral Scientist
Centers for Disease Control and Prevention
Division of Diabetes Translation, NCCDPHP
Atlanta, Georgia

Daniel J. Pilowsky, MD, MPH
Assistant Professor of Epidemiology and Psychiatry
Mailman School of Public Health
Columbia University
New York, New York

Joyce C. Pressley, PhD, MPH
Associate Professor of Epidemiology and Health Policy and
    Management
Mailman School of Public Health
Columbia University
New York, New York

Victoria H. Raveis, PhD
Research Professor and Director
Psychosocial Research Unit on Health, Aging & the Community
New York University
New York, New York

Linda Richter, PhD
Associate Director, Policy Research and Analysis
The National Center on Addiction and Substance Abuse
Columbia University (CASAColumbia)
New York, New York

Laura Robbins, DSW
Senior Vice President for Education & Academic Affairs
Associate Scientist, Research

Hospital for Special Surgery
New York, New York

Dara Rosenberg, DDS, MS, MPH, FACD
Director Department of Dentistry
St. Barnabas Hospital
Bronx, New York

Elizabeth Saenger, PhD
Director of Education
Center for Environmental Therapeutics
New York, New York

Julia Sheehy, PhD
Barnard College
Associate Director, Counseling Center
Adjunct Assistant Professor, Barnard College and Teachers College
Columbia University
New York, New York

William A. Sheremata, MD
Professor Emeritus of Clinical Neurology
Miller School of Medicine
University of Miami
Miami, Florida

David A. Sleet, PhD, FAAHB
National Center for Injury Prevention and Control
Centers for Disease Control and Prevention
Atlanta, Georgia

Laura Stadler, MS, RD
Irving Institute for Clinical and Translational Research
Columbia University Medical Center
New York, New York

Zena Stein, MA, MB, BCh, Dr Med Sc (Hon) Witwatersrand, Dr Sc (Hon) Columbia University
Professor of Epidemiology and Psychiatry Emerita
Mailman School of Public Health
Columbia University
HIV Center for Clinical and Behavioral Studies
New York State Psychiatric Institute
New York, New York

Judy A. Stevens, PhD, MPH
National Center for Injury Prevention and Control
Centers for Disease Control and Prevention
Atlanta, Georgia

Susan R. Sturgeon, DrPH, MPH
Associate Professor
School of Public Health and Health Sciences
University of Massachusetts Amherst
Amherst, Massachusetts

Eun Jung Suh, PhD
Assistant Professor of Clinical Psychology
Department of Psychiatry
Columbia University Medical Center
New York State Psychiatric Institute
New York, New York

Mervyn Susser, MB BCh, Dr Med Sc (Hon) Witwatersrand, FRCP (Edinburgh), FRCP (London)
Sergievsky Professor of Epidemiology Emeritus
Columbia University
New York, New York

Archana Vasudevan, MD
Consultant in Rheumatology
Department of General Medicine
Changi General Hospital
Singapore

Julie C. Will, PhD, MPH
Senior Epidemiologist
Centers for Disease Control and Prevention
Division of Heart Disease and Stroke Prevention
Atlanta, Georgia

Sidney J. Winawer, MD
Paul Sherlock Chair in Medicine
Gastroenterology and Nutrition Service, Department of Medicine
Memorial Sloan-Kettering Cancer Center
New York, New York

Ann G. Zauber, PhD
Member, Memorial Sloan-Kettering Cancer Center
Attending Biostatistician
Department of Epidemiology and Biostatistics
Memorial Sloan-Kettering Cancer Center
New York, New York

Zuo-Feng Zhang, MD, PhD
Professor, Department of Epidemiology
Fielding School of Public Health
University of California, Los Angeles
Los Angeles, California

Introduction to Epidemiology of Women's Health

An Overview of Women's Health: From the Past to the Future

Ruby T. Senie, PhD

Introduction

Women's health encompasses a continuum of biologic, psychologic, and social challenges that differ considerably from those of similarly aged men. These challenges significantly influence gender-specific longevity and quality of life. From conception, during in utero development, and continuing throughout the life course, women experience diverse health challenges influenced by genetic susceptibility interacting with changing endogenous hormone levels, environmental exposures, therapeutic interventions, and gender-specific cultural and psychosocial pressures.

Although most physical and mental conditions women experience do not specifically involve reproduction, endogenous hormones essential for childbearing significantly influence women's susceptibility to infectious diseases, autoimmune and rheumatologic disorders, and cancer. Compared with men and the clinical challenges they face, women experience disparities in health outcomes frequently affected by social, economic, and political inequities, especially among some American racial and ethnic groups.

The organization of this textbook reflects the concepts of life-course epidemiology in which health behaviors established at young ages have a significant impact on health status and quality of life in senior years. The topics selected represent some of the major infectious and chronic conditions women face across the life span from exposures in utero, activities during youth, development during puberty, reproductive decisions, and health patterns following menopause.

Each chapter presents findings from epidemiologic and psychosocial research primarily conducted among Americans; the focus is on studies that consider patterns of health and disease among groups rather than individual patients. The material should alert students and professionals, regardless of gender, to the unique health challenges women experience. Some of the conditions and diseases affect only women, others are more prevalent or serious among women, and some have risk factors or require interventions that differ for women compared with men with similar clinical problems.

Although women comprise more than 50% of the U.S. population, their healthcare needs had received limited research attention until recent years; women were often excluded from studies of diseases that affect both genders simply because changing levels of endogenous hormones complicated studies or because exposures might endanger a developing fetus. This discriminatory pattern changed as more women were successfully elected to leadership positions, forcing expansion of federally supported research to require the inclusion of women in every appropriate study.

This opening chapter provides a brief description of the changing political climate in the United States during the past 4 decades that significantly improved the lives of women, reviews three historical health transitions of the 20th century, and provides an overview of the diseases and conditions discussed in each section.

Politics Associated with Women's Health

A landmark event affecting women's health occurred in 1971 with the publication of *Our Bodies, Ourselves* by the Boston Women's Health Book Collective. Initially the text was prepared for a course "by and for women" to provide accurate and accessible information about female anatomy and physiology in addition to encouraging gender-relevant health policy changes. Since the publication of the first book, multiple additional texts with more detailed information have been published. The women's movement provided the impetus for women to demand inclusion in policymaking locally, resulting in more women being elected to state and federal government positions, including both houses of Congress.

The Congressional Caucus for Women's Issues, initially formed in 1977 by 15 representatives, significantly influenced the legal, economic, and health status of American women.[1] These representatives were aware that major clinical research had excluded women; therefore, one of their early campaigns led to legislation encouraging all federally funded clinical studies to include women unless the health conditions exclusively affected men. Caucus members ultimately recognized that stronger oversight was required for the policy to change.[1,2]

The nonprofit Women's Research and Education Institute (WREI), also established in 1977, contributed to the changing view of the health needs of women. The WREI staff provided synthesized data collected from many sources, which they formatted for presentation by federal and state policymakers, scholars, and advocates.[3] WREI's current mission includes identifying issues and contributing to policy decisions affecting women at home, in the workplace, and in the broader community through policy-establishing meetings, online publications, and internship positions for college students.[3]

Twenty years ago, the visibility of women's health received increased attention when Dr. Bernadine Healy was nominated as the first female director of the National Institutes of Health (NIH). That same day in 1990, NIH announced the establishment of the Office of Research on Women's Health (ORWH). The purpose of the new agency was to monitor and guide the *required* inclusion of women in NIH-funded studies that addressed medical conditions common to both women and men.[4]

The Women's Health Initiative (WHI), one of the primary health research programs developed by Dr. Healy, was the largest study ever conducted by NIH. More than 150,000 middle- and older-aged women were enrolled in one or more components of the initiative, including the randomized clinical trials and observational studies designed to identify risk and protective factors associated with heart disease, breast cancer, osteoporosis, and other clinical conditions. The first of many publications in 2002 reported increased risk of both heart disease and breast cancer among women randomized to received estrogen combined with progestin in contrast to placebo, necessitating early termination of one component of the WHI clinical trial.[5] After publication of these unanticipated results, hormone use by many postmenopausal women declined rapidly and incidence rates of breast cancer declined.[6] Follow-up of WHI study participants has provided important data on health effects of various exposures as referenced in this textbook.

By Executive Order in March 2009, President Obama created the White House Council on Women and Girls with a mandate that each federal agency account for the needs of women and girls when formulating policies in the programs they created and the legislation they support.[7] Although many women have been selected to chair and direct the activities of several federal agencies, the president was expressing concern for the needs of all American women when the Council on Women and Girls was created.[7]

In anticipation of its 20th anniversary, ORWH held public workshops in 2009–2010 in several regions of the country to review past accomplishments and set goals for the next decade. Members of scientific, medical, public health, and advocacy organizations, as well as the public, presented their action items for consideration. In addition to defining gender-specific health needs, disparities in health outcomes among subgroups were discussed and interventions proposed. At the ORWH anniversary meeting in the fall of 2010, the report, *A Vision for 2020*, was unveiled. Six broad goals were included in the strategic plan (Table 1-1); these goals provide a comprehensive framework aimed at stimulating research planning by multidisciplinary researchers and students interested in women's health.[4]

One goal of ORWH is to increase the number of women recruited to senior-level decision-making positions in order to leverage an expansion of federal funding for gender-specific health research. Career choices for women have expanded in the last several decades, requiring women to balance career options with childbearing demands; these personal goals often coincide in terms of timing. Reproductive decisions may create emotional turmoil, generating long-term physical and psychologic health challenges. Such life decisions were clearly described in Elsa Walsh's *Divided Lives*, a biographical account of three accomplished women, one of whom chose to become a breast surgeon but not a parent as she feared the conflicting time demands of each role.[8] Although a more supportive environment for women has been evolving, childbearing decisions continue to require compromises. Leadership by women is essential to appropriately guide research addressing gender-specific career choices, related health issues, and employment policies to enable childbearing by career-oriented women.

In July 2011 the Institute of Medicine (IOM) released the report *Clinical Preventive Services for Women, Closing the Gap* in response to a charge by the U.S. Department of Health and Human Services to review current preventive practices for women and to identify necessary additions.[9] The IOM report has guided policy decisions included in

Table 1-1
Goals defined in the Office of Research on Women's Health strategic plan for 2020
• Increase the study of sex and gender differences in basic biomedical and behavioral research
• Incorporate findings of sex and gender differences into the design and application of new technologies, medical devices, and therapeutic drugs
• Actualize personalized prevention, diagnostics, and therapeutics for women and girls
• Create strategic alliances and partnerships to maximize the domestic and global impact of women's health research
• Develop and implement new communication and social networking technologies to increase understanding and appreciation of women's health and wellness research
• Employ innovative strategies to build a well-trained, diverse, and vigorous women's health research workforce
Source; Data from Pinn VW, Clayton JA, Begg L, Sass SE. Public partnership for a vision for women's health research in 2020. *J Women's Health*. 2010;19:1603–1607.

the controversial Patient Protection and Affordable Care Act (ACA), which focuses on preventive services oriented to increasing optimum health status among Americans while reducing the burdens of long-term, debilitating illnesses.[10] Women are expected to benefit more than men from the focus on prevention given their longer life expectancy, reproductive health needs, gender-specific health problems, and higher incidence of chronic and disabling conditions. Contraception, a preventive service identified by the IOM, has enabled reduced family size with longer intervals between births, significantly improving the health and longevity of all women although disparities remain when rates are compared by racial/ethnic and economic subgroups as noted in Chapter 3.[12] The IOM report is briefly reviewed in Chapter 4.

Historical Perspective

The lives of American women were significantly influenced by three historical public health challenges of the 20th century, challenges that continue to have an impact on the goals established by ORWH for the next decade.

Epidemics of Infectious Diseases

Uncontrolled infectious diseases, especially in crowded urban areas, were major recurring threats early in the 20th century until public health interventions reduced exposures and prevented transmission of infectious agents (Figure 1-1). Longer life expectancy resulted from the dramatic reductions in death from infectious diseases, a major cause of maternal and infant mortality. Among the greatest public health achievements in the last century was the significant impact on women's lives of the decline in deaths during childbirth from a frighteningly high 1 per 100 in 1900 to

1 per 10,000 in 2000.[12] Similarly, the greatly reduced neonatal mortality rate increased life expectancy an average of 30 years for babies born in 2000 compared with newborns in 1900, only 40% of whom reached age 65.[11] In 1916, just 2 years before the influenza pandemic noted on Figure 1-1, maternal mortality was the second most common cause of death among women, after tuberculosis.[12] Infection control and improved clinical management of pregnancy, childbirth, and infant care enabled women to achieve their desired family size with fewer pregnancies.

Recalling the high mortality in 1918 when 500,000 Americans died, a rate of 1,000 per 100,000 population, has kept scientists focused on the potential emergence of virulent bacterial or viral infectious agents that might suddenly trigger another pandemic.[12] Life expectancy has significantly increased since World War II, driven primarily by medical innovations, especially drug discoveries. Antibiotics, vaccines, enhanced clinical devices, and procedures have greatly lowered mortality. However, infectious outbreaks continue to occur, challenging the need for rapid development and distribution of vaccines to address newly identified infectious agents, as occurred most recently with H1N1 influenza.[13] The diversity of facilities offering the vaccine greatly increased during the 2010–2011 season, enabling more than 37 million to be vaccinated.[14] Many public health workers and researchers urge continued vigilance as the potential for emerging infections are an ever-present concern given globalization of commerce and tourism and the ability of diseases to be transmitted from animals to humans.[15]

The Tobacco Epidemic

As high rates of mortality from infectious diseases were declining during the first 50 years of the 20th century, another lethal "epidemic" was growing. Figure 1-2 notes

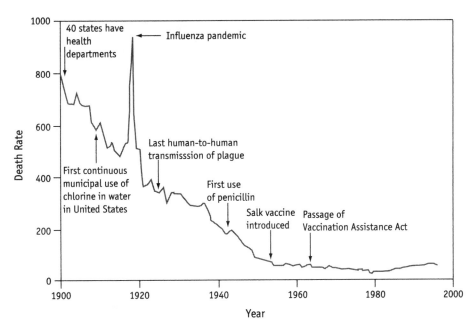

Figure 1-1 Trends in infectious disease mortality. Crude death rate per 100,000 population per year—United States 1900–1996.

Source: Reproduced from Centers for Disease Control and Prevention. Achievements in Public Health, 1900–1999. *MMWR* 1999;48(29):621.
The figure also appears in Levitt AM, Drotman DP, Ostroff S. Control of infectious diseases: a twentieth-century public health achievement. In: Ward JW, Warren C, eds. *Silent Victories. The History and Practice of Public Health in Twentieth-Century America*. New York, NY: Oxford University Press;2007: 3–17.

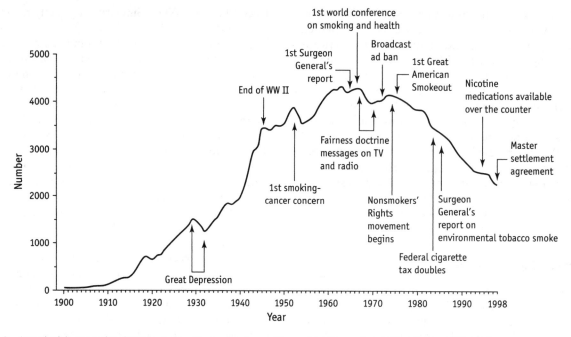

Figure 1-2 Annual adult per capita cigarette consumption and major smoking and health events—United States, 1900–1998.

Reproduced from Centers for Disease Control and Prevention. Achievements in Public Health, 1900–1999. *MMWR* 1999;48:986–993. Data from United States Department of Agriculture and 1986 Surgeon General's Report.

the rapid increase in cigarette sales, which reached a peak in the 1960s and has slowly declined in response to repeated warnings of major health risks by the Surgeon General and many researchers who linked smoking to most major chronic conditions.[16] Brandt stated in his historical review, *The Cigarette Century*, that one of the most important public health accomplishments of the 20th century was "to demonstrate scientifically that cigarette smoking causes *serious* disease and death."[17]

As maternal and infant mortality declined and improved contraceptive options became available, women's lives expanded to encompass higher education, employment, and community involvement, including election to influential positions in education, government, and other fields. Involvement in broader social networks influenced reproductive decisions and other health behaviors such as cigarette smoking, which gradually became acceptable as tobacco companies targeted women with carefully crafted advertisements.[17,18]

A multitude of public health measures have succeeded in reducing the sale of cigarettes and diminishing interest in smoking, including controls on cigarette advertising, increased taxes making cigarettes less affordable, and laws prohibiting smoking in most public indoor and outdoor settings, including parks and beaches.[19] An advertisement from the Centers for Disease Control and Prevention (CDC) program Tips from Former Smokers (Figure 1-3) suggests children have encouraged their mothers to quit. Smoking, a self-induced exposure, has caused high rates of mortality from many respiratory conditions, heart disease, and cancers among men and women; smokers also adversely affect the health of nonsmokers including children who passively inhale secondhand smoke. Both active and passive smoking have now been strongly associated with premature

mortality, as well as adverse birth outcomes. Lung cancer mortality during the past several decades has declined as men quit smoking, but reduced mortality from lung cancer among women has only recently been detected after years of increasing smoking-related deaths (Figure 25-1). In 2011, smoking remained the primary preventable cause of morbidity and premature mortality among women and

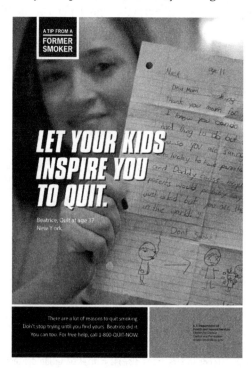

Figure 1-3 An advertisement from the CDC program Tips from Former Smokers.

Source: Courtesy of the CDC.

men, although men reduced their rate of smoking earlier than women (discussed in Chapter 4).[20]

Public health efforts to reduce cigarette sales have shown success (Figure 1-2) with data indicating that fewer Americans are smoking and that mortality due to cardiovascular disease, stroke, and respiratory conditions has been declining during the past 50 years. Unfortunately, the long latency between initiation of smoking and smoking-related diseases does not readily deter young people from developing the habit as they remain the target of tobacco advertisements.

Epidemic of Obesity

Public health improvements in sanitation reduced infection rates, advances in medical treatments increased longevity, and technologically enhanced agricultural production increased availability of low-cost, high-calorie foods. All these factors and many others encouraged the third epidemic, obesity, to emerge in the last decades of the 20th century (Figure 1-4). The availability of an overabundance of fresh and processed foods, some of which were fortified to enhance their nutritional value, encouraged overconsumption by a growing percentage of Americans. Their dietary intake exceeded the nutrients essential for growth during childhood, for successful reproduction,

and for health maintenance during adult years. As U.S. markets offered increasing varieties of processed foods containing excessive fats and sugars with limited nutritional value, the obesity epidemic evolved. Overconsumption coupled with limited physical activity has resulted in obesity and increased susceptibility to many conditions and diseases affecting women. Olshansky et al. predicted a reversal of the recently achieved longer life expectancy if this expanding epidemic continues among America's youth.[21] Chapter 5 discusses essential nutrients required for optimum health of women across the life span.

Less than 16% of female participants in the National Health Examination Study of 1960–62 had a body mass index of 30 or more; by 2005-2008, 36% of women were obese and 58% were overweight.[22] Prevalence rates of obesity, initially higher in southern and western states, have now increased across the United States and distinguish Americans when they travel abroad. National survey data document the changing prevalence of obesity (Figure 1-5). Since the rapid rise in obesity began in 1988, a corresponding increasing pattern of chronic diseases, cancer, and rheumatologic conditions has occurred as noted in subsequent chapters.

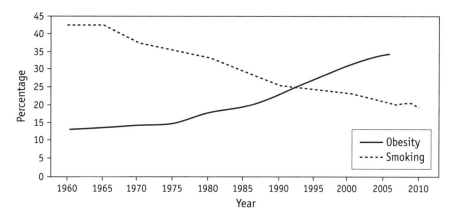

Figure 1-4   Trends in the prevalence of smoking and obesity—United States, 1960–2010.

Source: Reproduced from Fifty Years of Progress in Chronic Disease Epidemiology and Control. Morbidity Mortality Weekly Report 2011;60:70–77.

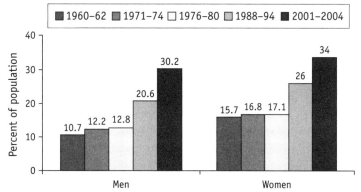

Note: Obesity is defined as a BMI (body mass index) of 30.0 and higher.

Figure 1-5   Age-adjusted prevalence of obesity among adults ages 20–74 NHES 1960–62, NHANES 1971–74, 1976–80, 1988–94, and 1999–2002.

Source: Reproduced from National Center for Health Statistics. Health, United States, 2010: With Special Feature on Death and Dying. Hyattsville, MD. 2010. Available at www.cdc.gov/nchs/data/hus/hus10.pdf.

Cohort studies of nurses and other health professionals have identified multiple lifestyle changes that led to gradual weight gain, with the strongest influences pertaining to dietary components, duration and types of physical activity, and hours spent sleeping.[23] Research among more diverse populations has suggested the prevalence of obesity is due to a complexity of personal health behaviors, genetics, and community and governmental policies.[24] Across a woman's life course, age at onset of obesity may be an important predictor of adverse health outcomes affecting childbearing, onset of chronic diseases, autoimmune conditions, and cancer. Recent estimates indicate that 1 in 10 deaths among women are due to obesity.[25]

About This Text

This section gives an overview of the contents of the book and the overall approach of the chapters.

Life-Course Epidemiology

Most chapters reveal a life-course approach to epidemiology research indicating many health conditions that develop among adults were initiated by physical and social exposures that occurred years earlier.[26] Life-course approaches provide an important perspective for studying health patterns over a woman's life span that recognizes the long latency between some exposures and disease onset.[27] Researchers identified disease-specific critical windows of exposure during youth initiating cellular changes that ultimately lead to adult diseases.

This book provides important information for students, professionals, and public health workers in meeting 21st century goals for health promotion to guide avoidance of disease and increase the probability of longevity free of activity limitations. Health education is needed to establish healthful behaviors during childhood in order to enhance the quality of life at older ages. Although genetic factors may influence risk, a more informed healthcare workforce has the potential to affect health behaviors in addition to encouraging access to appropriate medical interventions, to reduce risk associated with inherited susceptibility, and delay disease onset.

Each individual woman carries a person-specific trajectory across her life span including health outcomes related to biologic, behavioral, social, and psychologic events.[27] Recognized disparities influence disease development and survival among subsets of women whose exposures have differed significantly by socioeconomic status, education, personal lifestyle, and access to high-quality health care from early life through senior years. The federal ACA[10] and state-specific legislation mandate availability of health care for all Americans; measurements of successful changes in access to health care will be monitored by consistent data collection including race/ethnicity and other variables that may identify some causes of health disparities and opportunities for improving health outcomes.[28] The ACA identifies prevention as a national priority with financial support for many state and community-based health promotion and educational programs.[29] The following sections describe the chapter contents that provide baseline information to further these national priorities.

I. Introduction to Epidemiology of Women's Health: Chapters 1 to 3

In Chapter 1, the historical perspective and changing political influences of women provide background information that describes the great progress achieved in the 20th century and the many public health challenges that remain.

Chapter 2 addresses the primary goal of epidemiologic research: to identify risk factors associated with diseases, providing opportunities for prevention. Specialized research methods are required to accomplish these goals and to produce reliable results. Multiple investigations conducted in diverse populations often using different study designs are desirable to confirm new findings or identify different outcomes. Statistical procedures have been evolving to handle the extensive data now accumulating from gene-environment interaction studies. To overcome the hazards of conflicting findings, meta-analyses are conducted combining data from prior epidemiologic studies or randomized clinical trials, considered the "gold standard." Each study methodology has positive and negative influences on the accumulated results and all require careful assessment before firm conclusions are drawn and policy changes are considered.

Changing demographics of the U.S. population by age and race/ethnicity are provided in Chapter 3, enabling some predictions of the population distributions in coming decades. The diverse cultural and sociologic aspects associated with these changes have major implications for educational, research, and community-based services that will promote health and prevent injury throughout the life span. These data provide the foundation for subsequent chapters. Three of the five leading causes of death in young adult to middle-aged women are unintentional injury, suicide, and homicide; among women, an estimated 22% of premature deaths before age 65 are due to fatal injuries rather than health conditions such as heart disease or cancer that generally occur at later ages. The burden of injuries among women differs from that of men by age, race/ethnicity, types of injuries, and resulting disabilities.

II. Health Promotion and Morbidity Prevention: Chapters 4 to 7

The chapters in this section identify long-standing cohort studies in which basic health behaviors have been strongly associated with reduced morbidity and prolonged life expectancy. With more women surviving to older ages, higher rates of chronic conditions are anticipated to cause considerable morbidity but not high mortality while adding to healthcare costs. As the rates of disabilities increase, the quality of life during elder years may decline.[30] However, the early work of Breslow, Fries, and others indicates that onset of chronic and disabling conditions may be prevented or delayed by healthy lifestyles during youth and early adulthood.[31,32] Krieger emphasized the impact of diverse social factors on health and disease onset from neighborhood exposures, access to high-quality health care, and availability of healthy foods. She noted that patterns of social networking at young ages and especially during adolescence may contribute to subsequent inequalities in adult health and mortality.[33]

Among basic preventive services is maintenance of oral health for maximum benefit from preventive nutrition. Chapter 7 addresses complementary and alternative therapies that many women have found helpful and preferable for reducing physical and psychologic discomforts. Successful behavior changes through well-designed intervention programs expand the disease prevention goals of public health.

III. Sexual Health Across the Life Span: Chapters 8 to 11

American data indicate that changes in nutrition, physical activity, and social factors have influenced declining ages of menarche over the last century. The physical and psychosocial changes young girls experience before puberty and during adolescence significantly influence the emotional health of young women. Some of the studies discussed in Chapter 8 indicate maternal exposures to estrogen-disrupting chemicals may be transmitted during critical windows of fetal growth, potentially resulting in accelerated onset of puberty. As women mature and become emotionally involved with sexual partners, their reproductive health needs shift to include contraception, avoidance of unplanned pregnancy, appropriate timing of childbearing, treatment for infertility, etc. Chapter 9 addresses aspects of sexuality, contraception, and preparation for childbearing including new contraceptive options available in the 21st century.

Childbearing presents specific health burdens for women as epidemiology research has revealed some environmental and psychosocial exposures during pregnancy may adversely affect fetal development potentially influencing lifelong health risks.[34] More than 50 years ago the world learned of two medications tragically affecting pregnant women and their offspring with very different outcomes; the birth defects caused by one prescribed medication were recognized at the instant of birth, whereas the adverse effect of the other drug remained hidden until the exposed daughters experienced the hormonal surges of puberty. Both in utero exposures caused lifelong changes to the offspring and kindled the concept of life-course epidemiology research identifying influences of early life exposures on subsequent diseases. Treatment during pregnancy with thalidomide to control nausea[35] and diethylstilbestrol (DES)[36] to reduce preterm births are discussed in Chapter 10. Thalidomide produced developmental deformities of legs and arms; DES caused pelvic organ anomalies that complicated reproductive health and increased risks of several types of cancer. Cohorts of DES-exposed daughters and sons and their children (third generation) continue to be monitored.[37]

Women's health is often discussed politically with a primary focus on abortion rights; however, insurance coverage for contraceptive services to assist in avoidance of unplanned pregnancies remained limited. With prevention a focus of the new federal health care program, the ACA has mandated that contraceptives be covered by insurance without patient copay, a major accomplishment for women's health equity.[9] Although progress has been accomplished in reproductive health, some U.S. parameters lag far behind other industrialized countries in rates of maternal mortality, premature and low birth weight infants, and related reproductive health indicators, especially among low-income and minority women. Delayed childbearing has generated needs for assisted reproduction, a costly process enabled by new technology and willing young women. Life-course changes associated with menopausal symptoms present confusing options for women given the diversity of research findings that affect the quality of life at older ages. Ageism, prejudice toward older members of the population whose mental capacities are assumed to be in decline, has influenced the availability of employment and other activities for older women. With more females elected to political office and directing corporations, these images are slowly changing.

IV. Sexually Transmitted Infections: Chapters 12 to 14

Although the 20th century witnessed a sharp decline in infectious diseases through sound public health policies improving sanitation, development of antibiotics and vaccines for primary prevention, sexually transmitted diseases have remained a major public health issue for affected women and their offspring for centuries as discussed in Chapter 12. A new infectious disease was detected in 1981 shortly after the CDC declared smallpox totally eradicated. The first report described an unusual type of pneumonia diagnosed among five previously healthy men; subsequently, the disease was diagnosed in men and women across the globe. Thirty years later, the human immunodeficiency virus (HIV) infection is no longer inevitably fatal. The history of the acquired immune deficiency syndrome (AIDS) epidemic and research being conducted in the United States and elsewhere are discussed in Chapter 13 and 14.

The magnitude of the AIDS crisis grew rapidly in the United States, with rising mortality solidifying the activist community that demanded funding for research and treatment. Public and private funds enabled researchers with the benefit of technologic advances to rapidly identify the infectious agent, human immunodeficiency virus (HIV), and modes of transmission.[38] By 2008, an estimated 1.2 million Americans were living with HIV infection and almost 600,000 had died of AIDS. Figure 13-2 indicates that incidence rates among women vary considerably within the United States.

Treatment has changed the life-course trajectory of people living with AIDS and HIV infection. Although avenues for primary prevention of HIV infections are not yet available, Figure 1-6 indicates the changing patterns of the disease as the numbers of new diagnoses and deaths have declined and survival rates have continued to increase. Women and men with access to appropriate medication are able to live relatively normal lives

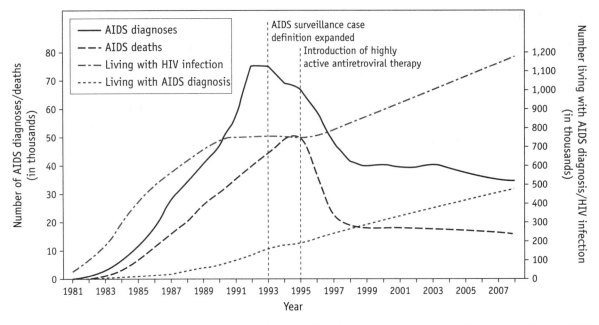

Figure 1-6 Estimated number of AIDS diagnoses and deaths and estimated number of people age > 13 living with diagnosed or undiagnosed HIV infection, United States 1981–2008.

Source: Reproduced from HIV surveillance – United States, 1981–2008. Morbidity and Mortality Weekly Report 2011;60:689–693.

and will subsequently be at risk for diseases common among older Americans without a history of HIV infection. Early in the history of AIDS, the focus on women was limited to potential maternal transmission during pregnancy or delivery; now the unique needs of female HIV/AIDS patients are also being addressed. The demands of activists resulted in the development of lifesaving antiretroviral therapies that have prolonged the lives of millions of Americans, although access to treatment is limited in some segments of the American population.

V. Psychologic and Psychosocial Conditions: Chapters 15 to 20

The six chapters in this section present psychologic conditions that are experienced with greater frequency among women than men. Women are more likely to be diagnosed with episodes of depression and anxiety disorders, and greater than 90% of eating disorder patients are female. Although more men succeed in taking their own lives, among women, suicide is the fifth cause of death between ages 25 and 44 and the fourth cause of death at younger ages. Fluctuating ovarian hormones following puberty may precipitate emotional responses triggering some mental health conditions. Partner violence is a highly prevalent risk to women's physical and mental health and is closely associated with depression, posttraumatic stress disorder, and alcohol and substance use. Partner violence is the primary cause of intentional death to women; in 2007, intimate partner violence resulted in more than 1,600 female deaths in the United States.[39] Understanding the epidemiology of psychologic and psychosocial conditions has led researchers to appreciate the need for integrated care joining clinical and socioecologic public health approaches

to prevent and to lessen the impact of these risks. Bipolar disease is among the most serious psychologic conditions affecting women owing to the difficulty in diagnosis, especially differentiating bipolar disorders from major depression. Suicide is more frequent among these bipolar patients than among women with other psychologic conditions. Alcohol use is a greater problem among men than women, although substance use disorders have adversely affected the physical and mental health of both women and men.

VI. Endocrine and Autoimmune Conditions: Chapters 21 to 24

According to the NIH, 23.5 million Americans have symptoms of an autoimmune disease. Among the more than 80 conditions influenced by women's endocrine system are lupus, diabetes, multiple sclerosis, and asthma, discussed in the chapters in this section. Autoimmune diseases are among the top 10 causes of death of women ages 15 to 64. Although these conditions may also affect men, more than 75% of those affected are female, and for some conditions the ratio is as high as 9:1. Research has not fully explained the gender differences in autoimmune disorders but hormonal influences appear to have a major role. Every organ system of the body is affected by these autoimmune conditions; symptoms vary widely among affected women and change over the life course, which often complicates diagnosis. Endocrine and autoimmune conditions producing long-term disability and requiring complex monitoring and treatment with multiple drugs are frequently diagnosed among younger women.[40] Pregnancy may exacerbate the course of some autoimmune conditions while improving the course of others; however, autoimmune diseases are a major cause of infertility and pregnancy loss. Hereditary patterns of some autoimmune conditions have been noted within affected families; however, a wide range of environmental exposures have also been studied among clusters of cases, especially those with sudden onset of symptoms.

VII. Malignancies: Chapters 25 to 30

Responding to public demands, Congress passed the National Cancer Act in 1971 launching the "War on Cancer," which directed the National Cancer Institute (NCI) to "collect, analyze and disseminate all data useful in the prevention, diagnosis and treatment of cancer."[41] The knowledge gained from the vast amount of research conducted with federal funding has enhanced understanding of carcinogenesis, enabling improved detection, treatment, and avenues for prevention. Over the past 50 years, technologic advances have clarified the role of damaged DNA as a critical first step initiating malignant transformation, although the biologic mechanisms of carcinogenesis remain incompletely understood. Now the focus of research has shifted to identifying inherited genetic variations that increase cancer risk by interacting with environmental exposures that induce multiple genetic alterations, which ultimately initiate a malignancy.[42] The once-normal cell with controlled cell division becomes a growing cluster of rapidly dividing cancer cells. Genetic alterations may begin in utero followed by multiple exposures during youth, leading to diagnosis many years later. People with increased genetic susceptibility often develop more aggressive cancers at earlier ages.

Many epidemiology investigations rely on national data collected through the NCI-funded Surveillance, Epidemiology, and End Results (SEER) program, which has documented regional incidence and mortality patterns reflecting differences within the American population by race/ethnicity, culture, environmental exposures, immigration patterns, etc. The addition of state tumor registries has expanded data sources to include incidence and mortality information from hospital pathology departments, laboratories, treatment centers, and clinicians, enhancing researchers' ability to identify high-incidence regions and monitor mortality rates. Site-specific cancer rates vary considerably across the country by age, race/ethnicity, education level, and socioeconomic status, providing important clues to disease etiology. The chapters in Section VII each review recognized and suspected risk factors that have been studied in relation to cancer development of different organs.

CDC data from 1960 to 2007 (Figure 1-7)[43] indicated dramatic reductions in deaths from heart disease and stroke. During the past 50 years, heart disease mortality declined more than 60% and stroke more than 75%. If the death rates of 1960 had remained unchanged, more than 1.5 million more deaths from these two conditions would be occurring annually. Compared with the more limited success in cancer, progress has been more rapid in controlling heart disease, although research was initiated with the Framingham Study several decades before the war on cancer was launched. However, several chapters note that national data confirm results from small, targeted studies that reported modest declines in cancer mortality during the past decade.

Table 1-2 notes site-specific risk for women by age 85; the six chapters address specific risk factors and available screening methods for lung, breast, ovarian, colon, endometrial, and cervical cancer. Multidisciplinary research has recently identified specific bacterial and viral causes of some malignancies, including the association of *H. pylori* with stomach cancer[44] and human papillomavirus (HPV) with cervical cancer.[45] Development of HPV vaccines enables primary prevention and the potential for dramatic reductions of cervical cancer incidence and mortality in the United States and especially in developing countries if vaccines are provided to those at highest risk.[45] However, investigators have cautioned that susceptibility to these

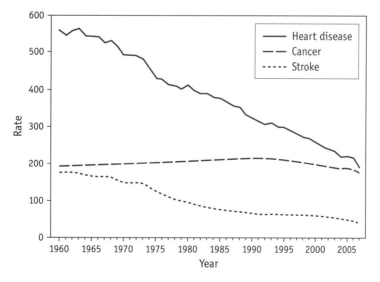

Figure 1-7   Age-adjusted death rates for heart disease, cancer, and stroke. United States, 1960–2007.

Data from National Center for Health Statistics. Health, United States, 2010: With Special Feature on Death and Dying. Hyattsville, MD. 2010. Available at www.cdc.gov/nchs/data/hus/hus10.pdf

Table 1-2

Estimated lifetime probability of developing cancer, by site, women by age 85, US, 2010

Site	Risk
All sites	1 in 3
Breast	1 in 8
Lung & bronchus	1 in 16
Colon & rectum	1 in 22
Uterine—endometrial	1 in 39
Non-Hodgkin lymphoma	1 in 56
Ovary	1 in 72
Melanoma	1 in 78
Pancreas	1 in 81
Urinary bladder	1 in 88
Uterine cervix	1 in 147

Data from Cancer Facts & Figures 2010, American Cancer Society http://www.cancer.org/acs/groups/content/@epidemiologysurveilance/documents/document/acspc-026238.pdf

cancers and many others is more complex than identification of single etiologic agents as social factors also affect disease risk.

Cancer develops through the interaction of genetic susceptibility and environmental exposures; risk may also vary due to person-specific time points of vulnerability. Social determinants interact with physiologic, emotional, and behavioral patterns to influence risk. Most epidemiologic research cannot predict cancer risk for specific individuals, but notes patterns to guide public health programs affecting the population at large.[24]

VIII. Chronic Conditions: Chapters 31 to 35

Significant declines in cardiovascular disease mortality compared with more limited reductions in cancer mortality are noted in Figure 1-7. Research conducted over the past 50 years identified factors associated with heart disease that led to changes in personal health behaviors associated with dietary patterns and diminished smoking that significantly reduced mortality. Preventive medications have lowered risks, and major advances in therapeutic interventions (discussed in Chapter 31) have greatly improved survival after cardiovascular events. Because symptoms of heart disease differ for women and men, the disease was often not recognized from the symptoms women reported, and some researchers have suggested women were not treated as aggressively as their conditions warranted, resulting in higher mortality. Greater public health attention needs to be focused on the known risk factors, including sedentary behavior, high body mass index, smoking, hypertension, and high cholesterol levels.

Chronic conditions are often characterized by musculoskeletal pain requiring medical treatment. The National Health Interview Survey of 2009 included a question about migraine-type pain lasting at least 24 hours; 22% of women compared with 10% of men reported they experienced migraine headaches that frequently affected their quality of life at varying ages from early adolescence to elder years. In contrast, back pain was almost equally reported by men and women as noted in Figure 1-8. Arthritis and fibromyalgia cause significant pain and disability for women; risk factors and treatment options are discussed in Chapters 33 and 34. Osteoporosis, a major cause of morbidity and mortality, affects many older females; hip fracture, specifically, has been found to be a final debilitating illness among a significant number of older women, as noted in Chapter 35. Comorbidity, diagnosis, and treatment of several simultaneous health conditions is a frequent occurrence complicating clinical options, especially at older ages.

IX. Aging: Chapters 36 to 39

As presented in several chapters, life expectancy has significantly lengthened, especially in the past few decades, increasing the importance of health maintenance during younger ages to preserve wellness and prevent illness at older ages. Health behaviors initiated during youth and maintained over time, especially practices such as exercise and weight control, are essential to maintaining mobility at older ages even in the face of increasing disabilities.

Many older women experience comorbid conditions that result in dependence on clinicians and healthcare providers. Researchers have been considering optimum approaches for providing clinical care with the greatest efficiency and compassion. The psychologic and emotional burdens associated with needing assistance, especially when performing activities of daily living, often precipitate depressive episodes. Bereavement associated

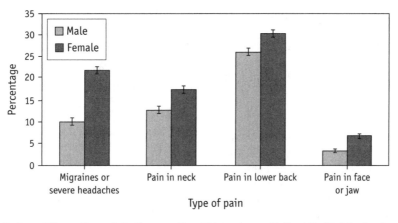

Figure 1-8 Percentage of adults [age >18] reporting pain lasting more than 24 hours by sex. National Health Interview Survey, 2009.

Source: Reproduced from QuickStats: Percentage of adults who had migraine or severe headaches, pain in the neck, lower back, or face/jaw, by sex – National Health Interview Survey, 2009. Morbidity and Mortality Weekly Report 2010;59:1557.

with the deaths of loved relatives or friends also takes its toll. Community-based organizations may provide important resources for social support and practical assistance.

New therapeutic interventions have reduced mortality from many chronic, disabling conditions that affect women more than men. As the media steadily report increasing prevalence of Alzheimer's disease, many older women fear developing this condition and the associated deterioration of mental functioning. Social interaction is essential for maintenance of an alert mind, although normal aging and genetic susceptibility may influence mental clarity. The four chapters in this section address clinical aspects of aging, psychosocial perceptions of aging women, prevention of unintentional injuries from falls, and Alzheimer's disease.

X. Impact of Research: Lessons from the Past, Future Challenges: Chapters 40 and 41

Cancer screening continues to command the attention of healthcare providers, advocacy organizations, and voluntary agencies; however, as Sackett stated more than 40 years ago, routine screening of the public is costly and may limit funds available for other programs that may offer greater health benefits for more people.[46] He also indicated that early detection modalities have both protective and harmful effects because minimally invasive screening occasionally detects suspicious findings that require more aggressive interventions to determine the true nature of the lesion, causing both physical and emotional harm.[46] These concerns have been debated for more than 60 years and continue to receive attention in the 21st century, as costs of unnecessary or harmful medical care are a pressing issue.[47] The history of mammography screening in Chapter 40 addresses these complex issues.

Studies referenced throughout the text note the role of family history and inherited risk associated with many conditions. Among the goals of the future often discussed in the media and among healthcare providers is personalized medical care based primarily on genetic analyses.

Researchers recognize that genetic variations are not all equally likely to cause diseases; therefore, complex technologic methodology is required to identify genetic patterns and to interpret genetic test results. Criteria have been developed for genetic testing for inherited susceptibility to various conditions. The field is expanding as direct-to-consumer genetic analyses are now available. Chapter 41 presents an overview of some aspects of genetic testing and the role of genetic analyses in the future health of American women. Healthcare providers may consider epidemiologic research results when planning preventive modalities and treatment decisions with their female patients based on family history and genetic testing. However, population-based results may not pertain to individuals whose person-specific risk characteristics extend beyond gender, age, and family history categories. Inherited susceptibility, personal health behaviors, reproductive decisions, and environmental exposures are among the many others factors that influence an individual's risk of disease and age at onset.[24]

Summary

This textbook aims to identify and promote public health efforts that may lower premature morbidity and mortality among women by emphasizing avenues for health maintenance and identifying common causes of disease among American women. Many factors are believed to contribute to poor health of some segments of the population, including those with limited access to health care who often lack health insurance or have inadequate coverage.[48] Studies indicate health outcomes are improved when clinical care is synchronized by a team of concerned providers after establishing a trusting relationship with their patients. Currently, the U.S. healthcare system limits opportunities for consistent and personalized care. The potential for change exists under provisions of the 2010 Affordable Care Act or other legislation. Patients and healthcare providers may have unique opportunities to reduce disparities through greater access to health education, coordinated care, and improved opportunities for disease prevention.

We planned this book to provide undergraduates, graduate students, and health professionals with baseline understanding of many conditions that affect women's health, hoping to stimulate career development among those using the text. Chapter topics were selected based on their frequency of occurrence, severity of symptoms, and effects on quality of life. Some normal health transitions across the life span as well as the effects of aging received attention, in addition to diseases requiring aggressive therapy. Although most health issues included in the text have a significant impact on the quality of women's lives, many other important problems could not be presented and may be explored by interested faculty and students. The collaborating authors are drawn from diverse public health and allied backgrounds, including clinicians and researchers. This overview of women's health across the life span should also be valuable for students entering fields outside of public health and the health professions who should benefit professionally and personally from greater understanding of some health issues women experience across the life span.

Discussion Questions

1. Why does women's health require special attention? What are some major health differences between women and men from early ages through the life course?

2. How has medical history in the 20th century influence health status of women in the 21st century? What role has reproduction played in overall health status?

3. How has treatment for HIV/AIDS, heart disease, and other conditions differed when men and women are compared?

4. Has the political climate in the United States influenced women's health or women's health research? Why women were often excluded for clinical trials that enrolled and studied only men?

5. How do psychologic and social factors interact with personal health behaviors to influence health status? In planning a public health intervention, how might the psychological and social issues contribute to the planning?

References

1. Schroeder P, Snowe O. The politics of women's health. In: Costello C., Stone A, eds. *The American Woman 1994-1995: Where We Stand. Women and Health.* New York, NY: W W Norton & Co; 1994.
2. Palca J. Women left out at NIH. *Science.* 1990;248:1601–1602.
3. Women's Research & Education Institute. www.wrei.org.
4. Pinn VW, Clayton JA, Begg L, Sass SE. Public partnership for a vision for women's health research in 2020. *J Women's Health.* 2010;19:1603–1607.
5. Rossouw JE, Anderson GL, Prentice RL, et al.; Writing Group for the Women's Health Initiative Investigators. Risks and benefits of estrogen plus progestin in healthy postmenopausal women: principal results from the Women's Health Initiative randomized controlled trial. *JAMA.* 2002;288:321–333.
6. Clarke CA, Glaser SL, Uratsu CS, et al. Recent declines in hormone therapy utilization and breast cancer incidence: clinical and population-based evidence. *J Clin Oncol.* 2006;24:e49–50.
7. Executive Order March 11, 2009. Council on Women and Girls. http://www.whitehouse.gov/the_press_office/President-Obama-Announces-White-House-Council-on-Women-and-Girls/.
8. Walsh E. *Divided Lives.* New York, NY: Simon & Schuster; 1995.
9. Institute of Medicine. *Clinical Preventive Services for Women: Closing the Gaps.* Washington, DC: National Academies Press; 2011. http://www.iom.edu/Reports/2011/Clinical-Preventive-Services-for-Women-Closing-the-Gaps.aspx.
10. Affordable Care Act. http://www.whitehouse.gov/healthreform#healthcare-menu.
11. Fuchs VR. New priorities for future biomedical innovations. *N Engl J Med.* 2010;363:704–706.
12. Levitt AM, Drotman DP, Ostroff S. Control of infectious diseases: a twentieth-century public health achievement. In: Ward JW, Warren C, eds. *Silent Victories. The History and Practice of Public Health in Twentieth-Century America.* New York, NY: Oxford University Press; 2007:3–17.
13. National Center for Immunization and Respiratory Diseases, CDC. Use of influenza A (H1N1) 2009 monovalent vaccine. *MMWR Morb Mortal Wkly Rep.* 2009;58:108.
14. Kennedy ED, Santibanez TA, Bryan LN, et al. Place of influenza vaccination among adults—United States 2010-11 influenza season. *MMWR Morb Mortal Wkly Rep.* 2011;60:781–785.
15. Feldmann H. Truly emerging—a new disease caused by a novel virus. *N Engl J Med.* 2011;1561–1563.
16. Eriksen MP, Green LW, Husten CG, et al. Thank you for not smoking: the public health response to tobacco-related mortality in the United States. In: Ward JW, Warren C, eds. *Silent Victories. The History and Practice of Public Health in Twentieth-Century America.* New York, NY: Oxford University Press; 2007:423–436.
17. Brandt AM. *The Cigarette Century: The Rise, Fall, and Deadly Persistence of the Product that Defined America.* New York, NY: Basic Books; 2009.
18. Howe HL. An historical review of women, smoking and advertising. *Health Education.* 1984; 15:3–8.
19. Cosgrove J, Bayer R, Bachynski KE. Nowhere left to hide? The banishment of smoking from public spaces. *N Engl J Med.* 2011;364:2375–2377
20. Preston SH, Wang H. Sex mortality differences in the United States: The role of cohort smoking patterns. *Demography.* 2006;43:631–646.
21. Olshansky SJ, Passaro DJ, Hershow RC, et al. A potential decline in life expectancy in the United States in the 21st century. *N Engl J Med.* 2005;352:1138–1145.
22. Ogden CL, Carroll MD. *Prevalence of Overweight, Obesity, and Extreme Obesity among Adults: United States, Trends 1960–1962 through 2007–2008.* Hyattsville, MD: National Center for Health Statistics; 2010.
23. Mozaffarian D, Hao T, Rimm EB, et al. Changes in diet and lifestyle and long-term weight gain in women and men. *N Engl J Med.* 2011;364:2392–2404.
24. Galea S, Riddle M, Kaplan GA. Causal thinking and complex system approaches in epidemiology. *Int J Epidemiol.* 2010;39:97–106.
25. Danaei G, Ding EL, Mozaffarian D, et al. The preventable causes of death in the United States: Comparative risk assessment of dietary, lifestyle, and metabolic risk factors. *PLoS Med.* 2009;6: e1000058. doi:10.1371/journal.pmed.1000058
26. Kuh D, Ben-Shlomo Y, Lynch J, et al. Life course epidemiology. *J Epidemiol Community Health.* 2003; 57:778–783.
27. Lynch J, Smith GD. A life course approach to chronic disease epidemiology. *Annu Rev Public Health* 2005;26:1–35.
28. Weissman JS, Hasnain-Wynia R. Advancing health care equity through improved data collection. *N Engl J Med.* 2011; 364:2276–2277.
29. Koh HK, Sebelius KG. Promoting prevention through the Affordable Care Act. *N Engl J Med.* 2010;363:1296–1299.
30. McKenna MT, Zohrabian A. US burden of disease-past, present and future. *Ann Epidemiol.* 2009;19:212–219.
31. Breslow L, Breslow N. Health practices and disability: Some evidence from Alameda County. *Prevent Med.* 1993;22:86–95.
32. Fries JF. Aging, natural death, and the compression of morbidity. *N Engl J Med.* 1980;303:130–135.
33. Krieger N. A glossary for social epidemiology. *J Epidemiol Community Health.* 2001;55:693–700.
34. Kotelcheck M. Safe mothers, healthy babies: Reproductive health in the twentieth century. In: Ward JW, Warren C, eds. *Silent Victories. The History and Practice of Public Health in Twentieth-Century America.* New York, NY: Oxford University Press; 2007: 105–134.
35. Leck IM, Millar ELM. Incidence of malformations since the introduction of thalidomide. *BMJ.* 1962:2:16–20.
36. Herbst AI, Ulfelder H, Poskanzer DC. Adenocarcinoma of the vagina. Association of maternal stilbestrol therapy with tumor appearance in young women. *N Engl J Med.* 1971;284:878–881.
37. Goodman A, Schorge J, Greene MF. The long-term effects of in utero exposures—the DES story. *N Engl J Med.* 2011;364:2083–2085.
38. Torian L, Chen M, Rhodes P. HIV surveillance-United States, 1981-2008. *MMWR Morb Mortal Wkly Rep.* 2011;60:689–691.
39. Karch DL, Lubell KM, Friday J, et al. Surveillance for violent deaths—National Violent Death Reporting System, 16 states, 2005. *MMWR Morb Mortal Wkly Rep.* 2008;57(SS03):11–43,45.
40. Ricker PP, Bird CE. Rethinking gender differences in health: why we need to integrate social and biological perspectives. *J Geront.* 2005;60B (special issue II): 40–47.

41. National Cancer Act of 1971, Pub L No. 92-218. http://legislative.cancer.gov/history/phsa/1971. Accessed August 4, 2012.

42. Loeb LA, Harris CC. Advances in chemical carcinogenesis: a historical review and prospective. *Cancer Res.* 2008;68:6863–6872.

43. Remington PI, Brownson RC. Fifty years of progress in chronic disease epidemiology and control. *MMWR Morb Mortal Wkly Rep.* 2011;60:70–77.

44. Brown LM. *Helicobacter pylori*: Epidemiology and routes of transmission. *Epidemiol Rev.* 2000;22:283–297.

45. Markowitz LE, Sternberg M, Dunne EF, et al. Seroprevalence of human papillomavirus types 6,11,16, and 18 in the United States: National Health and Nutrition Examination Survey 2003-2004. *J Infect Dis.* 2009;200:1059–1067.

46. Sackett DL. Screening for early detection of disease: to what purpose? *Bull NY Acad Med.* 1975;51:39–52.

47. Welch HG, Schwartz LM, Woloshin S. *Overdiagnosed.* Boston, MA: Beacon Press;.2011:14.

48. Bickell NA, Shastri K, Fei K, et al. A tracking and feedback registry to reduce racial disparities in breast cancer care. *J Natl Cancer Inst.* 2008;100: 1717–1723.

Epidemiologic Research Methods

Ruby T. Senie, PhD

Introduction

The field of epidemiology evolved during the 19th century as researchers developed methods to track disease by neighborhoods in order to control cholera epidemics and other infectious conditions in their communities. John Snow (1813–1858), who practiced medicine in London, has been credited with founding epidemiology. Through careful investigations, he suspected contaminated water was transmitting an agent that caused the massive outbreak of cholera in 1842. When residents were forced to obtain clean water from other sources, the epidemic subsided.[1]

In 1846 in Vienna, Ignac Semmelweiss (1818–1865), another 19th century physician epidemiologist, observed higher mortality rates from puerperal (childbed) fever among new mothers attended by doctors compared to women whose babies were delivered by midwives. When his colleague, a pathologist, developed the same infection and subsequently died, Semmelweiss hypothesized that the disease was transmitted to patients by doctors from the autopsy laboratory. After requiring doctors to wash their hands in chlorinated water before attending women in labor, maternal mortality from puerperal fever rapidly declined from 12% to 1%.[1]

Among the most notable contributions of epidemiology to public health in the 20th century was the link between increased cigarette smoking and rising incidence of lung cancer. In 1964, the U.S. Surgeon General reported that lung cancer risk was more than 10 times greater among smokers than nonsmokers. Few epidemiologic studies have observed risk associations of similar magnitude until the recently identified susceptibility genes that strongly predict hereditary cancer syndromes. Recent etiologic studies are benefitting by use of new technology that enables analysis of biospecimens, including blood, urine, saliva, and tissue samples, to search for potential disease-causing organisms, exposures, and biomarkers of disease. The resulting multidisciplinary collaborative studies have stimulated creative and more sophisticated approaches to understanding the causes of complex diseases.[2]

This chapter reviews established epidemiologic research methods used in many of the studies referenced in this text. Epidemiologists study risk factors for specific conditions and diseases affecting women across the life span. Recent innovative research has identified early life exposures, especially during periods of rapid growth, from prenatal development through early childhood to adolescence, as critical intervals when exposures may influence risk of adult onset diseases. A major public health goal of epidemiologic studies is identification of opportunities for preventing or delaying the development of disabling conditions, thus improving the quality of life among seniors.

Epidemiologic Parameters

Epidemiology is based on the belief that diseases do not occur randomly and opportunities for disease prevention may be provided by identifying potential etiologic agents. Investigations of disease patterns in humans are far more complex to design and conduct than laboratory-based animal studies in which genetic and environment exposures can be controlled. Among humans, our primary goal is to identify factors that differentiate groups of people with a disease from those within the same population who remain unaffected. To adequately study associations between diseases and potential risk factors, multidisciplinary teams are needed to design data collection instruments for measuring biologic, social, and environmental factors and to monitor changes in these parameters over time.[2] Although small clinic-based studies may provide etiologic clues, sophisticated statistical methods have been developed to analyze extensive data collected from study participants and collaborating laboratories. Through these challenging investigations, epidemiology has identified public health interventions that are contributing to improved health of all Americans.

Incidence and Prevalence

Essential for public health planning and resource allocation is an understanding of the magnitude of different clinical conditions affecting populations over their life course. Data are collected to determine the **incidence of a disease**, the number of newly diagnosed cases of disease in a specified interval of time in a defined population. The **prevalence of a disease** reflects the total number of affected women at one point in time including newly diagnosed cases and those with longer histories of the disease. An example is prevalence estimates of multiple sclerosis among American women. Distinguishing between incident and prevalent cases is essential; prevalent cases may have unique characteristics that enable long-term survival and, therefore, may not represent the full spectrum of the condition.

Person, Place, and Time

Traditional descriptive epidemiology has focused on disease patterns in relation to personal characteristics of the people affected, their geographic diversity and the timing of disease onset.[3] These basic features are addressed in most epidemiology studies of potential causal relationships.

Person. Epidemiologic studies classify individuals into groups according to their gender, race/ethnicity, age at disease onset, current knowledge of genetic status, and health behavior patterns among other factors. An example of gender-specific patterns pertains to breast cancer, which primarily affects women. Although differences in incidence and mortality rates have been associated with race/ethnicity, advances in genetic testing and identification of molecular markers may more accurately define person-specific risk patterns,[4] especially among multiracial families.[5]

Place. Geographic differences in incidence, prevalence, and clinical course of diseases have been studied for etiologic clues. One example is provided by ecologic studies of multiple sclerosis; the north-south gradient suggests risk may be influence by climate patterns.[6] Rates of death from coronary heart disease (CHD) among Americans ages 35 and older vary considerably by state. CHD mortality rates in some counties of southern states are more than double rates in western and northern sections of the country. The counties with the highest CHD deaths are characterized by disproportionally higher levels of poverty, obesity, and diabetes in addition to sedentary lifestyle.[7]

Migration studies have documented changes in disease patterns among succeeding generations of immigrants who adopt social–cultural patterns, are exposed to new environments, and assume health behaviors prevalent in their new residential and occupational settings. The study of rising breast cancer incidence rates among Hispanic women with each succeeding generation was reported by John and colleagues in California to be among women who immigrated at young ages and had longer residence in the United States.[8]

Geographic assessments have identified disparities associated with close proximity to toxic waste sites and polluting industries primarily affecting residential and employment settings of low-income and minority populations.[5] Some studies have linked environmental contaminants with neurodegenerative conditions detected decades after in utero exposures;[9] children are the most vulnerable members of the population due to their rapid rate of growth.[10] Therefore, research assessing risk factors for adult onset diseases often requires knowledge of early residential exposures.

Timing of exposures may critically influence risk of disease, especially at recognized transition intervals when susceptibility is increased due to rapid cell division. Across the life cycle, women are most vulnerable during prenatal development, puberty, pregnancy, and menopause.[10,11] Examples include in utero thalidomide exposure that was noted decades ago to cause tragic interruption of fetal limb development.[12] Another drug prescribed to pregnant women, an estrogen called diethylstilbestrol (DES) thought to prevent miscarriage, increased the risk of cancer in both mothers and daughters years later.[13] Risk of breast cancer is increased among mothers more than 30 years after use of DES and among daughters after age 40.[14] In addition, some daughters exposed in utero were prematurely diagnosed with vaginal or cervical cancer soon after puberty, whereas others have experienced gynecologic abnormalities, including infertility.[13]

Levels of Prevention

The major goal of public health education is to prevent disease through promotion of healthy lifestyles and avoidance of adverse environmental exposures. Early detection modalities through screening are advocated to avoid diagnosis of diseases at advanced stages. Once a condition has developed, subsequent goals address reduction of disabilities and maintenance of quality of life. These levels of prevention guide public health interventions.

Primary Prevention

Avoiding onset of a disease or condition is the goal of primary prevention. Vaccines provide such protection by stimulating the immune system, producing antibodies against an etiologic agent to prevent diseases such as poliomyelitis and measles.[15] Major concerns caused by fear of adverse health effects, especially from erroneous links to autism, have caused some parents to refuse immunizations for their children. Although vaccination is mandated by most states, some provide religious and/ or philosophic exemptions.[16] Recently developed vaccines have protected the public against infectious conditions such as flu (H1N1), diseases with infectious and chronic components including liver cancer (HepB)[17] and cervical cancer (human papillomavirus or HPV).[18] Eradication of the bacterial etiologic agent, *H. pylori*, through population-based administration of antibiotic therapy could provide primary prevention of gastric cancer.[19] Personal behaviors such as increased physical exercise and avoidance of smoking may prevent heart disease or delay disease onset.[20]

Secondary Prevention

Although screening to identify some diseases or conditions at early stages is often referred to as "prevention," such secondary prevention procedures do not protect against disease development. However, by altering the natural history through early detection followed by appropriate treatment, risk of death may be reduced or prevented. An example is provided by Berry and colleagues who used national data to document improved breast cancer survival due to a combination of screening mammography and adjuvant chemotherapy.[21] A potentially adverse effect of screening is overdiagnosis and unnecessary, aggressive treatment of clinically insignificant disease or borderline conditions.

Tertiary Prevention

The goals of tertiary prevention include prolonging survival and reducing symptoms to improve the quality of life after a condition is diagnosed and appropriate therapy has been received. Self-care guidelines for women with diabetes help lower the risk of blindness or kidney damage by daily monitoring and administration of insulin, which may slow the natural course of the disease.[22] Therefore, tertiary prevention may provide opportunities for rehabilitation through comprehensive and coordinated therapy.

Types of Epidemiologic Studies

Observational studies are conducted when knowledge of a condition or disease is limited. They provide data on the natural history of diseases, incidence rates by ages at diagnosis, race/ethnicity, gender, environmental exposures, and social class, which enable researchers to determine the need for targeted research and public health planning. Data from initial observational studies are essential for the development of hypotheses that are tested in more complex and costly analytic investigations. When appropriate and ethically feasible, randomized clinical trials may be designed to further test suggested avenues for disease interventions. Clinical observations often identify underlying causal factors that stimulate population-based research that may identify causal agents. The sequence of studies that identified the association of endometrial cancer with unopposed postmenopausal estrogen exposure provides an example as noted in Table 2-1.

Observational Studies

Ecologic

Population groups rather than individuals are the focus of ecologic investigations. Changes in disease patterns noted in national data or specific populations may provide important public health clues. For example, the ecologic study published by Austin and Roe in 1982 documented the previously suspected correlation between prescribing patterns of estrogen for menopausal symptoms and rising incidence rates of endometrial cancer. With discontinued use of these medications, diagnosis of endometrial cancer rapidly diminished.[23] A similar response was observed in 2007 as population-based breast cancer incidence rates declined for the first time after decades of steady increases. The authors attributed the downward trend to postmenopausal women discontinuing combined estrogen and progesterone therapy after the 2002 Women's Health Initiative reports.[24]

Another ecologic analysis of population-based data indicated an inverse association between annual sunlight exposure and breast cancer incidence. Compared with an annual incidence rate of 33 cases per 100,000 women in northern states, breast cancer affected 17–19 per 100,000 women in southern states, suggesting greater exposure to sunlight reduced risk of disease.[25] Although observed correlations identified in ecologic studies may not reflect causal risk factors among individuals, they often guide researchers in developing analytic investigations.[26] Caution is advised in relying on ecologic studies, as excess promotion of the results may result in an "ecologic fallacy," an inaccurate assumption based on correlations among populations rather than individuals.[27]

Cross-Sectional

The relationship of personal or clinical factors with disease status at one point in time is the focus of cross-sectional

---

Table 2-1

Evolution from a clinical observation to a causal association

Observation/concepts	Examples
Clinical observation between factor and condition—personal observation	Estrogen prescribed for menopausal symptoms—unexplained uterine bleeding
Etiologic studies—population level	Increased menopausal estrogen use was followed by elevated endometrial cancer rates
Analytic studies using personal data from research participants, consistency of results from numerous studies	Association confirmed in case/control, cohort and nested case control studies
Understanding the biologic mechanism led to discontinued hormone use that stimulated malignant growth	Rapid decline in endometrial cancer confirmed estrogen as a tumor promoter
Control of biologic mechanism with additional hormonal treatment	Addition of progesterone to estrogen caused shedding of the endometrial lining of the uterus
Lower incidence of endometrial cancer in other western countries	Lower frequency of hormone use for menopause in these countries

studies; however, the sequence of disease onset in relation to exposure cannot be determined. A cross-sectional study by Stewart et al. describes a survey mailed to randomly selected households in order to estimate the lifetime incidence of migraine by gender and age group.[28] Repeated cross-sectional surveys provide estimates of changes in disease patterns over time. Individuals with newly diagnosed disease (incident cases) and people who have survived for long intervals after diagnosis (prevalent cases) are included in cross-sectional studies. Although cross-sectional surveys can be useful, prevalent cases may have unique characteristics including more indolent disease enabling longer survival, which may compromise the usefulness of some cross-sectional studies. Tanner and Whitehouse used cross-sectional assessments to identified individual variability of age-specific growth patterns of girls during puberty. However, they supplemented their research with repeated longitudinal assessments of a subset of girls to detect any abnormalities in the rate of maturation.[29]

Analytic Studies

Hypotheses generated by results of descriptive studies guide the design of more complex and costly analytic investigations of individuals. Extensive data collection and appropriate biospecimens are collected from willing study participants. Careful calculations are required to estimate the optimum number of participants to assure adequate statistical power to provide meaningful results. A balanced assessment of study size is essential to achieve precision while being a cost effective research design. To address some research questions, smaller, targeted investigations that include clinical measurements and genotyping are often more manageable and informative than larger, population-based studies.[30] Appropriate selection of a specific analytic study designs to address an epidemiologic question depends on the frequency of the condition, the efficiency of recruitment procedures and data collection, and ethical issues affecting biospecimens collection, among other issues.

Case-Control Studies (Retrospective)

A classic study design repeatedly represented in epidemiologic literature referenced in this text is the case-control comparison. Data are collected uniformly from women with a newly diagnosed condition (cases) and unaffected women (controls) by either a personal interview (in person or by phone) or extensive mailed questionnaire. Questions based on prior research or hypotheses ask about exposures and life events preceding diagnosis among cases and during a comparable time interval for controls. These retrospective investigations rely heavily on the cooperation, memory, and honesty of the study participants.

Case-Case Studies (Retrospective)

Case-only studies are a convenient means for understanding risk and/or prognostic factors associated with differing forms of a condition or disease; studies may focus on etiologic or prognostic factors associated with pathologic features, ages at diagnosis, menopausal stage, etc.[31]

Research addressing specific case questions such as the impact of maintenance of fertility after breast cancer treatment on prognosis requires case-only recruitment.[32]

Cohort Studies

Cohorts are composed of prospectively recruited healthy women who are followed over time after completing baseline questionnaires, often also providing biosamples and possibly having clinical examinations. Cohort participants are requested to agree to repeated data collection over extended, occasionally undefined, time frames. A famous community-based investigation of heart disease was initiated in Framingham, Massachusetts, in 1948 with approximately one-third of all households represented among the original 15,000 male and female participants.[33] Development of birth cohorts, recruiting pregnant women or women planning to become pregnant, has become a valuable design for epidemiologic studies of prenatal exposures and pregnancy outcomes.[34]

Harvard researchers began recruitment of two cohorts of registered nurses in 1976, focusing on two different age brackets to include pre- and postmenopausal women. Participants in the Nurses' Health Study cohorts have been followed for several decades by questionnaires mailed biannually. Data collection has included changes in health status and personal behaviors including smoking, hormone use, diet, alcohol intake, and other exposures, providing resources for hundreds of publications on diverse health outcomes affecting women.[35] Some researchers have questioned the representativeness of the nurses enrolled in these cohorts. They may represent a female population biased by the "healthy worker effect" as well as higher education and health consciousness compared with women of similar ages in the general population.[36] Given these concerns, results based on data from the Nurses' Health Study may be generalizable only to females of similar ages, race/ethnicity, education level, and employment status.[3]

The American Cancer Society (ACS) has created three "prevention cohorts" recruited by county-based ACS volunteers beginning in 1959 with a second cohort added in 1982 and a third currently being planned to assess changes in cancer risk factors over time and among diverse populations. Participants provided baseline and follow-up questionnaire data and are contacted routinely by the ACS volunteers to maintain records of health status changes. Critics of the publications based on data from these cohorts noted that participants were often better educated and less diverse than other members of their communities. Despite these concerns, investigations using ACS-collected data have documented a significant number of cancer risk factors including the changing nature of family history of cancer as relatives grow older and cancer risk increases.[37]

Retrospective Cohort Studies

Cohorts have been created retrospectively through employment records, medical charts, site-specific exposures, birth records, etc. Although the data available on members of a retrospective cohort may be limited, women with specific exposures assembled retrospectively may be very important for identifying etiologic causes of disease. One study identified radium as the cause of oral cancer among women who painted watch faces many decades ago.[38] Another retrospective cohort that provided important research results was composed of infants exposed to radiation of the thymus in New York State who were found to be at increased risk of breast cancer more than 36 years later.[39]

Experimental Studies Randomized Controlled Trials (RCT)

The primary scientific method for reliable, unbiased assessment of an etiologic factor, diagnostic technique, behavioral intervention, or treatment modality is the randomized controlled trial (RCT). Randomization minimizes imbalance of measured and unmeasured personal and behavioral characteristics, a classic means for ensuring comparability of study participants. Women meeting entry criteria and agreeing to participate must be randomly assigned to intervention or control status. Exclusion criteria must be specifically defined and compliance with assignment must be carefully monitored. In order to ensure unbiased study results not influenced by study investigators, neither participants nor research coordinators should know the assigned treatment of participants. An external data monitoring panel must routinely assess study results, applying preset stopping criteria, in order to provide the public with benefits of the research as soon as possible and ensuring safety by prematurely interrupting the trial if negative results are detected, as occurred in a beta carotene trial among smokers.[40]

There may also be limitations in conducting RCTs. Inaccurate results may be recorded if participants fail to adhere to study protocols. For example, inconsistent use of a prescribed medication or placebo may incorrectly suggest a new medication or therapeutic intervention is ineffective. Public health programs may be developed based on inaccurate conclusions. Therefore, carefully designed RCTs should include detective measures for assessing compliance. The RCT conducted by researchers at the Chicago Lying-In Hospital in 1953 reported that diethylstilbestrol did not prevent miscarriage. The prescribed treatment and placebo tablets included an inert chemical marker that was detectable in urine samples collected at each prenatal visit documenting level of adherence to daily pill use.[41]

Randomized controlled trials may be the gold standard for research; however, some questions of special interest cannot be addressed by random assignment due to ethical consideration, willingness of participants to be randomized, etc. Interventions found to be effective in one population may not live up to expectations in other community settings (Table 2-2).

One of the most important RCTs recently conducted among American women assessed the effect of estrogen with and without progestin on several health outcomes. The Women's Health Initiative (WHI) included several RCTs and observational studies. Hundreds of research reports have been generated and have influenced clinical decisions by many women and their healthcare providers. As previously noted, a downturn in breast cancer has paralleled the reduced hormone use by postmenopausal women.[24]

Selection and Recruitment of Study Populations

Identifying and recruiting appropriate women to address a research question is of critical importance in epidemiologic research. Regardless of study design, characteristics of individuals who agree to participate compared to those who refuse are a potential source of bias that may adversely affect study results. Systemic differences in groups of women willing to be included in research projects are likely to influence the validity and generalizability of results.[3] As epidemiologic studies have grown in complexity with biospecimen collection and lengthy interviews or complex questionnaires, decisions to participate may be influenced by personal concerns for the disease being studied. Unbiased representative study populations are essential for valid research with participation response rates considered one measure of successful recruitment. To assess representativeness of participants in relation to the community of "at-risk women," investigators often compare baseline characteristics of the recruited study subjects with those who refused enrollment.[42] Major significant differences are a source of concern requiring specialized statistical methods.

Table 2-2

Factors that may influence generalizability of clinical trial results

Diversity of study participants: age distribution, race/ethnicity diversity, comorbid conditions

Geographic distribution: regional differences in disease patterns, risk factors, environmental exposures

Nature of available clinical settings, including access to health care

Interest and willingness of local healthcare providers to recruit participants or permit patients to enter proposed clinical trials

Knowledgeable staff with expertise availability to adequately conduct clinical trials to meet research standards

Relevance of the intervention to the needs, priorities, and values of study participants and research community

Local cultures influencing acceptance of trial results

Hospital-Based Recruitment

In the past, hospitalized patients were the primary research subjects, especially for studies of less common clinical conditions. Medical records provide documentation of disease status, portions of biospecimens collected for clinical care may also contribute to research, and personal interviews are readily accepted by hospitalized patients.[43] Studies of highly lethal conditions require rapid case ascertainment most conveniently accomplished during initial hospitalization. Medical centers also provide access to women unaffected by the specific conditions being studied to serve as controls. However, hospitalized control subjects may have unique characteristics and comorbid conditions that differ significantly from the larger non-institutionalized female population.[3] Therefore, epidemiologists have avoided hospitalized patients, preferring to recruit population-based study participants. However, recent interest in molecular epidemiology research has stimulated renewed interest in hospital-based recruitment, providing easier access to biospecimens, including tissue.[36]

Birth cohorts provide an opportunity to study the impact of genetic, cultural, and environmental exposures on physical growth and emotional development. Recruitment of pregnant women provides access to information on prenatal exposures; women and babies can be followed through delivery including birth experiences, postnatal exposures, infant feeding, growth rate, psychological development, etc.[34] A unique example is provided by the Dutch birth cohort of babies exposed prenatally to the German-imposed food embargo causing severe malnutrition during pregnancy. Adverse health effects are still being documented in the affected population after 5 decades of follow-up for health outcomes.[11] Diversity of study populations can be ensured by multisite collaborations including mothers of varying races–ethnicities and socioeconomic levels from rural and urban medical centers.

Population-Based Recruitment

Population-based study recruitment is preferred for epidemiologic studies as the study population is more representative of women at risk. Data representative of the broad U.S. population are provided by the National Center for Health Statistics (NCHS), a division of the Centers for Disease Prevention and Control (CDC). The NCHS annually conducts the National Health and Nutrition Examination Survey (NHANES). Using a complex, multistage probability design with oversampling of selected demographic subgroups to provide health and nutrition information from more than 20,000 American women and men of diverse heritages.

In the United States, infectious diseases must be reported to state health departments and the CDC, providing information public health workers use to develop prevention and control programs. Similarly, most states have mandated reporting of all newly diagnosed malignancies. These data enable calculation of incidence and mortality rates by cancer site, gender, age at diagnosis, and length of survival. Researchers, with approval of local institutional review boards and treating physicians, often seek participation of newly diagnosed cancer patients in etiologic and treatment studies. Protection of patient privacy is ensured by mandated procedures, including study descriptions provided in consent to participate forms.

To provide comparison populations for epidemiologic studies, unaffected members of the community are invited to contribute to research as control subjects. Unbiased recruitment of controls is essential. Controls must be drawn from the same base population as the cases. Several appropriate sources of population-based controls include Medicare enrollees, licensed drivers, or individuals contacted by random-digit dialing within specific area codes.

The Internet has provided a means for recruitment of a diverse, interested study population; although self-selected, the subjects are willing to respond to study protocols. This recruitment method provided Lieberman and colleagues with a diverse study population of women and men with a history of bipolar disorder, a serious mental condition of low frequency, who were not readily accessible through alternative recruitment avenues.[44]

Community and Geographic Recruitment

The Framingham Heart Study, noted previously in the discussion of cohort study design, included more than 30% of the population in 1948.[33] Federal funds continue to support the project, enabling follow-up of the original participants and their descendents. Results of the hundreds of studies conducted on data collected during comprehensive physical exams conducted every 4 years and analyses of biospecimens and questionnaire data have identified precursors of heart disease, stroke, and aging. Using these extensive research findings, guidelines for personal health behaviors have been established.[45] In addition to recommended health promotion guidelines, the study findings led to development of medications that have contributed to reduced heart disease mortality over the past 50 years.[46] Recent studies by several social scientists have observed maintenance of healthy behavior patterns among lifelong Framingham friends including smoking cessation, increased physical activity, and optimum weight for height, suggesting a "contagious" nature for healthy lifestyles within the social network of this aging population.[47]

Community-based research became a major component of the American response to the human immunodeficiency virus (HIV)/acquired immune deficiency syndrome (AIDS) epidemic as the CDC supported local interventions that successfully changed behaviors and contributed to reduced risk of HIV transmission.[48] Concern about localized environmental exposures has increased as incidence rates vary considerably among American cities and states. Investigators have targeted some studies in specific high-risk areas in order to detect potential community-based exposures associated with disease development that may compound individual-level risk factors. New technology has enabled measurement of some adverse exposures, providing scientific evidence of neighborhood contaminants that may increase disease risk many years after initial exposures.[49]

Recruitment Based on Clinical Characteristics

Characteristics of case subjects must be clearly defined and clinically confirmed before they are recruited to case-control studies or are identified in cohort studies. Many clinical factors require consideration when recruiting women for research including reproductive history, menstrual status, genetic susceptibility, among others. Menopausal status may be quite complex to define given the high proportion of hysterectomy at varying ages, accuracy of recall among women reporting natural menopause (not due to radiation, surgery, or medication) and indeterminate status of women using hormone replacement and experiencing menstrual-type bleeding.[50] To correlate self-reported menopausal status with hormonal changes, some studies use biologic measures obtained from serum[51] or vaginal smear cytology.[52]

Twin studies (both monozygotic and dizygotic) provide powerful means for identifying gene-environment interactions. When concordance of a condition is greater among monozygotic than dizygotic twins, the etiologic role of inheritance is strengthened as noted in some studies of social behaviors.[53] Recruitment of families at elevated risk for some diseases has provided resources for identifying specific susceptibility genes and family-specific genetic mutations.[54] Family-based registries provide unique opportunities for gene-environment interaction studies when paired siblings, who shared early life exposures, are discordant for adult onset diseases.[55] Genetic studies must recruit diverse populations to avoid population stratification, a form of bias that may occur when a genotype and a specific disease both vary by race, causing study results to be either false positive or false negative.[56] Many international collaborative studies have predicted gene-specific cancer risk from incidence patterns observed among members of highly selected families, which may overestimate the likelihood of disease development compared with mutation carriers from larger, more diverse populations.[57]

Data and Biologic Sample Collection

The quality of data collected is a primary determinant of valid epidemology studies. Descriptive research is often conducted using information routinely collected by federal agencies, vital statistics, state-based health departments, cancer registries, and hospital admissions (Table 2-3). Most analytic studies collect data directly from study participants by in-person interview, telephone, or mailed questionnaire. Among the data sources noted in Table 2-3 is the Behavioral Risk Factor Surveillance System (BFRSS) created by the CDC in 1984 to routinely assess personal health status and risk behaviors known to affect morbidity and mortality. Increased use of new communication technology has adversely affected BRFSS participation rates as contact is attempted only through landline telephones potentially limiting the representativeness of the data. To overcome these obstacles, the CDC has enhanced the system enabling annual BRFSS cross-sectional surveys to provide reliable data to guide public health policies (Table 2-3).[58]

Accurate recall of the frequency and duration of some important health behaviors is difficult to obtain reliably. Therefore, carefully developed and tested data collection instruments are used to collect information on personal behavior such as physical activity. A team of California investigators designed a self-report questionnaire to capture the broad range and complexity of exercise detailing the frequency, duration, and intensity of the activity which is now routinely used in epidemiologic studies.[59]

Reliability of self-reported data has been a constant concern as studies have shown inconsistent recall by women, regardless of their disease status, when asked about specific exposures such as use of prenatal medications,[60] frequency of screening procedures,[61] and extent of family history.[62] In response to questions addressing clinical events, occupational exposures, and other potentially important factors, study subjects must often rely on their memory as efforts to obtain documentation have rarely been successful. The Cancer and Steroid Hormone Study initiated in 1980 by the CDC included a women's health study calendar on which participants recorded dates of major life experiences to facilitate recall of reproductive events, use of contraceptives, etc. In addition, a book of photographs presenting all available brands and dosages of birth control pills were shown to study participants.[63]

Wording of questionnaires may influence the accuracy of responses as noted by Mitchell and colleagues[64] in a pilot study prior to a multisite investigation of an

Table 2-3

Sources of population-based data used in epidemiology studies

Sources of Data	Examples Referenced in This Textbook
Phone surveys, in-person interviews or phone contacts, mailed questionnaires	Behavioral Risk Factor Survey System [BRFSS], Health Interview Survey, investigator-initiated research
Mandatory laboratory reports	Newly diagnosed HIV & AIDS, sexually transmitted infections
Health maintenance organizations	Kaiser Permanente, Mayo Clinic, Puget Sound Cooperative
Federal and state-based cancer registries	Surveillance, Epidemiology and End Results [SEER], State Registries
Hospital and medical care statistics	Medicare, Medicaid, hospital admissions records
National health surveillance	National Health Center for Health Statistics [NHANES]

association between birth defects and prenatal drug exposure. Responses to open-ended inquiries about drug use generated fewer affirmative responses in contrast to questions naming specific drugs prescribed for common symptoms.[64] Consistent wording of questionnaires used for more than 40 years by the American Cancer Society Prevention Studies has enabled detection of changing health practices and disease outcomes across decades.[65]

The source of data, collection methods, and willingness of the study participants have a significant impact on the reliability, completeness, and usefulness of the information collected. When appropriate and feasible, biosamples have been used to compare self-reported behaviors with biochemical measures of exposure. One study measured levels of cotinine in saliva to compare with smoking history reported by adolescent study subjects.[66] A second technique for detecting inconsistent self-reported smoking by adolescents involved data collected during school and at home from the same participants; 20% who reported smoking on the school-based study denied ever smoking on the survey completed at home.[67]

Retrospective versus Prospective Data Collection

The prospective nature of cohort study data collection is designed to avoid "recall bias" that may influence responses, such as newly diagnosed women blaming specific exposures for their disease.[3] The potential long latency between enrollment of healthy women and disease detection during follow-up requires cohort studies to include large populations at risk for the condition(s) of interest who are willing to provide baseline data and biospecimens and to be repeatedly contacted for updated personal information.[33]

Data collected retrospectively during a single interview or survey from participants in case-control studies may result in findings that conflict with analyses of data collected prospectively during years of follow-up after initial cohort recruitment. Factors contributing to the divergent findings should be carefully explored and potentially resolved to avoid miscommunications with healthcare providers and the public. Moffitt and colleagues noted recall bias was avoided when mental health status was assessed prospectively among subjects ages 18 to 32; rates were doubled compared with retrospective reporting.[68] Although *falsely negative* findings may appear inappropriately reassuring, *falsely positive* epidemiologic studies may misguide public health decision making and future governmental funding.[69] Multiple factors contribute to the frequency of false-positive epidemiologic research, including numerous studies in different populations of potential risk factors leading inevitably to a proportion of false-positive findings, overinterpretation of minimally significant findings, and biased preference for reporting positive findings, among others.[69]

Epidemiologic Criteria of Causation

Epidemiologists conducting etiologic studies search for factors that explain differences in disease incidence

between groups of individuals, evaluating potential risk factors, assessing individual susceptibility, and environmental cofactors. Most clinical conditions have multiple causes including both genetic and environmental factors. Some genetic markers or environmental exposures may be *necessary* for disease to be initiated but may not be *sufficient* causes without additional adverse events. Analytic assessment of potential etiologic agents is complicated by the long latency known to exist between initial adverse exposures and detection of disease through screening or symptoms. Although risk factors may strongly predict disease in groups with specific characteristics, these may not readily translate to person-specific risk of each individual of the group as genetic and behaviors factors may strongly modify the likelihood of a disease developing.[27] In 1965, Hill developed the following criteria to guide evaluation of causal inference in epidemiologic studies; one or more of the following criteria are routinely noted in most investigations.[70]

Strength of the Association

The disease must occur with greater frequency among exposed than unexposed women; a larger difference between the groups increases the likelihood of a causal relationship. The first Surgeon General's report of 1964 based on hundreds of studies stated smoking was the cause of lung cancer, one of the strongest causal associations in public health literature.[71] The 2010 Surgeon General's report stated that exposure to active smoking and passive inhalation of cigarette smoke damages coronary arteries, lung tissue, and other organs.[72]

Biologic Gradient

When the frequency of a disease is positively correlated with increasing levels of exposure, a dose-response effect may be detected, strengthening the probability of a causal relationship. Early studies revealed that the risk of lung cancer significantly increased with the number of cigarettes smoked per day and total number of pack years of smoking.[43]

Temporality

Exposure to a potential causal factor must precede the onset of disease. For some conditions with long latency between exposures and disease, accurate timing of exposure may be difficult to document. However, timing may be crucial, as was learned with in utero exposure to DES. Use during the first few weeks of pregnancy was found to cause gynecologic abnormalities not detected until 15 or 20 years after birth.[13] In contrast to the long latency from administration to detection of adverse effects, the week of gestation when thalidomide was used had specific deforming effects on the developing fetus detected at birth.[11]

Specificity

If an exposure is associated with the emergence of a clinical condition at an unexpected age or frequency, a causal interpretation is strengthened. One historical example is provided by a small matched case-control study that identified prenatal exposure to DES as the cause of vaginal cancer diagnosed soon after puberty among young women.[13] Other adverse gynecologic effects of this hormonal exposure have complicated the lives of thousands of exposed women.

Consistency

When etiologic studies conducted among different populations repeatedly produce similar findings, the probability of a causal effect is increased. Multiple studies associated lack of pregnancy with increased risk of ovarian cancer. A 1955 report noted ovarian cancer deaths were 50% higher among never-married compared to married women. Subsequent research conducted 20 years later indicated nulliparity rather than marital status was associated with development of ovarian cancer.[73]

Biologic Plausibility

The suspected association must be biologically plausible in relation to the natural history of the disease. In DES-exposed women vaginal carcinoma appeared after onset of puberty, when increasing levels of endogenous estrogens stimulated tumor growth in previously initiated vaginal tissue.[13] Cramer suggested the biologic explanation for increased ovarian cancer among nulliparous women was associated with uninterrupted menstrual cycles that raise estrogen levels and potentially stimulate cancer development.[74]

Coherence of Evidence

When temporal trends indicate corresponding changes in a disease and an exposure, a causal relationship is more likely to exist, as in the correlation of estrogen use for menopausal symptoms and incidence rates of endometrial cancer observed first in ecologic studies and subsequently in analytic evaluations.[23] Similarly, a decline in both breast cancer incidence and exogenous hormone use has followed the 2002 publication of the Women's Health Initiative clinical trial results that clearly linked combined estrogen and progestin with estrogen-positive breast cancer.[24]

Statistical Assessment of Early Detection Modalities

The continuing development of new and costly modalities for early detection of disease has been heralded as a major advance in clinical medicine. Reduction in mortality has led to some screening methods being referred to as "preventive" modalities; however, these procedures meet secondary prevention criteria. Risk of disease is not reduced by screening. Detection at early, asymptomatic stages *increases* incidence rates, as can be noted in data from the cancer registries of the Surveillance, Epidemiology and End Results (SEER), a National Cancer Institute program, following expansion of cancer screening programs.[75] Early detection methods have been assessed in case-control studies[76] and among cohorts enrolled in

the Breast Cancer Detection Demonstration Project[77] that offered free screening to American women, although the gold standard for unbiased assessment is the randomized controlled trial.[75,78] Some screening modalities, such as the Pap test for detection of cervical cancer, have been adopted by healthcare providers without confirmatory studies.[79]

To assess the benefit of treatment after screening in contrast to therapy at a later stage after onset of symptoms, investigators must address two potential sources of error: *lead-time bias* and *length bias*.[75,79] **Lead-time** bias describes a time interval between earlier detection of a condition by screening among presumably healthy women and a diagnostic procedure detecting the condition after clinical evidence or symptoms develop. The duration of lead time varies in relation to the nature of the developing condition as well as personal characteristics of study subjects, including age, hormonal status, immune function, presence of comorbid conditions, etc. Although screen-detected cases may appear to benefit from longer survival time than cases diagnosed with symptoms, the possibility exists for the screened individual to have lived longer with the disease without benefit of improved length of survival.[75,78] Therefore, the statistic noting the proportion of people with screen-detected cancers surviving 5 years or longer includes the lead time obtained through earlier diagnosis by screening.

Length bias described the recognized problem that screening often detects diseases with long presymptomatic phases; the length of this phase varies considerably with the natural history of the diseases as well as specific patient characteristics. Clinical conditions with short preclinical phases are least likely to benefit from screening. Given that screening detects slower growing lesions, many of which may never become symptomatic, Welch and Black have suggested overdiagnosis has occurred. Highly sensitive screening methods applied to subclinical cases of disease using methods such as mammography and newer procedures, including magnetic resonance imaging (MRI), detected conditions that may not have surfaced during the woman's lifetime in the absence of screening.[80] In such settings, early diagnosis through screening may be harmful; women potentially receive detrimental treatment for conditions not clinically lethal.[75] Molecular markers are being identified to enable separation of more indolent disease from potentially aggressive lesions in order to avoid morbidity from unnecessary invasive screening and treatment.[81]

Screening tests must meet acceptable standards of accuracy before being applied to presumably healthy women. Four measures used to describe the level of accuracy of screening tests are calculated by comparing the true health status in relation to the test result as noted:[75]

1. Sensitivity: the probability of screened women with the condition who test positive

$$\frac{\text{True positives}}{\text{true positives} + \text{false negatives}}$$

2. Specificity: the probability of screened women who do not have the condition and test negative

$$\frac{\text{True negatives}}{\text{false positive} + \text{true negative}}$$

3. Positive predictive value: the proportion of screened women testing positive who have the condition

$$\frac{\text{True positive}}{\text{true positive} + \text{true negative}}$$

4. Negative predictive value: The proportion of screened women testing negative who do not have the condition

$$\frac{\text{True negative}}{\text{true negative} + \text{false negative}}$$

Statistic Measures of Association— Quantifying Risk of Disease

Carefully designed epidemiologic research requires appropriate analytic methods to address specific research questions. An essential component of each investigation is clearly defined statistical procedures that will be applied to assess relationships between "independent" variables and specific disease "outcomes." Estimates of association are calculated with 95% confidence intervals.

Absolute Risk, Relative Risk, Odds Ratio, and Attributable Risk

Absolute risk (AR) defines the probability of diagnosing a disease in members of a cohort over a defined interval of time. A descriptive example is the incidence of hypertension detected at initial assessment and at a follow-up examination 24 months later in relation to obesity. The strength of the absolute risk of an exposure depends upon its biologic effect and the prevalence of the disease in question.

Relative risk (RR), the ratio of two absolute risks, estimates the strength of the relationship, if one exists, between a defined risk factor and a disease.

$$\text{Relative Risk} = \frac{\text{Absolute risk of hypertension among obese women}}{\text{Absolute risk of hypertension among nonobese women}}$$

For example, to determine if obesity, defined as body mass index > 30, is associated with newly detected hypertension 24 months after enrollment of a cohort of older women, the rate of hypertension among obese participants is compared with the rate of among cohort members who were not obese when initially assessed.

Odds ratio (OR) is an alternative measure to RR. Because recruitment for case-control studies begins with disease status, estimates of absolute risk and RR are not possible. Statisticians have proven that ORs provide reliable and valid estimates of RRs when case/control studies enroll incident (newly diagnosed) cases and unbiased representative controls.[82] In this example, appropriately selected controls are assumed to represent normotensive members of the population at large.

$$\text{Odds Ratio} = \frac{\text{Obesity among newly identified hypertensive (cases) women}}{\text{Obesity among normotensive (control) women}}$$

Rather than a single measure, obesity can also be defined by differing levels: normal weight, overweight, obese, and morbidly obese. Using graduated categories of obesity enables calculations of ORs potentially indicating a dose response association with hypertension.

A **confounding** factor may be associated with obesity but may also be an independent risk factor for hypertension such as a diet high in salt. When confounding factors are suspected, studies require data collection and analyses designed to address potential confounding.

Population Attributable Risk (PAR) is an estimate of the number of cases of a condition that might have been avoided if exposure to a causal factor had not occurred. The magnitude of attributable risk is correlated with the RR or OR associated with the risk factor and the prevalence of the exposure in the population; therefore, the PAR for lung cancer associated with smoking increased in parallel with increasing prevalence of cigarette sales. Although cigarette smoking has declined in recent decades, the residual adverse effect of the behavior continues to influence lung cancer incidence rates, which are beginning to decline in the 21st century.

Interpreting Measures of Association

If the rates of disease are comparable in the exposed and unexposed groups, the relative risk would be approximately 1.0, indicating the exposure is not associated with risk of the disease in the population studied. Calculated relative risks greater than 1.0 indicate an increased likelihood of disease associated with the risk factor, and RR less than 1.0 suggests a decreased probability of disease or a potential protective factor. When the 95% confidence interval (CI) describing the range of possible relative risk or odds ratio estimates includes 1.0, no statistically significant difference exists between exposed and unexposed in relation to the factor being studied.[27]

Some studies may produce relative risks or odds ratios that satisfy the usual criteria of statistical significance denoted by a *P* value less than 0.05 indicating a low probability (less than 1 in 20) of the result being due to chance and the confidence interval does not include 1.0. However, other factors must be considered before research findings are considered important for public health. The magnitude of the estimate, the width of the confidence interval, and the biologic plausibility must be considered before a research result is considered a true and important contribution to public health.[83]

False-positive results may occur due to bias in study design, selection of the study population, instruments used for data collection, etc. Publication bias, the tendency of investigators to submit positive results and the tendency of journals to preferentially publish statistically significant findings, increases attention paid to potentially false-positive results.[83] Therefore, replication studies are essential, as they rarely confirm false-positive findings that were due to chance; however, confirmatory studies may produce false-positive results if similar study subjects and data collection materials are used. For these reasons, the diverse results from studies of differing designs must be considered. Greater confidence in research findings should be associated with mutually compatible results obtained from several differently designed studies conducted among diverse populations.[82] Many epidemiologists are skeptical of weak relative risks or odds ratios less than 3.0 if the finding is new and unexpected (Table 2-4).[2]

When the results of some investigations meet the expectations or beliefs of advocates and concerned members of the public, the study findings may receive inappropriate overly enthusiastic coverage by the media, often stimulating demands for further research.[27,83] Although the magnitude of the risk is vital to assess, relatively small differences in adverse exposures may affect the health of many people when a large percentage of the population is exposed.

Examples of risk assessments are included in Table 2-5.

Table 2-4

Interpreting statistical associations—possible explanations for results

Cause-effect	Risk factor is significantly associated with disease, meets one or more causal criteria
Bias	Systematic errors distort results – ex. Recall bias, biased study population selected
Confounding	Finding due to an independent exposure related to the risk factor & condition being studied
Chance	P-value >0.05 or $P<0.05$ large study population with small, biologically meaningless finding

Table 2-5

Assessment of the magnitude of the relative risks estimates

Relative Risk	Impact of Risk on Disease	Change in Risk	RR/OR [95% CI]*	Examples from Text Factor & Disease	Chapter & Ref
10.00 <	Extremely increased	≥ 600 – 1000% increase	RR–10.0 to RR 32.0	Risk of breast &/ or ovarian cancer associated with a BRCA mutation	Ch 41; Ref 16
5.00 – 9.99	Very great increase	≥ 500% increase	RR=7.4 [CI=3.3–16.3]	Alcohol abuse increased risk of bipolar disease in women	Ch 17; Ref 51
3.00 – 4.99	Large increase	200 – 399% increase	RR=3.9 [CI=2.0–7.7]	Daughter's risk of ovarian cancer following mother's diagnosis	Ch 27; Ref 44
2.00 – 2.99	Moderate increase	100 – 299% increase	RR=2.38 [CI=1.79–3.18]	Diabetes increased the risk of vascular dementia	Ch 24; Ref 91
1.35 – 1.99	Small increase	35 – 99% increase	RR=1.43 [CI=1.1–1.9]	Poor oral health increased risk of malnutrition in the elderly	Ch 36; Ref 62
1.21 – 1.34	Minimal increase	10 – 34% increase	RR=1.33 [CI=1.2–1.5]	Secondhand smoke increased risk of lung cancer among nonsmokers	Ch 25; Ref 23
1.01 – 1.20	Slight increase	1 – 9% increase	RR=1.13 [CI=1.02–1.24]	Early menarche (age<12 yrs) increased risk of adult hypertension	Ch 8; Ref 69

(continues)

Table 2-5

Assessment of the magnitude of the relative risks estimates (*continued*)

Relative Risk	Impact of Risk on Disease	Change in Risk	RR/OR [95% CI]*	Examples from Text Factor & Disease	Chapter & Ref
1.00	No influence on risk	No association	RR=1.0 [CI=0.9–1.01]*	Oral contraceptive use did not affect breast cancer risk (CARE study)	Ch 26; Ref 156
0.91 – 0.99	Slight nonsignificant decrease	1 – 9% decrease	RR=0.97 [CI=0.9–1.01]*	No association between Vitamin D supplementation and breast cancer risk	Ch 26; Ref 268
0.71 – 0.90	Small decrease	10 – 24% decrease	RR=0.81 [CI=0.74–0.88]	Cigarette smoking reduced risk of endometrial cancer	Ch 28; Ref 95
0.51 – 0.70	Moderate decrease	25 – 49% decrease	RR=0.54 [CI =0.47–0.63]	RCT of Tai Chi; lowered risk of falls in the elderly population	Ch 38; Ref 69
0.21 – 0.50	Large decrease	50 – 79% decrease	RR=0.33 [CI=0.16–0.64]	Tubal ligation significantly lowered ovarian cancer risk	Ch 27; Ref 79
≤ 0.20	Very great decrease	≥ 85% decrease	RR=0.15 [CI=0.0–0.2]	Prophylactic bilateral mastectomy significantly lowered breast cancer risk	Ch 26, Ref 299

*CI=Confidence Interval, results are nonsignificant when 95% CI includes 1.0

Multifactorial Research

Early in the 20th century research efforts focused on identifying specific bacterial and viral causes of infectious disease, which eventually enabled vaccines to be developed and diseases prevented. Recently, similar study designs have heralded the discovery of infectious components of several chronic conditions, providing the opportunity to dramatically change the incidence and mortality associated with cervical cancer[18] and stomach cancer[19] among other conditions. Although these single agents may be necessary in the causal pathway to disease development, increased susceptibility is dependent upon more complex cofactors, including physiologic, emotional, and behavioral patterns of women at risk. Therefore, appropriate research must be multidisciplinary, using new measurement technologies and analytic techniques.[2] As biospecimens are relied upon for measurements of exposures and genetic differences among study subjects, ethical and legal issues must be addressed to ethically obtain informed consent while protecting the privacy of research subjects whose invaluable resources are selected for analysis.[84]

Research has repeatedly shown that exposure-disease associations vary among different populations depending on host characteristics such as gender, age at time of exposure, nutrition status, inherited risk, and epigenetic factors. Genetic factors may differ even within families in which inheritance of the susceptibility genotype varies among parents and siblings; differing environmental exposures also contribute to disease risk among blood relatives.[85] Such variation, referred to as interaction or effect modification, raises important questions about the etiologic factors being investigated and emphasizes the individual nature of disease risk and the future of personalized medicine.

Conflicting Epidemiologic Research Findings

Epidemiologic studies of varying designs conducted among diverse populations often produce inconsistent or conflicting findings that confuse the public. Since epidemiologic research often addresses clinically important aspects of health and disease in diverse populations, the findings may not pertain to specific study participants with person-specific genetic and environmental risks of disease. However, clinicians guide individuals based on research results, and the public often responds to media presentations of newly published findings.[86] Therefore, some investigators and journalists caution against quick acceptance of early study results and may suggest that the public delay major health behavior changes until additional data are published.[86]

Differences may be anticipated when results of case-control studies are compared with associations reported from cohort studies in which women are followed over varying intervals of time. Data obtained from newly diagnosed cases may be influenced by disease status and not recalled accurately in comparison to controls; in contrast, cohort studies collect data over time as exposures are experienced reducing the likelihood of distorted recall.

Unique susceptibility or protective factors may be active among some members of study populations partially contributing to divergent outcomes, although study methodology may also influence the consistency of results when comparing studies of similar design including: data collection methods, self-reported health status vs. physical examination, conflicting definitions of specific conditions or clinical events, varying dosages and frequency of medication use, etc. Additional larger investigations may be required to accurately determine potential etiologic factors.[87]

Statistical Power

Before a study is launched or funding sought, the number of participants required to ensure adequate power must be determined. The size of the population influences the probability of finding a statistically significant relationship between risk factors and disease outcomes if one truly exists. In a case-control study, the number of women needed for each group is determined by the prevalence of the exposures being studied and their expected effect on risk factors of disease. Similarly, when establishing a cohort study, the frequency and magnitude of exposures to the risk factors and their impact on study outcomes all affect the number of participants required for baseline and follow-up data collection. In addition, the width of the confidence interval from a cohort study provides the range of the true effect and a measure of the study's power.[82]

Meta-Analyses and Reviews

Many epidemiologic studies are of limited sample size and are conducted in diverse settings often producing weak correlations. To obtain a summary estimate from individual published studies, the statistical technique called meta-analysis was developed and has been frequently applied to major topics of interest. The selection of published investigations to include in these composite analyses may be difficult because not all research reports may have provided adequate information for assessment of several important evaluation measures including study design, composition of the population, selection, and exclusion criteria. Meta-analyses provide a means for combining research findings from diverse study populations; however, publication bias may influence such studies given that positive, including falsely positive research, has a greater chance of being published and, therefore,

available for inclusion in meta-analyses. To address additional biases that may influence results of meta-analyses, guidelines to improve the quality of these important contributions to epidemiology research were published by a concerned team of investigators.[88] Although well-designed studies of adequate size are preferred to detect meaningful associations of risk factors and disease, pooled analyses can provide meaningful information when collaborators are able to combine raw data from multiple investigations that were similarly conducted providing comparable measures of exposures and disease outcomes.[89]

Future of Epidemiology Studies

Some critics have suggested epidemiologic methods are too imprecise to adequately measure subtle adverse or protective effects of low-level exposures.[90] Others have questioned the reliance on self-reported personal information including imprecise measures of environmental contaminants, which often produce conflicting or falsely positive results.[83] Recently, epidemiology has been accused of creating unnecessary anxiety after repetitive studies produce inconsistent findings that receive extensive attention by the media.[27,90] However, observational studies remain essential for assessment of health behaviors and clinical outcomes that ethically cannot be randomly assigned for experimental investigations.[88] New technology is being developed to measure endogenous factors as well as past and current environmental exposures. These developing tools have encouraged investigators to assemble data from diverse sources, stimulating development of causal inferences and potentially guiding future public health interventions. As this field of research matures aided by new scientific approaches and techniques, studies will be able to produce more consistent and valuable findings, which will increase respect for and reliance on epidemiology.

Summary

Well-designed epidemiologic studies, whether observational or experimental, contribute to understanding factors associate with disease development and prognosis. Statistical methods enabling assessment of the strength of causal or protective associations have evolved to accommodate multifactorial exposures of interest. The magnitude and biologic plausibility of identified etiologic agents contribute to causal hypotheses. Caution is advised when unexpected results are first presented; replication in different settings is essential to confirm newly identified risk factors. Technology advances have provided less costly molecular studies of biosamples, including blood and tissue specimens, fostering multidisciplinary investigations requiring complex analytic procedures. Gene-environment studies are providing new opportunities for more personalized assessment of health risks with the potential for disease prevention.

Discussion Questions

1. What are the major goals of epidemiology research? What study designs are most useful? Describe the strengths and weaknesses of each.

2. Describe the benefits and risks of early detection. Discuss the conflicts associated with screening methods.

3. To consider a factor an etiologic agent of disease causation, what criteria are used? Provide an example of each.

4. Methods of selection and recruitment of study participants is extremely important for epidemiologic studies. Describe the most desirable methods.

5. How does assessment of relative risk (RR) differ from calculation of an odds ratio (OR)?

6. When are statistical findings considered significant? How do you determine their public health significance?

References

1. Susser M, Stein Z. Contagion, infection, and the idea of specific agents. In: *Eras in Epidemiology*. New York, NY: Oxford University Press;2009:73–97.
2. Galea S, Riddle M, Kaplan GA. Causal thinking and complex system approaches in epidemiology. *Int J Epidemiol*. 2010;39:97–106.
3. Grimes DA, Schulz KF. Bias and causal associations in observational research. *Lancet*. 2002;359:248–252.
4. Tang H, Quertermous T, Rodriguez B, et al. Genetic structure, self-identified race/ethnicity, and confounding in case-control association studies. *Am J Hum Genet*. 2005;76:268–275.
5. Freeman HP. Commentary on the meaning of race in science and society. *Cancer Epidemiol Biomarkers Prev*. 2003;12(supp):232s–236s.
6. Marrie RA. Environmental risk factors in multiple sclerosis aetiology. *Lancet Neurol*. 2004;3:709–718.
7. Brown JR, O'Connor GT. Coronary heart disease and prevention in the United States. *N Engl J Med*. 2010;362:2150–2153.
8. John EM, Phipps AI, David A, Koo J. Migration history, acculturation, and breast cancer risk in Hispanics. *Cancer Epidemiol Biomarkers Prev*. 2005;14:2905–2913.
9. Perera FP, Li Z, Whyatt R, et al. Prenatal airborne polycyclic aromatic hydrocarbon exposure and child IQ at age 5 years. *Pediatrics*. 2009;124:e195–e202.
10. Landrigan PJ, Sonawane B, Butler RN, et al. Early environmental origins of neurodegenerative disease in later life. *Environ Health Perspect*. 2005; 113:1230–1233.
11. Heijmans BT, Tobi EW, Stein AD, et al. Persistent epigenetic differences associated with prenatal exposure to famine in humans. *PNAS*. 2008;105:17046–17049.
12. Leck IM, Millar ELM. Incidence of malformations since the introduction of thalidomide. *BMJ*. 1962;2:16–20.
13. Herbst AI, Ulfelder H, Poskanzer DC. Adenocarcinoma of the vagina. Association of maternal stilbestrol therapy with tumor appearance in young women. *N Engl J Med*. 1971;284:878–881.
14. Palmer JR, Wise LA, Hatch EE, et al. Prenatal diethylstilbestrol exposure and risk of breast cancer. *Cancer Epidemiol Biomarkers Prev*. 2006;15: 1509–1514.
15. McElligott JT, Darden PM. Are patient-held vaccination records associated with improved vaccination coverage rates? *Pediatrics*. 2010;125:e467–e472.
16. Parmet WE. Pandemic vaccines- The legal landscape.*N Engl J Med*. 2010;362:1949–1952.
17. Centers for Disease Control and Prevention (CDC). The Adult Hepatitis Vaccine Project—California, 2007–2008. *MMWR Morb Mortal Wkly Rep*. 2010;59:514–516.
18. Centers for Disease Control and Prevention (CDC). FDA licensure of bivalent human papillomavirus vaccine (HPV2, Cervarix) for use in females and updated HPV vaccination recommendations from the advisory committee on immunization practices (ACIP). *MMWR Morb Mortal Wkly Rep*. 2010;59:626–629.
19. Greenberg ER, Alberts DS, Potter JD. Introduction: what should we do now about *H. pylori*? *Cancer Epidemiol Biomarkers Prev*. 2005;14:1851–2.
20. Haskell WL, Lee IM, Pate RR, et al. Physical activity and public health. Updated recommendation for adults from the American College of Sports Medicine and the American Heart Association. *Circulation*. 2007;116:1081–1093.
21. Berry DA, Cronin KA, Plevritis SK, et al. Effect of screening and adjuvant therapy on mortality from breast cancer. *N Engl J Med*. 2005;353:1784–92.
22. American Diabetes Association. Standards of medical care in diabetes-2009. *Diabetes Care*. 2009;32(suppl1):S13–S61.
23. Austin DF, Roe KM. The decreasing incidence of endometrial cancer: public health implications. *Am J Public Health*. 1982;72:65–68.
24. Ravdin PM, Cronin KA, Howlader N, et al. The decrease in breast-cancer incidence in 2003 in the United States. *N Engl J Med*. 2007;356:1670–1674.
25. Garland FC, Garland CF, Gorham ED, Young JF. Geographic variation in breast cancer mortality in the United States: a hypothesis involving exposure to solar radiation. *Prev Med*. 1990;19:614–122.
26. John EM, Schwartz GG, Dreon DM, Koo J. Vitamin D and breast cancer risk: The NHANES I epidemiologic follow-up study, 1971–1975 to 1992. *Cancer Epidemiol Biomarkers Prev*. 1999;8:399–406.
27. Kabat GC. Hyping Health Risk. Environmental Hazards in Daily Life and the Science of Epidemiology. New York, NY: Columbia University Press;2008: 19–46.
28. Stewart WF, Wood C, Reed ML, et al. Cumulative lifetime migraine incidence in women and men. *Cephalalgia*. 2008;28:1170–1178.
29. Tanner JM, Whitehouse RH. Clinical longitudinal standards for height, weight, height velocity, weight velocity, and stages of puberty. *Arch Diseases Childhood*. 1976;51:170–179.
30. Wong MY, Day NE, Luan JA, et al. The detection of gene-environment interaction for continuous traits: should we deal with measurement error by bigger studies or better measurements? *Int J Epidemiol*. 2003;32:51–57.
31. Senie RT, Rosen OO, Rhodes P, et al. Obesity at diagnosis of breast carcinoma influences duration of disease-free survival. *Ann Internal Med*. 1992;116:26–32.
32. Petrek JA, Naughton MJ, Case LD, et al. Incidence, time course, and determinants of menstrual bleeding after breast cancer treatment: A prospective study. *J Clin Oncol*. 2006;24:1045–1051.
33. Oppenheimer GM. Becoming the Framingham study 1947–1950. *Am J Public Health*. 2005;95:602–610.
34. Susser E, Terry MB. A conception-to-death cohort. *Lancet*. 2003;361: 797–798.
35. Chiuve SE, Rimm EB, Mukamal KJ, et al. Light-to-moderate alcohol consumption and risk of sudden cardiac death in women. *Heart Rhythm*. 2010;7:1374–1380.
36. Schwartzbaum J, Ahlbom A, Feychting M. Berkson's bias reviewed. *Europ J Epidemiol*. 2003;18:1109–1112.
37. Jacobs EJ, Rodriguez C, Newton CC, et al. Family history of various cancers and pancreatic cancer mortality in a large cohort. *Cancer Causes Control*. 2009;20:1261–1269.
38. Clark C. A "Hitherto unrecognized" occupational hazard. In: *Radium Girls. Women and Industrial Health Reform, 1910–1935*. Chapel Hill, NC: University of North Carolina Press;1997:87–111.
39. Hildreth NG, Shore RE, Dvoretsky PM. The risk of breast cancer after irradiation of the thymus in infancy. *N Engl J Med*. 1989;321:1281–1284.
40. Omenn GS, Goodman GE, Thornquist M, Brunzell JD. Long-term Vitamin A does not produce clinically significant hypertriglyceridemia: results from CARET, the B-Carotene and retinol efficacy trial. *Cancer Epidemiol Biomarkers Prev*. 1994;3:711–713.
41. Dieckmann WJ, Davis ME, Rynliewicz LM, Pottinger RE. Does the administration of diethylstilbestrol during pregnancy have therapeutic value? *Am J Obstet Gynecol*. 1953;66:1063–1081.
42. Gammon MD, Neugut AI, Santella RM, et al. The Long Island Breast Cancer Study Project: description of a multi-institutional collaboration to identify environmental risk factors for breast cancer. *Breast Cancer Res Treat*. 2002;74:235–54.
43. Stellman SD, Muscat JE, Hoffmann D, Wynder EL. Impact of filter cigarette smoking on lung cancer histology. *Prev Med*. 1997;26:451–56.
44. Lieberman DZ, Massey SH, Goodwin FK. The role of gender in single vs married individuals with bipolar disorder. *Compr Psychiatry*. 2010;51:380–5.
45. Oppenheimer GM. Framingham Heart Study: The first 20 years. *Prog Cardiovasc Dis*. 2010;53:55–61.
46. Fox CS. Cardiovascular disease risk factors, type 2 diabetes mellitus, and the Framingham Heart Study. *Trends Cardiovasc Med*. 2010;20:90–95.
47. Fowler JH, Christakis NA. Dynamic spread of happiness in a large social network: longitudinal analysis over 20 years in the Framingham Heart Study. *BMJ*. 2008;337:a2338.
48. CDC AIDS Community Demonstration Projects Research Group. Community-level HIV intervention in 5 cities: final outcome data from CDC AIDS community demonstration projects. *Am J Public Health*. 1999;89:336–345.
49. Gammon MD, Santella RM. PAH, genetic susceptibility and breast cancer risk: An update from the Long Island Breast Cancer Study Project. *Europ J Cancer*. 2008;44:636–640.
50. Whittemore AS, Harris R, Itnyre J, et al. Characteristics relating to ovarian cancer risk: collaborative analysis of 12 US case-control studies. 1. Methods. *Am J Epidemiol*. 1992;1175–1183.
51. Garcia CR, Sammel MD, Freeman EW, et al. Defining menopausal status: creation of a new definition to identify the early changes of the menopausal transition. *Menopause*. 2005;12:128–135.
52. Senie RT, Lobenthal SW, Rosen PP. Association of vaginal smear cytology with menstrual status in breast cancer. *Breast Cancer Res Treat*. 1985;5: 301–310.
53. Fowler JH, Dawes CT, Christakis NA. Model of genetic variation in human social networks. *PNAS*. 2009;106:1720–1724.

54. Siegmund KD, Whittemore AS, Thomas DC. Multistage sampling for disease family registries. *Monogr Natl Cancer Inst*. 1999;26:43–8.

55. John EM, Hopper JL, Beck JC, et al. The Breast Cancer Family Registry: an infrastructure for cooperative multinational, interdisciplinary and translational studies of the genetic epidemiology of breast cancer. *Breast Cancer Res*. 2004;6:R375–389.

56. Rebbeck TR. Inherited genetic markers and cancer outcomes: Personalized medicine in the postgenome era. *J Clinical Oncol*. 2006;24:1972–1974.

57. Antoniou A, Pharoah PDP, Narod S, et al. Average risks of breast and ovarian cancer associated with *BRCA1* or *BRCA2* mutations detected in case series unselected for family history: a combined analysis of 22 studies. *Am J Hum Genet*. 2003;72:1117–1130.

58. Behavioral Risk Factor Surveillance System (BFRSS), National Center for Chronic Disease Prevention and Health Promotion. Prevalence and trends data. Nationwide (States and DC)—2008 tobacco use. http://apps.nccd.cdc.gov/BRFSS/sex.asp?cat=TU&yr=2008&qkey=4394&state=UB. Accessed January 17, 2011.

59. Mai PI, Sullivan-Halley J, Ursin G, et al. Physical activity and colon cancer risk among women in the California Teachers Study. *Cancer Epidemiol Biomarkers Prev*. 2007;16:517–525.

60. Tilley BC, Barnes AB, Bergstralh E, et al. A comparison of pregnancy history recall and medical records. *Am J Epidemiol*. 1985;121:269–281.

61. Caplan LS, McQueen DV, Qualters JR, et al. Validity of women's self-reports of cancer screening test utilization in a managed care population. *Cancer Epidemiol Biomarkers Prevent*. 2003;12:1182–1187.

62. Glanz K, Grove J, Le Marchand L, Gotay C. Underreporting of family history of colon cancer: Correlates and implications. *Cancer Epidemiol Biomarkers Prev*. 1999;8:635–639.

63. Wingo PA, Ory HW, Layde PM, Lee NC. The evaluation of the data collection process for a multicenter, population-based, case-control design. *Am J Epidemiol*. 1988;128:206–17.

64. Mitchell AA, Cottler LB, Shapiro S. Effect of questionnaire design on recall of drug exposure in pregnancy. *Am J Epidemiol*. 1986;123:670–6.

65. Shopland DR, Eyre HJ, Pechacek TF. Smoking attributable cancer mortality in 1991: is lung cancer now the leading cause of death among smokers in the United States? *J Natl Cancer Inst*. 1991;83:1142–48.

66. Kandel DB, Schaffran C, Griesler PC, et al. Salivary cotinine concentration versus self-reported cigarette smoking: Three patterns of inconsistency in adolescence. *Nicotine Tob Res*. 2006;8:525–537.

67. Griesler PC, Kandel DB, Schaffran C, et al. Adolescents' inconsistency in self-reported smoking. a comparison of reports in school and in home settings. *Public Opin Q*. 2008;72:260–290.

68. Moffitt TE, Caspi A, Taylor A, et al. How common are common mental disorders? Evidence that lifetime prevalence rates are doubled by prospective versus retrospective ascertainment. *Psychol Med*. 2010;40:899–909.

69. Boffetta P, McLaughlin JK, La Vecchia C, et al. False-positive results in cancer epidemiology: A plea for epistemological modesty. *J Natl Cancer Inst*. 2010;100:988–995.

70. Hill AB. The environment and disease: Association or causation? *Proceedings of the Royal Society of Medicine*. 1965;58:295–300.

71. Surgeon General, Advisory Committee of the USPHS. *Smoking and Health*. PHS Publication No. 1103. Washington, DC: US Department of Health, Education, and Welfare; 1964.

72. US Department of Health and Human Services. *How Tobacco Smoke Causes Disease: The Biology and Behavioral Basis for Smoking-Attributable Disease: A Report of the Surgeon General*. Atlanta, GA: US Department of Health and Human Services, Centers for Disease Control and Prevention, National Center for Chronic Disease Prevention and Health Promotion, Office on Smoking and Health; 2010.

73. Beral V, Fraser P, Chilvers C. Does pregnancy protect against ovarian Cancer? *Lancet*. 1978;1:1083–1087.

74. Cramer DW, Welch WR. Determinants of ovarian cancer risk. II. Inferences regarding pathogenesis. *J Natl Cancer Inst*. 1983;71:717–21.

75. Brawley OW, Kramer BS. Cancer screening in theory and in practice. *J Clin Oncol*. 2005;23:293–300.

76. Newcomb PA, Norfleet RG, Storer BE, et al. Screening sigmoidoscopy and colorectal cancer mortality. *J Natl Cancer Inst*. 1992;84:1572–1575.

77. Bryne C, Smart CR, Chu KC, Hartmann WH. survival advantage by age. Evaluation of the extended follow-up of the Breast Cancer Detection Demonstration Project. Cancer 1994;74(Suppl):301–310.

78. Morabia A, Zhang FF. History of medical screening: from concept to action. *Postgrad Med J*. 2004;80:463–469

79. Foltz AM, Kelsey JL. The annual Pap test: a dubious policy success. *Milbank Mem Fund Q Health Soc*. 1978;56:426–62.

80. Welch HG, Black WC. Overdiagnosis in cancer. *J Natl Cancer Inst*. 2010;102:605–613.

81. Esserman L, Thompson I. Solving the overdiagnosis dilemma. *J Natl Cancer Inst*. 2010;102:582–583.

82. Hennekens CH, Buring JE. Measures of disease frequency and association. In: Mayrent SL, ed. *Epidemiology in Medicine*. Boston, MA. Little, Brown and Company; 1987:54–97.

83. Boffetta P, McLaughlin JK, La Vecchia C, et al. False-positive results in cancer epidemiology: a plea for epistemological modesty. *J Natl Cancer Inst*. 2008;100:988–995.

84. Vaught JB, Lockhart N, Thiel KS, Schneider JA. Ethical, legal, and policy issues: dominating the biospecimen discussion. *Cancer Epidemiol Biomarkers Prev*. 2007;16:2521–2525.

85. Ottman R. Gene-environment interaction: Definitions and study designs. *Preventive Med*. 1996;25:764–770.

86. Angell M. Interpreting EPI studies. *N Eng J Med*. 1990;323:823–825

87. Bailar JC. When research results are in conflict. Editorial. *N Engl J Med*. 1985;313:1080–1081.

88. Stroup DF, Berlin JA, Morton SC, et al. Meta-analysis of observational studies in epidemiology. a proposal for reporting. *JAMA*. 2000;283:2008–2012

89. Collaborative Group on Epidemiological Studies of Ovarian Cancer. Ovarian cancer and oral contraceptives: collaborative reanalysis of data from 45 epidemiological studies including 23,257 women with ovarian cancer and 87,303 controls. *Lancet*. 2008;371:303–314.

90. Taubes G. Epidemiology faces its limits. *Science*. 1995;269:164–9.

Personal and Community-Based Health Promotion and Morbidity Prevention

Intentional and Unintentional Injury Mortality and Morbidity

Joyce C. Pressley, PhD, MPH and Patrick Dawson, BA, MPH

Introduction

Approximately 4.7% (57,063) of the total deaths in U.S. women in 2007 were due to an injury-related cause, including suicide and homicide.[1] Although women account for slightly less than one-third (31.3%) of all injury deaths each year, injury is important in the spectrum of diseases and conditions affecting women due to the timing of these events in the life course: contributions to mortality, morbidity, and disability, and in later life, threats to independent living. Injury exerts both direct and indirect effects on the lives of women. Despite men having higher mortality, injury continues to be the leading cause of death in women aged 1 to 39 years. During peak childbearing and childrearing years, three of the five leading causes of death in women aged 15 to 39 years are injury related—suicide, homicide, and unintentional injury. In addition, injury has an indirect impact through the disruption of women's lives and added stress as women frequently serve as caregivers to injured children, spouses/partners, and parents of both sexes.

The relative rank of the injury burden among all conditions and diseases affecting the health of women varies depending on 1) the indicator measures used to describe the burden of disease; 2) the fineness of categories of injury intent and mechanisms or causes; and 3) the composition of the population in terms of age, race/ethnicity, socioeconomic and educational status. Within these categories, the relative importance of types of injuries varies considerably across the age span. For example, injury ranks fourth among causes of mortality, but first in years of potential life lost (YPLL) before age 65 among all women (Figure 3-1). This difference is accounted for primarily by differences in the younger ages at which injury exerts its most profound influence compared with older ages at onset of major chronic diseases and conditions.[2,3]

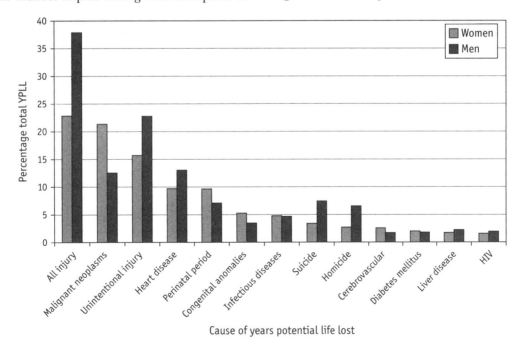

Figure 3-1 Percent of Years of Potential Life Lost in women and men by leading cause of death.

Source: Data from Web-based Injury Statistics Query and Reporting System (WISQARS) [Online]. (2007). National Center for Injury Prevention and Control, Centers for Disease Control and Prevention. www.cdc.gov/ncipc/wisqars. [2011 Feb 18].

In this chapter, the relative rank of injury is demonstrated among other prevalent diseases and health conditions women experience across the life span. The distribution of America's aging population by gender and age can be expected to affect the relative importance of several injury mechanisms. Research has tended to give greater emphasis to injuries among men who generally present with greater mortality risk; in contrast, the frequency of injury among women is handled statistically by controlling for gender.[4] In preparation of this chapter limited data were found for specific types of injury among women by age and race. Such information is key to addressing injury in an aging population. Therefore, this chapter largely presents original data analyses of injury mortality and morbidity across the age span among women. Except where otherwise stated, analyses use online data provided by the Centers for Disease Control and Prevention's web-based injury statistics query and reporting system (WISQARS).[1]

The Relation of Injury to the Age and Gender Structure of the U.S. Population

Females comprise a larger proportion of the U.S. population beginning in their late 20s for non-Hispanic whites (whites) and non-Hispanic blacks (blacks) and by age 30 for Hispanics (Figure 3-2). The disproportionate age-specific gender distribution is accelerated in the elderly years as women live longer lives than men.[5,6] This has implications for the magnitude of population-level injury, the types of injury observed, and caregiving demands.

The "baby boom" and the general trend toward longer life expectancy over the last several decades are leading to record numbers of older Americans in the total population (Figure 3-2a).[7,8] The race/ethnic specific population pyramids presented in Figures 3-2 b-d enable an appreciation of diverse composition of the American population by 5-year age intervals and the variability across race and ethnicity.[5] The composite of four pyramids indicates the

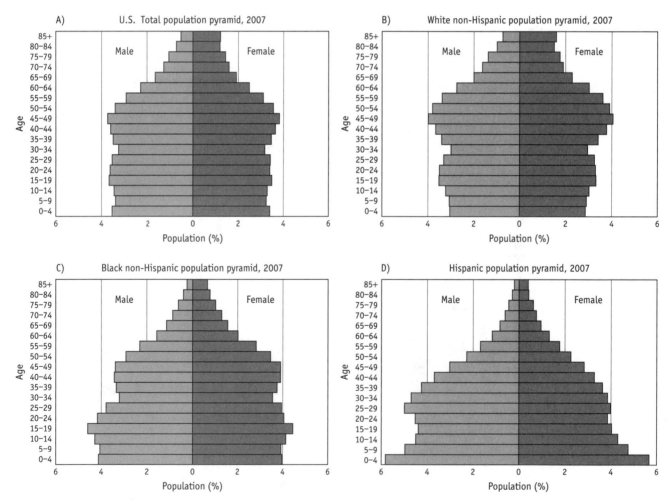

Figure 3-2 U.S. population pyramids by sex and 5 year age groups, 2007.

Source: Data from Web-based Injury Statistics Query and Reporting System (WISQARS). (2007). National Center for Injury Prevention and Control, Centers for Disease Control and Prevention.

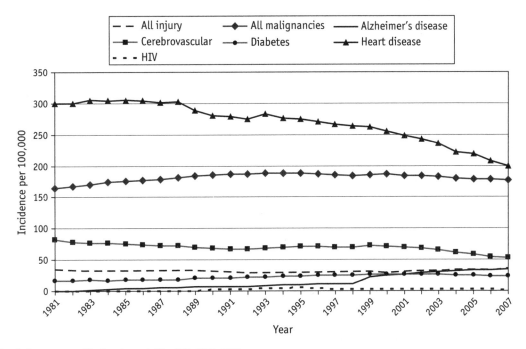

Figure 3-3 Trends in cause-specific female mortality, U.S. 1981–2007.

Source: Data from Web-based Injury Statistics and Reporting System [WISQARS] 2007. National Center for Injury Prevention and Control, Centers for Disease Control and Prevention.

population age structure varies considerably by race and ethnicity, with a "broad-based, slender and pointed pyramid" for Hispanics reflecting a relatively younger population structure. In contrast, whites have a more "rectangular bulging belt-line shape" indicating more older men and women, the baby boom generation (bulging belt-line). As they advance toward older ages, their incidence of injury mechanisms is changing with the emergence of frailty-influenced injury risk factors that contrast with younger generations.[9,10]

The shape of these pyramids, together with the age-specific injury and mortality rates in later sections of this chapter enable a glimpse into future 1) key injury risks and the relative importance of injuries among women; 2) injury prevention strategies to reduce the cost of injury-related care; 3) demands on women as the principal informal caregivers; and 4) demands on health and long-term care facilities to provide rehabilitation to injured women.

Magnitude of Injury Relative to the Total Disease Burden in the United States

For the last 25 years, mortality from all types of injury has ranked below heart disease, cancer, and cerebrovascular disease and higher than death due to human immunodeficiency virus (HIV), diabetes, and Alzheimer's disease (Figure 3-3).[1,11] The relative contribution to female mortality has narrowed between injury and both heart disease and cerebrovascular disease as the latter two causes of death have declined while total injury has remained fairly constant.

Table 3-1	
Percent of all deaths due to injury among females by age group, United States, 2007	
Age Group	**Percent of Deaths Due to Injuries (All Intents)**
< 1 year	6%
1–4 years	38%
5–9	39%
10–14	42%
15–19	67%
20–24	58%
25–34	42%
35–44	25%
45–54	13%
55–64	5%
65+	2%
All ages	4%

Data from Web-based Injury Statistics Query and Reporting System (WISQARS). (2007). National Center for Injury Prevention and Control, Centers for Disease Control and Prevention.

The proportion of injury mortality to all mortality is shown in Table 3-1. Injury is the cause of 6% of deaths in females under 1 year of age, but by age 15–19, accounts for two-thirds of all-cause deaths in that age category. The leading cause of injury death and YPLL in women is motor vehicle traffic (Table 3-2).

Table 3-2

Relative rank of injuries in females by Years of Potential Life Lost (YPLL) before age 65, cause of death, hospitalization, and emergency department visits (2007)

Mechanism of Injury	YPLL	Death	Hospitalization, Nonfatal	Emergency Department Visits, Nonfatal
Motor vehicle traffic, all	1	1	3	4
Fall, unintentional	8	2	1	1
Poisoning, unintentional	2	3	4	9
Suicide (fatal)/self-harm (nonfatal), all	3	4	2	11
Homicide (fatal)/assault (nonfatal), all	4	5	8	7
Suffocation, unintentional	5	6	13	15
Fire/burn, unintentional	6	7	14	12
Drowning, unintentional	7	8	16	17
Pedestrian, unintentional	9	9	9	14
Other transport, unintentional	10	10	6	8
Struck by/against, unintentional	11	11	5	3
Firearms, unintentional	12	12	17	16
Pedal cyclist, unintentional	13	13	12	13
Cut/pierce, unintentional	14	14	15	5
Overexertion, unintentional	15	15	7	2
Bites and stings, all	-	-	10	6
Foreign body, unintentional	-	-	11	10

Data from Web-based Injury Statistics Query and Reporting System (WISQARS). (2007). National Center for Injury Prevention and Control, Centers for Disease Control and Prevention.

Morbidity

Injury accounted for 3.8% of the 20.5 million hospitalizations of women each year and 29.1% of the 63.2 million emergency department visits in women in 2007.[12] Unintentional falls, which ranked second among leading causes of injury death and eighth in YPLL, are the leading cause of morbidity as measured by either injury-related hospitalizations or emergency department visits (Table 3-2).

Overexertion emerges as an important cause of emergency department (ED) use among women.[13] Its low rank in both YPLL and deaths indicate that overexertion is generally a nonfatal cause of injury in women. This and the large difference in costs for overexertion between nonfatal ED visits and nonfatal hospitalizations indicate that it is generally managed in the emergency department without requiring hospitalization. In contrast, motor vehicle traffic-related injury, the leading cause of injury-related death and YPLL, is also important for its contribution to nonfatal hospitalization and emergency department visits (Table 3-2).

Women continue to experience considerable morbidity following traumatic injury and are reported to have higher symptoms of acute stress, diminished quality of life, and more depression following trauma than men.[14–17]

Years of Potential Life Lost

The relative rank of injury-related YPLL before age 65 is shown in Table 3-2. The burden of total YPLL for all-cause injury is slightly higher than all malignancies (21.8% and 21.3% respectively) and more than double that of heart disease. Unintentional injuries ranked second (15.7%) among YPLL and intentional injury (homicide and suicide) ranked fifth. Injury deaths concentrated among older aged women contribute fewer YPLL; as noted in Table 3-2, unintentional falls rank tenth in YPLL but second in cause of mortality that occur primarily among the elderly.

Healthcare Costs

The relative rank of the injury burden using direct healthcare costs noted in Table 3-3 indicates the importance of type of injury. Frequently, these injury mechanisms exert their influence on healthcare costs through high incidence of emergency department visits. For example, care of

Table 3-3

Estimated costs of all causes of injury from emergency department visits, hospitalizations and deaths, 2005

	Mechanism	Nonfatal ED Visits	Nonfatal Hospitalizations	Total Direct Medical Costs	Total Estimated Cost
1	Fall	$4,286,127,000	$7,653,412,000	$12,152,862,000	$30,050,354,000
2	Motor vehicle traffic	$1,637,264,000	$3,418,625,000	$5,189,246,000	$22,968,021,000
3	Poisoning	$32,897,000	$1,190,792,000	$1,280,723,000	$9,715,677,000
4	Struck by/against	$1,949,903,000	$628,157,000	$2,579,618,000	$7,941,347,000
5	Overexertion	$2,023,851,000	$286,149,000	$2,310,009,000	$6,859,898,000
6	Firearms	$3,123,000	$42,807,000	$58,741,000	$3,446,835,000
7	Cut/pierce	$388,417,000	$242,697,000	$633,456,000	$3,062,935,000
8	Suffocation	$6,923,000	$81,429,000	$135,856,000	$2,642,835,000
9	Bites and stings	$634,411,000	$125,790,000	$760,201,000	$2,416,596,000
10	Pedestrian	$57,167,000	$419,122,000	$499,376,000	$2,303,000,000
11	Other transport	$294,732,000	$419,862,000	$719,203,000	$2,188,079,000
12	Fire/burn	$216,707,000	$116,568,000	$368,198,000	$1,799,436,000
13	Pedal cyclist	$162,056,000	$184,456,000	$348,153,000	$1,079,811,000
14	Drowning	$78,000	$34,202,000	$38,546,000	$876,688,000
15	Foreign body	$89,629,000	$204,070,000	$293,699,000	$678,484,000
16	Natural/environmental	$6,706,000	$30,973,000	$43,719,000	$417,609,000

Source: Table shows the estimated costs (in USD) of all intent injury by top mechanisms for nonfatal emergency department visit medical costs, nonfatal hospitalization medical costs, total direct medical costs (ED visits, hospitalizations, and deaths), and total combined costs (direct medical costs and work loss). Data from Web-based Injury Statistics Query and Reporting System (WISQARS) [Online]. (2007). National Center for Injury Prevention and Control, Centers for Disease Control and Prevention. www.cdc.gov/ncipc/wisqars. Accessed February 18, 2011.

women for overexertion and for animal bites or insect stings ranked fifth and ninth among injuries contributing to healthcare costs due to emergency department visits (Table 3-3).[12,13,18]

Age- and Race-Specific Injury Mortality Among Women

The type of injuries occurring among women differs by age and intent, necessitating assessment by age-specific causes of injury to accurately capture the impact among women across the life span. Examining total injury in summary form for all ages and race/ethnic groups masks important differences in incidence and modifiable risk factors across age and race, impeding identification of gaps in progress among specific ages with considerable disparity remaining among race/ethnic groups.[19,20]

All-cause injury deaths are shown in Figure 3-4 by age group and race/ethnicity. Very young black female children have higher all-cause injury mortality than Hispanic or white children until adolescence.[21] Disparities differ considerably with both intentional and unintentional injuries contributing to the observed racial disparities observed in young children.[22–25] All older women, regardless of race/ethnicity, experience escalating injury mortality. Several types of injuries demonstrate age-specific increases, but mortality associated with falls exceeds all others; deaths due to falls among older American women are potentially misclassified on emergency room records and death certificates.[26]

Intentional Injury Mechanisms

Approximately one-fourth (23.1%) of injury deaths of women are intentional—primarily suicide and homicide, which rank below unintentional injury, cancer, heart disease, and perinatal conditions in their contribution to YPLL. Intentional injury deaths are higher in YPLL than infectious diseases, cerebrovascular disease, or diabetes.

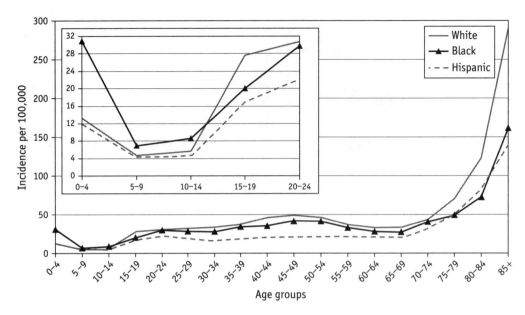

Figure 3-4 All injury deaths of females by age group and race/ethnicity.

Source: Data from Web-based Injury Statistics Query and Reporting System [WISQARS]. National Center For Injury Prevention and Control, Centers for Disease Control and Prevention.

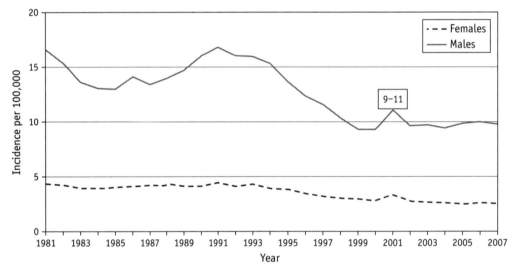

Figure 3-5a Homicide deaths per 100,000 by sex and year, United States 1981–2007.

Source: Data from Web-based Injury Statistics Query and Reporting System [WISQARS]. National Center for Injury Prevention and Control, Centers for Disease Control and Prevention.

Homicide

Figure 3-5a notes the decline in homicides beginning early in the 1990s among males and females that followed increases in the 1980s associated with the crack drug epidemic.[21,27,28] Although deaths associated with September 11, 2001 have been variously categorized over the last 10 years, the current classification in WISQARS is homicide, accounting for the 2001 blip observed in Figure 3-5a.[1] Commonly employed mechanisms of homicide in rank order include firearms, cut/pierced, suffocation, fire/burn, and poisoning.

Homicide rates are highly age specific and vary by gender, race, and ethnicity (Figure 3-5a and Figure 3-5b).

Women have rates of homicide that are just over 25% those of males, but otherwise show similar patterns by age and race. Black female infants and children have elevated rates compared to Hispanics and whites. Black female homicide rates are approximately 12% those of black males but are significantly higher than those of white females (Figure 3-5b). Homicide rates decline for elementary school aged children but increase among adolescents and teens, where they peak at the highest observed lifetime rates. Young Hispanic females have higher rates than young white females beginning in adolescence and continuing through middle age before narrowing in elderly ages (Figure 3-5b).[1]

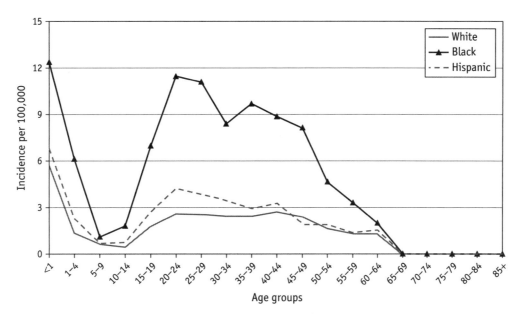

Figure 3-5b Homicide deaths among females per 100,000 by age group and race.

Source: Data from Web-based Injury Statistics Query and Reporting System [WISQARS]. 2007. National Center For Injury Prevention and Control, Center for Disease Control and Prevention.

Suicide

More than 7,300 American women die annually by suicide; only modest improvements have been documented over the last 25 years.[29,30] Between 1999 to 2007, suicide rates among white women increased 25% in contrast to 7.5% among Hispanic and 9.3% among black women. In 2007, the rate of suicide in white women was 3.5 times that of Hispanic and black women.

Although male rates of suicide are three to four times higher than those of females, rates among women are highly age dependent with distinctively different patterns by race and ethnicity (Figure 3-6). Rates for white women increase in the teen years, peak in middle age, begin to decline in the early 50s, and level off around age 70. Hispanic and black women show similar patterns with lower incidence. Among women dying by suicide in 2007, poisoning was the leading mode, followed by firearms, suffocation, falls, and drowning.[1]

Women are at higher risk of depression and experience more atypical symptoms of depressive illnesses and increased seasonal affective disorder than men. Although women are more likely to attempt suicide than men, they are less likely to die.[31] Depression is present in about half of all suicides,[32] but screening for warning signs has had limited success as a strategy for suicide prevention.[22,23]

Unintentional Injury

Among the nearly 44,000 women who died of unintentional injuries in 2007, the rate varied by age, race, and ethnicity over the life span. Preadolescent black females have higher unintentional injuries than Hispanic or white children. The recent increases observed for total

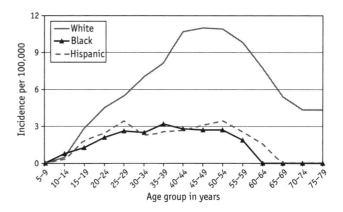

Figure 3-6 Suicide deaths among females per 100,000 by age group and race.

Source: Data from Web-based Injury Statistics Query and Reporting System [WISQARS] 2007 National Center for Injury Prevention and Control, Centers for Disease Control and Prevention.

unintentional injury mortality is related to poisonings and falls in adults over age 45 years.[33,34]

Motor Vehicle Traffic Deaths

Motor vehicle deaths peak in the teenage years and fall by age 30, followed by increases after age 65 (Figure 3-7). Greater mortality among the elderly appears to be due to age-related deficits despite fewer miles driven annually. Elderly drivers have the lowest crash rates per 100,000 licensed drivers but the highest traffic fatality rates per 100,000 miles traveled.[45] Vehicle occupant injury contributes disproportionately in very young black children, a finding that is reportedly associated with lower use of occupant restraints.[46–50] White adolescent females have motor vehicle occupant death rates that are one-third

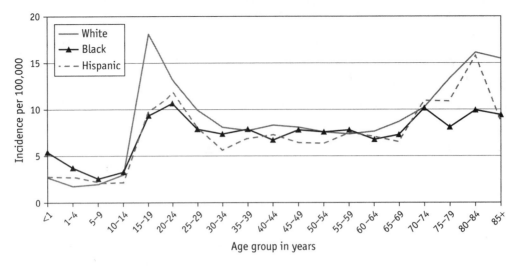

Figure 3-7 Motor vehicle deaths among females per 100,000 by age group and race.

Source: Data from Web-based Injury Statistics Query and Reporting System (WISQARS) [Online]. (2007). National Center for Injury Prevention and Control, Centers for Disease Control and Prevention. www.cdc.gov/ncipc/wisqars. [2011 Feb 18].

higher than in Hispanics and nearly double those of black teens. Adolescent teens, particularly adolescent black teens, are less likely to use seat belts as an occupant than as a driver.[51]

Occupant injury deaths increase as white females grow older with rates rising from mid to late 50s, a trend that continues through age 85. Women and blacks are more likely to die as passengers than as drivers. Older drivers tend to drive fewer miles and have lower crash rates per mile traveled but have higher case fatality rates than younger drivers. This pattern has been attributed to the presence of comorbid conditions and frailty.[52]

Risk factors for motor vehicle occupant mortality include failure to wear a seat belt, presence of alcohol, and being teenage or elderly drivers.[35,36] Trends in declining motor vehicle mortality rates have been variously attributed to a wide range of improvements including driver behavior, legislation, engineering, and enforcement.[37–40] Graduated driver licensing has been shown to lower teen driver mortality.[41] Alcohol laws have been extended beyond the drinking driver to include the seller, server, and host of underage drinking.[42–44] Legislation requiring in-person license renewal for older adults has been reported to reduce motor vehicle related fatality rates in elderly drivers.[40]

Pedestrian

Pedestrian injury accounts for approximately 12% of all motor vehicle deaths of women but is highly variable by age and race/ethnicity. Among Hispanic and black preschool-aged female children, pedestrian deaths are double those of white children, accounting for more than one-quarter of all motor vehicle traffic fatalities. Among elderly women, pedestrian deaths account for 50% of all motor vehicle deaths of Asian women, 35% of Hispanic women, 23% of black women, and 12% of white women. Pedestrian-related injury reduction has been achieved by providing better illumination, creating pedestrian islands, and installing clear warning signs.[53] Increasing attention

is being given to the environment in which older women and children reside. Many major cities, including New York, have transformed their approach to pedestrian safety through identification, targeted modification, and redesign of the highest risk crossings. Redesigns include increased use of pavement markings, electronic signage, adjustments in the timing allowed for pedestrian crossing at wide intersections, addition of timing signals for crossing, and midway raised median pedestrian stopping points.

Falls

Approximately 11,000 women die of falls each year. Unlike many other injuries, fall-related deaths tend to occur at older ages among women. This chapter focuses primarily on falls in younger age groups. Falls on the same level or on stairs significantly contribute to hospitalization among younger age groups, although serious pediatric injury and death occur after falls from height, particularly from windows in urban settings.[54,55] In some cities regulations requiring installation of window guards have virtually eliminated preventable falls from windows as a major cause of pediatric mortality.[54] Serious playground-related fall injuries have been diminished by lowering maximum fall heights in equipment design and installing rubberized ground cover.[56]

Preventing falls in younger populations is one of injury prevention's success stories. Various efforts have included successfully addressing falls on stairs with baby gates at the top and bottom in addition to redesigning baby furniture and baby walkers.[22,23] This emphasis on reducing pediatric mortality due to falls has resulted in gradual mortality declines among very young children.

Unintentional Poisoning

Both female and male preschool black children tend to have higher mortality rates from unintentional poisoning than Hispanic or white children.[57] Among women, deaths due to unintentional poisoning peak around age

40 for whites and by the mid-50s for black and Hispanic women (Figure 3-8). Hispanic women have rates that are approximately one-third those of black and white women. After age 50, white and black women show nearly identical rates and patterns of unintentional poisoning deaths. The low death rates observed for young Hispanic women persist through the elderly years.

Although unintentional poisoning deaths, particularly from opioids, have received considerable attention, questions have been raised regarding potential misclassification of unintentional poisonings that may have been intentional.[57] Additional studies are underway to investigate whether declining suicide rates and rising unintentional poisoning represent related phenomena.[57]

Federal legislation requiring medicines and poisonous household products to be placed in childproof containers has contributed to injury prevention.[22] In addition, the storage of household products out of reach or in locked cabinets has been effective, in contrast to placement of Mr. Yuk pictures on poison items, which did not deter poisoning among small children.[22-23] For seniors and older adults many medication-related poisonings can be avoided by careful delineation of dosages and schedules by doctors and healthcare professionals.[24]

Fire and Burn Deaths

Large disparities in fire and burn deaths are noted among American women; black females are at three to four higher times risk compared with white women across most of their life span with the largest disparities found among very young (aged 0–4 years) and the elderly (aged 65 years and older). Hispanic rates are closer to those of white rates (Figure 3-9).

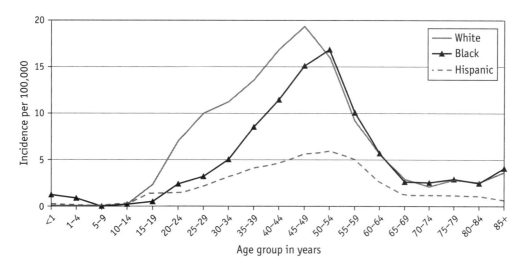

Figure 3-8 Unintentional poisoning deaths of females by age group and race/ethnicity.

Source: Data from Web-based Injury Statistics Query and Reporting System [WISQARS] 2007. National Center for Injury Prevention and Control, Centers for Disease Control and Prevention.

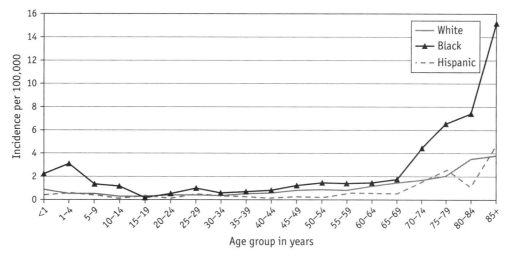

Figure 3-9 Fire/burn deaths of females by age group and race/ethnicity.

Source: Data from Web-based Injury Statistics and Reporting System [WISQARS] 2007 National Center For Injury Prevention and Control, Centers for Disease Control and Prevention.

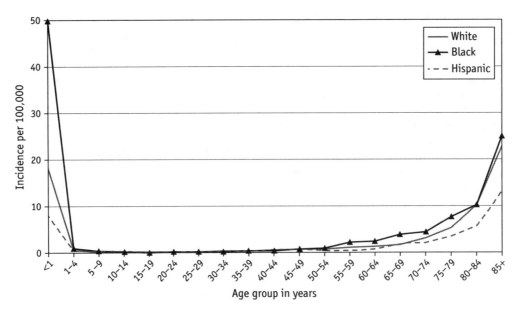

Figure 3-10 Suffocation deaths among females by age group and race/ethnicity.

Source: Data from Web-based Injury Statistics Query and Reporting System [WISQARS] 2007. National Center for Injury Prevention and Control, Centers for Disease Control and Prevention.

Several factors have been posited to explain the differences in deaths due to fire and burns: black women may live in older or substandard housing, in inner-city multi-family dwellings, in lower socioeconomic neighborhoods, or in more crowded conditions where auxiliary heating units may be more frequently used. Cigarette smoking, the most frequent cause of home fires and burn fatalities, often ignites bedding, furniture, or clothing.[20,22,58,59] More older black women than similarly aged white women die from fires, possibly because more white women reside in long-term care facilities[60] whereas more blacks living at home may have disabilities. Prevention efforts to decrease fire and burn injuries focus primarily on risk modification through safety code alterations, smoke detectors, and sprinkler installations in addition to home safety education.[61]

Suffocation

Unintentional suffocation deaths of females are highest among infants younger than 1 year and adults aged 80 and older (Figure 3-10). Deaths are higher in black women compared to Hispanic and white women (50 per 100,000 vs 20 per 100,000 deaths). Hispanic rates are less than half that of white rates. Rates of suffocation mortality among females are low between ages 5 to 44, but increase among women aged 50 and older.

Risk factors for suffocation have shifted over time as regulatory and educational approaches addressed contributing causes, such as unsafe baby products and plastic bags.[23] Current risk factors include women sleeping with their infants, infant bedding, toys and objects in infant sleep areas, and infant sleep position.[23,62,63] In a multiethnic study of home safety among young children, sleep position was shown to vary by race/ethnicity, with black parents more frequently placing children on their stomach.[64] Many cases of suffocation can be prevented among children by removal of small toys that may cause choking.[63] Among

unintentional injuries of very young children, suffocation was the only injury that increased, and only among infants under age 1 year. This temporal shift raises the questions of a potential change in diagnostic classifications from sudden infant death syndrome (SIDS) to suffocation.

Firearm Injury, All Intents

Of the 31,213 persons who died in the United States from firearm injury in 2007, women accounted for 4,177 (13.4%). Despite being a relatively small portion of total firearm deaths, women are nearly three times more likely to die from a firearm than from a traffic-related pedestrian injury. The distribution differed by age, race and ethnicity (Figure 3-11) with higher rates per 100,000 women being among black women (4.1) than whites (2.9), American Indians (2.5), or Hispanics (1.5). The majority of deaths in women occur between the ages of 15 and 69. Very few of the 76 (1.8%) firearm deaths of females classified as unintentional in 2007 were among young children and adolescents (n = 14) or very young children (n = 4).

Firearms were used by women in 52% of all suicides and nearly 2,000 women were victims of firearm-related homicide. Strategies for prevention of firearm deaths have variously included gun licensing and carrying laws, safe locked storage of guns in the homes, gun buyback programs, and other means to remove guns from homes. Drug control enforcement, firearm training and education, trigger locks, and loading indicators have all been used as preventive measures.[24,65,66] Approximately 90% of gun deaths occur indoors, the majority in the home. Prevention strategies to reduce unintentional firearm injury in children include establishing safety skills that teach children to immediately leave and inform an adult upon finding a firearm.[67]

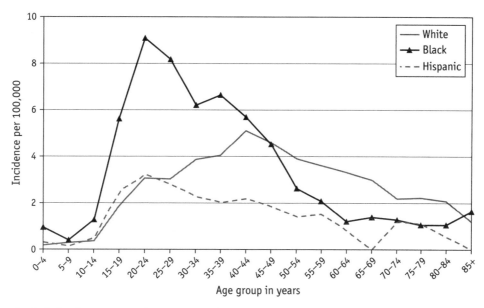

Figure 3-11 Firearm deaths in females per 100,000 by age group and race.

Source: Data from Web-based Injury Statistics Query and Reporting System [WISQARS] 2007. National Center for Injury Prevention and Control, Centers for Disease Control and Prevention.

Drowning and Environmental and Human-Caused Disasters

Over 4,000 Americans die from drowning each year. Women account for about one-fourth of all drowning deaths, including very young children and the elderly whose risk is two to three times greater than among women of other age groups. Risk of drowning varies by geographic region and across age, gender, race, and ethnicity.[20,68,69] Preventive strategies vary by age. Among children aged less than 5, drowning frequently occurs in bathtubs and swimming pools while being supervised by a parent.[23,24,68] Several strategies have been proposed for prevention: educational strategies with improved adult supervision, elimination of unattended standing water, swimming lessons, cardiopulmonary resuscitation training, regulations regarding fencing of swimming pools, installation of self-closing and locking gates, and redesign of pool drains.[23,24,68]

Environmental and natural disasters, such as the Gulf Coast Hurricane Katrina in 2005, have contributed to the higher mortality among elderly men and women. Natural and environmental deaths among those aged 85 and older reached as high as 191 and 265 per 100,000 for women and men, respectively. Rates were higher in men, but older women comprised a larger proportion of the population (Figure 3-2) and contributed larger absolute numbers of deaths. Preventive strategies for natural disaster deaths have included early warning systems; use of newer electronic social media to notify those at risk; public education; evacuations; improved highway, building, and environmental designs for earthquakes, hurricanes, and flooding; improved organized disaster management plans, facilities, and personnel; and other approaches.[70]

Historically, human-caused disasters have affected younger or working age populations more than the elderly and tended to be gender neutral or to affect greater numbers of men. One-fourth of deaths related to September 11, 2001 were of women, 97% of whom were aged 20–64 years. Similarly, after the Oklahoma City bombing in 1995, the Oklahoma state vital statistics indicated that over 80% of victims were of working age with approximately 39% women.[1] Some of the many preventive strategies include increased public education, screening, surveillance, and disaster preparedness at the individual, community, and governmental levels.[70,71]

Injury Caused by Adverse Effects of Medical Care and Drugs

Mortality and morbidity associated with adverse effects of medical care are the "iceberg" of unintentional injury among women.[72] Most experts in the field note that the problem is underreported in relation to its contribution to mortality, morbidity, and healthcare costs.[73] Of the nearly 1,400 deaths in women, 88% were recorded as attributal to adverse effects of medical care and 12% to adverse drug events (Figure 3-12).

Recreational and Sports Injury Morbidity

Although recreational injury is an infrequent cause of mortality, sports and recreational injuries contribute significantly to morbidity in young women. The knee and ankle are the most common sites of sports and recreational injury in both males and females. Gender differences in exposure to football, the leading sport for injury, account for a large portion of increased injuries among males compared to females. The second leading sport for

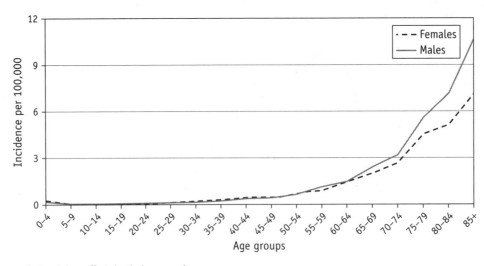

Figure 3-12 Adverse medical and drug effect deaths by sex and age group.

Source: Data from Web-based Injury Statistics Query and Reporting System [WISQARS] 2007. National Center for Injury Prevention and Control, Centers for Disease Control and Prevention.

injury is basketball where approximately 60% of all injury is to the knee.[74]

Two types of knee injury-related conditions are noted to be higher in females: patellofemoral pain syndrome and noncontact anterior cruciate ligament (ACL) injury, the latter of which occurs two to eight times more frequently in females.[74] Although factors contributing to these differences are still under investigation, several studies in humans and animals have suggested menstrual cycle hormonal changes may affect knee laxity and stiffness;[75] male-female differences in neuromuscular preactivity during side-cutting that contributes to lower knee stability in women.[74] Animal studies have identified sex-specific characteristics in landing, jumping, and running;[76–79] biomechanic and kinematic differences at the hip, knee, and ankle;[76] and differences associated with collagen mRNA expression in Type 1 collagen (T1C) and type 3 collagen (T3C) in rats with increased ACL stiffness and failure load in female rats.[77]

Occupational Injury

Despite a steady increase in workforce participation by women, the risk of occupational injury among women remains at approximately half that of men in all sectors except service, education, and agriculture.[80] Women make up approximately half of the workforce, but differ significantly by job sector. The type and severity of workforce injury, disability, and death vary by occupation and job classification. differentials in the healthy worker effect limit detection of adverse events experienced by working women.[81] Following occupational injuries, women may take longer to return to work.[80,81]

Although more women are nurses or nursing aides, men working in these positions are nearly twice as likely as women to be injured on the job. Compared to male occupational injury, women are less likely to experience toxic exposures but are more likely to be injured due to falls. Among occupation injuries, women are reported to

have higher rates of carpal tunnel syndrome, burns, and musculoskeletal injury including sprains and fractures.[80] Despite the fact that women comprise nearly half of the workforce, workstations are often designed to meet the needs of men with implications for injury prevention among women.[80]

Home and Homelessness Injury

Very young children and the elderly have higher exposure to and increased risk of home-related injury and death. Women and children living in poverty are at higher injury risk than those in wealthier families.[23] The home mortgage crisis with the accompanying home foreclosures is reported to have had a larger impact on families and mothers in lower income strata, minority women, and single mothers.[81] Homelessness is associated with higher fall-related injury in homeless children and adolescents. Falls from furniture are higher in homeless children aged less than 5 years.

Burns are a major cause of morbidity and mortality among very young children and among elderly women (Figure 3-9). The majority of fire-related deaths are due to residential fires, but two-thirds of burns in homeless, sheltered children are from hot liquids and vapors.[82] Among home injury success stories are the widespread legislation mandating smoke alarm installations, which have reduced fire and burn mortality; childproof closures on household poisons and medicines, leading to reduced home poisonings;[23] and fall prevention strategies such as installation of baby gates on stairs and window guards in urban housing, which have produced significant declines in falls from height including baby walkers, stairs, and windows.[23,24,54]

Summary

Although injury mortality in women contributes a smaller proportion to total mortality than injuries of men, injury remains the leading cause of death among women during peak childbearing and childrearing ages. Three of the five leading causes of death in young adult to middle-aged women are unintentional injury, suicide, and homicide. A major underrecognized impact of injury on the lives of women is the increased stress of caring for an injured child, spouse/partner, or aging parents. Although the data in this chapter primarily report injury occurring directly to females, injury to family members has a significant impact on the lives of mothers. Whereas some types of injuries have been declining, population aging is contributing to larger numbers of injured elderly females and males and is a major contributor to the loss of independent living while increasing healthcare costs.

Discussion Questions

1. Despite the higher mortality burden of chronic and infectious disease in women, injury is the highest contributor to YPLL in women. Explain this phenomenon and discuss how future epidemiologic research might address the impact of YPLL in women's health.

2. Motor vehicle injury comprises a significant portion of the injury burden in women, particularly in older ages. What factors might contribute to the observed elevated motor vehicle related mortality rates in older women, despite their having the lowest crash rates per 100,000 licensed drivers?

3. The injury burden varies depending on the measure used. Discuss the commonly used measures and explain how they differ and their strengths and weaknesses. Do you think it is helpful to have multiple measures? Why or why not?

4. Firearm injury in women is fragmented across mechanisms and intent, partially masking its importance in the health of women. Discuss the role of firearms in unintentional injury, suicide and homicide. Explain how preventive strategies might be expected to influence rates across intents.

5. Fall-related injury is the second leading cause of death in women and the highest contributor to morbidity as measured by hospitalizations and emergency department visits, but ranks tenth in YPLL. Explain.

6. How do individual-level factors like race and ethnicity manifest in injury risks? What are potential strategies to reduce such disparities in injury prevention efforts?

References

1. Centers for Disease Control and Prevention, National Center for Injury Prevention and Control. Web-based Injury Statistics Query and Reporting System (WISQARS). (2007). www.cdc.gov/ncipc/wisqars. Accessed April 28, 2011.
2. Centers for Disease Control and Prevention. Premature mortality in the United States: public health issues in the use of years of potential life lost. *MMWR Morb Mortal Wkly Rep.* 1986;35:1s–11s.
3. Gardner JW, Sanborn JS. Years of Potential Life Lost (YPLL)—What does it measure? *Epidemiology.* 1990;1:322–9.
4. Mack KA. Fatal and nonfatal unintentional injuries in adult women, United States. *J Women's Health.* 2004;13:754–63.
5. Wingard DL. The sex differential in morbidity, mortality, and lifestyle. *Annu Rev Publ Health.* 1984;5:433–458.
6. Oeppen J, Vaupel JW. Broken limits to life expectancy. *Demography.* 2002;296:1029–31.
7. Lee R, Skinner J. Will aging baby boomers bust the federal budget? *J Econ Perspect.* 1999;13:117–40.
8. Keehan S, Sisko A, Truffer C, et al. The baby-boom generation is coming to Medicare. *Health Affairs.* 2008;27:w145–w155.
9. Pressley JC, Patrick CH. Frailty bias in co-morbidity risk adjustments of community-dwelling elderly populations. *J Clin Epidemiol.* 1999;52: 753–760.
10. Awadzi KD, Classen S, Hall A, et al. Predictors of injury among younger and older adults in fatal motor vehicle crashes. *Accid Anal Prev.* 2008;40: 1804–10.
11. Ross JA, ed. *International Encyclopedia of Population.* New York: Macmillan Library Reference; 1982.
12. Niska R, Bhuiya F, and Xu J. *National Hospital Ambulatory Medical Care Survey: 2007 Emergency Department Summary,* Tables 2 and 11. National Health Statistics Reports; no 26. Hyattsville, MD: National Center for Health Statistics; 2010.
13. Niska R, Bhuiya F, and Xu J. *National Hospital Ambulatory Medical Care Survey: 2007 Emergency Department Summary,* Table 13. National Health Statistics Reports; no 26. Hyattsville, MD: National Center for Health Statistics; 2010.
14. Holbrook TL, Hoyt DB. The impact of major trauma: quality-of-life outcomes are worse in women than in men, independent of mechanism and injury severity. *J Trauma.* 2004;56:284–90.
15. Scheidt PC, Harel Y, Trumble AC, et al. The epidemiology of nonfatal injuries among US children and youth. *Am J Public Health.* 1995;85:932–8.
16. Ballesteros MF, Schieber RA, Gilchrist J, et al. Differential ranking of causes of fatal versus non-fatal injuries among US children. *Inj Prev.* 2003;9:173–6.
17. Powell EC, Tanz RR. Adjusting our view of injury risk: The burden of nonfatal injuries in infancy. *Pediatrics.* 2002;110:792–6.
18. Weiss HB, Friedman DI, Coben JH. Incidence of dog bite injuries treated in emergency departments. *JAMA.* 1999;281:232–3.
19. US Department of Health and Human Services. Chapter 15: Injury and violence prevention. In: *Healthy People 2010.* Vol 2. McLean, VA: International Medical Publishing, Inc.; 2000.
20. US Preventive Services Task Force. *Guide to Clinical Preventive Services: Report of the US Preventive Services Task Force.* 3rd ed. Philadelphia: Lippincott Williams and Wilkins; 2002.
21. Anderson CL, Agran PF, Winn DG, Tran C. Demographic risk factors for injury among Hispanic and non-Hispanic white children: an ecologic analysis. *Inj Prev.* 1998;4:33–8.
22. Institute of Medicine, Bonnie RJ, Fulco CE, Liverman CT, eds. *Reducing the Burden of Injury: Advancing Prevention and Treatment.* Washington, DC: National Academy Press; 1999.
23. Hemenway D. *While We Were Sleeping.* Los Angeles, CA: University of California Press; 2009.
24. Jones PR, Sheppard MA, Snowden CB, et al. Impact of poison prevention education on the knowledge and behaviors of seniors. *J Health Educ.* 2010;41:139–46.
25. Pressley JC, Barlow B, Kendig T, et al. Twenty-year trends in fatal injuries to very young children: the persistence of racial disparities. *Pediatrics,* 2007;119;e874–84.
26. Koehler SA, Weiss HB, Shakir A, et al. Accurately assessing elderly fall deaths using hospital discharge and vital statistics data. *Am J Forensic Med Pathol.* 2006;27:30–5.
27. Blumstein A, Rivara FP, Rosenfeld R. The rise and decline of homicide—and why. *Annu Rev Public Health.* 2000;21:505–41.
28. Cerdá M, Messner SF, Tracy M, et al. Investigating the effect of social changes on age-specific gun-related homicide rates in New York City during the 1990s. *Am J Public Health.* 2010;100:1107–15.
29. Phillips JA, Robin AV, Nugent CN, Idler EL. Understanding recent changes in suicide rates among the middle-aged: period or cohort effects? *Public Health Rep.* 2010;125:680–8.
30. Hu G, Baker SP. Reducing black/white disparity: changes in injury mortality in the 15–24 year age group, United States, 1999–2005. *Inj Prev.* 2008;14: 205–8.
31. Gorman, JM. Gender differences in depression and response to psychotropic medication. *Gend Med.* 2006;3:93–109.
32. Weissman MM, Klerman GL. Sex differences and the epidemiology of depression. *Arch Gen Psychiatry.* 1977;34:98–111.
33. Hu G, Baker SP. Trends in unintentional injury deaths, U.S., 1999–2005: age, gender, and racial/ethnic differences. *Am J Prev Med.* 2009;37:188–94.
34. Dessypris N, Dikalioti SK, Skalkidis I, et al. Combating unintentional injury in the United States: Lessons learned from the ICD-10 classification period. *J Trauma.* 2009;66:519–25.
35. Winston FK, Kallan MJ, Senserrick TM, Elliott MR. Risk factors for death among older child and teenaged motor vehicle passengers. *Arch Pediatr Adolesc Med.* 2008;162:253–60.
36. Plurad D, Demetriades D, Gruzinski G, et al. Motor vehicle crashes: The association of alcohol consumption with the type and severity of injuries and outcomes. *J Emerg Med.* 2010;38:12–7.
37. Pressley JC, Benedicto CB, Trieu L, et al. Motor vehicle injury, mortality, and hospital charges by strength of graduated driver licensing laws in 36 states. *J Trauma.* 2009;67:S43–S53.
38. Carpenter CS, Stehr M. The effects of mandatory seatbelt laws on seatbelt use, motor vehicle fatalities, and crash-related injuries among youths. *J Health Econ.* 2008;27:642–62.

39. Adekoya N. Motor vehicle-related death rates—United States, 1999–2005. *MMWR Morb Mortal Wkly Rep.* 2009;58:161–5.

40. Grabowski DC, Campbell CM, Morrisey MA. Elderly licensure laws and motor vehicle fatalities. *JAMA.* 2004;291:2840–6.

41. Longthorne A, Subramanian R, Chen CL. *An Analysis of the Significant Decline in Motor Vehicle Traffic Fatalities in 2008.* DOT HS-811 346. Washington, DC: US Department of Transportation, National Highway Traffic Safety Administration; June 2010.

42. Li G, Braver ER, Chen LH. Fragility versus excessive crash involvement as determinants of high death rates per vehicle-mile of travel among older drivers. *Accid Anal Prev.* 2003;35:227–35.

43. Dills AK. Social host liability for minors and underage drunk-driving accidents. *J Health Econ.* 2010;29:241–9.

44. Fell JC, Fisher DA, Voas RB, et al. The relationship of underage drinking laws to reductions in drinking drivers in fatal crashes in the United States. *Accid Anal Prev.* 2008;40:1430–40.

45. McGwin J Jr., Brown DB. Characteristics of traffic crashes among young, middle-aged, and older drivers. *Accid Anal Prev.* 1999;31:181–98.

46. Pressley JC, Trieu L, Barlow B, Kendig T. Motor vehicle occupant injury and related hospital expenditures in children aged 3 years to 8 years covered versus uncovered by booster seat legislation. *J Trauma.* 2009;67:S20–S29.

47. Rice TM, Anderson CL. The effectiveness of child restraint systems for children aged 3 years or younger during motor vehicle collisions: 1996 to 2005. *Am J Public Health.* 2009;99:252–7.

48. Trowbridge MJ, Kent R. Rear-seat motor vehicle travel in the U.S.: using national data to define a population at risk. *Am J Prev Med.* 2009;37:321–3.

49. Rangel SJ, Martin CA, Brown RL, et al. Alarming trends in the improper use of motor vehicle restraints in children: implications for public policy and the development of race-based strategies for improving compliance. *J Pediatr Surg.* 2008;43:200–7.

50. Greenspan AI, Dellinger AM, Chen J. Restraint use and seating position among children less than 13 years of age: is it still a problem? *J Saf Res.* 2010;41:183–5.

51. Briggs NC, Lambert EW, Goldzweig IA, et al. Driver and passenger seatbelt use among US high school students. *Am J Prev Med.* 2008;35:224–9.

52. *Drive Well: Promoting Older Driver Safety and Mobility in Your community.* DOT HS-809 838. Washington, DC: US Department of Transportation, National Highway Traffic Safety Administration and the American Society on Aging; 2007.

53. Malek M, Guyer B, Lescohier I. The epidemiology and prevention of child pedestrian injury. *Accid Anal Prev.* 1990;22:301–13.

54. Pressley JC, Barlow B. Child and adolescent injury as a result of falls from buildings and structures. *Inj Prev.* 2005;11:267–73.

55. Mosenthal AC, Livingston DH, Elcavage J, et al. Falls: Epidemiology and strategies for prevention. *J Trauma.* 1995;38:753–6.

56. Chalmers DJ, Marshall SW, Langley JD, et al. Height and surfacing as risk factors for injury in falls from playground equipment: a case-control study. *Inj Prev.* 1996;2:98–104.

57. Rockett IRH, Hobbs G, De Leo D, et al. Suicide and unintentional poisoning mortality trends in the United States, 1987–2006: two unrelated phenomena? *BMC Public Health.* 2010;10:705.

58. Adhikari B, Kahende J, Malarcher A, et al. Smoking-attributable mortality, years of potential life lost, and productivity losses—United States, 2000–2004. *MMWR Morb Mortal Wkly Rep.* 2008;57:1226–8.

59. Ballesteros MF, Jackson ML, Martin MW. Working toward the elimination of residential fire deaths: The Centers for Disease Control and Prevention's Smoke Alarm Installation and Fire Safety Education (SAIFE) program. *J Burn Care Rehabil.* 2005;26:434–9.

60. Salive ME, Collins KS, Foley DJ, George LK. Predictors of nursing home admission in a biracial population. *Am J Public Health.* 1993;83:1765–7.

61. Atiyeh BS, Costagliola M, Hayek SN. Burn prevention mechanisms and outcomes: Pitfalls, failures and successes. *Burns.* 2009;35:181–93.

62. Drago DA, Dannenberg AL. Infant mechanical suffocation deaths in the United States, 1980–1997. *Pediatrics.* 1999;103:e59–67.

63. LeBlanc JC, Pless IB, King WJ, et al. Home safety measures and the risk of unintentional injury among young children: a multicentre case-control study. *CMAJ.* 2006;175:883–7.

64. Pressley JC, Kiragu A, Lapidus G, et al. Race and ethnic differences in a multicenter study of home safety with vouchers redeemable for free safety devices. *J Trauma.* 2009;67:S3–S11.

65. Hemenway D. *Private Guns, Public Health.* Ann Arbor: University of Michigan Press; 2004.

66. US General Accounting Office. *Accidental Deaths: Many Deaths and Injuries Caused by Firearms Could Be Prevented.* Pub No PEMD-91-9. Washington, DC: US General Accounting Office; 1991.

67. Miltenberger RG. Teaching safety skills to children: prevention of firearm injury as an exemplar of best practice in assessment, training, and generalization of safety skills. *Behav Anal Pract.* 2008;1(1):30–6.

68. Quan L, Cummings P. Characteristics of drowning by different age groups. *Inj Prev.* 2003;9:163–8.

69. Cummings P, Quan L. Trends in unintentional drowning. *JAMA.* 1999;281:2198–202.

70. Cicero MX, Baum CR. Pediatric disaster preparedness: best planning for the worst-case scenario. *Pediatr Emerg Care.* 2008;24:478–81.

71. Brandeau ML, Zaric GS, Freiesleben J, et al. An ounce of prevention is worth a pound of cure: improving communication to reduce mortality during bioterrorism responses. *Am J Disaster Med.* 2008;3:65–78.

72. Phillips DP, Bredder CC. Morbidity and mortality from medical errors: an increasingly serious public health problem. *Annu Rev Public Health.* 2002;23:135–50.

73. Phillips DP, Barker GE. A July spike in fatal medication errors: a possible effect of new medical residents. *J Gen Intern Med.* 2010;25:774–9.

74. Bencke J, Zebis MK. The influence of gender on neuromuscular pre-activity during side-cutting. *J Electromyogr Kinesiol.* 2011;21:371–5.

75. Park SK, Stefanyshyn DJ, Loitz-Ramage B, et al. Changing hormone levels during the menstrual cycle affect knee laxity and stiffness in healthy female subjects. *Am J Sports Med.* 2009;37:588.

76. Joseph MF, Rahl M, Sheehan J, et al. Timing of lower extremity frontal plane motion differs between female and male athletes during a landing task. *Am J Sports Med.* 2011. (Epub ahead of print)

77. Romani WA, Langenberg P, Belkoff SM. Sex, collagen expression, and anterior cruciate ligament strength in rats. *J Athl Train.* 2010;45:22–8.

78. Ireland ML. Anterior cruciate ligament injury in female athletes: epidemiology. *J Athl Train.* 1999;43:150–4.

79. Hewett TE, Lindenfeld TN, Riccobene JV. The effect of neuromuscular training on the incidence of knee injury in female athletes: a prospective study. *Am J Sports Med.* 1999;27:699–706.

80. Islam SS, Velilla AM, Doyle EJ, et al. Gender differences in work-related injury/illness: Analysis of workers compensation claims. *Am J Ind Med.* 2001;39:84–91.

81. National Urban League, Jones SJ, Malveaux J, Height DI, eds. *State of Black America 2008: The Black Woman's Voice.* New York, NY: National Urban League; 2008.

82. Frencher SK, Benedicto CMB, Kendig TK, et al. A comparative analysis of serious injury and illness among the homeless and low SES housed living in New York City. *J Trauma.* 2010;69:S191–199.

Health Promotion, Disease Prevention

Ruby T. Senie, PhD

Introduction

The 20th century witnessed major achievements and transitions in public health and clinical medicine, from controlling infectious diseases to addressing the growing prevalence of smoking followed by increased sedentary lifestyles leading to the obesity epidemic. Greater life expectancy has been achieved through reduced maternal and infant mortality, significantly improving the quality of American lives. Additional public health achievements include development of antibiotic therapy, fluoridation of water supplies, therapy for mental health disorders, less invasive surgical techniques, organ transplantation, and kidney dialysis.[1] Of major importance has been development of vaccines providing primary prevention of infectious conditions, including polio and other lethal childhood diseases. Vaccines have eliminated the causes of morbidity and mortality among children that were frequently experienced by earlier American generations and remain prevalent in many developing countries.

Among the most significant accomplishments of epidemiologic research was identification of cigarette smoking as a leading cause of death from lung cancer, heart disease, and respiratory conditions. Scientific progress has continued in the past 25 years with the identification of the human papilloma virus as the cause of cervical cancer, and development of a vaccine providing primary prevention of the malignancy.[2] The identification of human immunodeficiency virus (HIV) as the cause of acquired immune deficiency syndrome (AIDS) and development of effective therapy rank among many other successes. Although effective treatment has turned this infectious disease into a chronic condition with greatly reduced mortality,[3] the continuing rate of new infections emphasizes the urgent need for an effective vaccine to provide primary prevention.[4]

Behavioral and environmental risks associated with chronic conditions such as heart disease, stroke, cancer, and diabetes are now the focus of primary prevention research. However, 21st century lifestyles, including worldwide travel, changes in environmental exposures, climate patterns, and other factors enable new diseases and health conditions to emerge.[5] Fauci and Morens advised that infectious diseases remain a perpetual challenge, requiring monitoring of pathogens that may evolve to more aggressive strains creating new infectious threats.[3] Therefore, constant surveillance and preparation by clinicians and public health workers are essential,[3] as are programs to prevent or delay onset of chronic conditions, such as the Million Heart project[6] and Tips from Former Smokers.[7] This chapter addresses some of the personal and community-based activities promoted by public health workers to improve quality of life, reduce health disparities, and lower healthcare costs.

Health Maintenance and Avoidance of Disease

In 1948, the constitution of the newly formed World Health Organization (WHO) stated: "Health is a state of complete physical, mental and social well-being and not merely the absence of disease or infirmity."[8] The WHO constitution also noted that the highest attainable standard of health was a fundamental right of every person regardless of race, religion, economic or social condition, or political belief. Among Americans, health issues became a focus when the federal government established the National Institutes of Health in 1948 and the National Science Foundation in 1950. With considerable federal support, the United States developed an enviable biomedical research environment, recognized internationally as a primary source of scientific discoveries, new therapies, and medical devices.[1]

In 1965 stimulated by the WHO goals, Breslow et al. launched one of the earliest research projects assessing the role of personal behaviors in health maintenance.[8] Although advances in clinical medicine increased life expectancy in the United States, epidemiologic studies conducted over many decades identified health behaviors that prevented major disabilities and premature mortality. In an early study by Breslow et al., physical, mental, and social well-being at baseline were found to correlate with mortality 5 and 10 years after recruitment of more than

7,000 residents of Alameda County, California.[8] Seven health practices contributed to health status: never smoking cigarettes, routine physical exercise, moderate or no alcohol intake, sleeping 7-8 hours, maintaining proper weight for height, eating breakfast, and not eating between meals.[8] Women in the cohort with positive health behaviors lived 7 years longer than those who were less health conscious. Based on the continued follow-up of the cohort, Breslow predicted that health promotion would be the focus of public health efforts in the 21st century designed with a two-pronged approach: 1) primary prevention through personal and community efforts to reduce or eliminate risk factors of chronic diseases and 2) secondary prevention by monitoring biomarkers predictive of disease to detect diseases at early, treatable stages.[8]

Few "magic bullets" exist to remedy medical conditions resulting from years of smoking, lack of routine exercise, overeating of inappropriate foods, inadequate rest, overindulgence in alcoholic beverages, etc. Therefore, the combination of personal behaviors and community health promotion efforts became the public health model for chronic disease prevention[10] reflected in several new federal health programs discussed in this chapter.[6,7]

Between 1935 and 2010, significant changes in mortality were recorded in the United States, an indicator of public health successes.[11] Analyses of data from the National Vital Statistics System presented in Figure 4-1 indicate significantly decreased death rates over the 75-year interval among children younger than age 15, although mortality also fell more than 50% for all except the oldest age group (Figure 4-1).[11] In 2008, several causes of mortality, including heart disease, stroke, and cancer, remain among the top five although age-related differences in rank exist. Chronic lung disease has become a relatively new cause of death related to long-term smoking. Women have benefitted more than men from the declining rates of mortality. Over the 75 years mortality trends have differed. Between 1935 and 1954, introduction of antibiotics was credited with lowering death rates by 29%. More recent progress in prevention, diagnosis, and treatment of heart disease has lowered mortality by 41%.[11]

The public continues to expect major discoveries to enhance disease prevention and improve clinical care as a result of federal support of scientific research. However, expectations may lead to misconceptions, as complaints about the slow progress have been noted in the media. Much time is required for scientific discoveries to be appropriately tested for safety and efficacy before translation from the laboratory to clinical practice. Substantial reforms of biomedical research efforts and U.S. health systems were proposed by Moses and Martin.[1] Healthcare costs in the United States far exceed other developed nations, although achievements are lower compared with others when assessed by traditional measures noted in Table 4-1, which provides a comparison of the United States health measures with superior ranking of other industrialized countries.[12] Additionally, clinical improvements are not equally distributed within the United States; disparities in health outcomes by economic and social status have a long history. The heterogeneity of Americans has been suggested as a contributing factor to the nation's inferior ranking[12] primarily attributable to large immigrant populations, which often lack access to clinical care due to limited financial resources, low education level, and language barriers that impede health-seeking behaviors.[13] Inadequate health care, specifically of women in these populations, also adversely affects the health status of their children. Multidisciplinary community-based programs have been developed by public health workers to address the unique health needs of culturally diverse communities.

Recent projections of greater longevity have focused attention on aging and potential increases in morbidity due to higher incidence of chronic conditions among the elderly. As the rates of disabilities increase, the quality

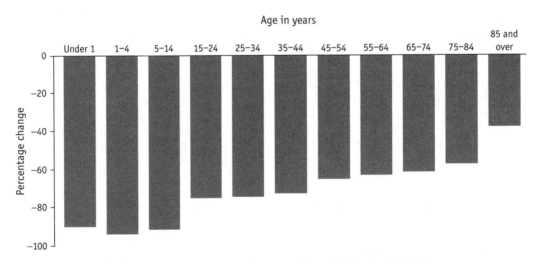

Figure 4-1 The percent decline in mortality by age group over 75 years between 1935 and 2010 in the United States.

Source: Reproduced from Hoyert DL. 75 years of mortality in the United States, 1935–2010 NCHS data brief, no 88. Hyattsville, MD: National Center for Health Statistics. 2012.

AGE	35–44	45–54	55–64	65–74	75–84	85+
1	Cancer 25.7%	Cancer 35.8%	Cancer 41.0%	Cancer 36.1%	Heart disease 25.9%	Heart disease 33.9%
2	Accidents 16.5%	Heart disease 15.3%	Heart disease 18.1%	Heart disease 20.6%	Cancer 23.1%	Cancer 10.2%
3	Heart disease 12.0%	Accidents 8.4%	Chronic lung diseases 5.3%	Chronic lung diseases 8.2%	Stroke 7.5%	Stroke 8.5%
4	Suicide 4.9%	Stroke 4.1%	Diabetes 4.2%	Stroke 5.2%	Chronic lung diseases 7.1%	Alzheimer's disease 7.4%
5	HIV/AIDS 3.8%	Chronic liver disease 3.1%	Stroke 4.1%	Diabetes 4.2%	Alzheimer's disease 4.3%	Chronic lung diseases 4.0%
6	Stroke 3.4%	Diabetes 3.1%	Accidents 3.2%	Kidney disease 2.1%	Diabetes 3.4%	Influenza and pneumonia 3.6%
7	Chronic liver disease 2.9%	Chronic lung diseases 2.8%	Chronic liver disease 1.9%	Accidents 1.9%	Influenza and pneumonia 2.5%	Diabetes 2.1%
8	Diabetes 2.6%	Suicide 2.6%	Kidney disease 1.7%	Septicemia 1.8%	Kidney disease 2.1%	Kidney disease 2.0%
9	Homicide 2.4%	HIV/AIDS 1.6%	Septicemia 1.7%	Influenza and pneumonia 1.6%	Accidents 1.9%	Accidents 1.9%
10	Chronic lung diseases 1.4%	Septicemia 1.5%	Influenza and pneumonia 1.1%	Alzheimer's disease 1.2%	Septicemia 1.7%	Hypertension 1.6%

Rank

Figure 4-2   The 10 leading causes of death among women by age group in 2008.

Source: Modified from Heron M. Deaths: Leading causes for 2008. National vital statistics reports; vol 60 no 6. Hyattsville, MD: National Center for Health Statistics. 2012.

Table 4-1

Selected health measures in the US compared with top ranking countries in 2010

Assessed Health Factor	In America	In Top Ranking Country	Country with Top Ranking
Female life expectancy from birth	81.1 years	86.4 years	Japan
Female life expectancy from age 65	20.3 years	23.9 years	Japan
Infant mortality rate	6.1 per 1000 live births	2.2 per 1000 live births	Iceland
Low birth weight infants [<2500 g]	8.2%	4.1%	Sweden
Cesarean Section	329 per 1000 live births	161 per 1000 live births	Finland
Obesity [BMI >30] self-reported weight & height	27.8%	13.4%	France
Clinically measured obesity	36.3%	3.2%	Japan
Current female smokers ages <15	13.6%	8.4%	Japan
Diabetes among adults ages 20-79	10.3%	3.6%	Norway & United Kingdom

Data From: Organization for Economic Cooperation and Development (OECD).
http://www.oecd-ilibrary.org/social-issues-migration-health/health-key-tables-from-oecd_20758480.

of life during elder years may decline.[14] However, early research by Breslow, Fries, and others indicated that onset of chronic and disabling conditions may be prevented or delayed by healthy lifestyles during youth and early adulthood.[10,15] Krieger emphasized that healthy choices may be impeded by diverse social factors, including continuing racial discrimination that adversely affects health status beginning at birth into a low-income setting in a segregated neighborhood with limited recreational facilities and lack of access to high-quality health care.[16]

Focus on Primary Prevention

Preventive care became the major focus of health legislation in 2010, shifting from treatment targeted for acute symptomatic disease to the admirable goal of improving quality of life by reducing disease risk and reserving funds for essential clinical care.[17] In 2011 the Institute of Medicine (IOM) published a landmark review of effective preventive services specifically addressing the needs of women between ages 10 and 65. The IOM report emphasized that the reproductive role of women creates the need for specific preventive services because pregnancy and childbirth carry health risks.[18] The independent panel of IOM reviewers included nonfederal primary care clinicians, health behavior specialists, and methodologists whose role was to 1) evaluate the benefits and harms of preventive services for asymptomatic women for specific conditions based on age and personal risk factors, and 2) recommend inclusion of specific preventive services in routine primary care. The grading system guiding recommended services was based on scientific evidence from A (advised to include) to D (discouraged from inclusion) or insufficient research for classification.

In addition to U.S. Preventive Services Task Force recommendations, the IOM reviewers relied upon published studies of programs that significantly decreased or delayed onset of diseases and disabling conditions.[18] Criteria for inclusion of evidence-based preventive services were set high to ensure benefits would exceed any potential harms because preventive services are targeted to healthy women.[18] Table 4-2 lists preventive services recommended by the IOM reviewers; these and many others were included in the Affordable Care Act (ACA) of 2010. Before the ACA, preventive services were not standardized and insurance coverage varied considerably among policies. The ACA defined required preventive health services for all insured Americans without copayments, and the law included funding for prevention programs developed by state and community-based health departments.[17]

Epidemiology research has as its major focus identification of modifiable causes of disease to guide personal health decisions, community-based activities, and appropriately scheduled clinical care. However, epidemiologic studies are complicated due to interactions among biological, behavioral, and societal factors.[19] Potential causal factors frequently influence one another; therefore, the challenge for researchers is to identify the specific genetic and environmental aspects that explain, modify, or mediate causal relationships.[19] Primary prevention of an infectious condition requires identifying the common sources of an etiologic agent by analyzing biospecimens in order to interrupt its transmission from mother to child, person to person, carried by an insect, or indirectly by contaminated food or water.[20] HIV provides an interesting example of an infectious disease transformed by new therapeutic modalities to a become chronic condition, lowering risks of transmission of the virus to sexual partners, lowering risk of progression to AIDS, and reducing mortality.[21] Development of a vaccine that stimulates immunity against the infectious agent is the ultimate avenue for primary prevention but remains a work in progress. Although new therapies prolong life, the Centers for Disease Contol and Prevention (CDC) reported in 2011 that a considerable percentage of HIV-infected women and men were not receiving appropriate therapy. Therefore, community-based efforts to remove barriers to HIV testing and increase treatment adherence are needed in addition

---

Table 4-2

Institute of Medicine identified gaps and recommended inclusion of specific services

- Improved screening for cervical cancer, counseling to prevent sexually transmitted infections, including counseling and screening for HIV

- A full range of contraceptive education, counseling, methods, and services enabling women to avoid unwanted pregnancies and space their pregnancies to promote optimal birth outcomes

- Services for pregnant women, including screening for gestational diabetes, lactation counseling, and funds for equipment to help women choose to breastfeed successfully

- At least one well-woman preventive care visit annually to receive comprehensive services including screening of blood pressure, cholesterol, fecal occult testing, diabetes, mental health, alcohol abuse, obesity, physical activity, tobacco use, and osteoporosis

- Screening and counseling of women and adolescent girls for interpersonal and domestic violence in a culturally sensitive and supportive manner

- The preventive healthcare services provided in a clinical setting specified in the ACA will be fully covered without requiring a patient copayment for women ages 10 to 65.

Reproduced from the Institute of Medicine at the National Academy of Sciences, 2011. *Clinical Preventive Services for Women: Closing the Gaps.* Washington, DC: The National Academies Press.

to counseling patients about personal behaviors to avoid disease transmission.[22]

In contrast to infectious disease research, studies focusing on chronic diseases search for risk factors reported more frequently by affected women compared with unaffected controls. After specific factors are consistently reported in multiple studies, public health programs are designed to lower the prevalence of risk factors with the goal of reducing disease incidence.[20] Epidemiologic research incorporating serologic testing of biomarkers contributes to recognition of subclinical diseases, and monitoring changes of molecular markers has become a major component of cohort studies.

During the 20th century, the CDC shifted their public health focus from communicable to chronic conditions as morbidity and mortality rates from infectious diseases were surpassed by disabilities and deaths from heart disease, stroke, diabetes, and cancer. The centers expanded their mission with a new focus on prevention and a commitment to develop programs addressing smoking cessation, reducing risks of diabetes and its complications, assessing illness due to environmental contaminants, studying patterns of mortality due to gun violence, etc., while continuing to protect the nation from the potential challenges of emerging infections.[22]

Preventive Measures Targeted to Personal Risks

Technologic advances enabled the decoding of the human genome 12 years ago, enabling clinicians and researchers to translate newly identified genetic information into customized person-specific health messages with opportunities for individualized medical care. The possible contribution of genetic inheritance to determining personal risk of diseases stimulated the search among molecular markers leading to the identification of susceptibility genes such as *BRCA1* and *BRCA2*.

Before genetic testing became available in medical practice, most clinicians began their clinical assessment inquiring about a patient's family history in order to guide recommendations for appropriate disease screening, health behaviors, and advice about preventive measures. Although a positive family history for a condition is a complex issue given that disease patterns vary by family size, age distributions, environmental influences, and accuracy of past diagnoses,[23] this traditional assessment provided the basis for studies of hereditary cancer syndromes initially identified by Lynch and others decades ago.[24]

Although identifying susceptibility genes holds great promise, most affected individuals are found to be negative for inherited susceptibility. Therefore, geneticists are searching for additional genetic markers and epidemiologists investigate potential nongenetic causes of diseases. Two approaches commonly used to identify avenues for disease prevention include experimental and observational studies. Experiments are conducted in the laboratory with animal models, cell cultures, or human volunteers in randomized trials such as the Women's Health Initiative.[25] In some settings experimental studies may not be practical

or the proposed intervention may not be ethically acceptable for random assignment such as use of fertility drugs. Therefore, to answer specific risk factor questions epidemiologists conduct observational cohort studies following healthy women over time or by designing case-control studies to compare exposures that occurred before diagnosis among women with a disease compared to those without the condition. Factors identified through observational studies cannot be classified as causal because multiple complex environmental exposures do not occur randomly and are rarely independent events; however, the results provide direction for future targeted research of larger more varied populations.

The public became increasingly aware of the role of genetics through reports in the media of the Human Genome Project,[26] which has now been heralded as enabling personalized medicine. As the cost of genetic testing has fallen, interest has grown in personal testing, which has led to the development of a new unregulated industry including direct-to-consumer marketing of genotyping without external standards to ensure accuracy.[1] In addition, the value of the newly acquired personal knowledge will depend upon research linking inherited susceptibilities with potential interventions that may prevent or delay disease development. A person's risk and responses to preventive interventions may depend on an individual's unique genetic characteristics; therefore, the risk–benefit balance will be unique for each person.[27] As studies identify effective interventions for individuals with specific genetic susceptibilities, research will be required to quantify anticipated benefits. The focus of epidemiologic studies will be to stratify populations into subgroups of individuals using genetics and disease-specific biomarkers in order to evaluate the risks and benefits of targeted interventions.[27] Ames provided an example of a potential targeted intervention addressing unique genetic profiles of individuals. He suggested that technology will soon mature to provide person-specific assessment of micronutrient deficiencies through a single finger prick blood sample that will generate guidance for diet adjustments or nutrient supplements in order to achieve optimum health, disease prevention, and greater longevity.[28]

Research is also needed to link genetic risk differences with personal and environmental exposures that may modify inherited susceptibilities. Each individual woman carries a person-specific trajectory affecting her health status during her life course related to biologic, behavioral, social, and psychologic influences. Therefore, health counseling may be the most important physician–patient interaction occurring during periodic medical encounters. Schroeder among others noted that health status is influenced disproportionately by five domains: behavioral patterns (40%), genetics (30%), social circumstances (15%), health care (10%), and environmental exposures (5%).[12] He suggested that access to medical care contributes only minimally to preventing premature mortality. In contrast, personal health behaviors especially smoking, physical inactivity, and obesity account for a major component of reduced life expectancy among Americans. Although technology was crucial for accomplishing the major public health successes of the past and will continue to enhance clinical care, behavioral changes are essential to improve the health of Americans in the 21st century.[12]

Primary Prevention in Communities

Following the recognition of disease-associated risk factors public health researchers faced challenges when applying the knowledge to educate diverse communities about health risks. Although chronic diseases most often occur among adults, epigenetic studies have provided scientific evidence that some risk patterns that become established early in life, in utero or prior to puberty, may have an impact on adult health. Therefore, parents and teachers have been encouraged to focus on establishing healthy lifestyles among youngsters.

Social, economic, and cultural factors influence health-related decisions among families affecting dietary choices, frequency of physical activity, and general health behaviors. Community programs may influence these decisions when multisite collaborative programs are coordinated among schools, clinical settings, markets, and local government policies. The Million Hearts, a collaboration of government and private sector health facilities, was designed to expand a core of standardized practices based on scientifically proven preventive efforts for heart disease in clinical settings and community-based health promotion programs. The goal is to avoid 1 million heart attacks and strokes during the next 5 years.[6] The program emphasizes four primary clinical interventions based on the proven efficacy of the ABCS protocol: aspirin therapy, blood pressure control, cholesterol management, and smoking cessation.[6] Data from the National Health and Nutrition Examination Survey (NHANES) indicated almost 50% of the American public has at least one risk factor for heart disease—including untreated hypertension, smoking, and/or elevated cholesterol—and many had more than one untreated risk factor, leaving many Americans at risk for heart disease and stroke. Electronic medical records will identify individuals requiring enhanced care and digital monitoring of health changes will indicate the value of clinical interventions and community-based programs. The project is directed to high-risk populations who will receive appropriate preventive treatment, whereas community-based efforts will promote healthful behaviors to lower heart disease risk, diabetes, and obesity in the broader population.[6]

Many federal, state, and local initiatives are coordinating their efforts by addressing healthy diets, smoking cessation, increased exercise, and weight control. Communities have received funding for tobacco control and chronic disease prevention efforts, including reduced use of sodium and elimination of trans fats. Media messages and package labeling are included to educate the public about health risks of smoking, counteracting tobacco advertising that often targets women.[6] ACA emphasizes prevention by eliminating cost sharing by patients for preventive services such as blood pressure and cholesterol screening and smoking cessation services; ACA also facilitates increased access to care for many who have lacked medical coverage. Team-based care by multidisciplinary providers is being encouraged to work closely with individuals to address their specific needs.[6] Other community-based programs are discussed later in this chapter.

Primary Prevention Associated with Adult Vaccinations

Vaccines are among the greatest public health achievements of the 20th century, credited with significant reduction of morbidity and mortality from many diseases caused by bacteria and viruses.[29] Many conditions that were lethal in the past, causing massive outbreaks, are now prevented.[30] However, the public has questioned the safety of vaccines, and some have resisted vaccine protection for their children. In addition, fewer than expected adults have received annual protection from influenza or pneumonia.[29] Much of the fear has been associated with a retracted study published in *Lancet* that erroneously linked the measles-mumps-rubella (MMR) vaccine with increased risk of autism and created a worldwide controversy, although multiple additional studies found no association.[31]

To address these public concerns, the IOM was again requested by the CDC to review the epidemiologic, clinical, and biologic evidence regarding any **adverse** health effects associated with specific vaccines; the effectiveness of the vaccines was not addressed in the requested review published in the 2012 report.[30] The authors carefully noted that among the vaccines studied, very rare adverse events were reported in publications and these occurred only among individuals whose immune deficiencies or unique susceptibility left them at increased risk of an adverse response. The review committee encouraged continued reporting of cases by clinicians to the Vaccine Adverse Event Reporting System, which they recommended for posting on the Web. They also encouraged use of electronic medical records for monitoring rare adverse health events.[30]

Vaccination for primary prevention of influenza was received by 40.5% of adults in 2010–2011 with coverage among states varying widely, from 56% in South Dakota to 33% in Nevada.[32] Children aged 17 and younger as well as adults over age 65 were more likely to receive the seasonal vaccine than middle-aged Americans. Vaccine coverage was significantly below the public health goals during the past two flu seasons, although heightened awareness of the H1N1 pandemic was associated with a small increase in coverage during 2009–2010.[32]

Pneumococcal vaccination is recommended for adults diagnosed with diabetes, emphysema, coronary heart disease, and other conditions associated with heightened susceptibility. Less than 19% of adults aged 19–64 at high risk have ever received pneumococcal vaccine in contrast to 59.7% of adults aged 65 and older, although percentages varied by race/ethnicity. Zoster vaccine is advised for primary prevention of a painful blistering skin rash condition, shingles (herpes zoster), which occurs among older immune-suppressed adults, but only 20% to 30% of eligible elders have received the vaccine.[33]

The recently developed human papillomavirus (HPV) vaccine to prevent cervical cancer and malignancies of other organs has been targeted to young women prior to potential exposure to HPV.[33] Although preventing a malignancy has been heralded as a major breakthrough in cancer prevention, some parents have questioned the timing, cost, number of doses, and appropriateness of the target population. However, as research continues, new findings now recommend HPV vaccine for young males, and studies suggest fewer than three doses may be equally effective.[2]

CDC and other federal agencies continue to educate the public regarding the safety of vaccines and their essential contribution to the nation's health. Many Americans lack personal knowledge of or experiences with the severe morbidity and mortality associated with many preventable conditions.[30] Public health workers have promoted the importance of adult vaccines and encouraged their availability at low cost in multiple locations, including clinical settings, employee health services, and pharmacies, which has increased acceptance although at rates that are still considered far lower than optimum.

Prevention by Not Smoking

The health hazards of smoking were recognized by clinicians as the incidence of lung cancer increased and epidemiologic studies documented the risks. Ecologic data linking cigarette consumption and mortality from lung cancer noted in Figure 4-3 confirmed clinical evidence of a national trend.[34] The first American studies indicating smoking was contributing to risk of lung cancer were published in 1950 and were confirmed by many investigators, leading to the First Surgeon General's report of 1964[35] linking smoking with multiple adverse health outcomes. Cigarette sales continued to climb until finally beginning to decline in 1980 (Figure 4-3).

Figures 4-4 and 4-5 present data on differences in smoking patterns among women and men during the 20th century in relation to the year of birth, noting the percentage of smokers who began smoking before age 20 and the number of years they smoked before age 40.[34] Women were slower to become regular smokers, but in more recent years they began smoking at an earlier age than men and are more resistant to quitting. In the past, cigarette advertising targeting women strongly influenced habit formation as adolescent females were influenced by seductive, slender female smokers.[36] Brandt described the deceptive cigarette advertising based on scientific misinformation that tobacco companies used to compete for smokers. He strongly encouraged greater public health attention to tobacco control.[37]

The prevalence of smoking among Americans decreased from 42.4% in 1965 to 19.3% in 2010, when the number of former smokers exceeded current smokers. To counteract continued tobacco advertising, the American Legacy Foundation created a campaign revealing the deceptive antismoking messages of the tobacco industry.[38] The combined effect of state and local laws creating smoke-free public environments while increasing cigarette taxes have encouraged many people to stop smoking. The ACA will cover the cost of smoking cessation programs, which have had a significant impact of reduced smoking in Massachusetts. Effective avenues for quitting smoking include advice from personal healthcare providers; individual, group, and telephone counseling; and medications. Data indicate former smokers are less likely to die from any cause and have longer years of life with lower risks of tobacco-associated disabilities than women and men who continue smoking.[39]

Although diminished in prevalence, smoking has remained the primary preventable cause of premature mortality in 2011 among women and men although the decline among men occurred more rapidly than among women. Gritz et al. noted the significant burden of tobacco-related disability and death associated with smoking that grew during the 20th century.[40] Figure 4-4 and Figure 4-5 indicate smoking grew faster early in the century among men than women. In 1924, 6% of women were smokers, rising to 16% only 5 years later, but more than 50% of men were smokers during these years. The sex differences reached a high of 28% before declining to less than 5%, suggesting that gender differences in longevity, so strongly influenced by smoking, may diminish in coming decades.[41]

Data from a national random-digit-dialing study, the American Smoking and Health Survey (ASHES), funded by the American Legacy Foundation, revealed that women lacked adequate knowledge of causes of tobacco-related mortality.[42] Many women identified breast cancer rather than lung cancer as the leading cause of cancer death among women, which Healton et al. related to the greater attention of the public, media, and government agencies to health risks associated with breast compared with lung

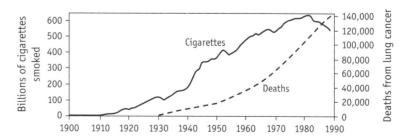

Figure 4-3 Cigarette consumption and number of lung cancer deaths, United States 1900–1990.

Source: Reproduced from Smoking, Tobacco, and Cancer Program, US Dept of Health and Human Services, NIH Pub No. 90-3107, 1990.

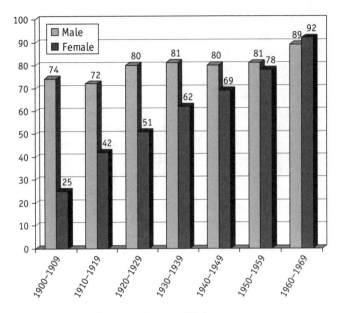

Figure 4-4 Percent of smokers who began smoking before age 20 by year of birth.

Source: Reproduced from Smoking, Tobacco, and Cancer Program, US Dept of Health and Human Services, NIH Pub No. 90-3107, 1990.

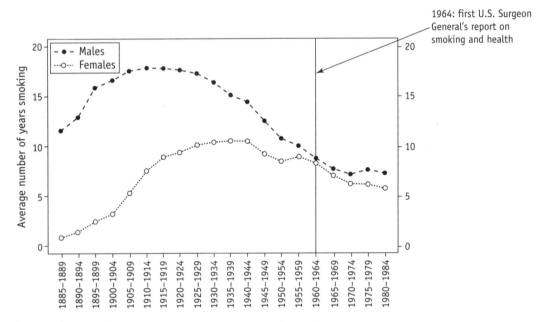

Figure 4-5 Average years of smoking before age 40 among women and men by birth cohort.

Source: Reproduced from Wang H, Preston S. Forecasting United States mortality using cohort smoking histories. PNAS 2009;106:393–398.

cancer. Women are repeatedly confronted with messages stressing annual mammography and any new research findings are featured.[42] Some investigators have suggested the more limited attention to lung cancer results from the stigma associated with the belief that the disease is self-imposed.[42]

For every woman who dies as a result of smoking, 20 others suffer serious chronic, painful disease such as arthritis, osteoporosis, and heart disease. Smoking also adversely affects fetal growth and newborn babies exposed to secondhand smoke are more likely to develop asthma.

Almost all medical problems experienced by women across the life span discussed in this text have an association with smoking. Given the magnitude of health risks associated with smoking, the CDC has launched a new program, Tips from Former Smokers, which features individuals whose quality of life and longevity have been threatened by their smoking histories or exposures to secondhand smoke.[7] This campaign is another major commitment of the federal government to prevent young people from beginning smoking and to convince adults to quit. The 12-week program will include messages on television, radio, newspaper, billboards, the internet, in movie theaters, magazines, and newspapers. The campaign is timely given that the cigarette package warnings have been contested in court by tobacco companies.

Reports indicate that 90% of men and women dying from tobacco-related illnesses began smoking as adolescents. Many studies have noted that smoking by parents and peers influences early onset of smoking in youth[43] and a new study reported exposures to smoking in films during early adolescents was linked with higher probability of young adolescents becoming established smokers at young ages. Films designed for young audiences should reconsider inclusion of smoking by their actors and potentially cigarette smoking could be included as a youth-rating criterion.[44]

Aspirin for Primary Prevention

Cardiovascular disease differs among women compared with men. Women tend to be older with a first cardiac event and the lifetime risk of stroke is higher than for men. After reviewing new research findings, the U.S. Preventive Services Task Force in 2009 recommended regular use of aspirin by women between the ages of 55 and 79 to reduce the risk of stroke when the estimated benefits for the individual exceeded risks of gastrointestinal bleeding.[45,46] Other studies indicating that aspirin lowered risk of heart disease included a wider spectrum of ages and was especially beneficial in reducing recurrence after a first myocardial infarction. The double-blind randomized trial, the Women's Health Study, reported reduced risks of stroke (RR = 0.83, 95% CI = 0.69 – 0.99), although no significant benefit in combined cardiovascular events including myocardial infarction or death for cardiac causes was found.[47] Many studies conducted over more than 2 decades have reported daily aspirin protected against several forms of cancer as well as lowering the risk of metastases.[48,49] The use of aspirin as a chemopreventive agent to lower cancer risk has been associated with suppression of inflammation and inhibition of COX-2, an enzyme that promotes tumor growth. Health behaviors that protected against infectious agents are repeatedly being found to also protect against chronic conditions; for example, recent reports suggest that daily aspirin may be protective against inflammation associated with heart disease and some forms of cancer.[50]

Clinical guidance has been complicated for patients at average risk by potential adverse health outcomes from aspirin studies that differ by dosages and frequency of use. The Million Heart project of the federal government previously discussed includes routine aspirin use as one preventive component of four recommendations to reduce heart disease among Americans.[6] However, some public health researchers hesitate to recommend expanded use of aspirin due to potential side effects, which include gastrointestinal bleeding, ulcers, and hemorrhagic stroke.[51] The risk of gastrointestinal bleeding requiring transfusion was more frequent among women randomized to aspirin than placebo in the Women's Health Study (RR = 1.4, 95% CI = 1.07 – 1.83).[47] Future genetic analyses may identify individuals with inherited bleeding disorders

for whom routine low-dose aspirin may increase susceptibility to bleeding disorders.

Risks and Benefits of Alcohol Consumption

Alcohol drinking among women has major risks and some benefits varying by quantity consumed, frequency of drinking, age, pregnancy status, underlying health risks, social circumstances, cultural patterns, and other factors. Although some studies suggest women who consume a **maximum** of one alcoholic beverage per day may benefit from diminished risk of cardiovascular disease, heavy drinking (three or more drinks per day) and binge drinking (four or more alcoholic drinks consumed on one occasion) increases risks of death from injuries, cirrhosis of the liver, suicide, hypertension, myocardial infarction, sexually transmitted diseases, unplanned pregnancy, and several types of cancer.[52] CDC's Behavioral Risk Factor Surveillance System (BRFSS) data indicated the 11% of female respondents who reported binge drinking were between ages 18 and 34; frequency and intensity varied by economic status.[53] Driving while alcohol impaired has been associated with an estimated 11,000 crash fatalities annually in the United States, with 4.5% of adults who reported binge drinking four or more times a month accounting for 55% of all alcohol-impaired driving episodes, often without use of seat belts.[54] Alcohol consumption during pregnancy has been associated with fetal alcohol syndrome, miscarriage, premature birth, sudden infant death syndrome, and birth defects.[53] To curb excess alcohol consumption some public health workers have encouraged higher taxes, greater regulation of the number of stores selling alcohol in a community, maintaining limits for sale of alcohol, and monitoring retail outlets for sales to minors.[53]

In contrast to these adverse effects of excess consumption, several studies indicated light to moderate drinking provided protection against cardiovascular disease by counteracting harmful effects of high cholesterol from high-saturated fat diets. Protective effects have been attributed to antioxidant and antithrombotic components primarily found in red wine. Goldberg et al. published a review of potential benefits for the American Heart Association.[55] The authors noted the difficulty of comparing and summarizing diverse studies that employed differing research methods, with varying definitions for drinking quantities and lack of control for other health-related factors. They advised that women should drink no more than one glass of wine per day, which could potentially increase high-density lipoprotein (HDL) cholesterol by 10%, a benefit that they considered comparable to routine exercise or niacin therapy.[55] In limited quantities alcoholic beverages also reduce platelet aggregation, they noted, providing antithrombotic action similar to aspirin. These authors concluded that the data from observational studies did not provide clear evidence of a protective role for wine and/or other alcoholic beverages, warning of the potential for abuse and development of addiction.[55]

Several large cohort studies have identified a modest protective role of alcohol. Among the 85,000 participants ages 34 to 59 in the Nurses' Health Study, light to moderate drinking (1.5 to 29.9 grams/day), compared with nondrinkers, was associated with decreased risk of death from cardiovascular disease especially among older members of the cohort. Women who drank more heavily were at increased risk of death from multiple causes.[56] Another report from Nurses' Health Study I followed the older cohort to age 70 or beyond and reported moderate alcohol consumed daily was an independent contributor to successful aging.[57] Postmenopausal women ages 50 to 79 at entry to the Women's Health Initiative (WHI) who indicated low to moderate alcohol consumption (one to six drinks per week) benefitted from reduced total mortality (HR = 0.81, 95% CI = 0.72 – 0.91) and lower incidence of hypertension (HR = 0.76, 95% CI = 0.65 – 0.87).[58] Moderate drinking also lowered mortality of Caucasian and African American WHI participants with a history of hypertension.[58] Among 72,000 female subscribers of Kaiser Permanente in Oakland, California, who were followed for more than 12 years after enrollment when drinking behaviors were recorded on entry health appraisals, either red or white wine but not liquor or beer was related to lower mortality from coronary heart disease and respiratory conditions.[59] A national project of the American Cancer Society, Cancer Prevention Study II, with more than 250,000 women enrolled, also noted lower risk of mortality associated with one alcoholic drink per day, although alcohol drinking did not compensate for the doubling of mortality risk associated with smoking.[60] In summary, the 2010 U.S. Department of Agriculture dietary guidelines suggested **moderate** alcohol intake up to one drink per day for women to provide health benefits. However, genetic differences influencing alcohol metabolism may alter the benefits and risks of drinking among women of different ages.

Preventing or Controlling Hypertension

Hypertension is among the nation's most common chronic conditions with nearly one-third of American adults having elevated blood pressure. Data from NHANES examinations of a representative sample of the U.S. population has suggested that nearly one in three Americans has hypertension and 43 million women and men are unaware of their elevated blood pressure.[61] Definitions of hypertension vary among clinicians, although antihypertensive medication is generally recommended for individuals with a blood pressure reading of 140 systolic or 90 diastolic or greater. The risk of women and men over age 50 developing hypertension is nearly 90%. Hypertension is a key risk factor for stroke, heart attack, and heart failure among other health problems; therefore, this condition requires routine monitoring and appropriate treatment.[61]

The CDC has recently advised a population-based strategy for blood pressure control that would benefit entire communities. The program, planned in collaboration with states and local communities as well as healthcare providers, emphasizes consumption of a healthful diet that excludes excessive salt, encourages increased physical activity, and maintenance or regaining an appropriate weight for height.[62] Collection of dietary data during

NHANES interviews indicated a majority of respondents were consuming more salt than recommended and an estimated 75% of salt is added during commercial food processing or in restaurant meals, preventing individual controls on consumption. To prevent the adverse effect of high dietary sodium on blood pressure, several public health programs and reports from the CDC have focused on dietary salt reduction.[61]

The Institute of Medicine recommended the United States adopt new strategies already established in other countries to establish sodium limits on foods and to improve sodium quantity labeling.[63] Recommendations for salt restriction were based on many studies, including the results reported by Bibbins-Domingo et al., who constructed a Markov model using national data from several sources to estimate reductions in morbidity and mortality following a dietary salt reduction of 3 g per day.[64] The number of new cases of coronary heart disease would be reduced by 60,000 to 120,000, stroke by 32,000 to 66,000, and myocardial infarction by 54,000 to 99,000 and the annual number of deaths from any cause would decline by 44,000 to 92,000. Figure 4-6 notes the benefit of salt dietary reduction among women and men by age and race. Modest salt restrictions would be especially beneficial among black women and men whose rates of hypertension are 50% higher than whites. Reduced sodium could potentially lower mortality disparities. The authors estimated 3 g per day salt reduction provided disease reduction comparable to a 50% decline in smoking, a 5% reduction in body mass index among obese people, or use of statin drugs to lower individual risk of heart disease. Salt reduction would reduce risk of stroke more than other interventions.[64] The Million Hearts project needs to convince food manufacturers to reduce sodium in processing to help accomplish the successes predicted.[6]

Primary Prevention Drug Interactions

The pharmaceutical industry has achieved many successes in treatment of heart disease, cancer, and infectious conditions including HIV/AIDS, which have significantly lowered mortality. Use of prescription drugs rose steadily between 1999 and 2008 in the United States with 48% of Americans reporting at least one prescribed drug and 11% using five or more medications. NHANES data indicated treatment with multiple prescribed drugs during the month prior to interview increased significantly with age (Figure 4-7). High rates of drug use have increased adverse interactions among prescribed medications as well as potentially lethal effects of their combination with over-the-counter products, illegal drugs, and alcohol, resulting in emergency visits.[65] Among the 41,000 deaths from poisoning in 2008, almost 90% were associated with combinations of legal and illegal drugs; 40% were specifically prescribed opioid analgesics.[66] Paulozzi et al. reported 100 deaths occurred per day from drug overdoses, a rate of 11.8 per 100,000 population.[67] Rates were higher among men (14.8/100,000) than women (9.0/100,000).[66] Drug poisoning associated with natural and semisynthetic opioid analgesics such as morphine,

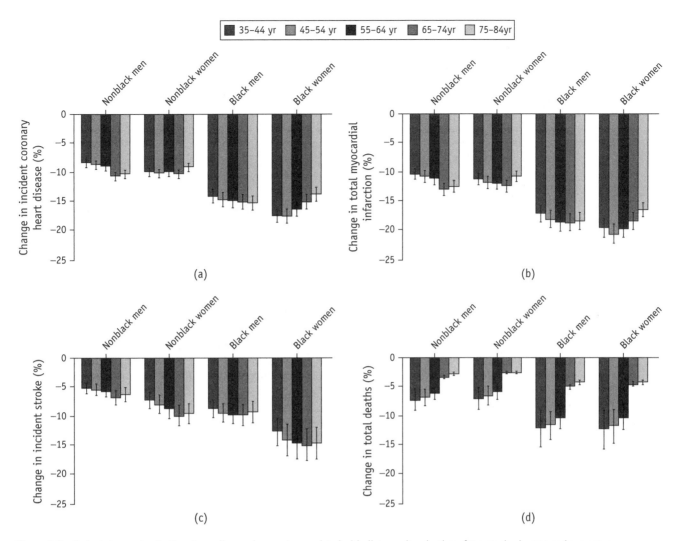

Figure 4-6 Projected annual reductions in cardiovascular events associated with dietary salt reduction of 3 g per day by race and age group.

Source: Reproduced from Bibbins-Domingo K, Chertow GM, Coxson PG, et al. Projected effect of dietary salt reductions on future cardiovascular disease. N Engl J Med 2010;362:590-599. © 2010 Massachusetts Medical Society. All rights reserved.

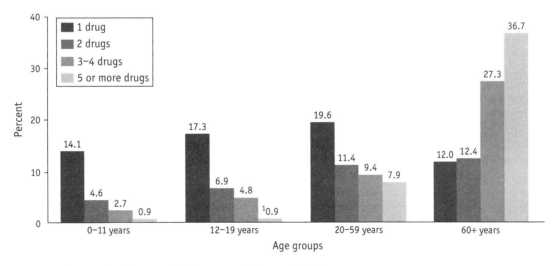

Figure 4-7 Percentage of prescription drugs used within past month, by age, United States, 2007-2008.

Data from Centers for Disease Control and Prevention, National Center for Health Statistics, National Health and Examination Survey. Reproduced from Gu Q, Dillon CF, Burt VL. Prescription drug use continues to increase: U.S. prescription drug data for 2007–2008. NCHS data brief, no 42. Hyattsville, MD: National Center for Health Statistics. 2010.

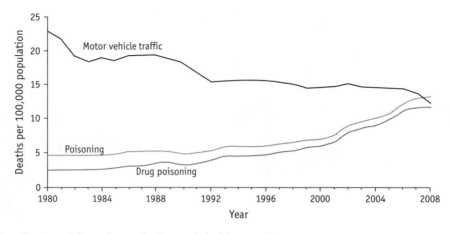

Figure 4-8 Motor vehicle, poisoning and drug poisoning death rates: United States, 1980–2008.

Source: Reproduced from Warner M, Chen LH, Makuc DM, Anderson RN, Miniño AM. Drug poisoning deaths in the United States, 1980–2008. NCHS data brief, no 81. Hyattsville, MD: National Center for Health Statistics. 2011.

hydrocodone, and oxycodone totaled more than 14,800 in 2008, triple the rate reported in 1999.[66,68] Over 5 million Americans reported use of prescription drugs for nonmedical purposes obtained from family and friends without personally receiving a doctor's order.[68]

To raise public awareness and focus attention on poison prevention, the CDC annually designates National Poison Prevention Week, which celebrated its 50th anniversary in March 2012.[69] However, the announcement included the sobering data tabulated from 2008 that indicated deaths from poisoning had become the leading cause of injury-related mortality in the United States, exceeding motor vehicle deaths (noted in Figure 4-8).[66] Unintentional and intentional injuries place a heavy burden on the lives of women, their families, and communities. Significant progress in lowering motor vehicle injury risk has been accomplished through driver education programs, required use of seat belts, improved technology including airbags, and sight testing before driving license renewal. Guided by their successes, these programs are being used as a model for comprehensive, multidisciplinary approaches to reversing the trend in drug poisoning. Among the planned approaches are recommendations to physicians to prescribe opioid medications exclusively for pain relief when nonopioid drugs are inadequate.

Public health interventions to reduce prescription drug overdose must be balanced between misuse and abuse while protecting the appropriate access for patients requiring pain relief.[67] Studies have indicated that 40% of opioid overdoses occurred among patients receiving care from multiple doctors; therefore, one avenue proposed to reduce risks would combine state-based monitoring of drug sales and insurance restrictions preventing early refills and multiple prescriptions for the same medications.[68] Additional proposals to control the current epidemic include advocating for improved legislation and greater enforcement of current laws and addressing issues raised during clinical care by encouraging physicians to follow evidence-based drug treatment guidelines.[68]

During the more than 4 decades since Congress passed the Poison Prevention Packaging Act requiring child-resistant caps on medication and toxic substances, progress has been achieved, although medication poisoning of children remains a significant problem. Annual estimates include 60,000 emergency department visits and more than 500,000 calls to poison control centers following potential poisoning of children from medications.

Prevention Through Physical Exercise and Weight Control

Studies of the increasing obesity epidemic have identified multiple interrelated contributing factors including genetic or familial susceptibility, personal diet and exercise behaviors, and aspects of residential neighborhoods such as availability of safe outdoor recreation facilities and sources of healthy foods.[19] For individuals, weight control relies on balancing food consumption with amount of physical exercise. Changing portion sizes in restaurants, greater availability of high-calorie foods in some local stores, and limited financial resources may compromise personal plans for healthy eating and weight control. Many people claim to desire following a healthy lifestyle, but time commitments to employers, family responsibilities, and other barriers interfere.

Community-based efforts and government regulations have become essential components of epidemiologic studies to identify preventive behaviors to avoid chronic disease. For example, a sedentary lifestyle and resulting obesity have been studied among urban residents by linking personal health behaviors including physical activity, diet, and obesity with the individual's residential environment including recreational use of land and proximity to safe, walkable neighborhoods.[70] Geographic information systems were employed to assess proximity to well-maintained outdoor recreational areas including parks and hiking trails plus access to public transportation, which were positively associated with greater physical activity and lower body mass index. Collaborative studies have shown that city residents are by necessity more physically active and less likely to be obese than individuals living in suburban or rural environments. However, highly

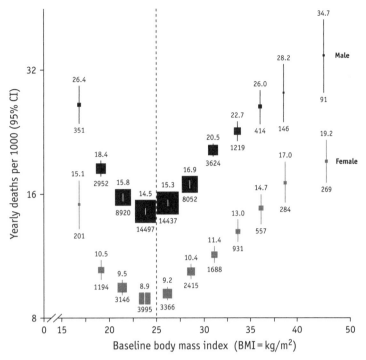

Figure 4-9 All cause mortality by BMI for males and females.

Source: Reproduced from Whitlock G, Lewington S, Sherliker P, et al. Body-mass index and cause-specific mortality in 900,000 adults: collaborative analyses of 57 prospective studies. The Lancet 2009;373:1083–1096 with permission from Elsevier.

dense areas of low-income families were found to have fewer amenities for exercise and recreation and those that existed were poorly maintained. In addition, higher crime rates may also inhibit outdoor activities. These characteristics resulted in residents reporting higher rates of obesity and less physical exercise than people living in more affluent sections where parks and trails are well maintained.[70]

Research has documented the importance of physical exercise at all ages across the life span, especially among the elderly; however, recently more Americans have become sedentary as they watch television, play computer games, or communicate for hours over the Internet. Studies have repeatedly indicated a minimum of 30 minutes per day of moderately intense exercise can reduce risks of several types of cancer, diabetes, heart disease, and depression. Regular exercise also enhances the quality of sleep, reduces stress, and helps control weight. A well-rounded exercise program provides for aerobic activity, strength training, flexibility, and balance training, each of which benefits the body in different ways.

Obesity

The prevalence of obesity has significantly increased in the United States with resulting higher incidence rates of diabetes, hypertension, heart disease, stroke, breast and endometrial cancers, among other chronic conditions. Olshansky et al. have predicted that obesity may cause a decline in life expectancy during the 21st century.[71] Figure 4-9 reflects the analyses from 57 international collaborative studies with data indicating cause-specific mortality from more than 900,000 women and men with body mass index (BMI) measurements recorded at

enrollment. Figure 4-9 indicates that the lowest mortality occurred between 22.5 and 25.0 BMI. Each 5 kg/m² higher weight was associated with 30% greater mortality.[72] Compared with the ideal BMI of 25, increasing BMI was associated with higher mortality than women or men closer to the ideal, whereas very low BMI, possibly due to preexisting disease, was also associated with more deaths.[72] The J-shaped curve is striking for the high mortality at either BMI extreme.

Being overweight or obese at older ages increases the risk of developing type 2 diabetes. This major health threat often develops in childhood, when food consumption and physical activity are out of balance. Excess consumption and limited strenuous exercise establish an unhealthful pattern affecting long-term health risks. In addition to diabetes, overweight and obese women increase their probability of developing cardiovascular disease, cancer, sleep apnea, arthritis, and other conditions that cause disabilities limiting mobility. Walking at a steady pace 30 to 60 minutes per day enhances health maintenance without straining muscles, maintains joint flexibility, strengthens bone, and controls weight while controlling risks of heart disease, hypertension, and other chronic conditions associated with aging.

Preventing Excess Exposure to Radiation

Epidemiologic data from atomic bomb survivors[73] and medical exposures[74] have established that moderate to high exposures to radiation, especially at young ages, may increase risks of cancer development years later. For this reason individualized screening recommendations have been proposed.[75] Several new powerful technologies provide significantly advanced diagnostic information guiding essential clinical care; however, these modalities also carry risks of high levels of radiation exposure.[76] As of 2010 an estimated 75 million computed tomography (CT) scans have been performed on approximately 10% of the population. CT scanning is a unique technology that produces three-dimensional images although at 100 to 500 times the radiation exposure of conventional X-rays. Therefore, a balance of the benefits and risks of CT scans is essential and the Food and Drug Administration (FDA) encourages clinicians to appropriately justify ordering CT scans for specific clinical problems and to carefully monitor radiation doses during the procedures.[76] Patients are being advised to retain a record of medical imaging in addition to the physician and/or hospital record as radiation is cumulative and risk–benefit ratio estimates per scan may be warranted.[77] Radiation is a known carcinogen documented through extensive epidemiologic research especially when exposures occur at young ages. Therefore, the FDA and professional organizations are committed to reducing unnecessary use of CT testing and protecting patients from excessive, unnecessary exposures.[77] Few evidence-based guidelines for CT use or the optimum radiation doses per scan have been developed. Although the FDA has approved CT scanners, the agency has no authority to oversee the use of the machines in clinical practice. Physicians often request imaging for legal protection, as failure to diagnose a serious problem may initiate a lawsuit, whereas overuse of scanning is rarely questioned.[78]

Physicians and technologists must be educated to limit radiation exposure and patients should question the necessity of the imaging. Currently, no agency is monitoring CT-dose information although some clinicians have suggested programs comparable to the Mammography Quality Standards Act of 1992 controlling breast screening programs.[77] However, the planning currently does not include standardization of appropriate use of the imaging equipment because the agency lacks that authority. Instead the FDA is encouraging professional organizations to standardize appropriate guidelines. Brenner and Hall anticipated increased use of CT-based screening of asymptomatic patients for lung and colon cancer as well as cardiac and whole body scanning. These investigators noted lifetime risk of cancer associated with CT scanning was relatively small on an individual level but given the increased exposure of Americans to ionizing radiation during the past 2 decades, the public health implications of CT exposure could be significant in future years.[79]

Prevention Through Public Health Education

Goals of the Office of Research on Women's Health (ORWH) during the next decade include studies to personalize prevention, diagnostics, and therapeutics for women and girls.[80] An essential component of that goal is health literacy, which has been strongly associated with health outcomes.[81] Although the focus has often been on reading and comprehension skills of the public, now health professionals including clinicians are held responsible for removing literacy-related barriers to improve health. Recent statistics indicate that almost 50% of Americans have difficulty reading and understanding printed health brochures and data have linked literacy level with health outcomes; therefore, health materials have been redesigned and presentations on the Web and mobile devices are providing preventive health concepts in simpler more direct language.[81]

Human biology classes enabling adolescents to understand body changes necessary for successful reproduction and the birth of healthy babies have been recommended for all high school students. Avoidance of unplanned or poorly timed pregnancies and sexually transmitted infections including HIV should be incorporated into these programs; however, data recently collected by CDC indicate a high percentage of high schools lack classes addressing these important health topics.[82] Young mothers may be unaware that their developing fetus may experience lifelong adverse health consequences from maternal exposures occurring very early in pregnancy, shortly after conception, when many women are not aware they are pregnant. Recommendations for primary prevention of adverse birth outcomes include improving preconception health care by developing interventions that identify biomedical, behavioral, and social risks that may cause harm to a developing baby.[83] Improved age-appropriate health education during childhood will provide benefits to the child and family throughout the life course. Health information must be designed to meet the intellectual levels and cultural understanding of all members of the population, especially the most vulnerable. The outcomes of meaningful public health efforts should result in delaying or avoiding the onset of disease and disability.[15]

Over the past few decades mass media campaigns have been conducted among large populations with the goal of encouraging healthful behaviors such as recently launched programs from CDC including Million Hearts, Tips from Former Smokers, and Text4Baby, which provides helpfully timed suggestions for pregnant women and new mothers. New electronic technology has expanded the ability of mass media campaigns to reach younger members of the population by targeting different subgroups with culturally appropriate messages including familiar music and language. The great public health promise resulting from mass media campaigns is based on the ability of messages to reach large audiences repeatedly over time often with subtle messages that encourage personal behavior changes. By influencing cognitive or emotional responses the health concepts may indirectly enhance norms developed and shared among social networks.[84] These avenues may reinforce specific health behaviors among individuals who did not personally observe advertisements.[84] More mass media campaigns have been directed to reducing smoking than any other primary prevention behavior and their success is documented by evidence of reduced smoking among adults. Greater success has been achieved when advertising is coordinated with other community-level policies such as higher cigarette taxes, smoke-free regulations, and messages targeted to specific segments of the population.[84]

Prevention of Disparities in Health Outcomes

Each woman carries her own unique life-course trajectory influenced by biologic, behavioral, social, and psychologic factors including health related events.[85] Health status at various stages of life is known to differ significantly by economic status, race/ethnicity, geographic environment, and personal lifestyle. Risk factors, incidence of diseases, and causes of mortality vary considerably by region in the United States as noted in two examples: HIV/AIDS and cardiovascular disease. Although major advances in biomedical sciences have contributed to improved health and greater life expectancy for most Americans, benefits are not shared equally among all segments of the U.S. population many of whom experience higher disease incidence, less successful treatment outcomes, and greater premature mortality.[13]

Access to high-quality health care is essential for treatment of symptomatic conditions; however, Danaei et al. reported disparities in risk factors were strongly related to disparities in mortality by race/ethnicity and income.[86] Health literacy may be a barrier for low-income and poorly educated members of communities to understand the health risks associated with specific behaviors. Skilled clinicians who are able to communicate complex issues in simple terms will be able to meet the specific needs of patients with low literacy skills.[81]

Although disparities have been recognized for decades and extensive research has been directed to defining the causes, statistics continue to reflect limited improvements in several critical health indicators such as perinatal mortality, frequency of infectious diseases, rates of nutrition-related conditions, and survival following diagnosis of chronic diseases including cancer.

Although high-risk behaviors identified by many public health researchers are associated with poor health statistics, other factors also contribute to health disparities. Research directed by Freeman, a breast surgeon, in the Harlem section of New York City identified several critical determinants of disparities affecting his patient population including social position, economic status, culture beliefs and practices, and residential environment.[87] Freeman focused on the lack of education and limited health literacy of patients who were unable to navigate the complex environment of Harlem Hospital and proposed a "patient navigator" program to reduce barriers to timely and appropriate clinical care.[87] Each patient was assigned a trained health navigator who provided assistance with scheduling appointments, enhancing patient–physician communication, ensuring timely diagnosis and treatment, and identifying available services and supportive care. The program has been mandated as a required service for accreditation of cancer centers by the American College of Surgeons' Commission on Cancer beginning in 2015. This program was tested in many settings and found

to significantly improve care provided to low-income patients of diverse racial/ethnic origin.[87] Epidemiologic studies emphasize the necessity of interventions appropriately meeting the needs of targeted populations and encouraging community awareness of available resources.

An avenue to address health disparities suggested by Moses and Martin included use of electronic data files in the clinical setting to provide objective assessment of the effectiveness of existing drugs and devices, greater participation in clinical trials within teaching hospitals and medical centers, collaborative arrangements for financing healthcare research and clinical care, cost-effective targets for basic health care for common diseases, and greater recognition of the important role of social and economic factors in disease development and health improvement.[1]

The Commission on Social Determinants of Health of the WHO noted that economic status has been a major source of disparity in health outcomes among rich and poor populations across countries and within nations including the United States.[13] Woolf et al. estimated almost 900,000 deaths could have been averted between 1991 and 2000 if white and black individuals had equal mortality rates.[88] Data collected during national surveys conducted between 1999 and 2010 identified a potential contributor to these disparities, increasing inability of low-income working-age adults to purchase high-cost prescribed medications. In 2010, 21.5% of those below the poverty level did not obtain medications compared to 3.9% of respondents with higher income.[89] Some progress is evident by the change in the ratio of black to white deaths between 1988 and 1996 was 1:4 and has declined to 1.2:1 between 2008 and 2010.[11]

Marmot and Bell suggested that the health gradient within a society is responsive to changing political, social, and economic status as occurred in Russia when adult mortality increased during the economic upheaval in 1992 that led to the demise of the Soviet Union.[13] Health status in the United States has declined since the 1980s as the economic gap between rich and poor significantly widened.[90] These challenges cannot be corrected simply through improved access to medical care.

Limited education including low health literacy may prevent some women from appreciating the importance of health messages regarding nutrition, early detection modalities, clinical instructions, or timely treatment.[91] Appropriate health education is essential among young women before pregnancy to ensure their children have a healthy environment during early development in utero. Healthful patterns established following birth, during childhood and adolescence will enhance the quality of life throughout the life course.

Recommendations from federal health agencies and professional organizations published in 2006 were designed to promote optimal health throughout the life span of women, children, and their families based on clinical care and population-focused public health strategies.[83] Programs that are culturally and linguistically appropriate are being developed to ensure maximal use and impact on the diverse American female population. The report encouraged greater education of consumers beginning among high school students to increase awareness of factors associated with adverse reproductive health outcomes especially among populations known to experiences health disparities.[83] The guidance for preconception health planning defines a continuum of clinical care addressing women's needs during differing stages of their reproductive years. Recognized disparities influence disease development and survival among subsets of women whose exposures have differed significantly by socioeconomic status, education, personal lifestyle, and access to high-quality health care from early life through senior years.

Summary

A life-course approach has guided the organization of this text reflecting the recent understanding of critical growth periods that may affect long-term health outcomes. At all ages, beginning with 9 months in utero to elder years, females undergo continual development and change requiring age-related protective behaviors to minimize risks of adverse clinical events while maximizing disease-free years. Focused studies are assessing prenatal development, factors associated with rapid growth before puberty, timing of sexual maturation, reproductive decisions, and the menopausal transition to better quantify beneficial preventive behaviors. These life phases are characterized by differing rates of cell replication and organ-specific susceptibility. Hormonal influences create the unique setting for preventive health services needed by women; environmental, medical, and behavioral factors influence personal decisions; and community programs increase awareness of health promotion activities. In addition, the heterogeneity of responses among women to disease-related risk factors and options for prevention will be modified when genetic analyses provide information to guide individuals. By identifying those at highest risk who carry specific susceptibility mutations, clinicians may be able to develop personalized medical care, encouraging preventive strategies and recommending early detection modalities to ultimately reduce morbidity along the life course and enable greater longevity free of disabilities. Health promotion and disease prevention are major aspects of public health efforts that must also continue to address the burden of disparities in health outcomes.

Discussion Questions

1. Describe a community health promotions objective and the design of community-wide interventions to achieve the objects.
2. What controls would be needed to adequately control prescribed medications that have recently been associated with increased emergency events and deaths?
3. How do epidemiologic studies of infectious conditions differ from chronic diseases? Describe come complex conditions that overlap infectious and chronic statuses?
4. Disparities in health outcomes have been present for many decades. Describe causes and some remedies.

References

1. Moses H, Martin JB. Biomedical research and health advances. *N Engl J Med.* 2011;364:567–571.
2. Kreimer AR, Rodriguez AC, Hildesheim A, et al. Proof-of-principle evaluation of the efficacy of fewer than three doses of a bivalent HPV 16/18 vaccine. *J Natl Cancer Inst.* 2011;103:1444–1451
3. Fauci AS, Morens DM. The perpetual challenge of infectious diseases. *N Engl J Med.* 2012;366:454–461.
4. Johnson MI, Fauci AS. HIV vaccine development—Improving on natural immunity. *N Engl J Med.* 2011;365:873–875.
5. Morse SS. Public health surveillance and infectious disease detection. *Biosecur Bioterror.* 2012;10:6–16.
6. Frieden TR, Berwick DM. The "Million Hearts" initiative—Preventing heart attacks and strokes. *N Engl J Med.* 2011;e27:1–4.
7. Centers for Disease Control and Prevention. CDC Launches national tobacco education campaign. *MMWR Morb Mortal Wkly Rep.*2012;61:178.
8. World Health Organization Constitution. 22 July 1946 basic documents. Geneva, Switzerland: WHO; 1985. http://www.who.int/governance/eb/who_constitution_en.pdf.
9. Breslow L, Enstrom JE. Persistence of health habits and their relationship to mortality. *Prev Med.* 1980;9:469–483.
10. Breslow L. From disease prevention to health promotion. *JAMA.* 1999;281:1030–1033.
11. Hoyert DL. 75 Years of mortality in the United States, 1935–2010. *NCHS.* 2012;no 88.
12. Schroeder SA. We can do better—Improving the health of the American people. *N Engl J Med.* 2007;357:1221–1228.
13. Marmot MG, Bell R. Action in health disparities in the United States. *JAMA.* 2009;301:1169–1171
14. McKenna MT, Zohrabian A. US burden of disease-past, present and future. *Ann Epidemiol.* 2009;19:212–219.
15. Fries JF. Aging, natural death, and the compression of morbidity. *N Engl J Med.* 1980;303:130–135.
16. Krieger N. Embodiment: a conceptual glossary for epidemiology. *J Epidemiol Community Health.* 2005;59:350–355.
17. Koh HK, Sebelius KG. Promoting prevention through the Affordable Care Act. *N Engl J Med.* 2010;363:1296–1299.
18. Institute of Medicine. *Clinical Preventive Services for Women: Closing the Gaps.* Washington, DC: The National Academies Press; 2011.
19. Galea S, Riddle M, Kaplan GA. Causal thinking and complex system approaches in epidemiology. *Int J Epidemiol.* 2010;39:97–106.
20. Kuller LH. Relationship between acute and chronic disease epidemiology. *Yale J Biol Med.* 1987;60:363–376.
21. Cohen SM, Van Handel MM, Branson BM, et al. Vital signs: HIV prevention through care and treatment—United States. *MMWR Morb Mortal Wkly Rep.* 2011;60:1618–1622.
22. Rosner D, Fried LP. Traditions, transitions, and transfats: new directions for public health. *Public Health Rep.* 2010;125:3–7
23. Freedman RA, Garber JE. Family cancer history: healthy skepticism required. *J Natl Cancer Inst.* 2011;103:776–777.
24. Lynch HT, Watson P, Bewira C, et al. Hereditary ovarian cancer. Heterogeneity in age at diagnosis. *Cancer.* 1991;67:1460–66.
25. Chlebowski RT, Anderson GL. Changing concepts: menopausal hormone therapy and breast cancer. *J Natl Cancer Inst.* 2012;104:517–527.
26. Lander ES, .Llinton LM, Birren B, et al. Initial sequencing and analysis of the human genome. *Nature.* 2001;409:860–921. (Errata, *Nature.* 2001;411:720, 412:565)
27. Whittemore AS. Evaluating health risk models. *Statist Med.* 2010;29:2438–2452.
28. Ames BN. Prevention of mutation, cancer and other age-associated diseases by optimizing micronutrient intake. *J Nucleic Acids.* 2010;2010:725071
29. Parmet WE. Pandemic vaccines—the legal landscape. *N Engl J Med.* 2010;362:1949–1952.
30. Institute of Medicine. *Adverse Effects of Vaccines: Evidence and Causality.* Board on Population Health and Public Health Practices. Washington, DC: The National Academies Press; 2012.
31. Poland GA, Jacobson RM. The age-old struggle against the antivaccinationists. *N Engl J Med.* 2011;364:97–99.
32. Centers for Disease Control and Prevention. Recommended adult immunization schedule—United States, 2012. *MMWR Morb Mortal Wkly Rep.* 2012;61:1–7.
33. Williams WW, Lu PJ, Singleton JA, et al. Adult vaccination coverage—United States, 2010. *MMWR Morb Mortal Wkly Rep.* 2012;61:66–72.
34. Smoking, Tobacco, and Cancer Program. *1985–1989 Status Report.* NIH Pub. No 90–3107. Washington, DC: US Department of Health and Human Services; , 1990.
35. Surgeon-General's Advisory Committee on Smoking and Health. *Smoking and Health.* Pub. no 1103. Washington, DC: Public Health Service;.., 1964.
36. Howe HL. An historical review of women, smoking and advertising. *Health Education.* 1984; 15:3–8.
37. Brandt AM. FDA regulation of tobacco—Pitfalls and possibilities. *N Engl J Med.* 2008;359:445–448.

38. Farrelly MC, Healton CH, Davis KC, et al. Getting to the truth: evaluating national tobacco countermarketing campaigns. *Am J Public Health*. 2002;92:901–907. (Erratum, *Am J Public Health*. 2003;93:703.)

39. Woloshin S, Schwartz LM, Welch HG. The risk of death by age, sex, and smoking status in the United States: putting health risks in context. *J Natl Cancer Inst*. 2008;100:845–853.

40. Gritz ER, Sarna L, Dresler C, Healton CG. Building a united front: aligning the agendas for tobacco control, lung cancer research, and policy. *Cancer Epidemiol Biomarkers Prev*. 2007;16:659–663.

41. Wang H, Preston SH. Forecasting United States mortality using cohort smoking histories. *PNAS*. 2009;106:393–398.

42. Healton CG, Gritz ER, Davis KC, et al. Women's knowledge of the leading causes of cancer death. *Nicotine Tob Res*. 2007;9:761–768.

43. Simons-Morton B, Haynie DL, Crump AD, et al. Peer and parent influences on smoking and drinking among early adolescents. *Health Educa Behav*. 2001;28:95–107.

44. Primack BA, Longacre MR, Beach ML, et al. Association of established smoking among adolescents with timing of exposure to smoking depicted in movies. *J Natl Cancer Inst*. 2012;104:549–555.

45. Wolff T, Miller T, Ko S. Aspirin for the primary prevention of cardiovascular events: An update of the evidence for the US Preventive Services Task Force. *Ann Intern Med*. 2009;150:405–410.

46. US Preventive Task Force. Aspirin for the prevention of cardiovascular disease: US Preventive Task Force recommendation statement. *Ann Intern Med*. 2009;150:396–404.

47. Ridker PM, Cook NR, Lee IM, et al. A randomized trial of low-dose aspirin in the primary prevention of cardiovascular disease in women. *N Engl J Med*. 2005;352:1293–1304.

48. Rothwell PM, Wilson M, Price JF, et al. Effect of daily aspirin on risk of cancer metastasis: a study of incidence cancers during randomised controlled trials. *Lancet* 2012;379:1591–1601

49. Rothwell PM, Price JF, Fowkes GR, et al. Short-term effects of daily aspirin on cancer incidence, mortality, and non-vascular death: analysis of the time course of risks and benefits in 51 randomised controlled trials. *Lancet*. 2012; 379:1602–1612.

50. McKeown RE. The epidemiologic transition: changing patterns of mortality and population dynamics. *Am J Lifestyle Med*. 2009;3(1 suppl):19S–26S.

51. Chan AT, Cook NR. Are we ready to recommend aspirin for cancer prevention? *Lancet*. 2012; (Pub ahead of print)

52. Bouchery EE, Harwood HJ, Sacks JJ, et al. Economic costs of excessive alcohol consumption in the US, 2006. *Am J Prev Med*. 2011;41:516–524.

53. Kanny D, Liu Y, Brewer RD, et al. Vital signs: Binge drinking prevalence, frequency, and intensity among adults—United States, 2010. *MMWR Morb Mortal Wkly Rep*. 2012;61:14–19.

54. Bergen G, Shults RA, Rudd RA. Vital signs: Alcohol-impaired driving among adults-united States, 2010. *MMWR Morb Mortal Wkly Rep*. 2011; 60:1–6.

55. Goldberg IJ. Mosca L, Piano MR, Fisher EA. Wine and your heart. a science advisory for healthcare professionals from the Nutrition Committee, Council of Epidemiology and Prevention, and Council on Cardiovascular Nursing of the American Heart Association. *Circulation*. 2001;103:472–475.

56. Fuchs CS, Stampfer MJ, Colditz GA, et al. Alcohol consumption and mortality among women. *N Engl J Med*. 1995;332:1245–1250.

57. Sun Q, Townsend MK, Okereke OI, et al. Alcohol consumption at midlife and successful ageing in women: a prospective cohort analysis in the Nurses' Health Study. *PLoS Med*. 2011;8:e1001090.

58. Freiberg MS, Chang YF, Kraemer KL, et al. Alcohol consumption, hypertension, and total mortality among women. *Am J Hypertens*. 2009;22:1212–1218.

59. Klatsky AL, Friedman GD, Armstrong MA, Kipp H. Wine, liquor, beer, and mortality. *Am J Epidemiol*. 2003;158:585–595.

60. Thun MJ, Peto R, Lopez AD, et al. Alcohol consumption and mortality among middle-aged and elderly US adults. *N Engl J Med*. 1997;337:1705–1714.

61. Gunn JP, Blair NA, Cogswell ME, et al. CDC Grand Rounds: Dietary sodium restriction—time for choice. *MMWR Morb Mortal Wkly Rep*. 2012;61:89–91.

62. Institute of Medicine. *Informing the Future: Critical Issues in Health*. Washington, DC: The National Academies Press; 2011

63. Institute of Medicine. *Strategies to ReduceSodium Intake in the United States*. Washington, DC: The National Academies Press; 2010.

64. Bibbins-Domingo K, Chertow GM, Coxson PG, et al. Projected effect of dietary salt reductions on future cardiovascular disease. *N Engl J Med*. 2010;362:590–599.

65. Cai R, Crane E, Poneleit K, Paulozzi L. Emergency department visits involving nonmedical use of selected prescription drugs—United States, 2004–2008. *MMWR Morb Mortal Wkly Rep*. 2010;59:705–709.

66. Warner M, Chen LH, Makuc DM, et al. Drug poisoning deaths in the United States, 1980–2008. *NCHS Data Brief*. 2011;81.

67. Paulozzi LJ, Jones CM, Mack KA, Rudd RA. Vital signs: overdoses of prescription opioid pain relievers—United States, 1999–2008. *MMWR Morb Mortal Wkly Rep*. 2011;60:1487–1492.

68. Paulozzi LJ, Baldwin G, Franklin G, et al. CDC Grand Rounds: prescription drug overdoses—a US epidemic. *MMWR Morb Mortal Wkly Rep*. 2012;61: 10–13.

69. Centers for Disease Control and Prevention. Announcements: National Poison Prevention Week, 50th Anniversary. March 18–24, 2012. *MMWR Morb Mortal Wkly Rep*. 2012;61:177.

70. Weiss CC, Purciel M, Bader M, et al. Reconsidering access: park facilities and neighborhood disamenities in New York City. *J Urban Health*. 2011;88: 297–310

71. Olshansky SJ, Passaro DJ, Hershow RC et al. A potential decline in life expectancy in the United States in the 21st century. *N Engl J Med*. 2005;352: 1138–45.

72. Whitlock G, Lewington S, Sherliker P, et al. Body-mass index and cause-specific mortality in 900,000 adults: collaborative analyses of 57 prospective studies. *Lancet*. 2009;373:1083–1096.

73. Land CE. Studies of cancer and radiation dose among atomic bomb survivors: the example of breast cancer *JAMA*. 1995;274:402–407.

74. Elkin EB, Klem ML, Gonzales AM, et al. Characteristics and outcomes of breast cancer in women with and without a history of radiation for Hodgkin's lymphoma: a multi-institutional, matched cohort study. *J Clin Oncol*. 2011;29:2466–2473.

75. Kerlilowske K. Evidence-based breast cancer prevention: The importance of individual risk. *Ann IntMed*. 2009;151:750–752.

76. US Food and Drug Administration. Radiation-emitting products. Initiative to reduce unnecessary radiation exposure from medical imaging. http://www.fda.gov/Radiation-EmittingProducts/RadiationSafety/RadiationDoseReduction/ucm2007191.htm

77. Smith-Bidman R. Is computed tomography safe? *N Engl J Med*. 2010;363:1–4.

78. Hillman BJ, Goldsmith JC. The uncritical use of high-tech medical imaging. *N Engl J Med*. 2010;363:4–6.

79. Brenner DJ, Hall EJ. Computed tomography—an increasing source of radiation exposure. *N Engl J Med*. 2007;357:2277–2284.

80. Pinn VW, Clayton JA, Begg L, Sass SE. Public partnership for a vision for women's health research in 2020. *J Women's Health*. 2010;19:1603–1607.

81. Rudd RE. Improving Americans' health literacy. *N Engl J Med*. 2010;2283–2285.

82. Kann L, Brener N, McManus T, Wechsler F. HIV, other STD, and pregnancy prevention education in public secondary schools—45 states, 2008–2010. *MMWR Morb Mortal Wkly Rep*. 2012 61;222–228.

83. Johnson K, Posner SF, Bierman J, et al. Recommendations to improve preconception health and health care—United States. *MMWR Morb Mortal Wkly Rep*. 2006;55:1–23.

84. Wakefield M, Loken B, Hornik RC. Use of mass media campaigns to change health behaviour. *Lancet*. 2010;376:1261–1271.

85. Lynch J, Smith GD. A life course approach to chronic disease epidemiology. *Annu Rev Public Health*. 2005;26:1–35.

86. Danaei G, Rimm EB, Oza S, et al. The promise of prevention: the effects of four preventable risk factors on national life expectancy and life expectancy and life expectancy disparities by race and county in the United States. *PloS Med*. 2010;7:e1000248.

87. Freeman HP, Rodriguez RL. History and principles of patient navigation. *Cancer*. 2011;117(15 suppl):3539–3542.

88. Woolf SH, Johnson RE, Fryer GE, Rust G, Satcher D. The health impact of resolving racial disparities: An analysis of US mortality data. *Am J Public Health*. 2004;94:2078–2081; *Am J Public Health*. 2008;98(9 suppl);S26–S28.

89. QuickStats. National Center for Health Statistics. Percentage of adults aged 16–64 years who did not get needed prescription drugs because of cost, by poverty status—National Health Interview Survey, 1999–2010. *MMWR Morb Mortal Wkly Rep*. 2011;60:1495.

90. Krieger N, Rehkopf DH, Chen JT, et al. The fall and rise of US inequalities in premature mortality: 1960–2002. *PLoS Med*. 2008;5:e46.

91. Institute of Medicine. *Health Literacy: A Prescription to End Confusion*. Board of Neuroscience and Behavioral Health. Washington, DC: The National Academy Press; 2004.

Preventive Nutrition: Public Health Implications

Laura Stadler, MS, RD and Wahida Karmally, DrPH, RD, CDE, CLS, FNLA

Introduction

This chapter addresses the specific nutrition needs of women, both physiologic and social, throughout the life cycle, to inform and support a preventive health perspective. The global increase in overweight and obesity and consequent rise in related chronic diseases make nutrition a critical component of public health initiatives. The nourishing properties of food extend beyond the provision of essential nutrients. The act of sharing food is a social activity, uniting people as families and friends and across cultures. Food behaviors incorporate social norms, reflect religious and cultural preferences, and are affected by environment, access, and socioeconomic status. Women's nutrition status affects that of their children and despite a shifting gender paradigm, women continue to be responsible for feeding their families. Healthcare professionals can empower women and have a positive impact on health outcomes by providing guidance among the deluge of health information in the media, changing food consumption patterns, and societal pressures. The evidence-based nutrition recommendations in this chapter are significant tools to use in supporting women's health through preventive nutrition.

Maternal Nutrition

Healthful lifestyle choices in pregnancy can optimize short- and long-term health of the mother and fetus.

Maternal physical changes and fetal growth requirements affect essential nutritional intake during pregnancy. Healthcare providers should be aware of the nutritional requirements during pregnancy as well as cultural and regional traditions that influence dietary practices during pregnancy. During pregnancy women may be motivated to improve their diet and make healthful lifestyle changes.

Body Weight and Pregnancy

Relative weight categories are classified by body mass index (BMI), a measure of weight for height expressed as kg per meter^2 that provides an estimate of body fat. Being at a healthy BMI (Table 5-1) prior to pregnancy reduces risks during pregnancy for both the mother and her fetus. Underweight and overweight are associated with pregnancy complications such as higher miscarriage rates, birth defects, perinatal death, and postnatal maternal anemia.[1-3] Overweight and obese women are more likely to retain excess weight postpartum and continue to gain weight with successive pregnancies;[3] therefore, women with BMI greater than 25 kg/m^2 planning to begin childbearing should lose weight prior to conception.[1,3,4]

Weight gain during pregnancy is necessary for fetal growth and development including the placenta, amniotic fluid, increased maternal blood volume and extracellular fluid, growth of maternal uterine and

Table 5-1	
Classification of body mass index[5]	
Weight Classification	**BMI Range in kg/m²**
Underweight	< 18.5
Healthy	18.5–24.9
Overweight	25–29.9
Obese	30–39.9
Severely obese	≥ 40

Reproduced from NIH, NHLBI Obesity Education Initiative. *Clinical Guidelines on the Identification, Evaluation, and Treatment of Overweight and Obesity in Adults.* Bethesda, MD: National Heart, Lung, and Blood Institute, National Institutes of Health; 1998.

mammary glands, and maternal fat stores. The most recent recommendations for weight gain published by the Institute of Medicine (IOM) are based on prepregnancy BMI (Table 5-2). The midwife, obstetrician, nurse, or dietitian should discuss appropriate weight gain guidelines before conception or at the first prenatal visit, as there are risks associated with inadequate weight gain as well as excessive weight gain.

Women with prepregnancy BMI greater than 29 are at risk for serious complications during pregnancy because excess weight adversely affects hormonal metabolic regulation. Pregnancy increases the burden, creating increased risk of gestational diabetes mellitus (GDM), gestational hypertension (GHTN), and preeclampsia due to the extensive hormonal and metabolic changes.[1,7,8] Women with a BMI > 29 often require cesarean delivery, which is associated complications such as bleeding, deep vein thrombosis, and poor wound healing.[3,8,9] Independent of self-reported folic acid supplementation, children born to women with a BMI > 29 are at a greater risk for neural tube defect, oral clefts, heart anomalies, and hydrocephaly.[10] The metabolic mechanism responsible for these risk factors is unknown but may be related to poor blood glucose control. Maintaining a healthy prepregnancy weight and gaining weight as recommended by the IOM are the best preventive measures to reduce risk for GHTN and preeclampsia.[3] For women with low calcium intakes, supplementation has been shown to reduce the risk of preeclampsia by 50%.[11]

To achieve the recommended weight gain, women need to increase their daily calorie intake starting in the second trimester by approximately 300 calories per day and in the third trimester by approximately 450 calories.[12] Women are "eating for two" in the sense that the nutrients the mother eats will support fetal growth, but women should not double food intake. Additional calories should come from nutrient-rich foods that are low in added sugar and fat. Focusing on fruits, vegetables, low-fat or fat-free dairy foods, beans, nuts, lean protein, and whole grains will not only benefit the mother and fetus but may also help establish healthy eating habits to support lactation by increasing caloric intake and nutrient needs during pregnancy.

Caffeine consumption may negatively affect the health of the fetus, potentially increasing the risk of miscarriage and low birth weight. Academy of Nutrition and Dietetics recommendations advise pregnant women to limit caffeine intake to less than 300 mg per day.[12,15]

Pregnant women should not drink alcohol due to the association with neurologic and developmental birth defects. As few as one to two alcoholic drinks per day can cause fetal alcohol syndrome and risks increase with greater quantities of alcohol intake.[12] There is no safe amount or type of alcohol to consume during pregnancy. Estimates from the CDC indicate between one and two babies of every 1,000 births is affected by fetal alcohol syndrome.[16]

Eating for optimal health may be especially challenging during pregnancy due to common discomforts such as bloating, nausea, acid reflux, and constipation, making it hard to eat certain foods that can enhance overall diet quality. Pregnant women require 8 to 10 cups of fluids per day.[12] Consumption of fruits, vegetables, whole grains, and adequate fluids will help alleviate constipation. Avoiding greasy, fried, and high-fat foods and caffeine may ease gastric reflux. Women should eat small meals at regular times throughout the day to alleviate potential discomforts.[12]

Nutrient Requirements in Pregnancy

Requirements for specific nutrients increase in pregnancy to support the growth of the placenta, maintain healthy rate of cell division, and increased maternal blood volume. These added requirements are partially met by increased capacity for absorption in the intestines and more efficient use of nutrients during pregnancy.[12] Depending on diet quality, a multivitamin may or may not be advisable. Women who have not been following a balanced diet should begin taking a multivitamin supplement prior to conception or as soon as they know they are pregnant. Supplemental iron during pregnancy avoids maternal anemia, improves neonatal iron status, and reduces the risk of small for gestational age babies.[15] The recommended daily iron intake during pregnancy is 27 mg, which is difficult to meet through diet alone;[16] therefore,

Table 5-2

Recommendations for weight gain during pregnancy, Institute of Medicine 2009

| Prepregnancy BMI | Total Weight Gain | | Rates of Weight Gain 2nd & 3rd Trimester | |
	Range [Kg]	Range [lbs]	Range [Kg]	Range [lbs]
Underweight [< 18.5 kg/m²]	12.5–18.0	28–40	0.51 [0.44–0.58]	1–1.3 lbs/week
Normal Weight [18.5–24.9 kg/m²]	11.5–16.0	25–35	0.42 [0.35–0.50]	0.8–1 lbs/week
Overweight [25.0–29.9 kg/m²]	7.0–11.5	15–25	0.28 [0.23–0.33]	0.5–0.7 lbs/week
Obese [≥ 30.0 kg/m²]	5.0–9.0	11–20	0.22 [0.17–0.27]	0.4–0.6 lbs/week

Reproduced from the Institute of Medicine at the National Academy of Sciences. *Weight Gain during Pregnancy: Reexamining the guidelines.* Washington, DC: National Academies Press; 2009.

daily supplemental iron is recommended during pregnancy.[12] Table 5-3 describes the recommended nutrients consumed by pregnant and nonpregnant women of childbearing age.

Fetal neural tube growth and closure happen within the first 8 weeks of pregnancy, often before women are aware of their pregnancy. For this reason women of childbearing age are encouraged to supplement their diet with 400 mcg/day of folic acid in order to reduce the risk of neural tube defects in the fetus by 50–75%.[17,18] During pregnancy, 600 mcg/day of folic acid are required; prenatal vitamin supplements typically contain 800 to 1000 mcg/day of folic acid.[16,19] There are several good dietary sources of folic acid including spinach, romaine, broccoli, lentils, black beans, and peanuts. Increased needs in pregnancy and inability to eat healthfully due to nausea will require vitamin and mineral supplements.

Omega-3 fatty acids are important to human health because of the protective effects they have against heart disease, inflammation, and mental health. The main three omega-3 fatty acids are eicosapentanoic acid (EPA), docosahexanoic acid (DHA), and alpha-linolenic acid (ALA). The body partially converts ALA to EPA (approximately 10%) or DHA (approximately 2%), which offer some protective benefits associated with omega-3 fatty acids. ALA comes from plant sources such as flaxseed, walnuts, canola oil, and soybean oil. Oily fish and fish-derived omega-3 fatty acid supplements are the best source of EPA and DHA. DHA is particularly important to fetal development because it is a major structural fat in the brain and the retina.[20] Limited research has assessed supplementation with omega-3 fatty acid during pregnancy; therefore, guidance from an obstetrician or midwife is recommended.[21] Fish that should not be eaten due to the high levels of PCB contaminates are wild striped bass, bluefish, wild sturgeon, bluefin tuna, king mackerel, swordfish, shark, and tilefish.[22,23] Smaller, nonpredatory fish such as anchovies and sardines are good sources of EPA and DHA and are less likely to be sources of contamination.[22] Other fish are safe to eat during pregnancy in six-ounce portions twice a week and should be cooked thoroughly.

Body Weight and Gestational Diabetes

Gestational diabetes (GDM) presents specific risks to both the mother and the fetus. Infants born to women with GDM have a greater prevalence of macrosomia (babies weighing more than 4,500 grams) complicating delivery and risking the health of the mother and fetus.

Table 5-3
Comparison of nutrient requirements of nonpregnant and pregnant women[15]

Nutrient	Nonpregnant Women 19–50 years old	Pregnant Women 19–50 years old
Vitamin A	700 mcg/day	700 mcg/day
Vitamin C	75 mg/day	85 mg/day
Thiamin	1.1 mg/day	1.4 mg/day
Riboflavin	1.1 mg/day	1.4 mg/day
Niacin	14 mg/day	18 mg/day
Vitamin B_6	1.3 mg/day	1.9 mg/day
Folate	400 mcg/day	600 mcg/day
Vitamin B_{12}	2.4 mcg/day	2.6 mcg/day
Pantothenic Acid	5 mg/day	6 mg/day
Choline	425 mg/day	450 mg/day
Chromium	25 mcg/day	30 mcg/day
Copper	900 mcg/day	1000 mcg/day
Iodine	150 mcg/day	220 mcg/day
Iron	18 mg/day	27 mg/day
Magnesium	Age 19–30 310 mg/day Age 31–50 320 mg/day	Age 19–30 350 mg/day Age 31–50 360 mg/day
Manganese	1.8 mg/day	2 mg/day
Molybdenum	45 mcg/day	50 mcg/day
Selenium	55 mcg/day	60 mcg/day
Zinc	8 mg/day	11 mg/day

Data from Cogswell ME, Parvanta I, Ickes L, et al. Iron supplementation during pregnancy, anemia, and birth weight: a randomized controlled trial. *Am J Clin Nutr.* 2003;78:773-81.

The children of women with GDM are at a greater risk for type 2 diabetes and obesity in childhood and later in life.[6,24] Women who are diagnosed with GDM should receive counseling from a registered dietitian to discuss lowering carbohydrate intake and to ensure optimum nutrition to reduce need for insulin, hospital admission, and perinatal complications. If there are no obstetric contraindications for exercise, physical activity can improve glucose control and reduce the risk of GDM. Women should allocate 30 minutes of moderate physical activity three times per week.[25]

Nutrient Needs in Childhood

Breastfeeding

Academy of Nutrition and Dietetics and the American Academy of Pediatrics recommend exclusive breastfeeding for 6 months, which has benefits for mothers (Table 5-4) and babies.[26] Exclusive breastfeeding means breastmilk should be the only food provided to the infant without any supplemental liquids or solids other than vitamins or minerals. Human milk is ideally suited for human infants, providing the optimal ratio of macronutrients in the most absorbable forms.[27] Maternal caloric, protein, and calcium intake does not affect the nutrient content of breast milk.[28-38] This ensures that the infant will receive the necessary nutrients for growth and development; however, the mother may not be receiving adequate nutrients for herself if she does not consume a varied diet rich in fruits, vegetables, whole grains, and lean protein, and dairy requirements. Women who are breastfeeding should not drink alcohol and should check with their physician about the use of prescription and over-the-counter medications. Lactation requires good hydration and women need to drink plenty of water. Women with a BMI over 30 have lower rates of successful breastfeeding initiation.

Benefits of Breastfeeding for Infants
Breastfeeding has numerous short- and long-term health benefits for infants. If breastfeeding is not successfully initiated or a mother chooses not to breastfeed, she should

Table 5-4
Maternal benefits of breastfeeding[38-53]
Establish emotional bonding and attachment
Opportunity for rest
Improved sleep quality
Lower blood pressure
Fewer depressive symptoms
Promotes uterine involution
Decreased risk postpartum hemorrhage
Improved iron status from lactational amenorrhea
Reduced risk of breast and ovarian cancers
Decreased risk of type 2 diabetes
Greater fat and weight loss in postpartum period

be provided with support and education on optimal formula-feeding practices. Breastmilk transfers mother's bacterial and viral immunoprotection to the infant, whose immune system is not yet functioning. Breastmilk is safe, fresh, and nutritionally complete except for vitamin D. Breastfed infants should receive vitamin D supplementation daily from birth.[55] By 6 months, infants should be introduced to iron-enriched, age-appropriate solid foods. Breastfed infants have greater control over intake and learn self-regulation of hunger and satiety. Bottle-fed infants are more likely to be encouraged to finish a certain volume of formula or expressed milk. The benefits in infancy from breastfeeding include proper development of the oral cavity and hard palate, decreased atopic dermatitis, reduced risk of sudden infant death syndrome, and a reduced incidence of necrotizing enterocolitis in premature infants[56-58] The health benefits of breastfeeding after infancy continue through childhood and into adulthood. Formula-fed infants have higher weight gain before age 2, which is associated with an increased risk of being overweight later in life, increased fat deposits, and increased risk of type 2 diabetes.[59] Being breastfed has a positive effect on systolic and diastolic blood pressure and reduces cholesterol levels later in life.[60]

Nutrition during Childhood, Adolescence, and Teen Years

Children need varied diets that are nutrient rich to support growth and social development. Food preferences are a common way for children to assert independence. Giving validity to child's needs and ensuring they have a balanced diet is a challenge for parents. In addition to the demands of busy family life, there are many aspects of American society that have changed quantitatively in just one generation, making healthful eating a challenge. In the United States between 1977 and 2001, the number of calories consumed from sweetened beverages and fruit drinks increased by 135%.[61-62] The U.S. Department of Agriculture Continuing Surveys of Food Intake by Individuals (CSFII) found that by 1996 children consumed almost 35% of their calories daily from meals eaten outside the home, an increase from 24% in 1977.[63] Most food eaten away from home offers menu items that are calorically dense yet nutrient poor. Analysis from National Health and Nutrition Examination Survey (NHANES) 1999–2002 shows that for children ages 2 to 18, fried potatoes accounted for over 28% of vegetable intake.[64] These statistics provide evidence indicating public health education and interventions are needed to support a healthy environment for children at school, in restaurants, and at home.

Children and adolescents who are overweight or obese are more likely than their healthy-weight peers to be overweight or obese as adults.[65,66] Self-esteem and confidence during adolescence can be adversely affected by being overweight. Girls are at particular risk of negative body image and eating disorders, which can have long-term health consequences for bone mineralization, growth, menstruation, and fertility. Being overweight has a negative impact on joint health, limiting physical activity, and potentially resulting in the need for joint replacements in adulthood. Children who are overweight or obese are at risk for adult chronic diseases such as dyslipidemia, hypertension, cardiovascular disease, diabetes, and for girls, polycystic ovary syndrome (PCOS). The heterogeneous symptoms of PCOS often emerge at menarche and may include oligomenorrhea or amenorrhea, hirsutism, and acne. PCOS is associated with metabolic complications such as hyperinsulinemia, sleep apnea, hypertension, dyslipidemia, and increased risk for type 2 diabetes. Weight reduction is an important part of treatment for overweight or obese girls and women with PCOS.[67]

Boys and girls have similar nutrient needs until puberty as noted in Table 5-5. After menarche, girls require more iron because of the blood loss from menstruation at an

Table 5-5

Institute of Medicine dietary reference nutrients[17]

	Children 1–3 years	Children 4–8 years	Females 9–13 years	Females 14–18 years	Males 9–13 years	Males 14–18 years
Vitamin A	300 mcg/d	400 mcg/d	600 mcg/d	700 mcg/d	600 mcg/d	900 mcg/d
Vitamin C	15 mg/d	25 mg/d	45 mg/d	65 mg/d	45 mgd	75 mg/d
Vitamin D	5 mcg/d	5 mcg/d	5 mcg/d	5 mcg/d	5 mcg/d	5 mcg/d
Vitamin E	6 mg/d	7 mg/d	11 mg/d	15 mg/d	11 mg/d	15 mg/d
Vitamin K	30 mcg/d	55 mcg/d	60 mcg/d	75 mcg/d	60 mcg/d	75 mcg/d
Thiamin	0.5 mg/d	0.6 mg/d	0.9 mg/d	1 mg/d	0.9 mg/d	1.2 mg/d
Riboflavin	0.5 mg/d	0.6 mg/d	0.9 mg/d	1 mg/d	0.9 mg/d	1.3 mg/d
Niacin	6 mg/d	8 mg/d	12 mg/d	14 mg/d	12 mg/d	16 mg/d
Vitamin B_6	0.5 mg/d	0.6 mg/d	1 mg/d	1.2 mg/d	1 mg/d	1.3 mg/d
Folate	150 mcg/d	200 mcg/d	300 mcg/d	400 mcg/d	300 mcg/d	400 mcg/d
Vitamin B_{12}	0.9 mcg/d	1.2 mcg/d	1.8 mcg/d	2.4 mcg/d	1.8 mcg/d	2.4 mcg/d
Pantothenic Acid	2 mg/d	3 mg/d	4 mg/d	5 mg/d	4 mg/d	5 mg/d
Biotin	8 mcg/d	12 mcg/d	20 mcg/d	25 mcg/d	20 mcg/d	25 mcg/d
Choline	200 mg/d	250 mg/d	375 mg/d	400 mg/d	375 mg/d	550 mg/d
Calcium	700 mg/d	800 mg/d	1300 mg/d	1300 mg/d	1300 mg/d	1300 mg/d
Chromium	11 mcg/d	15 mcg/d	21 mcg/d	24 mcg/d	25 mcg/d	35 mcg/d
Copper	340 mcg/d	440 mcg/d	700 mcg/d	890 mcg/d	700 mcg/d	890 mcg/d
Fluoride	0.7 mg/d	1 mg/d	2 mg/d	3 mg/d	2 mg/d	3 mg/d
Iodine	90 mcg/d	90 mcg/d	120 mcg/d	150 mcg/d	120 mcg/d	150 mcg/d
Iron	**7 mg/d**	**10 mg/d**	**8 mg/d**	**15 mg/d**	**8 mg/d**	**11 mg/d**
Magnesium	80 mg/d	130 mg/d	240 mg/d	360 mg/d	240 mg/d	410 mg/d
Manganese	1.2 mg/d	1.5 mg/d	1.6 mg/d	1.6 mg/d	1.9 mg/d	2.2 mg/d
Molybdenum	17 mcg/d	22 mcg/d	34 mcg/d	43 mcg/d	34 mcg/d	43 mcg/d
Phosphorus	460 mg/d	500 mg/d	1250 mg/d	1250 mg/d	1250 mg/d	1250 mg/d
Selenium	20 mcg/d	30 mcg/d	40 mcg/d	55 mc/g	40 mcg/d	55 mc/g
Zinc	3 mg/d	5 mg/d	8 mg/d	9 mg/d	8 mg/d	11 mg/d
Potassium	3 g/d	3.8 g/d	4.5 g/d	4.7 g/d	4.5 g/d	4.7 g/d
Sodium	1 g/d	1.2 g/d	1.5 g/d	1.5 g/d	1.5 g/d	1.5 g/d
Chloride	1.5 g/d	1.9 g/d	2.3 g/d	2.3 g/d	2.3 g/d	2.3 g/d

Adapted from the Institute of Medicine at the National Academy of Sciences. Dietary Reference Intakes: The Essential Guide to Nutrient Requirements. Washington, DC: National Academies Press; 2006.

age when teenagers begin to eat less nutritional diets due to increased time spent away from home and when they increasingly assert independence in dietary choices. The combination of social and physiologic factors increases risk of low iron status or iron-deficiency anemia among adolescent girls. Good dietary sources of iron include red meat, mollusks, poultry, fortified breakfast cereals, lentils, beans, spinach, chard, and collard greens. Animal-source iron is heme iron, which is more absorbable than non-heme iron from plant-based foods. Nonheme iron is converted to a more bioavailable form when consumed with vitamin C rich foods such as tomatoes, peppers, and citrus fruits or juices.

Adulthood

Overweight and Obesity

As estimated by BMI (Table 5-1) being overweight or obese increases a woman's risk of many chronic diseases and disabling conditions. In addition to BMI, waist circumference and waist-to-hip ratio are additional weight assessments of abdominal adiposity, which is positively correlated with obesity-related disease risk.[68] For non-pregnant women, a waist circumference > 35 inches and a waist to hip ratio > 0.8 significantly increase risk of diseases.[69] Rates of overweight and obesity are increasing around the world as are the associated chronic conditions. NHANES 2003–2006 reports that 60% of women aged 20–74 were overweight or obese, 34.3% were obese, and 7.2% were severely obese. These data represent significantly increased rates from data collected between 1988 and 1994 when 51% of women aged 20–74 years old were overweight or obese, 26% were obese, and 3.3% were severely obese.[70] This increasing trend of excess weight for height has augmented the percentage of American women at risk for coronary heart disease, type 2 diabetes, endometrial cancer, breast cancer, colon cancer, hypertension, dyslipidemia, stroke, liver and gallbladder disease, sleep apnea, respiratory problems, and osteoarthritis.[5] Figure 5-1 emphasizes the importance of healthy BMI and the adverse effects of BMI greater than 25.

Weight Management Approaches

Weight loss and weight maintenance require a multi-disciplinary approach including behavior therapy, diet modifications, and appropriate levels of exercise. Nutrition counseling as part of weight loss should increase knowledge and encourage behavioral changes to improve food choices by including lessons on food label reading, portion control, recipe modification, and cooking instruction.[71–91] Weight change is determined by the difference between caloric intake and caloric expenditure; excess caloric intake without comparable caloric expenditure results in weight gain. Only by lowering caloric intake while increasing caloric expenditure can weight loss be achieved. Calories from fat and carbohydrate should be reduced to create a caloric deficit for weight loss purposes. A daily caloric deficit of 500 to 1,000 calories should result in an optimal one- to two-pound weight loss per week

Be Fit to Be'ne'fit℠

Very Unhealthy	**≥30** Obese
Unhealthy	**25-29.9** Overweight
Healthy	**18.5-24.9**
Unhealthy	**<18.5** Underweight

If your BMI is ≥25 you are at increased risk for...
- Heart disease
- Diabetes
- Hypertension
- High cholesterol
- High triglycerides
- Low HDL cholesterol
- Stroke
- Cancers (Endometrial, breast, colon, prostate)
- Pregnancy complications
- Osteoarthritis
- Gallbladder disease
- Liver disease
- Depression
- Increased surgical risk
- Menstrual irregularities
- Hirsutism
- Incontinence
- Sleep apnea
- Back pain

EVEN A SMALL AMOUNT OF WEIGHT LOSS, 5-10% OF BODY WEIGHT, WILL IMPROVE WEIGHT RELATED PROBLEMS.

Figure 5-1 Be Fit to Be'ne'fit.

Courtesy of New York-Presbyterian Hospital & Columbia University Medical Center. Artwork by Megan Tubman, MS, R.D.

with an initial goal of losing 10% of weight in 6 months.[5] Caloric intake should be spread throughout the day. The consumption of four to five meals or snacks per day and eating breakfast are inversely related to obesity risk.[92–99] To achieve weight loss and maintenance of a lower weight, moderate physical activity for 30 minutes daily is advised unless medically contraindicated.[5]

Diets and Weight Loss Strategies

Healthcare providers should be knowledgeable regarding the risks and benefits of popular fad diets and should refer patients to a registered dietitian for individual nutrition counseling for weight loss. The Atkins, Ornish, Zone, and Weight Watcher's diets are equally effective for weight loss.[100–103] However, these diets may not meet individual nutrient needs and are may be difficult to maintain as they are very restrictive, time consuming, tedious, and costly. Low glycemic index diets restrict the quantity and type of carbohydrates eaten to moderate the impact on blood sugar levels. Although these diets may be helpful for managing blood sugar levels, they may be less effective for weight loss.[104–111] The effect of low-fat dairy products and calcium on weight loss is inconclusive, although low-fat dairy products (three to four servings per day) should be included as part of a balanced diet for weight management.[112–122] Low-carbohydrate diets may be more successful for some individuals; however, the weight loss benefits after 6 months are more limited than diets reduced in calories from fat and carbohydrate.[123–135] Bariatric surgery may be appropriate for some individuals whose weight loss goals have not been achieved through diet, physical activity, and behavior therapy.

To lose weight the focus should be on portion control, balance, variety, and moderation; a personalized diet based on individual preferences and health needs will be most successful. For weight maintenance, the Dietary Approaches to Stop Hypertension (DASH) diet described in Table 5-6 and the Mediterranean dietary patterns noted in Table 5-7 support nutrition strategies for chronic disease prevention and are appropriate for all women throughout the life cycle. The DASH dietary pattern focuses on intake of vegetables and fruit (5 to 10 servings daily), unsalted nuts, and low-fat dairy products contributing to an overall diet that is high in potassium and low in sodium, saturated fat, trans fat, and cholesterol.[136–142] The Mediterranean diet is also plant based and low in saturated and trans fats; it can improve cholesterol levels, lower body weight, and reduce blood pressure, protecting against risk of coronary heart disease.[143,144]

Cardiovascular Disease and Stroke

Cardiovascular disease is the leading cause of death in America, especially among older adults.[147] Modifiable risk factors for cardiovascular diseases include lowering total cholesterol (low-density lipoprotein or LDL-C, high-density lipoprotein or HDL-C), BMI, waist circumference, waist-to-hip ratio, physical activity, and stress level. Medical Nutrition Therapy (MNT) provided by a dietitian has effectively guided patients in reducing total and LDL-C and triglycerides and achieving a healthy weight.[96,148–159]

A cardioprotective diet optimizes the quality of macronutrients and recommends a balanced ratio of energy from macronutrients. The components of the Therapeutic Lifestyle Change (TLC) diet noted in Table 5-8 include recommendations specifically to lower cholesterol. Fat calories should come from mono- and polyunsaturated fatty acids found in unsalted nuts, seeds, and nut and seed oils.[96,160–175] Consumption of foods containing saturated and trans fats should be limited. Common dietary sources of saturated fat are butter, full-fat dairy products, and red meat. Trans fats are less common in the American food supply since labeling regulation were mandated in 2006. Some trans fats occur naturally in dairy products and meat; however, the majority of trans fats in the American diet still come from processed and fried foods. Intake of omega-3 fatty acids from marine and plant sources, either as dietary intake or supplements, is associated with a reduced risk of both fatal and nonfatal cardiac events. Fatty fish such as mackerel, salmon, herring, trout, sardines, and tuna provide EPA and DHA whereas plant-based foods such as ground flaxseeds, chia seeds, canola oil, soybean oil, and walnuts provide ALA.[175–188]

Carbohydrates should provide 50 to 60% of daily caloric intake from a variety of grains, fruits, and vegetables. The American Heart Association recommends 25 to 30 grams of fiber daily, including 7 to 13 grams of soluble fiber.[189] Total cholesterol can be lowered 2 to 3% and LDL-C can be lowered up to 7% by consuming a diet high

Table 5-6		
The DASH diet[140]		
Food Group	**Servings Per Day**	**Serving Size**
Grains and Whole Grain Products	6–8	1 slice bread; 1/2 cup cooked, rice, pasta, or cereal
Fruits	4–5	1 medium fruit, 1/4 cup dried fruit, 1/2 cup fruit juice
Vegetables	4–5	1 cup raw leafy vegetables, 1/2 cup raw or cooked vegetables
Nonfat or Low-Fat Dairy Foods	2–3	1 cup milk or yogurt; 1 1/2 oz cheese
Lean Meats, Fish, Poultry	6 or less	1 oz cooked meats, poultry, fish
Nuts, Seeds, Legumes (unsalted)	4–5 per week	1/3 cup nuts, 2 Tbsp peanut butter, 2 Tbsp seeds, 1/2 cup cooked legumes
Sweets and Foods with Added Sugars	5 or less per week	1 Tbsp sugar, 1 Tbsp jelly or jam, 12 oz cup sorbet, gelatin, 1 cup lemonade
Fats and oils	2–3	1 tsp soft trans fat free margarine, 1 tsp vegetable oil, 1 Tbsp mayonnaise, 2 Tbsp salad dressing

Data from Appel LJ, Moore TJ, Obarzanek E, et al. A clinical trial of the effects of dietary patterns on blood pressure. DASH Collaborative Research Group. *N Engl J Med.* 1997;336:117-124.

Table 5-7

The Mediterranean Diet[143]

Fruits, vegetables, breads, cereals, potatoes, beans, nuts, and seeds as foundation of diet

Olive oil as main fat source

Low to moderate intake of dairy products, fish, and poultry

Very limited red meat consumption

Eggs consumed no more than four times per week

Wine consumed in low to moderate amounts

Data from Scarmeas N, Luchsinger JA, Mayeux R, et al Mediterranean diet and mortality in a US population. *Arch Intern Med.* 2008;168:1823-1824.

Table 5-8

NHLBI therapeutic lifestyle change (TLC) diet recommendations[172]

Saturated fat	< 7% of calories
Dietary cholesterol	< 200 mg per day
Soluble fiber	Add 5 to 10 grams per day
Plant sterols/stanols	Add 2 grams per day
Weight	Lose 10 pounds if overweight

Data from Lichtenstein AH, Ausman LM, Jalbert SM, et al. Efficacy of a Therapeutic Lifestyle Change/Step 2 diet in moderately hypercholesterolemic middle-aged and elderly female and male subjects. *J Lipid Res.* 2002 43:264-273.

Table 5-9

NHLBI diagnostic criteria for metabolic syndrome[216]

Diagnostic criteria: Presence of at least 3 risk factors

Waist circumference	> 35 inches for women
Triglycerides	≥ 150 mg/dL
HDL-cholesterol	< 50 mg/dL for women
Blood pressure	≥ 130/85 mmHg
Fasting blood glucose	≥ 100 mg/dL

Data from Grundy SM, Cleeman JI, Daniels SR, et al. Diagnosis and management of the metabolic syndrome: an American Heart Association/National Heart, Lung, and Blood Institute scientific statement. *Circulation.* 2005;112;2735-52.

Diabetes Mellitus

As of 2007, an estimated 11.5 million American women have been diagnosed with diabetes, increasing their risk of death due to heart disease and stroke by two to four times compared with nondiabetic similarly aged women.[197] An additional 25% of American adults who have prediabetes (fasting blood glucose 100–125 mg/dL) could achieve glycemic control by losing weight through diet and physical activity preventing or delaying the onset of type 2 diabetes.[197] Nutrition counseling included in preventive health care can save medical costs and improve quality of life by guiding individuals to appropriate management of their nutritional intake. Dietitians provide nutrition education regarding carbohydrate counting, exchange system, healthy food choices, reduced energy and fat intake if appropriate, insulin-to-carbohydrate ratios, meal planning, behavioral strategies, and physical activity.[198–215] Losing weight and maintaining a healthy weight reduces risk of cardiovascular disease and can lower blood pressure, reducing the risk for microvascular complications such as eye, kidney, and nerve disease. The lifestyle changes that promote healthy outcomes and reduce risk are comparable for cardiovascular disease and diabetes.[198–215] Metabolic Syndrome describes the diagnosis or risk of multiple metabolic disorders in an individual; the criteria are noted in Table 5-9.

Nutrition, Body Weight, Cancer, and Cancer Risk

Consistent evidence has been published indicating an association between obesity and some types of cancer, including colorectal, pancreatic, esophageal, postmenopausal breast, kidney, and endometrial cancers. In addition, abdominal deposits have been linked with endometrial, pancreatic, and postmenopausal breast cancer.[217] Obesity has also been associated with poor survival among women diagnosed with breast cancer, especially those with early stage disease.[218] Recent research has suggested weight loss may provide some protection.[219]

in total and soluble fiber.[190–195] Most plant-based foods provide both soluble and insoluble fibers. Good sources of soluble fiber include oats, legumes, citrus fruits, apples, pears, and okra.

Hypertension

Achieving and maintaining a healthy weight can help maintain blood pressure within normal limits (< 120/80 mmHg with or without comorbidities). For overweight and obese individuals a weight loss of 22 pounds lowers systolic blood pressure by 5–20 mmHg.[136–138] Reducing dietary sodium can also help maintain a healthy blood pressure. Restricting sodium intake to 2,300 mg daily can reduce systolic blood pressure 2 to 8 mmHg. The DASH eating pattern can reduce systolic blood pressure by 8 to 15 mmHg (see Table 5-6). In addition to the DASH diet, the Joint National Committee on Prevention, Detection, Evaluation, and Treatment of High Blood Pressure recommends weight reduction, dietary sodium reduction, physical activity, and moderation of alcohol consumption as lifestyle modifications to prevent and manage hypertension.[196]

No specific diet has been recommended for cancer prevention; however, diets rich in fruits and nonstarchy vegetables (5 to 10 servings per day) have been associated with decreased risk of esophageal, mouth, stomach and other cancers.[217] Although limited alcohol may provide some health benefits, alcohol consumption has been found to have a dose-dependent association with increasing breast cancer risk.[220]

In patients diagnosed with cancer, individualized nutrition counseling is generally focused on increasing calorie and protein intake, ensuring adequate nutritional status for repair, and improving quality of life by mitigating anorexia, nausea, vomiting, and diarrhea.[221–225] Weight control remains a high priority as the hormonal levels associated with obesity may stimulate recurrence of cancer after primary treatment.

Aging

Food supports physical health and social well-being, both of which contribute to successful aging. Successful aging is defined as the ability to maintain three key behaviors: low risk of disease and disease-related disability, high mental and physical function, and active engagement of life.[226] A healthy weight is important for disease prevention and management at all stages in the life cycle. Following a healthful, balanced diet can help to prevent or manage chronic disease. After menopause women are at increased risk for osteoporosis and heart disease. In addition to following the TLC dietary recommendations or the DASH diet for cardiovascular health promotion, women require adequate calcium and vitamin D to maintain bone density, avoid bone loss, and decrease risk of osteoporosis. Good food sources of calcium include nonfat or low-fat milk, yogurt, cheese, and cottage cheese, as well as fortified cereals, soy milk, tofu, kale, broccoli, bok choy, and brussels sprouts. Vitamin D can be synthesized in the body from ultraviolet light and can be obtained through diet. Dietary sources of vitamin D include mackerel, tuna, and salmon and fortified dairy products, juice, and cereals. Vitamin D is essential for calcium absorption; vitamin D deficiency may cause muscle weakness increasing the risk for falls and fractures.[227]

Frailty, functional decline, and disability in older adults are caused by age-related loss of muscle mass and strength, known as sarcopenia.[228] Regular physical activity and adequate protein intake may help prevent sarcopenia, increasing strength, preventing falls, and improving quality of life.[229] Unintentional weight loss in older adults negatively influences health outcomes and quality of life. Regular nutrition assessment followed by individualized counseling and intervention can improve weight and nutrition status.[230–231] Research on centenarians has identified biomarkers associated with longevity including elevated HDL and high serum levels of vitamins A and E.[232–234] These are diet-mediated biomarkers supported by a diet rich in plant foods such as recommended by the DASH diet and the Mediterranean diet.

Summary

Proper nutrition and a healthy lifestyle are significant preventive health behaviors in all stages of the life cycle. Being at a healthy BMI prior to pregnancy as well as gaining weight within the recommended range during pregnancy improves short- and long-term health outcomes for both the mother and fetus. Adequate nutrition and a healthy weight during childhood and adolescence promotes proper growth and physical and social development. Women's unique nutritional needs for optimal health and reduced chronic disease risk factors can be met with informed choices. Popular diets may help women achieve weight loss and improve biomarkers, but the diets are not easily sustainable nor have they been shown to improve long-term health. The DASH diet and the Mediterranean diet are substantially researched nutrition approaches to promote optimal health outcomes. The risk of cardiovascular disease, stroke, hypertension, type 2 diabetes, and some cancers is reduced by maintaining a healthy weight. Referral for counseling by a registered dietitian for medical nutrition therapy is recommended as part of disease management. All aspects of aging, cognitive function, physical and mental health, and quality of life are positively influenced by continuation of a healthy weight, balance diet, and active lifestyle.

Discussion Questions

1. How is BMI calculated and what are the benefits of maintaining a healthy BMI at different times in the life cycle?
2. What are the risks of overweight and obesity during pregnancy?
3. State three benefits of breastfeeding on chronic disease risk for the infant.
4. What are the three specific nutrition concerns in adolescence?
5. What are the dietary principles of diets for disease-risk prevention?

References

1. Catalano P. Management of obesity in pregnancy. *ACOG.* 2007;109:419–33.
2. Bodnar LM, Siega-Riz AM, Cogswell ME. High prepregnancy BMI increases the risk of postpartum anemia. *Obes Res.* 2004;12:941–948.
3. Siega-Riz AM, King JC. Position of the America Dietetic Association and American Society for Nutrition: obesity, reproduction, and pregnancy outcomes. *J Am Diet Asso.* 2009;109:918–927.
4. Committee on Obstetric Practice. Obesity in pregnancy. *Obstet Gynecol.* 2005;106:671–5.
5. NIH, NHLBI Obesity Education Initiative. *Clinical Guidelines on the Identification, Evaluation, and Treatment of Overweight and Obesity in Adults.* Bethesda, MD: National Heart, Lung, and Blood Institute, National Institutes of Health; 1998. http://www.nhlbi.nih.gov/guidelines/obesity/ob_gdlns.pdf. Accessed December 2, 2009.
6. Institute of Medicine. *Weight Gain During Pregnancy: Reexamining the Guidelines.* Washington, DC: National Academies Press; 2009.
7. Chu SY, Callaghan WM, Kim SY, et al. Maternal obesity and risk of gestational diabetes mellitus. *Diabetes Care.* 2007;30:2070–76.
8. Weiss, JL, Malone FD, Emig D, et al. Obesity, obstetric complications and cesarean delivery rate—a population-based screening study. *Am J Obstet Gynecol.* 2004;190:1091–1097.
9. Vahratian A, Zhang J, Troendle JF, et al. Maternal prepregnancy overweight and obesity and the pattern of labor progression in term nulliparous women. *Obstet Gynecol.* 2004;104:943–51.

10. Waller DK, Shaw GM, Rasmussen SA, et al. Prepregnancy obesity as a risk factor for structural birth defects. *Arch Pediatr Adolesc Med.* 2007;161:745–750.

11. Hofmeyr GJ, Atallah AN, Duley L. Calcium supplementation during pregnancy for preventing hypertensive disorders and related problems. *Cochrane Database Syst Rev.* 2006:CD001059.S

12. Kaiser L, Allen LH. Position of the American Dietetic Association: nutrition and lifestyle for a healthy pregnancy outcome. *J Am Diet Assoc.* 2008;108:553–561.

13. Higdon JV, Frei B. Coffee and health: a review of recent human research. *Crit Rev Food Sci Nutr.* 2006;46:101–123.

14. Centers for Disease Control and Prevention (CDC). Fetal Alcohol Spectrum Disorders (FASDS). www.cdc.gov/ncbddd/fasd/index.html. Accessed January 28, 2010.

15. Cogswell ME, Parvanta I, Ickes L, et al. Iron supplementation during pregnancy, anemia, and birth weight: a randomized controlled trial. *Am J Clin Nutr.* 2003;78:773–81.

16. Institute of Medicine. *Dietary Reference Intakes: The Essential Guide to Nutrient Requirements.* Washington, DC: National Academies Press; 2006.

17. Centers for Disease Control and Prevention (CDC). Folic Acid. www.cdc.gov/ncbddd/folicacid/index.html/ Accessed December 2, 2009.

18. Berry RJ, et al. Prevention of neural tube defects with folic acid in China. *N Eng J Med.* 1999;341:1485–1490.

19. Standing Committee on the Scientific Evaluation of Dietary Reference Intakes, Food and Nutrition Board, Institute of Medicine. *Dietary Reference Intakes: Folate, Other B Vitamins, and Choline.* Washington, DC, National Academy Press; April 17, 1998.

20. Martinez M. Tissue levels of polyunsaturated fatty acids during early human development. *J Pediatr.* 1992;120:S129–138.

21. Makrides M, Duley L, Olsen SF. Marine oil, and other prostaglandin precursor, supplementation for pregnancy uncomplicated by pre-eclampsia or intrauterine growth restriction (Cochrane Review). In: *The Cochrane Library,* Issue 4. Chichester, UK: John Wiley & Sons, Ltd.; 2009.

22. Environmental Defense Fund. Contaminated fish: how many meals are safe per month? http://www.edf.org/documents/7534_Health_Alerts_seafood.pdf. Accessed December 8, 2009.

23. US Department of Agriculture. Food safety: Eating fish while you are pregnant or breastfeeding. http://www.choosemyplate.gov/pregnancy-breastfeeding/eating-fish.html. Accessed August 5, 2012.

24. Gillman MW, Rifas-Shiman S, Berkey CS, et al. Maternal gestational diabetes, birth weight, and adolescent obesity. *Pediatrics.* 2003;111:e221–226.

25. Metzger BE, Buchanan TA, Coustan DR, et al. Summary and recommendations of the Fifth International Workshop-Conference on Gestational Diabetes Mellitus. *Diabetes Care.* 2007;30:S2:S251–60.

26. James DCS, Lessen R. Position of the American Dietetic Association: promoting and supporting breastfeeding. *J Am Diet Assoc.* 2009;109:1926–42.

27. World Health Organization. *The Optimal Duration of Exclusive Breastfeeding: A Systematic Review.* Geneva, Switzerland: World Health Organization; 2002. http://www.who.int/nutrition/publications/optimal_duration_of_exc_bfeeding_review_eng.pdf. Accessed November 30, 2009.

28. Barbosa L, Butte NF, Villalpando S, et al. Maternal energy balance and lactation performance of Mesoamerindians as a function of body mass index. *Am J Clin Nutr.* 1997;66:575–583.

29. Damanik R, Wahlqvist M, Wattanapenpaiboon N. Lactagogue Effects of Torbangun, a Bataknese Traditional Cuisine. *Asia Pac J Clin Nutr.* 2006;15(2):267–274.

30. Dusdieker LB, Hemingway DL, Stumbo PJ. Is milk production impaired by dieting during lactation? *Am J Clin Nutr.* 1994;59:833–840.

31. Dusdieker LB, Stumbo PJ, Booth BM, Wilmoth RN. Prolonged maternal fluid supplementation in breast-feeding. *Pediatrics.*1990;86:737–740.

32. Laskey MA, Prentice A, Hanratty LA, et al. Bone changes after 3 mo of lactation: influence of calcium intake, breast-milk output, and vitamin-D receptor genotype. *Am J Clin Nutr.* 1998;67:685–692.

33. McCrory MA, Nommsen-Rivers LA, Mole PA, Lonnerdal B, Dewey KG. Randomized trial of the short-term effects of dieting compared with dieting plus aerobic exercise on lactation performance. *Am J Clin Nutr.* 1999;69:959–967.

34. Morse JM, Ewing G, Gamble D, Donahue P. The effect of maternal fluid intake on breast milk supply: a pilot study. *Can J Public Health.* 1992;83(3):213–216.

35. Motil KJ, Montandon CM, Hachey DL, et al. Relationships among lactation performance, maternal diet, and body protein metabolism in humans. *Eur J Clin Nutr.* 1989;43:681–691.

36. Motil KJ, Thotathuchery M, Bahar A, Montandon CM. Marginal dietary protein restriction reduced nonprotein nitrogen, but not protein nitrogen, components of human milk. *J Am Coll Nutr.* 1995;14(2):184–191.

37. Okamura T, Takeuchi T, Nishi O, et al. Effects of low-caloric diet in puerperium on prolactin, TSH, estradiol and milk secretion. *Acta Obst Gynaec Jpn.* 1987;39(11):2059–2055.

38. Strode MA, Dewey KG, Lonnerdal B. Effects of short-term caloric restriction on lactational performance of well-nourished women. *Acta Paediatr Scand* 1986;75:222–229.

39. Doan T, Gardiner A, Gay C, Lee K. Breastfeeding increases sleep duration of new parents. *J Perinat Neonat Nurs.* 2007;21:200–206.

40. Jonas W, Nissen E, Ransjö-Arvidon L, et al. Short- and long-term decrease of blood pressure in women during breastfeeding. *Breastfeed Med.* 2008;3:103–109.

41. Dennis CL, McQueen K. The relationship between infant-feeding outcome and post-partum depression: a qualitative systematic review. *Pediatrics* 2009;123:e736–51.

42. Dewey KG, Cohen RJ, Brown KH, Rivera LL. Effects of Exclusive Breastfeeding for 4 vs 6 months on maternal nutritional status and infant motor development: results of two randomized trials in Honduras. *J Nutr.* 2001;131:262–7.

43. Wang IY, Fraser IS. Reproductive function and contraception in postpartum period. *ObstetGynecol Surv.* 1994;49:56–63.

44. Kennedy KI, Visness CM. Contraceptive efficacy of lactation amenorrhea. *Lancet* 1992;339:227–30.

45. Collaborative Group on Hormonal Factors in Breast Cancer. Breast cancer and breastfeeding: collaborative reanalysis of individual data from 47 epidemiological studies in 30 countries, including 50,302 women with breast cancer and 96,973 without the disease. *Lancet* 2002;360:187–95.

46. Zheng T, Holford TR, Mayne ST, et al. Lactation and breast cancer risk: a case-control study in Connecticut. *Br J Cancer.* 2001;84:1472–6.

47. Trggvadóttir L, Tulinius J, Jórunn EE, Sigurvinsson T. Breastfeeding and reduced risk of breast cancer in an Icelandic cohort study. *Am J Epidemiol.* 2001;154:36–42.

48. Tung KH, Wilkens LR, Wu AH, et al. Effect of anovulation factors on pre- and postmenopausal ovarian cancer risk: revisiting the incessant ovulation hypothesis. *Am J Epidemiol.* 2005;161:321–9.

49. Food and Nutrition Board and Institute of Medicine. *Dietary Reference Intakes for Energy, Carbohydrate, Fiber, Fat, Fatty Acids, Cholesterol, Protein and Amino Acids (Macronutrients)* Washington DC: National Academies Press; 2002.

50. Hatsu IE, McDougald DM, Anderson AK. Effect of infant feeding on maternal body composition. *Int Breastfeed J.* 2008;3:18.

51. Kac G, Benicio MH, Velasquez-Melendez G, et al. Breastfeeding and postpartum weight-retention in a cohort of Brazilian women. *Am J Clin Nutr.* 2004;79:487–93.

52. Rooney BL, Schauberger SW. Excess weight gain and long-term obesity: one decade later. *Obstet Gynecol.* 2002;100:245–52.

53. Olson CM, Strawderman MS, Hinton PS, Pearson TA. Gestational weight gain and postpartum behaviors associated with weight change from early pregnancy to 1 yr postpartum. *Int J Obes.* 2003;27:117–27.

54. Sichieri R, Field AE, Rich-Edwards J, Willett WC. Prospective assessment of exclusive breastfeeding in relation to weight change in women. *Int J Obes Relat Metab Disord.* 2003;28:815–20.

55. Wagner CL, Greer FR. Section on Breastfeeding and Committee on Nutrition. Prevention of rickets and vitamin D deficiency in infants, children, and adolescents. *Pediatrics.* 2008;122:1142–52.

56. Ip S, Chung M, Raman G, et al. *Breastfeeding and Maternal and Infant Health Outcomes in Developed Countries. Evidence Report/Technology Assessment.* AHRQ Publication No, 07-E007. Rockville, MD: Agency for Healthcare Research and Quality; 2007.

57. Vennemann MM, Bajanowski T, Brinkmann B, et al. Does breastfeeding reduce the risk of sudden infant death syndrome? *Pediatrics.* 2009;123:e406–10.

58. Schanler R, Shulman R, Lau C. Feeding strategies for premature infants: beneficial outcome of feeding fortified human milk vs preterm formula. *Pediatrics.* 1999;103:1150–7.

59. Koletzko B, Von Kries R, Monasterolo RC, et al. Can infant feeding choices modulate later obesity risk? *Am J Clin Nutr.* 2009;89:1502–1508S.

60. Horta BL, Bahl R, Martines JC, Victora CG. Evidence on the Long-Term Effects of Breastfeeding. systematic reviews and meta-analyses. Geneva, Switzerland: World Health Organization; 2007. http://whqlibdoc.who.int/publications/2007/9789241595230_eng.pdf. Accessed December 1, 2009.

61. Bleich SN, Wang YC, Wang Y, Gortmaker SL. Increasing consumption of sugar-sweetened beverages among US adults: 1988–1994 to 1999–2004. *Am J Clin Nutr.* 2009;89:372–81.

62. Nielsen SJ, Popkin BM. Changes in beverage intake between 1977 and 2001. *Am J Prev Med.* 2004;27:205–10.

63. Nielsen SJ, Siega-Riz AM, Popkin BM. Trends in energy intake in US between 1977 and 1996: similar shifts seen across age groups. *Obes Res.* 2002;10:370–8.

64. Lorson BA, Melgar-Quinonez HR, Taylor C. Correlates of fruit and vegetable intakes in US children. *J Am Diet Assoc.* 2009;109:474–8.

65. Field AE, Cook NR, Gillman MW. Weight status in childhood as a predictor of becoming overweight or hypertensive in early adulthood. *Obesity Research.* 2005;13:163–9.

66. Magarey AM, Daniels LA, Boulton TJ, Cockington RA. Predicting obesity in early adulthood from childhood and parental obesity. *Int J Obes Relat Metab Disord.* 2003;27:505–13.

67. Ehrman DA. Polycystic ovary syndrome. *N Engl J Med.* 2005;352:1223–36.

68. Folsom AR, Kaye SA, Sellers TA, et al. Body fat distribution and 5-year risk of death in older women. *JAMA.* 1993;269:483–94.

69. Huxley R, Mendis S, Zheleznyakov E, et al. Body mass index, waist circumference and waist:hip ratio as predictors of cardiovascular risk-a review of the literature. *Eur J Clin Nutr.* 2010;64:16–22.

70. National Center for Health Statistics, Centers for Disease Control and Prevention.. Mean energy and macronutrient intake among persons 20–74 years of age, by sex and age: United States, 1971–1974 through 2001–2004. www.cdc.gov/nchs/data/hus/hus08.pdf#073. Accessed November 25, 2009.

71. Birkett D, Johnson D, Thompson JR, Oberg D. Reaching low-income families: focus group results provide direction for a behavioral approach to WIC services. *J Am Diet Assoc.* 2004; 04:1277–1280.

72. Capps O, Cleveland L, Park J. Dietary behaviors associated with total fat and saturated fat intake. *J Am Diet Assoc.* 2002;102:490–496, 501–502.

73. Cavallaro V, Dwyer J, Houser RF, et al. Influence of dietitian presence on outpatient cardiac rehabilitation nutrition services. *J Am Diet Assoc.* 2004;104:611–614.

74. Keller-Olaman SJ, Edwards V, Elliott SJ. Evaluating a food bank recipe-tasting program. *Can J Diet PractRes.* 2005;66:183–186.

75. Masley S, Phillips S, Copeland JR. Group office visits change dietary habits of patients with coronary artery disease: the dietary intervention and evaluation trial (DIET). *J Fam Pract.* 2001;50:235–239.

76. Newman VA, Thomson CA, Rock CL, et al for the Women's Healthy Eating and Living (WHEL) Study Group. Achieving substantial changes in eating behavior among women previously treated for breast cancer—an overview of the intervention. *J Am Diet Assoc.* 2005;105:382–391.

77. Bushman BJ. Effects of warning and information labels on consumption of full-fat, reduced-fat and no-fat products. *J Appl Psychol.* 1998; 83: 97–101.

78. Kessler H, Wunderlich SM. Relationship between use of food labels and nutrition knowledge of people with diabetes. *Diabetes Educ* 1999; 25(4): 549–559.

79. Kral TVE, Roe LS, Rolls BJ. Does nutrition information about the energy density of meals affect food intake in normal-weight women? *Appetite.* 2002;39:137–145.

80. Kreuter MW, Brennan LK, Scharff DP, Lukwago SN. Do nutrition label readers eat healthier diets? Behavioral correlates of adults' use of food labels. *Am J Prev Med.* 1997;13:277–283.

81. Kristal AR, Levy L, Patterson RE, et al. Trends in food label use associated with new nutrition labeling regulations. *Am J Public Health.* 1998;88:1212–1215.

82. Lin CTJ, Lee JY, Yen ST. Do dietary intakes affect search for nutrient information on food labels? *Soc SciMed.* 2004;59:1955–1967.

83. Macon JF, Oakland MJ, Jensen HH, Kissack PA. Food label use by older Americans: data from the Continuing Survey of Food Intakes by Individuals and the Diet and Health Knowledge Survey 1994–1996. *J Nutr Elder.* 2004;24:35–52.

84. Marietta AB, Welshimer KJ, Anderson SL. Knowledge, attitudes, and behaviors of college students regarding the 1990 Nutrition Labeling Education Act food labels. *J Am Diet Assoc.* 1999;99:445–449.

85. Miller CK, Jensen GL, Achterberg CL. Evaluation of a food label nutrition intervention for women with type 2 diabetes mellitus. *J Am Diet Assoc.* 1999;99:323–328.

86. Miller CK, Probart CK, Achterberg CL. Knowledge and misconceptions about the food label among women with non-insulin-dependent diabetes mellitus. *Diabetes Educ.* 1997;23:425–432.

87. Neuhouser ML, Kristal AR, Patterson RE. Use of food nutrition labels is associated with lower fat intake. *J Am Diet Assoc.* 1999;99:45–50,53.

88. Perez-Escamilla R, Haldeman L. Food label use modifies association of income with dietary quality. *J Nutr.* 2002;132:768–772.

89. Roefs A, Jansen A. The effect of information about fat content on food consumption in overweight/obese and lean people. *Appetite.* 2004;43:319–322.

90. Smith SC, Taylor JG, Stephen AM. Use of food labels and beliefs about diet-disease relationships among university students. *Public Health Nutr.* 2000;3(2):175–182.

91. Westcombe A, Wardle J. Influence of relative fat content information on responses to three foods. *Appetite.* 1997;28:49–62.

92. Forslund HB, Torgerson JS, Sjostrom L, Lindroos AK. Snacking frequency in relation to energy intake and food choice in obese men and women compated to a reference population. *Int J Obes.* 2005;29:711–9.

93. Drummon SE, Crombie NE, Cursiter MC, Kirk TR. Evidence that eating frequency is inversely related to body weight status in male, but not female, non-obese adults reporting valid dietary intake. *Int J Obes.* 1998;22:105–12.

94. Basdevant A, Craplet C, Guy-Grand B. Snacking patterns in obese French women. *Appetite* 1993;21:11–23.

95. Ma Y, Bertone ER, Stanek EJ, et al. Association between eating patterns and obesity in a free-living US adult population. *Am J Epidemiol.* 2003;158:85–92.

96. Cho S, Dietrich M, Brown CJ, et al. The effect of breakfast type on total daily energy intake and body mass index: results from the Third National Health and Nutrition Examination Survey (NHANES III). *J Am Coll Nutr.* 2003;22:296–302.

97. Song WO, Chun OK, Obayashi S, et al. Is consumption of breakfast associated with body mass index in US adults? *J Am Diet Assoc.* 2005;105:1373–82.

98. Martin A, Normand S, Sothier M, et al. Is advice or breakfast consumption justified? Results from a short-term dietary and metabolic experiment in young healthy men. *Br J Nutr.* 2000;84:337–44.

99. Schlundt DG, Hill JO, Sbrocco T, et al. The role of breakfast in the treatment of obesity: a randomized clinical trial. *Am J Clin Nutr.* 1992;55:645–51.

100. Katcher HI, Hill AM, Lanford JL, et al. Lifestyle approaches and dietary strategies to lower LDL-cholesterol and triglycerides and raise HDL-cholesterol. *Endocrinol Metabl Clin North Am.* 2009;38:45–78.

101. Academy of Nutrition and Dietetics. Evidence Analysis Library. http://www.adaevidencelibrary.org/default.cfm?auth=1. Accessed August 6, 2012.

102. Gardner CD, Kiazand A, Alhassan S, et al. Comparison of the Atkins, Zone, Ornish, and LEARN Diets for change in weight and related risk factors among overweight premenopausal women. *JAMA.* 2007;297:969–77.

103. Dansinger ML, Gleason JA, Griffith JL, Selker HP, Schaefer EJ. Comparison of the Atkins, Ornish, Weight Watchers, and Zone diets for weight loss and heart disease risk reduction: a randomized trial. *JAMA.* 2005;293(1):43–53.

104. Alfenas RCG, Mattes RD. Influence of glycemic index/load on glycemic response, appetite, and food intake in healthy humans. *Diabetes Care.* 2005;28:2123–2129.

105. Bouche C, Rizkalla SW, Luo J, et al. Five-week, low-glycemic index diet decreases total fat mass and improves plasma lipid profile in moderately overweight nondiabetic men. *Diabetes Care.* 2002;25:822–828.

106. Carels RA, Darby LA, Douglass OM, et al. Education on the glycemic index of foods fails to improve treatment outcomes in a behavioral weight loss program. *Eating Behaviors.* 2005;6:145–150.

107. Ebbeling CB, Leidig MM, Sinclair KB, et al. Effects of an ad libitum low-glycemic load diet on cardiovascular disease risk factors in obese young adults. *Am J Clin Nutr.* 2005;81:976–982.

108. Frost GS, Brynes AE, Bovill-Taylor C, Dornhorst A. A prospective randomized trial to determine the efficacy of a low glycemic index diet given in addition to healthy eating and weight loss advice in patients with coronary heart disease. *Eur J Clin Nutr.* 2004;58:121–127.

109. Pereira MA, Swain J, Goldfine AB, et al. Effects of a low-glycemic load diet on resting energy expenditure and heart disease risk factors during weight loss. *JAMA.* 2004;292:2482–2490.

110. Sloth B, Krog-Mikkelsen I, Flint A, et al. No difference in body weight decrease between a low-glycemic-index and a high-glycemic-index diet but reduced LDL cholesterol after 10-wk ad libitum intake of the low-glycemic-index diet. *Am J Clin Nutr.* 2004;80:337–347.

111. Thompson WG, Rostad Holdman N, Janzow DJ, et al. Effect of energy-reduced diets high in dairy products and fiber on weight loss in obese adults. *Obes Res.* 2005;13:1344–1353.

112. Cifuentes M, Riedt CS, Brolin RE, et al. Weight loss and calcium intake influence calcium absorption in overweight postmenopausal women. *Am J Clin Nutr.* 2004;80:123–130.

113. Davies KM, Heaney RP, Recker RR, et al. Calcium intake and body weight. *J Clin Endocrinol Metab.* 2000;85;4635–4638.

114. Jacqmain M, Doucet E, Despres J-P, et al. Calcium intake, body composition, and lipoprotein-lipid concentrations in adults. *Am J Clin Nutr.* 2003;77:1448–1452.

115. Lin Y-C, Lyle RM, McCabe LD, et al. Dairy calcium is related to changes in body composition during a two-year exercise intervention in young women. *J Am College Nutr.* 2000:19;754–760.

116. Lovejoy JC, Champagne CM, Smith SR, et al. Ethnic differences in dietary intakes, physical activity, and energy expenditure in middle-aged, premenopausal women: the Healthy Transitions Study. *Am JClin Nutr.* 2001;74: 90–95.

117. Pereira MA, Jacobs, Jr. DR, Van Horn L, et al. Dairy consumption, obesity, and the insulin resistance syndrome in young adults: the CARDIA study. *JAMA.* 287:16:2081–2089.

118. Thompson WG, Rostad Holdman N, Janzow DJ, et al. Effect of energy-reduced diets high in dairy products and fiber on weight loss in obese adults. *Obes Res.* 2005;13(8):1344–1353.

119. Venti CA, Tataranni PA, Salbe AD. Lack of relationship between calcium intake and body size in an obesity-prone population. *J Am Diet Assoc.* 2005;105:1401–1407.

120. Zemel MB, Richards J, Mathis S, et al. Dairy augmentation of total and central fat loss in obese subjects. *Int J Obes Relat Metab Disord.* 2005;29(4):391–397.

121. Zemel MB, Shi H, Greer B, et al. Regulation of adiposity by dietary calcium. *The FASEB Journal.* 2000;14:1132–1138.

122. Zemel MB, Thompson W, Milstead A, et al. Calcium and dairy acceleration of weight and fat loss during energy restriction in obese adults. *Obes Res.* 2004;12;582–590.

123. Aude YW, Agatston AS, Lopez-Jimenez F, et al. The National Cholesterol Education Program diet vs a diet lower in carbohydrates and higher in protein and monounsaturated fat: a randomized trial. *Arch Intern Med.* 2004;164:2141–2146.

124. Brehm BJ, Seeley RJ, Daniels SR, D'Alessio DA. A randomized trial comparing a very low carbohydrate diet and a calorie-restricted low fat diet on body weight and cardiovascular risk factors in healthy women. *J Clin Endocrinol Metab.* 2003;88:1617–1623.

125. Brehm BJ, Spang SE, Lattin BL, et al. The role of energy expenditure in the differential weight loss in obese women on low-fat and low-carbohydrate diets. *J Clin Endocrinol Metab.* 2005;90:1475–1482.

126. Dansinger ML, Gleason JA, Griffith JL, et al. Comparison of the Atkins, Ornish, Weight Watchers, and Zone diets for weight loss and heart disease risk reduction. *JAMA.* 2005;293:43–53.

127. Foster FD, Wyatt HR, Hill JO, et al. A randomized trial of a low-carbohydrate diet for obesity. *N Engl J Med.* 2003;348:2082–2090.

128. Landers P, Wolfe MM, Glore S, et al. Effect of weight loss plans on body composition and diet duration. *J Okla State Med Assoc.* 2002;95:329–331.

129. Lean MEJ, Han TS, Prvan T, Richmond PR, Avenell A. Weight loss with high and low carbohydrate 1200 kcal diets in free living women. *Eur J Clin Nutr.* 1997;51(4):243–248.

130. Luscombe-Marsh ND, Noakes M, Wittert GA, Keogh JB, Foster P, Clifton PM. Carbohydrate-restricted diets high in either monounsaturated fat or protein are equally effective at promoting fat loss and improving blood lipids. *Am J Clin Nutr.* 2005;81:762–772.

131. Meckling KA, O'Sullivan C, Saari D. Comparison of a low-fat diet to a low-carbohydrate diet on weight loss, body composition, and risk factors for

diabetes and cardiovascular disease in free-living, overweight men and women. *J Clin Endocrinol Metab.* 2004;89(6):2717–2723.

132. Nickols-Richardson SM, Coleman MD, Volpe JJ, Hosig KW. Perceived hunger is lower and weight loss is greater in overweight premenopausal women consuming a low-carbohydrate/high-protein vs high-protein/low-fat diet. *J Am Diet Assoc.* 2005;105:1433–1437.

133. Samaha FF, Iqbal N, Seshadri P, et al. A low-carbohydrate as compared with a low-fat diet in severe obesity. *N Engl J Med.* 2003;348:2074–2081.

134. Stern L, Iqbal N, Seshadri P, et al. The effects of low-carbohydrate versus conventional weight loss diets in severely obese adults: one-year follow-up of a randomized trial. *Ann Intern Med.* 2004;140:778–785.

135. Yancy WS, Olsen MK, Guyton JR, et al. A low-carbohydrate, ketogenic diet vs. a low-fat diet to treat obesity and hyperlipidemia: a randomized controlled trial. *Ann Intern Med.* 2004;140:769–777.

136. Appel LJ, Champagne CM, Harsha DW, et al.; Writing Group of the PREMIER Collaborative Research Group. Effects of comprehensive lifestyle modification on blood pressure control: main results of the PREMIER Clinical Trial. *JAMA.* 2003;289:2083–2093.

137. Miller ER III, Erlinger TP, Young DR, et al. Results of the Diet, Exercise and Weight Loss Intervention Trial (DEW-IT). *Hypertension.* 2002;40(5): 612–618.

138. Stevens FJ, Obarzanek E, Cook NR, et al. Long-term weight loss and changes in blood pressure: results of the Trials of Hypertension Prevention, Phase II. *Ann Intern Med.* 2001;134:1–11.

139. Appel LJ, Espeland MA, Easter L, et al. Effects of reduced sodium intake on hypertension control in older individuals: results from the trial of non-pharmacologic interventions in the Elderly (TONE). *Arch Intern Med.* 2001;161:685–693.

140. Appel LJ, Moore TJ, Obarzanek E, et al. A clinical trial of the effects of dietary patterns on blood pressure. DASH Collaborative Research Group. *N Engl J Med.* 1997;336:1117–124.

141. Obarzanek E, Sacks FM, Vollmer WM, et al; DASH Research Group. Effects on blood lipids of a blood pressure-lowering diet: the Dietary Approaches to Stop Hypertension (DASH) Trial. *Am J Clin Nutr.* 2001;74:80–89.

142. Sacks FM, Svetkey LP, Vollmer WM, et al. Effects on blood pressure of reduced dietary sodium and the dietary approaches to stop hypertension (DASH) diet. *N Engl J Med.* 2001;344:3–10.

143. Scarmeas N, Luchsinger JA, Mayeux R, et al. Mediterranean Diet and mortality in a US population. *Arch Intern Med.* 2008;168:1823–1824.

144. Shaie I, Schwarzfuchs D, Henkin Y, et al. Dietary Intervention Randomized Controlled Trial (DIRECT) Group. Weight loss with a low carbohydrate, Mediterranean, or low-fat diet. *N Engl J Med.* 2008;359:229–41.

145. National Institutes of Health, National Heart, Lung, and Blood Institut.. *DASH Eating Plan.* Bethesda, MD: US Department of Health and Human Services; 2006; http://www.nhlbi.nih.gov/health/public/heart/hbp/dash/new_dash.pdf. Accessed December 15, 2009.

146. American Heart Association. Mediterranean diet. http://www.heart.org/HEARTORG/GettingHealthy/NutritionCenter/Mediterranean-Diet_UCM_306004_Article.jsp. Accessed August 7, 2012.

147. Centers for Disease Control and Prevention. Deaths and mortality. http://www.cdc.gov/nchs/fastats/deaths.htm. Accessed December 2, 2009.

148. Dalgård C, et. al. Saturated fat intake is reduced in patients with ischemic heart disease 1 year after comprehensive counseling but not after brief counseling. *J Am Diet Assoc.* 2001;101:1420–14229.

149. Dallongeville J, Leboeuf N, Blais C, et al. Short-term response to dietary counseling of hyperlipidemic outpatients of a lipid clinic. *J Am Diet Assoc.* 1994;94:616–621.

150. Delahanty LM, et.al. Clinical and cost outcomes of medical nutrition therapy for hypercholesterolemia: a controlled trial. *J Am Diet Assoc.* 2001;101:1012–1023.

151. Elson RB, Splett PL, Bostick RM, et al. Dietitian practices for adult outpatients with hypercholesterolemia referred by physicians. The Minnesota Dietitians Survey. *Arch Fam Med.*1994;3:1073–1080.

152. Geil P, Anderson JW, Gustafson NJ. Women and men with hypercholesterolemia respond similarly to an American Heart Association step 1 diet. *J Am Diet Assoc.* 1995;95:436–441.

153. Hebert JR, Ebbeling CB, Ockene IS, et al. A dietitian-delivered group nutrition program leads to reductions in dietary fat, serum cholesterol and body weight: The Worcester area trial for counseling in hyperlipidemia (WATCH). *J Am Diet Assoc.* 1999;99:544–552.

154. Henkin Y, Shai I, Zuk R, et al. Dietary treatment of hypercholesterolemia: do dietitians do it better? *Am J Med.* 2000;109:549–555.

155. McGehee MM, Johnson EQ, Rasmussen HM, Salryoun N, Lynch MM, Carey M. Benefits and costs of medical nutrition therapy by registered dietitians for patients with hypercholesterolemia. *J Am Diet Assoc.* 1995;95:1041–1043.

156. Plous S, Chesne RB, McDowell AV. Nutrition knowledge and attitudes of cardiac clients. *J Am Diet Assoc.* 1995;95:442–446.

157. Prosser LA, Stinnett AA, Goldman PA, et al. Cost-effectiveness of cholesterol-lowering therapies according to selected patient characteristics. *Ann Intern Med.* 2000;132:769–779.

158. Sheils JF, Rubin R, Stapleton DC. The estimated costs and savings of medical nutrition therapy: the Medicare population. *J Am Diet Assoc.* 1999;99:428–435.

159. Thompson RL, Summerbell CD, Hooper L, et al. Dietary advice given by a dietitian versus other health professional or self-help resources to reduce blood cholesterol (Cochrane Review). In: *The Cochrane Library,* Issue 3, 2004. Chichester, UK: John Wiley & Sons, Ltd.

160. National Heart, Lung, and Blood Institute; National Institutes of Health. *Third Report of the National Cholesterol Education Program Expert Panel on Detection, Evaluation and Treatment of High Cholesterol in Adults (Adult Treatment Panel III).* National Cholesterol Education Program, , NIH Publication no 02–5215. Bethesda, MD: US Department of Health and Human Services; September 2002.

161. Bautista LE, Herran OF, Serrano C. Effects of palm oil and dietary cholesterol on plasma lipoproteins: results from a dietary crossover trial in free-living subjects. *Europ J Clin Nutrition.* 2001;55:748–54.

162. Brunner E, White I, Thorogood M, et al. Can dietary interventions change diet and cardiovascular risk factors? A meta-analysis of randomized controlled trials. *Am J Pub Health.* 1997;87:1415–1422.

163. De Lorgeril M, Salen P, Martin JL, et al. Mediterranean Diet, traditional risk factors, and the rate of cardiovascular complications after myocardial infarction, final report of the Lyon Diet Heart Study. *Circulation.* 1999; 99:779–785.

164. Denke MA, Sempos CT, Grundy SM. Excess body weight. An under recognized contributor to high blood cholesterol levels in white American men. *Arch Int Med.* 1993;153:1093–1103.

165. Ginsberg HN, Kris-Etherton P, Dennis B, et al. The effects of reducing saturated fatty acids on plasma lipids and lipoproteins in healthy subjects. *Atherioscler Thromb Vasc Biol.* 1998;18:441–449.

166. Howell WH, McNamara DJ, Tosca MA, et al. Plasma lipid and lipoprotein responses to dietary fat and cholesterol: meta-analysis. *Am J Clin Nutr.* 1997;65:1747 1764.

167. Jenkins DJ, Kendall CW, Marchie A, et al. The effect of combining plant sterols, soy protein, viscous fibers, and almonds in treating hypercholesterolemia. *Metabolism.* 2003;52(11):1478–83.

168. Johnson CL, Rifkind BM, Sempos CT, et al. Declining serum cholesterol levels among US adults: National Health and Nutrition Examination Surveys. *JAMA.* 1993;269:3002–3008.

169. Judd JT, Baer DJ, Kris-Etherton P et al. Dietary cis and trans monounsaturated and saturated FA and plasma lipids and lipoproteins in men. *Lipids.* 2002;37:123–31.

170. Kris-Etherton PM, Zhao G, Pelkman CL, et al. Beneficial effects of a diet high in monounsaturated fatty acids on risk factors for cardiovascular disease. *Nutr Clin Care.* 2000;3:153–162.

171. Kris-Etherton PM. Summary of the Scientific Conference on Dietary Fatty Acids and Cardiovascular Health: Conference Summary from the Nutrition Committee of the American Heart Association. *Circulation.* 2001;103:1034–1039.

172. Lichtenstein AH, Ausman LM, Jalbert SM, et al. Efficacy of a Therapeutic Lifestyle Change/Step 2 diet in moderately hypercholesterolemic middle-aged and elderly female and male subjects. *J Lipid Res.* 2002;43:264–273.

173. Mensink RP, Zock PL, Kester AD, Katan MB. Effects of dietary fatty acids and carbohydrates on the ratio of serum total to HDL cholesterol and on serum lipids and apolipoproteins: a meta-analysis of 60 controlled trials. *Am J Clin Nutr.* 2003;77:1146–1155.

174. Obarzanek E, Sacks FM, Vollmer WM, et al; DASH Research Group. Effects on blood lipids of a blood pressure-lowering diet: the Dietary Approaches to Stop Hypertension (DASH) Trial. *Am J Clin Nutr.* 2001;74:80–89.

175. Yu-Poth S, Zhao G, Etherton T, Naglak M, Jonnalagadda S, Kris-Etherton PM. Effects of the National Cholesterol Education Program's Step I and Step II dietary intervention programs on cardiovascular disease risk factors: a meta-analysis. *Am J Clin Nutr.* 1999;69:632–646.

176. Albert CM, Campos H, Stampfer MJ, et al. Blood levels of long-chain n-3 fatty acids and the risk of sudden death. *N Engl J Med.* 2002;346:1113–1118.

177. Albert CM, Hennekens CH, O'Donnell CJ, Ajani UA, Carey FJ, Willett WC, Riskin JN, Manson JE. Fish consumption and risk of sudden cardiac death. *JAMA.* 1998;279:23–28.

178. Baylin A, Kabagambe EK, Ascherio A, Spiegelman D, Campos H. Adipose tissue a-linolenic acid and nonfatal acute myocardial infarction in Costa Rica. *Circulation.* 2003;107:1586–1591.

179. Bucher HC, Hengstler P, Schindler C, Meier G. N-3 polyunsaturated fatty acids in coronary heart disease: a meta-analysis of randomized controlled trials. *Am J Med.* 2002;112:298–304.

180. Daviglus ML, Samler J, Orencia AJ, Dyer AR, Liu P et al. Fish consumption and the 30-year risk of fatal myocardial infarction. *N Engl J Med.* 1997;336:1046–1053.

181. De Lorgeril M, Salen P, Martin JL, et al. Mediterranean Diet, traditional risk factors, and the rate of cardiovascular complications after myocardial infarction, final report of the Lyon Diet Heart Study. *Circulation.* 1999;99:779–785.

182. Erkkila AT, Lehto S, Pyorala K, Uusitupa MI. N-3 fatty acids and five-year risks of death and cardiovascular disease events in patients with coronary artery disease. *Am J Clin Nutr.* 2003;78:65–71.

183. Hu FB, Stampfer MJ, Manson JE, et al. Frequent nut consumption and risk of coronary heart disease in women: prospective cohort study. Nurses Health Study. *BMJ.* 1998;317:1341–1345.

184. Kris-Etherton PM, Harris WS, Appel LJ for the Nutrition Committee. AHA Scientific Statement: Fish Consumption, Fish Oil, Omega-3 Fatty Acids, and Cardiovascular Disease. *Arterioscler Thromb Vasc Biol.* 2003;23(2):e20-e30.

185. Lemaitre RN, King IB, Mozaffarian D, et al. N-3 polyunsaturated fatty acids, fatal ischemic heart disease, and nonfatal myocardial infarction

in older adults: the Cardiovascular Health Study. *Am J Clin Nutr.* 2003;77:319–325.

186. Nilsen DW, Albrektsen G, Landmark K, et al. Effects of a high-dose concentrate of n-3 fatty acids or corn oil introduced early after an acute myocardial infarction on serum triacylglycerol and HDL cholesterol. *Am J Clin Nutr.* 2001;74:50–56.

187. Oomen CM, Feskens EJ, Rasanen L, et al. Fish consumption and coronary heart disease mortality in Finland, Italy, and The Netherlands. *Am J Epidemiol.* 2000;151:999–1,006.

188. National Institutes of Health, National Heart, Lung, and Blood Institute. *Lowering Your Cholesterol with TLC.* Bethesda, MD: US Department of Health and Human Services; 2005. http://www.nhlbi.nih.gov/health/public/heart/chol/chol_tlc.pdf. Accessed December 21, 2009.

189. Bazzano LA, He J, Ogden LG, et al. Dietary fiber intake and reduced risk of coronary heart disease in US men and women: the National Health and Nutrition Examination Survey I Epidemiologic Follow-up Study. *Arch Intern Med.* 2003;163:1897–1904.

190. Liu S, Stampfer MJ, Hu FB, et al. Whole-grain consumption and risk of coronary heart disease: Results from the Nurses' Health Study. *Am J Clin Nutr.* 1999;70:412–419.

191. Liu S, Buring J, Sesso H, et al. A prospective study of dietary fiber intake and risk of cardiovascular disease among women. *J Am Coll Cardiol.* 2002;39:49–56.

192. Pereira MA, O'Reilly E, Augustsson K, et al. Dietary fiber and risk of coronary heart disease. *Arch Intern Med.* 2004;164:370–376.

193. Van Horn L. Fiber, lipids, and coronary heart disease. a statement for healthcare professionals from the Nutrition Committee, American Heart Association. *Circulation* 1997;95:2701–2704.

194. Wolk J, Mason JE, Stampfer MJ, et al. Long-term intake of dietary fiber and decreased risk of coronary heart disease among women. *JAMA.* 1999;281:1998–2004.

195. Karmally W, Montez MG, Palmas W, et al. Cholesterol-lowering benefits of oat-containing cereal in Hispanic Americans. *J Am Diet Assoc.* 2005;105:967–70.

196. NHLBI. The Seventh Report of the Joint National Committee on Prevention, Detection, Evaluation, and Treatment of High Blood Pressure. *Hypertension* 2003;42:1206.

197. National Diabetes Fact Sheet, 2007. http://www.cdc.gov/diabetes/pubs/pdf/ndfs_2007.pdf. Accessed August 7, 2012.

198. Ash S, Reeves MM, Yeo S, et al. Effect of intensive dietetic interventions on weight and glycaemic control in overweight men with Type II diabetes: a randomised trial. *Int J Obesity.* 2003;27:797–802.

199. Banister NA, Jastrow ST, Hodges V, et al. Diabetes self-management training program in a community clinic improves patient outcomes at modest cost. *J Am Diet Assoc.* 2004;104:807–10.

200. Bray P, Thompson D, Wynn JD, et al. Confronting disparities in diabetes care: The clinical effectiveness of redesigning care management for minority patients in rural primary care practices. *J Rural Health.* 2005;21:317–21.

201. Chima CS, Farmer-Dziak N, Cardwell P, Snow S. Use of technology to track outcomes in a diabetes self-management program. *J Am Diet Assoc.* 2005;105(12):1933–8.

202. DAFNE Study Group. Training in flexible, intensive insulin management to enable dietary freedom in people with type 1 diabetes: dose adjustment for normal eating (DAFNE) randomised controlled trial. *BMJ.* 2002;325:746–751.

203. The Diabetes Control and Complications Trial Research Group. The effect of intensive treatment of diabetes on the development and progression of long-term complications in insulin-dependent diabetes mellitus. *N Engl J Med.* 1993;329:977–986.

204. Franz MJ, Monk A, Barry B, et al. Effectiveness of medical nutrition therapy provided by dietitians in the management of non-insulin-dependent diabetes mellitus: a randomized controlled clinical trial. *J Am Diet Assoc.* 1995;95:1009–1017.

205. Gaetke LM, Stuart MA, Truszczynska H. A single nutrition counseling session with a registered dietitian improves short-term clinical outcomes for rural Kentucky patients with chronic disease. *J Am Diet Assoc.* 2006;106(1):109–112.

206. Goldhaber-Fiebert JD, Goldhaber-Fiebert SN, Tristan ML, Nathan DM. Randomized controlled community-based nutrition and exercise intervention improves glycemia and cardiovascular risk factors in type 2 diabetic patients in rural Costa Rica. *Diabetes Care.* 2003;26:24–29.

207. Graber AL, Elasy TA, Quinn D, et al. Improving glycemic control in adults with diabetes mellitus: shared responsibility in primary care practices. *South Med J.* 2002;95(7):684–90.

208. Laitinen JH, Ahola IE, Sarkkinen ES, et al. Impact of intensified dietary therapy on energy and nutrient intakes and fatty acid composition of serum lipids in patients with recently diagnosed non-insulin-dependent diabetes mellitus. *J Am Diet Assoc.* 1993;93:276–283.

209. Lemon CC, Lacey K, Lohse B, et al. Outcomes monitoring of health, behavior, and quality of life after nutrition intervention in adults with type 2 diabetes. *J Am Diet Assoc.* 2004;104(12):1085–15.

210. Maislos M, Weisman D, Sherf M. Western Negev Mobile Diabetes Care Program: a model for interdisciplinary diabetes care in a semi-rural setting. *Acta Diabetol.* 2002;39(1):49–53.

211. Miller CK, Edwards L, Kissling G, Sanville L. Nutrition education improves metabolic outcomes among older adults with diabetes mellitus: results from a randomized controlled trial. *Prev Med.* 2002;34:252–9.

212. Wilson C, Brown T, Acton K, Gilliland A. Effects of clinical nutrition education and educator discipline on glycemic control outcomes in the Indian Health Service. *Diabetes Care.* 2003;26:2500–04.

213. Wolf AM, Conaway MR, Crowther JQ, et al. Translating lifestyle intervention to practice in obese patients with type 2 Diabetes: Improving control with activity and nutrition (ICAN) study. *Diabetes Care.* 2004;27:1570–1576.

214. Delahanty LM, et al. Clinical Significance of medical nutrition therapy in achieving diabetes outcomes and the importance of the process. *J Am Diet Assoc.* 1998;98:28–30.

215. Monk A, Barry B, McClain K, et al. Practice guidelines for medical nutrition therapy provided by dietitians for persons with non-insulin-dependent diabetes mellitus. *J Am Diet Assoc.* 1995;95:999–1006.

216. Grundy SM, Cleeman JI, Daniels SR, et al. Diagnosis and Management of the Metabolic Syndrome: an American Heart Association/National Heart, Lung, and Blood Institute Scientific Statement. *Circulation.* 2005;112;2735–52.

217. World Cancer Research Fund/American Institute for Cancer Research. Food, nutrition, physical activity and the prevention of cancer: a global perspective. Washington, DC: World Cancer Research Fund International, American Institute for Cancer Research, 2007. http://www.dietandcancerreport.org/. Accessed December 5, 2009.

218. Senie RT, Rosen PP, Rhodes P, et al. Obesity at diagnosis of breast carcinoma influences duration of disease-free survival. *Ann Int Med* 1992;116:26–32.

219. Wolin KY, Colditz GA. Can weight loss prevent cancer? *Br J Cancer.* 2008;99:995–9.

220. National Cancer Institute. Breast Cancer Prevention. www.cancer.gov/cancertopics/pdq/prevention/breast/healthprofessional/allpages. Accessed December 15, 2009.

221. Ravasco P, Monteiro-Grillo I, Vidal P, Camilo M. Dietary counseling improves patient outcomes: a prospective, randomized, controlled trial in colorectal cancer patients undergoing radiotherapy. *J Clin Oncol.* 2005;23:1431–1438.

222. Goncalves Dias MC, de Fatima Nunes Marucci, Nadalin W, Waitzberg DL. Nutritional intervention improves the caloric and protein ingestion of head and neck cancer patients under radiotherapy. *Nutr Hosp.* 2005;20:320–325.

223. Isenring E, Capra S, Bauer J, Davies PS. The impact of nutrition support on body composition in cancer outpatients receiving radiotherapy. *Acta Diabetol.* 2003 Oct;40(suppl 1):S162–4.

224. Dawson ER, Morley SE, Robertson AG, Soutar DS. Increasing dietary supervision can reduce weight loss in oral cancer patients. *Nutr Cancer.* 2001;41:70–74.

225. Ravasco P, Monteiro-Grillo I, Vidal PM, Camilo ME. Impact of nutrition on outcome: A prospective randomized controlled trial in patients with head and neck cancer undergoing radiotherapy. *Head and Neck.* 2005 27:659–668.

226. Rowe JW, Kahn RL. *Successful Aging.* New York, NY: Pantheon Books; 1998.

227. Holick MF. Vitamin D deficiency. *Engl J Med.* 2007;357:266–81.

228. Kim J-S, Wilson JM, Lee S-R, Dietary Implications on mechanisms of sarcopenia: roles of protein, amino acids and antioxidants. *J Nutr Biochem.* 2010;21:1–13.

229. Maltais ML, Desroches J, Dionne IJ. Changes in muscle mass and strength after menopause. *J Musculoskelet Neuronal Interact.* 2009;9:186–97.

230. Payette H, Boutier V, Coulombe C, et al. Benefits of nutritional supplementation in free-living, frail, undernourished elderly people: a prospective randomized community trial. *J Am Diet Assoc.* 2002;1002:1088–95.

231. Splett PL, Roth-Yousey LL, Vogelzang JL. Medical nutrition therapy for the prevention and treatment of unintentional weight loss in residential healthcare facilities. *J Am Diet Assoc.* 2003;103:352–362.

232. Jeune B. Living longer—but better? *Aging Clin Exp Res.* 2002;14:72–93.

233. Barzilai N, Gabriely I, Gabriely M, et al. Offspring of centenarians have a favorable lipid profile. *J Am Geriat Soc.* 2001;49:76–9.

234. Rabini RA, Vigini A, Martarelli D, et al. Evidence for reduction of pro-atherosclerotic properties in platelets from healthy centenarians. *Exp Gerontol.* 2003;38:367–71.

Oral and Dental Health

Dara Rosenberg, DDS, MS, MPH, FACD

Introduction

Oral health is inextricably linked to overall health maintenance and well-being across the life span. Among children dental decay is the leading infectious, chronic disease.[1] In adults, periodontal infections are among the most significant oral influences on systemic health, including cardiovascular diseases, stroke, respiratory diseases and diabetes—conditions that are all significant causes of mortality in women.[2] These infections may also contribute to premature delivery and low birth weight babies. Only a few longitudinal studies of oral diseases have looked specifically at gender differences.[3] Although causation has been difficult to prove, inadequate maintenance of oral health has been associated with diagnosis of various systemic conditions.[4–16] Oral diseases both lead to and contribute to other medical conditions as well as adversely affecting their clinical course.

Oral health is influenced by economic, demographic, psychological, social, and behavioral factors. Donahue states, "a disproportionate number of women live in poverty, many women are uninsured or underinsured, and women comprise the larger proportion of the aging population. These factors adversely affect (oral) health outcomes" and place women at increased risk for developing oral diseases.[17]

The 60th World Health Assembly (World Health Organization, Geneva, Switzerland, May 2007) proposed a resolution calling for oral health to be integrated into chronic disease prevention programs. Preventive measures, in the form of improved oral health education of women, healthcare workers, and clinicians, should stress the importance of home care, diet, professional checkups to limit and control oral infections, and use of fluoride. This chapter examines the impact on women's health of compromising oral conditions at each life stage on the progression, treatment, and prevention of systemic diseases.

Figure 6-1 graphically demonstrates that there are interrelationships between oral health, systemic health, genetic, sociodemographic, and economic factors, and preventive actions. This chapter describes those interrelationships and in particular highlights those issues important to women.

Historical Milestones in Women's Oral Health

Historically, oral health, especially women's oral health, has not had the recognition or extent of study that other medical fields have received. The body of information concerning women's health had its origins in 1975 with the creation of the National Women's Health Network, which brought to the forefront gender-specific health issues. In 1999 the Executive Summary of volume 8: *Agenda for Research on Women's Health for the 21st Century*, a listing of priorities for research on women's oral health included the use of oral exams in the detection of domestic violence; child abuse and eating disorders; investigation of gender-controlled transcription differences that influence autoimmune disease; female stress responses to pain; the relationship of oral disease in HIV-infected women and their children; the relationship among periodontal disease, alveolar bone loss, and osteoporosis; and periodontal disease and the risk of preterm births.[18]

Sources of Data in Women's Oral Health

Although limited data identifying women's oral health conditions are available, the National Survey of Oral Health in U.S. Employed Adults and Seniors was conducted in 1985–86 in response to the Public Health Service Task Force on Women's Health Issues of 1983. Redford and Gift analyzed this oral health data set for tooth loss patterns, dental caries, and periodontal diseases.[19] Subsequent national surveys have included only a few dental parameters.

The 1989 National Health Interview Survey analyzed by Lipton et al. reported higher prevalence rates among women for all types of orofacial pain within the prior 6 months. The female-to-male ratio of orofacial pain was found to be as high as 20:1.[20] Using the same database, Gift et al. found that women experience more restricted days (inability to perform usual activities, including all forms of work) as a consequence of their dental visits and dental pain.[21]

In 1998, four states (Arkansas, Illinois, Louisiana, and New Mexico) began collecting oral health data under the Pregnancy Risk Assessment Monitoring System (PRAMS). Analysis of this data indicated that between 12% and 25%

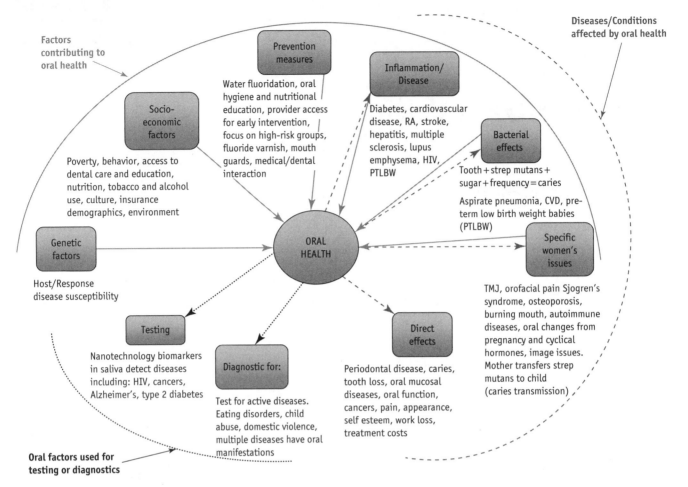

Figure 6-1 Relationship of oral health to overall health.

of pregnant women reported dental problems, but only 50% actually sought dental treatment. Women with dental problems who did not obtain treatment were also more likely to have delayed receiving prenatal care and were covered by public health insurance.[22]

Women's Oral Heath by Life Stages

Women report higher rates than men of temporomandibular joint (TMJ) disorders, orofacial pain, Sjögren's syndrome, and burning mouth syndrome, in addition to oral changes associated with pregnancy.[23] The main risk factors for poor oral health include poverty, inadequate nutrition, poor oral hygiene, and the use of tobacco and alcohol.[24] Differences in prevalence between males and females may result from the interactions of genetic, hormonal, environmental, behavioral (access to dental care, education, culture), and/or socioeconomic factors. There are clear socioeconomic disparities in health-related behaviors.[23]

The intricate link between oral health and general health supports the need for adoption of healthy lifestyles for health preservation and disease prevention. Demographic, genetic, biological, and behavioral risk factors have been identified that predict the development of oral problems;[25–28] however, maintenance of oral health depends upon improved self-care, and regular professional interventions as well as proper nutrition are necessary throughout all life stages.

From Conception Through Childhood

Mothers, both genetically and behaviorally, control and guide the oral health status of their children. A review of twin studies identified genetic factors as the basis for caries in 40% of paired siblings. Women carrying alleles at the HLA_DRB1 locus were more heavily colonized with *Streptococcus mutans* (a gram positive bacteria associated with caries development) than the control group.[29] Infants were colonized with the identical strains of strep mutans as their mothers. Among children ages 2 to 3, 66% were colonized with strep mutans and 88% of those children had been breastfed. Longer contact time with their mothers during breastfeeding provided greater opportunity to acquire these bacteria. In addition, breastmilk may contain immune components that suppress the infants' response to bacteria found in milk.[30] A discrete window of infectivity is believed to exist; although cariogenic bacteria may be present from birth, colonization cannot occur until the first tooth erupts at 6 to 7 months. Strep mutans is also spread in nursery environments between children during the early colonization time frame.[31] Prevention strategies for mothers have been reinforced by studies of antibacterial agents such as sodium fluoride, chlorhexidine rinses, and xylitol gum, which delay or reduce transmission of the bacteria to infants.[29] A major goal is to decrease bacterial load in mothers prenatally and to retain low bacterial levels post partum.

Girls experience growth spurts at earlier ages and over a briefer interval, reaching skeletal maturity about 2 years earlier than boys. Girls have attained 90% facial growth by menarche.[38] The implications of these differences are related to potential orthodontic treatment and management of malocclusions in girls and boys, as well as earlier and longer exposure to cariogenic bacteria that promote decay. The oral cavity is colonized with indigenous microflora, which are usually benign and essential for well-being. The longer teeth are exposed to carbohydrates and specific oral bacteria that metabolize carbohydrates, producing acids that demineralize tooth enamel, the greater the possibility of tooth decay.

Caries in children may affect eating, sleeping and school work in addition to undernutrition, weight loss, and short stature. Oral pain is one of the most common reasons for school absenteeism. Children should be seen by a dentist by 6 months, or 1 month after the eruption of the first tooth. New mothers need to be educated about appropriate oral hygiene regimens for themselves as well as their children, the effects of sugars and oral bacteria, early fluoride application, proper brushing, nutritional support, and the importance of professional dental care.

Role of Genetics in Oral Health

The field of genomics is beginning to clarify the complexity of factors related to chronic diseases. Gingival inflammation (gingivitis), an oral condition affecting over 50% of the adult population, had been considered a condition primarily controlled by individual oral hygiene. However, one recent study found a large number of genes in humans are expressed during the initiation and resolution of gingivitis. Activation of the immune system was noted to be the major pathway from plaque build-up on teeth to gingival inflammation.[32] Periodontal disease susceptibility has been related to multiple gene variations.[29] New technology enabling development of markers for gum disease may improve treatment options and provide avenues for prevention of periodontal disease. The Periodontal Susceptibility Test (PST, Interleukin Genetics Genotype Inc., Waltham, Massachusetts) the only commercially available genetics susceptibility test, uses genetic analysis to determine the likelihood of periodontal disease in an individual which may guide disease management in the future.

Genes have also been associated with oral cancer susceptibility, development, and prognosis. Genetic mutations identified in the mitochondria have been associated with risk of head and neck cancers are linked specifically to females, as mitochondria are only maternally inherited.[33] Genetic aspects also contribute to taste preferences for sweets, salivary flow rates, and immune functioning, all of which have implications for oral and systemic health.

Genomics will enable expansion and improvement in public health approaches including screening for disease susceptibility as well as identifying early and subclinical disease conditions. Genetics may direct elimination of specific types of bacteria as some individuals are hyperreactors. Microbiota do not cause oral diseases; instead, the individual's response to the presence of bacteria creates the environment for development of the chronic conditions. Genetics can have an impact on host susceptibility, but genetics and the environment together determine host response. The interaction of the two factors determines disease risk; changing environmental exposures can alter the expression of genetic mediated disease.[34] Thus, simply stressing improvement in oral hygiene may not provide the preventive response predicted.

Biomarkers found in saliva also provide exciting technologic screening techniques that will soon be used for surveillance of general health and disease.[35] These biomarkers are salivary proteomes (protein components), which circulate from all parts of the body and have been associated with multiple sclerosis, cancers, Alzheimer's disease, type 2 diabetes, and alveolar bone loss. They have also been found to change as women age.[36] Saliva promises to be a diagnostic tool for detecting diseases through nanotechnology.

Cleft palate (1:2500 births) and cleft lip (1:1000 births) are among the most frequently occurring craniofacial defects resulting from both genetic susceptibility and environmental exposures. The female palatal shelves fuse 1 week later than in the male, providing additional time for adverse environmental effects (drugs, etc.) to alter the developmental process.[37] Females with isolated clefts (clefts that exist on only one side) have been found to be at greater risk for an associated Bloch-Sulzberger syndrome.[29] Some oral conditions that develop at young ages may increase risk of cancer many years later among those with known genetic syndromes. Knowledge of these relationships enables early detection/suspicion of many cancers.[29]

Adolescence

The cyclical changes in hormones increase the severity of pubertal gingivitis and enhance host-bacteria interactions in the oral cavity.[37] Menstrual gingivitis beginning several days before menstruation may afflict adolescent girls despite their efforts to maintain good oral hygiene. During teen years, overconsumption of sodas and high-carbohydrate/sugar foods leads to increased risk of caries. An additional negative impact on oral tissues is smoking; a 2007 survey found that by 10th grade, 29% of girls are regular smokers.[19] Smoking increases the risk and results in earlier onset of severe periodontal disease resistant to successful treatment.[37] Smoking is a very strong risk factor for periodontal disease, cardiovascular conditions, and, in conjunction with alcohol consumption, is a risk factor for oral cancer. Smoking cessation counseling is equally effective when provided by dentists or physicians.[39]

The use of oral contraceptives adversely affects oral soft tissues. Becoming sexually active also increases risk of human immunodeficiency virus (HIV) infection. Women tend to display oral manifestations of HIV and acquired immune deficiency syndrome (AIDS), such as *Candida* infections, linear gingival erythema, necrotizing ulcerative gingivitis, and severe periodontitis, at lower viral levels than men.[40] Dentists may be the first healthcare providers to diagnose the disease.

Young Adulthood

Young women focus on body image issues to a much greater extent than young men. As a result, orthodontic care is sought more often by young women although they do not have higher rates of malocclusion.[37] Women at this age are prone to eating disorders such as anorexia nervosa, bulimia nervosa, and binge eating, which can result in several oral health problems. For women with anorexia or bulimia who engage in self-induced vomiting, the hydrochloric acid from the vomit in conjunction with the action of the tongue erodes the teeth, causing the smooth, glossy erosive pattern called perimylolysis. The extent of erosion is related to the duration and frequency of purging incidents per day, the amount of acid dilution (i.e., drinking after purges), and oral hygiene habits (brushing after purging).[41] Consumption of highly acidic, low-calorie foods, such as raw citrus fruits, can also create dished-out defects on the buccal and facial surfaces of teeth when eaten in excess. Individuals who purge as part of their eating disorder may also experience enlargement of the parotid glands, which are located on both sides of the lower jaw. The glands are soft and painless and continue to produce saliva at the normal flow rates. There is a direct relationship between the size of the glands and the duration and frequency of purging.[41]

Increased tooth decay in this population may result from the use of antidepressants prescribed for anorexia, which cause xerostomia, a reduction in the amount or chemical composition of saliva. In addition, fluid imbalance following overuse of diuretics and laxatives may also create xerostomia.[42] Saliva, which physically washes away food substrate, also contains enzymes that kill oral bacteria. Significant increases in caries may occur among women who have binge eating disorder, because they eat high-calorie foods throughout the day, increasing the opportunity for bacteria to produce acids that dissolve the enamel of the teeth.[41] Frequent toothbrushing tends to work with the acids to erode the enamel further instead of providing protection. Rinsing with a basic solution of 0.05% sodium fluoride will neutralize the acid.[28] The use of fingers or other objects to induce the gag reflex may result in soft tissue trauma of the palate, mucous membranes, and pharynx.

Image issues, societal pressures, and environmental stresses become more pronounced during young adulthood. Stress creates physiologic responses including raised serum cortisol levels that reduce inflammatory response to infection followed by an increase in oral bacteria levels. Periodontal disease has been related to increased stress as well as depression.[43] Increased stress also manifests as bruxism (grinding of teeth), temporomandibular disorder (TMD) causing pain and jaw muscle problems, and recurrent apthous stomatitis (canker sores).[17] Several cross-sectional studies have found significantly higher prevalence of TMD among young females, suggesting the role of estrogen receptors in these joints.[44] Chronic pain and depression are frequently manifestations of sexual abuse or trauma. Willumsen reported that women who have been exposed to abuse may feel especially vulnerable during dental visits.[45] The vulnerability experienced during a dental exam (from supine position, objects placed in the mouth, loss of control) may be related to the abusive experience as the majority of abuse victims suffer head and neck trauma.[25]

Data collected with the Corah Dental Anxiety Scale (PASS) indicated women experience higher dental anxiety than men; females, especially those who reported being physically or sexually abused, report more pain than men. Almost 50% of the women at a facial pain center had a history of abuse.[17] Most dentists do not question female patients about abuse. Dentists and physicians should create an environment conducive to discussion of potential abuse through targeted questioning.

More than 10 million American women are on oral contraceptives, which mimic the hormonal condition of pregnancy through the combination of synthetic estrogen and progesterone to prevent ovulation.[46] Developing a dry socket (localized alveolar osteitis) as a result of the surgical tooth extraction is increased 2.6 times among women using oral contraceptives.[47] The blood clot in the tooth socket dissolves too quickly (2 to 3 days after the extraction), exposing the bone. Healing is delayed by 1 to 2 weeks and severe pain is typically experienced. More than 30% of women with a dry socket had an extraction performed during day 1 through 22 of the pill, whereas none occurred during days 23–28 of the cycle.[47] Careful scheduling by women is essential to avoid this problem.

Contact sports participation increased by 700% among women in the 1980s, resulting in dental trauma and orofacial injuries associated with many sports including basketball, soccer, field hockey, lacrosse, softball, and volleyball.[48] Injuries result from lack of protective mouth guards, which prevent fractured teeth, intraoral lacerations, jaw fractures, and dislocations. Females of all ages who participate in sports should be advised to wear a properly fitted athletic mouth guard.

Reproductive Years—Pregnancy

During pregnancy, gingivitis, the most common oral tissue response to elevated ovarian hormones, occurs in 35% to 100% of women, depending upon the study.[46] Controlling plaque by brushing and flossing reduces the biofilm on teeth, which is primarily composed of microorganisms, proteins, and polysaccharides. Steroid hormones alter the gingival tissues thereby changing the types of bacteria present and their effects on and around the teeth. The most extreme oral tissue response to pregnancy hormones is growth of a "pregnancy tumor" that presents as a spongy, blood-filled mass. In most cases, after pregnancy, the gingival tissues recede to prepregnancy levels with no bone loss.

Russell investigated the long-held belief that a tooth is lost for every pregnancy by analyzing data from the third National Health and Nutrition Examination Survey (NHANES III) and noted predictors of tooth loss including socioeconomic level, race, parity, frequency of dental visits, smoking, diabetes, age at most recent live birth, and length of time since most recent live birth. Parity, the number of births, had a greater impact on tooth loss than smoking. Higher parity may also be related to increased stress and anxiety, which have been shown to modulate health behaviors that adversely affect the immune system and lead to compromised oral health.[27]

Rates of preterm deliveries have increased over the last 20 years from 9% in 1980 to 12% in 2004. Approximately 50% of infection induced preterm births are caused by subclinical anaerobes and mycoplasmas. Cytokines, pro-inflammatory mediators produced as a result of periodontal infections, are known to interfere with fetal growth and to induce labor. Oral bacteria have been found in amniotic fluid and have been identified in association with preterm and low birth weight babies.[49,50] A recent study found that women with perinatal loss were more than twice as likely to have periodontal disease, and those with extreme prematurity perinatal loss were more than four times as likely to suffer from periodontal disease, compared to women with full-term liveborn infants.[51]

Some studies that provided treatment of periodontal disease during pregnancy did not find a reduction in pre-term births compared to the untreated group; however, there was a decrease in spontaneous abortion and still-birth in the group receiving antenatal periodontal treatment. Other investigations have found women whose periodontal disease was not treated successfully were more likely to have preterm births.[52] A complicating factor in determining the effect of periodontal infection is the immune response of mothers to inflammation. Some women are hyperreactors to the inflammatory process. Hs-CRP (high-sensitivity C-reactive protein) or other inflammatory markers should be used in these studies to distinguish between these women in future studies. The intervention should ideally be initiated before pregnancy, because the inflammatory response may continue systemically after the initial infection has been treated.

There have been great strides in clinical care of preterm babies; however, little has been accomplished to prevent premature delivery. The California Dental Association Foundation in collaboration with the American College of Obstetricians and Gynecologists released the first perinatal guidelines in 2010 titled *Oral Health during Pregnancy and Early Childhood: Evidence-Based Guidelines for Health Professionals*. Although this professional document does not state that periodontal disease causes preterm births, the text stresses the importance of oral health prior to, during, and post pregnancy to ensure the health of both mother and child. Reducing the prevalence of periodontal disease in all young women prior to pregnancy is a primary public health goal. Programs should be designed to integrate oral health education into prenatal classes, health maintenance programs, and other social support services. The use of educational materials should be culturally sensitive and encourage facility referrals to a dentist as early in the pregnancy as possible. It is important to receive initial dental care to remove all sources of infection and then follow up with preventive care throughout the pregnancy. Provider partnerships between obstetricians/gynecologists and dentists, the Special Supplemental Nutrition Program for Women, Infants, and Children (WIC), Head Start and Healthy Start programs and the dental professionals should be encouraged.

Midlife—Peri and Post Menopause

Estrogen levels begin to diminish several years before menopause and continue to decline as women age. Diminishing hormone levels are associated with increased risk of autoimmune diseases which have their peak incidence between ages 40 and 60.[37] Oral bacteria may also exacerbate autoimmune diseases such as multiple sclerosis and lupus. Periodontitis and rheumatoid arthritis are characterized by destruction of hard and soft tissue as a result of inflammation. Clinical trials have indicated that treatment of periodontal disease significantly reduced severity of rheumatoid arthritis.[53]

Salivary quantity and quality change with alterations in estrogen. The decrease in salivary flow rate (SFR) may not only be initiated by a reduction in estrogen levels, but may also be manifested by diseases including diabetes, vitamin B deficiency, Parkinson's disease, and over 400 medications including diuretics, antidepressants, and anticonvulsive medications.[45] One of the most common conditions of middle-aged women is Sjögren's syndrome, characterized by severe xerostomia (dry mouth), keratoconjunctivitis sicca (dry eyes), and rheumatoid arthritis, which is far more prevalent in women than men.[10] Reduction of salivary flow results in increased caries development, gingival inflammation, and *Candida* infection.

Another condition, Burning Mouth Syndrome (BMS), often develops in conjunction with xerostomia. This burning syndrome has no known cause, is experienced in the mouth and lips, and occasionally alters taste sensation.[44] In a multisite study by Lamey et al. participants with BMS (88% female with a mean age of 65 years) had a significantly higher number of adverse life experiences including anxiety, depression, cancer phobia, gastrointestinal problems, and chronic fatigue than did the women without BMS.[54] Scleroderma, another autoimmune disease, affects the oral cavity through collagen deposition causing reduced motility of the muscles of the face and throat.[37]

Decreased estrogen and elevated cortisol levels predispose women to develop osteoporosis, which is frequently associated with tooth loss.[41] Bone loss is rapid and may make the jaws more susceptible to accelerated loss of alveolar bone (bone that holds teeth).[41] Periodontitis and osteoporosis have several of the same risk factors: increasing age, smoking, and medications that interfere with healing.[39] Osteoporosis, periodontal disease, estrogen levels, oral bacterial infections, and tooth loss are linked in multiple ways.[39,48–54] Women with higher 17β-estradiol (E2) levels had a mean net gain in alveolar bone density over a 1-year longitudinal study, whereas those who were E2 deficient showed a mean net loss in alveolar bone density.[55] The Women's Health Initiative Oral Ancillary Study found significant correlations between mandibular basal bone mineral density and hip bone density (r = 0.74, P < 0.001).[39] Estrogen replacement therapy is associated with greater tooth retention and preservation of alveolar bone.[56] A number of studies among postmenopausal women have found an association between obesity, periodontal disease, and tooth loss.[57] There are several implications of these findings. The analysis of alveolar bone height during dental visits may signal the first signs of a reduction in full-body bone density. Postmenopausal women diagnosed with osteoporosis may not be good candidates for dental implants. In addition, therapy given to slow the loss of BMD, such as hormone replacement, calcium, sodium fluoride and vitamin D supplements, and drug therapy, may in fact also preserve alveolar bone and thus teeth.[39] Panoramic radiographs taken in dental offices have also been found to be a good diagnostic tool for identifying women who are at high risk for fractures.[58]

Bisphosphonates, which inhibit osteoclastic (bone-building) activity, that remodel bone, have been prescribed for severe osteoporosis, severe hypercalcemia in malignancy, and bone-resorption diseases such as multiple myeloma and Paget's disease. An estimated 50% of Caucasian postmenopausal women over the age of 50 will experience osteoporotic fractures.[59] Bisphosphonate use has significantly reduced the incidence of vertebral fractures by 40%–50% and nonvertebral fractures by 20%–40%.[59] However, case findings starting in 2003 have shown that bisphosphonate use may result in osteonecrosis of the jaws (BON).[45] Symptoms of BON include difficult wound healing, bony sequesters, and pain. Loss of significant sections of the mandible has occurred because of the decreased healing potential. Although 25% of BON occurred spontaneously, 38% resulted from tooth extraction, 29% resulted from periodontal disease, 11% was from periodontal surgery, 3% from implant placement, and 1% from apical surgery.[45] In 2004, 27 million bisphosphonate prescriptions were written for treatment of osteoporosis in the United States; only 30 cases of BON have been directly related to oral bisphosphonates.[61]

Diabetes, a disease that compromises immune function, increases vulnerability to oral infection as a result of increasing salivary glucose levels, which in turn supports bacterial growth. Concomitantly, periodontal disease has been shown to inhibit the body's ability to control blood sugar levels. Among diabetics, periodontal disease has been shown to be an independent predictor of death from ischemic heart disease and myocardial infarction.[61] How can a periodontal infection have such a systemic impact? The total tissue surface of an individual with moderate to severe periodontal disease can range from 8 to 20 cm^2, depending upon the number of teeth involved. This large overall surface area becomes a significant source of inflammation.[13]

Although periodontal disease is increased among diabetes, survey data indicate that diabetics report lower use of dental services than nondiabetics. Hispanics and non-Hispanic blacks have higher rates of diabetes and also access the dental care system to a lesser extent. The National Health Objectives for 2010 contain a goal to increase the proportion of adults with diabetes who have an annual dental exam to at least 71% (Objective 5-15). This underscores the need to increase awareness of oral health in diabetic care management.

Moise Desvarieux, leading the INVEST program in upper Manhattan, firmly established the relationship of periodontal and cardiovascular disease (CVD). The study discovered that people who have suffered from past periodontal disease and tooth loss will continue to develop systemic manifestations (CVD) from the original oral inflammatory disease. Those with periodontal disease and those who were edentulous have the same high chance for CVD. This relationship holds for stroke outcomes as well.[62,63] Grau reported a 400% increase in stroke risk associated with periodontal disease but found no relationship between caries and stroke.[16]

Periodontists and cardiologists acknowledged the fact that inflammation is a major risk factor for heart disease and periodontal disease may increase the level of inflammation throughout the body. They developed clinical guidelines in 2009 with recommendations including the following: patients with periodontitis and at least one major atherosclerotic CVD risk factor such as smoking or family history for CVD should have a medical evaluation. Cardiac patients should have a periodontal evaluation if they exhibit gingival disease, tooth loss, or unexplained elevation of Hs-CRP. The cardiologist and periodontist should cooperate in order to optimize CVD risk reduction by increasing access to periodontal care.[64]

Participants in NHANES III, which was conducted between 1991 and 1994, included 2,300 men and women who were tested for periodontal disease and completed a thinking skills test that revealed greater memory problems among adults aged 60 and older, with the highest compared to the lowest levels of *Porphyromonas gingivalis*, bacteria that causes periodontal disease. Studies have indicated a linkage between brain function and maintenance of oral health that reduces periodontal disease and potential systemic inflammation.[65]

A 2009 study in the *Journal of the American Dental Association* reported that participants with all types of arthritis, obesity, CVD, diabetes, emphysema, hepatitis C (HCV) liver condition, or stroke were significantly more likely to report having poor oral health or to have more missing teeth than were participants without a chronic disease. They were also significantly more likely to be referred for an urgent periodontal problem. Periodontitis is reported to be associated with higher systemic inflammatory burden including among patients with end-stage renal disease requiring hemodialysis maintenance.[66] Improved communication between physicians and dentists may lead to earlier dental intervention in these populations. Smoking was the strongest predictor of dental disease followed by belonging to a racial or ethnic minority and having a low income. Arthritis, CVD diabetes, obesity, and HCV were associated with oral health after controlling for sociodemographic factors and smoking. Decreased dental function can decrease the quality of life even further among people with chronic diseases.[67] A study investigating the effect of periodontal treatment on per member per month costs for diabetes, coronary artery disease, and cerebrovascular disease found that periodontal care reduced the cost of medical care for these three medical conditions.[68] In response to these findings CIGNA Dental has developed a Periodontal Disease Risk Assessment tool to encourage their insured population to seek early dental intervention.

Older Years

The increase in oral disease in older women may be a reflection of the decreased visual and manual (arthritis) dexterity required to cleanse the mouth. Medication-induced reduction in salivary flow may also encourage caries development. Medications may also induce taste disorders, bleeding, oral lesions, erythema multiforma, gingival enlargement, recurrent oral viral infections, and allergic ulcerations.[69] Diet changes due to tooth loss, taste alteration due to medications, and psychologic components may result in more processed and highly cariogenic foods being consumed, which leads to higher caries rates.[70] The incidence of oral cancers rises with age; two-thirds of all cases are diagnosed after age 65. The risk increases with smoking and alcohol use.[70]

Anaerobic bacteria found in the mouth are the usual pathogens associated with aspirate pneumonia, the primary cause of death from infectious disease. Aspirate pneumonia occurs in 250 cases per 1,000 long-term care residents with prevalence in nursing homes of 2.1%.[71] An oral hygiene interventional study was conducted among half the nursing home population of 366 residents; over a 2-year period residents who did not receive oral care experienced almost 2.5 times (RR = 2.45) the number of febrile days, were 1.5 times (RR = 1.67) more likely to develop pneumonia, and were 2.5 times (RR = 2.4) more likely to die from the pneumonia that occurred, suggesting that preventive oral hygiene may decrease risk of infection and death in nursing home settings.[72]

By age 65, almost 30% of the adults are edentulous (have no teeth). Dentures are often difficult to wear because of poor construction, minimal remaining jaw bone, and poor quality and quantity of saliva. Dentures often require a change in diet to softer foods, most of which are less nutritious. Semba et al. followed 826 community dwelling women (mean age of 74 years) for 5 years; women with dentures had a higher risk of malnutrition, frailty, and mortality.[73] This study indicates the importance of good oral health for healthy aging.

The geriatric population also suffers from strokes and dementia. The mouth is often a primary source of pain in these patients because oral hygiene is not always provided, enabling dental infections to develop. Many women with these conditions suffer from oral pain without being able to express the source of the pain. The importance of oral health care is critical at this stage of life; medical and dental collaboration is particularly important for seniors. This collaboration can enhance healthcare delivery and improve patient outcomes.

Water Fluoridation

No review of oral health would be complete without mention of water fluoridation, which has been heralded as one of the 10 most effective public health efforts of the 20th century.[74] In the 1930s low rates of tooth decay were noticed to occur in areas where the water had natural fluoride. Studies conducted in communities in the 1940s to 1950s confirmed that the addition of low levels of fluoride (0.7–1.2 mg/L, levels established by the U.S. Public Health Service) to the water supply resulted in the same reductions in decay as naturally occurring fluoride. Tooth decay is reduced when fluoride comes in direct contact with teeth from infancy through adulthood as well as systematically during childhood when teeth are developing. Currently, 69% of Americans (184 million people) have access to fluoridated water at levels sufficient to prevent tooth decay.[75]

The benefits of fluoridation have diffused into non-fluoridated communities as a result of the use of fluoridated water in food processing.[76] Cost savings of fluoridation have been determined to range from $15.95 to $18.62 per person per year.[77] The Environmental Protection Agency (EPA) regulates fluoride as a drinking water contaminant. EPA's maximum contaminant level goal (MCLG); the level at which no adverse health effects occur, is 4 mg/L. The National Research Council's March 2006 report, *Fluoride in Drinking Water: A Scientific Review of EPA's Standard*, concluded "the available evidence [referring to the association of fluoride with numerous conditions including: osteosarcoma in boys, bone fractures, effects on hormones, the gastrointestinal system, immune system, and reproductive and developmental outcomes] was tentative and mixed and no recommendations were made for revising fluoride levels." Fluorosis, a dose-related condition resulting in white or brown staining of the teeth or pitting of the enamel, may occur at higher levels of fluoride exposure; however, this report addressed fluoride levels greater than the 0.7–1.2 mg/L used to prevent tooth decay.[78]

Data indicate that fluoride exposure levels among the population have increased in the last 40 to 50 years resulting in an increase in some effects. The impact of the overexposure on the risk for severe dental fluorosis in one or more teeth depends on the frequency and duration of the overexposures. EPA has proposed a reference dose (RfD) of 0.08 mg/kg/day for protection against pitting of the tooth enamel (severe dental fluorosis) and concluded that this value is also protective against fractures and skeletal effects in adults.

The new assessments have clarified what we know about the relationships between fluoride exposure and dental fluorosis, bone fractures, and skeletal fluorosis. The new assessments also reflect updated exposure estimates that account for changes in fluoridation practices and use of consumer dental products since the original drinking water standard was set. At this time and with the finalization of the new risk assessment, the Agency has not yet made a decision about revising the drinking water standard for fluoride.[79]

Summary

The destructive periodontal pathogens acquired early in life increase with age and can enter the systemic circulation and potentially stimulate a variety of medical conditions. Chronic periodontal disease may potentially alter the function of the vasculature and health of tissues throughout the body. Poor dental health may increase the risk of developing chronic conditions such as cardiovascular disease, stroke, and diabetes. In addition, women with chronic conditions including rheumatoid arthritis, diabetes, respiratory disease, cardiovascular disease, liver disease, and stroke have been found to have very poor oral health with considerable tooth decay and/or missing teeth. The association of oral health with chronic conditions has common risk factors including inadequate nutrition, tobacco use, low income, and lack of dental insurance. Minority and low-income women have the greatest need for improved oral health and are least likely to access the healthcare system. Numerous public health preventive responses may reduce the number of women afflicted with dental diseases, thus improving oral health, systemic health, and quality of life. Women's oral health issues should be included in future epidemiologic studies.

Discussion Questions

1. What are the oral conditions most prevalent in women by life stages?
2. How does periodontal disease affect oral as well as systemic health?
3. What are the chronic medical diseases and conditions that have been connected with poor dental health?
4. What are the strategies to reduce the risk of dental disease?
5. What emerging diagnostic tools will enhance public health strategies for early diagnosis and intervention of systemic diseases related to oral disease?
6. How can the coordination of medical and dental care lead to improved health outcomes?

References

1. United State Public Health Service, Office of the Surgeon General. *Oral Health in America: A Report of the Surgeon General.* Rockville, MD: Department of Health and Human Services, US Public Health Service; 2000.
2. Clemmens D, Kerr R. Improving oral health in women: nurses' call to action. *Am J Matern Child Nurs.* 2008;33:10–14.
3. Gift HC. Editorial. Needed: a research agenda for women's oral health. *J Dent Res.* 1993;72:552–553.
4. Scannapieco FA. Periodontical inflammation: from gingivitis to systemic disease? *Compend Cont Educ Dental.* 2004;25:16–25.
5. Genco R, Offenbacher S, Beck J. Periodontal disease and cardiovascular disease: epidemiology and possible mechanisms. *J Am Dent Assoc.* 2002;133 (suppl):14S–22S.
6. Amabile N, Susini G, Pettanati-Soubayrous I, et al. Severity of periodontal disease correlates inflammatory systemic status and independently predicts the presence and angiographic extent of stable coronary artery disease. *J Intern Med.* 2008;263:644–652.
7. Behekar AA, Singh S, Saha S, Molinar J, Arora R. The prevalence and incidence of coronary heart disease is significantly increased in periodontitis: A meta-analysis. *Am Heart J.* 2007;154:830–837.
8. Desvarieux M, Demmer RT, Rundek T, et al. Periodontal microbiota and carotid intima-media thickness: the oral infections and vascular disease epidemiology study (INVEST). *Circulation.* 2005;111:576–82.
9. Taylor GW, Burt BA, Becker MP, et al. Severe periodontitis and risk for poor glycemic control in patients with non-insulin-dependent diabetes mellitus. *J. Periodontol.* 1996;67:1085–93.
10. Grossi SG, Skrepcinski FB, DeCaro T, et al. Treatment of periodontal disease in diabetics reduces glycated hemoglobin. *J Periodontol.* 1997;68:713–9.
11. Scannapieco FA, Bush RM, Paju S. Associations between periodontal disease and risk for nosocomial bacterial pneumonia and chronic obstructive pulmonary disease: a systematic review. *Ann Periodontol.* 2003;8:54–69.
12. Jeffcoat MK, Guers NC, Reddy MS, et al. Periodontal infection and preterm birth: results of a prospective study. *J Am Dent Assoc.* 2001;132:875–80.
13. Hujoel PP, White BA, Garcia RI, et al. The dentogingival epithelial surface area revisited. *J. Periodontal Res.* 2001;36;48–55.
14. D'Aiuto F, Parkar M, Andreuou G, et al. Periodontitis and systemic inflammation: control of the local infection is associated with a reduction in serum inflammatory markers. *J Dent Res.* 2004;83:156–60.
15. Paquette DW. The periodontal-cardiovascular link. *Compend Cont Educ Dent.* 2004;25:681–92.
16. Grau AJ, Becher H, Ziegler CM, et al. Periodontal disease as a risk factor for ischemic stroke. *Stroke.* 2004;35:496–501.
17. Gardiner DM; Raigrodski AJ. Psychosocial issues in women's oral health. *Dent Clin North Am.* 2001;45:479–90.
18. Studen-Pavlovich D, Ranalli DN. Evolution of women's oral health. *Dent Clin North Am.* 2001;45:433–42.
19. Redford M. Beyond pregnancy gingivitis: brining a new focus. *J Dent Educ.* 1993;57:742–8.
20. Marbach JJ, Varoscak JR. Treatment of TMJ and other facial pains: a critical review. *NY State Dent J.* 1980;46:181–188.
21. Gift HC, Reisine ST, Larach DC. The social impact of dental problems and visits. *Am J Public Health.* 1992;82:1663–1668.
22. Gaffield ML, Colley Gilbert B, Malvitz D, Romaguera R. Oral health during pregnancy. An analysis of information collected by the Pregnancy Risk Assessment Monitoring System. *J Am Dent Assoc.* 2001;132:1009–1016.
23. Pihlstrom BL, Michalowicz, BS, Johnson NW. Periodontal diseases. *Lancet.* 2005;386:1809–1820.
24. Weintraub JA. Gender differences in oral health research: beyond the dichotomous variable. *J Dent Educ.* 1993;57:753–758.
25. Steinberg BJ, Minsk L, Gluch JI, Giorgio SK. Women's oral health issues. In: Clouse, AL, Sherif, K, eds. *Women's Health in Clinical Practice.* Current Clinical Practice. Totowa, NJ: Humana Press; 2008:273–293.
26. Copeland LB, Krall EA, Brown LJ, Garcia RI, Streckfus CF. Predictors of tooth loss in two US adult populations *J Public Health Dent.* 2004;64:31–37.
27. Russell S, Ickovics J, Yaffee R. Exploring potential pathways between parity and tooth loss among American women. *Am J Public Health.* 2008;98:1263–1270.
28. Slavkin, H. Distinguishing Mars from Venus: emergence of gender biology differences in oral health and systemic disease. *Compendium.* 2002;23:29–31.
29. Verbin S. Genetic influences in women's oral health. *Dent Clin North Am.* 2001;45:443–67.
30. Li Y, Wang W, Caufield PW. The fidelity of mutans streptococci transmission and caries status correlate with breast-feeding experience among Chinese families. *Caries Res.* 2000;34:123–132.
31. Alves A, Nogueira R, Stipp R, Pampolini F, Moraes A, Goncalves R, Hofling J, Li Y, Mattos-Graner R. Prospective study of potential sources of Streptococcus mutans transmission in nursery school children. *J Med Microbiol.* 2009;58:476–481.
32. Offenbacher S, Barros SP, Paquette DW, Winston JL, Biesbrock AR, Thomason RG, Gibb RD, Fulmer AW, Tiesman JP, Juhlin KD, Wang SL, Reichling TD, Chen KS, Ho B. Gingival transcriptome patterns during induction and resolution of experimental gingivitis in humans. *J Periodontol.* 2009;80:1963–82.
33. Cottrell DA, Blakely EL, Borthwick GM, et al. Role of mitochondrial DNA mutations in disease and aging. *Ann NY Acad Sci.* 2000;908:199–207.
34. Ebersole JL, Steffen MJ, Gonzalez-Martinez J, Novak MJ. Effects of age and oral disease in systemic inflammatory and immune parameters in nonhuman primates. *Clin Vaccine Immunol.* 2008;15:1067–1075.
35. Scannapieco FA, Ng P, Hovey K, et al. Salivary biomarkers associated with alveolar bone loss. *Ann NY Acad Sci.* 1098:496–497.
36. Ambatipudi K, Lu, B, Hagen F, et al. Quantitative analysis of age specific variation in the abundance of human female parotid salivary proteins. *J Proteome Res.* 2009;8:5093–5102.
37. Markovic N. Women's oral health across the lifespan. *Dent Clin North Am.* 2001;45:513–521.
38. Studen-Pavlovich D, Ranalli D. Women's oral health across the lifespan. Part two. *Northwest Dent.* 2002;81:19–23, 62.
39. Jeffcoat M, Lewis C, Reddy M, Wang C, Redford M. Post-menopausal bone loss and its relationship to oral bone loss. *Periodontology.* 2000;23:94–102.
40. Riley C, London JP, Burmeister JA. Periodontal health in 200 HIV-positive patients. *J Oral Pathol Med.* 1992;21:124–127.
41. Studen-Pavlovich D, Elliott MA. Eating disorders in women's oral health. *Dent Clin North Am.* 2001;45:491–511.
42. Bartlett DW, Smith BGN. The dental impact of eating disorders. *Dental Update.* 1994;21:404–407.
43. Morse DR, Schacterle GR, Furst L, et al. The effect of stress and meditation on salivary protein and bacteria: a review and pilot study. *J Human Stress.* 1982;8:31–39.
44. Covington P. Women's oral health issues: an exploration of the literature. *Probe.* 1996;30:173–177.

45. Willumsen T. Dental fear in sexually abused women. *Eur J Oral Sci* 2001;109:291–296.

46. Zachariasen R. The effect of elevated ovarian hormones on periodontal health: oral contraceptives and pregnancy. *Women Health*. 1993;20:21–30.

47. Catellani JE, Harvey S, Erickson SH, Cherkin D. Effect of oral contraceptive cycle on dry socket. *J Am Dent Assoc*. 1980;101:777–780.

48. Randalli, DN, Rye LA. Oral health issues for women athletes. *Dent Clin North Am*. 2001;45:523–39.

49. Han YW, Shen T, Chung P, et al.. Uncultivated bacteria as etiologic agents of intra-amniotic inflammation leading to preterm birth. *J Clin Microbiol*. 2009;47:38–47.

50. Han YW, Shen T, Chung P, et al. Uncultivated bacteria as etiologic agents of intra-amniotic inflammation leading to preterm birth. *J Clin Microbiol*. 2009;47:38–47.

51. Shub A, Wong C, Jennings B, et al. Maternal periodontal disease and perinatal mortality. *Aust N Z J Obstet Gynecol*. 2009;49:130–136.

52. Xiong X, Buekens P, Fraser WD, et al. Periodontal disease and adverse pregnancy outcomes: a sytematic review. *Br J Obstet Gynaecol*. 2006;113:135–143.

53. Ortiz P, Bissada NF, Palorno L, et al. Periodontal therapy reduces the severity of active rheumatoid arthritis in patients treated with or without tumor necrosis factor inhibitors. *J Periodont*. 2009;80:535–540.

54. Lamey PJ, Freeman R, Eddie S, et al. Vulnerability and presenting symptoms in burning mouth syndrome. *Oral Surg Oral Med Oral Pathol Radiol Endod*. 2005;99:48–54.

55. Brennan RM, Genco RJ, Wilding GE, et al. Osteoporosis and oral infection: independent risk factors for oral bone loss. *J Dent Res*. 2008;87:323–327.

56. Krall EA, Dawson-Hughes B, Hannan MT, et al. Postmenopausal estrogen replacement and tooth retention. *Am J Med*. 1997;102:536–542.

57. Taguchi A, Tsuda MS, Ohtsuka M, et al. Interaction of obesity and skeletal bone mineral density in tooth retention in Japanese postmenopausal women. *Menopause*. 2007;14:500–504.

58. Taguchi A, Ohtsuka M, Makamoto T, Suei Y, Kudo Y, Tamimoto K, Bollen, AM. Detection of post-menopausal women with low bone mineral density and elevated biochemical markers of bone turnover by panoramic radiographs. *Dentomaxillofacial Radiol*. 2008;37:433–437.

59. Basu N, Reid D. Bisphosphonate associated osteonecrosis of the jaw. *Menopause International*. 2007;13:56–59.

60. Woo SB, Helstein JW, Kalmar JR. Narrative review. Bisphosphonates and osteonecrosis of the jaws. *Am Intern Med*. 2006;144:753–761.

61. Compston J. Oral bisphosphonates and osteonecrosis of the jaw: are the MHRA recommendations appropriate? *Menopause International*. 2007;13:54–55.

62. Desvarieux M, Demmer R, Rundek T, et al. Relationship between periodontal disease, tooth loss, and carotid artery plaque: The Oral Infections and Vascular Disease Epidemiology Study. *Stroke*. 2003;34:2120–2125.

63. Demmer R, Desvarieus M. Periodontal infections and cardiovascular disease: the heart of the matter. *J Am Dent Assoc*. 2006;137;14S–20S.

64. Friedewald, V, Kornman K, Beck J, et al. The American Journal of Cardiology and Journal of Periodontology Editor's Consensus: periodontitis and atherosclerotic cardiovascular disease. *J Periodontol*. 2009;80:1021–1032.

65. Noble JM, Borrell LN, Papapanou PN, et al. Periodontitis is associated with cognitive impairment among older adults: analysis of NHANES-III. *J Neurol Neurosurg Psychiatry*. 2009;80:1206–1211.

66. Craig R, Kotanko P, Kamer A, Levin N. Periodontal diseases—a modifiable source of systemic inflammation for the end-stage renal disease patient on haemodialysis therapy? *Nephrol Dial Transpl*. 2007;22:312–315.

67. Griffin S, Barker L, Griffin P, Cleveland J, Kohn W. Health needs among adults in the United States with chronic diseases. *J Am Dent Assoc*. 140:1266–1274.

68. Albert DA, Sadowsky D, Papapanou P, et al. Research article. An examination of periodontal treatment and per member per month medical costs in an insured population. *BMC Health Services Res*. 2006;6:103.

69. Ghezzi E, Ship J. Systemic diseases and their treatments in the elderly: impact on oral health. *J Public Health Dent*. 2000;60:289–296.

70. Mulligan R The three phases of Eve: exploring the common and unique findings in oral and systemic health of differently aging women. *Compendium*. 2002;23:32–40.

71. Terpenning MS, Taylor GW, Lopatin DE, et al. Aspiration pneumonia: dental and oral risk factors in an older veteran population. *J Am Geriatr Soc*. 2001;49:557–563.

72. Yoneyama T, et al. Oral care reduces pneumonia in older patients in nursing homes. *J Am Geriatr Soc*. 2002;50:430–433.

73. Semba RD, Blaum CS, Bartali B, et al. Denture use, malnutrition, frailty, and mortality among older women living in the community. *J Nutr Health Aging*. 2006;10:161–167.

74. Achievements in Public Health 1900–1999-Fluoridation of drinking water to prevent dental caries. *MMWR Morb Mortal Wkly Rep*. 1999;48:933–940.

75. Centers for Disease Control and Prevention, Community water fluoridation. www.cdc.gov/fluoridation/benefits/background.htm. Accessed September, 1, 2009.

76. Griffin SO, Gooch BF, Lockwood SA, Tomar SL. Quantifying the diffused benefit from water fluoridation in the United States. *Community Dent Oral Epidemiol*. 2001;29:120–129.

77. Griffin SO, Jones K, Tomar SL. An economic evaluation of community water fluoridation. *J Public Health Dent*. 2001;61:78–86.

78. *Fluoride in Drinking Water: A Scientific Review of EPA's Standards*. Board on Environmental Studies and Toxicology. National Research Council of the National Academies., Washington, DC: The National Academies Press; 2000:1–446.

79. United States Environmental Protection Agency. Six-Year Review of Drinking Water Standards. http://water.epa.gov/lawsregs/rulesregs/regulatingcontaminants/sixyearreview/index.cfm. Accessed November 2012.

Epidemiology of Women's Use of Complementary and Alternative Medicine

Heather Greenlee, ND, PhD; Judith S. Jacobson, DrPH, MBA; and Fredi Kronenberg, PhD

Introduction

In 1993, a report published in the *New England Journal of Medicine* received widespread publicity because it revealed that, according to the findings of a national telephone (random digit dialing) survey of English-speaking adults (N = 1,539) conducted in early 1991, one-third of respondents, both female and male, had used at least one "unconventional therapy" in the past year (Table 7-1) and had made more visits to "providers of unconventional therapy" than to primary care doctors.[1] Among the aspects of the report that caused concern in the medical community was the observation that only 38.5% of respondents who used such therapies had informed their doctors.

However, although 83% of respondents reported having a medical condition, the conditions for which the therapies were most commonly used were minor chronic complaints rather than serious illnesses (Table 7-2).

Virtually all those who saw an unconventional therapy provider for cancer, diabetes, hypertension, or lung, skin, urinary tract, or dental problems also saw a medical doctor. Few commentators acknowledged that most of the therapies surveyed, with the possible exceptions of chiropractic and acupuncture, were more likely to have represented wellness care than treatment for a medical condition.

By the winter of 1997–1998, when a follow-up survey using similar sampling methods was conducted (N = 2,055), the prevalence of use of what was then termed "alternative medicine" had risen to 42%.[2] The same 16 modalities were included in the second survey.[3] As noted previously, respondents who reported using alternative therapies were most frequently doing so for chronic conditions, including back problems, anxiety, depression, and headaches, and only 39.8% had mentioned their use of "alternative medicine" to their doctors. Use was found to be more common among women (48.9%) than men (37.8%) in the second survey. The use of herbal medicines and "megavitamins," as well as the proportion of respondents using an alternative therapy while seeing a medical doctor for the same condition, increased substantially. Hence, the authors expressed concern about possible unrecognized (because the physician was uninformed) adverse interactions of herbal medicines and/or vitamins with conventional medication.[3]

In 2002, the National Health Interview Survey (NHIS, N = 31,044) added an alternative health/complementary and alternative medicine supplement to the survey to assess the prevalence of use of "complementary and alternative medicine" (CAM). Several people analyzed these data and, though they used slightly different combinations of modalities in their calculation, CAM use seemed to

Table 7-1

"Unconventional therapies" surveyed in 1993[1]

Relaxation techniques	Chiropractic
Massage	Imagery
Spiritual healing	Commercial weight-loss programs
Herbal medicine	Self-help groups
Lifestyle diets (e.g., macrobiotics)	Energy healing
Biofeedback	Hypnosis
Homeopathy	Megavitamin therapy
Folk remedies	Acupuncture

Data from Eisenberg DM, Kessler RC, Foster C, et al. Unconventional medicine in the United States. Prevalence, costs, and patterns of use. *N Engl J Med*. 1993;328:246-252.

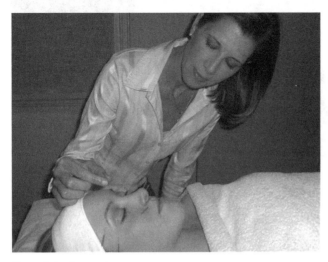

Figure 7-1 Acupuncture.

Courtesy of Shellie Goldstein, M.S., L.Ac., 928 Broadway, Suite 1104, NY, NY 10010.

Table 7-2

The top 10 conditions for which unconventional therapies were used in a 1993 survey[1]

Back problems	Allergies
Arthritis	Insomnia
Sprains or strains	Headaches
High blood pressure	Digestive problems
Anxiety	Depression

Data from Eisenberg DM, Kessler RC, Foster C, et al. Unconventional medicine in the United States. Prevalence, costs, and patterns of use. *N Engl J Med*. 1993;328:246-252.

---

have stabilized at about 35%, depending on the analysis.[4–6] CAM use was associated with being aged 40–64 years (rather than older or younger), female gender, nonblack/non-Hispanic race, and an annual income of $65,000 or greater.[6] Although these surveys asked about common health problems, none asked about health conditions specific to women.

Since 1993, the field of CAM research has grown exponentially. Many studies have analyzed patterns of CAM use, predictors of CAM use, and effects of specific CAM therapies. Investigators also began to examine CAM therapies used specifically by women for women's health conditions.[7–9] This chapter provides an overview of women's CAM use based on surveys of general population samples and highlights CAM use for menopause, acquired immune deficiency syndrome (AIDS), sexually transmitted diseases (STDs), and breast cancer; those conditions were selected because they are important to the quality of women's lives and because several surveys have focused on CAM use in those conditions. In addition, the chapter explores some of the methodologic issues inherent in CAM research.

Definitions of CAM

The U.S. National Center for Complementary and Alternative Medicine (NCCAM), part of the National Institutes of Health (NIH), defines CAM as "a group of diverse medical and health care systems, practices, and products that are not generally considered to be part of conventional medicine." NCCAM distinguishes complementary modalities that are used *in addition to* conventional medicine from alternative therapies that are used *instead of* conventional medicine. An additional category, "integrative medicine," has recently been defined as health care that "combines treatments from conventional medicine and CAM for which there is evidence of safety and effectiveness." NCCAM often groups many CAM modalities into four distinct but overlapping domains that have been incorporated into some CAM survey questionnaires and analyses:[10]

- *Mind-body medicine*: techniques to enhance the mind's capacity to affect bodily function and symptoms, such as yoga, meditation, prayer, art therapy, and dance therapy;
- *Natural products*: healing and disease prevention through the intake of natural substances, such as botanicals, vitamins, minerals, and food;
- *Manipulative and body-based practices*: spinal manipulation and massage; acupuncture
- *Other CAM practices*:
  - Movement therapies, such as Feldenkrais method, Alexander technique, Pilates, and Trager psychophysical integration
  - Traditional healers, such as Native American healers/medicine men/women and curanderas
  - Energy medicine, encompassing energy biofield therapies, such as qi gong, reiki, and therapeutic touch, which draw on energy fields that are believed to surround and permeate the human body, and bioelectromagnetic-based therapies, which use devices that create or apply pulsed, magnetic, and/or alternating- or direct-current fields

Whole medical systems, such as naturopathic medicine, homeopathic medicine, traditional Chinese medicine, Tibetan medicine, and Ayurveda, are complete systems of theory and practice that cut across all four CAM practice domains and are often included as a fifth domain in surveys of CAM use.

Among these whole systems, the traditional systems of medicine are often considered separately, particularly in the international arena. In 2008, the World Health Organization defined "traditional medicine [as] the sum total of knowledge, skills and practices based on the theories, beliefs and experiences indigenous to different cultures that are used to maintain health, as well as to prevent, diagnose, improve or treat physical and mental illnesses." WHO also noted that "traditional medicine adopted by other populations (outside its indigenous culture) is often termed alternative or complementary medicine."[11] The term *traditional complementary and alternative medicine (T/CAM)* is sometimes used, particularly internationally, to focus on the traditional medical systems of other cultures, especially when those systems are significantly used in a particular culture, and to include CAM as described in western countries.

This chapter primarily focuses on a U.S. perspective on CAM. However, many people living in the United States come from other countries and continue to use the medicines and health-related practices common in their country of origin. Immigrants and their families may view their own traditional system of medicine as conventional and other systems, including western or allopathic medicine, as alternative or complementary.

Reasons for CAM Use

Women (and men) use CAM therapies for a variety of reasons, including health maintenance, health promotion, disease prevention, disease treatment, and relief of symptoms or side effects of conventional treatment.[12] Women are motivated to use CAM by personal belief in natural therapies, dissatisfaction with conventional medicine, family/social influences, and (least frequently) medical advice.[13] Women who use CAM are also more likely to engage in other health-promoting behaviors, such as not smoking, having a lower body mass index, eating more fruits and vegetables, engaging in higher levels of physical activity, and having regular health checkups.[14–16] However, some CAM users are less likely to engage in conventional public health vaccination efforts.[17] CAM use was found to be related to personality, social supports, and physical and mental health in a national survey.[18] The CAM modality and the health-related context in which it is used may influence a patient's decision about mentioning it to her medical doctor. For example, it may be important for a breast cancer patient to notify her oncologist that she is using a dietary supplement to promote general well-being during her chemotherapy treatment,[12,19] but it may not be important for a woman who is experiencing job-related stress to disclose to her provider that she is taking a yoga class. Not all forms of CAM need to be medicalized.

Epidemiology of Women's Use of CAM in the United States

In the United States as well as other countries, women use more conventional health care than men,[20,21] and most studies find that they use more CAM as well.[2,4,6,22,23–25] Women use CAM for health conditions across the life cycle, for chronic conditions as well as serious illness.[26–29]

The national surveys conducted in the United States in the 1990s made the biomedical research community aware of the increasing prevalence of CAM use but did not compare women's patterns of CAM use to those of men or ask about particular health conditions for which women used CAM. Moreover, only English speakers were eligible to participate, and the questions dealt with broad categories of CAM. Hence, the investigators could not relate gender, race/ethnicity, or national origin to the use of specific CAM therapies for particular conditions.

In 2001, Kronenberg and colleagues conducted a national telephone interview survey of CAM use among 3,068 women in 4 race/ethnic groups (747 non-Hispanic whites, 1,081 African Americans, 1,057 Mexican Americans, and 1,021 Chinese Americans), in English, Spanish, Mandarin, and Cantonese.[8] More than 40% of the respondents reported having used at least 1 of 11 CAM modalities in the prior year (51.6% of non-Hispanic Whites, 37.9% of African Americans, 36.4% of Mexican Americans, and 40.8% of Chinese Americans). The types of CAM used and the conditions for which they were used CAM varied by ethnicity. Non-Hispanic white women were the most likely to use vitamins and to see chiropractors and used CAM most often for joint pain or arthritis, back pain, or headaches. Mexican American women were the least likely to have seen a medical doctor, and they used CAM (mainly medicinal herbs) most often for cancer, heart disease, or osteoporosis treatment. African American women were the least likely to have seen a CAM practitioner, and used CAM (mainly medicinal herbs) most often for joint pain, back pain, or osteoporosis.[8]

Most women who used botanicals and other dietary supplements also used prescription and over-the-counter drugs such as aspirin and commercial allergy medications; the prevalence of concurrent use varied by condition.[13] For example, almost all cancer patients who used dietary supplements also used conventional medications, but fewer women used conventional medications (e.g., hormone replacement therapy) simultaneously with supplements for menopausal symptoms. Few respondents who used CAM for conditions such as back pain, headaches, insomnia, pregnancy-related discomfort, menstrual symptoms, and weight loss consulted a medical doctor regarding those symptoms. However, most of those who both used CAM and saw a medical doctor did report their CAM use to the doctor (52–96%, depending on the condition).[13] This finding differs from studies that included both men and women, which concluded that most people did not inform their medical doctor of their CAM use.[1]

Chao and colleagues analyzed data from the 2002 National Health Interview Survey and the 2001 Health Care Quality Survey (HCQS) on 10,759 respondents who reported any CAM use in the prior year.[30] Survey participants who used provider-based rather than self-selected CAM modalities were more likely to report use to their medical providers. In contrast to CAM users who relied on self-care, members of minority populations who lacked a consistent provider were less likely to discuss CAM use with a clinician.

Epidemiology of CAM Use for Specific Conditions

Menopause

Women's experiences of menopause vary greatly both within and across cultures. Contributing factors include genetics, diet, exercise, other lifestyle factors, and environmental exposures. Symptoms such as hot flashes, often experienced through the period of transition to and through menopause, prompt many women to seek relief from physicians, pharmacists, and health food practitioners. Women approaching menopause also may seek medical advice or take preventive measures to lower their perceived risk of cardiovascular disease and osteoporosis.

For decades, many physicians in western countries prescribed hormone replacement therapy (HRT) to treat the short-term symptoms commonly associated with menopause and longer-term problems associated with the menopausal decline in estrogen, including osteoporosis. HRT was also thought to prevent cardiovascular disease. This recommendation was prevalent despite studies that indicated HRT use increased risk for breast cancer and unopposed estrogen replacement therapy increased the risk of endometrial cancer. In 2002, the NIH-funded Women's Health Initiative (WHI) reported that HRT actually increased the risk of cardiovascular disease and breast cancer.[31] In response to the WHI findings, many physicians advised patients to discontinue hormone use. As menopausal symptoms returned, many women sought alternative methods for symptom control. Others had never taken HRT due to fear of side effects, contraindications, or preferences for natural products. Many turned to botanicals, dietary supplements, and other CAM therapies, such as acupuncture.

Newton and colleagues surveyed 866 menopausal women ages 45–65 enrolled in a Washington State health maintenance organization (HMO) to specifically question their use of eight CAM therapies for menopausal symptoms.[32] More than 68% of women reported using at least one of the eight therapies for hot flashes, 75% for night sweats, and 80% for sleep problems. Herbal, homeopathic, and naturopathic remedies were the therapies most commonly used to treat hot flashes or night sweats. About 22% of respondents were using both CAM and hormonal therapy.

A longitudinal, multiethnic, multicenter cohort study of midlife women conducted in 2002–2003, the Study of Women's Health Across the Nation (SWAN), examined the relationships of use of 21 CAM modalities among 5 race/ethnicity groups by menopausal status and symptoms. Overall, 52.7% reported use of CAM, not including diet, exercise, vitamins, or prayer. Although CAM use varied little across broad symptom categories (vasomotor, psychological, somatic), use of particular modalities differed by type of symptom. Compared with women who did not report troubling menopausal symptoms, those who frequently experienced vasomotor symptoms (i.e., hot flashes) were significantly more likely to obtain relief by using black cohosh and soy supplements in addition to following healthful eating patterns and relying on prayer.[33]

Analyses of the SWAN data provided CAM use by race/ethnicity in relation to reported symptoms. At baseline, 49.5% of Hispanic women, 48.3% of African Americans, 37.7% of Japanese women, 37.3% of white women, and 30.4% of Chinese women reported vasomotor symptoms. Japanese and white women were significantly more likely to use any CAM modality than other groups (Japanese 64.2%. white 57.6%. Chinese 46%. African American 38.8%. Hispanic 20%). Japanese women, followed by white women, were also more likely to use nutritional remedies. Herbal

and physical remedies were preferred by Japanese women in contrast to more psychologic remedies (e.g., meditation, imagery, relaxation) used by white women. Japanese and Chinese women used more herbal therapies and less psychologic therapies than other groups. More white and African American women with symptoms used CAM than did Chinese and Japanese women, and those with vasomotor symptoms were more likely than asymptomatic women to use CAM.[34]

The 2002 NHIS included 17,295 white, black, Hispanic, and Asian women who were asked about their use of 27 CAM modalities spanning 5 CAM domains.[35] In this nationally representative sample, 40% of women reported any CAM use. Use varied by race/ethnicity and age: Asian women were the most likely to report CAM use, and CAM use was highest among women in their 50s and almost as high among women in their 40s. Biologically based therapies were those most frequently reported in all groups, and mind-body therapies were the next most widely used. CAM was used most commonly for back pain (15.4%), colds (10.2%), neck pain (7.2%), and arthritis (5.8). Only 1.6% of respondents used any CAM for menopause and 1.5% used them for menstrual disorders. Women without insurance were less likely to use manipulative therapies and more likely to use alternative medical systems (acupuncture, naturopathy, homeopathy) than women with insurance. Most women thought that using CAM plus conventional therapy was most helpful and that "pursuit of wellness" was an important reason for such use. In a smaller study of 500 women aged 40–60 years (47% African American, 40% Caucasian, 12% Hispanic, and 2% Asian) attending clinics at the University of Illinois at Chicago, 79% reported using botanical/dietary supplements for menopausal symptoms.[36] In this study CAM was used by most women (68%) to treat disease or prevent disease (24%). The most commonly used botanicals were soy, green tea, other herbal teas, chamomile, gingko, ginseng, echinacea, St. John's wort, and black cohosh. Women who took prescription medications were more likely to take botanic dietary supplements than others; however, only 30% of supplement users reported their CAM use to their physician.

Clearly, patterns of use vary by race/ethnicity, region, subpopulations sampled, and CAM modalities included in the survey questionnaire. However, CAM use, especially of natural products, is common although information about the safety and efficacy is not readily available.

AIDS/STDs

For both biologic and social reasons, young women of color are more likely to develop a sexually transmitted disease than men or white women. In addition to HIV/AIDS, the Centers for Disease Control and Prevention (CDC) monitor three reportable STDs: chlamydia, gonorrhea, and syphilis. Screening tests are available for all three, and all can be effectively treated with antibiotics. In the United States an estimated 55,400 new HIV infections were diagnosed in 2006, 24% of them among women, and 9,579 AIDS cases were diagnosed among women, representing about 27% of the total for that year.[37] More than 1.2 million cases of chlamydia, 336,742 cases of gonorrhea, and 13,500 cases of primary and secondary syphilis were reported to the CDC in 2008, at least half among women, but approximately 70% of chlamydia infections and 50% of gonorrhea infections are asymptomatic; therefore, the actual number of affected women is likely to be considerably higher. Because sexually transmitted human papilloma virus, genital herpes, and hepatitis are not reportable, accurate estimates of incidence and possible coinfections are not known.

Studies of CAM use among individuals with STDs other than HIV/AIDS are sparse, but patterns are consistent with those observed in HIV/AIDS. In a cohort of 391 HIV-positive women in Alabama and Georgia, of whom 85% were African American, 58.6% reported using CAM including vitamin supplements (36%), religious healing (27%), dietary modification (22%), and herbal agents (16%).[38] CAM use was more prevalent among women aged ≥ 35 years than younger women, as well as among women with higher education, uninsured women, and women who had been HIV-positive for over 4 years compared with those who had been diagnosed more recently. Vitamin users were more likely than nonusers to be white. Women with a history of three or more HIV-related infections were also more likely to be CAM users than those with fewer infections.

In a more recent survey, 914 (618 male and 296 female) HIV-infected participants in the HIV Research Network in the eastern, midwestern, southern, and western United States were asked, "Did you receive treatment from any alternative therapist, for example a massage therapist, acupuncturist, herbalist, or other alternative practitioner in the past 6 months?" Only 16% responded affirmatively. In a model including gender, race/ethnicity, HIV risk factors, CD4 count, illicit drug use, HIV-1 RNA, insurance, employment, education, Highly Active Antiretroviral Therapy (HAART) and mental healthcare visits, the factors that predicted having received treatment from a CAM practitioner were illicit drug use, having at least a college education, and seeing a mental healthcare provider.[3]

Another study explored strategies to cope with fatigue among 100 HIV-positive individuals (two-thirds male), aged 50 years or older. About 45% of those who reported fatigue used herbal agents, special juices, meditation, massage, or acupuncture, along with more conventional treatments, to control that symptom.[39]

Breast Cancer

Breast cancer is the most commonly diagnosed cancer among American women.[40] Among cancer patients, those with breast cancer are the most likely to use CAM therapies in conjunction with their conventional treatment.[41] The modalities most commonly used included vitamins, minerals, botanicals, and other dietary supplements.[14,15,41,42]

Numerous studies in the United States[14,15,42–58] and in other countries[28,59–73] have examined CAM use by breast cancer patients. Most surveys have asked about general categories of CAM use (vitamins/minerals, herbal therapies, special diets, homeopathy, acupuncture, energy

healing, etc.), with very few reporting use of specific dietary supplements. The majority of these studies use convenience samples (e.g., clinic populations); few are population based. Some studies examine patterns of CAM use before and after breast cancer diagnosis and some examine patterns of CAM use concurrent with different types of conventional breast cancer therapy.

Demographic characteristics associated with use of any CAM therapies among breast cancer patients include younger age, higher education in most studies but not all, higher household income, type of medical insurance, not being married, engaging in regular exercise, and not smoking. Disease and treatment characteristics associated with general CAM use among breast cancer patients include having a recent diagnosis with more advanced disease. Most patients received chemotherapy treatment, radiation therapy, and breast-conserving surgery. CAM use was associated with breast cancer-related symptoms and pain.

Among breast cancer patients enrolled in the Nurses' Health Study use of different types of CAM was associated with demographic, disease, and behavioral characteristics.[44] For example, specific characteristics associated with dietary supplement use include older age, higher education, being white (as compared to nonwhite), having a lower BMI, moderate alcohol consumption, being physically active, receiving radiation therapy, and having had breast reconstruction. The investigators concluded that future studies should focus on predictors of individual categories of CAM use although few such studies have as yet been published.

The Pathways Study is recruiting newly diagnosed female breast cancer patients who are members of Kaiser Permanente Northern California; a prepaid integrated healthcare program to participate in a cohort study of prognosis.[74] Recruitment is ongoing with an expected enrollment of 4,300 participants by 2014. Data collection by phone interview includes detailed baseline and follow-up information on medical history, diet, physical activity, use of complementary and alternative therapies, and quality of life for linkage with detailed pathology data and treatment records. The study aims are to investigate effects of lifestyle and molecular factors, including diet, CAM use, and genetic polymorphisms, on breast cancer recurrence and survival. Baseline analyses have shown that use of pharmacologic and nonpharmacologic forms of CAM before and after diagnosis is highly prevalent in the ethnically diverse cohort of Pathways Study participants.[14,15]

Methodologic Issues Related to Studying CAM Use

Inconsistencies in the literature describing CAM use among women may be due to methodologic issues. In epidemiologic studies, a CAM therapy may be considered an "exposure" (i.e., a therapy that increases or decreases the risk of developing a disease) or an "outcome" (i.e., a therapy whose use may or may not result from having a disease). The research design of the study and its purpose will affect the results, as will the underlying disease patterns and distribution of CAM use in the study population. No two studies have asked women exactly the same questions about their CAM use. Questionnaires differ in the broad CAM categories identified and the descriptions of the specific modalities. They range from 5 broad domains (as per NCCAM) to 36 specific modalities. Among nutritional supplements, botanicals, and other biologicals, the items listed vary, and the questionnaires differ in assessment of individual doses, duration, and frequency of use. Data collection instruments also differ in timing of use in relation to specific needs such as before or after diagnosis of a condition or disease, and, if after diagnosis, during treatment for that disease. Study results may also vary due to secular trends in CAM and dietary supplement use among U.S. and non-U.S. populations. For example, mistletoe extract as a breast cancer therapy is common, even mainstream, in Europe, but rarely used in the United States.

A separate methodologic issue relates to the variability in the delivery or administration of specific CAM practices and differences in contents of substances used. Some observational epidemiologic studies examine the effects of use of a CAM modality on risk of developing a disease. For example, a study may examine the use of green tea on

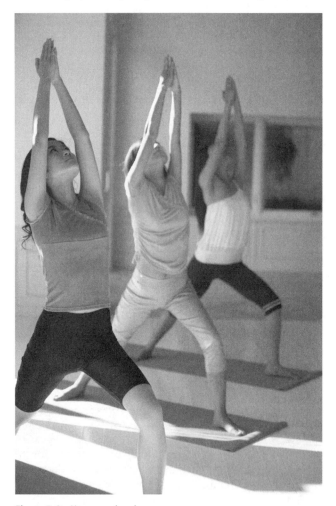

Figure 7-2 Yoga exercise class.

© Motoyuki Kobayashi/Digital Vision/Thinkstock

the risk of developing breast cancer. However, green tea is no longer just a hot drink made from boiled water and tea leaves as it is also available in the form of powdered extracts, liquid extracts, and food additives. These commercial preparations are known to vary in composition and quality. In addition, people vary in their habitual intake of traditionally brewed green tea, which may vary from several cups per day to infrequent consumption such as less than one cup per month. Their tea drinking habit may be long-standing over many years or a more recently established pattern. Similar variability exists in association with dietary supplements, mind-body practices including yoga, tai chi, and reiki as well as the training and practices of CAM providers. The research findings are strongly influenced by the methods developed by investigators who define the variables and collect data on specific CAM modalities.

Access to CAM and Conventional Care

Like conventional medicine, many CAM modalities, especially those that involve a practitioner or provider, have costs that are rarely covered by public or private health insurance. A few hospitals and other facilities offer CAM services supported by philanthropists or research funding enabling CAM modalities to be offered without charge. Cost, therefore, is often a barrier to use of certain types of CAM.

However, for some uninsured individuals, CAM and/ or traditional therapies may be less expensive and/or more culturally acceptable than conventional medical care. Cultural or religious traditions may give some individuals relatively easy access to CAM modalities in contrast to barriers to conventional care. In some communities, traditional values, especially those involving women's bodies and modesty, may limit use of mammographic or cervical cancer screening, diagnostic testing, or treatment.[50] Instead, women may resort to prayer or other traditional practices for conditions ranging from a breast lump to vaginal discharge.

One concern expressed by some clinicians concerns CAM use by individuals who need and would benefit from conventional medical care but instead rely on alternatives that may be less effective or potentially harmful. Cases have been reported in which patients died because they chose alternative medicine over conventional care or used a supplement that was either intrinsically harmful or contaminated.[75,76] However, this is not the norm; most patients do not forego conventional treatments. Instead they use both CAM and conventional medicine. Adverse events are not unique to CAM. Patients have died of iatrogenic causes and from being prescribed one form of standard medication rather than another form of the drug.[77] Some CAM users are explicitly motivated by distrust of conventional medicine and concerned about adverse effects of clinical treatments. However, others are generally health conscious and are more likely than non-CAM users to receive routine preventive services including screening. Paradoxically CAM users are more likely to use conventional practitioners than non-CAM users.[14,15,78] Most CAM users who have access to conventional medicine use both; few use only CAM, and few adverse events have been reliably linked to interactions of CAM combined with conventional treatment.

CAM from a Public Health Perspective

From a public health perspective, many CAM modalities may be beneficial for particular communities or a larger public and thus should be evaluated for their efficacy and cost-effectiveness in promoting health and preventing disease. Given their widespread use, it seems reasonable to assume that some benefit must result from CAM use and many appear to cause little harm. However, clinical trials of certain CAM modalities may be more challenging to conduct than assessment of a single pharmaceutical agent. Complex botanic agents require the knowledge of their source and quality before designing a study to determine appropriate doses and regimens. Approaches such as traditional Chinese medicine and other whole-systems approaches are complex treatments that may involve multiple modalities, some of which may change with the course of the disease. In addition, CAM modalities should be evaluated, at least initially, in the context in which they have been traditionally prepared and used. It is also important to consider population differences between those who traditionally used a CAM modality compared with those who are newly using the modality as biologic traits may influence the effects of the CAM modality. For example, clinical trials of soy for menopausal hot flashes have provided mixed results. We now know that Asian women, who have eaten soy for years as part of their traditional diet, have different intestinal flora than American women, and American women do not have the specific bacterial species that convert soy to estrogenic metabolites. Reproducing the conditions of use of an herbal agent, for example, outside its traditional setting is challenging. Even growing an herb in larger volume or in slightly different soil may affect its chemical composition, and investigators may not be able to correctly identify the active component or components or extract them without affecting their biologic properties. Testing the agent on study participants whose lifestyle is radically different from that of the traditional users also may affect the results and interpretation of research assessing the agent.

In the United States and other countries, urban areas such as New York City, San Francisco, and Los Angeles have large immigrant communities in which many people use the medicines of their home countries. Because these T/CAM modalities are in use among human populations, it is theoretically possible to conduct observational studies of their effects. But such studies require collecting voluminous demographic and behavioral data on users and nonusers, as well as on the patterns and contexts of their use of the modality of interest. Bodeker and colleagues[79] described a growing trend in which some highly publicized T/CAM modalities such as acupuncture are incorporated into the dominant medical system and now available in many western hospitals and medical settings. Other modalities are available in parallel health systems, operating largely outside the mainstream western medical system. Few physicians, nurses, or other allied health professionals are trained to ascertain use of CAM modalities by their patients. Some questionnaires ask only about self-medication whereas others question patients about visits to CAM practitioners. T/CAM categories may range from 5 broad domains to 36 or more individual therapies/modalities, or the instrument may use open-ended questions leaving respondents to define what they use and consider relevant to the interviewer's interest. Recall periods may be 12 months, 2 weeks, or a lifetime. And interviewing techniques (phone, face to face, postal questionnaire) and the language of the interview may yield different responses.

Some efforts have been made in the United States, Europe, and elsewhere to develop policy guidelines.[80,81] Standards of practice, licensing, and regulation have been developed for a small number of practices (e.g., massage, acupuncture, chiropractic, naturopathy). These developments may make it easier to find a practitioner and to determine his or her level of competence. But regulation and credentialing can also have a downside. They may create barriers to practice for some CAM providers, barriers to CAM access for low-income patients, and barriers to disclosure of CAM use in the conventional setting. If the potential of T/CAM for improved public health and health economics is to be evaluated, it will be necessary to develop policies regarding the assessment of safety, efficacy, quality, and access.

Summary

Traditional, complementary, integrative, and alternative medicines, however defined, are used by large numbers of women in the United States and throughout the world in developed and developing countries. These modalities are perceived as being of value and importance to those using them. Women use CAM for the promotion of wellness and health maintenance in addition to treatment of health conditions throughout their own lives. Women also mediate the CAM use of their families, as they do their family's conventional health care. Not all CAM use warrants "medicalization." However, it does behoove society to safeguard and possibly enhance public health by understanding the effects of CAM therapies, ensuring that products on the market are safe and contain the ingredients as labeled, that they are manufactured in conformity with good safety practices, that practitioners meet some standards of training and expertise, and that the underserved can obtain necessary and cost-effective care, be it conventional or CAM.

Discussion Questions

1. "Unconventional therapy" has been defined in several ways by several different organizations. Name the organizations and define the modalities in their terms.
2. Use of complementary and alternative health modalities have been used by many women for various clinical problems. Name some of the conditions and the therapies used.

3. Menopause is a time of transition for women. Recent research findings have added a level of anxiety and greater interest in CAM modalities. Describe the recent research on women's health, briefly note the findings that have created fear and resulted in alternatives to traditional therapies relied upon in the past.

4. Why do women fail to advise their treating physicians of the "unconventional" and self-selected therapies? What problems could arise for women deciding not to disclose their use of various alternative modalities?

5. CAM methodologies are diverse. How might physical movements such as yoga and tai chi provide a positive effect? Nutritional supplements vary in composition and dosages. Should the use of these preparations be discussed with treating clinicians? If so, why?

References

1. Eisenberg DM, Kessler RC, Foster C, et al. Unconventional medicine in the United States. Prevalence, costs, and patterns of use. *N Engl J Med.* 1993;328:246–252.

2. Eisenberg DM, Davis RB, Ettner SL, et al. Trends in alternative medicine use in the United States, 1990–1997: results of a follow-up national survey. *JAMA.* 1998;280:1569–1575.

3. Josephs JS, Fleishman JA, Gaist P, Gebo KA; HIV Research Network. Use of complementary and alternative medicines among a multistate, multisite cohort of people living with HIV/AIDS. *HIV Med.* 2007;8:300–305.

4. Barnes P, Powell-Griner E, McFann K, Nahin RL. Complemenary and alternative medicine use among adults. *Advance Data.* 2004:1–19.

5. Graham RE, Ahn AC, Davis RB, et al. Use of complementary and alternative medical therapies among racial and ethnic minority adults: results from the 2002 National Health Interview Survey. *J Natl Med Assoc.* 2005;97:535–545.

6. Tindle HA, Davis RB, Phillips RS, Eisenberg DM. Trends in use of complementary and alternative medicine by US adults: 1997–2002. *Altern Ther Health Med.* 2005;11:42–49.

7. Bair Y, Gold EB, Zhang G, et al. Use of complementary and alternative medicine during the menopause transition: longitudinal results from the Study of Women's Health Across the Nation. *Menopause.* 2008;15:32–43.

8. Kronenberg F, Cushman LF, Wade CM, et al. Race/ethnicity and women's use of complementary and alternative medicine in the United States: results of a national survey. *Am J Public Health.* 2006;96:1236–1242.

9. Newton KM, Buist DS, Keenan NL, et al. Use of alternative therapies for menopause symptoms: results of a population-based survey. *Obstet Gynecol.* 2002;100:18–25.

10. National Centers for Complementary and Alternative Medicine NIH. What is CAM? 2010. http://nccam.nih.gov/health/whatiscam/. Accessed November 16, 2010.

11. World Health Organization. Traditional medicine. Fact sheet no 134. 2008. http://www.who.int/mediacentre/factsheets/fs134/en/. Accessed December 1, 2010.

12. Fugh-Berman A, Ernst E. Herb-drug interactions: review and assessment of report reliability. *Br J Clin Pharmacol.* 2001;52:587–595.

13. Wade C, Chao M, Kronenberg F, et al. Medical pluralism among American women: results of a national survey. *J Womens Health.* 2008;17:829–840.

14. Greenlee H, Gammon MD, Abrahamson PE, et al. Prevalence and predictors of antioxidant supplement use during breast cancer treatment: the Long Island Breast Cancer Study Project. *Cancer.* 2009;115:3271–3282.

15. Greenlee H, Kwan ML, Ergas IJ, et al. Complementary and alternative therapy use before and after breast cancer diagnosis: the Pathways Study. *Breast Cancer Res Treat.* 2009;117:653–665.

16. McNaughton SA, Mishra GD, Paul AA, et al. Supplement use is associated with health status and health-related behaviors in the 1946 British birth cohort. *J Nutr.* 2005;135:1782–1789.

17. Jones L, Sciamanna C, Lehman E. Are those who use specific complementary and alternative medicine therapies less likely to be immunized? *Prev Med.* 2010;50:148–154.

18. Honda K, Jacobson JS. Use of complementary and alternative medicine among United States adults: the influences of personality, coping strategies, and social support. *Prev Med.* 2005;40:46–53.

19. Saxe GA, Madlensky L, Kealey S, et al. Disclosure to physicians of CAM use by breast cancer patients: findings from the Women's Healthy Eating and Living Study. *Integr Cancer Ther.* 2008;7:122–129.

20. Brett KM, Burt CW. Utilization of ambulatory medical care by women: United States, 1997–98. *Vital Health Stat.* 2001;13:1–46.

21. Green CA, Pope CR. Gender, psychosocial factors and the use of medical services: a longitudinal analysis. *Soc Sci Med.* 1999;48:1363–1372.

22. Druss BG, Rosenheck RA. Association between use of unconventional therapies and conventional medical services. *JAMA.* 1999;282:651–656.

23. Ni H, Simile C, Hardy AM. Utilization of complementary and alternative medicine by United States adults: results from the 1999 national health interview survey. *Med Care.* 2002;40:353–358.

24. Paramore LC. Use of alternative therapies: estimates from the 1994 Robert Wood Johnson Foundation National Access to Care Survey. *J Pain Symptom Manage.* 1997;13:83–89.

25. Thomas K, Coleman P. Use of complementary or alternative medicine in a general population in Great Britain. Results from the National Omnibus survey. *Am J Public Health.* 2004;26:152–157.

26. Astin JA, Reilly C, Perkins C, Child WL. Breast cancer patients' perspectives on and use of complementary and alternative medicine: a study by the Susan G. Komen Breast Cancer Foundation. *J Soc Integr Oncol.* 2006;4:157–169.

27. Mansky PJ, Wallerstedt DB. Complementary medicine in palliative care and cancer symptom management. *Cancer J.* 2006;12:425–431.

28. Nagel G, Hoyer H, Katenkamp D. Use of complementary and alternative medicine by patients with breast cancer: observations from a health-care survey. *Support Care Cancer.* 2004;12:789–796.

29. Wells M, Sarna L, Cooley ME, et al. Use of complementary and alternative medicine therapies to control symptoms in women living with lung cancer. *Cancer Nurs.* 2007;30:45–55; quiz 56-47.

30. Chao MT, Wade C, Kronenberg F. Disclosure of complementary and alternative medicine to conventional medical providers: variation by race/ethnicity and type of CAM. *J Natl Med Assoc.* 2008;100:1341–1349.

31. Women's Health Initiative Investigators. Risks and benefits of estrogen plus progesterone in healthy postmenopausal women: principal results from the Women's Health Initiative randomized controlled trial. *JAMA.* 2002;288:321–333.

32. Newton KM, Buist DS, Keenan NL, et al. Use of alternative therapies for menopause symptoms: results of a population-based survey. *Obstet Gynecol.* 2002;100:18–25.

33. Gold E, Bair Y, Zhang G, et al. Cross-sectional analysis of specific complementary and alternative medicine (CAM) use by racial/ethnic group and menopausal status: the Study of Women's Health Across the Nation (SWAN). *Menopause.* 2007;14:612–623.

34. Bair Y, Gold, EB, Zhang, G, et al. Use of complementary and alternative medicine during the menopause transition: longitudinal results from the Study of Women's Health Across the Nation. *Menopause.* 2008;15:32–43.

35. Upchurch DM, Chyu L, Greendale GA, et al. Complementary and alternative medicine use among American women: findings from The National Health Interview Survey, 2002. *J Womens Health.* 2007;16:102–113.

36. Mahady GB, Parrot J, Lee C, et al Botanical dietary supplement use in peri- and postmenopausal women. *Menopause.* 2003;10:65–72.

37. Hall HL, Song R, Rhodes P, et al. Estimation of HIV incidence in the United States. *JAMA.* 2008;300:520–529.

38. Mikhail IS, DiClemente R, Person S, et al. Association of complementary and alternative medicines with HIV clinical disease among a cohort of women living with HIV/AIDS. *J Acquir Immune Defic Syndr.* 2004;37:1415–1422.

39. Siegel K, Brown-Bradley CJ, Lekas HM. Strategies for coping with fatigue among HIV-positive individuals fifty years and older. *AIDS Patient Care.* 2004;18:275–288.

40. American Cancer Society. Breast Cancer Facts & Figures 2009–2010.

41. Gansler T, Kaw C, Crammer C, Smith T. A population-based study of prevalence of complementary methods use by cancer survivors: a report from the American Cancer Society's studies of cancer survivors. *Cancer.* 2008;113:1048–1057.

42. Patterson RE, Neuhouser ML, Hedderson MM, et al. Types of alternative medicine used by patients with breast, colon, or prostate cancer: predictors, motives, and costs. *J Altern Complement Med.* 2002;8:477–485.

43. Ashikaga T, Bosompra K, O'Brien P, Nelson L. Use of complimentary and alternative medicine by breast cancer patients: prevalence, patterns and communication with physicians. *Support Care Cancer.* 2002;10:542–548.

44. Buettner C, Kroenke CH, Phillips RS, et al. Correlates of use of different types of complementary and alternative medicine by breast cancer survivors in the nurses' health study. *Breast Cancer Res Treat.* 2006;100:219–227.

45. Burstein HJ, Gelber S, Guadagnoli E, Weeks JC. Use of alternative medicine by women with early-stage breast cancer. *N Engl J Med.* 1999;340:1733–1739.

46. Carpenter CL, Ganz PA, Bernstein L. Complementary and alternative therapies among very long-term breast cancer survivors. *Breast Cancer Res Treat.* 2009;116:387–396.

47. Demark-Wahnefried W, Peterson B, McBride C, et al. Current health behaviors and readiness to pursue life-style changes among men and women diagnosed with early stage prostate and breast carcinomas. *Cancer.* 2000;88:674–684.

48. Henderson JW, Donatelle RJ. Complementary and alternative medicine use by women after completion of allopathic treatment for breast cancer. *Altern Ther Health Med.* 2004;10:52–57.

49. Lafferty WE, Tyree PT, Devlin SM, et al. Complementary and alternative medicine provider use and expenditures by cancer treatment phase. *Am J Manag Care.* 2008;14:326–334.

50. Lee MM, Lin SS, Wrensch MR, et al. Alternative therapies used by women with breast cancer in four ethnic populations. *J Natl Cancer Inst.* 2000;92:42–47.

51. Lengacher CA, Bennett MP, Kip KE, et al. Frequency of use of complementary and alternative medicine in women with breast cancer. *Oncol Nurs Forum.* 2002;29:1445–1452.

52. Morris KT, Johnson N, Homer L, Walts D. A comparison of complementary therapy use between breast cancer patients and patients with other primary tumor sites. *Am J Surg.* 2000;179:407–411.

53. Navo MA, Phan J, Vaughan C, et al. An assessment of the utilization of complementary and alternative medication in women with gynecologic or breast malignancies. *J Clin Oncol.* 2004; 22:671–677.

54. Newman V, Rock CL, Faerber S, et al. Dietary supplement use by women at risk for breast cancer recurrence. The Women's Healthy Eating and Living Study Group. *J Am Diet Assoc.* 1998;98:285–292.

55. Rock CL, Newman VA, Neuhouser ML, et al. Antioxidant supplement use in cancer survivors and the general population. *J Nutr.* 2004;134:3194S–3195S.

56. Shen J, Andersen R, Albert PS, et al. Use of complementary/alternative therapies by women with advanced-stage breast cancer. *BMC Complement Altern Med.* 2002;2:8.

57. VandeCreek L, Rogers E, Lester J. Use of alternative therapies among breast cancer outpatients compared with the general population. *Altern Ther Health Med.* 1999;5:71–76.

58. Wyatt G, Sikorskii A, Wills CE, Su H. Complementary and alternative medicine use, spending, and quality of life in early stage breast cancer. *Nurs Res.* 2010;59:58–66.

59. Balneaves LG, Kristjanson LJ, Tataryn D. Beyond convention: describing complementary therapy use by women living with breast cancer. *Patient Educ Couns.* 1999;38:143–153.

60. Boon H, Stewart M, Kennard MA, et al. Use of complementary/alternative medicine by breast cancer survivors in Ontario: prevalence and perceptions. *J Clin Oncol.* 2000;18:2515–2521.

61. Boon HS, Olatunde F, Zick SM. Trends in complementary/alternative medicine use by breast cancer survivors: comparing survey data from 1998 and 2005. *BMC Womens Health.* 2007;7:4.

62. Chen Z, Gu K, Zheng Y, et al. The use of complementary and alternative medicine among Chinese women with breast cancer. *J Altern Complement Med.* 2008;14:1049–1055.

63. Downer SM, Cody MM, McCluskey P, et al. Pursuit and practice of complementary therapies by cancer patients receiving conventional treatment. *BMJ.* 1994;309:86–89.

64. Ezeome ER, Anarado AN. Use of complementary and alternative medicine by cancer patients at the University of Nigeria Teaching Hospital, Enugu, Nigeria. *BMC Complement Altern Med.* 2007;7:28.

65. Gray RE, Fitch M, Goel V, et al. Utilization of complementary/alternative services by women with breast cancer. *J Health Soc Policy.* 2003;16:75–84.

66. Helyer LK, Chin S, Chui BK, et al. The use of complementary and alternative medicines among patients with locally advanced breast cancer—a descriptive study. *BMC Cancer.* 2006;6:39.

67. Maher EJ, Young T, Feigel I. Complementary therapies used by patients with cancer. *BMJ.* 1994;309:671–672.

68. Moschen R, Kemmler G, Schweigkofler H, et al. Use of alternative or complementary therapy in breast cancer patients—a psychological perspective. *Support Care Cancer.* 2001;9:267–274.

69. Rees RW, Feigel I, Vickers A, et al. Prevalence of complementary therapy use by women with breast cancer. A population-based survey. *Eur J Cancer.* 2000;36:1359–1364.

70. Risberg T, Lund E, Wist E, et al. Cancer patients use of nonproven therapy: a 5-year follow-up study. *J Clin Oncol.* 1998;16:6–12.

71. Salminen EK, Lagstrom HK, Heikkila S, Salminen S. Does breast cancer change patients' dietary habits? *Eur J Clin Nutr.* 2000;54:844–848.

72. Salminen E, Bishop M, Poussa T, et al. Dietary attitudes and changes as well as use of supplements and complementary therapies by Australian and Finnish women following the diagnosis of breast cancer. *Eur J Clin Nutr.* 2004;58:137–144.

73. Yap KP, McCready DR, Fyles A, et al. Use of alternative therapy in postmenopausal breast cancer patients treated with tamoxifen after surgery. *Breast J.* 2004;10:481–486.

74. Kwan ML, Ambrosone CB, Lee MM, et al. The Pathways Study: a prospective study of breast cancer survivorship within Kaiser Permanente Northern California. *Cancer Causes Control.* 2008;19:1065–1076.

75. Chiu J, Yau T, Epstein RJ. Complications of traditional Chinese/herbal medicines (TCM)—a guide for perplexed oncologists and other cancer caregivers. *Support Care Cancer.* 2009;17:231–240.

76. Meijerman I, Beijnen JH, Schellens JH. Herb-drug interactions in oncology: focus on mechanisms of induction. *Oncologist.* 2006;11:742–752.

77. Nerich V, Limat S, Demarchi M, et al. Computerized physician order entry of injectable antineoplastic drugs: an epidemiologic study of prescribing medication errors. *Int J Med Inform.* 2010;79:699–706.

78. Garrow D, Egede LE. Association between complementary and alternative medicine use, preventive care practices, and use of conventional medical services among adults with diabetes. *Diabetes Care.* 2006;29:15–19.

79. Bodeker G, Kronenberg F, Burford G. Policy and public health perspectives on traditional, complementary and alternative medicine: an overview. In: Bodeker G, Burford G, eds. *Traditional, Complementary & Alternative Medicine: Policy & Public Health Perspectives.* London: Imperial College Press; 2007:9–38.

80. House of Lords Select Committee on Science and Technology. Sixth Report: Complementary and Alternative Medicine. 2000. www.publications.parliament.uk/pa/ld199900/ldselect/ldsctech/123/12301.htm. Accessed November 15, 2010.

81. White House Commission on Complementary and Alternative Medicine Policy. Final Report of the White House Commission on Complementary and Alternative Medicine Policy. 2002. (http://www.whccamp.hhs.gov/. Accessed November 16, 2010.

Sexual Health Across the Life Span

Puberty

Tamarra James-Todd, PhD, MPH

Introduction

Much research has been dedicated to the study of puberty in women. The importance of puberty as a health outcome lies in its variability at onset, which serves as a proxy for lifetime estrogen exposure. As such, early puberty, or longer exposure to endogenous estrogen, is associated with a number of chronic diseases and conditions, including breast cancer. For centuries, geographic, ethnic, and socioeconomic variations in puberty have been documented. Onset of puberty has changed over time, suggesting that puberty is not regulated simply by genetics but also by environmental factors. These factors include nutrition, exposure to certain types of chemicals, and socioeconomic position.

Puberty is defined as the beginning of the period in which an individual is capable of reproducing. However, puberty includes the entire process of sexual maturation, culminating in menarche in girls. Since the earlier measures of puberty are often less pronounced, many epidemiologic studies have primarily focused on the terminal end of puberty—menarche—as the main outcome. Fewer studies have evaluated earlier pubertal events as the primary outcome, such as height velocity, breast development (thelarche), or pubic hair development (adrenarche). Although earlier research suggest a high correlation between earlier pubertal events and age at menarche, as high as 0.86,[1–2] recent studies suggest that the correlation between the early and late events of puberty are weaker, approximately r = 0.3.[1] A number of factors may be contributing to this phenomenon, including secular changes in earlier pubertal events, along with stabilization of later pubertal events. Alternatively, different sensitivities of early and late pubertal events to environmental and social factors could be contributing to the lower correlation between early and late pubertal events. As such, it may be important to consider the benefits and limitations to using particular pubertal measurements in epidemiologic studies of puberty and particular health outcomes.

In Table 8-1, an overview of the benefits and limitations of the use of specific pubertal measurements in

Table 8-1

Pubertal events and measurement issues

	Thelarche	Andrenarche	Height Velocity	Menarche
Gold Standard	Tanner Staging for breast development	Tanner Staging for pubic hair development	Height measurements each year	Assessed prospectively through follow-up of girls prior to onset
Alternative Assessment Method	Recall age at breast development	Recall age at pubic hair development	Recall height	Recalled or status quo
Reliability	Recall is poor;[6] Gold standard is observer dependent	Recall is poor; Gold standard is observer dependent	Recall is poor; Gold standard is observer dependent	Most studies have shown moderate reliability of recalled age at menarche
Main Issues or Concerns About Using Measures in Epidemiologic Studies	Without palpation, adipose tissue may lead to misclassification	Dependent on adrenal androgens in girls, so does not provide information about pituitary-ovarian maturity	Need for repeated measurements may be expensive and lead to loss to follow-up	Distant from the onset of puberty, depends on tempo, and may involve entire axis

epidemiologic studies is provided. Age at menarche is obtained either through asking participants whether they have reached menarche, asking if they can recall their age at menarche, or evaluating the onset of menarche prospectively. Typically, breast and pubic hair development are assessed by a physician using Tanner staging, which was developed in 1962.[3] With this process, five stages ranging from preadolescent to mature stage are documented by an independent physician reader. Figure 8-1 shows stages 2–5 (stage 2 typically denotes the first pubertal stage). These stages are typically identified visually, which has led to some concerns regarding thelarche misclassification due to lack of palpation to distinguish between breast and fat tissue.[4]

An additional concern about which pubertal measure to use when designing a study includes whether the particular question of interest is sensitive to the pathway leading to a given pubertal event. For example, thelarche may arise from a relatively complex set of events that ultimately lead to the development of breast, whereas menarche may be initiated from the activation of estrogen.[5] Specific issues surrounding data collection and sources of confounding should also be considered when determining the specific measure of puberty to use. Other measurements of puberty that may be important to consider are the length of time between the early and late events of puberty, as well as the coefficient of variation in a given measurement of puberty.

Tanner Stage	Breast	Pubic Hair
Stage 2	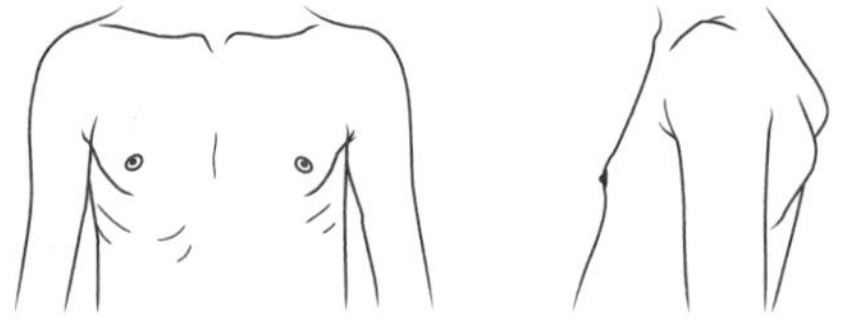 Breast bud stage and elevation of breast and papilla as small mound, enlarged areola diameter	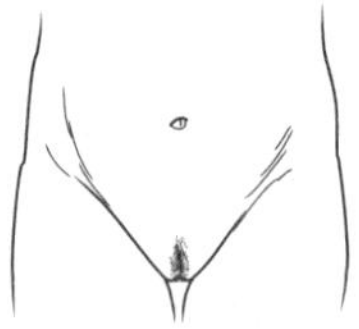 Sparse growth of long, slightly pigmented, downy hair along labia
Stage 3	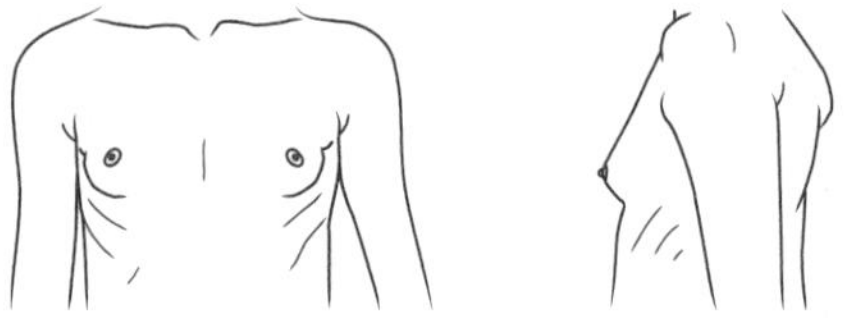 Further enlargement of breast and areola with no separation of contours	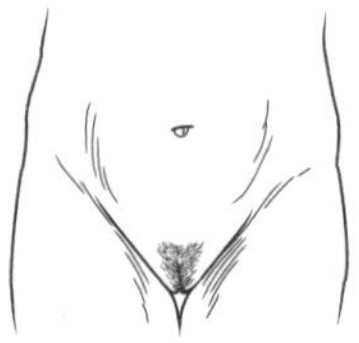 Darker, coarser, and more curled hair spreads to the junction of the pubes
Stage 4	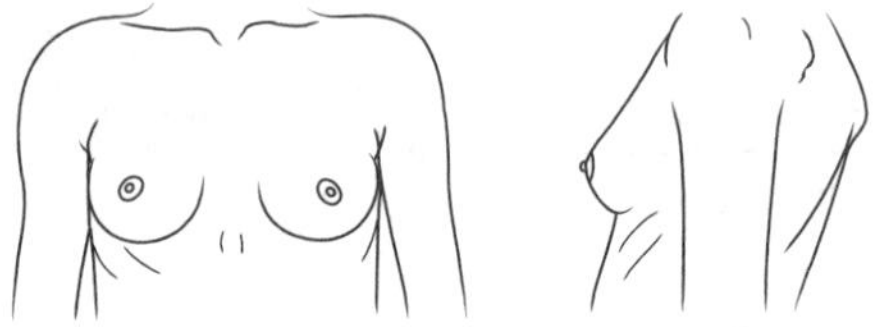 Projection of the areola and papilla to form a secondary mound above the level of the breast	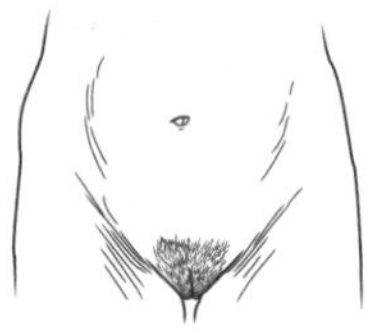 Adult hair, but covers a smaller area than most adults
Stage 5	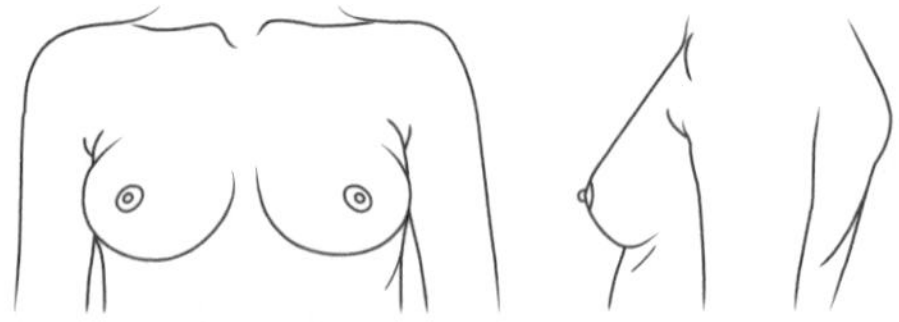 Mature stage with projection of papilla only; areola has recessed to general contour of breast	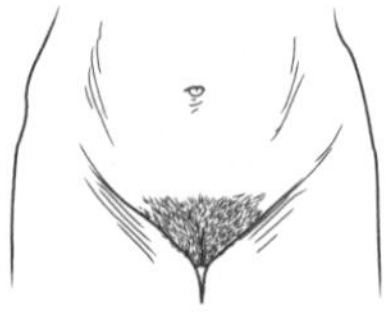 Adult quantity and type of hair with a triangular distribution

Figure 8-1 Tanner Developmental Staging.

Source: Courtesy of Jonathan Todd. Adapted from Marshall WA, Tanner JM. Variations in pattern of pubertal changes in girls. *Arch Dis Child*. 1969;44: 291–303.

Secular Trends in Puberty in the United States

Age at Menarche in the United States

In 1982, Grace Wyshak and Rose Frisch published an article showing secular trends in age at menarche declining over the past 150 years.[6] Although the average age at menarche was between 15 and 17 years of age around the 1800s in Europe, by 1960 the average age at menarche in most European countries and in the United States was between 13 and 13.5 years of age.[6] This decline in age at menarche has been mainly attributed to improvements in nutrition and social conditions[2].

Although the decline in age at menarche during the early part of the 20th century was steady and has been consistently reported,[5] conflicting evidence exists for a decline in age at menarche during second half of the 20th century and early portion of the 21st century. In particular, inconsistent data exist on whether age at menarche has continued to decline from 1960 to present.[7] Data from the National Health and Nutrition Examination Survey third cycle (NHANES III, 1988–1994) analyzed approximately 7,000 girls from the ages of 1–16 years. The average age at menarche was 12.54 years, a slight decrease since the National Health Examination Survey (NHES) cycle one.[8] In 2005, the NHANES 1999–2002 was published showing a mean age at menarche to be 12.34 years.[9] However, blacks and Mexican Americans were overrepresented in this sample and may have contributed to a decrease in age at menarche.[9] The 1997 Pediatric Research in Office Settings (PROS) study reported a mean age at menarche of 12.88 years, which was similar to the age at menarche reported 25 years earlier in the NHES.[10] Interestingly, the largest decline in age at menarche was reported between 1973 and 1994 with a 2- month decline in age at menarche in white girls and a 9.5 month decline in age at menarche in black girls who participated in the Bogalusa Heart Study.[11] With the exception of black girls in the Bogalusa study, most U.S. studies of menarche suggest either a modest decline or a plateau of age at menarche in the later 20th century. However, these mixed conclusions coupled with possible geographic and racial/ethnic variations still make it difficult to concretely state whether a secular trend exists. If one does, it is not nearly as drastic as that which occurred in the earlier portion of the 20th century.

Breast Development

Although age at menarche still serves as a primary outcome in many studies, an increasing number of researchers are evaluating thelarche as a primary endpoint. Part of the increasing use of thelarche rather than age of menarche has resulted from prospective studies by Danish researchers who found significantly earlier breast development among girls born between 2006 and 2008 compared with those born twenty years earlier.[12] Evidence that age at thelarche has declined comes from a number of studies.

In 1969, Marshall and Tanner reported the mean age at stage 2 (B2) for breast development as 11.15 years.[13]

This study concluded that the onset of puberty occurred sometime between 8.5 years and 13 years in girls.[13] In 1997, the PROS study reported a substantially earlier age for B2 in black girls compared to white girls—8.9 years and 10.0 years, respectively.[10] This finding along with several other studies suggests that girls may be developing breasts a full year earlier in recent years, compared to 40 years ago. In fact, a 2008 expert panel concluded that there were sufficient data to suggest or establish a secular trend in the onset of breast development,[7] which was a public health concern.

Pubic Hair Development

In conjunction with breast development, pubic hair development has become an increasing primary pubertal outcome of interest. Differing from breast development, appearance of pubic hair is a response to increases in adrenal androgens in girls, providing no information for the maturing pituitary-ovary axis.[5] That said, age at onset of breast development and age at first appearance of pubic hair are moderately correlated.[14] In fact, almost 70% of pubic hair and breast development was concordant in a large U.S.-based probability sample.[15] However, the order of these events varies, with some girls developing breast first, whereas others develop pubic hair first.[13]

In the United States, a limited number of studies have evaluated growth of pubic hair over time, making it difficult to determine whether secular trend changes have occurred. However, the Bogalusa Heart Study reported 10.86 years for whites and 10.13 years for blacks entering puberty stage 2 (PH2) for pubic hair development in the 1970s.[16] The 1990s PROS study reported a slightly earlier age at PH2 in whites and a much more drastic decline in age at PH2 in blacks, 10.51 and 8.78 years, respectively.[10] However, with little data available before the 1980s and a limited number of studies using this as a primary measure, there is insufficient evidence to determine whether a secular trend toward earlier pubic hair development in girls exists[7] although existing data has suggested appearance of pubic hair has occurred at younger ages among black compared with white girls living in the United States.

Height and Height Velocity

Rapid growth or height is another hallmark of puberty in girls. As such, girls who reach menarche earlier tend to be of shorter stature compared to girls who reach menarche later. Height increased dramatically between 1800 and 1950, with height in European countries increasing by > 10 cm.[17] Children who ranged in age from 10–14 years had the greatest height increase.[17] Like other pubertal measures, it is more difficult to determine whether trends in height have continued to change since the mid-20th century. However, recent studies from Belgium, Australia, and England have shown an increase of up to 2.5 cm for children born since 1960.[18–21] A study from Bogalusa, Louisiana, also noted an increase in height between the period of 1973 and 1992.[17] The greatest increase occurred in preadolescents, blacks, and boys.[17] However, girls between the ages of 9 and 12 years experienced a significant increase in height of 0.8 cm for white girls and 1.5 cm for black girls during this time interval.[17] This may suggest that height is still increasing, even during the more recent decades, which would parallel with decreases in age at onset for other pubertal events. However, more data are needed in this area to confirm secular changes in height during the last half of the 20th century.

Racial and Ethnic Variations in Puberty

In a well-cited 1969 *New England Journal of Medicine* article on age at menarche, Zacharias and Wurtman noted that:

> "It is virtually impossible to isolate the effects of racial factors on sexual development. In the first place, very few populations exist that are racially pure; most commonly, many constitutional types are present in each person. Secondly, racial factors, like climate, cannot be separated from socioeconomic influences such as habitat and nutrition."[22]

Racial/Ethnic Differences in Age at Menarche

Racial/ethnic differences in age at menarche have been well-documented in epidemiologic research. In the 1930s Nicholas Michelson conducted a study comparing 1,397 black girls to 1,922 white girls in the United States. He found that black girls reached menarche later than white girls (13.4 years and 13.1 years, respectively).[23] Although the black participants in his study were born earlier than the white participants, Michelson concluded that the 4-month difference in age at menarche noted between blacks and whites was primarily attributed to socioeconomic differences.[23] Specifically, he reported that blacks in the study had poorer nutrition than whites, which led to a delay in menarche.

By the mid-20th century, age at menarche had declined somewhat and was more similar between blacks and whites. For example, data from the National Health and Examination Study (1960–1962) showed that black and white women between 18 and 34 years of age reported a mean age at menarche of 12.85 years and 12.72 years, respectively. However, overall mean values for all women in the study showed that blacks reached menarche earlier than whites possibly due to biased recall by women age 34 years and/or possibly secular changes had occurred in age at menarche of girls younger than age 18.

By the late 20th century, black girls showed a significantly earlier age at menarche compared to white girls. In fact, black girls had a 40% increased likelihood of reaching menarche earlier than white girls in the Bogalusa Heart Study.[11] Results were similar in both NHANES III and the Bogalusa Heart Study.[17, 24] Limited data are available on Hispanic girls in the United States; however, a study by Anderson et al. found only a 3-week difference in age at menarche between NHANES III (1988–1994) participants and NHANES 1999–2002 among Mexican American participants, with respective mean ages at menarche of 12.45 and 12.39 years.[9] Despite the limited data on Hispanic girls, it appears that black and white girls have reached menarche earlier throughout the 20th century, with a more pronounced decrease and earlier age at menarche seen in blacks. Reasons for this decline in age at menarche are unknown. Genetic differences between blacks and whites have been implicated as the main factor; however, the relatively short time interval during which this downward shift in age has occurred suggests environmental influences are more likely, especially recent racial/ethnic changes in diet and body size.

Racial/Ethnic Differences in Breast and Pubic Hair Development

More recent studies have documented racial/ethnic differences in the onset of earlier pubertal events. In the NHES cycle III (1966–1970), the 50th percentile age for B3 was 10.29 years for black girls, 11.52 years for white girls.[25] Approximately 20 years later, NHANES III found that the 50th percentile for B3 was almost a full year earlier in black girls but stable for white girls.[25] Pubic hair development in these two populations was similar to breast development, with black girls reaching Tanner stage 3 of pubic hair development earlier than white girls.[25] The hallmark PROS study also noted differences in breast and pubic hair development among black and white girls. In particular, 77.4% of black girls had reached B2 or PH2 by age 9 years, whereas only 38.2% of white girls had reached either B2 or PH2 by age 9.[10] This study, along with others highlighted a potential need to consider setting the normal age for breast and pubic hair development at 8 years of age or earlier, as well as considering earlier cut points for different racial/ethnic groups.[2] However, these data should be taken with caution, as the reasons for these differences could be affected not only by genetic variations but also social and environmental factors, which may be difficult to tease apart in most epidemiologic studies. Of particular concern is the substantial overlap between race/ethnicity and socioeconomic status,[26] discussed next. In addition, tempo of puberty may explain some of these differences.

Socioeconomic Status and Puberty

Socioeconomic status (SES) is a multifaceted determinant of health, which includes education, income, and parental occupation.[26] SES also incorporates nutrition, healthcare access, and overall living environment.[22] As such, SES is indirectly related to many health outcomes, including sexual maturation of children. In fact, many studies have found an association between socioeconomic status and age at menarche.[22] However, the direction of this association varies between countries and seems to be highly dependent on industrialization and nutritional factors specific to particular populations. For example, higher SES is associated with early age at menarche in developing countries.[27–28] On the other hand, in developed countries such as the United States, higher SES is associated with later age at menarche compared to girls of lower SES. [29–30]

SES is thought to operate primarily through nutrition status,[22] especially in developing countries, where malnutrition affects growth and development of lower SES girls. In developed countries, it has been proposed that overnutrition, leading to childhood obesity, explains earlier age at menarche.[31] In the United States, lower SES is associated with larger body size.[32] In fact, body size is known to be associated with age at menarche, with heavier girls being more likely to reach menarche earlier. More detail on this association is provided later. Despite the inverse association between lower SES and increased body size, one study found that body size did not explain the association between SES and age at menarche in a racially diverse population of girls.[30]

Several other ways in which SES could operate to influence age at menarche have been explored including father's absence from the home as a potential stressor and the weathering effect on developing girls.[33–34] These studies show that father's absence is associated with earlier age at menarche as the absence could have an adverse economic impact on the environment in which a girl is reaching sexual maturity. More research is needed to understand the influence of SES and stress on age at menarche. Yet, there appears to be a fairly strong association between age at menarche and allostatic load,[35] an indicator of cumulative stress due to chronic or repeat exposure to stress hormones. Future studies must elucidate the specific pathways in which SES can operate to alter age at menarche. In addition, more studies are needed to determine the association between SES and age at earlier pubertal events. Prospective study designs should be used to evaluate SES markers of stress and their association with the onset of puberty.

Nutrition, Body Size, and Puberty

Along with the increase of earlier age at puberty in girls, there has also been an increase in childhood obesity. In fact, rates of obesity among children between ages 6 and 11 years have tripled in the United States over the past 30 years from 6.5% in 1980 to 19.8% in 2008.[36] One reason for the rise in obesity is increased fat and sugar intake, including increased consumption of sugar sweetened beverages.[37] In addition, changes in cultural activity levels have limited physical exercise with children engaged in more sedentary behaviors.[38] As such, more children are at increased risk of adult chronic diseases including dyslipidemia, diabetes, and heart disease.[39]

The parallel trends of childhood obesity and earlier age at puberty have not gone unnoticed by researchers. In fact, multiple studies have evaluated the association of body size and age at puberty (typically menarche), with consistent results. For example, in the National Heart, Lung, and Blood Institute's National Growth and Health Study, white girls who reached menarche earlier were 3.5 kg heavier compared to girls who reached menarche at midonset (12–13 years) and 6.5 kg heavier compared to girls with late-onset menarche (age 14 or older).[40] Skinfold thickness had a similar association with puberty in this study.

Patterns are similar for black girls, which is particularly important to note given their earlier age at menarche and increased risk of being overweight and obese compared to white girls ages 6–11 years.[41] Other research, including the PROS study, had similar findings with girls who had not started breast development having a –0.029 body mass index (BMI) Z-score compared to girls who were at B2 or higher, who had a BMI Z-score of 0.551.[31] A study using data from NHANES III found that early maturers had a twofold increased odds of obesity compared to normal weight girls (95% CI = 1.1–3.5).[42] However, it remains unclear as to whether increased adiposity is a direct cause of earlier age at puberty. More specifically, the question still remains whether increased adiposity initiates puberty earlier in girls with higher BMI or if earlier puberty causes increased adiposity.

In 1971, Frisch and Revelle proposed the answer to this question—that a critical body weight of 48 kg must be reached in order to initiate and maintain menarche.[43] This theory was modified due to limited variability in this study and a range of actual weights at which the girls reached menarche. The modified theory stated that there was a critical fat mass needed for the initiation and maintenance of menarche.[44] However, this specific theory remains controversial.

A recent study from Sweden suggested that Frisch may be correct in thinking that higher body fatness precedes menarche; peak height velocity was negatively correlated with BMI in children ages 2–8 years.[45] In a separate study, increased BMI during early childhood was associated with earlier average age at puberty.[46] Higher body fatness also appears to initiate appearance of pubic hair although this operates under the adrenal androgen mechanism.[47]

Body size could be linked to puberty through leptin, a protein that controls body weight and signals to the brain the body's energy stores. In fact, leptin provides a permissive signal to allow puberty to progress.[48] Since leptin levels are highly correlated with body fatness (r = 0.88), children who have greater body fatness would be expected to have higher leptin levels and be more likely to enter puberty earlier.[48] Several studies have shown an association between increased serum leptin concentrations in girls during puberty. A study conducted in Great Britain reported that leptin levels increased as girls progressed from stages B2 to B5 of breast development.[49] Increased leptin levels has been shown to occur as early as 2 years prior to increases in serum lutenizing hormone (LH) or estradiol levels, which is consistent with the idea that a certain level of energy stores is needed to allow puberty to progress.[48] This finding is another piece of evidence supporting the hypothesis that a certain amount of weight or body fat must be obtained to permit puberty to progress. However, assessment is complicated given the potential role of estrogen and progesterone to promote storage of body fat resulting in subsequent weight gain or conversely, the early signs of puberty including increased body fat and weight gain may be due to activation of hormones, such as estrogen and progesterone.

Prenatal and Early Childhood Exposures and Age at Puberty

Early life factors have been linked to alterations in pubertal growth and development. One association that has been consistently found is that of small for gestational age (SGA) and earlier age at menarche. Many studies have concluded that girls who were SGA reach menarche approximately 5–10 months earlier than normal birth weight girls.[50] Many children who are born SGA experience rapid weight gain during early childhood, which is thought to be one of the mechanisms through which birth size leads to alterations in the timing of puberty.[50] Together, SGA and rapid weight gain may be operating through changes in follicular stimulating hormone (FSH), insulin, and other hormones that can alter the onset of puberty.[51] In addition, changes in leptin levels could alter body fatness and ultimately age at menarche. In fact, SGA is associated with hyperinsulinemia, lower levels of sex-hormone binding globulin, and excess central fat.[52] As such, SGA may simply be a marker for insulin sensitivity and leptin levels, which can interact with other hormones and lead to the onset of puberty.

Other factors that have been studied include in utero and early childhood exposure to cigarette smoke, with inconclusive results. A recent study reported girls who had been exposed during fetal development to 10 or more cigarettes per day experienced menarche 2.8 months earlier than unexposed girls.[53] Girls whose mothers quit smoking while pregnant reached menarche 4.1 months earlier compared to unexposed girls.[53] Passive smoke exposure during childhood also appears to increase the risk of earlier age at menarche.[54] On the other hand, heavy smoking has been associated with delayed menarche.[55] It is possible that dose and timing of cigarette exposure could lead to different associations with menarche as exposures early in pregnancy may coincide with fetal ovary development. Although the association of active and passive exposure in utero to cigarette smoke with age of menarche of daughters remains uncertain, the frequency of cigarette smoking among women has significantly declined improving the health of mothers and their children.

Endocrine-Disrupting Chemicals

Declines in puberty and age at menarche have raised concerns about exposure to environmental chemicals, particularly a class of chemicals known as endocrine disruptors (EDCs). Used in a variety of processes, including food packaging, cosmetics, and pesticides, EDCs mimic circulating endocrine hormones and may have agonistic and/or antagonistic effects on basic biologic processes.[56] Chemicals may have multiple modes of action depending on dose, duration, frequency, and the developmental stage at the time of exposure. In fact, EDCs could affect the onset of puberty by influencing the neuroendocrine hypothalamic-pituitary axis as well as ovaries, breast, and vaginal tissue.[56]

EDCs have been shown in several case series to be associated with early puberty. For example, a case series reported that children exposed to estrogen in hair products developed pubic hair and breast tissue as early as 14 months.[57] When these products were no longer used, breast and pubic hair regressed. In 2001, a study linked suspected EDC exposure with early breast development and ovarian cysts.[58] A recent report indicated an association between the use of certain types of hair products and earlier age at menarche; these products are thought to contain multiple EDCs, including phthalates and parabens.[59]

More definitive evidence for an association of EDCs with modifications to puberty has been noted in studies evaluating EDC exposure in utero and early life. A study in Michigan of anglers and their wives found an increase of in utero DDE (a metabolite of the insecticide DDT) levels of 15 µg/liter reduced age at menarche by 1 year ($P = 0.04$).[60] In a similar region of the United States, PBBs (polybrominated biphenyls) contaminated the Michigan food chain and were also associated with earlier age at menarche.[61] Specifically, girls with high levels of PBB in utero exposure reached menarche almost 6 months earlier than girls with low levels of PBB.[61] Similar findings existed for PBB exposure through breastmilk.[61] On the other hand, a number of studies have not found an association between early life exposures to dioxin or persistent organochlorine pollutants and age at menarche.[62–63] Nevertheless, certain chemicals may lead to earlier puberty if exposure occurs during a critical or sensitive period in development.

Although exposure to some EDCs may initiate earlier age at puberty, others may delay puberty. For example, exposure to toxic metals, including lead, has been shown to delay puberty. Also, high levels of dioxin have been associated with delayed breast development in girls.[64] These studies indicate EDCs have the potential to alter pubertal timing; however, more studies are needed to better understand which chemicals influence onset of puberty. Furthermore, the effect of exposures at differing stages of development and by routes of exposure need to be determined.

Long-Term Sequelae of Age of Menarche

As mentioned earlier, age at puberty is of particular interest because of its association with several health outcomes. Perhaps the most noted association is of early menarche and breast cancer.[65] More specifically, early age at menarche is associated with greater lifetime exposure to estrogen, which subsequently has been associated with increased risk of breast cancer.[66] However, age at menarche is a relatively moderate breast cancer risk factor, conferring a 5–20% increased risk for each earlier year at menarche compared with ages 12–13.[67]

Another chronic disease associated with early menarche is asthma; women with menarche between ages 8 and 11 had increased risk of asthma compared with those who were older at menarche (OR = 1.80; 95% CI = 1.09–2.97).[68] Early menarche is also associated with cardiovascular disease (CVD).[69] For example, a Danish study reported an increased risk of hypertension (HR = 1.13, 95% CI = 1.02–1.24) and cardiovascular mortality (HR = 1.28, 95% CI = 1.02–1.62) among women with early menarche compared to women whose menarche occurred at age 12 or older.[69] An association has also been found between early puberty and increased lipid levels in adulthood, which provides further evidence for an association between menarche and CVD.[70] Of interest, a report from the Australian Longitudinal Study of Ageing found an association between early menarche and all-cause mortality, with respondents who reported reaching menarche before age 12 having a 28% increased risk of mortality over the follow-up period compared to women who reached menarche at age 12 or older.[71] An inverse association between early menarche and all-cause mortality has also been found.[72]

One of the strongest and most consistent associations is the relationship of age at menarche and adult body size.[73] In fact, a European study suggests that the association between early age at menarche and type 2 diabetes almost purely arises from increased postmenarcheal body size.[74] Girls who reach menarche earlier are shorter and heavier than girls who reach menarche later. However, disentangling body size as either a precursor to age at menarche or an intermediary on the pathway between menarche and a particular disease outcome is challenging. Further complicating this association is that body size could operate both as an antecedent and as an intermediate factor. This complex association requires special modeling techniques when considering research questions that assess age at menarche and outcomes associated with body size. Interestingly, recent findings from the Nurses' Health Study showed an association between early age at menarche and type 2 diabetes, despite body size.[75] Regardless, age at menarche appears to be a predictor of subsequent poor health outcomes, whether mediated through body size or not. As such, it is important to consider menarche and possibly other pubertal events as potentially modifiable risk factors that could alter subsequent risk of chronic diseases.

Summary

Puberty is an important public health measure as the sexual maturation resulting in menarche spans several years and is influenced by both genetic aspects and environmental exposures. Although genetic factors account for approximately half of the variation in age at menarche,[76] decreasing age at the onset of puberty over the past century suggests that environmental changes play a major role. Nutrition, physical inactivity, and chemical exposures are just a few potential risk factors that have been examined. In addition, researchers have investigated racial/ethnic and socioeconomic variations in age at puberty, noting that African Americans and girls of lower SES are more likely to reach puberty earlier. Furthermore, timing and route of environmental exposures are important factors to consider.

Earlier age at puberty has implications for long-term health status including increased susceptibility to a number of chronic diseases or conditions in adulthood, such as obesity, breast cancer, and possibly CVD. Although much research has been dedicated to documenting differences across generations and specific populations, new research is needed to identify potential environmental exposures associated with decreases in age at puberty during our modern era. Also, more research is required to understand the racial/ethnic and socioeconomic variations in developmental stages. By identifying these factors and understanding the mechanisms through which they alter puberty, we can reduce the burden of disease among adults associated with earlier age at puberty.

Discussion Questions

1. How has the timing of sexual development changed over the past century?
2. What body changes are indicators of puberty?
3. What chemicals are being studied in relation to trends in age of menarche?
4. Define the importance of characteristics associated with earlier age at sexual development.

References

1. Biro FM, Huang B, Crawford PB, et al. Pubertal correlates in black and white girls. *J Pediatr.* 2006;148:234–240.
2. Kaplowitz P. Pubertal development in girls: secular trends. *Curr Opin Obstet Gynecol.* 2006;18:487–491.
3. Tanner JM, ed. *Growth at Adolescence.* Oxford: Blackwell Scientific Publications; 1962.
4. Kaplowitz PB, Oberfield SE. Reexamination of the age limit for defining when puberty is precocious in girls in the United States: implications for evaluation and treatment. Drug and Therapeutics and Executive Committees of the Lawson Wilkins Pediatric Endocrine Society. *Pediatrics.* 1999;104:936–941.
5. Parent AS, Teilmann G, Juul A, et al. The timing of normal puberty and the age limits of sexual precocity: variations around the world, secular trends, and changes after migration. *Endocr Rev.* 2003;24:668–693.
6. Wyshak G, Frisch RE. Evidence for a secular trend in age of menarche. *N Engl J Med.* 1982;306:1033–1035.
7. Euling SY, Herman-Giddens ME, Lee PA, et al. Examination of US puberty-timing data from 1940 to 1994 for secular trends: panel findings. *Pediatrics.* 2008;121:S172–191.
8. Anderson SE, Dallal GE, Must A. Relative weight and race influence average age at menarche: results from two nationally representative surveys of US girls studied 25 years apart. *Pediatrics.* 2003;111:844–850.
9. Anderson SE, Must A. Interpreting the continued decline in the average age at menarche: results from two nationally representative surveys of US girls studied 10 years apart. *J Pediatr.* 2005;147:753–760.
10. Herman-Giddens ME, Slora EJ, Wasserman RC, et al. Secondary sexual characteristics and menses in young girls seen in office practice: a study from the Pediatric Research in Office Settings network. *Pediatrics.* 1997;99:505–512.
11. Freedman DS, Khan LK, Serdula MK, Dietz WH, Srinivasan SR, Berenson GS. The relation of menarcheal age to obesity in childhood and adulthood: the Bogalusa heart study. *BMC Pediatr.* 2003;3:3.
12. Aksglaede L, Sorensen K, Petersen JH, et al. Recent decline in age at breast development: the Copenhagen Puberty Study. *Pediatrics.* 2009;123:e932–939.
13. Marshall WA, Tanner JM. Variations in pattern of pubertal changes in girls. *Arch Dis Child.* 1969;44:291–303.
14. Christensen KY, Maisonet M, Rubin C, et al. Characterization of the correlation between ages at entry into breast and pubic hair development. *Ann Epidemiol.* 2010;20:405–408.
15. Schubert CM, Chumlea WC, Kulin HE, et al. Concordant and discordant sexual maturation among US children in relation to body weight and BMI. *J Adolesc Health.* 2005;37:356–362.
16. Foster TA, Voors AW, Webber LS, et al. Anthropometric and maturation measurements of children, ages 5 to 14 years, in a biracial community—the Bogalusa Heart Study. *Am J Clin Nutr.* 1977;30:582–591.
17. Freedman DS, Khan LK, Serdula MK, et al. Secular trends in height among children during 2 decades: The Bogalusa Heart Study. *Arch Pediatr Adolesc Med.* 2000;154:155–161.
18. Gerver WJ, De Bruin R, Drayer NM. A persisting secular trend for body measurements in Dutch children. The Oosterwolde II Study. *Acta Paediatr.* 1994;83:812–814.
19. Hitchcock NE, Gracey M, Maller RA, Wearne KL. The Busselton children's survey, 1983. Body size from five to 16 years of age. *Med J Aust.* 1986;145:373–376.

20. Vercauteren M, Susanne C. The secular trend of height and menarche in Belgium: are there any signs of a future stop? *Eur J Pediatr.* 1985;144:306–309.

21. Chinn S, Rona RJ. Secular trends in weight, weight-for-height and triceps skinfold thickness in primary schoolchildren in England and Scotland from 1972 to 1980. *Ann Hum Biol.* 1987;14:311–319.

22. Zacharias L, Wurtman RJ. Age at menarche. Genetic and environmental influences. *N Engl J Med.* 1969;280:868–875.

23. Michelson N. Studies in the physical development of Negroes. IV. Onset of puberty. *Am J Physical Anthropol.* 1943;1:417–424.

24. Chumlea WC, Schubert CM, Roche AF, et al. Age at menarche and racial comparisons in US girls. *Pediatrics.* 2003;111:110–113.

25. Sun SS, Schubert CM, Liang R, et al. Is sexual maturity occurring earlier among US children? *J Adolesc Health.* 2005;37:345–355.

26. Williams DR, Collins C. US Socioeconomic and Racial Differences in Health. In: LaViest TA, ed. *Race, Ethnicity, and Health: A Public Health Reader.* San Francisco, CA: Jossey-Bass; 2000.

27. Pasquet P, Biyong AM, Rikong-Adie H, et al. Age at menarche and urbanization in Cameroon: current status and secular trends. *Ann Hum Biol.* 1999;26:89–97.

28. Qamra SR, Mehta S, Deodhar SD. A mixed-longitudinal study on the pattern of pubertal growth: relationship to socioeconomic status and caloric-intake—IV. *Indian Pediatr.* 1991;28147–156.

29. Braithwaite D, Moore DH, Lustig RH, et al. Socioeconomic status in relation to early menarche among black and white girls. *Cancer Causes Control.* 2009;20:713–720.

30. James-Todd T, Tehranifar P, Rich-Edwards J, Titievsky L, Terry MB. The impact of socioeconomic status across early life on age at menarche among a racially diverse population of girls. *Ann Epidemiol.* 2010;20:836–842.

31. Kaplowitz PB, Slora EJ, Wasserman RC, Pedlow SE, Herman-Giddens ME. Earlier onset of puberty in girls: relation to increased body mass index and race. *Pediatrics.* 2001;108:347–353.

32. Popkin BM, Gordon-Larsen P. The nutrition transition: worldwide obesity dynamics and their determinants. *Int J Obes Relat Metab Disord.* 2004;28:S2–9.

33. Belsky J, Steinberg L, Draper P. Childhood experience, interpersonal development, and reproductive strategy: and evolutionary theory of socialization. *Child Dev.* 1991;62:647–670.

34. Belsky J, Steinberg LD, Houts RM, et al. Family rearing antecedents of pubertal timing. *Child Dev.* 2007;78:1302–1321.

35. Allsworth JE, Weitzen S, Boardman LA. Early age at menarche and allostatic load: data from the Third National Health and Nutrition Examination Survey. *Ann Epidemiol.* 2005;15:438–444.

36. Childhood Overweight and Obesity. *Overweight and obesity* 2010; http://www.cdc.gov/obesity/childhood/. Accessed February 7, 2011.

37. Bleich SN, Wang YC, Wang Y, Gortmaker SL. Increasing consumption of sugar-sweetened beverages among US adults: 1988–1994 to 1999–2004. *Am J Clin Nutr.* 2009;89:372–381.

38. Anderson PM, Butcher KE. Childhood obesity: trends and potential causes. *Future Child.* 2006;16:19–45.

39. Freedman DS, Mei Z, Srinivasan SR, Berenson GS, Dietz WH. Cardiovascular risk factors and excess adiposity among overweight children and adolescents: the Bogalusa Heart Study. *J Pediatr.* 2007;150:12–17 e12.

40. Biro FM, McMahon RP, Striegel-Moore R, et al. Impact of timing of pubertal maturation on growth in black and white female adolescents: The National Heart, Lung, and Blood Institute Growth and Health Study. *J Pediatr.* 2001;138:636–643.

41. CDC Grand Rounds: Childhood Obesity in the United States. *MMWR Morb Mortal Wkly Rep.* 2011;60:42–46.

42. Wang Y. Is obesity associated with early sexual maturation? A comparison of the association in American boys versus girls. *Pediatrics.* 2002;110:903–910.

43. Frisch RE, Revelle R. Height and weight at menarche and a hypothesis of menarche. *Arch Dis Child.* 1971;46:695–701.

44. Frisch RE. Body fat, menarche, fitness and fertility. *Hum Reprod.* 1987;2:521–533.

45. He Q, Karlberg J. BMI in childhood and its association with height gain, timing of puberty, and final height. *Pediatr Res.* 2001;49:244–251.

46. Lee JM, Appugliese D, Kaciroti N, Corwyn RF, Bradley RH, Lumeng JC. Weight status in young girls and the onset of puberty. *Pediatrics.* 2007;119:e624–630.

47. Charkaluk ML, Trivin C, Brauner R. Premature pubarche as an indicator of how body weight influences the onset of adrenarche. *Eur J Pediatr.* 2004;163:89–93.

48. Kaplowitz PB. Link between body fat and the timing of puberty. *Pediatrics.* 2008;121:S208–217.

49. Ahmed ML, Ong KK, Morrell DJ, et al. Longitudinal study of leptin concentrations during puberty: sex differences and relationship to changes in body composition. *J Clin Endocrinol Metab.* 1999;84:899–905.

50. Hernandez MI, Mericq V. Pubertal development in girls born small for gestational age. *J Pediatr Endocrinol Metab.* 2008;21:201–208.

51. Hernandez MI, Mericq V. Impact of being born small for gestational age on onset and progression of puberty. *Best Pract Res Clin Endocrinol Metab.* 2008;22:463–476.

52. Ibanez L, Ong K, Dunger DB, de Zegher F. Early development of adiposity and insulin resistance after catch-up weight gain in small-for-gestational-age children. *J Clin Endocrinol Metab.* 2006;91:2153–2158.

53. Shrestha A, Nohr EA, Bech BH, Ramlau-Hansen CH, Olsen J. Smoking and alcohol use during pregnancy and age of menarche in daughters. *Hum Reprod.* 2011;26:259–265.

54. Windham GC, Bottomley C, Birner C, Fenster L. Age at menarche in relation to maternal use of tobacco, alcohol, coffee, and tea during pregnancy. *Am J Epidemiol.* 2004;159:862–871.

55. Ferris JS, Flom JD, Tehranifar P, Mayne ST, Terry MB. Prenatal and childhood environmental tobacco smoke exposure and age at menarche. *Paediatr Perinat Epidemiol.* 2010;24:515–523.

56. Mouritsen A, Aksglaede L, Sorensen K, et al. Hypothesis: exposure to endocrine-disrupting chemicals may interfere with timing of puberty. *Int J Androl.* 2010;33:346–359.

57. Tiwary CM. Premature sexual development in children following the use of estrogen- or placenta-containing hair products. *Clin Pediatr (Phila).* 1998;37:733–739.

58. Larriuz-Serrano MC, Perez-Cardona CM, Ramos-Valencia G, Bourdony CJ. Natural history and incidence of premature thelarche in Puerto Rican girls aged 6 months to 8 years diagnosed between 1990 and 1995. *P R Health Sci J.* 2001;20:13–18.

59. James-Todd TM, Terry MB, Rich-Edwards JW, Deierlein AL, Senie RT. Childhood hair product use and earlier age at menarche in a racially diverse study population: a pilot study. *Ann Epidemiol.* 2011;21(6):461–465.

60. Vasiliu O, Muttineni J, Karmaus W. In utero exposure to organochlorines and age at menarche. *Hum Reprod.* 2004;19:1506–1512.

61. Blanck HM, Marcus M, Tolbert PE, et al. Age at menarche and Tanner stage in girls exposed in utero and postnatally to polybrominated biphenyl. *Epidemiology.* 2000;11:641–647.

62. Axmon A. Menarche in women with high exposure to persistent organochlorine pollutants in utero and during childhood. *Environ Res.* 2006;102:77–82.

63. Warner M, Samuels S, Mocarelli P, et al. Serum dioxin concentrations and age at menarche. *Environ Health Perspect.* 2004;112:1289–1292.

64. Den Hond E, Roels HA, Hoppenbrouwers K, et al. Sexual maturation in relation to polychlorinated aromatic hydrocarbons: Sharpe and Skakkebaek's hypothesis revisited. *Environ Health Perspect.* 2002;110:771–776.

65. Apter D, Vihko R. Early menarche, a risk factor for breast cancer, indicates early onset of ovulatory cycles. *J Clin Endocrinol Metab.* 1983;57:82–86.

66. Vihko RK, Apter DL. The epidemiology and endocrinology of the menarche in relation to breast cancer. *Cancer Surv.* 1986;5:561–571.

67. Bernstein L, Teal CR, Joslyn S, Wilson J. Ethnicity-related variation in breast cancer risk factors. *Cancer.* 2003;97:222–229.

68. Macsali F, Real FG, Plana E, et al. Early age of menarche, lung function and adult asthma. *Am J Respir Crit Care Med.* 2010;183: 8–14.

69. Lakshman R, Forouhi NG, Sharp SJ, et al. Early age at menarche associated with cardiovascular disease and mortality. *J Clin Endocrinol Metab.* 2009;94:4953–4960.

70. Pierce MB, Kuh D, Hardy R. Role of lifetime body mass index in the association between age at puberty and adult lipids: findings from men and women in a British birth cohort. *Ann Epidemiol.* 2010;20:676–682.

71. Giles LC, Glonek GF, Moore VM, Davies MJ, Luszcz MA. Lower age at menarche affects survival in older Australian women: results from the Australian Longitudinal Study of Ageing. *BMC Public Health.* 2010;10:341.

72. Jacobsen BK, Heuch I, Kvale G. Association of low age at menarche with increased all-cause mortality: a 37-year follow-up of 61,319 Norwegian women. *Am J Epidemiol.* 2007;166:1431–1437.

73. Ong KK. Early determinants of obesity. *Endocr Dev.* 2010;19:53–61.

74. Lakshman R, Forouhi N, Luben R, et al. Association between age at menarche and risk of diabetes in adults: results from the EPIC-Norfolk cohort study. *Diabetologia.* 2008;51:781–786.

75. He C, Zhang C, Hunter DJ, et al. Age at menarche and risk of type 2 diabetes: results from 2 large prospective cohort studies. *Am J Epidemiol.* 2010;171:334–344.

76. Towne B, Czerwinski SA, Demerath EW, Blangero J, Roche AF, Siervogel RM. Heritability of age at menarche in girls from the Fels Longitudinal Study. *Am J Phys Anthropol.* 2005;128;210–219.

Sexuality and Sexual and Reproductive Health

Leslie M. Kantor, MPH and Gina Gambone, MPH

Introduction

Sexuality, an integral component of our humanity, includes physical, emotional, interpersonal, social, and spiritual aspects that can be approached from a variety of disciplinary perspectives, including historical, medical, psychologic, biologic, anthropologic, sociologic, demographic, religious, and epidemiologic. According to the World Association of Sexual Health:

Sexuality is an integral part of the personality of every human being. Its full development depends upon the satisfaction of basic human needs such as the desire for contact, intimacy, emotional expression, pleasure, tenderness and love. Sexuality is constructed through the interaction between the individual and social structures. Full development of sexuality is essential for individual, interpersonal, and societal well being."[1]

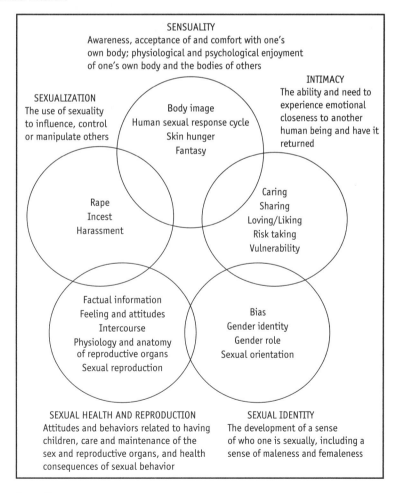

Figure 9-1 Interacting circles of sexuality.

Modified from Life Planning Education. Advocates for Youth, Washington DC. www.advocatesforyouth.org. Circles of Sexuality created by Dennis M. Dailey, Professor Emeritus, University of Kansas, based on the initial work of Harvey Gochros.

Another way to conceptualize sexuality is via the five overlapping circles of sexuality as presented in Figure 9-1 illustrating the various aspects of sexuality.

Sexuality Throughout the Life Course

People are sexual beings from birth until death, and their life trajectories are greatly influenced by their sexual decisions, including with whom to partner, whether and when to have children, and how much to conform to or resist gender expectations. Frequently in our society, the word sexuality is equated with sexual behavior, which is only one aspect of sexuality.

Sexuality is shaped by many forces and theories that may emphasize one set of influences over the others. For example, one view of sexuality, often referred to as "essentialism," suggests that biologic instincts and reproduction are dominant forces shaping sexuality. Another important theory, first posited by Freud and then developed by many other scholars, suggested that psychological processes, particularly early experiences with primary caretakers and within the family, were the major forces shaping sexual development. In addition, sexuality has been shaped by social forces.[2] Although a full exploration of the various approaches to thinking about sexuality is beyond the scope of this chapter, it is important to understand that myriad forces that shift over time and vary by culture shape sexuality.

The National Guidelines Task Force developed a set of concepts and topics related to sexuality that should be included in the curriculum from kindergarten through 12th grade. These guidelines suggested that sexually healthy adults exhibit the following life behaviors:[3]

- Appreciate one's own body.
- Be informed about reproduction as needed.
- Affirm that human development includes sexual development with or without reproduction and sexual experience.
- Interact with all genders in respectful and appropriate ways.
- Affirm one's own sexual orientation and respect the sexual orientations of others.
- Express love and intimacy in appropriate ways.
- Develop and maintain meaningful relationships.
- Avoid exploitative or manipulative relationships.
- Make informed choices about family options and relationships.
- Exhibit skills that enhance personal relationships.
- Identify and live according to one's own values.
- Take responsibility for one's own behavior.
- Practice effective decision making.
- Develop critical thinking skills.
- Communicate effectively with family, peers, and romantic partners.
- Enjoy and express one's sexuality throughout life.
- Express one's sexuality in ways that are congruent with one's values.
- Enjoy sexual feelings without necessarily acting on them.

- Discriminate between life-enhancing sexual behaviors and those that are harmful to self and/or others.
- Practice health-promoting behaviors and early identification of potential problems.
- Express one's sexuality while respecting the rights of others.
- Seek new information to enhance one's sexuality.
- Engage in sexual relationships that are consensual, honest, pleasurable, and protected.
- Use contraception effectively to avoid unintended pregnancy.
- Avoid contracting or transmitting a sexually transmitted disease, including human immunodeficiency virus (HIV).
- Act consistently with one's own values when dealing with an unintended pregnancy.
- Seek early prenatal care.
- Help prevent sexual abuse.
- Demonstrate respect for people with different sexual values.
- Exercise democratic responsibility to influence legislation dealing with sexual issues.
- Assess the impact of family, culture, media, and societal messages on one's thoughts, feelings, values, and behaviors related to sexuality.
- Critically examine the world around them for biases based on gender, sexual orientation, culture, ethnicity, and race.
- Promote the rights of all people to accurate sexuality information.
- Avoid behaviors that exhibit prejudice and bigotry.
- Reject stereotypes about the sexuality of different populations.
- Educate others about sexuality.

People learn about sexuality from their primary caregivers, other relatives and peers, and from the broader culture including media, schools, and religious institutions. Some life behaviors of sexually healthy adults are enhanced by what is learned from these sources whereas others are more challenging in the face of contradictory or confusing messages. For example, cultural ideas about beauty and sexiness frequently suggest that one must be young, thin, and white to be "hot." For people who do not fit into these categories, these pervasive cultural ideas are a challenge to maintaining good body image.

Body Image

Different cultures sexualize different parts of the body. In the United States, breasts are highly sexualized body parts whereas in many African countries, breasts are viewed more pragmatically for their role in feeding infants. Historically, various women's body parts have been seen as more or less sexualized—in early 20th century America legs were highly sexualized and kept concealed.[4] Today, women's clothing has changed, but body parts and their display continue to be seen as sexual or as nonerotic; these ideas are communicated through media, parents, and peers.

Body image is influenced by a range of factors with much critical attention focused on media's influences on girls and women. Poor body image may lead to a continuum of problems ranging from simple dissatisfaction to significant eating disorders such as bulimia and anorexia. Population-based studies of girls indicate a high level of dieting; approximately 45% of girls in grades 5 through 12 reported having been on a diet at least once compared to 20% of boys.[5] Not being overweight is "very important" to 69% of girls and 54% of boys.[5] Changing appearance is a multibillion dollar industry in the United States.

Adolescent Sexual Development

Adolescence is second to infancy as a life stage characterized by rapid physical, emotional, intellectual, interpersonal, and social changes. During adolescence, young people undergo the physical changes of puberty when they spend more time with and are more greatly influenced by peers. They receive extensive messages about gender, sexual orientation, sexual behavior and relationships from friends, family, religious institutions, and the media and generally form their first sexual relationship. Although most young people navigate the many challenges of adolescence successfully, others experience significant familial, social, and health challenges, some of which can have long-term implications.

From a public health perspective, key concerns for adolescents include helping young people develop and maintain close relationships with parents, family, and peers. Once they begin to engage in relationships including sexual expression, they need to be certain that sexual encounters are consensual, mutual, and pleasurable and include use of protection against sexually transmitted diseases and unplanned pregnancy.

Data on adolescent sexual behavior are available from two main sources: the National Survey of Adolescent Health (Add Health) and the Youth Risk Behavior Survey (YRBS). The Add Health program began with a nationally representative sample of 7th–12th graders in 1994–1995; the cohort of young people has been followed longitudinally with four in-home interviews, the most recent in 2008 when the cohort was ages 24–32. The YRBS cross-sectional survey is conducted every 2 years by the Centers for Disease Control and Prevention and provides data representative of grades 9 through 12. Both surveys include a variety of questions related to health including several pertaining to sexual behavior. However, neither study includes questions related to masturbation, most likely the first sexual behavior experienced by young people, which is discussed later in this chapter.

According to the YRBS of 2002, nearly half (48%) of 9th through 12th graders have had sexual intercourse at least once; 35% of students were sexually active (sex during the 3 months before the survey).[7] Among these 35% who indicated they were sexually active, 61.5% used condoms and 22.5% reported using alcohol or drugs before last sexual intercourse.[6] The average age of first intercourse among young women is 17.4 years and among young men it is 17 years.[7]

Another key issue for adolescents is development of a sexual identity and orientation, a key developmental task regardless of whether one is gay, lesbian, bisexual, or heterosexual. Unfortunately, pressures to be heterosexual combined with discrimination and harassment of young people who are or are perceived to be nonheterosexual can lead to serious problems for adolescents. According to the Gay, Lesbian and Straight Education Network's 2007 National School Climate Survey, 86.2% of lesbian, gay, bisexual, and transgender students indicated they had been verbally harassed, 44.1% reported physical harassment, 22.1% reported being physically assaulted at school in the past year because of their sexual orientation, 60.8% of students stated they felt unsafe in school because of their sexual orientation, and more than one-third (38.4%) felt unsafe because of their gender expression.[8]

Masturbation

Even prior to birth, there is evidence that fetuses may touch their genitals although no information exists on any sensations experienced. Touching the genitals is common among young children although the behavior is stigmatized in some cultures. Masturbation is often omitted from research on sexual behavior, which primarily is focused on partnered forms of sexual expression. The largest and most comprehensive study of sexual behavior among people ages 18–59 in the United States published in 1995 found that 60% of men and 40% of women masturbated in the year before the survey.[9] Among teens ages 14–17, 73.8% of males and 48.1% of females had masturbated. The likelihood of ever masturbating increased with age: at age 14, 62.6% of boys had masturbated compared to 79.8% at age 18. Among girls, 42.3% had masturbated at age 14 compared to 58% at age 17.[10] A study of older adults found that 63% of men and 32% of women ages 57–64 and 32% of men and 16% of women ages 75–85 masturbated in the past year.[11] A nationally-representative survey noted that among women ages 18–50, 52.5% had used vibrators in the past year.[12] Those reporting vibrator use were more likely to have had a recent gynecological exam and to report higher sexual functioning than women who had not used vibrators.

Adult Sexual Behavior

There have been few population-based studies of sexual behavior in the United States. The most comprehensive study undertaken to date was the National Health and Social Life Survey (NHSLS) in 1992 with 3,432 adult participants who were asked to provide detailed information about behaviors with all their sexual partners.[9] The NHSLS found that vaginal intercourse was the only nearly universal behavior engaged in by adults ages 18–59. Questions included oral and anal sex: among men 77% had engaged in active oral sex over their lifetimes (27% in their last sexual event). Among women, 68% had ever engaged in active oral sex (19% in their last sex event). When asked about having oral sex performed on them, 79% of men responded positively (28% at their last sex event) and 73% of women (20% at their last sex event).

Anal sex was reported by 26% of men at some point in their sexual history with 10% noting anal sex in the last year; among women, 20% indicated ever engaging in anal sex with 9% reporting anal sex in the last year.[9]

More recent data on sexual behavior from the National Survey of Family Growth (NSFG) focused on reproduction and included questions on a variety of sexual behaviors among men and women. The NSFG was conducted 10 years after the NHSLS and showed that 97% of males ages 25–44 had experienced vaginal intercourse, 90% reported oral sex with a female partner and 40% had engaged in anal intercourse at some point in their sexual experience.[13] Six percent of men reported oral or anal sex with a male partner. Among females aged 25–44, 98% had engaged in sexual intercourse, 88% had engaged in oral sex with a male partner, and 35% had engaged in anal intercourse. Eleven percent of women report sexual experience with another woman. The question asked of women on the NSFG related to sexual behavior with a same sex partner was: Have you ever had any sexual experience of any kind with another female?" In contrast, the questions asked of men regarding sexual contact with a male partner were specific about oral or anal sex behaviors.[13]

Fewer data are available regarding sexual behavior among adults older than reproductive age because most research funding is related to pregnancy. The aging of the population is bringing increased attention to sexuality among older adults. A recent study conducted on a nationally representative probability sample of people ages 57–85 showed that sexual activity remains prevalent among the elderly but declines with age (sex and sexual activity were defined for the study as "any mutually voluntary activity with another person that involves sexual contact, whether or not intercourse or orgasm occurs").[14] The percentage indicating sexual activity declined from 73% among 57- to 64-year-old men and women to 53% among 65- to 74-year-olds and 26% among women and men ages 75–85. Further, there were great gender disparities in the likelihood of having a spousal or intimate partner in the oldest age group surveyed. Among men aged 75–85, 78% had a spouse or intimate partner whereas only 40% of women had a spouse or intimate partner.[14] Among sexually active older adults age 57-85, a significant minority reported sexual problems including, for women, low desire (43%), difficulty with vaginal lubrication (39%), and inability to have an orgasm (34%). Among sexually active men, 37% noted erectile difficulties.

Sexual Relationships

There are a variety of types of relationships within which sexual activity takes place: between people who just met, people who define their relationship as "casual," people who define themselves as "just friends" but also engage in sexual behavior regularly, or within relationships that are longer term and may include cohabitation or marriage.

Marriage

Historically, among most societies and religions, marriage is the one setting in which sexual behavior was clearly sanctioned, but there is no evidence that any society has existed in which sexual behavior took place only within marriage. Reasons for marriage have shifted historically from largely economic or societal expectations to an emphasis on love and the quality of relationships between partners, including a satisfying sexual relationship.[15]

In the United States at any given time, about half the population lives in households led by married partners. In the 2000 census, 52% reported they were married and 26% were living alone. The American Community Survey for 2006–2008 showed that among people age 15 and older, 50.2% were married, 10.6% were divorced, 2.2% were separated and 30.8% were never married.[16] Across the life span, about 90% of women will marry at least once and this trend is predicted to continue.[17] In 2008, the marriage rate was 7.1 per 1,000 and the divorce rate was 3.5 per 1,000.[18]

Very few people marry as teenagers—by age 18, only 6% of women and 2% of men in the United States have married. However, 50% of American women have married by age 25 and 50% of American men by age 27.[19] Married men and women have lower mortality rates than their unmarried peers and are less likely to experience cancer, heart attacks, and surgery.[20] The positive relationships associated with marriage suggest healthier people are more likely to marry and remain married. Married partners provide emotional support and encourage healthful lifestyle choices that reduce morbidity and mortality although marriage can also contribute to a number of health problems when conflicts are frequent or marital satisfaction is low.

In a review of 64 articles, Kiecolt-Glaser and Newton examined associations between marital conflict and negative immunologically mediated disease outcomes; adverse physiologic changes resulting from marital conflict were greater for women and lasted longer.[20] Women experienced depression, pain, and poor oral health including development of periodontal disease associated with spousal conflict. A positive marital relationship for women linked with greater longevity was characterized by companionship and equal influence in making major decisions.[20]

Human Sexual Response Cycle

The first model of human sexual response—presented in 1966 by Masters and Johnson—proposed a linear four-stage physiological response to sexual stimuli for men and women: arousal, plateau, orgasm, and resolution.[21] In 1979, Kaplan added desire to the model, modifying it into what is now considered the traditional human sexual response cycle: desire, arousal, orgasm, and resolution (Figure 9-2).[21,22]

In the last decade, recognition that women's sexual response may be different from men's and not necessarily linear has challenged the traditional model. Whipple and Brash-McGreer proposed a circular model for women, including seduction (encompassing desire), sensations (excitement and plateau), surrender (orgasm), and reflection (resolution).[23] These authors suggested that

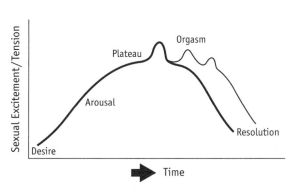

Figure 9-2 Traditional human sexual response.

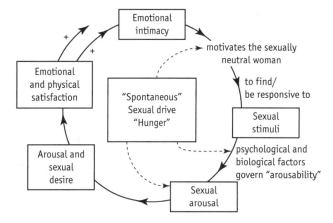

Figure 9-3 Non-linear female sexual response cycle.

Source: Reproduced with permission from Basson R. Female sexual response: the role of drugs in the management of sexual dysfunction. Obstet Gynecol 2001;98:350–353.

pleasure and satisfaction during a sexual experience can lead to the seduction phase of the next sexual experience, although dissatisfaction may hinder the next sexual experience. More recently, Basson proposed a nonlinear model of female sexual response that illustrated that the goal of sexual activity for women is physical and/or emotional satisfaction, which may or may not include orgasm (Figure 9-3).[22] Emotional intimacy and sexual stimuli play key roles, and many psychosocial factors (e.g., low self-image, past negative experiences, lack of safety) and biologic factors (e.g., hyperthyroidism, depression) can significantly affect a woman's sexual response.

Sexual Dysfunction

Sexual dysfunction in women includes a range of possible problems including lack of desire for sex, inability to achieve orgasm, problems with lubrication, pain during sex, anxiety during sex, or not finding sex pleasurable.[24] For men, sexual dysfunction includes lack of desire for sex, inability to achieve orgasm, inability to get or maintain an erection, ejaculating too quickly, pain during sex, anxiety during sex, or not finding sex pleasurable.[24] Treatment for sexual dysfunction may include education about sexuality, medication, counseling, or therapy. The development and marketing of Viagra and other medications designed to help men get and maintain erections has made pharmacological intervention a popular method for addressing sexual concerns. Indeed, some scholarly work is now examining how makers of Viagra and other treatments for erectile dysfunction are exaggerating the prevalence of erectile dysfunction in order to create markets for their products.[25] Clinical trials have also been undertaken to assess whether Viagra could be used as a treatment for low sexual desire or lack of orgasm among women. Thus far, treatments for male sexual dysfunction did not show any effectiveness in women. The working group on A New View of Women's Sexual Problems consisting of scholars, sexuality therapists, sexuality educators, and feminist activists has brought important attention to the ways sexual dysfunction has been defined so that normal variations in sexual desire, arousal, and response over the

life cycle have been pathologized: "Because there are no magic bullets for the socio-cultural, political, psychological, social or relational bases of women's sexual problems, pharmaceutical companies are supporting research and public relations programs focused on fixing the body, especially the genitals. The infusion of industry funding into sex research and the incessant media publicity about 'breakthrough' treatments have put physical problems in the spotlight and isolated them from broader contexts. Factors that are far more often sources of women's sexual complaints—relational and cultural conflicts, for example, or sexual ignorance or fear—are downplayed and dismissed."[26] As with all issues related to sexuality, it is important to understand the interplay of ideas about biology, gender, appropriate sexual behavior, and, indeed, the way that economics may influence ideas about sexuality in order to understand the ways that sexuality is framed and dealt with throughout society.

Pregnancy and Pregnancy Prevention in the United States

Women between the ages of 15 and 44 are considered to be of "reproductive age" because of typical physical development. Most women ovulate (begin to release eggs from the ovaries) by age 15 and begin to enter perimenopause by age 44. Perimenopause is the period before ovulation and menstruation cease when fertility declines as ovulation becomes more sporadic.

Puberty and the Menstrual Cycle

Girls experience puberty generally between ages 10 and 14 when the hormones produced by the hypothalamus (a gland located at the base of the brain that regulates temperature, sleep, emotions, sexual function, and behavior) stimulate the pituitary gland and the ovaries to produce estrogen and progesterone. Growth of pubic and underarm hair, breast enlargement, vaginal and uterine growth, widening hips, and increased height, weight, and fat distribution (secondary sexual characteristics) gradually occur during early phases of puberty. The composite of hormonal changes result in ovulation (release of an egg from the ovary) and menstruation (shedding of the lining of the uterus when no pregnancy occurs). Females are born with all of the ova (eggs) that they will ever have. At birth, ovaries generally contain about 400,000 ova, many more than will ever be released.[27]

Male puberty, which generally occurs between the ages of 13 and 15, includes secretion of the male hormone testosterone, which stimulates spermatogenesis (sperm production), and the development of secondary sexual characteristics (increased height and weight, broadening shoulders, growth of the testes and penis, pubic and facial hair growth, voice deepening, and muscle development).[27]

The external genitalia in girls and women are properly called the vulva and includes the mons pubis (a fatty mound that covers the pubic bone), the labia majora (outer lips of the vagina), the labia minora (the inner lips of the vagina), the vaginal opening, the urethral opening (opening of the urethra, a tube that carries urine from the bladder outside of the body), the clitoris (a small structure with sensitive nerve endings located within the labia minora),and the perineum (the space between the rectal opening and the vaginal opening). Stimulation of the clitoris is what leads to orgasm in girls/women (Figure 9-4).[27]

The internal reproductive anatomy includes the uterus, two ovaries, two fallopian tubes, the urethra, the pubic bone, and the rectum. Once ovulation begins, the lining of the uterus, the endometrium, proliferates and sheds monthly in response to hormonal changes. The lower portion of the uterus is called the cervix, and the opening to the cervix is called the os. Menstrual blood flows through the os into the vagina during menstruation (Figure 9-5).[27]

There are four phases to the menstrual cycle: the follicular phase, the ovulatory phase, the luteal phase and the menstrual phase.[28] The first day of menstruation is considered day 1 of the menstrual cycle; days 1-5 the first half of the follicular phase, involve several follicles containing oocytes (immature ova/egg cells) beginning to develop in response to the release of follicle stimulating hormone (FSH). In general, one follicle becomes "dominant" and produces increasing amounts of estrogen, which stimulates the release of luteinizing hormone (LH) and inhibits FSH, which suppresses development of other ova. During the ovulatory phase, LH levels are highest and the ovarian follicle "ruptures" and releases one ovum, which is moved into the fallopian tube by hairlike projections called cilia. This process is called ovulation (Figure 9-6). Increasing estrogen levels cause cervical mucus to become clear and profuse and the os to dilate. These two actions may facilitate pregnancy by encouraging the passage of sperm into the fallopian tubes. At other times in the menstrual cycle, the opening to the cervix (the os) closes, and cervical mucus becomes thicker, impeding progress of sperm through the os.[27]

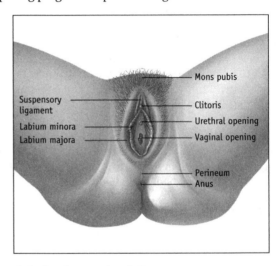

Figure 9-4 Female external genitalia.

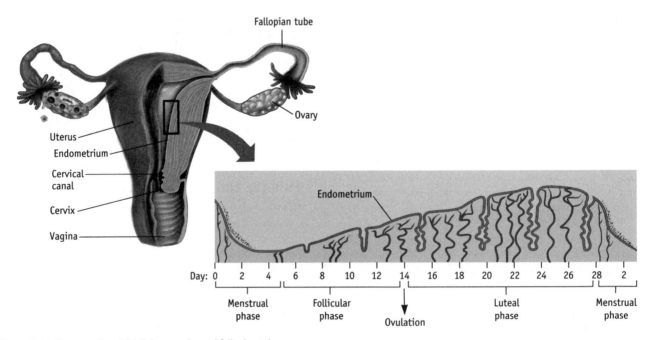

Figure 9-5 Uterus, endometrial lining, ovaries and fallopian tubes.

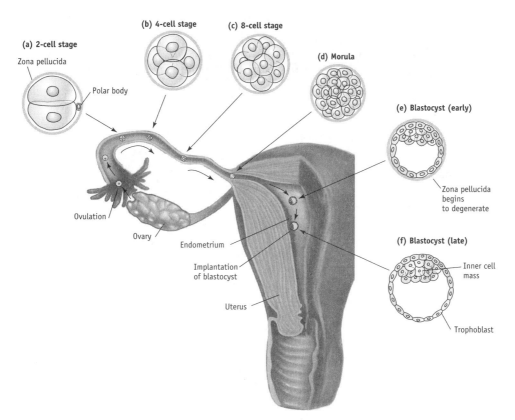

Figure 9-6 Ovulation.

The luteal phase of the cycle follows ovulation when the ruptured follicle is transformed into the corpus luteum, producing high levels of progesterone that cause the endometrium to thicken in preparation for possible implantation of a fertilized egg. If fertilization does not occur, the menstrual phase begins in which the corpus luteum shrinks and levels of both estrogen and progesterone drop. The withdrawal of estrogen and progesterone results in disintegration of the endometrial lining producing menstruation. The average menstrual cycle is 28–35 days, and menstrual flow varies from 3 to 7 days. Following menstruation, estrogen and progesterone levels are low, triggering release of cyclical hormones beginning the next cycle. If fertilization does take place, menstruation will not recur for the duration of the pregnancy.[27]

Menopause, the end of routine ovulation and menstruation, generally occurs between the ages of 45 and 55, with the average age 51.3.[29] Menopause is an entirely normal process but can be accompanied by bothersome symptoms including hot flashes, fatigue, moodiness, insomnia, decreased libido and sexual response, changes in memory, weight gain, and vaginal dryness. Until cessation of ovarian function is confirmed through a blood test and/or 1 year of no menses, women may continue to ovulate and, therefore, require contraception to prevent unintended pregnancy.[27]

During sexual intercourse between a male and a female, when a male ejaculates, semen is released into the vagina and transported through the uterus into the fallopian tubes. Fertilization can be successful only if intercourse depositing fresh semen is timed to ovulation, midcycle, when the ovum is transported down the fallopian tube.[28]

Ectopic pregnancy, a rare event, occurs when a fertilized egg becomes implanted outside the uterus, most often in a fallopian tube. Scarring of fallopian tubes caused by untreated sexually transmitted infections may impede the transport of a fertilized egg from the fallopian tubes to the uterus. If left undiagnosed or untreated, the fertilized egg grows in the fallopian tube and may result in tubal rupture. Without medical or surgical intervention, ectopic pregnancy may result in infertility, severe infection, or even death. Symptoms of ectopic pregnancy include pain in the vagina, abdomen, or lower back, vaginal bleeding or spotting, dizziness, fainting, and low blood pressure.[27]

Contraception

Women have several options to avoid unplanned pregnancy including hormonal and barrier methods in addition to male and female sterilization. In the United States, almost 9 in 10 women who are at risk for pregnancy (of reproductive age, sexually active, and not currently pregnant) are using a method of contraception.[30] However, not all couples use a contraceptive method correctly and consistently with each intercourse. When calculating the effectiveness rates of contraception, level of effectiveness in preventing pregnancy depends upon the shared experience of the partners because "perfect use" may differ from "actual use" (Table 9-1).[31]

Hormonal Methods

Hormonal methods deliver synthetic forms of the naturally occurring ovarian hormones estrogen and progesterone either in combination or progestin-only preparations that function effectively by preventing ovulation and thickening

Table 9-1

Percentage of women who experience an unintended pregnancy during the first year of typical use and the first year of perfect use of different forms of contraception. United States.

Method	Typical Use	Perfect Use
No method	85	85
Spermicides	29	18
Withdrawal	27	4
Fertility awareness-based methods	25	
Standard days method		5
Two-day method		4
Ovulation method		3
Sponge		
Parous women	32	20
Nulliparous women	16	9
Diaphragm	16	6
Condom		
Female	21	5
Male	15	2
Combined pill and progestin-only pill	8	0.3
Patch (OrthoEvra)	8	0.3
Vaginal ring (NuvaRing)	8	0.3
Injection (Depo-Provera)	3	0.3
IUD		
ParaGuard (copper T)	0.8	0.6
Mirena (LNG-IUS)	0.2	0.2
Implant (Implanon)	0.05	0.05
Female sterilization	0.5	0.5
Male sterilization	0.15	0.1

Source: Reproduced from Trussell J. Contraceptive efficacy. In: Hatcher RA, Trussell J, Nelson AL, Cates W, Kowal D, and Policar M (eds). Contraceptive Technology: Twentieth Revised Edition. New York NY: Ardent Media; 2011. p. 779–863.

cervical mucus, which prevents sperm from entering the os entrance of the uterus. Hormonal methods come in several forms: pill, patch, vaginal ring, injection, and implant.

Oral Contraceptives

Combined oral contraceptives are designed to be taken at approximately the same time each day with 3 weeks of active preparation and 1 week of placebo pills. Prevention of pregnancy may be jeopardized when some users skip pills, vary the time of day, or do not restart their active pills after the week of placebo pills on time. Progestin-only pills are recommended for postpartum women and those who experience side effects from taking estrogen. With perfect use of oral contraceptives, 0.3% of women are expected to become pregnant but among typical users pregnancy occurs to 8%.[32,33]

Patch

The patch is commonly called by its brand name OrthoEvra. This small, plastic patch sticks to the skin and releases estrogen and progestin to prevent pregnancy. The patch is changed once a month and then worn for 3 weeks followed by one patch-free week. As with oral contraceptives, with perfect use the patch protects against pregnancy in all but 0.3% of women, but if not consistently used, 8% become pregnant.[34]

Vaginal Ring

The vaginal ring is commonly called by its brand name NuvaRing. A woman inserts the small, flexible ring into her vagina once a month and leaves it in place for 3 weeks, followed by 1 week without the ring. The ring releases estrogen and progestin to prevent pregnancy and if used correctly and consistently, the vaginal ring has similar success at preventing pregnancy as noted for the patch and oral contraceptives.[34]

Injection

Depo-Provera, the contraceptive injection of progestin effectively functions to prevent pregnancy for 3 months. When received every 3 months on schedule, 0.3% of women are expected to become pregnant, but if time elapses before another injection, 3% may become pregnant.[35]

Implant

The contraceptive implant, called Implanon, is a thin, flexible plastic rod about the size of a matchstick that is inserted under the skin of the upper arm and releases progestin for approximately 3 years to effectively prevent pregnancy. Less than 1 in 1,000 women is expected to become pregnant while using Implanon.[36]

Emergency Contraception

Another hormonal method of birth control can be taken after unprotected intercourse or after the failure of another method such as condom breakage or failure to take oral contraceptive pills for a few days. Emergency contraception, used immediately or up to 5 days after intercourse, is available over the counter in the United States to people age 17 and over. Those under age 17 need a prescription.[37]

There are two main formulations of oral contraceptive pills that are used for emergency contraception. Progestin-only emergency contraception, which is 89% effective in preventing pregnancy, is currently sold in the United States under the brand names Plan B, Plan B One-Step, and Next Choice. The other emergency contraception option is a higher dose of the combined estrogen and progestin daily pill; the recommended regimen reduces the risk of pregnancy by 74%. A third emergency contraceptive option is the insertion of an IUD.[37]

Intrauterine Device (IUD)

A long-term method of birth control is provided by an IUD, a small, T-shaped device that is inserted by a healthcare provider into a woman's uterus. IUDs prevent fertilization of an egg by altering the lining of the uterus and impairing sperm function. Two kinds of IUDs are available in the United States. The ParaGard IUD is wrapped with copper and is 99.4% effective for up to 10 years. The Mirena IUD releases a small amount of levonorgestrel and is 99.8% effective for up to 5 years. Both are designed to fit comfortably in the uterus. The ParaGard IUD is also 99% effective as a form of emergency contraception following unprotected intercourse if inserted by a healthcare provider within 120 hours (5 days).[38]

Barrier Methods

Barrier methods of pregnancy prevention create a physical or chemical barrier preventing sperm from reaching an egg. These methods rely on careful use and thus may be less effective at preventing pregnancy than hormonal methods; however, when used consistently and correctly, their effectiveness rates are still high.

Male Condom

Condoms are latex or polyurethane (a type of plastic) sheaths that are unrolled over an erect penis to collect semen when a man ejaculates, preventing semen from entering the vagina. In addition, condoms reduce the risk of sexually transmitted infections by covering the penis and keeping semen from entering the vagina, anus, or mouth. Male condoms must be used consistently and correctly with each act of intercourse to be effective. With perfect use, condoms are 98% effective and with typical use, 85% effective.[39]

Female Condom

The female condom is a loose-fitting polyurethane sheath that is inserted into the vagina before intercourse to collect semen when a man ejaculates. The pouch has two flexible rings at each end. The closed ring is inserted into the vagina to hold the pouch in place, while the open ring remains outside the vagina so that the penis enters the vagina or anus through the ring during intercourse (Figure 9-7a and Figure 9-7b). The female condom, like the male condom, reduces the risk of both pregnancy and STIs by preventing semen from entering the vagina and reducing skin contact between the penis and the vagina. Female condoms must be used consistently and correctly with each act of intercourse to be effective. Female condoms are 95% effective with perfect use and 79% effective with typical use.[40]

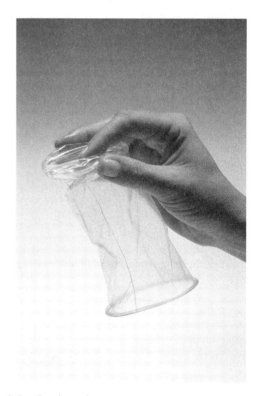

Figure 9-7a Female condom.

Source: © Jones & Bartlett Learning. Photographed by Kimberly Potvin

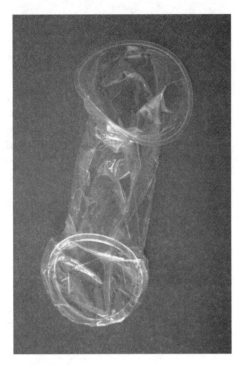

Figure 9-7b Female condom.

Source: © Photodisc

Diaphragm

The diaphragm is a reusable, flexible, latex dome-shaped cup that is inserted with spermicide lubrication before intercourse into the vagina behind the pubic bone to cover the cervix, restricting the movement of sperm from entering the vagina. Accurate fit of the diaphragm by a healthcare provider is essential to meet the physical requirements of the patient. Additional spermicide needs to be added to the vagina if more than one act of intercourse occurs before removal of the diaphragm, which should be left in place for at least 6 hours to prevent pregnancy. The diaphragm is 94% effective with perfect use and 84% effective with typical use.[40]

Cervical Cap

The cervical cap is a reusable, silicone bowl-shaped cap that is inserted into the vagina before intercourse and covers the cervix. The cervical cup prevents sperm from entering the uterus by sealing on to the cervix when appropriate size has been identified by a healthcare provider. Spermacide can be added to the inside or outside of the cap to increase the protection the cap provides. The cervical cap must be left in place for 8 hours following intercourse. For women who have never given birth vaginally, the cervical cap is 86% effective with perfect use or typical use. For women who have given birth vaginally, the cervical cap is 71% effective with perfect use. With typical use among women who have given birth vaginally, the cervical cap is substantially less effective than the diaphragm or female condom.[40]

Sponge

The sponge, made of soft polyurethane foam imbedded with spermicide, is inserted into the vagina covering the cervix. The sponge continuously releases spermicide and can be used only once. It is sold over the counter and is available in only one size. It protects for up to 24 hours and to be effective must be left in place for at least 6 hours after intercourse. For women who have never given birth vaginally, the sponge is 91% effective with perfect use and 84% effective with typical use. For women who have given birth vaginally, the sponge is 80% effective with perfect use and only 68% effective with typical use.[40]

Spermicides

Spermicides available as foams, creams, gels, suppositories, and film contain the chemical nonoxynol-9, which is lethal to sperm. These preparations are inserted in the vagina shortly before intercourse and can be used alone or preferably with other methods of birth control. With typical use, reported pregnancy rates range from less than 5% to more than 50% in the first year of use although perfect use data indicates they are 82% effective and effectiveness is 71% with typical use.[40]

Additional Methods

Withdrawal

Withdrawal is commonly referred to as "pulling out." To prevent sperm from entering the vagina during intercourse, a man removes his penis from the vagina before ejaculation. With a partner who is consistent, the annual rate of pregnancy is 4%. However, given the moment before ejaculation is often difficult to predict, withdrawal may not be effective, as noted by the 27% of women who become pregnant each year.[41]

Fertility Awareness-Based Methods

Fertility awareness-based methods—also called "natural family planning"—require tracking ovulation to avoid intercourse during a woman's fertile period. There are several methods to predict ovulation including charting menstrual cycles on the calendar, early morning temperature records before getting out of bed, and/or assessment cervical mucus. With perfect use, most methods are 95–97% effective. With typical use, methods range from 78–88% effective.[42]

Intended and Unintended Pregnancy

In the United States an estimated 6.4 million pregnancies occur annually, half of which are "intended" and half are "unintended" indicating that a large percentage of couples are not planning their pregnancies or have difficulty using effective contraception consistently and correctly.[43,44] However, unintended pregnancies may result in wanted births, as many women experiencing unplanned pregnancies may end up feeling happy about having a baby. Of all pregnancies, about two-thirds result in a live birth, about 20% end in abortion, and the remainder end in miscarriage.[43,44]

Among adolescents, 85% of pregnancies are unintended. Each year, 750,000 pregnancies occur among teens ages 15–19.[45] Rates of teen pregnancy and teen births in the United States are far higher than rates in other industrialized countries—the teen birth rate in the United States is 54 per 1,000 compared to 7.7 per 1,000 in Sweden, 10 per 1,000 in France, and 28 per 1,000 in England.[46] Among American females 18% will give birth at least once by age 20.[47] Adolescent pregnancy and childbearing result in life-course changes for teen mothers, their children, and their parents. Given increased efforts to secure child support and increasing societal expectations that males should be responsible for their children, additional life changes also occur for young fathers. Often educational attainment is curtailed for teenage mothers, diminishing opportunities for career development and economic stability.[48,49] Babies born to teen mothers are more likely to be low birth weight and to experience developmental and educational delays. Some evidence suggests that the children of teen mothers are more likely to experience teen pregnancies themselves and to end up incarcerated as adolescents or young adults.[48,49] Although approximately 27% of teen pregnancies end in abortion, the proportion of teens choosing abortion has declined over the past 15 years, suggesting life-course alterations associated with early parenting affect most teenage mothers.[50] Adolescent pregnancy can be prevented by either increasing the proportion of adolescents who abstain from sexual intercourse or ensuring that adolescents use an effective method of contraception when engaging in sexual behavior. Of note, those young people who fail to use a method of birth control at their first sexual experience are more than twice as likely to experience an unintended pregnancy and first birth during their teen years.[47] Analyses show that declines in adolescent pregnancy are mainly attributable to better contraceptive use.[51] Among teens, racial/ethnic differences in rates of pregnancy have been observed during the past decade as presented in Figure 9-8.

Contraception Use by Adolescents

Among teens ages 15–18 use of contraception, particularly condoms at first sex, is relatively high approximately 70%.[47] However, teens are less likely to use the most effective hormonal methods of birth control pill. Nationally, at first intercourse, 16% of teens age 15–16 and 23% of teens age 17–19 used the pill. The combined use of condoms and hormonal contraception is rare in the United States—only 8% of adolescents report dual use nationally.[52]

Contraception Use by Adults

In 2002, five of eight women in the United States ages 15–44 (62%) were currently using some method of contraception. The three most common methods were the pill (19%), female sterilization (17%), and the male condom (15%).[30] Leading methods vary by age, education, marital status, and income. The pill is most widely used by women in their 20s with at least a college degree who have never married.[53] In 2002, among women who were using contraception ("contraceptors"), 53% of those ages 20–24 and 38% of women ages 25–29 used the pill.[30] Female sterilization is most widely used by women age 35 and older, with higher education who were married.[53] Forty-one percent of contraceptors aged 35–39 and 50% of those aged 40–44 have been sterilized.[30] Poor and low-income women are more than twice as likely to use the 3-month injection method (Depo-Provera) than higher income women. Dual use of condoms with another more effective method is practiced by 15% of women using contraception.[53]

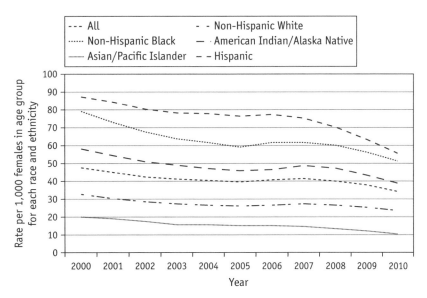

Figure 9-8 Birth rates (live births) per 1,000 females aged 15-19 Years, by race and Hispanic ethnicity, 2000–2010.

Modified from Hamilton BE, Martin JA, Ventura SJ. Births: Preliminary data for 2010. *Nat Vital Stat Rep* 2011;60: Table 2. Centers for Disease Control and Prevention. National Center for Health Statistics. http://www.cdc.gov/TeenPregnancy/AboutTeenPreg.htm

Abortion

About half of all pregnancies in the United States are unintended and 42% of these unplanned pregnancies end in abortion.[44] Pregnancy termination is one of the most common surgical procedures in the United States. Aspiration is the most common method for first-trimester surgical abortion. Using modest cervical dilation and an electric vacuum pump or handheld syringe, the contents of the uterus are removed through the os.[54] After the first trimester, dilation and evacuation (D&E) is the most common surgical procedure; it is typically performed between 13 and 16 weeks gestation although occasionally performed through 24 weeks. D&E combines vacuum aspiration and the use of forceps. Osmotic cervical dilating devices or misoprostol are used to prepare the cervix before D&E procedures.

Other second trimester abortion procedures include misoprostol induction, vaginal administration of dinoprostone, or intravenous administration of high-dose oxytocin.[54] Misoprostol is a medication that softens and dilates the cervix and may be used for medical abortion, a nonsurgical option for termination of pregnancy in the first trimester. Two medication regimes are available and can be used through 7–9 weeks gestation depending on the regime: methotrexate-misprostol and mifepristone-misoprostol. In both regimes, misoprostol facilitates the expulsion of the pregnancy by preparing the cervix and stimulating the uterus to contract. The methotrexate-misoprostol regime acts on rapidly dividing cells of the early placenta and is 92–96% effective in terminating pregnancy through 7 weeks of gestation.[54] This regime is less common since 2000 when the Food and Drug Administration approved mifepristone, also known as RU-486 and commonly referred to as "the abortion pill." Mifepristone is a synthetic steroid that blocks the action of progesterone, which is required for implantation of a fertilized egg.[54] Trials of mifepristone in the United States and United Kingdom indicated 92–95% efficacy for pregnancy termination through 7 weeks of gestation.[55] Women usually need to make two or three office visits to complete medical abortion.[54] In 2005, early medical abortions accounted for 14% of nonhospital procedures.[56] Mifepristone was expected to make abortion more widely accessible geographically; however, research shows no significant improvement in geographic availability although this may soon change.[60]

The number of abortions in the United States declined from 1.61 million in 1990 to 1.31 million in 2000 to 1.2 million in 2005.[56] Although the reasons for the decline are not clear, the reduction in abortion rates may be the result of more effective use of contraception. Geographic location, gestational limits, restrictive state policies, and cost are barriers to access for some women.[56]

Restricted Access to Abortion

Abortion services are concentrated in metropolitan areas; therefore, some women must travel 50–100 miles or more to obtain services. In 2005, the vast majority (87%) of U.S. counties did not have an abortion provider.[56] Depending on the week of pregnancy when a woman seeks an abortion, providers' willingness to perform the procedure varied: 40% of providers offered early abortions within 4–5 weeks since last menstrual period and 67% provided services at 13 weeks or later and 20% after 20 weeks, but only 8% at 24 weeks. The largest proportion of providers offering abortions (96%) is at 8 weeks.[56] Thirty-four states mandate waiting periods between counseling and obtaining abortion services.[57] Laws requiring parental consent and/or notification further impede minors' access to abortion in 34 states.[58] State laws continue to evolve with some recently adding a required sonogram before an abortion is performed.

Access to abortion has been restricted for over 3 decades by the Hyde Amendment, which banned federal funding of abortion services in 1976, except in the case of rape, incest, or life endangerment to the woman. Furthermore, 32 states and the District of Columbia have banned state Medicaid funding for abortion.[59,60] The burden of bans on federal and state funding falls heaviest on low-income women, many of whom obtain health coverage through Medicaid. A review of 38 studies published in 2009 indicated that roughly 25% of Medicaid-eligible women who wanted an abortion carried the pregnancy to term, in part, because of unavailable Medicaid funding.[60] In a 2004 study, 58% of women reported that they would have preferred having their abortion earlier; among these women, 26% cited the time necessary to raise funds to cover the cost as the main reason for delay.[61] This figure rose to 36% among women who obtained an abortion in the second trimester. The cost of abortion varies among providers and depends on gestational period. Ninety percent of abortions in the United States are performed in the first trimester; at 10 weeks the median charge was $430 in 2005.[56] However, the cost can exceed $1,200 for abortions performed after 20 weeks.[56]

Summary

Sexuality is much broader than sexual behavior and includes relationships, gender identity, sexual orientation, body image, and self-identity. People learn about sexuality from birth. A range of caregivers and sociocultural institutions, including parents, teachers, religious leaders, and the media, play important roles in educating or miseducating people about sexuality. Young women and their partners should be familiar with all forms of contraception before becoming sexually active and also need to have access to essential services if an unplanned pregnancy occurs. In order to help people become sexually healthy adults, society must become more willing and able to address issues of sexuality openly and honestly.

Discussion Questions

1. What is generally included and excluded from discussions about sexuality? Why do you think that is?

2. How do you think ideas about gender and sexual orientation influence women's and men's experience of their own sexuality?
3. Which contraceptive methods are best for women at various points in their sexual and reproductive lives?
4. What lessons about sexuality that are learned in childhood and adolescence may be helpful or harmful to sexual development?
5. What key messages are useful for people to know about sexual dysfunction?
6. How could society help children, adolescents, and adults to become more sexually healthy?

References

1. World Association of Sexology. Declaration of Sexual Rights. http://www.worldsexology.org/millennium-declaration. Accessed August 13, 2012.
2. Ross E, Rapp R. Sex and society: a research note from social history and anthropology. *Comparative Studies in Society and History.* 1981;23:51–72.
3. Sexuality Information and Education Council of the United States. *Guidelines for Comprehensive Sexuality Education: Kindergarten–12th Grade.*3rd ed. New York: National Guidelines Task Force; 2004.
4. Haug F. *Female Sexualization, A Collective Work of Memory.* New York: Verso Classics; 1999.
5. Neumark-Sztainer D, Hannan PJ. Weight-related behaviors among adolescent girls and boys: results from a national survey. *Arch Pediatr Adolesc Med.* 2000;154:569–577.
6. Centers for Disease Control and Prevention. Youth risk behavior surveillance—United States, 2007, Surveillance Summaries. *MMWR Morb Mortal Wkly Rep.* 2008;57(no SS-4). http://www.cdc.gov/mmwr/PDF/ss/ss5704.pdf. Accessed August 13, 2012.
7. Chandra A, Martinez GM, Mosher WD, et al. Fertility, family planning, and reproductive health of U.S. women: data from the 2002 National Survey of Family Growth. National Center for Health Statistics. *Vital Health Statistics.* 2005;23.
8. Kosciw JG, Diaz EM, Greytak EA. *2007 National School Climate Survey: The Experiences of Lesbian, Gay, Bisexual and Transgender Youth in Our Nation's Schools.* New York: GLSEN; 2008.
9. Michael RT, Gagnon JH, Laumann EO, Kolata G. *Sex in America: A Definite Survey.* New York: Warner Books; 1995.
10. Robbins CJ, Fortenberry D, Reece M, et al. Masturbation frequency and patterns among U.S. adolescents. *J Adolesc Health.* 2010;46:S36–S37.
11. Waite LJ, Laumann EO, Das A, Schumm LP. Sexuality: measures of partnerships, practices, attitudes, and problems in the National Social Life, Health, and Aging Study. *J Gerontol B Psychol Sci Soc Sci.* 2009;64(suppl 1):i56–66.
12. Herbenick D, Reece M, Sanders S, et al. Prevalence and characteristics of vibrator use by women in the United States: results from a nationally representative study. *J Sexual Med.* 2009;6:1857–1866.
13. Mosher WD, Chandra A, Jones J. Sexual behavior and selected health measures: men and women 15–44 years of age, United States, 2002. *Advance Data from Vital and Health Statistics.* 2005;no 362.
14. Lindau ST, Schumm LP, Laumann EO, et al. A study of sexuality and health among older adults in the United States. *N Engl J Med.* 2007;35:762–774.
15. Coontz, S. *Marriage, A History.* New York: Viking; 2005.
16. U.S. Census Bureau. American Community Survey. http://www.census.gov/acs/www/. Accessed August 13, 2012.
17. Goldstein JR, Kenney CT. Marriage delayed or marriage forgone? New cohort forecasts of first marriage for U.S. women. *Am Sociological Rev.* 2001;66:506–519.
18. Centers for Disease Control and Prevention. FastStats: Marriage and divorce. http://www.cdc.gov/nchs/fastats/divorce.htm. Accessed March 1, 2010.
19. Goodwin P, McGill B, Chandra A. Who marries and when? Age at first marriage in the United States: 2002. *National Center for Health Statistics Data Brief.* 2009;19:1–8.
20. Kiecolt-Glaser JK, Newton TL. Marriage and health: his and hers. *Psychol Bull.* 2001;127:472–503.
21. Berman JR, Bassuk J. Physiology and pathophysiology of female sexual function and dysfunction. *World J Urol.* 2002;20:111–118.
22. Basson R. Female sexual response: the role of drugs in the management of sexual dysfunction. *Obstet Gynecol.* 2001;98:350–353.
23. Association of Reproductive Health Professionals. What you need to know: female sexual response. March 2008. http://www.arhp.org/Publications-and-Resources/Clinical-Fact-Sheets/Female-Sexual-Response. Accessed October 25, 2009.
24. Laumann EO, Paik A, Rosen RC. Sexual dysfunction in the United States: prevalence and predictors. *JAMA.* 1999;281:537–44.
25. Lexchin J, Bero LA, Djulbegovic B, Clark O. Pharmaceutical industry sponsorship and research outcome and quality: systematic review. *BMJ.* 2003;326:1167–1170.
26. New View Campaign. Website. http://www.newviewcampaign.org. Accessed March 23, 2010.
27. Cohen BJ, Wood DL, Dena LW, Memmler RL. *Memmler's The Human Body in Health and Disease.* 9th ed. Philadelphia: Lippincott Williams & Wilkins; 2000.
28. Hatcher RA, Namnoun AB. The menstrual cycle. In: RA Hatcher et al., eds. *Contraceptive Technology.* 19th ed. New York: Ardent Media, Inc; 2008.
29. Nelson AL, Stewart, FH. Menopause and perimenopausal health. In: RA Hatcher et al., eds. *Contraceptive Technology.* 19th ed. New York: Ardent Media, Inc; 2008.
30. Mosher WD, Martinez GM, Chandra A, et al. Use of contraception and use of family planning services in the United States: 1982–2002. *Advance Data from Vital and Health Statistics.* 2004;no 350.
31. Trussel J. Choosing a contraceptive: efficacy, safety, and personal considerations. In RA Hatcher et al., eds. *Contraceptive Technology.* 19th ed. New York: Ardent Media, Inc; 2008.
32. Raymond EG. Progestin-only pills. In: RA Hatcher et al., eds. *Contraceptive Technology.* 19th ed. New York: Ardent Media, Inc; 2008.
33. Nelson AL. Combined oral contraceptives. In: RA Hatcher et al., eds. *Contraceptive Technology.* 19th ed. New York: Ardent Media, Inc; 2008.
34. Nanda K. Contraceptive patch and vaginal contraceptive ring. In: RA Hatcher et al., eds. *Contraceptive Technology.* 19th ed. New York: Ardent Media, Inc; 2008.
35. Goldberg AB, Grimes DA. Injectable contraceptives. In: RA Hatcher et al., eds. *Contraceptive Technology.* 19th ed. New York: Ardent Media, Inc; 2008.
36. Raymond EG. Contraceptive implant. In: RA Hatcher et al., eds. *Contraceptive Technology.* 19th ed. New York: Ardent Media, Inc; 2008.
37. Stewart F, Trussel J, Van Look PFA. Emergency contraception. In: RA Hatcher et al., eds. *Contraceptive Technology.* 19th ed. New York: Ardent Media, Inc; 2008.
38. Grimes DA. Intrauterine devices (IUDs). In: RA Hatcher et al., eds. *Contraceptive Technology.* 19th ed. New York: Ardent Media, Inc; 2008.
39. Warner L, Steiner MJ. Male Condoms. In: RA Hatcher et al., eds. *Contraceptive Technology.* 19th ed. New York: Ardent Media, Inc; 2008.
40. Cates W Jr, Raymond EG. Vaginal barriers and spermacides. In: RA Hatcher et al., eds. *Contraceptive Technology.* 19th ed. New York: Ardent Media, Inc; 2008.
41. Kowal D. Coitus interruptus (withdrawal). In: RA Hatcher et al., eds. *Contraceptive Technology.* 19th ed. New York: Ardent Media, Inc; 2008.
42. Jennings VH, Arevalo M. Fertility awareness-based methods. In: RA Hatcher et al., eds. *Contraceptive Technology.* 19th ed. New York: Ardent Media, Inc; 2008.
43. Ventura SJ, Abma JC, Mosher WD, Henshaw SK. Estimated pregnancy rates by outcome for the United States, 1990–2004. *National Vital Statistics Report* 2008;56.
44. Finer LB, Henshaw SK. 2006: Disparities in rates of unintended pregnancy in the United States, 1994 and 2001. *Perspect Sex Reprod Health.* 2006;38:90–96.
45. Guttmacher Institute. *Facts on American Teens' Sexual and Reproductive Health.In Brief.* 2010. http://www.guttmacher.org/pubs/FB-ATSRH.pdf. Accessed March 3, 2010.
46. Singh S, Darroch JE. Adolescent pregnancy and childbearing: levels and trends in developed countries. *Family Planning Perspectives.* 1999;32:14–23.
47. Abma JC, Martinez, GM, Mosher, WD, Dawson, BS. Teenagers in the United States: Sexual activity, contraceptive use, and childbearing, 2002. National Center for Health Statistics, *Vital Health Statistics* 2004;23.
48. Logan C, Holcombe E, Manlove J, Ryan S. *The Consequences of Unintended Childbearing. A White Paper.* Washington, D.C.: Child Trends, Inc; 2007.
49. Maynard R. *Kids Having Kids: Economic Costs and Social Consequences of Teen Pregnancy.* Washington, DC: National Campaign to Prevent Teen Pregnancy; 1997.
50. Guttmacher Institute. *U.S. Teenage Pregnancies, Births and Abortions: National and State Trends and Trends by Race and Ethnicity.* New York: Guttmacher Institute; 2010. Available at http://www.guttmacher.org/pubs/USTPtrends.pdf. Accessed March 1, 2010.
51. Santelli JS, Lindberg LD, Finer LB, Singh S. Explaining recent declines in adolescent pregnancy in the United States: the contribution of abstinence and improved contraceptive use. *Am J Public Health.* 2007;97:150–156.
52. Waddell EN, Labor N, VanWye G. Teen sexual activity and birth control use in New York City. *NYC Vital Signs.* 2007;6:1–4.
53. Guttmacher Institute. *Fact Sheet: Contraceptive Use in the United States.* New York: Author; 2008. http://www.guttmacher.org/pubs/fb_contr_use.html., Accessed March 1, 2010.
54. Paul M, Stewart FH. Abortion. In: RA Hatcher et al., eds. *Contraceptive Technology.* 19th ed. New York: Ardent Media, Inc; 2008.
55. Finer LB, Wei J. Effect of mifepristone on abortion access in the United States. *Obstet Gynecol.* 2009;114:623–630.
56. Jones RK, Zolna MR, Henshaw SK, Finer LB. Abortion in the United States: Incidence and Access to Services, 2005. *Perspect Sex Reprod Health.* 2008;40:6–16.

57. Guttmacher Insitute. Counseling and Waiting Periods for Abortion. *State Policies in Brief*. New York: Author; 2012. http://www.guttmacher.org/statecenter/spibs/spib_MWPA.pdf. Accessed August 21, 2012.

58. Guttmacher Institute. Parental Involvement in Minors' Abortions. *State Policies in Brief*. New York: Author; 2012. http://www.guttmacher.org/statecenter/spibs/spib_PIMA.pdf. Accessed August 21, 2012.

59. Guttmacher Institute. Facts on Induced Abortion in the United States. *In Brief*. New York: Author; 2011. http://www.guttmacher.org/pubs/fb_induced_abortion.html. Accessed August 21, 2012.

60. Henshaw SK, Joyce TJ, Dennis A, Finer LB, Blanchard K. *Restrictions on Medicaid Funding for Abortions: A Literature Review*. New York: Guttmacher Institute; 2009.

61. Finer LB, Frohwirth L, Dauphinee L, et al. Timing of steps and reasons for delays in obtaining abortions in the United States. *Contraception*. 2006;74:334–344

62. West C, Zimmerman DH. Doing gender. In: Plante RF, Maurer LM, eds. *Doing Gender Diversity: Readings in Theory and Real-World Experience*. Philadelphia: Westview Press; 2010.

63. Blackless M, Charuvastra A, Derryck A, et al. How sexually dimorphic are we? Review and synthesis. *Am J Hum Biology*. 2000;12:151–155.

64. Plante RF, Maurer LM, eds. *Doing Gender: Readings in Theory and Real-World Experience*. Philadelphia: Westview Press; 2010.

65. Weeks J. *Making Sexual History*. Malden, MA: Blackwell Publishers; 2000.

66. The Kinsey Institute. Kinsey's Heterosexual-Homosexual Rating Scale. http://www.kinseyinstitute.org/research/ak-hhscale.html. Accessed January 7, 2010.

67. Coleman, E. Assessment of sexual orientation. In: Coleman E, ed. *Psychotherapy with Homosexual Men and Women: Integrated Identity Approached for Clinical Practice*. New York: Haworth Press; 1988.

68. Diamond, L. *Sexual Fluidity: Understanding Women's Love and Desire*. Cambridge, MA: Harvard University Press; 2009.

69. Transgender Law Center. Peeing in peace: a resource guide for transgender Activists and Allies. In: Plante RF, Maurer LM, eds. *Doing Gender Diversity: Readings in Theory and Real-World Experience*. Philadelphia: Westview Press; 2010.

Epidemiology of Reproductive Health

Ruby T. Senie, PhD

Introduction

Endogenous hormone levels, essential for childbearing, launch women's unique health-related experiences from conception through prenatal development, accelerating during puberty to enable reproduction. Ovarian hormones influence and are influenced by genetics, personal behaviors, environmental exposures, infectious diseases, and therapeutic interventions. Over the life course the continuum of organ development and preparation for childbearing becomes evident with early indicators of puberty, extending from menarche to menopause. During the intervening years women's health needs are primarily related to menstrual function and reproductive decision making. Clinical care provides access to contraception and ensures healthy childbearing. Assisted reproduction technologies offer the possibility of pregnancy to infertile couples. During reproductive years, some women are diagnosed with autoimmune and chronic conditions that may complicate pregnancy, affect their ability to care for their children, and influence long-term health and emotional well-being.

Most women will successfully give birth to the number of children desired. Others may experienced unplanned pregnancies or find they are unable to conceive. Some gynecological conditions experienced during reproductive years, such as endometriosis, uterine fibroids, sexually transmitted infections, and abnormal development of pelvic organs, may cause discomfort, require invasive clinical procedures, and potentially impede fertility. As more women delay childbearing, the frequency of a first birth at an older age has risen, accompanied by greater risks of adverse pregnancy outcomes such as preterm birth, low birth weight babies, and a complicated deliveries. Advances in reproductive technology have provided opportunities for childbearing at older ages although with increased frequency of multiple gestations and associated infant health risks. During past decades as maternal and infant mortality declined, increased family planning options became available. Women's lives have expanded to include higher education, employment, and community involvement including election to influential positions in education, government, and industry. This chapter addresses some of the historical events that guided clinical care, reviews some reproductive epidemiologic studies, and presents challenges women continue to face during their reproductive years that may influence their health long after menopause.

Progress and Challenges in Reproductive Health

During the 20th century major public health efforts dramatically reduced maternal (Figure 10-1) and infant mortality by 97%, significantly increasing life expectancy.[1] Infection control coupled with improved clinical management of pregnancy, childbirth, and infant care enabled women to achieve their desired family size with fewer pregnancies. For centuries women experienced approximately 100 menstrual cycles during their reproductive years beginning with menarche between ages 13 and 15 followed by frequent pregnancies coupled with long intervals of breastfeeding, reducing the number of ovulatory cycles before menopause. In the 21st century many young women will experience 10 to 20 years of regular menstrual cycles before their first planned or unintended pregnancy. Decisions regarding reproduction may be influenced by a combination of cultural patterns, religious influences, and social norms, which may generate physical and psychological pressures.

Advances in recent decades have provided effective contraceptive options, ensuring fertility control and longer intervals between births. Although major improvements have enhanced the health of mothers and their newborns, disparities continue to adversely affect reproductive health of some American women. U.S. statistics lag far behind the significantly lower maternal and infant mortality rates achieved by other developed countries. Some of the factors known to contribute to adverse pregnancy-related and neonatal outcomes are discussed in this chapter; however, a considerable proportion of the higher rates of morbidity and mortality associated with pregnancy are known to be caused by pre-existing poor health conditions such as obesity and hypertension.

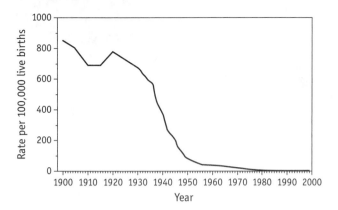

Figure 10-1 Maternal mortality rate by year per 100,000 live births, United States, 1900–1999.

Source: Reproduced from Division of Reproductive Health, National Center for Chronic Disease Prevention and Health Promotion, CDC. Achievements in Public Health, 1900–1999: Healthier Mothers and Babies. *Morbidity Mortality Weekly Report* 1999;48:849–858.

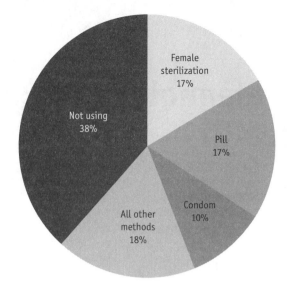

Figure 10-2 Percent distribution of women aged 15 to 44 by contraceptive use in the United States, 2006–2008.

Source: Reproduced from Mosher WD, Jones J. Use of contraception in the United States: 1982–2008. *Vital and Health Statistics* 2010; Series 23:29.

Contraception: Preventing Unintended Pregnancy

In 2011 the Institute of Medicine (IOM) published a landmark review, *Clinical Preventive Services for Women: Closing the Gap*, which included preventive services to avoid unintended pregnancy and healthy birth spacing.[2] Data from the National Survey of Family Growth (NSFG) guided the decisions noted in the IOM report. The NSFG, established in 1973, collects information on family growth and dissolution, marriage, divorce, and cohabitation through interviews of a random sample of Americans. Questions include contraceptive patterns, sterilization, infertility problems, births, and pregnancy outcomes. NSFG data have consistently indicated that 49% of U.S. pregnancies were unintended, either unwanted or poorly timed, and 42% of unwanted pregnancies ended in abortion.[3] American rates of unplanned pregnancies and abortions far exceed those of other developed countries.[4]

Following the IOM report recommendations, the Affordable Care Act (ACA) of 2010 requires health insurance plans to cover contraceptive costs without copayment.[5] Some studies have associated unintended pregnancy with women of low income lacking access to costly contraceptives.[3] By eliminating cost as a barrier, public health officials and family planning advocates anticipate this controversial aspect of the ACA will enable women to plan their pregnancies, reduce the number seeking an abortion, and lengthen the interval between births to a minimum of 18 months in order to limit risks of adverse maternal and fetal outcomes.[5] Shorter intervals between births have been associated with infants born at low birth weight, preterm, and small for gestational age, each associated with increased infant morbidity and mortality.[6] Women with chronic conditions such as obesity and diabetes may require longer intervals between pregnancies to control their complicating illnesses. For some women with serious health problems, pregnancy may be life threatening, increasing

their need for frequent monitoring.[7] Women's reproduction decisions significantly affect their lives, the lives of their partners, and their children.

The increased availability of Food and Drug Administration (FDA)-approved effective contraceptives including barriers, hormonal methods, emergency contraception, implanted devices and sterilization were noted in the IOM report.[2] Research cited by professional organizations considers family planning an essential preventive service for all sexually active adolescents and adult women to avoid unintended pregnancies and reduce dependency on abortion.[8] Given the most effective contraceptives do not rely on user compliance and are long lasting,[9] responsible family planning, a major public health goal, may be achieved with the options financially provided by the ACA law.

Use of birth control increased from 56% in 1982 to 62% in 2008 as the number of contraceptive methods increased; however, data from 2006–2008 presented in Figure 10-2 indicate 38% of sexually active women ages 15 to 44 reported no contraceptive use.[10] Among the 4 million births occurring annually in the United States, 400,000 are to teens aged 15 to 19, the highest incidence of any developed country. These poorly timed births often have lifelong negative effects on young mothers and their offspring. Their babies are frequently born at low birth weight, with greater morbidity during childhood. These children often experience lower educational achievements and are more likely to become teenage parents themselves.[11]

The Pregnancy Risk Assessment Monitoring System' (PRAMS) created by the Centers for Disease Control and Prevention (CDC) collects data on maternal attitudes and experiences before, during, and shortly after pregnancy from approximately 75% of all American births.[11] Data for 2004–2008 indicated 50% of teenage mothers were not using any birth control method when they became pregnant. More than 30% thought they "could not get pregnant," 13% stated they lacked access to birth control, and 25% claimed their partners refused contraception.[11] CDC has worked with healthcare providers, parents, and community leaders by encouraging adolescents to delay sexual activity, improving education about reproduction, and providing increased access to effective birth control including emergency contraception.[11]

Family planning considerations of individual women change over time; contraceptive needs of younger women may be less appropriate or desirable at older ages. Trussell reviewed contraceptive failures to estimate the probabilities of pregnancy for each available birth control method when used correctly and consistently. His data indicated conception was likely within 12 months in 85% of couples not using birth control in contrast to nearly 100% avoidance of unwanted pregnancy following female or male sterilization.[12] Trussell's research indicated that long-acting reversible hormonal implants and copper intrauterine contraceptives were 99% effective but remained underused due to their initial high cost.[12] However, elimination of financial barriers led more women to select a reversible but longlasting method, avoiding almost 2,000 unwanted pregnancies among Kaiser Permanente subscribers.[13] Access to contraceptive options was considered cost effective with almost $4 saved on pregnancy costs for each $1 spent on pregnancy prevention.[14] Many effective birth control options require the collaborative effort of women and their partners although the availability of emergency contraception without medical prescription provides an additional opportunity for women ages 17 and older to prevent unwanted pregnancy.[15] Data indicate 50% of all American women experience unplanned pregnancies at some time during their reproductive years and some are terminated by abortion. Preventing these unplanned pregnancies protects the health of mothers and their families and avoids pregnancy interruption.

Reproductive Potential

Fertility is controlled by ovulatory menstrual cycles. The number of oocytes that develop during fetal growth declines before birth by more than 75%[16] to approximately 400,000 present at puberty.[17] Cycle length varies after menarche although once routine timing has been established, the usual pattern may be disrupted by severe weight loss associated with strenuous exercise (described by Frisch et al.[18]) or illness such as anorexia.[19] Follicle-stimulating hormone (FSH) from the pituitary gland prepares several hundred eggs for ovulation during each cycle although only one is normally released. Viable oocytes decline with age; an estimated 20,000 are available at peak fertility around age 30.[20] Only a few thousand follicles remain at age 40,[21] with less than 1,000 present at menopause.[22] After peak fertility the number of follicles preparing for ovulation diminishes, creating less consistent and more frequent anovulatory cycles limiting opportunities for conception.[22,23] Impaired fertility may become a factor as women approach their 40s although

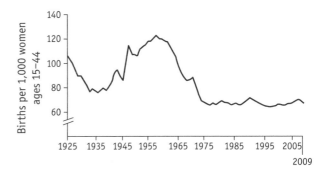

Figure 10-3 Fertility rate trends, 1925–2009, United States.

Source: Reproduced from Martin JA, Hamilton BE, Ventura SJ, et al. Births: Final data for 2009. *National Vital Statistics Reports* 2011;60:1.

the variability of oocytes released increases the risk of twin births.[23]

The general fertility rate in 2009 was 66.7 births per 1,000 women ages 15 to 44. Rates have varied considerably over the past decades in relation to economic and social conditions (Figure 10-3).[24] The decline in 2009 reported by the National Center for Health Statistics (NCHS) reflected the economic downturn of 2008, a pattern noted during the depression of the 1930s and in the 1970s during high inflation.[24] The fertility rate in 2009 was 45% lower than the peak in 1957. Between 1990 and 2002 declining fertility was greater among non-Hispanic black women (24%) than non-Hispanic white (9%) or Hispanic women (12%). When assessed by "replacement" rate, fertility among Hispanic and non-Hispanic black women continued to exceed replacement in contrast to non-Hispanic white women who have consistently fallen below replacement levels. "Replacement" describes the level of a given generation exactly replacing itself with an average of 2,100 births per 1,000 women.[24] Changes in the annual fertility rate are also influenced by the rate of legal induced abortion, which was 21.3 per 1000 women in 2005, a decline of 12% since 1980. Reduced abortions were reported among all race/ethnic groups although more non-Hispanic black than Hispanic or non-Hispanic white women obtained abortions in 2005.[25]

Between 1950 and 2000 the birth rate in the United States dropped from 24 live births per 1,000 women to 14.5 per 1,000 with approximately 10% of reproductive age women pregnant each year.[10] Births to unmarried women have increased by 40.6% with significant differences by race/ethnicity; rates among black (72.3%), Native American (65.8%), and Hispanic (52.5%) women were considerably higher than among white (28.6%) and Asian (16.9%) women.[10] In the absence of contraception, the probability of pregnancy was twice as high among young women ages 19 to 26 years compared with women older than age 35. In addition, fertility of older men declines although less strikingly than among older women.[26]

Across the United States regional patterns exist with distinctly different contraceptive methods used, ages at first and subsequent pregnancies, options for pregnancy interruption, and comorbid conditions affecting maternal health. Although the American Congress of Obstetricians and Gynecologists (ACOG) recommends the availability and use of emergency contraception to prevent unplanned pregnancy after unprotected sexual intercourse,[27] the medication is not equally available across the country. Many of these reproductive decisions influence subsequent physical and mental health of women as they mature through adulthood to older ages influencing regional differences in rates of cancer, heart disease, diabetes, etc.

Conception and Implantation

Among young, healthy couples the probability of conception during one ovulatory cycle of unprotected intercourse averages 20% to 25%, with 85% becoming pregnant after one year.[28] The complex sequence resulting in conception begins with a dominant follicle raising hormone levels, which trigger the uterine lining to prepare for implantation of a fertilized egg. As estradiol levels increase luteinizing hormone (LH) is released causing the follicle to rupture and ovulation to occur. The released egg is transported through the fallopian tube where fertilization can occur if intercourse has provided viable sperm within a few days of ovulation (see Figure 10-4).

Once the sperm enters the egg complex, the merged chromosomes create the genetically unique fertilized embryo that immediately begins to divide and travel toward the uterus for implantation. Cells in the dividing embryo form clusters of increasingly smaller cellular groupings before development of distinct organ systems.

Following ovulation the empty follicle is transformed into the corpus luteum, which produces progesterone, the hormone essential for stimulating uterine preparation and maintaining the pregnancy until the placenta begins progesterone production. After conception, the uniquely

modified maternal immune response prevents rejection of the embryo, which contains foreign DNA from the sperm.[29] During the first few days of development, the fertilized egg (zygote) may separate into two genetically identical parts, each becoming a separate, monozygous twin, or into a higher number of divisions. Fraternal (dizygotic) twins occur when two eggs are released at ovulation and fertilized during one menstrual cycle, which occurs more frequently among older women.

The free-floating embryo attaches to the prepared endometrium by invading the stroma and establishing the placenta. Once implantation has occurred, the lack of a normally timed menstrual cycle indicates to the woman that conception has taken place.[30] This complex sequence of events results in only 30% of fertilized eggs successfully implanting during the brief interval of receptivity of the endometrium.[31] In 1% to 2% an ectopic pregnancy occurs when the fertilized ovum implants in the fallopian tube before reaching the uterus. The dividing cells may die in the tube or cause the tube to rupture, creating a potentially life threatening condition responsible for 3% to 4% of pregnancy-related deaths.[32] Women are generally unaware when conception occurs; therefore, sudden sharp pelvic pain requires emergency care. Ectopic pregnancy-related deaths have declined in recent decades possibly associated with use of pregnancy tests, ultrasound diagnosis, and improvement in laparoscopic surgery and medical management.[32] The estimated mortality rate due to ectopic pregnancy, 31.9 per 100,000 pregnancies, is 4.5 times greater than death after a live birth.[33] Between 2003 and 2007 African American women were approximately 6.8 times more likely to die from an ectopic pregnancy and their all-cause maternity mortality was 2.7–3.7 times higher than that for white women.[34] A history of pelvic infection that may have damaged the fallopian tubes is

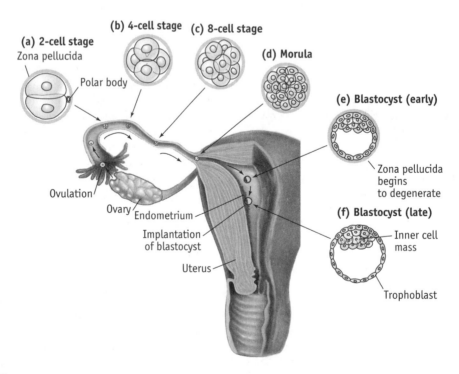

Figure 10-4 Ovulation.

associated with elevated risk of ectopic pregnancy. Although the rate has decreased in recent years,[33] a recent sudden increased incidence in Florida was found to be associated with illicit drug use accompanied by delayed medical care.[32] Women who have been treated for an ectopic pregnancy are at increased risk of another ectopic event.[34]

Since 1965 ACOG has defined pregnancy as beginning with implantation of the embryo and rising levels of human chorionic gonadotropin (HCG).[35] Some clinicians, politicians, and members of the public believe pregnancy begins with fertilization of the ovum by the sperm. These differences influence acceptance of contraceptive technologies; for example, the intrauterine device impedes implantation in contrast to oral contraceptives that prevent ovulation.

Conditions Contributing to Infertility

Infertility, the inability to conceive within 12 months of unprotected intercourse, is a common health problem affecting approximately 10% of women and their partners.[28] Most analyses suggest 50% of infertility results from problems of women, 30% due to the men alone, and 20% combined factors from both partners.[20] Tubal abnormalities, often caused by pelvic inflammatory disease, have been found responsible for 25% to 35% of female infertility. Among other major causes of infertility are increasing age, menstrual abnormalities, primary ovarian insufficiency, polycystic ovary syndrome, sexually transmitted infections, endometriosis, uterine fibroids, and some other conditions that are treated by hysterectomy.

Maternal Age

During the past few decades American women have delayed childbearing to complete their education and begin careers resulting in older maternal age at first birth.[28] In 1980 women aged 30 or older accounted for 20% of all births; by 2009 the proportion increased to 35%[36] and births to women older than age 40 have increased more than 70%.[37] Data comparing 1990 with 2005 in Figure 10-5 from the National Center for Health Statistics indicate a welcome

decline in teenage pregnancies and a significant increase in childbearing at ages 30 and older.[38]

Recent data indicate a 36% increase in first births among women ages 35 to 39 and 70% increase among women 40–44. In 2002, more than 260 women gave birth between ages 50 and 54.[37] Delayed childbearing has major implications for women's future health, socioeconomic status, family size, and a range of birth outcomes. Although age at first birth has increased in all states during the past 3 decades, major geographic differences exist by region with the oldest mean age recorded in the northeast and youngest in central and southern states.[38] Asian American women were oldest with a mean age of 28.5 years and American Indian/Alaskan Native women were youngest with a mean age of 21.9 years. In contrast to other developed countries, the ages at first birth among all segments of the American population were younger.[38]

In addition to higher rates of infertility, maternal age of 35 years or older carries increased risk of adverse neonatal events including preterm birth, low birth weight, or small for gestational age.[39] Some researchers note that older age during pregnancy increases risks of developmental abnormalities not readily detectable at birth including autism.[40] Age-related decline in female fertility is attributed to oocyte quality, decreased ovarian responsiveness to stimulation, and significantly increased aneuploidy (too few or too many chromosomes).[41] The uterus is less contributory to age-related infertility than the ovaries. Therefore, older women are able to carry a pregnancy achieved with eggs from a young donor. However, among some women pregnancy may be a health hazard necessitating gestational surrogacy.

Premenstrual Syndrome (PMS)

Premenstrual syndrome, experienced by millions of women, is among the most common disorders affecting quality of life.[42] More than 50% of menstruating women have pain with each cycle and an estimated 10% suffer from severe bleeding with cramps that limit normal activities. Others experience emotional and physical PMS symptoms of varying intensity that recur for 10 days to 2 weeks during the luteal phase.[42] PMS symptoms vary from mild, affecting 20% to 40%, to severe, a condition called premenstrual dysphoric disorder (PDD) affecting 3% to 8%.[43] Patients with PMS demonstrate a distinctive pattern with anxiety increasing progressively during the late luteal phase until the onset of menses brings rapid resolution and emotional stability until ovulation begins the next luteal phase (Table 10-1). The physical and emotional symptoms of PMS disrupt normal reproductive patterns resulting in delayed childbearing and subsequent infertility.

Compared with serum levels of controls, PMS patients had significantly lower levels of free estradiol and higher sex hormone-binding globulin (SHBG) specifically during the luteal phase. Thys-Jacobs et al. suggested the PMS hormonal patterns they identified adversely affected cognitive function.[42] In a Cochrane Review of controlled trials assessing PDD treatment, oral contraceptives containing drospirenone, a low-dose estrogen, reduced symptoms

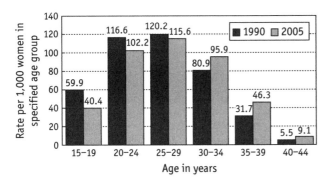

Figure 10-5 Birth rates by age of mother: United States, 1990 and 2005.

Source: Reproduced from Hamilton BE, Martin JA, Ventura SJ. Births: Preliminary data for 2005. *National vital Statistics Reports* 2005;55:11. http://www.cdc.gov/nchs/data/nvsr/nvsr55/nvsr55_11.pdf.

Table 10-1

Common symptoms occurring during the luteal phase of the menstrual cycle associated with premenstrual syndrome (PMS) and premenstrual dysphoric disorder (PDD)

- Depressed mood
- Anxiety
- Lability, emotional instability
- Irritability
- Decreased interest in usual activities
- Difficulty concentrating
- Marked lack of energy
- Change in appetite, overeating or food craving
- Hypersomnia or insomnia
- Sense of being overwhelmed
- Physical discomforts, breast tenderness, headaches, bloating

more effectively than a placebo.[43] Additional research suggested disturbances in calcium regulation may contribute to PMS with some relief provided by calcium supplements.[42]

Sexually Transmitted Infections (STIs)

Human reproduction creates opportunities for infections acquired during sexual intercourse to be transmitted from mother to offspring during pregnancy, at delivery, and while breastfeeding.[44] Major STIs may adversely affect reproduction, causing infertility of women and men. In addition, prenatal exposure of fetuses to STIs including human immunodeficiency virus/acquired immune deficiency syndrome (HIV/AIDS) may result in life-threatening birth defects. Recently developed HIV treatment for pregnant women now provides protection for the developing fetus and may reduce viral transmission during breastfeeding. Women receiving prenatal care and those with fertility problems should be screened for STIs as some infections acquired during vaginal intercourse may remain asymptomatic and untreated, able to persist and spread in the pelvis and beyond, potentially becoming life threatening for mother and baby.[45]

Chlamydia is commonly transmitted among sexual partners and when severe infection develops, tubal obstruction may result.[46] Chronic gonorrhea infection may cause painful pelvic inflammatory disease with damage to fallopian tubes causing sterility or risk of ectopic pregnancy.[45] During pregnancy some frequently diagnosed STIs include genital vaginosis and herpes.[44] At critical times of development, infections transmitted to the fetus may cause anatomical and/or functional abnormalities in the developing reproductive organs.[44] In addition, preterm delivery has been associated with some STI conditions including bacterial vaginosis.[45]

Polycystic Ovary Syndrome (PCOS)

Polycystic ovary syndrome, associated with anovulatory infertility, is a genetically complex endocrine disorder characterized by menstrual dysfunction, early pregnancy loss, and later pregnancy complications. Azziz et al. indicated two of the following three characteristics were considered diagnostic of PCOS: 1) very frequent ovulation or anovulatory cycles, 2) clinical or biochemical indications of excessive circulating androgens, and 3) polycystic ovaries assessed by ultrasound.[47] An estimated 6% to 8% of women of reproductive age are affected. In addition to experiencing eight or fewer menstrual cycles in 12 months that may be either very short, less than 26 days, or excessively long, more than 35 days, PCOS patients have been found to have low progesterone levels during the luteal phase of the menstrual cycle.[47] Additional characteristics of PCOS include premature puberty with early growth of pubic hair, elevated androgen levels, and excess circulating insulin. Factors contributing to PCOS include genetic susceptibility combined with adverse environmental exposures during embryonic and fetal development.[47] These patients are often obese with metabolic abnormalities including insulin resistance or diabetes.[48]

Uterine Leiomyomata (Fibroids)

In the United States an estimated 300,000 hysterectomies are performed annually for treatment of fibroids, a common benign gynecologic condition affecting 20%–30% of premenopausal women. In addition to causing infertility, fibroids have been associated with repeated miscarriage among women who are able to conceive.[49] Infertility may result from fibroid tumors protruding into the uterine cavity, interfering with embryo implantation, and obstructing normal fetal growth.[49] The tumors develop in the wall of the uterus causing excessive bleeding (menorrhagia) and iron-deficiency anemia. Additional prevalent symptoms include pelvic pain and pressure, pressure on the bladder causing urinary frequency and incontinence, constipation, and pain during sexual intercourse.[49] Many women who have delayed childbearing may require treatment for symptomatic fibroids and seek therapy enabling maintenance of fertility.

Multiple fibroids have differing genetic patterns indicating they develop independently. Compared with normal uterine tissue, fibroids have increased hormone receptors responding to circulating estrogens.[51] Therefore, earlier age at menarche providing longer lifetime exposure to estrogen[51] doubles the risk of fibroids compared to later menarche.[52] Fibroids were diagnosed five times more frequently among African American than white women in a case-control study in Baltimore, Maryland,[49] and in the Nurses' Health Study II fibroids developed at younger ages (mean 31 years) among black compared with white women (mean of 37 years).[53]

Treatment options depend on age, symptoms, coexisting conditions, desires for childbearing, and the nature of the fibroids.[53] Nonsteroidal anti-inflammatory drugs (NSAIDS) may provide some relief although these medications may increase blood loss. Reduced risk was associated with oral contraceptive use compared to contraceptives never being used (OR = 0.2, 95% CI = 0.1–0.6).[49] Some women avoid hysterectomy to retain reproductive potential electing myomectomy, a surgical procedure that removes fibroid tumors, leaving the uterus intact.[54] The procedure provides immediate symptom relief but fibroid tumors often regrow. For unknown reasons black women developed more severe symptoms with greater complications during or following myomectomy. Fibroids may also be diminished by treatment with progesterone inhibitors including RU486[55] although long-term use produces a hypoestrogenic environment increasing the risk of bone loss. Short-term regimens are preferred and often prescribed prior to myomectomy to shrink the tumor before surgery.[56]

Magnetic resonance imaging (MRI) has been used to guide high-intensity ultrasound beams to the tumors raising their temperature and destroying the outer layers. Regrowth is possible and ability to become pregnant is not ensured.[54] Although the uterus and ovaries are intact, impaired reproductive function has been reported.[54] However, a British study of 1,200 women treated by embolization noted 56 of 108 women became pregnant; 17 experienced miscarriages, 2 had stillbirths, one had an ectopic pregnancy, and 33 gave birth although 6 babies were preterm.[57] After embolization increased risk of miscarriage, preterm delivery, and postpartum hemorrhage requiring cesarean delivery occurred more frequently than in the general population.[57]

Family history of fibroids was linked to a twofold increased risk.[58] Obesity, independent of race/ethnicity,[59] and weight gain during adult years increased risk by 50%. Premenopausal obesity, associated with lower progesterone levels, enables unopposed estrogen to stimulate fibroid growth.[60] After controlling for body mass index (BMI), hypertension was also an adverse factor among premenopausal nurses; for each 10-mmHg elevation of blood pressure, risk was increased 8% to 10%.[61] Since smoking lowers estrogen levels, smokers were 20% to 50% less likely to develop fibroids in a large case-control study.[52] Some clinicians suggested cigarette smoking alters hormone receptors in uterine tissue, lowering cellular response to circulating estrogen.[60]

Exercise and dietary patterns have been studied. College athletes were less likely to develop fibroids than nonathletes reflecting the relationship of estrogen stimulation.[62] Faerstein et al. reported an association between fibroid development and sexually transmitted infections.[49] High consumption of red meat and ham was associated with increased risk, but a diet rich in green vegetables[63] and dairy products lowered the risk.[64]

Endometriosis

Studies suggest endometriosis is caused by misplaced endometrial tissue from retrograde menstrual discharge passing through fallopian tubes into the pelvic cavity. The resulting infection causes infertility and excessive menstrual and pelvic pain during intercourse.[65] The condition affects 6% to 10% of women during childbearing years; 30% of infertility patients have a history of endometriosis.[66] The extent of disease varies from severe morbidity causing distortion of pelvic organs to mild painless disease.[67] Adhesions due to inflammation distort pelvic structures causing mechanical and biochemical problems that impede conception.[68] Infertility was also associated with macrophages and cytokines in peritoneal fluid found to be toxic to sperm and the developing embryo.[69,70] A 2002 meta-analysis by Barnhart et al. of 22 studies assessing pregnancy after in vitro fertilization (IVF) among women with a history of endometriosis reported 54% achieved pregnancy but successful IVF declined with increasing severity of the disease.[68]

Suggested causes of the disease include genetics, environmental exposures, altered immune response, and higher than average estrogen levels. Development of endometriosis is sixfold greater among women with an affected first-degree relative compared to women with no family history.[71–73] Linkage analyses among affected sibling-pairs are being studied for candidate genes associated with endometriosis. Some studies have suggested compromised immune function with diminished natural killer cells increases vulnerability to endometriosis in addition to autoimmune and endocrine conditions.

Infertility Following Cancer Treatment

A systematic review of published quality of life studies of young breast cancer survivors by Howard-Anderson et al. found a majority expressed fear of treatment-induced premature menopause and subsequent infertility; 30% based their treatment decisions on anticipated impact on potential childbearing.[74] Before initiating treatment many young patients requested guidance from infertility specialists and sought ovarian stimulation to retrieve oocytes prior to chemotherapy. Robertson et al. suggest that patients scheduled for chemotherapy that may cause ovarian failure should be advised about options for fertility preservation including embryo banking. They noted some clinicians fail to refer cancer patients to infertility specialists, fearing the exposure to hormonal treatment.[75] The authors found the lack of significant complications after fertility preservation encouraging for patients and their healthcare providers. New technology has improved the success of IVF treatment that may now offer childbearing options to the growing number of young cancer survivors.[75]

Infertility Caused by Eating Disorders

Nutritional deficiencies resulting from eating disorders can also compromise reproduction by causing menstrual dysfunction leading to amenorrhea. One small study at an infertility clinic found that over one-third of the patients receiving ovulation induction had an active eating disorder.[19] If these patients become pregnant, they are at elevated risk for miscarriage, prenatal mortality, and preterm birth at low birth weight. Moreover, a study in Sweden noted infants of mothers with anorexia who were born at low birth weight had higher risks of developing anorexia later in life potentially associated with genetic and environmental factors.[76]

Infertility Associated with Prenatal Exposure to Diethylstilbestrol

Between the 1930s and the 1970s more than 2 million American women were prescribed diethylstilbestrol (DES) a hormone believed by clinicians to prevent pregnancy complications. A recently reported 40-year follow-up of more than 4,500 women exposed prenatally to DES has identified higher rates of infertility and adverse pregnancy outcomes compared with 2,000 unexposed controls as noted in Table 10-2.[77] This exposure is discussed more fully later in this chapter. The average age of the exposed daughters at last follow-up was 48 years.[77]

Shorter reproductive years for DES exposed women led to earlier menopause, which Steiner et al. hypothesized was associated with abnormal organ development and possibly reduced number of oocytes at birth leading to earlier depletion during the menopausal transition.[78]

Treatment of Infertility—Assisted Reproduction Technology (ART)

ART includes all fertility treatments in which eggs and sperm are handled with the goal of assisting patients to become parents preferably of one healthy child at a time but methods of treatment often produce multiple births. Although most twin births occur naturally, ovulation stimulation and assisted reproduction have increased the frequency of twin births more than 20 times during the past 3 decades.[36]

Ovarian Stimulation

In recent years drugs to induce ovulation are among the most frequently prescribed medications in the United States; use has doubled and continues to increase as the number of infertile women seeking ART climbs.[79] Clomiphene was first approved by the FDA in 1967 and gonadotropins in 1969. Long-term follow-up data of women who have used these medications in their 20s and 30s has not been consistently collected and many who used these drugs have only recently reached older ages when health problems could occur. Some evidence suggested use of clomiphene citrate and gonadotropins could increase risks of ovarian and breast cancer due to their effect of increasing estrogen and progesterone levels.[79] A single stimulation cycle may produce eggs equivalent to 24 natural ovulatory cycles and many women require several treatment cycles to achieve conception.[80] New data from a recent Dutch study of women treated by IVF compared with subfertile women found a twofold increased risk of borderline invasive and invasive ovarian tumors.[81] Additional follow-up of American women should be conducted.

Table 10-2

Risk of adverse reproductive health outcomes in women with and without prenatal exposure to diethylstilbestrol (DES)

Adverse Outcome	Risk among DES Exposed	Risk among Unexposed	Excess Risk [95% CI]	Hazard Ratio [95% CI]
Infertility	33.3%	15.5%	17.8% [14.5–20.9]	2.37 [2.05–2.75]
Spontaneous Abortion	50.3%	38.6%	11.7% [3.3–20.1]	1.64 [1.42–1.88]
Ectopic Pregnancy	14.6%	2.9%	11.7% [8.9–14.5]	3.72 [2.58–5.38]
Preterm Delivery	53.3%	17.8%	35.4% [27.3–43.6]	4.68 [3.74–5.86]
Preeclampsia	26.4%	13.7%	12.7% [4.5–20.9]	1.42 [1.07–1.89]
Stillbirth	8.9%	2.6%	6.3% [0.8–13.3]	2.45 [1.33–4.54]
Neonatal Death	7.8%	0.6%	7.2% [1.9–12.5]	8.12 [3.53–18.65]
Early Menopause	5.1%	1.7%	3.4% [2.1–4.7]	2.35 [1.67–3.13]

Source: Data from Hoover RN, Hyer M, Pfeiffer RM, et al. Adverse health outcomes in women exposed in utero to diethylstilbestrol. *N Engl J Med* 2011;365:1304–1314.

In-Vitro Fertilization (IVF)

In-vitro fertilization, a multistep and complex process, is increasingly being used by infertile couples to achieve childbearing. An estimated 12% of American women have obtained infertility services. The most frequent method to achieve pregnancy is through the transfer of fertilized eggs into the woman's uterus. To assist women and their partners in deciding about IVF treatment, a federal law was passed in 1992, the Fertility Clinic Success Rate and Certification Act, mandating CDC to publish pregnancy success rates for ART fertility clinics. These statistics are available on the Internet.[82] IVF is challenging for women as multiple hormone injections are required for ovarian stimulation to harvest oocytes.[83] Laboratory procedures combine eggs and sperm or by a newer procedure, intracytoplasmic sperm injection is applied providing special help for male fertility problems. Embryos are then transferred to the prepared uterus through the cervix.[28]

Age alone has an impact on fertility among women receiving IVF-embryo transfers as the probability of live births decreases progressively from 45% among women younger than age 35 to 37.3% for women 35 to 37 years, 27% among women ages 38 to 40 years, 15.2% ages 41–42 and 6.7% ages 43–44. In contrast, 54% of eggs obtained from young donors resulted in live births regardless of the age of the recipient.[82] Figure 10-6 notes the type of ART cycles completed in 2009 differed significantly by women's ages with the majority of women younger than 35 using their own eggs in contrast to 73% of women older than 44 who relied on donor eggs. Regardless of age, however, most cycles involved fresh eggs or embryos rather than frozen.[82] In 2009 more than 84,000 women received egg or embryo transfers, producing approximately 38,000

pregnancies, resulting in 30,787 live-birth deliveries of one or more babies; 62% of these births were singleton and 29% twins.[82]

Although clinicians and patients have been recommended to limit the number of embryos transferred during IVF to avoid adverse pregnancy outcomes, 40% of treatment cycles in the United States and 21% in Europe involve transfer of at least three embryos, and between 20% and 30% of IVF pregnancies produce twins or higher order multiple gestations.[28] In some countries with nationalized health care, the number of embryos permitted for transfer is restricted by patient age: women younger than 40 may transfer two embryos and older women may transfer three.

American physicians have freedom to individualize the number of embryos to be transferred and have noted that most partners undergoing assisted reproduction desire twins. IVF treatment must be concerned with the health of the infants who are often small for gestational ages, even among singleton births. The rate of live births among older women was significantly lower regardless of the number of embryos transferred.[84] Although transfer of two or three embryos increased the live birth rate more than transfer of only one, at any maternal age the transfer of three or more embryos was associated with a significantly higher risk of multiple pregnancies with severe complications including preterm birth and low birth weight. Therefore, transfer of two embryos is recommended for best birth outcomes.[84]

Another problem couples experience after ovarian stimulation or ART is the creation of more embryos than needed necessitating selective reduction, a procedure that may result in total pregnancy loss.[85] In addition, couples may have remaining embryos after completing their desired family size.[86] Sauer noted three options for use of the sur-

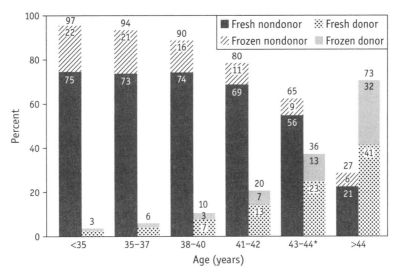

*Note: Total does not equal 100% due to rounding.

Figure 10-6 Types of assisted reproductive technology cycles by age group, United States—2009.

Source: Courtesy of Centers for Disease Control and Prevention. http://www.cdc.gov/art/artreports.htm.

plus harvested embryos: they can be donated for research, provided to another couple seeking in vitro assisted reproduction, or they can be discarded. For many couples this decision is emotionally difficult and partners may not agree.[87] Some storage facilities have reported couples may pay storage fees for many years. Other couples have been found to discontinue payment to avoid decision-making, leaving clinics to determine future disposal. In March 2009 President Obama issued an Executive Order removing barriers to responsible scientific research involving human stem cells ensuring federal funding for ethically responsible and scientifically worthy research using donated embryos from couples who have completed their desired family size.[88]

Donor Oocytes or Embryos

IVF technology including donor eggs provides opportunities for pregnancy and childbearing to women with diverse causes of infertility who are unable to conceive a child using their own eggs. The 2008 guidelines for gamete and embryo donation of the Practice Committee of the American Society for Reproductive Medicine recommended optimal screening for sexually transmitted infections, genetic diseases, and psychological assessments for the male and female donors and recipients.[89] The document notes "oocyte donation requires ovarian stimulation with monitoring oocyte retrieval, involving significant inconvenience, discomfort, and risks for the donor."[89] As of 2009 an estimated 100,000 young American women have sold or donated their oocytes through approximately 470 IVF clinics after one or more hormonally induced ovarian stimulations.[90] The ethical aspects of financial compensation for oocytes has generated a growing literature with scientists expressing discontent with the practice but accepting the necessity of payment for time, effort, and inconvenience.[91]

With diminishing quality of their remaining oocytes, older women have sought fresh donor eggs that provide greater opportunities for successful pregnancy.[93] Over age 45, 92% of IVF patients used donor eggs, increasing their probability of a live birth by almost 50% compared with using their own eggs.[82] A recent report by Kort et al. compared adverse outcomes following IVF with donor eggs among pregnant women age 50 and older with events experienced by IVF-donor patients age 42 or younger. Although older women are at greater risk for maternal complications, especially hypertensive disorders, the incidence difference by age was not significant.[92] Pregnancy among older women close to menopause may increase as studies indicate childbirth rates following oocyte cryopreservation are comparable to fresh IVF cycles with fewer congenital anomalies (1.2%) than reported in the general public (3%).[93] Technologic advances have improved oocyte retrieval and fertilization as reported below by Knopman et al.[93]

Oocyte donation is a significant contributor to ART treatment for older couples and technologic advances ease oocyte retrieval and improved endometrial preparation increasing implantation success.[41] Donors have been recruited by advertisements on websites and in college publications that generally specify financial arrangements and desired personal characteristics of donors including age range, race/ethnicity, college SAT score, physical activity level, and health behaviors.[90] Oocyte donors may be anonymous after screening by the ART facility or private agency with limited personal history of the donor provided to the intended parents or donors may be recruited by potential recipients followed by screening by the ART facility.[41]

Since IVF clinics do not maintain contact with donors, studies of postdonor health experiences have relied upon alternative avenues for data collection.[90] One small Internet-based study of 155 women reported 30% experienced ovarian hyperstimulation syndrome, painful enlargement of the ovaries, and 26% had subsequent menstrual or fertility problems. Study participants frequently lacked contact with the IVF clinic and rarely received information about pregnancy outcomes resulting from their donations.[90] The authors noted their data cannot be considered representative of the large number of women who have donated oocytes although they encouraged research to assess the long-term health and safety of oocyte donations.

Two unique IVF experiences provide personal examples of the impact of egg donation. Sills et al. reported a patient with premature ovarian failure, a genetic cause of infertility affecting 1% of women,[94] was unable to conceive and received oocytes from her nonidentical twin sister who had a 10-month-old child conceived without medical assistance. Her oocytes donated to her twin successfully produced twin male babies.[94]

Another IVF experience that has become a trend among some career oriented women was described by Knopman et al. A healthy 38-year-old patient requested cryopreservation of oocytes for her own potential future use. Her history included a terminated pregnancy 7 years earlier. Following ovarian stimulation, nine oocytes were obtained and cryopreserved. The patient subsequently married, spontaneously achieved pregnancy, and gave birth to a daughter.[93] However, when a second pregnancy was desired, the couple was unable to conceive. Following unsuccessful ovarian stimulation and a failed fresh IVF attempt, the cryopreserved oocytes were thawed and fertilized by intracytoplasmic sperm injection. While the developing embryos were monitored, the mother's endometrium was prepared for transfer. A singleton gestation developed and her full-term pregnancy was uncomplicated.[93]

Gestational Carriers

"Third-party reproduction" refers to donated oocytes, sperm, embryos, or uterus provided by donors to enable others to become parents.[41] Some women, whose health prevents their carrying a pregnancy, arrange with a surrogate who agrees to carry the developing embryo(s) for remuneration. Gestational carrier arrangements enable a younger woman to carry embryos created in vitro with sperm and egg and transferred to her uterus following hormonal preparation. Although the fetus has no genetic link to the surrogate, the immune status of pregnancy prevents rejection.[41] Many countries do not permit gestational surrogacy or have legal regulations. None exist in the United States where commercial surrogacy is permitted.[41] The complexity of egg retrieval and transfer to a gestational carrier is reviewed by Luk et al.[41] Long-term cohort studies of children born through different IVF procedures are required to fully understand the physical and psychological life-course effects of the complex procedures required for assisted reproduction.

Preimplantation Genetic Diagnosis (PGD)

Increased use of in vitro fertilization has enabled many couples to consider genetic testing of embryos before transfer to the uterus.[95,96] Women of childbearing age with a strong family history of hereditary disease are learning their mutation status providing the opportunity for genetic assessment of embryos prior to implantation relieving some of the emotional burden and fear of transmitting the genetic syndrome to the couple's offspring.[95] Among a random sample of IVF clinic websites, 70% provided information about genetic assessment and availability at the clinic; however, clinicians reviewing the websites considered the information provided by some clinics lacking adequate coverage of risks and benefits of PGD.[97] As oncologists have used genetic information to guide treatment of cancer patients, couples are opting to use genetic analyses as a component of assisted reproduction.[96] Prenatal testing indicates the status of a developing fetus providing the option of pregnancy termination.[96] However, genetic analysis of an early embryo following fertilization before implantation is being performed with increasing frequency for common cancer syndromes and other inherited conditions.

The American Medical Association defined the Code of Medical Ethics, which was updated in 1994 to provide for three primary areas of prenatal genetic testing to include:[98]

- Screening or evaluation of prospective parents for genetic disease before conception to predict the likelihood of conceiving an affected child;
- Analysis of embryos at the preimplantation stage of artificial reproductive techniques; and
- In utero testing after conception by ultrasound, amniocentesis, or chorionic villus sampling to determine the genetic status of the fetus.

IVF provides hope for pregnancy and childbearing with each cycle, although it is frequently followed by failed implantation, increasing risks of depression and anxiety.[95] However, being able to test the DNA before implantation has provided security after successful implantation. Figure 10-7 demonstrates the procedure; one or two cells are removed from each 3-day-old embryo for genetic analysis. The procedure does not adversely affect the viability of the fertilized egg.

A retrospective cohort study suggested preimplantation genetic analysis was associated with reduced rates of pregnancy loss before 20 weeks gestation especially among women older than age 40.[99] Studies noted no excess congenital anomalies detected among more than 1,000 births following PGD,[96] although Hansen et al. in 2002 reported birth defects were increased twofold among babies born after IVF. These defects were potentially associated with

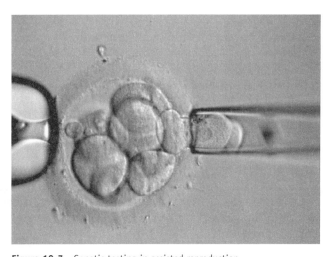

Figure 10-7 Genetic testing in assisted reproduction.

Source: Courtesy of M.R. Hughes, Genesis Genetics Institute, Detroit, MI.

one or more of the following: advanced ages of infertile couples, underlying cause of infertility, medications used to induce ovulation and to maintain the pregnancy, and risks associated with freezing and thawing of embryos.[100] Matched studies are needed with comparable maternal ages and duration of follow-up to uncover any potential increase in neonatal abnormalities. Noyes et al. indicated cryopreservation was not associated with increased congenital anomalies[101] and Klipstein suggested PGD may eventually reduce the number of pregnancy terminations.[83] Ethical considerations will influence the acceptance of all aspects of this newest component of assisted reproduction including the very controversial testing for sex selection.

Multiple Births

After decades of relatively stable annual incidence rates of multiple births at 2% per year, rates began to rise in 1980. By 2009, 1 of every 30 babies born in the United States was a twin compared to the 1 in 53 in 1980, an increase of 76% from 18.9 to 33.3 per 1,000 births.[36] A major contributor to the changed incidence is ART including IVF and ovulation stimulation without ART, which now account for 70% of all American twin births. Among American women seeking pregnancy through ART in 2009, 29% produced twins and 7% had triplets.[82] Frequency of twin births differed by maternal age as noted in Figure 10-8. Rates increased close to 100% among women ages 35 to 39 and more than 200% among women ages 40 and older.[36] If the 1980 rate pertained in 2009, 865,000 fewer twins would have been born in the past 3 decades.[36]

The rates vary considerably by state with the fewest twins born in New Mexico (2% of all births) and the highest percentage in Connecticut (5%). Twins were born with similar frequency among non-Hispanic white and black women (38 per 1,000 births) but lower among Hispanics (22.5 per 1,000 births). The probability of naturally occurring dizygotic twins rises eightfold between teenage years and ages 35 to 40 before declining rapidly. Some couples state they are pleased to create an instant family with twins although neonatal mortality and other adverse

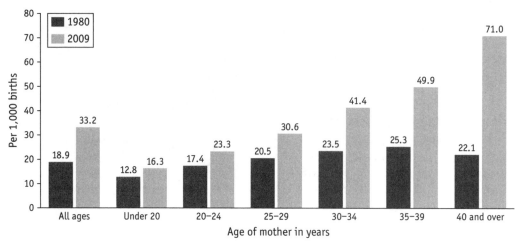

Figure 10-8 Twin birth rates, by age of mother: United States, 1980 and 2009.

Source: Reproduced from Martin JA, Hamilton BE, Osterman MJK. Three decades of twin births in the United States, 1980–2009. *NCHS Data Brief;* 2012; No. 80.

birth outcomes are significantly increased among twins compared with singleton births. In 2009 more than 50% of twins were born preterm or at low birth weight; 8% to 15% of twins are at risk of very premature birth (less than 33 weeks) and 7% to 11% at very low birth weight (less than 1,500 grams). Some research has suggested IVF twin births are at greater risk than twins conceived naturally.[36]

Newton et al. assessed patients' decisions regarding IVF transfer options and twin pregnancies at a university hospital in Ontario. After being informed of the potential risks associated with twin and higher order births (three or more offspring in one birth), couples favored transferring fewer embryos with a maximum of two, balancing the desire for pregnancy and accepting potential risks associated with twins.[102] Reductions from multiple to twin pregnancies were considered acceptable as higher order pregnancies carry greater risks. Compared with women carrying one fetus, women carrying twins or more fetuses have a greater need for bed rest and are more likely to experience premature labor, hypertension, postpartum hemorrhage, and cesarean delivery.[28]

Preconception and Prenatal Care

Although maternal and newborn health has been enhanced by routinely scheduled prenatal care enabling management of chronic diseases and monitoring of pregnancy-related health conditions, scientific evidence indicates the health of women *before* pregnancy will have the greatest impact on pregnancy outcomes.[103] Among preventive care practices advocated by the IOM report were annual examinations for adult women to receive recommended preventive services, including guidance and counseling regarding personal behaviors prior to pregnancy and between pregnancies. These stages of women's health have been found most successful times for modifications of biomedical, behavioral, and social risks that affect their health and that of their children.[2] Women experiencing unplanned or unintended pregnancies are often not aware

that conception has occurred, resulting in adverse exposures to the fetus during the earliest weeks of pregnancy from smoking, alcohol consumption, illegal drugs, etc. Women experiencing unplanned pregnancies are also at greater risk of depression, anxiety, and domestic violence.[2]

Federal health agencies and professional organizations have advised women of childbearing age to receive clinical preventive care during their reproductive years; however, the percentage of women receiving medical care before pregnancy is rarely tabulated.[104] Recent birth certificate data reported by CDC indicated more than 7% of women received no prenatal care or were monitored only in the third trimester. Prenatal care has increased in recent decades but continues to differ by race/ethnicity (Figure 10-9). This pattern has continued as noted in a recent CDC report; initiation of care during the first trimester was greatest among non-Hispanic white women (76%) and lower among non-Hispanic black women (59%) and Hispanic women (65%).[105]

Progress to reduce low birth weight, preterm birth, and infant mortality has slowed during the past decade.[104] The U.S. infant and maternal mortality rates exceed those of other industrialized nations and within the United States racial and ethnic disparities continue to plague reproductive health outcomes.[106] Therefore, many programs have encouraged preconception health care, pregnancy planning, and early prenatal care. Since a majority of Americans rely on mobile phones and related technology for health information, successful smoking cessation programs,[107] weight loss studies, and medication adherence efforts[108] are using these technologies to reach at-risk women. CDC has built on the concept by developing an innovative project, Text4baby (text4baby.org), an online health information service for pregnant women.[109] After registering with their anticipated date of delivery, vital health messages are provided and carefully timed to coincide with the specific stage of the individual's pregnancy.[109] Text4baby also identifies local public clinics for prenatal and infant care. The free service is available in Spanish and English, even if the woman does not have a text message plan.[109]

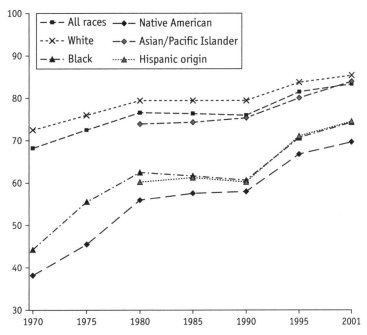

Figure 10-9 Prenatal care for mothers with live births by race and Hispanic origin, 1970–2001.

Source: Courtesy of Women's Research and Education Institute.

Targeted health interventions are also advised between pregnancies (interconception) for women with a history of previous adverse reproductive outcomes such as fetal loss, infant with a birth defect, or low birth weight baby. Past history may be a predictor of a repeated adverse event.[104] During postpartum care, clinicians have the opportunity to guide reduction of medical, dental, and psychosocial factors that may have contributed to any poor reproductive outcome.[104]

Exposures Complicating Pregnancy and Birth Outcomes

Influenza Infection during Pregnancy

Influenza causes more severe illness among pregnant than non-pregnant women, often resulting in hospitalization. In addition, high temperature early in pregnancy associated with the flu may cause birth defects.[110] Pregnant women with severe influenza who gave birth during their flu hospitalization were more likely to deliver a baby of low birth weight preterm than healthy delivering women. Since approximately 4 million births occur annually in the United States, a large proportion of women are likely to be pregnant during any flu epidemic. A New York City study of the 2009–2010 pandemic reported extremely high hospitalization rates with several deaths among pregnant compared to nonpregnant women.[111] The severity of H1N1 infections led to ethical concerns regarding prioritizing pregnant women for vaccine coverage and treatment when supplies were limited. An additional concern pertains to new drugs for resistant influenza viruses that may be inadequately tested for safety and efficacy for pregnant women and their fetuses.[112] Educational programs of the CDC and promoted by public health workers significantly increased flu vaccine coverage with doctors' recommendations a primary motivator of public acceptance, enhanced by expanded access at local pharmacies and clinics.[113]

Weight Gain during Pregnancy

Both excessive and insufficient weight gain during pregnancy can negatively influence maternal and infant health. Research indicates inappropriate maternal weight gain can result in cesarean delivery, preterm birth, small-for and large-for-gestational-age birth, and neonatal mortality.[114] The new IOM guidelines recommend a minimum weight gain of 11 pounds and maximum gain of 40 pounds for a woman having a singleton, term pregnancy regardless of her pre pregnancy BMI. Recommended weight gains for women with multiple-gestation pregnancies are higher.[114] The revised Institute of Medicine recommendations published in 2009 considered the increasing prevalence of overweight and obesity among American women of childbearing ages from diverse race/ethnicity groups when advising appropriate weight gain during pregnancy.[114]

Since prepregnancy BMI influenced birth outcomes in a meta-analysis of published research by Stothard et al.,[115] women planning pregnancies should be encouraged to lose weight including through bariatric surgery to protect the future health of their infant.[116] The meta-analysis revealed babies born to obese rather than normal weight mothers had higher incidence of congenital anomalies including spina bifida (OR = 2.2, 95% CI = 1.86–2.69), heart defects (OR = 1.20, 95% CI = 1.09–1.31), among other birth adverse events.[115] Overweight and obese nulliparous women are also at greater risk of a cesarean delivery with their first birth.[117]

Excess weight during pregnancy raised risks of chronic conditions including diabetes and hypertension that complicate pregnancies and increase morbidity during post-pregnancy years. A study of more than 1 million births in Michigan found a causal relationship between maternal weight gain and birth weight; each additional kg gained during pregnancy was associated with a 7.35 g increase in birth weight.[118] Infants of women who gained 24 kg during pregnancy compared to women who gained 8 to 10 kg were at more than twofold greater risk of weighing 4000 g at birth. Since birth weight predicts BMI during childhood and adult years, excess maternal weight gain predicts obesity-related condition in her offspring.[118]

Pregestational and Gestational Diabetes

A meta-analysis of 20 studies indicated gestational diabetes mellitus (GDM), diabetes diagnosis during pregnancy, is strongly associated with level of obesity increasing from a twofold risk among overweight women to almost ninefold among severely obese women compared with normal-weight pregnant women.[119] GDM generally occurs during the second or third trimester affecting between 2% and 10% of pregnancies annually. In addition to excess weight before pregnancy, GDM increases with maternal age with risk 7 to 10 times higher among women older than age 30. Mothers with GDM often deliver preterm and if untreated, GDM may increase risk of cardiac, neurologic, or vascular abnormalities in the fetus.[120] Women diagnosed with type 1 or type 2 diabetes are encouraged to plan childbearing with their physician to ensure the personal safety of pregnancy. Control of blood sugar levels during pregnancy provides some protection against the increased risk of birth defects, miscarriage, and stillbirth. Babies of women with diabetes tend to grow larger complicating delivery and increasing risk of cesarean section.[120]

Following delivery some women diagnosed with GDM will recover and others may require continued diabetes treatment for a condition that was not detected before pregnancy. The National Birth Defects Prevention Study has focused on specific defects found in babies of mothers with diabetes diagnosed prior to pregnancy and GDM. These children are at significant risk of being overweight and insulin resistant throughout childhood and at adult ages.

Preeclampsia

In a prospective study of more than 16,000 pregnant women, the risks of gestational hypertension and pre-eclampsia were strongly associated with obesity, especially severe obesity, threatening maternal and fetal health.[121] Compared with women whose BMI was less than 30, risks among obese women differed by degree; BMI of 30–34 was associated with an OR = 2.5 (95% CI = 2.1–2.0) for gestational hypertension and OR = 1.6 (95% CI = 1.1–2.3) for preeclampsia. Odds ratios were over three for severely obese women with BMI greater than 35.[121] Preeclampsia affects 3% to 5% of women during their first pregnancy but less than 2% during subsequent pregnancies.[122]

Although the condition may not cause symptoms, signs of preeclampsia are generally recognized during the second trimester characterized by hypertension, protein detectable in urine, and elevated risks of gestational diabetes. For some women symptoms may occur suddenly with severe headache and very high blood pressure creating a potentially life-threatening outcomes. When the condition is severe, fetal growth may be affected; however, prenatal development is normal among milder cases.[20] Chronic hypertension before and during pregnancy increases the risk of preeclampsia necessitating the need for blood pressure control, although some antihypertensive medications may adversely affect the developing fetus requiring careful prescribing patterns.[123] Risk is elevated twofold among women with a maternal family history. Daughters born of women who experienced preeclampsia are more likely to develop the condition themselves.[20]

Some researchers consider preeclampsia an immunologic process as changes in placental growth factors are predictive of onset.[124] Although the risk of a second pregnancy being affected by preeclampsia is lower than with the first gestation, risk rises with longer intervals between pregnancies supporting an immunologic hypothesis.[122] Neonatal mortality is twice as great among babies born to women with preeclampsia primarily associated with preterm delivery.[20]

Medication Exposures

The Centers for Disease Control and Prevention in January 2012 noted the following update in *Health Matters for Women*, "The safety of most medications taken by pregnant women is unknown and dependent on many factors."[125] Pregnant women are advised to discuss use of prescription, over-the-counter, or herbal medications with their doctor; however, physicians rely on the CDC regarding possibility of birth defects or other adverse outcomes of "exposures" during pregnancy. Although some pregnant women must take medications to control chronic conditions such as asthma, epilepsy, hypertension, and depression, specific effects on the developing fetus may not be known.[125]

Clinical decisions regarding medical treatment during pregnancy must weigh the potential adverse effects of interrupted therapy against the possible risks from fetal exposure to medications. Although pregnancy-induced physiologic changes affect maternal kidney and liver function thus modulating the action of some medications, limited research been conducted among pregnant women to guide safe drug use.[112] Since drug companies are not permitted to test medications on pregnant women, these companies have little information about potential effects of new drugs on the pregnant woman or her fetus. In an effort to collect data and provide more guidance in the future regarding potential adverse effects from medications, the Food and Drug Administration has created Pregnancy Registries, which are organized by drug categories and medical conditions such as asthma, autoimmune diseases, cancer, epilepsy, HIV/AIDS, and depression and specific medications.[126] The online registries collect treatment information from pregnant women about the effects of drugs on themselves and their babies. Researchers will use the data to compare pregnancy outcomes of women who have taken specific medications with those who have not used any drugs during pregnancy. Such studies may help provide much needed guidance for appropriate clinical care.

Treatment of preexisting health conditions are challenging for clinicians as failure to properly treat a pregnant woman's medical problem may negatively affect not only her well-being but also that of her fetus. For example, women using isotretinoins (e.g. Accutane) for acne are advised to avoid unplanned pregnancy as the treatment has been associated with birth defects and miscarriage. Similarly, some psychological illnesses are influenced by pregnancy or their treatments may adversely affect the neonate. Several conditions that may be prevalent in pregnant women include bipolar disease, eating disorders, depression, and posttraumatic stress disorder.

The adverse effects of medications on the developing fetus date from the 1950s when few clinicians thought drugs taken by pregnant women could cross the placenta until thalidomide caused severe limb deformities and organ malformations among thousands of babies. The critical windows of maternal use of thalidomide occurred during limb development.[127] The drug was prescribed primarily in Europe for nausea early in pregnancy but not approved by an astute researcher at the FDA, limiting exposure of American women and protecting developing children. To avoid such adverse events, an amendment to the 1962 FDA act required drug companies to demonstrate the efficacy and safety of a drug submitted for approval, identifying any risks and benefits of drug use, and reporting adverse reactions to the FDA.[126]

Another drug with long-term adverse effects, prescribed in the United States and abroad for pregnant women between the 1930s and 1970s was a synthetic nonsteroidal estrogen called diethylstilbestrol. The drug, formally approved in 1947 by the FDA to prevent recurrent miscarriage, was soon prescribed for many pregnant women regardless of their reproductive history. Advertisements such as Figure 10-10 in medical journals and women's magazines encouraged DES use for "health benefits." However, animal studies had revealed some adverse effects of DES. Therefore, a carefully designed randomized controlled trial was conducted by concerned clinicians

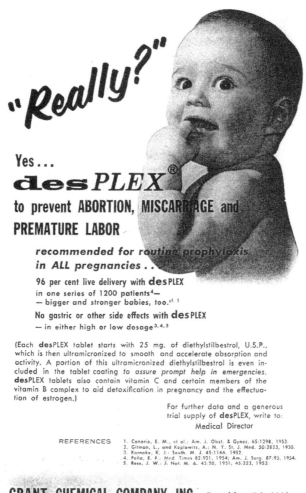

Figure 10-10 Advertisement for desPlex [DES] published in 1956.

Source: Courtesy of DES Action USA. www.desaction.org.

at Chicago Lying-In Hospital. The trial revealed DES did not prevent pregnancy problems but instead increased pregnancy loss compared to a placebo.[128] The results published in 1953 were strongly disputed and DES continued to be prescribed, affecting an estimated 2 million American women. Use was abruptly discontinued when Herbst et al. reported an association of prenatal DES exposure with vaginal cancer among young women.[129] Although subsequent increased screening of young DES daughters found few additional vaginal cancers, follow-up has identified abnormalities of reproductive organs including the fallopian tubes, resulting in more than a sevenfold increased risk of infertility.[130]

During more than 40 years of continuous monitoring, hazards associated with prenatal exposure to DES continue to be studied in relation to critical periods during in utero development with benign and malignant outcomes.[131] Table 10-2 notes the comparative risk among DES-exposed and unexposed women reported by Hoover et al. in 2011.[77] During early months of pregnancy maternal hormones orchestrate synchronized cell growth that ensures normal organ development of the fetus. DES exposure disrupted the normal continuum resulting in irreversible congenital abnormalities that differed by the timing and dosage during gestation. DES is now considered an "endocrine disruptor," one of many prevalent in the environment that are increasingly associated with risks of miscarriage and higher rates of preterm births. Many of the more than 80,000 chemicals approved for use in the United States are considered endocrine or estrogen disruptors and may be found in pesticides, plastics, household, and industrial products.[132] Maternal exposure to some of these chemicals is transmitted to the fetus with the potential for disruption of organ development.

Alcohol and Drug Abuse

Alcohol is a teratogen that interrupts normal fetal growth with a range of adverse effects depending on the timing and amount of consumption. One of the most clearly described effects of large amounts of maternal alcohol consumption is fetal alcohol syndrome, which is characterized by facial anomalies, retarded growth, and neurological abnormalities[20] with prevalence estimated at less than 2 babies affected per 1,000 births.[133] A Norwegian study assessed birth outcomes among binge drinkers (5 or more drinks at one sitting) and reported an OR = 2.2 (95% CI = 1.1–4.2) of cleft lip and cleft palate OR = 2.6 (95% CI = 1.2–5.6). The risk increased with number of binge drinking occasions.[134] The adverse effects of heavy alcohol consumption on fetal abnormalities occur early in the first trimester often before conception has been recognized. Risks associated with lower consumption are not known, but the high incidence of unplanned pregnancies increases the likelihood of fetal exposure. Contraceptive use followed by planned conception can avoid alcohol associated birth defects. Targeted preventive services during childbearing years should assist women planning childbearing to control their alcohol dependency. Pregnant women receive reminders of the risks associated with alcohol from posters displayed by law in restaurants and drinking establishments.

Smoking

Although smoking among women has declined in recent years, many adolescent girls and young women ignore the health messages; they begin smoking and may continue during their reproductive years. Smoking during pregnancy has been associated with birth defects, preterm delivery, and low birth weight as well as adverse health during youth and adult ages. Statistics indicate 10% to 12% of American women continue smoking during pregnancy.[135] A population-based case-control study, National Birth Defects Prevention Study (NBDPS), noted mothers of babies with septal heart defects were more likely to have smoked at the time of conception; the risk was positively associated with number of cigarettes smoked per day.[136] Another birth defect associated with maternal smoking in the NBDPS study was craniosynostosis, in which bones in a baby's skull close too early, altering the shape of the head and face and sometimes the brain. Mothers in the NBDPS who were heavy smokers during pregnancy (15 or more cigarettes per day) were at increased risk of having a baby with craniosynostosis, although the risk was not found when women quit smoking early in pregnancy and also avoided secondhand smoke.[137]

Maternal smoking has been associated with fetal growth restriction but a meta-analysis conducted by Oken and colleagues reported in utero exposure to cigarette smoke increased the rate of childhood obesity.[138] The association was unaffected by gestational weight gain, infant feeding, or child behaviors suggesting that exposures during prenatal development influenced health outcomes during youth and adulthood. Kandel and Udry reported maternal smoking was associated with future smoking by adolescent daughters but not male children.[139] The clearance of nicotine is elevated during pregnancy, which may increase the number of cigarettes needed to satisfy nicotine craving as well as dosages of patches used to help women quit.[135]

Environmental Exposures

During pregnancy, the placenta transfers nutrients and waste products between maternal and fetal circulation. In utero exposures are particularly damaging because of the unique vulnerabilities of the developing brain to toxic chemicals during critical windows of development resulting in permanent and irreversible brain and organ damage.[140]

Suggested explanations for greater vulnerability of the fetus include:[140]

- Rapid cell division, proliferation, and differentiation increases cellular susceptibility to environmental damage.
- Environmental exposures to the fetus are greater pound for pound than exposure to adults.
- Blood-brain barrier protecting adults is not fully developed until after birth.
- A developing fetus cannot detoxify and excrete chemicals as adults can.

The effects of prenatal exposures to common urban pollutants monitored during pregnancy by personal air sampling of the mother were studied by Perera et al. in relation to birth outcomes providing evidence of decreased birth weight and smaller head circumference associated with exposure to polycyclic aromatic hydrocarbons (PAHs).[141] Although these findings are provocative and in agreement with other less detailed research, the biologic mechanisms are not yet understood.[141] Additional studies included molecular and genetic evidence of widespread exposure to PAHs associated with chromosomal abnormalities during prenatal development, which may be associated with increased cancer risk years later.[142]

Fetal exposures to chemicals may cause immediate harm to the developing brain and other organ systems although for some substances the damage may never be overtly recognized or may not be detectable for years or decades. Scientists refer to this phenomenon as the "fetal basis of adult disease," a term created by British researchers who related malnourishment during pregnancy and postnatal years to higher risks of heart disease and diabetes at adult ages compared with well-fed infants.[143] Although use of DES in pregnancy has been discontinued due to its carcinogenic effects, other chemicals including bisphenol A (BPA), a similar compound, is widely used as a component of plastic in water bottles, baby bottles, dental sealants, and epoxy resin used in the lining of food cans. Phthalates are also estrogen-disrupting chemicals commonly used in consumer products, released into the environment, and detected in food. Metabolites of these chemicals are measurable in urine samples.[144] Recent studies have linked developmental problems of school-age children with prenatal exposures to phthalates.[144] Metabolite concentrations measured in maternal urine samples during pregnancy were significantly associated with decreases in psychomotor development among girls, and metabolite levels were associated with decreased mental development measured by the standardized test designed for early childhood assessment, the Bayley Scales of Infant Development II.[144]

Folic Acid Supplementation

Among the essential nutrition requirements during pregnancy for maximum maternal health and fetal development is folic acid to prevent neural tube defects in newborns. This defect may occur during the first weeks of gestation, a critical period when unalterable biologic developmental events are known to occur.[145] In 1992 the U.S. Public Health Service advised women of childbearing age to consume 400 µg of folic acid daily to protect any unplanned pregnancies. The Food and Drug Administration mandated adding folic acid to all enriched cereal grain products by January 1998; time trends indicated between 1996 and 2006 the incidence of spina bifida fell from 5.22 to 3.05 per 10,000, a decline of more than 30%.[145] The U.S. Preventive Services Task Force issued an update of their 1996 recommendations based on controlled trials and observational studies indicating that preconception folic acid supplements reduced neural tube defects by 11% to 65% and there was no evidence of harm from the exposure.[146]

Spina bifida is estimated to affect 1,500 births annually with rates varying by race/ethnicity. Hispanics are at highest risk (4.17 per 10,000 births), followed by non-Hispanic whites (3.22) and African Americans (2.64).[146] Anencephaly, another neural tube defect, results from developmental failure of parts of the brain and skull; death often follows shortly after birth. Neural tube birth defects of the brain and spine occur in the first weeks after conception, which may be several weeks before a woman recognizes she is pregnant.[146] Folic acid may also reduce the risk of cleft palate.[20] A recently published prospective study of more than 38,000 children conducted in Norway indicated folic acid supplements consumed during 4 weeks before conception and 8 weeks after confirmed pregnancy reduced the risk of delayed language development among 3-year-olds children.[147] Therefore, women of childbearing age are encouraged to consume 400 µg of folic acid daily to ensure adequate preconception treatment and protect a developing fetus should an unplanned pregnancy occur.[146]

Dental Care during Pregnancy

This section presents some research findings and recommendations for dental care essential for vulnerable women. Russell et al. used dental examination data from the National Health and Nutrition Examination Survey III, 1988–1994 including more than 2,500 white and black women ages 18 to 64 who reported one or more pregnancies. Their research indicated parity was significantly associated with untreated dental caries, regardless of socioeconomic status, race, or age. Women with higher parity were more likely to have untreated tooth decay and tooth loss.[148] Long-term adverse effects of pregnancy on dental health may be due to changes in saliva, oral flora, and immunosuppression.[148] A study conducted in North Carolina among pregnant women noted that limited access to dental care left racial and ethnic minority women at higher risk of dental caries, gingivitis, and periodontal infections than white women.[149] The authors suggested women's financial issues and childcare needs may limit access to dental care even among pregnant women with dental problems; therefore, those most in need are often least likely to receive dental treatment when they are pregnant.

Scans during Pregnancy

Ultrasound early in pregnancy can provide evidence of major fetal structural defects including Down syndrome, the presence of multiple fetuses, abnormal placental attachment, and estimates of fetal age based on size. In the United States and most other countries, sex selection based on ultrasound is illegal although reports indicate the practice continues.[20] Lazarus and colleagues conducted a retrospective review of pregnant women treated at a medical center in Rhode Island between 1997 and 2006 and found imaging reports from nuclear medicine for computerized tomography (CT), fluoroscopy, and plain film x-ray examinations increased more than 10% per year although CT exams, which deliver more radiation than other modalities, increased more than 25% per year.[150] Most CT exams did not involve the uterus, providing some protection from direct radiation exposure to the fetus although low-level radiation scatter remained a concern.[150] Later in pregnancy ultrasound provides assessment of fetal position and size in relation to the mother's pelvic dimensions. Other imaging modalities have led to concerns of potential harm to the fetus including MRI and CT. Regardless of potential risks, scanning is required when serious life-threatening conditions are suspected.[150]

Reproductive Outcomes

In the 21st century 99% of childbirth occurs in hospitals, the most common cause for hospital admission, and most deliveries are attended by physicians. However, home births were standard early in the 20th century until the frequency fell to 44% by 1940; in the 21st century all but 1% of babies are born in hospitals.[151] Some women are cared for by family doctors who refer their patients for obstetric care if necessary. In other settings the care is shared between physicians and nurses or nurse–midwives.[152] In 2007, approximately 12% of all births to American women were attended by certified nurse–midwives (CNMs) and 92% of those deliveries occurred in hospitals.[152] Rates differed considerably by state in relation to local laws and hospital policies controlling midwife practices; rates were highest in New Mexico (28.5% of all vaginal births) followed by Vermont with 18.3% attended by a CNM.[152] Midwives, acting as the lead professional, have provided maternity care in community or hospital settings to healthy women with uncomplicated or low-risk pregnancies and continue to provide care to women who experience complications and need medical intervention.[153] A recent Cochrane systematic review of midwifery-led care from 11 randomized trials noted deliveries by CNMs were more likely to be spontaneous vaginal births with women in greater control during labor.[153] ACOG considers hospitals and birthing centers the safest setting for childbirth but also recognized the recent renewed interest in home births, respecting the rights of women to make medically informed decisions regarding the benefits and risks.[154] Most home births are planned, for healthy women with low-risk profiles, and attended by certified nurse–midwives with availability of rapid transfer to hospital if an emergency were to develop.[154]

Vaginal Birth

The bony structure of the female pelvis and the increasing size of the fetus at time of birth have added to the painful aspects of labor and delivery. ACOG considers extreme pain many women experience an unacceptable circumstance given availability of safe medical interventions.[155] Options for pain relief include pharmaceutical methods including epidural, spinal block, and systemic and local analgesia or nonpharmaceutical options including Lamaze, acupuncture, and massage. More physician-attended births than deliveries by CNM include epidural/spinal anesthesia.[156] Data from vaginal deliveries of singleton births recorded in 27 states indicated 61% received epidural/spinal anesthesia

with first delivery. A history of chronic hypertension was a strong indicator for pharmaceutical intervention and evidence by monitoring of fetal distress increased the use of epidural/spinal anesthesia during labor.[156]

In recent decades rates of induced labor have increased from 9.5% in 1990 to 22.8% in 2007, a 140% increase, due to medical necessity associated with comorbid conditions or elective inductions. The data did not include the frequency of transition from induced labor to cesarean section.[105] However, a retrospective study conducted in Vienna, Austria, reported induction compared with spontaneous onset of labor between 38 and 42 weeks gestation doubled the risk of subsequent cesarean delivery.[157] One factor noted in U.S. data complicating vaginal birth and leading to cesarean was presentation. Breech presentation in 2007 was 55.9 per 1,000 births, which rose with maternal age to 82.5 per 1,000 births among women age 40 or older.[105]

Cesarean Delivery

Cesarean delivery, the most frequent surgical procedure in the United States, involves major abdominal surgery and may be associated with complications for mother and neonate. In the past, cesareans were performed primarily to protect the health of the mother. More recently the health of the fetus has been a major reason for surgery. Major obstetric indications for the rising rate of cesarean births include difficult childbirth or nonprogressive labor, fetal distress, breech presentation, and previous cesarean delivery specifically to protect the health of the fetus.[158] Ultrasound has provided assessment of fetal position and size in relation to the mother's pelvic dimensions; these assessments have become the standard of care. In addition, electronic fetal monitoring has alerted attending clinicians to heart rate irregularities potentially indicating life-threatening status of the fetus.[158]

In 2007 approximately 1.4 million American women had a cesarean birth, representing more than 32% of all deliveries. The trend to more than 3 births in 10 by cesarean section represents an increase of more than 50% over rates of 1996, reflecting both primary and repeat cesarean births with a decline in vaginal births after a surgical delivery (Figure 10-11).[159] Rates of cesarean section have increased among all women although they were highest among the oldest age group, 40 to 54 years, often associated with multiple births (Figure 10-12).[159] Cesarean deliveries for first child are most frequently followed by a second cesarean delivery rather than vaginal birth. Following a slight decline to 21% when vaginal births after cesarean were considered an option, the rate has steadily escalated, reaching the highest level in 2007.

Among women without any recognized medical risk having a singleton birth at full term, rates of cesarean deliveries increased for first time mothers to 11% and multiparous women by 4.4% regardless of age.[160] The rate for women age 40 or older was twice the rate among mothers younger than 20 and obesity increased the probability of cesarean delivery. These increases in recent years have occurred among all racial/ethnic groups with rates in 2007 highest for non-Hispanic black women (34%) although

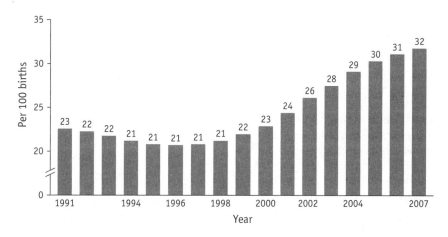

Figure 10-11 Cesarean delivery rates per 100 births. United States, 1991–2007.

Source: Reproduced from Menacker F, Hamilton BE. Recent trends in cesarean delivery in the United States. *NCHS Data Brief* 2010;35.

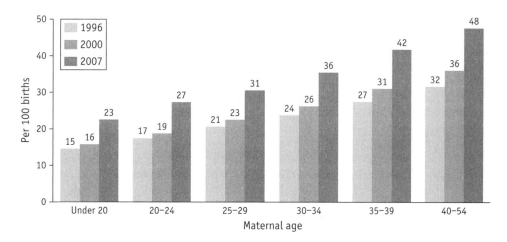

Figure 10-12 Cesarean delivery rates, by maternal age: United States, 1996, 2000, and 2007.

Source: Reproduced from Menacker F, Hamilton BE. Recent trends in cesarean delivery in the United States. *NCHS Data Brief* 2010; No. 35.

the rate was 28% or more among women of each ethnic group.[159] Rates of cesarean section deliveries differed significantly among the states for example the rate in New Jersey (38%) was 42% higher than in Utah (22%) and 50% in Puerto Rico.[159] Cesarean rates varied by gestational ages; the highest frequency was for early preterm infants (less than 34 completed weeks of gestation). Preterm birth is common at low birth weight and is more frequent with multiple than singleton births. In addition to age, physician practice patterns, maternal choice, and legal pressure may be influencing the rising cesarean delivery rates.[159]

The Consortium of Safe Labor, which includes 12 clinical centers (19 hospitals) with more than 250,000 births, found a cesarean rate of 30.5% varying among centers from 20% to 44%. Delivery was by cesarean section for 65% of the multifetal gestations without attempting vaginal delivery and 31% of nulliparous patients.[161] Cesarean delivery was twice as high after induced labor than spontaneous labor (21% vs 14%). Truly "elective" cesarean delivery with surgery preceding onset of labor was noted among 10% although the major contributor to surgical delivery was a prior cesarean section.[161] Repeated

cesarean births also limit total family size as risks increase with multiple surgical deliveries. Of concern to clinical members of the National Institute of Child Health and Human Development Maternal-Fetal Medicine Units Network were the elective repeat cesareans performed before 39 weeks gestation as the timing increased risk of adverse neonatal outcomes.[162] ACOG issued a revised practice bulletin indicating attempted vaginal birth after previous cesarean is appropriate for many women, contrary to the standard practice of many obstetricians.[163]

A national survey questioned new mothers about their experiences of childbirth. They reported pain associated with instrumental birth, incisional pain after cesarean section, and perineal pain following vaginal birth.[164] Declercq et al. also found new mothers were overwhelmed after cesarean section with incision pain remaining a major disabling problem for several months postpartum. Many women were unaware or had an incomplete understanding of potential complications from surgical births especially when the procedures were not medically indicated.[164] Some clinicians suggest research is needed to assess the long-term health outcomes of mothers and their infants following cesarean delivery for an uncomplicated pregnancy compared with vaginal birth.

Birth Defects

In the United States 1 in 33 babies is born with a birth defect, which is often a leading cause of infant mortality. Most birth defects occur without known cause although evidence suggests 10% are attributable to genetic abnormalities.[165] The Congenital Defects Program, initiated by the CDC in Atlanta in 1978, indicated prevalence rates have remained stable for decades (2.8 to 3.0 per 100 live births) with rates slightly higher among women age 35 and older.[165] Each year in the United States 40,000 infants are born with heart defects, the leading cause of infant deaths.

Preterm and Low Birth Weight

Although mortality rates associated with preterm birth have declined during the past several decades primarily associated with access to perinatal and pediatric intensive care units, the rate of preterm births continues to increase in the United States, reaching an estimated 12.7% of pregnancies in 2007, considerably higher than in Canada (7.6%), Australia (8.2%) or Ireland (4.4%). Multiple maternal factors have contributed to higher preterm birth rates among non-Hispanic black women (18.3%) compared with white (11.5%), Hispanic (12.3%) or Asians (10.9%) including low socioeconomic status, lack of prenatal care, being unmarried, being a cigarette smoker, poor nutrition before and during pregnancy, stress, and genetics.[166] Infection and inflammation including maternal history of chlamydia have been linked with a 50% increased risk of preterm birth and a history of gonorrhea is associated with a threefold increase.[44]

Research has noted that women delivering preterm are at greatly increased risk of a repeat preterm birth reflecting environmental exposures, genetics, and their combined effects.[132] Mothers who were born preterm are at increased risk of delivering their own babies preterm and having repeated preterm deliveries.[20] In addition, concordance of preterm delivery is higher in monozygotic than dizygotic twins.[167] Although some increased preterm births result from multiple gestations following assisted reproduction, other maternal factors may contribute to repeated preterm births including congenital abnormalities of maternal reproductive organs resulting from prenatal exposures during organ development.[132]

Maternal age is strongly associated with low birth weight among women delivering a singleton birth (Figure 10-13).[168] Babies born at low birth weight are at increased risk of developing type 2 diabetes and coronary heart disease in adulthood. Women with a history of prenatal exposure to DES were found to have significantly increased risk of preterm birth (OR = 2.97, 95% CI = 2.27–3.87) and a higher risk of small for gestational age (OR = 1.61, 95% CI = 1.31–1.98).[169] Low birth weight has also been linked to prenatal exposure to tobacco smoke. Preterm infants, born before completing 37 weeks gestation, are less likely to survive their first year compared with babies born later in pregnancy.[166] Babies who survive have higher risks of diagnosis with cerebral palsy and respiratory distress syndrome leading to chronic lung disease across the life span.[162] Length of gestation was also associated with cerebral palsy in a Norwegian follow-up study. Compared with delivery at 40 weeks, babies born at 37–38 weeks or at 42 weeks or later were more likely to be diagnosed with cerebral palsy by age 4.[170] Similar risk patterns associated with pre- and postterm deliveries have been found with other congenital anomalies involving cerebral function.[170] Premature birth is a common, serious, and costly problem that affects more than 500,000 babies in the United States annually, causing disability and death in too many cases.

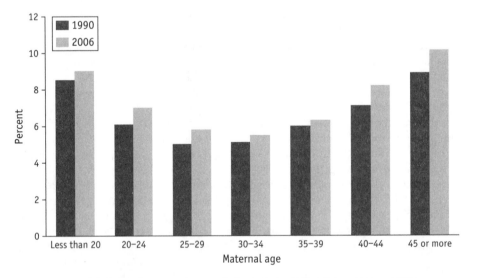

Figure 10-13 Percentage of low birthweight infants by maternal age at singleton births: United States, 1990 and 2006.

Source: Reproduced from Martin JA, Hamilton BE, Sutton PD, et al. Births: Final data for 2006. *National Vital Statistics Reports* 2009;57:7.

Miscarriage and Stillbirth

Early pregnancy loss is often undetectable as conception occurs without any specific signs until the hormonal signal provided by rising urinary excretion of human chorionic gonadotropin (hCG) at the time of implantation. Measurement of hCG provides estimates of pregnancy loss after implantation but the percentage of conceptions that do not result in implantation remains unknown. The annual rate of later pregnancy loss includes an estimated 1 million miscarriages and stillbirths. Miscarriage is defined as spontaneous pregnancy loss before the 20th week of gestation and stillbirth refers to death of a fetus at 20 weeks or older.[37]

Childbearing attempts among older women are more often affected by repeated miscarriage; risk is less than 10% among women age 20 but reaches as high as 90% among potential mothers age 45 or older unless donor eggs from younger women are used for IVF.[20] Karyotyping of the products of miscarriages has indicated 65% of the embryos were chromosomally abnormal.[37] Very early pregnancy losses before the 12th week of gestation may appear to the woman as heavy menstrual flow.[20] In a study by Lawson et al. of participants in the Nurses' Health Study II, occupational exposures increased miscarriage rates.[171] In contrast to early pregnancy loss, later miscarriages may require hospitalization and surgery to remove retained tissue from the uterus.[20]

An estimated 26,000 stillbirth occur annually, approximately 1 in 160 pregnancies, among the 4 million babies born in the United States. Stillbirths may occur during pregnancy but before labor begins or once labor has started; the causes differ by timing. Obesity and smoking are two behavioral factors that contribute to stillbirths.[172] The proportion of stillbirths due to genetics varies with the definition although data indicate 40% are due to single malformations, 40% multiple abnormalities, and the remaining 20% are associated with placental problems.[172] Stillbirths also increase with maternal age from a rate of 4 per 1,000 pregnancies among women younger than age 30 to 10 per 1,000 after age 40.[37] Differences were recorded by race with non-Hispanic blacks at 2.3 times greater risk than non-Hispanic white women and risk among Hispanic women was 14% higher than among non-Hispanic white women. Prospective population-based study findings from postmortem examinations of 512 neonates provided some clues to the causes of stillbirth including obstetrical conditions (30%), placenta or umbilical cord abnormalities (34%), fetal genetic or structural abnormalities (6%), infection (13%), or hypertension and other maternal illnesses (17%).[173] The higher rate of stillbirth among black women remains unexplained although obstetrical complications and infection seemed to be greater among these women than others and the same factors were associated with increased miscarriage among non-Hispanic blacks.[173]

Placental Abruption and Placenta Previa

In normal pregnancies the placenta separates from the uterus following delivery, but in 6 to 10 pregnancies per 1,000, the placenta separates prematurely, causing severe pain and massive vaginal bleeding that can be lethal for the mother and her fetus. Although placental abruption can occur without warning, the position of the placenta, detectable by sonogram, provides warning signs. Expert obstetrical care protects the mother although the risk to the fetus is extremely elevated.[20] Smoking was associated with an odds ratio of 2.36 (95% CI = 1.29–4.33). Additional risk factors linked to placenta abruption include multiple gestations, hypertension, abdominal trauma, illicit drug use, and previous abruptions.[174]

A similar potentially lethal problem occurs when the placenta grows over the cervical opening (placenta previa) and tears with contractions of labor.[20] The incidence is estimated at 3 to 5 per 1,000 pregnancies and can be detected by sonogram before onset of labor.[175] Risk was increased by 40% among twin births compared to singleton and older maternal age (greater than 35 years) was associated with an eightfold elevated risk.[176] Several studies noted a dose response relationship between smoking during pregnancy and increased risk of placenta previa, but the incidence was similar to never smokers when women quit smoking during pregnancy.[174]

Maternal and Infant Mortality

In 2006 approximately 550 women died from maternal causes with a rate of 13.3 per 100,000 live births; the rate among black women (32.7) was close to 3.4 times the rate among white women (9.5) and Hispanic women (10.2).[177] Although much progress has been accomplished in the United States to reduce maternal mortality, the rates in America continue to surpass those of other developed countries in which universal health care is provided. Three primary causes of maternal mortality include: postpartum hemorrhage, infection, and hypertensive disorders—toxemia or eclampsia. Comprehensive prenatal care monitors risk of maternal death due to hypertensive conditions but other obstetrical complications cannot be predicted or prevented.[20] Maternal mortality has declined significantly in the last 100 years although pregnancy-associated deaths remain a major public health concern.[178]

The decline in infant mortality in the United States from 100 deaths per 1,000 live births in 1900 to 6.9 in 2000 has not fallen significantly further during the first decade of the 21st century (Figure 10-14). Male infants were at 20% greater risk of death in the first year of life than female infants in each racial/ethnic group. Two-thirds of all infant deaths occur within 1 month of birth. Rates differed significantly by race and Hispanic origin; highest infant mortality was among non-Hispanic black women (13.4), a rate 2.4 times that of non-Hispanic white women (5.6). These infant mortality disparities may reflect maternal sociodemographic and behavioral risk factors including lower education level, lack of adequate prenatal care, maternal smoking, and birth to adolescent mothers. Lower income and more limited access to health care are adverse pregnancy outcome predictors.

Since preterm births are at increased risk of neonatal mortality, the results from a randomized trial of group prenatal care demonstrating a 33% reduction in preterm

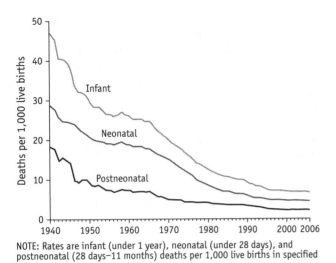

NOTE: Rates are infant (under 1 year), neonatal (under 28 days), and postneonatal (28 days–11 months) deaths per 1,000 live births in specified group.

Figure 10-14 Infant, neonatal, and postneonatal mortality rates: United States, 1940–2006.

Source: Reproduced from Heron M, Hoyert DL, Murphy SL, et al. Deaths: final data for 2006. *National Vital Statistics Reports* 2009;57:No. 14.

births and reduced mortality are noteworthy. The trial was conducted in two university-affiliated hospital prenatal clinics (New Haven, Connecticut, and Atlanta, Georgia) with a primarily young, vulnerable population with a mean age of 20.4 years, 49% younger than age 19, and 80% African American. Group care provided additional clinical and psychosocial advantages compared with individualized care with healthier planned, well-spaced pregnancies.[179]

New York City recently announced data for 2008 that indicated the lowest rate of infant mortality ever achieved, 5.3 deaths per 1,000 live births, a decline of 21% in the past decade.[180] However, disparities were also reported; higher infant mortality among black (9.5) and Puerto Ricans (6.3) babies in contrast to Hispanics (4.8), Caucasians (3.4) and Asians (2.8). The data alerted the New York City Health Department to geographic sections of the metropolitan area in need of special efforts to reduce these disparities.[180]

Maternal contributors to infant mortality include poor preconception health, infections, stress, racism, and detrimental cultural patterns.[151] However, national data indicate the causes of infant deaths after a live birth include congenital malformations (20%), premature delivery and low birth weight (17%), sudden infant death syndrome (8%), maternal complications affecting newborn (6%), accidents (4%), complications associated with the placenta (4%), respiratory distress of newborn (3%), neonate hemorrhage (2%), and circulatory system conditions (2%).[177] The U.S. infant mortality rate was five times greater for multiple births than for singleton births in 2006 when 3% of live births were multiple but 15% of all infant deaths were from multiple births.[181] The infant mortality rate among twins was 27.9 per 1,000 live births but increased greatly to 69.6 among triplets. The gestational age of the infant at birth is the

strongest predictor of the infant's subsequent health and survival. Infants born prematurely, even by a few weeks, have a significantly greater risk of disability and death than infants born at full term.[177] Collins et al. suggested the very low birth weight that accounts for 63% of the high neonatal mortality among African American reflects accumulated racial discrimination, an independent risk factor.[182] Rates of maternal and infant mortality are important national indicators reflecting maternal health, access to medical care, socioeconomic conditions, and public health practices.[181]

Postpartum Depression

Mood disorders occurring during pregnancy and postpartum affect 25% to 85% of women with the range depending upon the definitions and measurement tools applied. Women are at higher risk of depression than men at all ages; however, the hormonal impact of pregnancy stimulates unique emotional responses including depression and anxiety, which increase significantly after delivery when estrogen and progesterone levels fall. For most women, symptoms resolve within a few weeks of delivery.[183] The more severe condition, postpartum depression (defined as clinical depression lasting several months to 1 year after birth), is believed to affect 8% to 16% of postpartum women.

Depression and anxiety affect both mother and baby immediately after birth and over the child's life course. A study conducted among more than 25,000 women giving birth at Kaiser Permanente Medical Care Program in Northern California between 1997 and 1998 was designed to assess frequency of depression from treatment records and follow-up interviews with a random sample of patients.[183] Among those with clinical records indicating postpartum depression, only 25% were treated for a new episode of depression. Barriers to seeking clinical care and treatment reported during phone interviews with patients were personal or cultural. The authors promoted patient and clinician education about the risks associated with onset of depression and encouraged screening for signs of mood disturbances during prenatal and postpartum visits.[183]

Fitelson et al. noted postpartum depression requires prompt treatment as the disorder may adversely affect the mother's ability to care for her newborn child.[184] Women with postpartum depression have expressed concern about adverse effects on their infant from prescribed medications transmitted through their breastmilk. Limited research has been conducted to assess any potential harm associated with maternal medications transmitted during nursing. Infants may be vulnerable due to their immature liver and kidney function,[184] therefore, some physicians refer patients for nonpharmacologic treatment although alternatives may have limited benefits for some women. The alternatives therapies may include psychological treatment, cognitive behavior changes, nondirective counseling, and emphasis on partner support. Some patients benefit from acupuncture, massage, light therapy, and routine exercise programs.[184]

Breastfeeding

Increasing the number of new mothers electing to breast-feed and encouraging 6 months of exclusive nutrition with breastmilk has been a goal of the American Academy of Pediatrics[185] and the American Dietetic Association,[186] based on research that documents the health benefits for mothers and their newborns. The advantages include ideal nutritional support and psychological, social, and economic benefits.[185] Human milk is the preferable food for babies; therefore, if direct breastfeeding is not possible, mothers are advised to express milk.[114] A review of the nutritional aspects of nursing suggests that only vitamin and mineral supplements should be provided for the first 6 months followed by introduction of foods while continuing breastfeeding during the infant's first year. Breastfeeding forges maternal–infant bonding while protecting the infant from potential life-threatening respiratory and gastrointestinal infections as well as reducing the risk of sudden infant death syndrome.[185] Breastmilk contains anti-infective, anti-inflammatory, and immunoregulatory factors that provide passive immunity to the baby. These multiple immunologic factors produced by the mother's acquired and innate immune systems are conveyed through nursing to the infant whose own immune system remains immature for the first 2 years of life.[187]

When breastfeeding begins within an hour of delivery, maternal blood loss is diminished and more rapid uterine involution occurs. Frequent and exclusive breastfeeding results in lactation amenorrhea, which reduces the risk of premenopausal breast cancer while ensuring child spacing. However, ovulation will naturally resume within several months, requiring another birth control method to avoid unplanned children.[114] Infants who have received breastmilk have been found to have lower cholesterol levels and normal systolic and diastolic blood pressure compared to age-matched babies who were not breastfed. In addition, breastfeeding lowers the likelihood of children becoming obese during adolescence.[188]

Recently, interest in breastfeeding has increased with a majority of new mothers planning to breastfeed although the number maintaining breastfeeding after hospital discharge is more limited.[189] CDC data from 2007 indicated 75% of mothers began breastfeeding but only 43% reporting continuing for 6 months and only 22% at 12 months. In-hospital maternity experiences have been associated with future feeding behaviors.[190] Perrine et al. reported the experiences during the first few hours after childbirth influence initiation and continuation of breastfeeding. These CDC researchers recommended hospitals include prenatal breastfeeding classes, train staff to provide support for new mothers by encouraging breastfeeding within 1 hour of birth or recovery from cesarean delivery and by providing rooming-in 24 hours per day. The use of a pacifier, formula, or water supplements, and samples of formula at hospital discharge should be avoided.[191]

Taveras et al. found clinicians' perceptions of counseling about breastfeeding differed from those of their patients when they were linked.[190] Among doctors who said they always or usually discussed feeding methods, less than 20% of their patients agreed such a discussion had occurred.[190] Duration of breastfeeding depends on many factors including confidence and commitment.[192] Employment also complicates successful, prolonged breastfeeding. Women with longer maternity leaves and/or part-time employment are able to breastfeed longer although those who must return to work benefit from support programs offered by some employers who also provide protected private locations for use of breast pumps during the work day.[193] Low-income women may require financial support to purchase or rent a breast pump to enhance their ability to work while maintaining breastfeeding.[194] A recently reported randomized trial added another benefit to breastfeeding. The Promotion of Breastfeeding Intervention Trial (PROBIT), with long-term follow-up conducted by Canadian researchers in Belarus reported exclusive, prolonged breastfeeding was associated with cognitive benefits evident at 6 years based on IQ testing and teachers' academic rating.[195]

Pregnancy Termination

Surveys indicate that about one in three American women will have had at least one elective pregnancy termination during their reproductive years.[196] In 2008 an estimated 90% of the 1.2 million abortions were performed during the first trimester with a rate of 22 abortions per 100 pregnancies.[197] A small percentage was performed later in gestation necessitated by serious illness of the mother or fetal abnormalities detected by sonogram or genetic analysis. Another reason for pregnancy termination is rape;[20] women are at increasing risk for unplanned pregnancies after an intimate relationship becomes violent. More than 50% of women ages 16 to 29 seeking care at family planning clinics in Northern California revealed they had experienced physical or sexual partner violence preventing effective birth control and resulting in forced pregnancy.[198] At a family planning clinic in Iowa 30% of women seeking an abortion had experienced high rates of intimate partner violence[199] and 31% of male patients at three community health clinics in Boston responded to an anonymous computer-generated survey that they had perpetrated physical and sexual violence against a female partner involving unplanned pregnancy resulting in abortion.[200] With federal and state restrictions increasingly limiting women's access to family planning, emergency contraception, and abortion services, especially for low-income women, unplanned pregnancies will continue with tragic effects on the lives of women and their children.[201,202]

Although availability of facilities varies greatly across the country, surgical and medical procedures for pregnancy termination up to 9 weeks' gestation are federally legal. Suction curettage, a safe procedure with less than 1% complications, has been the primary abortion method since the 1970s although medical abortion was approved by the FDA in 2000 and is now provided by many clinics and physicians.[197] Neither method of pregnancy interruption adversely affects future childbearing differently than a continued pregnancy.[196] No increase in rates of ectopic pregnancy, placenta previa, infertility, or miscarriage have been identified, although some studies have suggested an increased risk of preterm birth associated with an increasing number of abortions.[196]

Some early epidemiologic studies had suggest risk of breast cancer was positively associated with the number of abortions. However, reanalysis of prospective studies involving 83,000 women, including breast cancer cases and controls, reported no association; the researchers advised that data collection retrospectively had provided biased results.[204] Although some clinicians have suggested mental health problems are diagnosed more often after an abortion, contrary reports found women expressed relief after the procedure.[203] Some women expressed lingering sadness or regret depending upon marital status, age, health, etc. Greater prevalence of postpartum depression follows live births as discussed previously. However, to avoid another unplanned pregnancy, clinicians suggest the insertion of an intrauterine device at time of abortion, providing reversible contraception.[203]

Access to safe pregnancy termination is being restricted by federal and state political action as well as health insurance policies. Extreme acts of violence against abortion providers have contributed to the limited geographic distribution of abortion services, which controls options available for many American women. In the United States 87% of counties lack an abortion provider.[197] Before legal facilities were available, American women sought alternative unsafe methods for interrupting pregnancy, which resulted in considerable mortality.[20] Death rates declined dramatically after abortion was legalized in 1973. With threats to financial support for women's reproductive health services, public health leaders fear the rates of maternal and infant mortality concentrated among disadvantaged populations will increase.[205] Political action by the public health community is essential to provide all American women with safe and effective reproductive health care.

Summary

The first decade of the 21st century has heralded renewed interest in women's health with a special focus on preventive services and reproductive events experienced during more than 30 years between menarche and menopause. Although a more supportive environment has been evolving, childbearing decisions carry health risks while continuing to require maternal compromises that are often dictated by financial status, educational goals, career options, employer controls, and other considerations. Recently, political debates have focused on controlling women's reproductive health decisions through access to and financial options for abortion. The political arguments expanded in response to the mandate of the federal Affordable Care Act requiring insurance policies to provide contraception and sterilization services without patient copay, an essential preventive service identified by the 2011 Institute of Medicine report. Although great progress was achieved during the 20th century in

lowering maternal and infant mortality, some U.S. health statistics lag far behind other industrialized countries especially in rates of unplanned pregnancies, preterm and low birth weight infants, and subsequent long-term adverse health outcomes. Aspects of maternal child care that must be addressed to improve pregnancy outcomes include elimination of racial and social inequalities in healthcare services, reduction of preterm births, and reduced comorbid conditions before conception to lower risks during pregnancy. Political leadership by women is necessary to ensure financial support for appropriate clinical care at critical stages across women's life span and to guide research addressing reproductive health needs of all American women.

Discussion Questions

1. From a historical perspective what aspects of public health contributed to reduced maternal and infant mortality? Since other industrialized nations report significantly superior reproductive health statistics compared to the United States, what changes are required to improve the health of American women during reproductive ages?

2. With increasing availability of contraceptive options, statistics continue to indicate that approximately 50% of pregnancies were unplanned, unwanted, or mistimed. What are the barriers to consistent family planning?

3. Infertility appears to be increasing among American women. Describe some health conditions and their treatment that affect infertility.

4. Technology has significantly contributed to improving reproductive health for women in the 21st century. Name some of the new options and the technology that have enhanced reproductive options for women and their partners.

References

1. Kotelcheck M. Safe mothers, healthy babies: Reproductive health in the twentieth century. In: Ward JW, Warren C, eds. *Silent Victories. The History and Practice of Public Health in Twentieth-Century America.* New York: Oxford University Press; 2007:105–134.
2. Institute of Medicine. *Clinical Preventive Services for Women: Closing the Gaps.* Washington, DC: National Academies Press; 2011. http://www.iom.edu/ Reports/2011/Clinical-Preventive-Services-for-Women-Closing-the-Gaps.aspx.
3. Finer LB, Henshaw SK. Disparities in rates of unintended pregnancy in the United States, 1994 and 2001. *Persp Sex Reprod Health.* 2006;38:90–96.
4. Trussell J, Wynn L. Reducing unintended pregnancy in the United States. *Contraception.* 2008;77:1–5.
5. Affordable Care Act. Pub L 111–148. http://www.healthcare.gov/law/full/ index.html.
6. Conde-Agudelo A, Rosa-Bermudez A, Kafury-Goeta AC. Birth spacing and risk of adverse perinatal outcome. *JAMA.* 2006;295:1809–1823.
7. Sui SC, Sermer M, Colman JM, et al. Prospective multicenter study of pregnancy outcomes in women with heart disease. *Circulation.* 2001;104:515–521.
8. Santelli JS, Melnikas AJ. Teen fertility in transition: recent and historic trends in the United States. *Ann Rev Public Health.* 2010;31:371–383.
9. Trussell J, Lalla AM, Doan QV, et al. Cost effectiveness of contraceptives in the United States. *Contraception.* 2009;79:5–14.
10. Mosher WD, Jones J. Use of contraception in the United States: 1982–2008. *Vital and Health Statistics.* 2010;Series 23:29.
11. Harrison AT, Gavin L. Hastings PA. Prepregnancy contraceptive use among teens with unintended pregnancies resulting in live births—Pregnancy Risk Assessment Monitoring System (PRAMS), 2004–2008. *MMWR Morb Mortal Wkly Rep.* 2012;61:25–29.

12. Trussell J. Contraceptive failure in the United States. *Contraception.* 2011;83:397–404.
13. Postlethwaite D, Trussell J, Zoolakis A, et al. A comparison of contraceptive procurement pre- and post-benefit change. *Contraception.* 2007;76:360–365.
14. Cleland K, Peipert JF, Westhoff C, et al. Family planning s a cost-saving preventive health service. *N Engl J Med.* 2011;364:e37.
15. Wood AJJ, Drazen JM, Greene MF. The politics of emergency contraception. *N Engl J Med.* 2012;366:101–102.
16. Lintern-Moore S, Peters H, Moore GPM, Faber M. Follicular development in the infant human ovary. *J Reprod Fert.* 1974;39:53–64.
17. Baker TG. A quantitative and cytological study of germ cells in human ovaries. *Proc R Soc Lond B Biol Sci.* 1963;158:417–433.
18. Frisch RE, Wyshak G, Vincet L. Delayed menarche and amenorrhea in ballet dancers. *N Engl J Med.* 1980;303:17–19.
19. Key A, Mason H, Bolton J. Reproduction and eating disorders: a fruitless union. *Eur Eat Disord Rev.* 2000;8,98–107.
20. Wilcox AJ. *Fertility and Pregnancy.* New York, Oxford University Press, Inc; 2010.
21. Thomford PJ, Jelovsek FR, Mttison DR. Effect of oocyte number and rate of atresia on the age of menopause. *Reprod Toxicol.* 1987;1:41–51.
22. Lambalk CB, van Disseldorp J, de Koning CH, Broekmans FJ. Testing ovarian reserve to predict age at menopause. *Maturitas.* 2009;63:280–291.
23. Snowdon DA, Kane RL, Beeson L, et al. Is early menopause a biologic marker of health and aging? *Am J Public Health.* 1989;79:709–714.
24. Martin JA, Hamilton BE, Ventura SJ, et al. Births: final data for 2009. *Nat Vital Stat Rep.* 2011;60:1–104.
25. Hamilton BE, Ventura SJ. Fertility and abortion rates in the United States, 1960–2002. *Int J Androl.* 2006;29:34–45.
26. Dunson DB, Colombo B, Baird DD. Changes with age in the level and duration of fertility in the menstrual cycle. *Hum Reprod.* 2002;17:1399–1403.
27. Armstrong C. ACOG recommendations on emergency contraception. *Am Fam Physician.* 2010;82:1278.
28. Van Voorhis BJ. In vitro fertilization. *N Engl J Med.* 2007;356:379–386.
29. Moffett A, Loke C. Immunology of placentation in eutherian mammals. *Nat Rev Immunol.* 2006;6:584–594.
30. Ben-Schlomo Y, Kuh D. A life course approach to chronic disease epidemiology: conceptual models, empirical challenges and interdisciplinary perspectives. *Int J Epidemiol.* 2002;31:285–293.
31. Sharkey AM, Smith SK. The endometrium as a cause of implantation failure. *Best Pract Res Clin Obstet Gynecol.* 2003;17:289–307.
32. Noell D, Delke I, Hill WC, et al. Ectopic pregnancy mortality—Florida, 2009–2010. *MMWR Morb Mortal Wkly Rep.* 2012;61:106–109.
33. Grimes DA. Estimation of pregnancy-related mortality risk by pregnancy outcome, United States, 1991–1999. *Am J Obstet Gynecol.* 2006;194:92–94.
34. Creanga AA, Shapiro-Mendoza CK, Bish CL, et al. Trends in ectopic pregnancy mortality in the United States. *Obstet Gynecol.* 2011;117:837–843.
35. American Congress of Obstetricians and Gynecologists. *Guidelines for Women's Health Care.* 3rd ed. Washington, DC: Author; 2007.
36. Martin JA, Hamilton BE, Osterman JK. Three decades of twin births in the United States, 1980–2009. *NCHS Data Brief.* 2012;no 80.
37. Heffner LJ. Advanced maternal age—How old is too old? *N Engl J Med.* 2004;351:1927–1929.
38. Matthews TJ, Hamilton BE. Delayed childbearing: more women are having their first child later in life. *NCHS Data Brief.* 2009;21:1–8.
39. Kathiresan ASQ, Roca LE, Istwan N, et al. The influence of maternal age on pregnancy outcome in nulliparous women with twin gestation. *Am J Perinatol.* 2011;28:355–359.
40. Durkin MS, Maenner MJ, Newschaffer CJ, et al. Advanced parental age and risk of autism spectrum disorder. *Am J Epidemiol.* 2008;168:1268–1276.
41. Luk J, Greenfield DA, Seli E. Third party reproduction and the aging couple. *Maturitas.* 2010;66:389–396.
42. Thys-Jacobs S, Starkey P, Bernstein D, et al. Calcium carbonate and the premenstrual syndrome: effects on premenstrual and menstrual symptoms. *Am J Obstet Gynecol.* 1998;179:444–452.
43. Lopez LM, Kaptein AA, Helmerhorst FM. Oral contraceptives containing drospirenone for premenstrual syndrome. *Cochrane Database Syst Rev.* 2012 Feb 15;2. CD006586.
44. Baecher-Lind LE, Miller WC, Wilcox AJ. Infectious disease and reproductive health. *Obstet Gynecol Surv.* 2010;65:53–65.
45. Centers for Disease Control and Prevention. Sexually transmitted diseases (STDs). STDs & pregnancy—CDC Fact Sheet. www.cdc.gov/std/pregnancy/STDFact-Pregnancy.htm.
46. Kodaman PH, Arici A, Seli E. Evidence-based diagnosis and management of tubal factor infertility. *Curr Opin Obstet Gynecol.* 2004;16:221–229.
47. Azziz R, Woods KS, Reyna R, et al. The prevalence and features of polycystic ovarian syndrome in an unselected population. *J Clin Endocrinol Metab.* 2004;89:2745–2749.
48. Legro RS, Barnhart HX, Schlaff WD, et al. Clomiphene, metformin, or both for infertility in the polycystic ovary syndrome. *N Engl J Med.* 2007;356:551–566.
49. Faerstein E, Szklo M, Rosenshein N. Risk factors for uterine leiomyoma: A practice-based case-control study. 1. African-American heritage, reproductive history, body size, and smoking. *Am J Epidemiol.* 2001;153:1–10.
50. Anderson J. Growth factors and cytokines in uterine leiomyomata. *Semin Reprod Endocrinol.* 1996;14:269–282.
51. Cramer SF, Patel A. The frequency of uterine leiomyomas. *Am J Clin Pathol.* 1990;94:435–438.
52. Samadi AR, Lee NC, Flanders WD, et al. Risk factors for self-reported uterine fibroids: a case-control study. *Am J Public Health.* 1996;86:858–862.
53. Catherino WH, Parrott E, Segars J. Proceedings from the National Institute of Child Health and Human Development Conference on the Uterine Fibroid Research Update Workshop. *Fertil Steril.* 2011;95:9–12.
54. Goodwin SC, Spies JB. Uterine fibroid embolization. *N Engl J Med.* 2009;361:690–697.
55. Murphy AA. RU486 in the treatment of leiomyomata uteri. *Infert Reprod Med Clin North Am.* 1996;7:57–68.
56. Davis KM, Schlaff WD. Medical management of uterine fibromyomata. *Obstet Gynecol Clin North Am.* 1995;22:727–738.
57. Walker WJ, McDowell SJ. Pregnancy after uterine artery embolization for leiomyomata: A series of 56 completed pregnancies. *Am J Obstet Gynecol.* 2006;1266–1271.
58. Baird DD, Dunson DB, Hill MC, et al. High cumulative incidence of uterine leiomyoma in black and white women: ultrasound evidence. *Am J Obstet Gynecol.* 2003;188:100–107.
59. Marshall LM, Spiegelman D, Barbieri RL, et al. Variation in the incidence of uterine leiomyoma among premenopausal women by age and race. *Obstet Gynecol.* 1007;90:967–973.
60. Westhoff C, Gentile G, Lee J, et al. Predictors of ovarian secretion in reproductive-age women. *Am J Epidemiol.* 1996;144:381–388.
61. Boynton-Jarrett R, Rich-Edwards JW, Malspeis S, et al. A prospective study of hypertension and risk of uterine leiomyoma. *Am J Epidemiol.* 2005;161:628–638.
62. Wyshak G, Frisch RE, Albright NL, et al. Lower prevalence of benign diseases of the breast and benign tumors of the reproductive system among former college athletes compared to nonathletes. *Br J Cancer.* 1986;54:841–845.
63. Chiaffarino F, Paraqzzini F, La Vecchia C, et al. Diet and uterine myomas. *Obstet Gynecol.* 1999;94:395–398.
64. Wise LA, Radin RG, Palmer JR, et al. A prospective study of dairy intake and risk of uterine leiomyomata. *Am J Epidemiol.* 2010;171:221–232.
65. Giudice L, Kao LC. Endometriosis. *Lancet.* 2004;364:1789–1799.
66. Houston DE. Evidence for the risk of pelvic endometriosis by age, race, and socioeconomic status. *Epidemiol Rev.* 1984;6:167–91.
67. Moen MH, Stokstad T. A long-term follow-up study of women with asymptomatic endometriosis diagnosed incidentally at sterilization. *Fertil Steril.* 2002;78:773–76.
68. Barnhart K, Dunsmoor-Su R, Coutifaris C. Effect of endometriosis on in vitro fertilization. *Fertil Steril.* 2002;77:1148–1155.
69. Oral E, Arici A, Olive DL, Huszar G. Peritoneal fluid from women with moderate or severe endometriosis inhibits sperm motility: the role of seminal fluid components. *Fertil Steril.* 1996;66:787–92.
70. Aeby TC, T Huang, RT Nakayama. The effect of peritoneal fluid from patients with endometriosis on human sperm function in vitro. *Am J Obstet Gynecol.* 1996;174:1779–83.
71. Simpson JL, Elias S, Malinak LR, Buttram VC Jr. Heritable aspects of endometriosis, I: genetic studies. *Am J Obstet Gynecol.* 1980;137:327–31.
72. Kennedy S, Mardon H, Barlow D. Familial endometriosis. *J Assist Reprod Genet.* 1995;12:32–34.
73. Stefansson H, Geirsson RT, Steinthorsdottir V, et al. Genetic factors contribute to the risk of developing endometriosis. *Hum Reprod.* 2002;17:555–59.
74. Howard-Anderson J, Ganz PA, Bower JE, Stanton AL. Quality of life, fertility concerns, and behavioral health outcomes in younger breast cancer survivors: a systematic review. *J Natl Cancer Inst.* 2012;104:1–20.
75. Robertson AD, Missmer SA, Ginsburg ES. Embryo yield in vitro fertilization in women undergoing banking for fertility preservation before chemotherapy. *Fertil Steril.* 2011;95:588–591.
76. Cnattingius C, Hultman M, Dahl M, Sparen P. Very pre-term birth, birth trauma, and the risk of anorexia nervosa among girls. *Arc Gen Psych.* 1999;56:634–638.
77. Hoover RN, Hyer M, Pfeiffer RM, et al. Adverse health outcomes in women exposed in utero to diethylstilbestrol. *N Engl J Med.* 2011;365:1304–1314.
78. Steiner AZ, D'Aloisio AA, DeRoo LA, et al. Association of intrauterine and early-life exposures with age at menopause in the Sister Study. *Am J Epidemiol.* 2010;172:140–148.
79. Brinton LA, Westoff CL, Scoccia B, et al. Causes of infertility as predictors of subsequent cancer risk. *Epidemiol.* 2005;16:500–507.
80. Fishel S, Jackson P. Follicular stimulation for high tech pregnancies: are we playing it safe? *BMJ.* 1989;299:309–311.
81. van Leeuwen FE, Klip H, Mooij TM, et al. Risk of borderline and invasive ovarian tumors after ovarian stimulation for in vitro fertilization in a large Dutch cohort. *Hum Reprod.* 2011;26:3456–3465.
82. Centers for Disease Control and Prevention. Assisted reproductive technology.ART reports and resources. CDC Assisted Reproductive Technology Success Rates, National Summary and Fertility Clinic Reports. http://www.cdc.gov/art/artreports.htm.

83. Klipstein S. Preimplantation genetic diagnosis: technological promise and ethical perils. *Fertil Steril*. 2005;83:1347–1353.

84. Lawlor D, Nelson SM. Effect of age on decisions about the numbers of embryos to transfer in assisted conception: a prospective study. *Lancet*. 2012 Jan 11 (Epub ahead of print)

85. Evans MI, Britt DW. Fetal reduction. *Semin Perinatol*. 2005;29:321–329.

86. Spar D. The egg trade—Making sense of the market for human oocytes. *N Engl J Med*. 2007;356:1289–1291.

87. Sauer M, Kavic SM. Oocyte and embryo donation 2006: reviewing two decades of innovation and controversy. *Reprod Biomed Online*. 2006;12: 153–162.

88. National Institutes of Health. National Institutes of Health guidelines on human stem cell research. 2009. http://stemcells.nih.gov/policy/2009guidelines.htm.

89. Practice Committee of the American Society for Reproductive Medicine and the Practice Committee of the Society for Assisted Reproduction Technology. 2008 guidelines for gamete and embryo donation: a Practice Committee report. *Fertil Steril*. 2008;90:S30–44.

90. Kramer W, Schneider J, Schultz N. US oocyte donors: a retrospective study of medical and psychosocial issues. *Hum Reprod*. 2009;3144–3149.

91. Klein JU, Sauer MV. Ethics in egg donation: past, present, and future. *Semin Reprod Med*. 2010;28:322–328.

92. Kort DH, Gosselin J, Choi JM, et al. Pregnancy after age 50: defining risks for mother and child. *Am J Perinatol*. 2012;29:245–250.

93. Knopman JM, Noyes N, Grifo JA. Cryopreserved oocytes can serve as the treatment for secondary infertility: a novel model for egg donation. *Fertil Steril*. 2010;93:2413.e7–e9.

94. Sills ES, Brady AC, Omar AB, et al. IVF for premature ovarian failure: first reported births using oocytes donated from a twin sister. *Reprod Biol Endocrinol*. 2010;8:31.

95. Offit K, Sagi M, Hurley K. Preimplanation genetic diagnosis for cancer syndromes. A new challenge for preventive medicine. *JAMA*. 2006;296: 2727–2730.

96. Offit K, Kohut K, Clagett B, et al. Cancer genetic testing and assisted reproduction. *J Clin Oncol*. 2006;24:4775–4782.

97. Klitzman R, Zolovska B, Folberth W, et al. Preimplanation genetic diagnosis on in vitro fertilization clinic websites: presentations of risks, benefits, and other information. *Fertil Steril*. 2009;92:1276–1283.

98. American Medical Association. E-2.12 AMA Code of Medical Ethics. Genetic counseling. AMA Policy Finder. http://www.ama-assn.org/ama/pub/physician-resources/medical-ethics/code-medical-ethics/opinion212.page.

99. Munne S, Fischer J, Warner A, et al. Preimplantation genetic diagnosis significantly reduces pregnancy loss in infertile couples: a multicenter study. *Fertil Steril*. 2006;85:326–332.

100. Hansen M, Kurinczuk JJ, Bower C, Webb S. The risk of major birth defects after intracytoplasmic sperm injection and in vitro fertilization. *N Engl J Med*. 2002;346:725–730.

101. Noyes N, Borini A, Porcu E. Over 900 oocyte cryopreservation babies born with no apparent increase in congenital anomalies. *Reprod Biomed Online*. 2009;18:769–776.

102. Newton CR, McBride J, Feyles V, et al. Factors affecting patients' attitudes toward single- and multiple-embryo transfer. *Fertil Steril*. 2007;87:269–78.

103. Antrash H, Jack BW, Johnson K, et al. Where is the "w"oman in MCH? *Am J Obstet Gynecol*. 2008;199(6 suppl 2);S259–265.

104. Johnson K, Posner SF, Bierman J, et al. Recommendations to improve preconception health and health care—United States. *MMWR Morb Mortal Wkly Rep*. 2006;55:1–23.

105. Martin JA, Hamilton BE, Sutton PD, et al. Births: final data for 2007. *Nat Vital Stat Rep*. 2010;58:No 24.

106. Krieger N, Rehkopf DH, Chen JT, et al. The fall and rise of US inequities in premature mortality: 1960–2002. *PLoS Med*. 2008;5:e46.

107. Zhu SH, Cummins SE, Wong S, et al. The effects of a multilingual telephone quitline for Asian smokers: a randomized controlled trial. *J Natl Cancer Inst*. 2012;104:299–310.

108. Eakin EG, Reeves MM, Marshall A, et al. Living well with diabetes: a randomized controlled trial of a telephone-delivered intervention for maintenance of weight loss, physical activity and glycaemic control in adults with type 2 diabetes. *BMC Public Health*. 2010;10:452.

109. Jordan ET, Ray EM, Johnson P, Evans WD. Text4Baby: using text messaging to improve maternal and newborn health. *Nurs Womens Health*. 2011;15: 206–212.

110. Newsome K, Williams J, Way S, et al. Maternal and infant outcomes among severely ill pregnant and postpartum women with 2009 pandemic influenza A (H1N1)—United States, April 2009—August 2010. *MMWR Morb Mortal Wkly Rep*. 2011;60:1193–1196.

111. Creanga AA, Johnson TF, Graiter SB, et al. Severity of 2009 pandemic influenza A (H1N1) virus infection in pregnant women. *Obstet Gynecol*. 2010;115:717–726.

112. Farrell RM, Beigi RH. Pandemic influenza and pregnancy: an opportunity to reassess maternal ethics. *Am J Public Health*. 2009;99:S231–S235.

113. Ahluwalia IB, Harrison L, Ding H, et al. Influenza vaccination coverage among pregnant women—29 states and New York City, 2009–2010 season. *MMWR Morb Mortal Wkly Rep*. 2012;61:113–118.

114. Institute of Medicine. *Weight Gain during Pregnancy: Reexamining the Guidelines*. Washington, DC: National Academies Press; 2009.

115. Stothard KJ, Tennant PWG, Bell R, Rankin J. Maternal overweight and obesity and the risk of congenital anomalies: A systematic review and meta-analysis. *JAMA*. 2009;301:636–650.

116. Smith J, Ciafione K, Biron S, et al. Effects of maternal surgical weight loss in mothers on intergenerational transmission of obesity. *J Clin Endocrinol Metab*. 2009;94:4275–4283.

117. Vahratian A, Siega-Riz M, Savitz DA, Zhang J. Maternal prepregnancy overweight and obesity and the risk of cesarean delivery in nulliparous women. *Ann Epidemiol*. 2005;15:467–474.

118. Ludwig DS, Currie J. The relationship between pregnancy weight gain and birth weight: a within family comparison. *Lancet*. 2010; 376:984–990.

119. Chu SY, Callaghan WM, Kim SY, et al. Maternal obesity and risk of gestational diabetes mellitus. *Diabetes Care*. 2007;30:2070–2076.

120. Correa A, Gilboa SM, Besser LM, et al. Diabetes mellitus and birth defects. *Am J Obstet Gynecol*. 2008;199:237.e1–9.

121. Weiss JL, Malone FD, Emig D, et al. Obesity, obstetric complications and cesarean delivery rate—A population-based screening study. *Am J Obstet Gynecol*. 2004;190:1091–1097.

122. Skjaerven R, Wilcox AJ, Lie RT. The interval between pregnancies and the risk of preeclampsia. *N Engl J Med*. 2002;346:33–38.

123. Seely EW, Ecker J. Chronic hypertension in pregnancy. *N Engl J Med*. 2011;365:439–446.

124. Levine RJ, Maynard SE, Qian C, et al. Urinary placental growth factor and risk of preeclampsia. *JAMA*. 2005;293:77–85.

125. Centers for Disease Control and Prevention. CDC Features. Medication use during pregnancy. http://www.cdc.gov/Features/MedicationsPregnancy/.

126. US Food and Drug Administration. List of pregnancy exposure registries. http://www.fda.gov/ScienceResearch/SpecialTopics/WomensHealthResearch/ucm134848.htm.

127. McBride WG. Thalidomide embryopathy. *Teratology*. 1977;16:79–82.

128. Dieckmann WJ, Davis ME, Rynkiewicz LM, Pottinger RE. Does the administration of diethylstilbestrol during pregnancy have therapeutic value? *Am J Obstet Gynecol*. 1953;66:1062–1081.

129. Herbst AL, Ufelder H, Poskanzer DC. Adenocarcinoma of the vagina. *N Engl J Med*. 1971;284:878–881.

130. Palmer JR, Hatch EE, Rao S, et al. Infertility among women exposed prenatally to diethylstilbestrol. *Am J Epidemiol*. 2001;154:316–321.

131. Newbold RR. Lessons learned from perinatal exposure to diethylstilbestrol. *Toxicol Applied Pharmacol*. 2004;199:142–150.

132. Goodman A, Schorge J, Greene MF. The long term effects of in utero exposures—The DES story. *N Engl J Med*. 2011;364:2083–2084.

133. May PA, Gossage JP. Estimating the prevalence of fetal alcohol syndrome. a summary. *Alcohol Res Health*. 2001;25:159–167.

134. DeRoo LA, Wilcox AJ, Drevon CA, Lie RT. First-trimester maternal alcohol consumption and the risk of infant oral clefts in Norway: a population-based case-control study. *Am J Epidemiol*. 2008;168:638–646.

135. Oncken C. Nicotine replacement for smoking cessation during pregnancy. *N Engl J Med*. 2012;366:846–847.

136. Malik S, Cleves MA, Honein MA, et al. National Birth Defects Prevention Study. Maternal smoking and congenital heart defects. *Pediatrics*. 2008;121:e810–816.

137. Carmichael SL, Ma C, Rasmussen SA, et al. Craniosynostosis and maternal smoking. *Birth Defects Res A Clin Mol Teratol*. 2008;82:78–85.

138. Oken E, Levitan EB, Gillman MW. Maternal smoking during pregnancy and child overweight: systematic review and meta-analysis. *Int J Obesity*. 2008;32:201–210.

139. Kandel DB, Udry JR. Prenatal effects of maternal smoking on daughters' smoking: nicotine or testosterone exposure? *Am J Public Health*. 1999; 89:1377–1383.

140. Grandjean P, Landrigan PJ. Developmental neurotoxicity of industrial chemicals. *Lancet*. 2006;368:2167–2178.

141. Perera FP, Rauh VA, Tsai WY, et al. Effects of transplacental exposure to environmental pollutants on birth outcomes in a multiethnic population. *Environ Health Perspect*. 2003;111:201–205.

142. Perera FP. Molecular epidemiology, prenatal exposure and prevention of cancer. *Environ Health*. 2011;10(suppl 1):55.

143. Tamashiro KLK, Moran TH. Perinatal environment and its influences on metabolic programming of offspring. *Physiol Behav*. 2010;100:560–566.

144. Whyatt RM, Liu X, Rauh VA, et al. Maternal prenatal urinary phthalate metabolite concentrations and child mental, psychomotor, and behavioral development at 3 years of age. *Environ Health Perspect*. 2012;120:290–295.

145. Boulet SL, Yang Q, Mai C, et al. Folate status in women of childbearing age, by race/ethnicity-United States, 1999–2000, 2001–2002, and 2003–2004. *MMWR Morb Mortal Wkly Rep*. 2007;55:1377–1380.

146. Wolff T, Witkop CT, Miller T, Syed SB. Folic acid supplementation for the prevention of neural tube defects: an update of the evidence for the US Preventive Service Task Force. *Ann Intern Med*. 2009;150:632–639.

147. Roth C, Magnus P, Schjølberg S, et al. Folic acid supplements in pregnancy and severe language delay in children. *JAMA*. 2011;306:1566–1573.

148. Russell SL, Ickovics JR, Yaffee RA. Parity & untreated dental caries in US women. *J Dent Res*. 2010;89:1091–1096.

149. Boggess KA, Urlaub DM, Massey KE, et al. Oral hygiene practices and dental service utilization among pregnant women. *JADA*. 2010;141:553–561.

150. Lazarus E, DeBenedectis C, North D, et al. Utilization of imaging in pregnant patients: 10 year review of 5270 examinations in 3285 patients—1997–2006. *Radiology*. 2009;251:517–524.

151. MacDorman MF, Matthews TJ. Infant deaths—United States, 2000–2007. *MMWR Morb Mortal Wkly Rep*. 2011;60:49–51.

152. Declercq E. Trends in midwife-attended births, 1989–2007. *J Midwifery Womens Health*. 2011;56:173–176.

153. Hatem M, Sandall J, Devane D, et al. Midwife-led versus other models of care for childbearing women (Review). *Cochrane Database Syst Rev*. 2008 Oct 8; (4):CD004667.

154. ACOG Committee on Obstetric Practice: ACOG Opinion No. 476, February 2011-Planned home birth. *Obstet Gynecol*. 2011;117:425–428.

155. American College of Obstetrics and Gynecologists. Pain relief during labor. ACOG Committee Opinion on Obstetric Practice No. 295. *Obstet Gynecol*. 2004;104:213.

156. Osterman MJK, Martin JA. Epidural and spinal anesthesia use during labor: 27-state reporting area, 2008. *Nat Vital Stat Reports*. 2011;59:no 5.

157. Kiesewetter B, Lehner R. Maternal outcome monitoring: induction of labor versus spontaneous onset of labor—a retrospective data analysis. *Arch Gynecol Obstet*. 2012 Feb 2 (ePub ahead of print).

158. Minkoff H. The ethics of cesarean section by choice. *Semin Perinatol*. 2006;30:309–312.

159. Menacker F, Hamilton BE. Recent trends in cesarean delivery in the United States. *NCHS Data Brief*. 2010;35.

160. Menacker F, Declercq E, Macdorman MF. Cesarean delivery: Background, trends, and epidemiology. *Semin Perinatol*. 2006;30:235–241.

161. Zhang J, Troendle J, Reddy UM, et al. Contemporary cesarean delivery practice in the United States. *Am J Obstet Gynecol*. 2010;203:326.e1–326.e10.

162. Tita ATN, Landon MB, Spong CY, et al. Timing of elective repeat cesarean delivery at term and neonatal outcome. *N Engl J Med*. 2009;360;111–120.

163. ACOG Committee on Obstetric Practice: Practice Bulletin No. 115, August 2010. Vaginal birth after previous cesarean delivery. *Obstet Gynecol*. 2010;116:450–463.

164. Declercq E, Cunningham DK, Johnson C, Sakala C. Mothers' reports of postpartum pain associated with vaginal and cesarean deliveries: results of a national survey. *Birth*. 2008;35:16–24.

165. Rynn L, Cragon J, Correa A, et al. Update on overall prevalence of major birth defect—Atlanta, Georgia, 1978–2005. *MMWR Morb Mortal Wkly Rep*. 2008;57:1–5.

166. Martin JA. Preterm births—United States, 2007. *MMWR Morb Mortal Wkly Rep*. 2011;60:78–79.

167. Weinberg CR, Shi M. The genetics of preterm birth: using what we know to design better association studies. *Am J Epidemiol*. 2009;170:1373–1381.

168. Martin JA, Hamilton BE, Sutton PD, et al. Births: Final data for 2006. *Nat Vital Stat Rep*. 2009;57:no 7.

169. Hatch EE, Troisi R, Wise LA, et al. Preterm birth, fetal growth, and age at menarche among women exposed prenatally to diethylstilbestrol. *Reproduct Toxicol*. 2011;31:151–157.

170. Moster D, Wilcox AJ, Vollset SE, et al. Cerebral palsy among term and post-term births. *JAMA*. 2010;304:976–982.

171. Lawson CC, Rocheleau CM, Whelan EA, et al. Occupational exposures among nurses and risk of spontaneous abortion. *Am J Obstet Gynecol*. 2012;206 (Epub ahead of print)

172. Wapner RJ. Genetics of stillbirth. *Clin Obstet Gynecol*. 2010;53:628–634.

173. The Stillbirth Collaborative Research Network Writing Group. Causes of death among stillbirths. *JAMA*. 2011;306:2459–2468.

174. Andres RL. The association of cigarette smoking with placenta previa and abruptio placentae. *Sem Perinatol*. 1996;20:154–159.

175. Ananth CV, Smulian JC, Vintzileos AM. The effect of placenta previa on neonatal mortality: a population-based study in the United States, 1989 through 1997. *Am J Obstet Gynecol*. 2003;188:1299–1304.

176. Ananth CV, Demissie K, Smulian JC, Vintzileos AM. Placenta previa in singleton and twin births in the United States, 1989 through 1998: a comparison of risk factor profiles and associated conditions. *Am J Obstet Gynecol*. 2003;188:275–281.

177. Heron M, Hoyert DL, Murphy SL, et al. Deaths: final data for 2006. *National Vital Statistics Reports*. 2009;57:no 14.

178. Hoyert DL. Maternal mortality and related concepts. *Vital Health Stat*. 2007;3:33.

179. Ickovics JR, Kershaw TS, Westdahl C, et al. Group prenatal care and perinatal outcomes: a randomized controlled trial. *Obstet Gynecol*. 2007;110:330–339.

180. New York City Department of Health and Mental Hygiene. Executive summary of the Annual Summary of Vital Statistics. New York: Author; 2009. www.nyc.gov/html/doh/downloads/pdf/vs/highlights2009.pdf.

181. Matthews TJ, MacDorman MF. Infant mortality statistics from the 2006 period linked birth/infant death data set. *Nat Vital Stat Reports*. 2010;58:17.

182. Collins JW, David RJ, Handler A, et al. Very low birthweight in African American infants: the role of maternal exposure to interpersonal racial discrimination. *Am J Public Health*. 2004;94:2132–2138.

183. Coates AO, Schaefer CA, Alexander JL. Detection of postpartum depression and anxiety in a large health plan. *J Behav Health Serv*. 2004;31:117–133.

184. Fitelson E, Kim S, Baler AS, Lright K. Treatment of postpartum depression: clinical, psychological and pharmacological options. *Int J Womens Health*. 2011;3:1–14.

185. American Academy of Pediatrics Section on Breastfeeding. Policy Statement. Breast feeding and the use of human milk. *Pediatrics*. 2005;115:496–506.

186. James DCS, Lessen R. Position of the American Dietetic Association: promoting and supporting breastfeeding. *J Am Diet Assoc*. 2009;109:1926–42.

187. Morrow AL, Rangel JM. Human milk protection against infectious diarrhea: implications for prevention and clinical care. *Semin Pediatr Infect Dis*. 2004;15:221–228.

188. Koletzko B, Von Kries R, Monasterolo RC, et al. Can infant feeding choices modulate later obesity risk? *Am J Clin Nutr*. 2009;89(suppl):1502–1508S.

189. DiGirolamo AM, Grummer-Srawn LM, Fein SB. Effect of maternity-care practice on breastfeeding. *Pediatrics*. 2008;122:S43–S49.

190. Taveras EM, Li RW, Grummer-Strawn L, et al. Mothers' and clinicians' perspectives on breast feeding counseling during routine preventive visits. *Pediatrics*. 2004;113:F405–F411.

191. Perrine CG, Shealy KR, Scanlon KS, et al. Vital signs: hospital practices to support breastfeeding—United States, 2007 and 2009. *MMWR Morb Mortal Wkly Rep*. 2011;60:1020–1025.

192. Blyth R, Creedy DK, Dennis CL, et al. Effect of maternal confidence on breastfeeding duration: an application of breastfeeding self-efficacy theory. *Birth-Issues Perinatal Care*. 2002;29:278–284.

193. Meek JY. Breastfeeding in the workplace. *Pediatr Clin North Am*. 2001;48: 461–474.

194. Chamberlain LB, McMahon M, Philipp BL, Merewood A. Breast pump access in the inner city: a hospital-based initiative to provide breast pumps for low-income women. *J Hum Lact*. 2006;22:94–98.

195. Kramer MS, Aboud F, Mironova E, et al. for the Promotion of Breast Feeding Intervention Trial (PROBIT) Study Group. *Arch Gen Psych*. 2008;65:578–584.

196. Templeton A, Grimes DA. A request for abortion. *N Engl J Med*. 2011;365: 2198–2204.

197. Jones RK, Kavanaugh ML. Changes in abortion rates between 2000 and 2008 and lifetime incidence of abortion. *Obstet Gynecol*. 2011;117:1358–1366.

198. Miller E, Decker MR, McCauley HL, et al. Pregnancy coercion, intimate partner violence and unintended pregnancy. *Contraception*. 2010;81:316–322.

199. Saftlas AF, Wallis AB, Shochet T, et al. Prevalence of intimate partner violence among an abortion clinic population. *Am J Public Health*. 2010;100: 1412–1415.

200. Silverman JG, Decker MR, McCauley HL, et al. Male perpetration of intimate partner violence and involvement in abortions and abortion-related conflict. *Am J Public Health*. 2010;100:1415–1417.

201. Whelan P. Abortion rates and universal health care. *N Engl J Med*. 2010;362:e45.

202. Annas GJ, Mariner WK. women and children last—the predictable effects of proposed federal funding cuts. *N Engl J Med*. 2011;364:1590–1591.

203. Raymond EG, Grimes DA. The comparative safety of legal induced abortion and childbirth in the United States. *Obstet Gynecol*. 2012;119:215–219.

204. Beral V, Bull D, Doll R, et al. Collaborative Group on Hormonal Factors in Breast Cancer. Breast cancer and abortion: collaborative reanalysis of data from 53 epidemiological studies, including 83,000 women with breast cancer from 16 countries. *Lancet*. 2004;363:1007–1016.

205. Rosenfield A, Charo RA, Chavikin W. Moving forward on reproductive health. *N Engl J Med*. 2008;18:1869–1871.

Menopause

Ruby T. Senie, PhD

Introduction

A major focus of women's clinical health needs across the life span links the rise and fall of hormones with physical, emotional, social, and cultural patterns that influence the quality of life. Between puberty and late middle age, health concerns are primarily related to menstrual function, contraception, pregnancy, and early onset of chronic conditions. Some women will have successfully given birth to the number of offspring desired; others may have experienced unplanned childbearing or were unable to achieve conception without medical intervention. With the end of reproductive potential, as hormone levels decline and menstrual cycles become more variable in frequency and duration, the health needs of most women shift to experiences associated with the menopausal transition and accompanying increases in chronic conditions.

Although questions have been raised about the "medicalization" of menopause, a naturally occurring life-course event, the complex, person-specific physical and psychosocial responses encourage many women to seek relief with pharmaceutical preparations or natural remedies. The variability of estrogen levels has systemic affects influencing nutrient absorption and metabolism, bone and mineral health, blood pressure, migraine headaches, memory and cognition, and urinary continence. Since menopause often triggers the onset of chronic conditions, researchers have focused on factors related to the variability of age at last menses, subsequent impact of hormone depletion, conditions leading to surgical menopause, and risks and benefits of bilateral oophorectomy. With increased life expectancy documented during the 20th century, women are now living more than a third of their lives after menopause when their health status may reflect behaviors established at earlier ages. This chapter provides a brief review of women's experiences during the transition to menopause from years characterized by reproductive potential and concludes with an overview of the role of exogenous hormone therapy and other health behaviors that influence the quality of life during and after menopause.

The Menopausal Transition

Women naturally experience changes in reproductive potential from highest fertility soon after puberty lasting 15–20 years through stages of subfertility before progressing to perimenopause and cessation of menses.[1] Treloar, using data collected prospectively from two cohorts, defined two transition time points when the greatest menstrual cycle variability was detected: following menarche for 2 to 3 years and several years prior to menopause.[2,3] Therefore, perimenopause or "premenopause" is characterized by menstrual cycles that are less predictable in length and frequency, reflecting declining quantity and quality of remaining ovarian oocytes.[4] Studies of surgically removed ovaries suggested the number of remaining follicles determined the transition between regularity of cycles to variability of the perimenopausal stage.[5]

Rising levels of follicle stimulating hormone (FSH) released by the pituitary gland without compensating increases in luteinizing hormone (LH) are predictive of loss of ovulatory function.[6] Levels of inhibin B and antimullerian hormone (AMH), both produced by ovarian follicles, reflect ovarian reserve including the number and quality of the remaining aging oocytes.[7] The function of inhibin B is to regulate FSH; therefore, increasing FSH levels and declining inhibin B and AMH have become important endocrine markers of age-related reduced reproductive capacity.[4]

Lack of standard criteria defining "menopause" has complicated epidemiologic research; however, advances in technology have recently enabled identification and measurement of hormones associated with declining reproductive potential providing a reasonable option for consistent classification of menopausal status in future studies. Currently, most researchers rely on self-reported dates to define "natural menopause" as 12 consecutive months of amenorrhea not induced by radiation, hysterectomy, or medications although some studies have used a 6-month interval.[4] With the addition of reproducible measurements of inhibin B, AMH, and other steroid hormones or maturation index of vaginal cytology,[8] future research will provide more reliable assessments of the menopausal transition.

153

The gradual reduction in ovarian hormones to postmenopausal status generally evolves over 2 to 8 years with daily premenopausal ovarian estradiol levels ranging from 80 to 500 μg and estrone from 80 to 300 μg to the reduced levels detected several years after last menses of 6 μg estradiol and 40 μg of estrone primarily produced by peripheral aromatization of androstenedione in adipose tissue.[9] The reductions affect organ systems throughout the body producing a variety of symptoms.[6]

Hot flashes, the most prevalent symptom, have been reported by 50% to 85% of perimenopausal women, often begin around the age of 40, an age when some women are attempting to have their first pregnancy.[10] Hot flashes may be intense and highly unpredictable, disrupting activities daily or only occasionally, at any hour of the day or night.[11] For most women these episodes last 3 to 10 minutes, causing flushing and sweating with a feeling of intense heat that produces red blotching on the face and upper chest, frequently associated with feelings of anxiety and palpitations.[11,12]

In addition to vasomotor symptoms, declining estrogen levels causes a wide variety of changes in tissues of many organs, resulting in thinning of the vaginal wall, urinary incontinence, sexual dysfunction, and interrupted sleep. Emotional changes include increased anxiety, depression, fatigue, headaches, and some memory lapses. Symptoms become more intense for a year or two as the variability of cycles increases before final menses (Table 11-1). Months of amenorrhea may be interrupted by resumption of occasional ovulatory cycles;[4] although fertility may be significantly diminished, some women remain at risk of an unplanned pregnancy[13] as studies indicate serum levels and vaginal cytology continue to reflect estrogen stimulation for several years after last menses.[8,9]

Data from the 1999 National Health Interview Survey (NHIS) was analyzed by Brett and Cooper to assess characteristics of a representative sample of American

women experiencing menopause compared with similarly aged premenopausal women.[14] Between ages 40 to 54, 18% were in transition, defined as the absence of routine menstrual cycles for at least 3 months but not more than 11 months, and 61% were premenopausal. These authors noted that smokers were more likely to be postmenopausal within each age group.[14] Irregular cycles were more common among obese young women potentially reflecting polycystic ovarian syndrome rather than approaching menopause.[15]

Freeman et al. followed a population-based cohort of more than 400 premenopausal African American and Caucasian women ages 35 to 47 from 1995 to 2007 in order to assess effects of declining hormone levels on weight gain and central adiposity.[16] Compared with thinner premenopausal women, obese women experienced more frequent irregular menstrual cycles associated with significantly lower levels of estradiol and inhibin B.[16] The authors suggested lower inhibin B levels among obese premenopausal women may reflect earlier decline in ovarian reserve compared with nonobese women.[16] The relationship between obesity and endogenous hormones reversed during the menopausal transition; obese postmenopausal women had significantly higher estradiol levels compared with thinner women reflecting a shift in the source of estrogen from the ovaries to adipose tissue.[16]

Age at Natural Menopause

Natural menopause generally occurs among American women between ages 45 and 55 with a mean age of 51 although an estimated 8% stop menstruating before age 40 and 5% continue until age 60. The variability in age at menopause has importance for public health given earlier age at menopause is known to increase risks of cardiovascular disease and osteoporosis although research documents that women experiencing menopause at younger ages are at lower risk of breast cancer.[17]

Family history of early onset menopause in a first- or second-degree relative (mother, sister, aunt or grandmother) was reported by 38% of young postmenopausal women compared with only 9% of similarly aged premenopausal women.[18] Having a sister with early menopause was associated with a significantly increased odds ratio (OR = 9.1, 95% CI = 3.1–26.5) for similarly early cessation of menses.[18] Family patterns have also noted similar ages at natural menopause among mother–daughter pairs suggesting heritability of menopausal age ranging from 30% to 85% depending up the study populations.[19] Women whose mothers experienced earlier menopause were found to have significantly higher levels of FSH, the biomarker of ovarian aging, linking genetic and environmental factors to age of last menses.[1] Single gene defects on the long arm of the X chromosome were implicated in premature ovarian failure in research conducted by Krauss et al. who studied hereditary patterns of a family reporting menstrual irregularities and menopause before age 40 over three generations.[20] Recent studies using genome-wide scans have identified candidate genes that may explain the natural variation in ovarian aging and variability of the reproductive life span.[19]

Table 11-1
Common symptoms reported by perimenopausal women
Hot flashes
Night sweats
Weight gain
Insomnia
Mood swings/irritability
Memory or concentration problems
Vaginal dryness
Heavy bleeding
Fatigue
Depression
Hair changes
Headaches
Heart palpitations
Sexual dysfunction
Urinary incontinence

Trends in menopausal age are influenced by diverse factors including genetic, social, environmental, and hormonal exposures. Secular changes in smoking habits, childbearing, body mass index (BMI), and educational attainment appeared to influence both age at menarche and menopause among data from birth cohorts reported by Nichols et al.[21] Compared with earlier birth cohorts of 1910–1914, women born between 1930 and 1935 were more likely to be parous, smoke cigarettes, drink alcohol, be college educated, have higher BMI, and have used oral contraceptives.[21] As these patterns continue to evolve potentially lengthening reproductive years, women may experience changes in chronic health conditions associated with greater exposure to endogenous hormones.

The Black Women's Health Study, based on a mailed survey to more than 64,000 American women ages 21 to 69, provided data on menopause and related health factors. Palmer et al. noted earlier age at natural menopause was positively associated with quantity of current and past smoking and inversely associated with body mass index among members of their black study population.[22] Significant differences in timing of menopause were also found among more than 90,000 racially and ethnically diverse women included in the collaborative Multiethnic Cohort Study from Los Angeles and Hawaii. Relative to non-Hispanic white women, older age at menopause was noted among Japanese Americans associated with body weight, nonsmoking history, and older age at first birth.[17] Hispanics women were younger at menopause than non-Hispanic white women, especially those born outside the United States. The results supported the hypothesis that age at menopause is associated with genetic, reproductive, environmental, and lifestyle factors.[17]

Kinney et al. noted the proestrogen effect of moderate alcohol drinking was associated with a 2 year later age at menopause in contrast to nondrinkers; however, in this study the antiestrogen effect of smoking reduced age of menopause in relation to number of cigarettes smoked per day.[23] Data from NHIS found smoking was significantly associated with being postmenopausal (OR = 2.2, 95% CI = 1.7–3.0) compared with similarly aged premenopausal women.[14] Some studies have reported that heavier smokers enter menopause almost 3 years earlier than nonsmokers.[24] Researchers have suggested aromatic hydrocarbon exposure from cigarette smoking may adversely affect the ovaries accelerating follicle aging. Data from the Study of Women's Health Across the Nation (SWAN), a multiethnic community-based cohort of approximately 3,000 women recruited in seven regions of the United States to study the menopausal transition, indicated natural menopause occurred at a median age of 51.4 years. Women smoking 10 cigarettes per day (half a pack) were 40% more likely to experience early menopause, limiting their reproductive years. Although smoking reduced the age at menopause,[25] others noted the association was small compared with the influence of family patterns among first-degree relatives including heritability detected among monozygotic twins compared with dizygotic twin pairs.[26]

Two major studies have recently correlated earlier age at menopause with exposure to diethylstilbestrol (DES) during fetal development. Data from the National Cancer Institute Combined Cohort Study of DES Exposed Women who have been followed for reproductive outcomes to age 45 and other health outcomes to age 55 indicate early menopause was more than twofold greater than among unexposed women (HR = 2.35, 95% CI = 1.67–3.31).[27] Similar findings were reported from the Sisters Study, a prospectively followed cohort of American and Puerto Rican women ages 35 to 74 recruited to study genetic and environmental breast cancer risk factors.[28] Information collected from more than 32,000 unaffected sisters indicated prenatal exposures to DES was the strongest factor associated with earlier age at menopause (HR = 1.45, 95% CI = 1.27–1.65).[28] Steiner et al. hypothesized that abnormal organ development experienced by some DES-exposed women may have limited the number of oocytes available at birth leading to earlier depletion during the reproductive years before the menopausal transition.[28]

Another prospectively followed cohort reported earlier menopause associated with greater frequency of ovulatory cycles. Women ages 20 to 35 with short menstrual cycles (less than 26 days) became menopausal more than a year earlier than women with longer cycles; a 2-year difference was noted when women with short cycles were compared with women whose cycles were 33 days or longer.[29] The association of greater number of ovulatory cycles and menopause before age 45 was also found among nulliparous women and those with low parity.[30] A study by Pines et al. noted earlier menopausal age (mean 46.4 years) among women with ovarian induction treatment for infertility compared with control subjects not requiring or desiring infertility treatment whose mean menopausal age was significantly older (50.0 years, P < 0.001). This finding suggested accelerated maturation of numerous oocytes may diminish ovarian reserve, shortening the transition to premature menopause.[31]

Most epidemiologic studies rely on self-reported menopausal age rather than obtaining biosamples to measure hormonal levels. However, research has indicated women tend to round their recalled age to 45, 50, or 55.[8] To assess reporting consistency and reliability, repeated responses to the same question from baseline to follow-up interviews were compared among participants in the first National Health and Nutrition Examination Survey (NHANES) I and Follow-up Study (1971–1984).[32] Ages at natural menopause reported at first and second interviews were within 1 year among 44% of participants; however, more consistent reporting of age was observed among the 59% of respondents who had experienced surgical menopause. The differences in recalled menopausal ages increased with age at interview and the time interval between the two interviews. Given the uncertainty, the authors suggested self-reported menopausal age may be less accurate than other health events.[32] To enhance recall of age-related health events, some researchers have created memory aides such as a personal calendars on which life events such as marriages, births, and diagnoses of chronic conditions are first recorded before the interview asks about the factors of interest.[33]

Hysterectomy—Surgical Menopause

Among American women of reproductive age, hysterectomy is the second most frequently performed surgery after cesarean section delivery.[34] An estimated 600,000 procedures are performed annually in the United States and 20 million women, one-third of the total female population under age 60, has had a hysterectomy. More than 70% were performed for benign conditions.[34] The Behavior Risk Factor Surveillance System (BRFSS) data indicated the mean age at hysterectomy in the United States was 46.5 years (S.D.=20.4). The clinical problems leading to hysterectomy vary but an estimated 22% of otherwise healthy perimenopausal women had experienced heavy menstrual bleeding (menorrhagia) causing anemia which adversely affected their quality of life. Although clinicians may initially prescribe medical therapy, the lack of improvement has often precipitated surgical menopause. National Hospital Discharge Survey (NHDS) data compiled by the Centers for Disease Control and Prevention (CDC) between 2000 and 2004 indicated 50% of hysterectomies were performed annually for treatment of uterine fibroids.[35]

National data indicated hysterectomy rates rose between 1965 and 1999 when one in nine women aged 35 to 45 had a hysterectomy. The rate in 2004 was 5.1 per 1,000 varying by age as with the highest frequency among women ages 40–44 (12.5 per 1,000) and secondarily among ages 45–49 (11.8 per 1,000) (Figure 11-1).[34] Rates differed geographically from the highest in southern states (6.3 per 1,000) to lowest in the northeast (3.7 per 1,000) (Figure 11-2).[34] Data from several studies indicate black women ages 30 to 54 had significantly higher rates of hysterectomy than white women of the same age primarily associated with higher incidence of uterine fibroids. The NHDS data noted southern women were 6 years younger at hysterectomy than the average age, 48 years, in the northeast.[35]

Recently the proportion of abdominal hysterectomies remained stable at 67.9% and 32.1% were performed vaginally with one-third of these less invasive procedures accompanied by laparoscopy.[35] In 2004 the primary indication for hysterectomy among women between ages

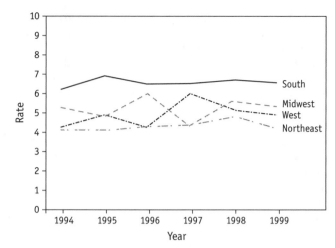

*Per 1,000 female, civilian residents aged ≥15 years.

†Regions are defined as follows: **Northeast** (Connecticut, Maine, Massachusetts, New Hampshire, New Jersey, New York, Pennsylvania, Rhode Island, and Vermont); **Midwest** (Illinois, Indiana, Iowa, Kansas, Michigan, Minnesota, Missouri, Nebraska, North Dakota, Ohio, South Dakota, and Wisconsin); **South** (Alabama, Arkansas, Delaware, District of Columbia, Florida, Georgia, Kentucky, Louisiana, Maryland, Mississippi, North Carolina, Oklahoma, South Carolina, Tennessee, Texas, Virginia, and West Virginia); and **West** (Alaska, Arizona, California, Colorado, Hawaii, Idaho, Montana, Nevada, New Mexico, Oregon, Utah, Washington, and Wyoming).

Figure 11-2 Hysterectomy rates by geographic region—United States, 1994–1999.

Source: Reproduced from Keshavarz H, Hillis SD, Kieke BA, Marchbanks PA. Hysterectomy surveillance—United States, 1994–1999. Morbidity Mortality Weekly Report 2002;51(SS05):1–8.

35 and 54 was treatment for fibroids in contrast to older women whose surgical menopause was more frequently treatment for uterine prolapse or cancer. As alternative treatments for fibroids were developed, hysterectomy rates significantly decreased from 44.2% in 2000 to 38.7% in 2004 (P < 0.001).[35]

Although hysterectomy generally relieves women of symptoms associated with benign gynecological conditions, some outcomes following surgery, including incontinence, decreased sexual function, and discomfort from early, rapid onset of vasomotor symptoms of menopause, may adversely affect subsequent quality of life.[36] African American women in the Multiethnic Cohort Study experienced surgical menopause more frequently than participants of other racial/ethnic groups.[17] Debate continues regarding overuse of hysterectomy for benign conditions as well as accompanying bilateral oophorectomy. Even if one or both ovaries are retained, the trauma of hysterectomy accelerates reduction in ovarian estrogen production resulting in earlier menopausal symptoms onset compared with women of similar ages without hysterectomy.[37]

Moorman et al. studied factors associated with premenopausal hysterectomy for benign conditions without bilateral oophorectomy among participants ages 30 to 47 in the Prospective Research on Ovarian Function (PROOF) study. Hysterectomy performed primarily for fibroids was more frequent among women with higher parity, history of tubal ligation, lower education level, and

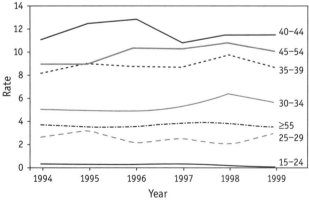

*Per 1,000 female, civilian residents in each age group.

Figure 11-1 Hysterectomy rates by age group—United States, 1994–1999.

Source: Reproduced from Keshavarz H, Hillis SD, Kieke BA, Marchbanks PA. Hysterectomy surveillance—United States, 1994-1999. Morbidity Mortality Weekly Report 2002;51(SS05):1–8.

higher BMI. Prospective data indicated weight gain was greater following hysterectomy even though ovaries were retained compared with women who did not undergo any surgery. The authors noted clinical efforts were necessary to avoid the development of obesity.[38]

Bilateral Oophorectomy—Risks and Benefits

Fear of ovarian cancer, an aggressive malignancy causing approximately 15,000 deaths annually, has led to bilateral oophorectomy at the time of hysterectomy for benign conditions even though age-specific ovarian cancer rates are low. Data from CDC indicated 55% of women younger than age 45 had concurrent bilateral oophorectomy at time of hysterectomy as did 78% of women ages 45 to 64. The rate of concurrent bilateral oophorectomy declined from 55.8% in 2000 to 49.5% in 2004 reflecting an increase in vaginal procedures with ovarian preservation.[35] Figure 11-3 presents the most recent data available noting age-related differences in hysterectomy with bilateral oophorectomy between 1994 and 1999.[34] Regional variations in rates were geographically similar to the hysterectomy rates noted in Figure 11-2 with highest frequency in southern states and lowest in the northeast.[34] Differences in clinical practice guidelines and patient requests may explain the regional patterns.

Parker et al. reviewed health benefits and risks of bilateral oophorectomy prior to natural menopause among almost 30,000 nurses who were followed after undergoing hysterectomy for benign conditions before age 50; 55.6% had bilateral oophorectomy and 44.4% ovarian conservation.[39] Although risks of breast and ovarian cancer were diminished after bilateral oophorectomy, an increase in all-cause mortality from coronary heart disease, stroke, and lung cancer was observed. Among the 13,305 who retained their ovaries, 34 (0.26%) died of ovarian cancer. In addition, women suffered from the sudden loss of hormone stimulation with rapid onset of menopausal symptoms including hot flashes, sleep disturbances,

mood alterations and vaginal dryness requiring medical treatment.[39] Therefore, Parker et al. recommended caution when considering elective bilateral oophorectomy among women younger than age 65 since loss of ovarian hormones may be accompanied by adverse health outcomes.[40] Shuster and colleagues advised women at genetic risk of breast and ovarian cancer due to a mutation of a BRCA gene, to avoid bilateral prophylactic oophorectomy before age 40, but encouraged those at high risk to have the surgery after age 55 with careful surveillance during intervening years.[41]

Cardiovascular Disease

Prior to menopause women experienced lower rates of heart disease compared with men of similar ages primarily associated with endogenous estrogen levels. Estrogen is believed to protects women by maintaining healthy levels of both low-density lipoprotein cholesterol (LDL) and high-density lipoprotein cholesterol (HDL).[42] To test the association and assess biochemical and physiological changes linked to the menopausal transition, Matthews et al. recruited a random sample of more than 500 premenopausal women ages 42 to 50 residing in Alleghany County, Pennsylvania, to a 5-year study that included baseline and follow-up data collection. Within 3 years of recruitment significant changes in biochemical measures of coronary heart disease risk were found among naturally menopausal participants who were not prescribed hormonal therapy: among women with earlier signs of menopause, especially among smokers, LDL levels increased and HDL levels decreased.[42] Data from the Nurses' Health Study analyzed by Colditz et al. found loss of hormonal stimulation following bilateral oophorectomy among nurses aged 40 to 44 resulted in a twofold increased risk of myocardial infarction compared with women of the same age group with intact ovaries.[43] The SWAN study also noted significantly higher rates of heart disease among younger women at natural menopause, a finding that was consistent with the protective role of later menopause against heart disease morbidity and mortality.[25]

Life Expectancy

Members of the Seventh-Day Adventists cohort had longer life expectancy with increasing age at natural menopause; the risk of death was twice as great during 6 years of follow-up among women with last menses before age 40 compared with women aged 50 to 54.[44] Snowdon et al. suggested that earlier age at natural menopause indicated ovarian aging, which might be associated with aging of other organs, predictive of earlier mortality.[44] A recent meta-analysis conducted by Atsma et al. linked increased mortality at young ages with early menopause and bilateral oophorectomy.[45] A statistical model estimated an 8.6% increase in mortality before age 80 associated with bilateral oophorectomy before age 55, but a prospective cohort study found mortality increased 67% following prophylactic surgery before age 45.[46] Therefore, bilateral oophorectomy reduced the risk of breast and ovarian cancer

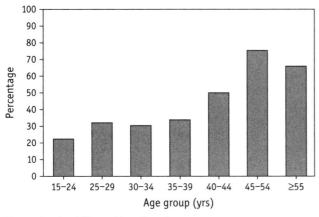

*Among female, civilian residents in each age group.

Figure 11-3 Percentage of hysterectomies with bilateral oophorectomy, by age group–United States, 1994–1999.

Source: Reproduced from Keshavarz H, Hillis SD, Kieke BA, Marchbanks PA. Hysterectomy surveillance—United States, 1994–1999. Morbidity Mortality Weekly Report 2002;51(SS05):1–8.

but these protective effects were countered by increased all-cause mortality as well as morbidity associated with osteoporosis, hip fracture, heart disease, and lung cancer.[46] The adverse effect of oophorectomy is related to the loss of ovarian production of androgens and androstenedione, which convert to estrogen in adipose tissue after menopause. Therefore, clinicians advising women must guide treatment decisions based on person-specific risk factors and concerns.[39]

Urinary Tract Infections and Urinary Incontinence

Many women experience stress-associated urinary incontinence—urine leakage during physical activity or involuntary coughing, sneezing, or laughing, which may reflect pelvic floor disorders. Risk of incontinence frequently follows urinary tract infection (UTI), which has been reported by an estimated 9% of women older than aged 50 resulting in more than 8 million women requiring medical treatment annually.[47] Among women who experienced premenopausal UTI associated with sexual intercourse, risk of postmenopausal recurrent asymptomatic UTI is increased due to declining hormonal levels result in thinning of the vaginal walls with loss of elasticity and lubrication.[48] Reduced lubrication increases mechanical irritation during sexual intercourse, enabling pathogens to invade vulnerable tissue and to enter the bladder. With menopause the vaginal pH increases enabling growth of diverse bacteria.[49] Hu et al. noted recurrent UTIs were more common among sexually active postmenopausal women, suggesting behaviors that predispose women to infection.[47] An additional contributor to UTI identified by Raz et al. was urine retention resulting from incomplete bladder emptying and obstructed urine flow; each problem enhanced bacterial growth.[48] An earlier randomized trial by these investigators indicated topical estrogen treatment dramatically lowered the incidence of UTI by decreasing vaginal pH and reducing the need for antibiotic therapy.[49] The authors noted that vaginal administration provided low estrogen exposure with limited systemic effects, which they documented by serum hormone levels.[49]

Urinary incontinence is increased among women following repeated UTIs.[48] Surveys indicate that rates of incontinence vary from 15% to 50% among community-dwelling postmenopausal women depending upon their age and health status.[50] Minassian et al. analyzed NHANES data from 2001–2002 to identify common characteristics of women experiencing incontinence including increasing perimenopausal stage and age, history of hysterectomy, obesity, and high parity.[50] Nygaard et al. also used data from 2005–2006 NHANES participants to assess the prevalence of urinary and fecal incontinence in relation to pelvic floor disorders.[51] Pressure on the bladder may cause urine to leak through the urethra as the sphincter muscle weakens following pregnancy and childbirth, with aging or after pelvic surgery including hysterectomy (Figure 11-4). A major cause of incontinence is pelvic organ prolapse, which may occur after labor and delivery when pelvic organs are inadequately supported by muscles of the pelvic

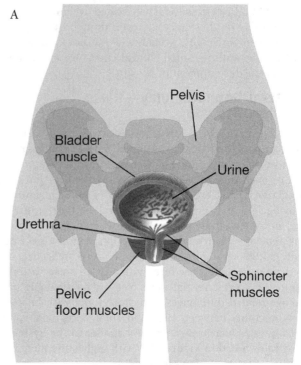

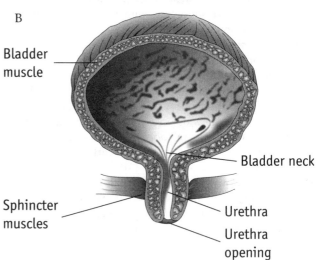

Figure 11-4 Bladder control organs affecting urinary incontinence.

Source: © Jones & Bartlett Learning

floor allowing the organs to protrude through the vaginal opening.[51] At least one pelvic floor problem was reported by 24% and the proportion significantly increased with age from 10% among women younger than 40 to more than 50% among those age 80 or older. Both high parity and obesity increased the risk of one or more pelvic floor abnormalities.[51]

Urgency urinary incontinence results from overactive muscle contractions during bladder filling, Nygaard stated. Due to the unexpected, sudden, and often large volumes of urine leakage, this problem is more disturbing with greater negative impact on quality of life than stress incontinence.[52] Bladder training by urinating on a schedule has been proposed as a means of reducing incontinence and controlling urinary urgency.[52] Women have been advised to perform Kegel exercises,[53] contracting and relaxing sphincter muscles, to strengthen the pelvic region and improve urine retention.

The Program to Reduce Incontinence by Diet and Exercise (PRIDE) was designed to compare incontinence among women randomly assigned to an intensive weight-loss intervention with usual clinical care. Self-help materials provided to all overweight and obese participants described the female anatomy enabling women to identify pelvic floor muscles and methods for performing daily exercises to control urinary urgency and reduce incontinence.[54] Among overweight and obese women in the PRIDE study, the 6-month behavioral intervention accomplished both weight loss and reduced weekly episodes of urinary incontinence by 70%. The investigators found successful symptom reduction and weight loss very encouraging and proposed expansion of behavioral programs.[54] The impressive results from the PRIDE study at 6 months were maintained at 12 months although the trend did not extend to 18 months when the outcomes of the intervention and control groups began to merge following improvement among the controls who benefited from self-help booklets.[55]

In the past doctors, recognizing the effect of estrogen on pelvic organs, had prescribed oral and/or vaginal hormonal therapy for postmenopausal women with urinary incontinence. However, several studies completed in recent decades indicated oral hormone use increased onset of incontinence; data from the Nurses' Health Study,[56] the Heart and Estrogen/progestin Replacement Study (HERS),[57] and the Women's Health Initiative (WHI) all found hormone exposure had an adverse effect on incontinence.[58] The WHI data also noted hormone use increased stress incontinence among those randomly assigned to either estrogen plus progestin (RR = 1.87, 95% CI = 1.61–2.18) or estrogen alone (RR = 2.15, 95% CI = 1.77–2.62), although the authors suggested these findings may not pertain to other hormonal therapies at other dosages.[58]

Electrical stimulation of the pelvic floor muscles by a probe placed in the vagina has provided inconsistent benefits for reducing incontinence and other nonsurgical efforts have been suggested with limited improvement.[52] Surgery to repair prolapsed organs can be accomplished either vaginally or abdominally; surgical mesh may be needed although its use may increase risk of complications including infection. Urinary incontinence is a very troubling and socially embarrassing condition experienced by many postmenopausal women; new pharmaceutical agents are being developed to potentially offer some relief.

Vaginal Symptoms

Reduced hormone levels cause dryness and itching of vaginal tissue, a distressing problem for some women that is rarely discussed with physicians even though 30% of women are either occasionally or permanently affected. In contrast to vasomotor symptoms that generally diminish over time, changes affecting the vagina and surrounding connective tissue are more permanent as changing blood flow reduces elasticity and secretions are diminished in response to declining estrogen levels.[59] As tissues become thinner and more fragile, the vaginal canal shortens, causing pain and bleeding during intercourse (dyspareunia) often noted by older women. After menopause, vaginal fluid is less acidic facilitating growth of bacteria and increasing risk of infections.[59] Grady noted vaginal estrogens in creams or estradiol-releasing rings provide relief for many patients. In addition, nonhormonal lubricants such as Replens, available over the counter, provide comparable relief especially during sexual activity.[59] Some women use nonhormonal lubricants regularly to relieve vaginal dryness.

Sexuality after Menopause

The effect of hormonal changes on vaginal tissue following natural or surgical cessation of menses, affect sexual desire, arousal, and orgasm.[60] Although many older women note greater freedom of sexual expression after menopause when pregnancy is no longer a risk, the physical changes resulting from diminished hormones require some supplemental lubrication to avoid painful intercourse.[61] Media often depict sexual behavior primarily among young members of society, implying that enjoyment of intimacy declines with age. Sexual expression may differ among older adults compared with patterns shared by the same individuals many years earlier; however, sexual intimacy remains a vital aspect of life for most women and men.[61] Sexual responses include a complex of emotional, cultural, and physical aspects that may necessitate differing methods of arousal and stimulation as women age.

Illness may affect desire or impede ease of familiar aspects of sexual expression for some women. Although some medications have controlled clinical problems enabling longer life expectancy, the side effects of drugs prescribed for women and men may interfere with or reduce sexual desires.[61] Chronic pain from arthritis or immobility after a stroke may require special consideration among partners to achieve a comfortable and satisfying sexual experience. Some older women may have lost their lifelong partner resulting in their need to explore sexual expression with new partners. This unfamiliar experience may rekindle fears from younger days of sexually transmitted infections as well as potential inability to adequately respond to sexual advances of a new partner. Older women who have experienced surgical procedures affecting their body image may feel less desirable and have difficulty becoming sexually aroused.

Physiologic changes occurring during the menopausal transition and through older ages may cause soreness during intercourse. These discomforts may be relieved with nonprescription lubricants. When applied by the woman's partner, lubricants may reduce discomfort while stimulating desire and enhancing feelings of healthy aging.[61] Given the high risk of sexual dysfunction among healthy women, Gast et al. conducted a randomized double-blind controlled trial (RCT) funded by a pharmaceutical company to assess the role of low-dose oral estrogen-progesterone therapy combined with estrogen cream. Compared with the control group who received placebo pills and cream, women randomized to combined therapy reported significantly improved comfort during sexual intercourse as well as reduction of other menopausal symptoms.[62]

Quality of Life

Although the physiologic changes associated with menopause have been extensively studied, the social, psychological, and functional well-being have been less fully addressed. Limited research has assessed the development of depression following the onset of menopause although some studies have indicated that women experience a negative quality of life during the menopausal transition associated with hot flashes and other vasomotor discomforts due to diminished hormone levels. In the RCT by Gast et al. hormonal therapy improved several essential quality of life aspects of menopause[62] although their results differed with recent reports from the Women's Health Initiative among an older study population.[63] Hayes et al. indicated that women randomized in the WHI trial to receive estrogen plus progestin experienced no significant adverse effects to their general health, vitality, mental health, depressive symptoms, or sexual desire.[63]

The prospective SWAN study followed women from premenopausal to postmenopausal status; after adjustment for a wide range of variables, menopausal status was independently related to physical functioning limitations but not strongly associated with other health-related quality of life measures.[64] As assessed by the RAND-36 questionnaire, quality of life was primarily associated with vasomotor symptoms, vaginal dryness, urine leakage, and difficulty sleeping. African American women were less likely to report reduced vitality than white women but more frequently reported body pain and reduced social functioning. Interestingly, the SWAN participants who reported current or past hormone therapy (HT) were more likely to report poor functioning then nonusers.[64]

Another investigation of more than 700 women recruited from a primary care setting for a longitudinal study of "stage transitions results in detectable effects" (STRIDE) included 5 years of follow-up to assess the impact of menopausal status separately from the experiences of hot flashes and vaginal symptoms.[65] The RAND-36 questionnaire quantified physical and mental health scales as estimates of health-related quality of life. When compared with premenopausal women and after controlling for vasomotor symptoms, the composite Rand-36 score reflected lower quality of life among women experiencing various stages of the menopausal continuum.[65] This study revealed a greater negative impact of menopause than others in the literature; the diminished quality of life reported by these women did not improve when vasomotor symptoms declined. Responses to menopause are very personal and reflect many interactions including physical, psychological, and social factors that may vary with age and health status.

Hormonal Therapy for Menopausal Symptoms

Over more than 5 decades as millions of peri- and post-menopausal American women experienced declining endogenous hormone production, doctors prescribed HT to relieve vasomotor symptoms and prevent osteoporosis and other chronic conditions. Historians noted that a growing industry was created by gynecologists prescribing estrogen and pharmaceutical companies promoting their products as "antiaging" treatment for women experiencing menopausal symptoms.[66] The drugs were claimed to enhance energy and improve mood, and to provide a "general sense of well-being." In addition, long-term treatment was recommended to avoid the chronic conditions known to be prevalent among older women.[67]

By the end of the 20th century more than 25% of all women age 40 and older had been prescribed HT, among the most frequently used medications by women.[68] Physicians considered HT appropriate for most postmenopausal women while acknowledging these medication carried some risks.[69] Numerous studies had documented 80% to 90% improvement in the frequency and severity of hot flashes associated with use of oral, vaginal, or more recently developed transdermal hormones.[59] Although limited scientific support existed defining benefits and risks of HT, pharmaceutical companies advertised frequently in medical journals and lay magazines to convince doctors and their patients that estrogen therapy would improve their quality of life. Epidemiological reports from observational studies noted reduced risk of bone fractures and coronary heart disease among patients prescribed HT. Thinner women reported greater menopausal discomfort and more frequent need for hormone supplements than heavier women whose enhanced conversion of androstenedione to estrogen in adipose tissue moderated their symptoms and lowered their risk of bone fractures.[70]

Routine prescribing of estrogen was initially halted when case-control and cohort studies identified "unopposed" estrogen as a major contributing risk factor associated with the rapid rise of endometrial cancer that was first reported in California.[71] A meta-analysis revealed a twofold greater risk of malignancy among estrogen users (RR = 2.3, 95% CI = 2.13–2.51) compared with nonusers and the relative risk rose sharply to RR = 9.5 after 10 years of use.[72] Estrogen exposure, without the moderating presence of progesterone or progestin, was found to stimulate uncontrolled endometrial-cell proliferation, increasing the likelihood of cancer development. To minimize this risk and mimic the normal menstrual cycle, progestin was added to the monthly protocol.[71]

In 1992 Grady et al. conducted a meta-analysis of numerous case-control and cohort studies to critically review the risks and benefits of disease prevention associated with long-term use of unopposed estrogen or estrogen plus progestin among asymptomatic postmenopausal women.[73] The authors concluded that hormone therapy "should probably be recommended for women who have had a hysterectomy and those with coronary heart disease or at risk for coronary heart disease. For other women, the best course of action is unclear."[73] This major publication by CDC researchers changed the primary focus of prescribing of HT to chemoprevention for heart disease, the leading cause of death among women. The known "small" increased risk of breast cancer was considered an acceptable tradeoff. This publication and many others encouraged clinicians to prescribe postmenopausal hormone therapy after consideration of a woman's family history of heart disease and breast cancer.[73]

The recommendations for use of HT were based on observational epidemiologic studies of current and past prescribed medications reported by study participants reflecting clinical decisions by physicians and acceptance by their patients. However, concerns persisted about the lack of randomized trials for appropriate assessment of any benefits and/or risks of HT among women after random assignment to treatment or placebo. Clinicians and researchers feared the available data may have been biased since hormone users were likely to differ from women not taking HT.[74] To address the possibility of biased prescribing, Matthews et al. studied HT use among their randomly recruited cohort of premenopausal women from Pennsylvania.[75] After several years of follow-up as women entered the menopausal transition, significant baseline differences were predictive of subsequent hormone use. Their findings indicated that combined therapy or estrogen alone after hysterectomy was prescribed to women with healthier biologic and psychological characteristics including better cardiovascular profiles, higher education level, more physical activity and were in the normal range for fasting insulin level, weight and blood pressure.[75] Sturgeon et al. reported another aspect of biased reporting of hormone use prevalent in case-control studies. Decreased mortality was noted among current HT users compared with never users but a higher mortality rate was found among women who had recently stopped hormone use.[76] These authors hypothesized that hormones did not prolong life but were discontinued when a life threatening condition was diagnosed.[76]

Regardless of cancer risk evident in animal models and lack of reliable studies among humans, hormones were initially prescribed as women experienced menopausal symptoms although physicians frequently advised continued HT use for many years. However, some clinicians questioned their safety. In her 1997 book Dr. Susan Love described potential risks associated with HT, especially increased risk of breast cancer.[74] Her concerns conflicted with the prescribing patterns that had become standard practice; her text generated considerable anger among clinicians and confused women. Pharmaceutical companies responded with "educational" advertising emphasizing the preventive aspects of HT use.[69]

Few RCTs of hormone exposure were conducted in the past as research often excluded women, a pattern that was corrected by Dr. Bernadine Healy, the first female director of the National Institutes of Health (NIH) who was appointed in 1991. During her 2-year tenure, women's health received increased attention resulting in two major accomplishments: inclusion of women was required in all appropriate research applications submitted to NIH and NIH funds

were allocated for the costly randomized trials and observational components of the Women's Health Initiative. The WHI was designed to investigate prevention, causes, and treatment of diseases affecting women including the impact of hormone therapy on the health of older women.

Estrogen replacement or combined estrogen and progestin for women without hysterectomy had been prescribed for peri- and postmenopausal women, including those without symptoms, by physicians believing the medication was protective against heart disease and would improve quality of life for their patients. However, a rapid change in practice occurred in 2002 when results of several RCTs were reported including the WHI, which questioned the benefits and identified risks of HT.[77] The trial of hormone therapy for women with established heart disease, the HERS Study, reported no benefit negating the use of hormone therapy for secondary protection against repeated cardiovascular events.[78]

The HERS trial findings were followed later in 2002 by results from the WHI randomized trial of combined estrogen and progestin therapy, which was terminated when the monitoring committee judged the risks exceeded any benefits.[79] The committee stated that combined therapy was not a viable primary prevention modality for healthy postmenopausal women between ages 50 and 79 with an intact uterus. The intervention was associated with increased risks of heart disease, stroke, breast cancer, and thromboembolic disease which outweighed benefits of fewer fractures and less colon cancer. These risks did not differ by age or racial/ethnic group according to the authors who indicated their results were applicable to the wider population of American women of similar ages.[79]

A national study of pharmaceutical sales between 1995 and July 2003 noted a sharp increase in HT use from 58 million prescriptions annually in 1995 to a peak in 1999 of 90 million, which remained the annual average until the rapid drop in 2003 following publication of the WHI results.[77] Before 2003 an estimated 42% of American women aged 50 to 74 were using HT; use declined by 44% as noted in Figure 11-5, which presents national data from a variety of ambulatory departments.[80] The rapid decline in HT prescribing responded to the extensive media coverage of the WHI results, patient pressure, and potential medical legal concerns.[81] Some women reported stopping hormone use without reviewing their health status with their physician.[68]

Incentives to discontinue hormone use increased as results of the unopposed estrogen RCT were published in 2004 after that trial was also terminated due to a 40% increased risk of stroke. Although breast cancer was slightly diminished, no beneficial effect on cardiovascular disease or overall mortality had occurred among women receiving unopposed estrogen compared with controls.[82] The lack of protective effect of estrogen against development of heart disease differed from observational studies but was consistent with the secondary prevention study HERS noted previously. Blood pressure elevation was detected among women receiving unopposed estrogen and may have been associated with the increased risk of stroke.[82] Based on the results of the two RCTs, the inves-

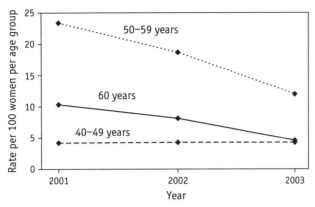

Figure 11-5 Rate of prescribed combined hormone therapy for women age 40 and older, United States, 2001–2003.

Reproduced from QuickStats: annual rate of visits to office-based physicians and hospital outpatient departments during which combined estrogen-progestin hormone therapy was prescribed for women aged >40 years, by age group. *Morbidity Mortality Weekly Report* 2006;55:1047. Data from Hing E, Brett K. Changes in U.S. prescribing patterns of menopausal hormone replacement therapy, 2001–2003. *Obstet Gynecol* 2006;108:33–40.

tigators stated that women and their providers now had useful risk estimates for personalized decision making.[82]

Table 11-2 notes the reported hazard ratios of estrogen plus progestin and unopposed estrogen reported from the two randomized trials of the WHI which was designed to assess long term health benefits.[79,82] However, some clinicians have suggested that publications have overestimated risks of either combined therapy or estrogen alone and have advised patients to consider use of non-oral

methods of hormone administration including vaginal rings, vaginal gel, intranasal estrogen delivery, and transdermal patch urging long-term studies to assess their efficacy.[83]

Prentice et al. assessed the WHI trial results in relation to age at onset of menopause and timing of initiation of hormone administration; these authors included comparisons with data from the observational component of the WHI.[84] The randomized WHI trials included some older women who used HT during their menopausal transition but discontinued use years before enrolling in the WHI. Other women of similar ages had never used HT. Another potential complicating factor suggested by Prentice et al. was the statistical procedures applied to data from observational studies may have biased the reported findings.[84] Willett et al. noted three primary differences when WHI trial results were compared with cohort studies such as the Nurses' Health Study: 1) observational studies enroll a cross-section of women, some of whom had been using hormones for years; 2) observational studies include women receiving standard treatment, which would have included hormone use close to the onset of the menopausal transition; and 3) elevation of coronary heart disease diagnosis in the WHI occurred soon after entry to the trial when potential subclinical disease among susceptible older participants may have been triggered by either estrogen or the combined hormone intervention. These authors noted that the randomized trial and observational data were quite similar when data were stratified by year of starting HT.[85]

Table 11-2

Risks of disease among women randomized to hormones compared with placebo: Results from the Women's Health Initiative Randomized Controlled Trials

Outcome	Estrogen plus Progestin[1]	Unopposed Estrogen[2]
	Hazard Ratio [95% CI]	Hazard Ratio [95% CI]
Coronary heart disease	1.29 [1.02–1.63]	0.91 [0.75–1.12]
Fatal MI	1.18 [0.70–1.97]	0.94 [0.65–1.36]
Nonfatal MI	1.32 [1.02–1.72]	0.89 [0.70–1.12]
Stroke	1.41 [1.07–1.85]	1.39 [1.10–1.77]
Fatal	1.20 [0.58–2.50]	1.13 [0.54–2.34]
Nonfatal	1.50 [1.08–2.08]	1.39 [1.05–1.84]
Pulmonary embolism	2.13 [1.39–3.25]	1.34 [0.87–2.06]
Deep vein thrombosis	2.07 [1.49–2.87]	1.47 [1.04–2.08]
Invasive breast cancer	1.26 [1.00–1.59]	0.77 [0.59–1.01]
Endometrial cancer	0.83 [0.47–1.47]	Post hysterectomy
Colorectal cancer	0.63 [0.43–0.92]	1.08 [0.75–1.55]
Hip fracture	0.66 [0.45–0.98]	0.61 [0.41–0.91]
Death due to other causes	0.92 [0.74–1.14]	1.08 [0.88–1.14]

CI = 95% Confidence Interval   MI = myocardial infarction CIs including 1.00 are not statistically significant

Sources:
1. Writing Group for the Women's Health Initiative Investigators. Risks and benefits of estrogen plus progesterone in healthy postmenopausal women: principal results from the Women's Health Initiative randomized controlled trial. *JAMA* 2002; 288:321–333.

2. Anderson GL, Limacher M, Assaf AR, et al. Effects of conjugated equine estrogen in postmenopausal women with hysterectomy: the Women's Health Initiative randomized controlled trial. *JAMA* 2004;291:1701–1712.

A telephone survey conducted between July and September 2003 among randomly contacted women aged 50 or older from a primary care practice assessed the prevalence of HT use, trust in medical recommendations, and future preventive behaviors.[86] Most responders discontinued use of HT within a year of the initial WHI publication. Among women who continued therapy, only estrogen or lower dosages of combined therapy were being used. Interestingly, after learning of the WHI results 26% of responders said they had lost trust in medical recommendations and 34% were less likely to take a new medication for heart disease prevention.[86] These authors, all clinicians, encouraged colleagues to provide patients with balanced presentations about risks and benefits of therapy and existing uncertainty when research had not provided definitive answers.[86]

Another survey conducted by the Slone Epidemiology Center of Boston University between 1998 and 2004 used random-digit dialing to obtain a nationally representative sample from 48 states to assess current medication use including menopausal hormones.[87] These investigators noted a decline in hormone use from 28% in 2002 before WHI results were released to 12% in 2004 for estrogen with or without progestin. Results were comparable among all study subjects regardless of race/ethnicity, age, education level, or region of the United States.[87] Among more than 24,000 women aged 50 to 79 enrolled in a health maintenance organization, a significant drop in prescriptions for HT followed the initial WHI trial results although many women had difficulty discontinuing use.[88] Records indicated that 24% resumed some hormone use of formulations other than Prempro used in the WHI studies. They were more likely to use products with less available information regarding effectiveness or long-term health consequences.[88]

A follow-up analysis of the RCT data of the WHI was conducted to assess potential differing effects of hormone exposure by age and years since menopause among women randomized to estrogen alone or combined therapy.[89] Although not statistically significant, differences in heart disease risk were evident; highest risk was associated with hormone exposure 20 or more years after menopause but risk was reduced among women on HT within 10 years of menopause.[89] The WHI writing team suggested exogenous estrogen may function differently depending upon the years since last menses; therefore, a critical window of benefit may exist.[79] When HT is used soon after menopause, lower blood lipid levels may limit development of early stages of atherosclerosis; however, among women who experienced menopause decades earlier, hormone use may trigger unanticipated acute coronary events through inflammatory mechanisms on preexisting, undetectable disease.[89] Rossouw speculated that estrogen use might trigger erosion or rupture of unstable plaque in arteries of older women in contrast to HT among younger menopausal women who might benefit from slower development of atherosclerosis, emphasizing the importance of timing and duration of hormonal therapy associated with menopause.[90]

An ancillary substudy of the WHI trial included measures of calcified-plague in coronary arteries assessed by computed tomography (CT) among more than 1000 women aged 50 to 59 with a history of hysterectomy who were randomized to unopposed estrogen or placebo; the estrogen treated group had 50% less coronary artery calcification than participants on placebo. Greater calcification is believed to increase risk of heart disease.[91] The authors found the results reassuring as estrogen use by younger menopausal women in their study was associated with fewer subsequent cardiac events although they encouraged additional research to confirm their findings.[91]

A group of historians, epidemiologists, clinicians, and women's health advocates met in 2004 to discuss the WHI research findings. Among the many important issues discussed were the initial study design given the older ages of many participants who ranged from 50 to 79 (mean age was 63.3 years), which limited assessment of health effects of hormone use during the menopausal transition.[81] The use of only one formulation and dose of estrogen and progestin limited WHI results that may not apply to other hormonal preparations, differing dosages, and methods of administration. Manipulation of women's health by the pharmaceutical industry was feared by advocates who noted research was targeted to detecting adverse outcomes required by the Food and Drug Administration rather than documenting health benefits. Industry, assisted by clinicians, has expanded the population requiring routine medication by developing "preventive agents" encouraging the belief that "treatment" would improve women's quality of life.[81]

The North American Menopause Society now advises women to limit the duration and dose of hormones used for symptom relief.[70] In her review of the WHI trials Warren noted that the results pertained primarily to older women and not necessarily applicable to those entering the menopausal transition. She expected the rapid discontinuation of HT to adversely affect women's quality of life during the years of strongest symptoms. In addition, she suggested transdermal hormonal patches provide absorption through the skin, avoiding the liver and providing greater benefit with fewer side effects. Lower doses of combined therapy were less likely to produce breast tenderness and also reduced irregular bleeding which frequently caused women to abandon combined hormonal therapy.[70] Grady reviewed the WHI results from studies of more than 27,000 women in relation to menopausal symptoms and suggested clinical interventions.[59] She noted that the WHI was focused not on symptom relief but on assessing long term health benefits. She addressed available remedies for menopausal symptoms including preparations that might provide symptom relief at lower hormonal doses or by differing routes of administration with potentially fewer adverse outcomes than the drugs used in the WHI. However, no studies have yet provided any scientific evidence of benefit from these suggested alternative interventions.[59]

Nonhormonal Therapy for Menopausal Symptoms

Following the publications of several studies indicating HT was associated with some adverse health effects and limited benefits, many women abruptly discontinued therapy, which triggered a return of vasomotor discomforts and a search for alternative remedies. Hot flashes again became one of the main reasons menopausal women were seeking help either from healthcare providers, dietary supplements, or over-the-counter remedies.[11] Although some advertised treatment options claimed to reduce hot flashes, the North American Menopause Society and clinicians have recommended lifestyle changes such as keeping the core body temperature cool by wearing loose clothing, sipping cold drinks, avoiding spicy food, and keeping room temperature low.[92]

In a review of several nonhormonal patient directed treatment options to reduce vasomotor symptoms that work for some women but not all, Grady noted that randomized trials are essential for evaluating improvement from diverse person-controlled modalities that may lower the frequency of hot flashes from exercise to acupuncture or slow-paced deep breathing. Modalities studied include acupuncture, yoga, Chinese herbs, dietary soy and phytoestrogen preparations. Although many women think of these treatments as "natural" and safe, some have adverse outcomes; therefore, Grady advised women to review treatment consideration with appropriate clinicians before use.[59]

Alternative options for symptom relief have been limited but the results of a multicenter randomized controlled trial conducted by Freeman et al. were welcomed, providing another potential treatment. The trial compared the effect of escitalopram, a selective serotonin reuptake inhibitor, and placebo in reducing the frequency and severity of menopausal hot flashes.[93] Escitalopram doses of 10 or 20 mg per day significantly reduced the frequency of hot flashes by 50% from baseline compared with 36% reduction among women randomized to placebo during the 8-week study. Placebo effects are common in clinical trials of treatment for hot flashes, Freeman et al. indicated. The clinical recommendation for escitalopram is for generalized anxiety and major depression; for women not reporting these psychological symptoms, escitalopram reduced hot flashes and study participants expressed satisfaction with the therapy.[93]

A symposium convened in 2011 by the North American Menopause Society reviewed the extensive literature assessing the therapeutic role of soy, soy isoflavones, and their metabolites on menopausal symptoms, cancer risk, bone loss, and cognition. Some of their findings included an analysis of soy use and action among pre- and post-menopausal women who consumed either dietary soy and soy isoflavones or isoflavones dietary supplements.[94] Although isoflavone content of soy foods are often listed on food labels, the researchers noted that levels varied considerably due to differences in growing and processing conditions. Diversity of available soy products has increased greater consumption by Americans who have noted health benefits associated with foods containing isoflavones. More than 30% of Americans now eat soy foods or beverages at least once a month. The symposium recommendations included the use of 50 mg isoflavones per day for relief of vasomotor symptoms since isoflavones were shown to have both estrogenic and antiestrogenic properties.

However, additional studies were recommended to assess benefits and any side effects since many published studies were small and had major limitations.[94] Some clinical trials indicated that the consumption of soy products in relation to onset of menopausal symptoms influenced efficacy similar to the "critical window" of benefit associated with HT use. Women's use of complementary and alternative medicine for menopausal symptoms vary by race/ethnicity but is common among a large percentage of American women.

Summary

The hormonal milieu of women across the life span undergoes a gradual transition as reproductive years end with the onset of the menopausal transition. Clinical care becomes refocused on vasomotor symptoms caused by diminishing hormone levels and on chronic conditions that become more prevalent during postmenopausal years. The misconception expressed by many clinicians over past decades that menopause had become an "estrogen-deficient disease" was corrected by reports early in the 21st century from clinical trials that indicated long-term hormonal treatment carried more risks than benefits. A review of past use of hormone therapy and new guidelines following the continuing reports from the Women's Health Initiate provide an understanding of the changing concepts regarding health during and following the menopausal transition. Public health achievements have provided greater longevity enabling women to live many years after menopause; therefore, the quality of life and productive energy of postmenopausal women are of major importance as future health care programs are established.

Discussion Questions

1. What are the leading biochemical and personal indicators of the transition from reproductive ages to menopause?
2. Historically women were prescribed hormonal therapy as endogenous ovarian hormone levels declined. Discuss the history of the past and current prescribing patterns.
3. What physiologic changes are associated with urinary tract infections and urinary incontinence? Name risk factors and studies addressing these issues.
4. The Women's Health Initiative is the largest series of studies ever conducted among women. Describe the goals, methodology, study designs, populations included, and their findings. What were the merits of the many components of the project and what are the major controversies?

References

1. Steiner AZ, Baird DD, Kesner JS. Mother's menopausal age is associated with daughter's early follicular phase urinary, follicle stimulating hormone level. *Menopause.* 2008; 15:940–944.
2. Treloar AE, Boynton RE, Behn BG, Brown BW. Variation of the human menstrual cycle through reproductive life. *Int J Fertil.* 1967;12:77–126.

3. Treloar AE. Menstrual cyclicity and the pre-menopause. *Maturitas.* 1981;3:249–264.

4. Burger HG, Hale GE, Dennerstein L, Robertson DM. Cycle and hormone changes during perimenopause: the key role of ovarian function. *Menopause.* 2008;15:603–612.

5. Richardson SJ, Senikas V, Nelson JF. Follicular depletion during the menopausal transition: evidence for accelerated loss and ultimate exhaustion. *J Clin Endocrinol Metab.* 1987;65:1231–1237.

6. Greendale GA, Lee NP, Arriola ER. The menopause. *Lancet.* 1999;353:571–580.

7. Visser JA, de Jong FH, Laven JS, Themmen AP. Anti-mullerian hormone: a new marker for ovarian function. *Reproduction.* 2006;131:1–9.

8. Senie RT, Lobenthal SW, Rosen PP. Association of vaginal smear cytology with menstrual status in breast cancer. *Breast Cancer Res Treat.* 1985;5:301–310.

9. Longcope C, Franz C, Morello C, et al. Steroid and gonadotropin levels in women during the peri-menopausal years. *Maturitas.* 1986;8:189–196.

10. Wise PM, Krajnak KM, Kashon ML. Menopause: the aging of multiple pacemakers. *Science.* 1996;273:66–70.

11. Kronenberg F. Menopausal hot flashes: a review of the physiology and biosociocultural perspective on methods of assessment. *J Nutr.* 2010;140:1380S–1385S.

12. Freedman RR. Physiology of hot flashes. *Am J Hum Biol.* 2001;13:453–464.

13. Kaunitz AM. Hormonal contraception in women of older reproductive age. *N Engl J Med.* 2008;358:1262–1270.

14. Brett KM, Cooper GS. Associations with menopause and menopausal transition in a nationally representative US sample. *Maturitas.* 2003;45:89–97.

15. Kato I, Toniolo P, Akhmedkhanov A, et al. Prospective study of factors influencing the onset of natural menopause. *J Clin Epidemiol.* 1998;51:1271–1276.

16. Freeman EW, Sammel MD, Garcia CR. Obesity and reproductive hormone levels in the transition to menopause. *Menopause.* 2010;17:718–726.

17. Henderson KD, Bernstein L, Henderson B, et al. Predictors of the timing of natural menopause in the Multiethnic Cohort Study. *Am J Epidemiol.* 2008;167:1287–1294.

18. Cramer DW, Xu H, Harlow BL. Family history as a predictor of early menopause. *Fertil Steril.* 1995;64:740–745.

19. Lambalk CB, van Disseldorp J, de Koning CH, Broekmans FJ. Testing ovarian reserve to predict age at menopause. *Maturitas.* 2009;63:280–291.

20. Krauss CM, Turksoy N, Atkins L, et al. Familial premature ovarian failure due to an interstitial deletion of the long arm of the X chromosome. *N Engl J Med.* 1987;317:125–131.

21. Nichols HB, Trentham-Dietz A, Hampton JM. From menarche to menopause: trends among US women born from 1912 to 1969. *Am J Epidemiol.* 2006;164:1003–1011.

22. Palmer JR, Rosenberg L, Wise LA, et al. Onset of natural menopause in African American women. *Am J Public Health.* 2003;93:299–306.

23. Kinney A, Kline J, Levin B. Alcohol, caffeine and smoking in relation to age at menopause. *Maturitas.* 2006;54:27–38.

24. Augood C, Duckitt K, Templeton AA. Smoking and female infertility: a systematic review and meta-analysis. *Hum Reprod.* 1998;13:1532–1539.

25. Gold EB, Bromberger J, Crawford S, et al. Factors associated with age at natural menopause in a multiethnic sample of midlife women. *Am J Epidemiol.* 2001;153:865–874.

26. Snieder H, MacGregor AJ, Spector TD. Genes control the cessation of a woman's reproductive life: a twin study of hysterectomy and age at menopause. *J Clin Endocrinol Metab.* 1998;83:1875–1880.

27. Hoover RN, Hyer M, Pfeiffer RM, et al. Adverse health outcomes in women exposed in utero to diethylstilbestrol. *N Engl J Med.* 2011;365:1304–1314.

28. Steiner AZ, D'Aloisio AA, DeRoo LA, et al. Association of intrauterine and early-life exposures with age at menopause in the Sister Study. *Am J Epidemiol.* 2010;172:140–148.

29. Whelan EA, Sandler DP, McConnaughey DR, Weinberg CR. Menstrual and reproductive characteristics and age at natural menopause. *Am J Epidemiol.* 1990;131:625–632.

30. Cramer DW, Xu H, Harlow BL. Does "incessant" ovulation increase risk for early menopause? *Am J Obstet Gynecol.* 1995;172:568–573.

31. Pines A, Shapira I, Mijatovic V, et al. The impact of hormonal therapy for infertility on the age at menopause. *Maturitas.* 2002;41:283–287.

32. Hahn RA, Eaker E, Rolka H. Reliability of reported age at menopause. *Am J Epidemiol.* 1997;146:771–775.

33. Wingo PA, Ory HW, Layde PM, Lee NC. The evaluation of the data collection process for a multicenter, population-based, case-control design. *Am J Epidemiol.* 1988;128:206–217.

34. Keshavarz H, Hillis SD, Kieke BA, Marchbanks PA. Hysterectomy surveillance—United States, 1994-1999. *MMWR Morb Mortal Wkly Rep.* 2002;51(SS05):1–8.

35. Whiteman MK, Hillis SD, Jamieson DJ, et al. Inpatient hysterectomy surveillance in the United States, 2000-2004. *Am J Obstet Gynecol.* 2008;198:34.e1–34.e7.

36. Jacoby VL, Fujimoto VY, Giudice LC, et al. Racial and ethnic disparities in benign gynecologic conditions and associated surgeries. *Am J Obstet Gynecol.* 2010;202:514–521.

37. Farquhar CM, Sadler L, Harvey SA, Stewart AW. The association of hysterectomy and menopause: a prospective cohort study. *Br J Obstet Gynecol.* 2005;112:956–962.

38. Moorman PG, Schildkraut JM, Iversen ES, et al. A prospective study of weight gain after premenopausal hysterectomy. *J Women Health.* 2009;18:699–708.

39. Parker WH, Jacoby V, Shoupe D, Rocca W. Effect of bilateral oophorectomy on women's long-term health. *Women's Health.* 2009;5:565–576.

40. Parker WH, Broder MS, Chang E, et al. Ovarian conservation at the time of hysterectomy and long-term health outcomes in the Nurses' Health Study. *Obstet Gynecol.* 2009;113:1027–1037.

41. Shuster LT, Gostout BS, Grossardt BR, Rocca WA. Prophylactic oophorectomy in premenopausal women and long term health—a review. *Menopause Int.* 2008;14:111–116.

42. Matthews KA, Meilahn E, Kuller LH, et al. Menopause and risk for coronary heart disease. *N Engl J Med.* 1989;321:641–646.

43. Colditz GA, Willett WC, Stampfer MJ, et al. Menopause and the risk of coronary heart disease in women. *N Engl J Med.* 1987;316:1105–1110.

44. Snowdon DA, Kane RL, Beeson L, et al. Is early menopause a biologic marker of health and aging? *Am J Public Health.* 1989;79:709–714.

45. Atsma F, Bartelink ML, Grobbee DE, van der Schouw YT. Postmenopausal status and early menopause as independent risk factors for cardiovascular disease: a meta-analysis. *Menopause.* 2006;13:265–279.

46. Rocca WA, Grossardt BR, de Andrade M, et al. Survival patterns after oophorectomy in premenopausal women: a population-based cohort study. *Lancet Oncol.* 2006;7:821–828.

47. Hu KK, Boyko EJ, Scholes D, et al. Risk factors for urinary tract infections in postmenopausal women. *Arch Intern Med.* 2004;164:989–993.

48. Raz R, Gennesin Y, Wasser J, et al. Recurrent urinary tract infections in postmenopausal women. *Clin Inf Dis.* 2000;30:152–156.

49. Raz R, Stamm WE. A controlled trial of intravaginal estradiol in postmenopausal women with recurrent urinary tract infections. *N Engl J Med.* 1993;329:753–756.

50. Minassian VA, Stewart WF, Wood GC. Urinary incontinence in women. *Obstet Gynecol.* 2008;111:324–331.

51. Nygaard I, Barber MD, Burgio KL, et al. Prevalence of symptomatic pelvic floor disorders in US women. *JAMA.* 2008;300:1311–1316.

52. Nygaard I. Idiopathic urgency urinary incontinence. *N Engl J Med.* 2010;363:1156–1162.

53. Kegel AH. Physiologic therapy for urinary stress incontinence. *JAMA.* 1951;146:915–917.

54. Subak LL, Wing R, West DS, et al. Weight loss to treat urinary incontinence in overweight and obese women. *N Engl J Med.* 2009;360:481–490.

55. Wing RR, Creasman JM, West DS, et al. Improving urinary incontinence in overweight and obese women through modest weight loss. *Obstet Gynecol.* 2010;116:284–292.

56. Grodstein F, Lifford K, Resnick NM, Curhan GC. Postmenopausal hormone therapy and risk of developing urinary incontinence. *Obstet Gynecol.* 2004;103:254–260.

57. Grady D, Brown JS, Vittinghoff E, et al. Postmenopausal hormones and incontinence: The Heart and Estrogen/Progestin Replacement Study. *Obstet Gynecol.* 2001;97:116–120.

58. Hendrix SL, Cochrane BB, Nygaard IE, et al. Effects of estrogen with and without progestin on urinary incontinence. *JAMA.* 2005;293:935–948.

59. Grady D. Management of menopausal symptoms. *N Engl J Med.* 2006;355:2338–2347.

60. Holzapfel S. Aging and sexuality. *Can Fam Physician.* 1994;40:748–766.

61. Carpenter LM, Nathanson CA, Kim YJ. Physical women, emotional men: Gender and sexual satisfaction in midlife. *Arch Sex Behav.* 2009;38:87–107.

62. Gast MJ, Freedman MA, Vieweg AJ, et al. A randomized study of low-dose conjugated estrogens on sexual function and quality of life in postmenopausal women. *Menopause.* 2009;16:1–10.

63. Hays J, Ockene JK, Brunner RL, et al. Effects of estrogen plus progestin on health-related quality of life. *N Engl J Med.* 2003;348:1839–1854.

64. Avis NE, Colvin A, Bromberger JT et al Change in health-related quality of life over the menopausal transition in a multiethnic cohort of middle-aged women: Study of Women's Health Across the Nation. *Menopause.* 2009;16:860–869.

65. Hess R, Thurston RC, Hays RD, et al. The impact of menopause on health-related quality of life: results from the STRIDE longitudinal study. *Qual Life Res.* 2011 Jul 14 (Epub ahead of print)

66. Seaman B. *The Greatest Experiment Ever Performed on Women.* New York: Hyperion; 2003.

67. Rothman SM, Rothman DJ. *The Pursuit of Perfection.* New York: Pantheon Books; 2003.

68. Hing E, Brett K. Changes in U.S. prescribing patterns of menopausal hormone therapy, 2001-2003. *Obstet Gynecol.* 2006;108:33–40.

69. Angier N. *Woman, An Intimate Geography.* New York: Houghton Mifflin Company; 1999.

70. Warren MP. Historical perspective in postmenopausal hormone therapy: defining the right dose and duration. *Mayo Clin Proc.* 2007;82:219–226.

71. Key TJ, Pike MC. The dose-effect relationship between "unopposed" oestrogens and endometrial mitotic rate: its central role in explaining and predicting endometrial cancer risk. *Br J Cancer.* 1988;57:205–212.

72. Grady D, Gebretsadik T, Kerlikowske K, et al. Hormone replacement therapy and endometrial cancer risk: a meta-analysis. *Obstet Gynecol.* 1995;85:304–313.

73. Grady D, Rubin SM, Petitti DB, et al. Hormone therapy to prevent disease and prolong life in postmenopausal women. *Ann Int Med.* 1992;117:1016

74. Love SM. *Dr. Susan Love's Hormone Book.* New York: Random House; 1997.

75. Matthews KA, Kuller LH, Wing RR, et al. Prior to use of estrogen replacement therapy, are users healthier than nonusers. *Am J Epidemiol.* 1996;143:971–978.

76. Sturgeon SR, Schairer C, Brinton LA, et al. Evidence of a healthy estrogen user survivor effect. *Epidemiology.* 1995;6:227–231.

77. Hersh AL, Stefanick ML, Stafford RS. National use of postmenopausal hormone therapy: annual trends and response to recent evidence. *JAMA.* 2004;291:47–53.

78. Grady D, Herrington D, Bittner V, et al. Cardiovascular disease outcomes during 6.8 years of hormone therapy: Heart and Estrogen/progestin Replacement Study follow-up (HERS II). *JAMA.* 2002;288:49–57.

79. Writing Group for the Women's Health Initiative Investigators. Risks and benefits of estrogen plus progesterone in healthy postmenopausal women: principal results from the Women's Health Initiative randomized controlled trial. *JAMA.* 2002; 288:321–333.

80. QuickStats: Annual rate of visits to office-based physician and hospital outpatient departments during which combination estrogen-progestin hormone therapy was prescribed for women aged > 40 years, by age group—United States, 2001–2003. *MMWR Morb Mortal Wkly Rep.* 2006;55:1047.

81. Krieger N, Lowy I, Aronowitz R, et al. Hormone replacement therapy, cancer, controversies, and women's health: historical, epidemiological, biological, clinical, and advocacy perspectives. *J Epidemiol Community Health.* 2005;59:740–748.

82. Anderson GL, Limacher M, Assaf AR, et al. Effects of conjugated equine estrogen in postmenopausal women with hysterectomy: the Women's Health Initiative randomized controlled trial. *JAMA.* 2004;291:1701–1712.

83. Sitruk-Ware R. New hormonal therapies and regimens in the postmenopause: routes of administration and timing of initiation. *Climacteric.* 2007;10:358–370.

84. Prentice RL, Manson JE, Langer RD, et al. Benefits and risks of postmenopausal hormone therapy when it is initiated soon after menopause. *Am J Epidemiol.* 2009;170:12–23.

85. Willett WC, Manson JE, Grodstein F, et al. Re: "Combined postmenopausal hormone therapy and cardiovascular disease: Toward resolving the discrepancy between observational studies and the Women's Health Initiative Clinical Trial." *Am J Epidemiol.* 2006;163:1067–1068.

86. Schonberg MA, Davis RB, Wee CC. After the Women's Health Initiative: decision making and trust of women taking hormone therapy. *Women's Health Issues.* 2005;15:187–195.

87. Kelly JP, Kaufman DW, Rosenberg L, et al. Use of postmenopausal hormone therapy since the Women's Health Initiative findings. *Pharmacoepidemiol Drug Saf.* 2005;14:837–842.

88. Wegienka G, Havstad S, Kelsey JL. Menopausal hormone therapy in a health maintenance organization before and after Women's Health Initiative hormone trials termination. *J Womens Health.* 2006;15:369–378.

89. Rossouw JE, Prentice RL, Manson JE, et al. Postmenopausal hormone therapy and risk of cardiovascular disease by age and years since menopause. *JAMA.* 2007;297:1465–1477.

90. Rossouw JE. Implications of recent clinical trials of postmenopausal hormone therapy for management of cardiovascular disease. *Ann NY Acad Sci.* 2006;1089: 444–453.

91. Manson JE, AllisonMA, Rossouw JE, et al. Estrogen therapy and coronary-artery calcification. *N Engl J Med.* 2007;356:2591–2602.

92. Love SM. *Dr. Susan Love's Menopause and Hormone Book, Making Informed Choices.* New York: Three Rivers Press; 2003.

93. Freeman EW, Guthrie KA, Caan B, et al. Efficacy of escitalopram for hot flashes in healthy menopausal women: a randomized controlled trial. *JAMA.* 2011;305:267–274.

94. North American Menopause Society. The role of soy isoflavones in menopausal health: report of the North American Menopause Society/Wulf H. Utian Translational Science symposium in Chicago, IL (October 2010). *Menopause.* 2011;18:732–753.

Sexually Transmitted Infections

Sexually Transmitted Infections

Stephen S. Morse, PhD

Introduction

We have all experienced infectious diseases at numerous times in our lives. Even in industrialized countries like the United States, where improved nutrition, sanitation, immunization, and antimicrobial therapy have reduced the deadly impact of infectious disease experienced in much of the world, these diseases remain a presence in all our lives causing much suffering. Women are subject to essentially all of the several hundred known infectious diseases. However, several diseases have particular significance for women, such as sexually transmitted diseases or diseases that may adversely affect pregnant women or the developing fetus. This chapter briefly surveys salient aspects of some of these infections. For further details of infections not covered in this chapter, texts and other references for further reading are provided.

A major exception to some of the generalizations presented in this chapter about infectious diseases is human immunodeficiency virus (HIV) infection. In recent years, HIV has become the foremost concern among sexually transmitted infections. HIV is not addressed in this chapter, which focuses on other infections of particular concern to women.

Sexually Transmitted Infections

A relatively large number of infections can be transmitted by sexual contact, but only some are traditionally considered "sexually transmitted diseases" (STDs) or "sexually transmitted infections" (STIs) (Table 12-1). The federal Centers for Disease Control and Prevention (CDC) lists the following diseases: bacterial vaginosis, chlamydia and lymphogranuloma venereum (LGV), gonorrhea, genital herpes, human papillomavirus (HPV), pelvic inflammatory disease (PID), syphilis, and trichomoniasis. Infectious conditions presented in this chapter include: gonorrhea, syphilis, herpes simplex type 2 (HSV-2), chlamydia (and lymphogranuloma venereum), and HPV and a brief discussion of PID. The terms, and concepts are convenient conventions, but as with all diseases, absolute statements must be viewed with caution. Many of the infections we usually call "sexually transmitted" are so termed because they are most often transmitted by sexual contact, but they can also be transmitted by other means. Although STI are usually transmitted by sexual intercourse and affect the reproductive tract, particularly in women, a number of these infections can be found in other parts of the body. Anal or oropharyngeal infections are no longer unusual, particularly with gonorrhea, syphilis and HSV, and anal warts caused by HPV have been recognized for many years. Conversely, a number of infections usually transmitted by other routes may also be sexually transmitted. One example is the recent report of sexual transmission of methycillin-resistant *Staphylococcus aureus* (MRSA).[1]

Medical literature regularly uses the terms "sexually transmitted diseases" and "sexually transmitted infections"; for most purposes, we can consider these terms virtually interchangeable. The CDC currently uses "STD." On the other hand, purists will object that STD is not entirely accurate, because the term "disease" implies the presence of symptoms, and many of these infections are often asymptomatic or very mildly symptomatic in many individuals. In addition, some noninfectious diseases can be sexually transmitted, such as "crab lice" (*Phthyris pubis*) or scabies (*Sarcoptes scabei*, a mite infestation of the skin). Others object to the term STD because they feel there is some stigma attached to this traditional term. For convenience, we use the term STI in addressing infections in women.

In addition to those infections traditionally classified as "STD" or "STI," a number of other infections can be transmitted sexually, as well as by other routes. Some would normally be considered "blood-borne" infections, such as hepatitis B or hepatitis C. In the case of hepatitis C, which is blood-borne, there is disagreement about the role of sexual transmission in the epidemiology of this infection.[2-4] Circumstantial evidence suggests that sexual transmission of hepatitis C can, and probably does, occur occasionally, but the risk of transmission by this route, and its relative importance in the epidemiology of this infection, are unclear.

Table 12-1

Common sexually transmitted infections

Infection	Name of Organism Causing Infection	Usual Signs and Symptoms	Estimated Prevalence per Year in U.S.*	Treatment**
Gonorrhea	*Neisseria gonorrheae*	May cause urethritis or pelvic inflammatory disease. Often asymptomatic in women (male sexual partners frequently symptomatic, with urethritis and discharge, and should be examined).	111.6/100,000 population	Antibiotics, e.g., ceftriaxone, (sensitivity testing usually recommended, as many strains are now resistant to many commonly used antibiotics)
Syphilis	*Treponema pallidum*	Primary infection: Skin lesions ("condylomata") at site of infection. If untreated, progresses to secondary stage (variable, usually about 2–8 weeks) with rash, often on palms and soles. Untreated cases can progress to tertiary syphilis later in life, often with central nervous system involvement. Congenital syphilis may involve liver, connective tissue (including heart valve), skeletal, or dental abnormalities.	Approx. 1.5/100,000 women (Congenital syphilis: 10.1/100,000 live births, 2007)	Antibiotics (usually penicillin)
Herpes simplex Type 2 (HSV-2)	Herpes simplex virus type 2 (Herpesvirus hominis 2)	Often asymptomatic in women. When symptomatic, typically small vesicular lesions on genitals or genital area, with inflammatory (red) background; itching or burning sensation common. Virus remains latent after primary infection and may show periodic reactivation (varies with different individuals; may or may not be symptomatic).	16.2% (seroprevalence)†	Acyclovir, famciclovir, or valacyclovir (usually treated only when symptomatic or just before delivery in a pregnant patient)
Chlamydia	*Chlamydia trachomatis*	Often asymptomatic. When symptomatic, typically urethritis, cervicitis (inflammation of cervix with discharge) or pelvic inflammatory disease.	401.3/100,000 population	Antibiotics (usually azithromycin or doxycycline)

| HPV | Human papillomavirus | Most commonly warts, including genital or anogenital warts; some HPV varieties cause cervical cancer. | Estimates vary. Primary care clinics: Estimated 15% | Treatment is symptomatic. For warts, usually removed by physical ablation when troublesome. A vaccine is now available for the virus subtypes (Types 16 and 18) that are most frequently associated with cervical carcinoma. |

*Source: Centers for Disease Control and Prevention. *Sexually Transmitted Disease Surveillance, 2008*. Atlanta, GA: U.S. Department of Health and Human Services; November 2009.

**Provided for general information only. Ref.: Gilbert, DN, Moellering Jr RC, Eliopoulos GM, Saag MS, eds. *The Sanford Guide to Antimicrobial Therapy 2010*. 40th ed. Sperryville, VA: Antimicrobial Therapy Inc.; 2010. For specific therapeutic advice, consult an authoritative clinical reference or health department.

†Seroprevalence (infection is lifelong)

Some Selected Diseases

Gonorrhea

Gonorrhea is probably one of the oldest sexually transmitted infections known. Its cause is the bacterium *Neisseria gonorrheae*. In males' urogenital tracts, gonorrhea is easily recognized, causing a painful urethritis with discharge. The incubation period is typically about 2–5 days. In females, however, the infection is often far less noticeable and may often be asymptomatic. When symptomatic, it usually causes urethritis or pelvic inflammatory disease. Unfortunately, it may escape detection until an episode of chronic pelvic inflammatory disease occurs, and by then the chronic inflammation may cause sterility. For this reason, gonorrhea should be considered when women present with another STI. Congenital gonorrhea was once a common cause of blindness in infants, and until very recently a drop of silver nitrate was instilled in the eyes of all newborns to prevent this complication. Gonorrhea is now less prevalent, but it remains a public health concern, and accounts for many visits to STD clinics. According to CDC, current overall prevalence in the United States is 111.6 per 100,000 population.[5] In 2008 the rate of gonorrhea in women was slightly higher (119.4 per 100,000 women) than the rate in men (103.0 per 100,000 men).[5] The prevalence of gonorrhea is higher in some populations as noted in the section on the epidemiology of sexually transmitted infections. With changing sexual practices, oral and anal infections, which are harder to recognize, have also increased as a proportion of total gonorrhea cases, although somewhat less so in women than in men who have sex with other men. In the past this infection was successfully treated with penicillin, but most strains are now resistant to this drug and many other antibiotics. Consequently, antibiotic sensitivity testing is recommended when feasible, as resistance is constantly evolving and many strains are now resistant to many commonly used antibiotics. The current drug of choice is ceftriaxone.

Syphilis

Another "classic" STI, syphilis was once a greatly feared disease. Syphilis is caused by the bacterium *Treponema pallidum*, a spirochete (so called because of its characteristic spiral, or "corkscrew" shaped, appearance on microscopy). Syphilis had been on the wane for a number of years (probably largely because of public health control measures but possibly also for other reasons that are not well understood), but has recently been increasing in industrialized countries.[6] The organism is fairly delicate and has not been successfully grown in culture. Diagnostic testing relies on traditional methods used for most of the 20th century, including serology to detect antibodies in the infected individual or microscopic detection of the bacterium.

In the 19th century, physicians devoted a great deal of attention to syphilis, which was then untreatable and poorly understood, referring to it as "the great imitator" or "great mimic" of diseases because of its many different manifestations. In most patients, after an incubation period of about 21 days (variable, from 3 to 90 days) the primary infection manifests as skin lesions ("condylomata") at the site of infection. The infection is easily treated if diagnosed at this stage. Many antibiotics are effective, and usually penicillin is the drug of choice. If untreated, the infection progresses to the secondary stage, usually in about 2 to 8 weeks, characterized by rash, often on palms and soles, and fever. The rash is often distinctive and is classically described as "florid." As most patients who receive any treatment are usually treated in the early stages, fortunately few clinicians today see cases of secondary syphilis. Untreated cases can progress to tertiary syphilis later in life, often with central nervous system involvement. In pregnant women with newly acquired or secondary syphilis, congenital syphilis can occur in the newborn. The disease may involve the liver, connective tissue (including heart valves), and skeletal or dental abnormalities.

The prevalence of syphilis, although increasing, is still relatively low. CDC estimates the prevalence as approximately 1.5 per 100,000 women (for congenital syphilis: 10.1 per 100,000 live births in 2007).[5] This rate slowly has been increasing since 2004. Like gonorrhea, and unlike most of the other STIs, contact tracing and examination of sexual partners is generally recommended. Syphilis is associated with HIV and contact tracing should be performed whenever feasible.

Chlamydia

Chlamydia and herpes simplex (HSV) are widely considered the most prevalent STIs (although similar increases in prevalence may be identified for other infections in the future as screening improves and diagnostic methods become more sensitive). Chlamydia was once the province of specialists, but in the last several decades there has been an increasing appreciation of its importance. Much of this increased emphasis on chlamydia is due to increased screening and greatly improved diagnostic tests.[8] Molecular tests, such as testing for chlamydial DNA by the polymerase chain reaction (PCR), have revolutionized the diagnosis and screening of chlamydia and made screening programs feasible but have also greatly increased estimates of the prevalence of this infection.

For specialists in tropical medicine, *Chlamydia trachomatis* is best known as the cause of trachoma, which causes millions of cases of infectious conjunctivitis and blindness in developing countries, due to *C. trachomatis* serovars (serotypes) A-C. Fortunately, this disease is not often seen in the United States or other industrialized counties. However, another group (serovars D-K) of *C. trachomatis* is sexually transmitted and is of great importance as an STI. These chlamydial infections are often asymptomatic. When symptomatic, typical signs and symptoms include urethritis, cervicitis (inflammation of cervix, accompanied by discharge) or pelvic inflammatory disease.[9] Congenital infection, sometimes persisting up to 2 to 3 years, has been identified.[10] Congenital infections may be asymptomatic or can manifest as conjunctivitis or pneumonia. Chlamydia may also cause miscarriage or other long-term sequelae in women, although the evidence is more limited.[11]

Estimates of prevalence vary somewhat, but in general chlamydia is considered one of the most common reportable infections and probably the most prevalent STI in the United States, with current prevalence estimates of 401.3 per 100,000 population.[5] Prevalence in 2001–2002 was 4.2% among young adults (18–26 years of age) in the "Add Health" study (National Longitudinal Study of Adolescent Health).[12] In the large National Health and Nutrition Examination Survey (NHANES), which tested adults 14–39 years old, the overall prevalence of chlamydia infection was 2.2% in 1999–2002, with a prevalence of 2.0% in males and 2.5% in females.[13] Studies in primary care clinics[14] in the early 1990s estimated median prevalence at about 15%. Epidemiologic data suggest that the prevalence of chlamydia has not decreased in recent years and in fact may be increasing, as noted in Figure 12-1; however, it is difficult to separate apparent increased prevalence from more complete ascertainment.

Although it is ubiquitous, chlamydia prevalence varies geographically within the United States, varying from a low of about 275–300 (per 100,000 women) in Maine, West Virginia, and Oregon, to 1,085 in Mississippi and 1,431 in Washington, D.C. (Figure 12-2). Many of the geographic differences are probably a combination of the quality of screening and ascertainment, together with some actual differences in distribution of the infection. CDC estimates that chlamydia rates are higher among women when compared to rates in men.[5] It is likely that chlamydia has long been ubiquitous and that the apparent increases in incidence are largely the result of better screening and testing in recent years.[5] Once diagnosed, chlamydia is treatable. Azithromycin or doxycycline are most widely used.

Other serotypes (serovars L1-3) of *Chlamydia trachomatis* cause lymphogranuloma venereum, which is not generally endemic to the United States but is found throughout parts of Asia, Africa, South America, and the

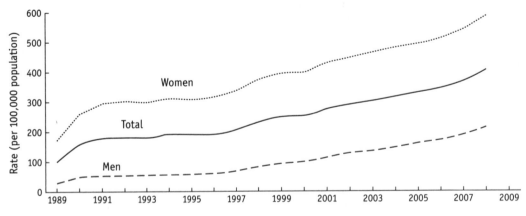

Figure 12-1 Chlamydia—Rates: Total and by gender, United States, 1989–2008.

Reproduced from Centers for Disease Control and Prevention. Sexually Transmitted Disease Surveillance, 2008. Atlanta, GA: U.S. Dept of Health and Human Services, November 2009.

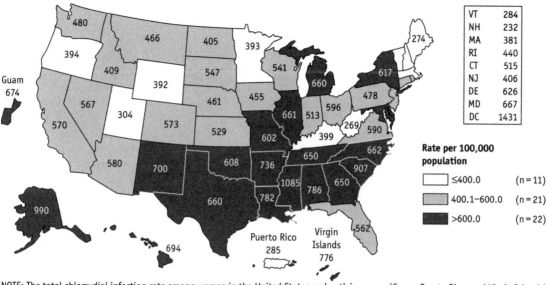

VT	284
NH	232
MA	381
RI	440
CT	515
NJ	406
DE	626
MD	667
DC	1431

Rate per 100,000 population

☐	≤400.0	(n = 11)
▨	400.1–600.0	(n = 21)
■	>600.0	(n = 22)

NOTE: The total chlamydial infection rate among women in the United States and outlying areas (Guam, Puerto Rico, and Virgin Islands) was 580.0 per 100,000 female population.

Figure 12-2 Chlamydia—Rates among women by state: United States and outlying areas, 2008.

Reproduced from Centers for Disease Control and Prevention. Sexually Transmitted Disease Surveillance, 2008. Atlanta, GA: U.S. Dept of Health and Human Services, November 2009.

Caribbean. After the small and often painless primary lesion at the site of infection, the disease progresses after several weeks to a very noticeable lymphadenopathy (usually in the groin), often with systemic symptoms that include fever and headache or meningitis. The disease is striking, largely because of the pronounced lymphadenopathy in the groin, but, as with other *Chlamydia trachomatis* infections, should resolve with appropriate treatment.

Herpes Simplex Type 2 (HSV-2)

Herpesviruses are among the most prevalent of all human viruses, and this large group of DNA viruses (eight human herpesviruses are known) includes varicella-zoster (VZV, the cause of chickenpox and, later in life, shingles), Epstein-Barr virus (EBV), and cytomegalovirus (CMV), which cause infectious mononucleosis, human herpesvirus 8 (the cause of Kaposi's sarcoma), and herpes simplex (HSV). After initial infection, herpesviruses usually remain dormant in the body and may reactivate at later times. Zoster (shingles), for example, is a reactivation later in life of a chickenpox infection that probably originally occurred in childhood. The infection is generally lifelong; therefore, most studies use seroprevalence, the prevalence in the population of antibodies to the virus, as an indication of infection. Adult seroprevalence for most herpesviruses is generally very high, approaching 98% for varicella-zoster virus and generally in a similar range for EBV, CMV, and HSV. Two serotypes of HSV are recognized. Type 1 (HSV-1, taxonomically Herpesvirus hominis 1) is the more common, and causes "cold sores" or "fever blisters," typically on the lips, when the virus reactivates. Prevalence has traditionally been very high, usually estimated to affected between 50 and 90% in healthy adults, with reactivation in about one-third.[15] Herpes simplex virus

type 2 (HSV-2, Herpesvirus hominis 2) is traditionally considered a sexually transmitted infection and is usually acquired sexually. However, it should be recognized that both HSV types can infect mucosal surfaces, the eye, and skin through small cuts or scratches occurring anywhere on the body. Therefore, HSV-1 is sometimes seen in the genital region and HSV-2 has been found above the waist. Both cause similar lesions when symptomatic, although HSV-2 lesions may be smaller. Infection is often asymptomatic, especially in women. When symptomatic, HSV-2 typically shows small vesicular lesions on the genitals or in the genital area, with inflammatory (red) background; an itching or burning sensation is common. The incubation period is typically about 2 to 3 weeks. As mentioned, the virus remains latent after primary infection and may show periodic reactivation. The probability and frequency of reactivation vary with different individuals and may be symptomatic or asymptomatic.[16] Primary infection or reactivations can be treated with acyclovir, famciclovir, or valacyclovir, although the clinical effectiveness of these therapeutic agents for mild reactivations is still unclear. As a result, most patients are usually treated only when symptomatic or just before delivery in a pregnant patient. Congenital HSV can be severe or fatal, with multiorgan involvement, although there is some disagreement about the frequency of maternal to child transmission and risk factors; Corey and colleagues have suggested that the risk is greater when HSV infection has been newly acquired during late pregnancy.[16]

Some studies suggest that regular use of antiviral medication may prevent transmission to sexual partners.[17] Although sexual transmission of HSV-2 is common, evidence suggests that transmission is not inevitable and couples can take precautions to reduce risk. In one study of HSV transmission in couples,[18] 125 HSV-2 seronegative women with HSV-2 seropositive partners were followed during the course of pregnancy; during this period, 17 (20% adjusted for gestation length) acquired HSV-2. The major risk factor identified was duration of partnership of 1 year or less, which accounted for 63% of incident infections.[18] Perhaps even more interesting, use of condoms by an infected male partner could prevent transmission, even in high-risk populations.[19] Therefore, condoms have a protective effect. Although the pores of latex condoms are larger than the size of the virus particle, condoms may reduce transmission by virus attached to tissue fragments and by greater care taken by a partner who regularly uses condoms. Use of condoms and refraining from sexual activity when active lesions are present or when the infected individual is aware of a reactivation are often recommended by clinicians and seem prudent risk reduction measures.

As for most other herpesviruses, prevalence of HSV-2 is high, although less than that of VZV or HSV-1. Based on the NHANES study, CDC has estimated the seroprevalence of HSV-2 in the United States is approximately 16.2% overall.[5] Corey and colleagues have tabulated prevalence in a number of populations, with similar results.[20] In most of these studies, women reportedly had a slightly higher seroprevalence than men (their overall figures were 22% for the general population, with 26% seroprevalence in women and 18% in men),[20] but this could reflect ascertainment bias. As would be expected, the prevalence is consistently higher among men and women attending STD clinics.[20]

In the past, there have been suggestions that prior infection with HSV or another STI may increase susceptibility to HIV infection. Although initial results seemed robust,[21] other studies (such as a thorough study in Rakai, Uganda) seemed to contradict this finding.[22] There is some evidence that treating HSV genital infection does reduce HIV load.[20] Thus, the issue is still unresolved,[23,24] as are the reasons. Does the recruitment of potential target cells, such as macrophages, in inflammatory genital infections make it easier for HIV to establish infection, or is the possible potentiation of HIV by HSV simply the result of common risk factors for several STIs, or is there another explanation? Although the relationship is still unclear, it does make the case that we should also think about STI as a general diagnostic group, recognize that coinfection is common, and therefore institute appropriate simultaneous testing and treatment for the range of STIs and encourage individual "safe sex" practices.[22]

Human Papillomaviruses (HPV)

The human papillomaviruses are small DNA viruses that are geographically ubiquitous. To the best of our knowledge, all grow in skin or surface epithelium. Although the viruses appear to be closely related, with similar overall genome organization and common structural proteins, over 150 HPV types have been described, of which over 90 have been molecularly characterized. Research suggests that some overlap exists among the diverse HPV types but

they also appear to differ in their biologic effects and predilections for specific tissues or anatomic locations.

Estimates of prevalence vary. Similar to Chlamydia and HSV, HPV is probably a very common infection. Prevalence was estimated at 15% in one study in primary care clinics[25] and at 26.8% in another study of U.S. females ages 14–59.[26] CDC reports prevalence (presumably in higher risk groups) of 35% in individuals 14–19 years old, 29% in 20 to 29-year-olds, and 13% in 30 to 39-year-olds.[5] Among women, being young and sexually active is associated with high prevalence rates.[5]

Traditionally, the best known sexually transmitted diseases caused by HPV have been genital warts (also often called condylomata). Anogenital warts, in both women and men, are a disfiguring and troublesome manifestation of HPV infection and have been known for many years. Treatment is symptomatic and usually involves chemical or physical ablation. Choice of treatment varies with site, type of lesion, and the practitioner's preferences, but common methods include cryotherapy (freezing), local treatment with certain acids or other chemicals, or surgery.

Most significantly, a major current issue is the role of HPV in causing cervical dysplasia (tissue abnormalities) and cervical cancer. There has been a long history of attempts to implicate various viruses in cervical carcinoma, and at one time HSV-2 was actively investigated as a possible cause.[27] However, in recent years it has become recognized that HPV is likely the major cause of cervical carcinoma and other neoplasias involving the female reproductive tract.[28–31] Certain HPV types have a greater predilection to cause cervical carcinoma.[29] Types 16 and 18 especially have been most frequently associated with cervical carcinoma and precancerous lesions of the cervix and apparently much less frequently with genital warts. On the other hand, Types 6 and 11 have been the HPV types most frequently identified in genital warts and in low-grade neoplasia. A vaccine is now available for several of the virus subtypes that are most frequently associated with cervical carcinoma (Types 16 and 18) and anogenital warts (Types 6 and 11). Two vaccines[32] are currently approved for use in the United States, a quadrivalent vaccine that includes both the two most prevalent carcinogenic types (Types 16 and 18) as well as Types 6 and 11, associated with anogenital warts; and a bivalent vaccine, containing Types 16 and 18. A recent study suggests that the vaccine appears effective in preventing cervical lesions and that immunity was still effective at 42 months, the end of the study period.[33]

The implications of HPV immunization are profound; research suggests that most cervical carcinoma can be prevented by immunizing a girl before she can acquire genital HPV infection, that is, before initiation of sexual activity. The CDC has recently recommended that HPV immunization be widely adopted.[34] However, as with any vaccine that is recommended for universal administration, various ethical questions have been raised; the sexually transmitted nature of the infection raises additional issues for some people.[35–37] Should all girls receive the vaccine? If so, at what age? What about the risk of adverse reactions, especially in individuals who may be at low risk? Recently males are also being considered for vaccination as they are at risk for some cancers caused by HPV. Research has indicated that the vaccine is effective and adverse reactions are few. The potential benefits greatly outweigh the risks, but these are all suitable subjects for broader discussion.

Pelvic Inflammatory Disease (PID) and Other Infections

There are a number of other sexually transmitted diseases of the female reproductive tract. Infections with *Trichomonas vaginalis* (a protozoan) usually present with vaginal pain or sensitivity, inflammation (e.g., redness), and a whitish or gray discharge. Trichomoniasis is common as an STI, and both the patient and her partner should be treated.

CDC Case Definition, Pelvic Inflammatory Disease

Pelvic Inflammatory Disease (Revised 9/96)
Clinical Case Definition

A clinical syndrome resulting from the ascending spread of microorganisms from the vagina and endocervix to the endometrium, fallopian tubes, and/or contiguous structures. In a female who has lower abdominal pain and who has not been diagnosed as having an established cause other than pelvic inflammatory disease (PID) (e.g., ectopic pregnancy, acute appendicitis, and functional pain), all the following clinical criteria must be present:

Lower abdominal tenderness, and

Tenderness with motion of the cervix, and

Adnexal tenderness

In addition to the preceding criteria, at least one of the following findings must also be present:

- Meets the surveillance case definition of C. trachomatis infection or gonorrhea
- Temperature > 100.4 F (> 38.0 C)
- Leukocytosis >10,000 white blood cells/mm3
- Purulent material in the peritoneal cavity obtained by culdocentesis or laparoscopy
- Pelvic abscess or inflammatory complex detected by bimanual examination or sonography
- Patient is a sexual contact of a person known to have gonorrhea, chlamydia, or nongonococcal urethritis

Case Classification

Confirmed: a case that meets the clinical case definition

Comment

For reporting purposes, a clinician's report of PID should be counted as a case.

Source: Reproduced from Centers for Disease Control and Prevention. Case definitions for infectious conditions under public health surveillance, 1997. MMWR 1997;46(No. RR-10;1).

Pelvic inflammatory disease (PID) is a clinical diagnosis for inflammatory disease of the female reproductive tract resulting from infection. Its incidence has been fairly high and constant (Figure 12-3). PID usually involves the fallopian tubes or uterine lining, but the ovaries or other adjacent structures can also be affected, possibly preceded by inflammation of the cervix. Inflammation and scarring of the fallopian tubes characteristic of chronic PID can cause reduced fertility or even inability to conceive. PID should therefore be properly diagnosed and promptly treated when identified. The condition may be noted on gynecological examination, or the patient may complain of abdominal tenderness, pain, or discharge, frequently accompanied by fever. Although a number of infections

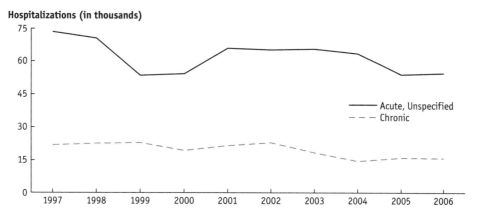

NOTE: The relative standard error for these estimates of the total number of acute unspecified PID cases ranges from 11.9% to 17.2%. The relative standard error for these estimates of the total number of chronic PID cases ranges from 11% to 18%. Data only available through 2006.

Figure 12-3   Pelvic inflammatory disease—Hospitalizations of women ages 15 to 44 years, United States, 1997–2006.

Reproduced from Centers for Disease Control and Prevention. Sexually Transmitted Disease Surveillance, 2008. Atlanta, GA. U.S. Dept of Health and Human Services, November 2009.

may cause PID, the classic (and probably most commonly identified) causes are gonorrhea or chlamydia. Because PID is the result of sexually transmitted infection, risk factors are usually the same as for most other STIs: PID is seen most frequently in young sexually active women. Although patients with PID may have had multiple partners or may have acquired the infection from a previous partner some time ago, the patient's regular partner or partners should be tested and treated for STIs as well. As PID can lead to tubal damage and resulting sterility, it should be treated immediately and effectively.

Other Infectious Disease Situations of Special Risk to Women

Although a discussion of infections that represent a hazard to the developing fetus is beyond the scope of this chapter, we can note that a number of infections fall into this category. In addition to some of the sexually transmitted infections mentioned already, well-known examples include *Toxoplasma* infection and rubella ("German measles"). Congenital rubella has now become rare, thanks to the development of an effective vaccine and aggressive public health efforts.

Several infection agents appear to manifest increased severity or mortality in pregnant women, including *Listeria*. Listeriosis is a bacterial infection that may be acquired through food or other sources, and, when symptomatic, often causes flulike illness (often with elevated white blood cell counts and sometimes with central nervous system involvement). Pregnant women, usually in the third trimester, have been reported to have a greatly increased risk of bacteremia (bacteria in the blood) with this organism.[38]

Oddly, at least two infections that normally have low mortality in healthy young adults have been associated with greatly increased mortality in pregnant women: Hepatitis E[39,40] and "swine" influenza,[41] including notoriously the recent pandemic H1N1 influenza.[42] The reasons remain unclear. The surprising result that pregnant women appeared to be at special risk of more severe disease during the last (H1N1 2009) influenza pandemic increased the recognition that the reasons for the increased virulence of some infectious diseases in pregnancy are poorly understood and is a fertile subject for further investigation. Subsequently, the Food and Drug Administration has suggested that further research in this area should be encouraged.[43]

Epidemiology of Sexually Transmitted Infections

Ascertainment and Data Sources

Accurately ascertaining the number of cases of disease is a challenging problem. For infectious diseases, there are several factors that greatly complicate this. Some infectious diseases can be recognized clinically, but many do not have sufficiently unique features to allow definitive diagnosis solely by clinical examination and therefore need to be diagnosed through laboratory tests. Many infectious diseases may be mild or asymptomatic and therefore may never come to the attention of a clinician. Many others are so familiar that medical care is rarely sought unless the disease becomes severe.

As might be expected, this problem is further complicated for sexually transmitted infections. Sexuality is a very personal and private aspect of women's lives, and people often feel uncomfortable seeking medical help for these infections or discussing them. Views of sexuality and communication about it differ by stage of life (e.g., motherhood, adolescence, middle age), cultural heritage and race, and physician communication styles. Even when a sexual disease is diagnosed, there may be great disparities in the likelihood that the infection will be reported. A number of sexually transmitted infections are notifiable; that is, they are required by law to be reported to the health department. Although these determinations are made individually by each state, and may vary somewhat in different states, there is a consensus list of Nationally Notifiable Infectious Conditions. All states have agreed to report these conditions to the CDC (http://www.cdc.gov/ncphi/disss/nndss/phs/infdis2010.htm). This list includes most of the traditionally known sexually transmitted diseases, including chancroid, chlamydia, gonorrhea, HIV, and syphilis. Hepatitis B, which is usually blood-borne but can be sexually transmitted, and hepatitis C, which is also usually blood-borne but possibly may be transmitted sexually at times, are also reportable.

As discussed previously, some diseases, like gonorrhea, are easily diagnosed in many patients. Others, like chlamydia, are often asymptomatic and may go undiagnosed. Social factors are also especially significant with STIs. It is almost proverbial that a person with symptomatic gonorrhea or syphilis is more likely to become a reported case if he or she seeks treatment at an STD clinic, many of which are staffed by local health departments, rather than from physicians in private practice.[5] Differences in reporting practices indicate the great difficulty of accurately ascertaining cases even when the disease is recognized and mandated for physicians to report, let alone the many cases that may go unreported because they are not recognized or the patient has not sought medical attention.

Recognizing that all infectious disease epidemiologic data are likely to have multiple sources of error and may be undercounted, and that this problem is further complicated in sexually transmitted diseases, nevertheless it is possible to obtain some reasonable estimates of disease occurrence and transmission. A number of sources of epidemiologic data are used for this purpose. Data are collected by state and local health departments from clinicians (under notifiable disease reporting) and from STD clinics or other health clinics (such as maternal health clinics) operated by health departments.[5] Many health departments also have various surveillance systems to target data collection for certain infections. At the national level, data are collected by CDC through a variety of mechanisms in addition to the National Notifiable Disease Surveillance System. Much of the information is compiled in publications such as the CDC's *Sexually Transmitted Disease Surveillance, 2008*, which is highly recommended as an indispensable source of information for all researchers interested in the epidemiology of STDs in the United States and the most accessible source of national epidemiologic data on these diseases.[5] CDC's National Center for HIV/AIDS, Viral Hepatitis, STD, and TB Prevention (NCHHSTP) maintains an STD Surveillance System (STDSS) for this purpose. However, in order to obtain more accurate estimates of disease frequency, a population-based system (rather than one based just on disease reporting) is necessary. Regular national surveys such as the flagship National Health and Nutrition Examination Survey, which the CDC describes as "a nationally-representative survey of the U.S. civilian, non-institutionalized 14- to 39-year old population," and the National Longitudinal Study of Adolescent Health as well as a number of others include items relating to infectious diseases. These studies are also included in the surveillance summaries published by CDC. Thus, the information on herpes simplex seroprevalence is based on serologic testing from samples taken as part of the NHANES study. Although there have been debates about herpes seroprevalence, CDC's results from NHANES represent the most extensive and dependable sample we have available, and is as close to a "gold standard" as we are likely to obtain. Last, but not least, there are a number of research projects to study specific diseases, and these targeted programs are also important sources of both biologic and epidemiologic data.[44–46]

Contact Tracing and Case Investigation

Contact tracing of STDs has figured prominently in the popular imagination over the years and to some may seem almost synonymous with the activities of the health department or infectious disease epidemiologists. Despite its hold on the popular imagination, contact tracing is employed in relatively limited circumstances. The purpose of contact tracing is to identify other infected individuals so that they may be appropriately treated and counseled. Its principal public health value is therefore to reduce additional cases. Contact tracing is still important for the acute sexually transmitted diseases, most notably gonorrhea, syphilis, and (when feasible) HIV. It is not routinely practiced for most of the other common STIs, such as HPV, herpes, and, in most cases, chlamydia; these infections tend to be very widespread and most people who present clinically may well have acquired these infections long ago, so that there is relatively little public health gain. However, there is great value in counseling and education of the patient and, when done appropriately, of sexual partners.

A number of studies have demonstrated the importance of testing for other STI whenever a patient presents with an STI, as many studies identify a relatively high frequency of coinfections.[22,44-46] Although exact figures are difficult to obtain, and the frequency of reported coinfections varies with the population being tested and the method of screening, this result is not surprising, as many of the risk factors and behaviors are similar.

Diagnostic methods have improved markedly in recent years, leading to improvements not only in clinical management but in understanding the epidemiology of these infections. In the past, culture was the standard method for most STI, with the exception of syphilis and HPV, which could not readily be cultured. Although culture remains useful, molecular methods, especially the polymerase chain reaction (PCR), are now the mainstay for all of the infections discussed except syphilis (where serologic methods are still most often used). Molecular methods such as PCR provide great sensitivity and can also give relatively rapid results (within a day or less). With current technologies, it is now possible to screen for several STIs at the same time, allowing coinfections to be better identified and appropriately treated. For screening, urine samples are frequently used. In clinical cases, a sample of the lesion or vaginal or cervical swab may be used. If testing can be done quickly (as is becoming increasingly possible with rapid PCR testing), patients could even be treated for the coinfections while still in the clinic.

Risk Factors and Disparities in STDs

Among women, the population at greatest risk for almost all STIs are young, sexually active women, ages 15–24 who represent only 25% of the sexually experienced population but acquire almost half of all new STIs.[5,47] It is tautologic to say that high-risk behaviors, such as multiple partners, sexual violence, or commercial sex work, can increase risk of exposure. Women of lower socioeconomic status, who often come from minority groups, also are often disproportionately at risk.[5] Although some of this disparity may reflect ascertainment bias, a number of other factors come into play. These include access to health care and possibly less access to public health prevention education or reduced ability to carry out recommended preventive modalities.

The prevalence of STI and the fact that many are treatable or that transmission can be limited through personal precautions (such as use of condoms by either partner, vaginal microbicides, or immunization for HPV) strongly support the importance of effective education and public health messaging. Unfortunately, the sensitivity of many sexual issues makes this especially challenging in the case of STIs. Finally, STIs are also occasionally seen in prepubertal children. Unfortunately, in some cases this may be the result of sexual abuse. Differentiating sexual abuse from congenital acquisition or precocious sexual activity is an especially knotty legal and ethical issue.[7,48,49]

Even in a field as thoroughly studied as STI, surprises can still occur. In what may be one of the most unusual examples, the CDC's *Morbidity and Mortality Weekly Report* described the case of a young woman who presented at a clinic with vaginitis and other classical signs of a sexually transmitted disease, but who tested negative for the usual infections. Her illness was eventually determined to be vaccinia (the smallpox vaccine virus), which she acquired from her sexual partner, a military recruit who had just been immunized.[49] We will leave it to the reader's imagination to speculate on a possible route of transmission, but the case demonstrates that the field of infectious diseases still has many surprises for the alert epidemiologist or clinician!

Summary and Prospects for the Future

There are a number of STIs, including some among the most ancient human infectious diseases (gonorrhea, perhaps herpes simplex), and others among the most recent (HIV). Sexual transmission remains an effective route of transmission for a number of organisms. Diagnosis, epidemiology, and control in women are complicated by the fact that many are asymptomatic and therefore detected only through screening or testing. These issues are further complicated by our difficulties in discussing and dealing with sexuality and sexually related matters. The incidence of STIs is strongly related to our social inhibitions regarding frank discussion of sexual matters and of the stigma associated with this mode of transmission. The burden of disease falls disproportionately on women, in part because of the greater risk and consequences of chronic infection.

Appropriate education and frank discussion are essential. Many STIs are treatable, and others can be controlled through public health measures and appropriate preventive actions by infected sexual partners. Success with reduction of congenital rubella (not sexually transmitted, but well known for its effects on the developing fetus) indicate what can be achieved. The development of a vaccine for HPV is another promising recent development with profound implications for preventing cervical carcinoma and other serious chronic gynecological conditions, potentially saving many lives at minimal cost.

Despite notable advances in reducing the burden of STI, there is still much to be done. Although some of the "classic" STIs, such as gonorrhea, have declined over the last century, these infectious diseases are still very much with us. We once thought syphilis would soon be eliminated, but Farhi and colleagues note that "since 2000, the incidence of syphilis has risen in developed countries."[6] Ramos and colleagues contrast progress in control of mother-to-child transmission of HIV in Brazil with "failure in congenital syphilis."[51]

A Coda: Emerging Infections

Although most of these infections have been prevalent for a long time, new infections enter the human population from time to time or rapidly spread from a geographically limited area. HIV is a prime example of an "emerging infection," defined as an infection that has newly appeared or is rapidly increasing in incidence or geographic range.[52] Unknown until the late 1970s, HIV has now become one of our greatest health concerns worldwide. To generalize, in addition to the known and currently familiar infections, in the last century we have witnessed the emergence of a number of previously unknown or unfamiliar infections. HIV is a foremost example, but there have been many others, including SARS (Severe Acute Respiratory

Syndrome) in 2003, hemolytic uremic syndrome caused by certain toxin-producing subtypes of the common bacterium *Escherichia coli*, and pandemic influenza (H1N1) in 2009. These infections, that have not previously been recognized but appear suddenly and rapidly increase in number of cases or geographic range are often called emerging infections.[52] They may often be infections that already exist in other species or in geographically limited human populations but are given an opportunity to come in contact with new human populations, or to spread. Such factors of modern life as agricultural or environmental change may put people in contact with a new and previously unfamiliar infectious agent in the environment. Thus, changes in the ecology and in the relationship of humans to the environment can result in the emergence of apparently "new" infectious diseases. This phenomenon is likely to grow as the pace of ecological change continues to increase worldwide, and as globalization continues.

Although many new infections may be geographically limited or have limited ability to transmit to humans (H5N1 avian influenza is a well-known recent example), others may be transmissible from person to person (examples include pandemic influenza, SARS, and HIV) and may be spread through human activities such as global travel and trade, sexual transmission, the healthcare system, or the blood supply. Among others. HIV is also an excellent demonstration of this aspect. Although the evidence remains largely circumstantial, studies indicate that the ancestor of HIV may have been introduced into the human population from another animal species, probably chimpanzees in central Africa,[53] and most likely through hunting and butchering or handling of the meat.[54] HIV then spread through sexual transmission, initially locally and regionally (in which truck drivers and the commercial sex trade probably played a large initial role),[55] and then globally.[56] Additional transmission occurred through contaminated blood products and injection equipment. HIV therefore became a major pandemic scourge, aided by its long duration of infectiousness (years) and social changes that provided numerous opportunities for transmission, despite the relatively poor transmissibility of HIV itself that would have made the virus an unlikely important infectious disease threat. This should be an object lesson that we need to avoid complacency and to recognize that sexually transmitted infections may spread widely while society struggles with their social complexities and stigma.

The microbes causing infections can also evolve. A classic example is the development of antibiotic resistance in bacteria. Therefore, we must bear in mind that although the discussion in this chapter is a snapshot of some infectious diseases currently affecting women, infectious diseases are dynamic and can reflect changes both in the infecting organisms and in the host. For example, with an aging population, infectious diseases rarely seen in the past, are becoming more prominent as control of other major health problems has prolonged life expectancy among older adults.

Further Reading

Due to the importance and variety of infectious diseases, it is impossible to cover all examples, even all sexually transmitted infections, in this chapter. Fortunately, there are a number of excellent standard references available on infectious diseases, and the interested reader should consult these for further information:

Clinical Aspects and Basic Science: Mandell GL, Bennett JE, Dolin R (eds.) *Principles and Practice of Infectious Diseases.* 6th ed. Philadelphia: Elsevier; 2005.

Public Health Aspects: Heymann DL (ed.) *Control of Communicable Diseases Manual.* 19th ed. Washington,DC: American Public Health Association; 2008. (Includes brief descriptions of the causative agents, as well as public health recommendations.)

Epidemiology: Centers for Disease Control and Prevention (CDC). *Sexually Transmitted Disease Surveillance, 2008.* Atlanta, GA: U.S. Department of Health and Human Services; November 2009. http://www.cdc.gov/std/pubs/.

Discussion Questions

1. Should all women be screened for chlamydia? Should all men be screened?
2. In general, have improved screening and diagnostic technology had an effect on the incidence of STIs in the United States? If so, what effects can be attributed to these improvements?
3. Identify and evaluate other actions that could be implemented to reduce the incidence of STI in the United States. Which do you think are most important? Which would be easiest to implement?
4. Some have argued that we have been more successful reducing mother-to-child transmission of HIV than of syphilis or gonorrhea. Do you agree or disagree? What evidence supports this view? If this is true, what could be done to change this?
5. Do you foresee changes in the incidence of sexually transmitted infections? Why or why not? If so, which ones do you think are most likely to increase and which will decrease?
6. Should all females receive HPV vaccine? If so, at what age should they first receive the vaccine? Should all boys also receive HPV vaccine?
7. If a vaccine were to be developed against chlamydia, what do you think would be the likely benefits and disadvantages (other than cost)? Who should receive it? What factors should be taken into consideration? Would you advocate the vaccine for your own family?

References

1. Cook HA, Furuya EY, Larson E, et al. Heterosexual transmission of community-associated methicillin-resistant *Staphylococcus aureus*. *Clin Infect Dis.* 2007;44:410–413.
2. Thomas DL, Cannon RO, Shapiro CN, Hook EW III, Alter MJ, Quinn TC. Hepatitis C, hepatitis B, and human immunodeficiency virus infections among non-intravenous drug-using patients attending clinics for sexually transmitted diseases. *J Infect Dis.* 1994;169:990–995.
3. Nakashima K, Kashiwagi S, Hayashi J, Noguchi A, Hirata M, Kajiyama W, Urabe K, Minami K, Maeda Y. Sexual transmission of hepatitis C virus among female prostitutes and patients with sexually transmitted diseases in Fukuoka, Kyushu, Japan. *Am J Epidemiol.* 1992;136:1132–1137.
4. Utsumi T, Hashimoto E, Okumura Y, et al. Heterosexual activity as a risk factor for the transmission of hepatitis C virus. *J Med Virol.* 1995;46:122–125.
5. Centers for Disease Control and Prevention. *Sexually Transmitted Disease Surveillance, 2008.* Atlanta, GA: U.S. Department of Health and Human Services; November 2009. http://www.cdc.gov/std/pubs/.
6. Farhi D, Zizi N, Grange P, Benhaddou N, et al. The epidemiological and clinical presentation of syphilis in a venereal disease centre in Paris, France. A cohort study of 284 consecutive cases over the period 2000–2007. *Eur J Dermatol.* 2009;19:484–489.
7. Hammerschlag MR, Guillén CD. Medical and legal implications of testing for sexually transmitted infections in children. *Clin Microbiol Rev.* 2010;23:493–506.
8. Bandea CI, Kubota K, Brown TM, et al. Typing of *Chlamydia trachomatis* strains from urine samples by amplification and sequencing the major outer membrane protein gene (omp1). *Sex Transm Infect.* 2001;77:419–422.
9. McCormack WM, Alpert S, McComb DE, et al. Fifteen-month follow-up study of women infected with *Chlamydia trachomatis*. *N Engl J Med.* 1979;300:123–125.
10. Bell TA, Stamm WE, Wang SP, Holmes KK, Grayston JT. Chronic *Chlamydia trachomatis* infections in infants. *JAMA.* 1992;267:400–402.
11. Gottlieb SL, Berman SM, Low N. Screening and treatment to prevent sequelae in women with *Chlamydia trachomatis* genital infection: how much do we know? *J Infect Dis.* 2010;201(suppl 2):S156–S167.
12. Miller WC, Ford CA, Morris M, et al. Prevalence of chlamydial and gonococcal infections among young adults in the United States. *JAMA.* 2004;291:2229–2236.
13. Datta SD, Sternberg M, Johnson RE, et al. Gonorrhea and chlamydia in the United States among persons 14 to 39 years of age, 1999 to 2002. *Ann Intern Med.* 2007;147:89–96.
14. Cates W, Jr., Wasserheit JN. Genital chlamydial infections: epidemiology and reproductive sequelae. *Am J Obstet Gynecol.* 1991;164:1771–1781.
15. Straus SE. Introduction to herpesviridae. In: Mandell GL, Bennett JE, Dolin R (eds.) *Principles and Practice of Infectious Diseases.* 6th ed. Philadelphia: Elsevier; 2005: 1756–1762.
16. Corey L, Wald A. Maternal and neonatal Herpes Simplex Virus infections. *N Engl J Med.* 2009;361:1376–1385.
17. Fuchs J, Celum C, Wang J, et al. HIV Prevention Trials Network 039 Protocol Team. Clinical and virologic efficacy of herpes simplex virus type 2 suppression by acyclovir in a multicontinent clinical trial. *J Infect Dis.* 2010;201:1164–1168.
18. Gardella C, Brown Z, Wald A, et al. Risk factors for herpes simplex virus transmission to pregnant women: a couples study. *Am J Obstet Gynecol.* 2005;193:1891–1899.
19. Wald A, Langenberg AG, Krantz E, et al. The relationship between condom use and herpes simplex virus acquisition. *Ann Intern Med.* 2005;143:707–713.
20. Corey L, Wald A, Celum CL, Quinn TC. The effects of herpes simplex virus-2 on HIV-1 acquisition and transmission: a review of two overlapping epidemics. *J Acquir Immune Defic Syndr.* 2004;35:435–445.
21. Abu-Raddad LJ, Magaret AS, Celum C, et al. Genital herpes has played a more important role than any other sexually transmitted infection in driving HIV prevalence in Africa. *PLoS One.* 2008;3:e2230.
22. Tobian AA, Ssempijja V, Kigozi G, et al. Incident HIV and herpes simplex virus type 2 infection among men in Rakai, Uganda. *AIDS.* 2009;23:1589–1594.
23. Grosskurth H, Gray R, Hayes R, et al. Control of sexually transmitted diseases for HIV-1 prevention: understanding the implications of the Mwanza and Rakai trials. *Lancet* 2000;355:1981–1987.
24. Haaland RE, Hawkins PA, Salazar-Gonzalez J, et al. Inflammatory genital infections mitigate a severe genetic bottleneck in heterosexual transmission of subtype A and C HIV-1. *PLoS Pathog.* 2009;5:e1000274.
25. Datta SD, Koutsky L, Ratelle S, et al. Human papillomavirus infection and cervical cytology in women screened for cervical cancer in the United States, 2003–2005. *Ann Intern Med.* 2008;148:493–500.
26. Dunne EF, Unger ER, Sternberg M, et al. Prevalence of HPV infection among females in the United States. *JAMA.* 2007;297:813–819.
27. Jones C. Cervical cancer: is herpes simplex virus type II a cofactor? *Clin Microbiol Rev.* 1995;8:549–556.
28. Gissmann L, Boshart M, Dürst M, Ikenberg H, Wagner D, zur Hausen H. Presence of human papillomavirus in genital tumors. *J Invest Dermatol.* 1984;83(1 suppl):26s–28s.
29. Muñoz N, Bosch FX, de Sanjosé S, et al. Epidemiologic classification of human papillomavirus types associated with cervical cancer. *N Engl J Med.* 2003;348:518–27.
30. Ferlay J, Bray F, Pisani P, Parkin DM. *GLOBOCAN 2002: Cancer Incidence, Mortality and Prevalence Worldwide.* IARC CancerBase no 5, ver 2.0. Lyons, France: IARC Press; 2004.
31. World Health Organization. Human papillomavirus infection and cervical cancer. http://www.who.int/vaccine_research/diseases/viral_cancers/en/index3.html. Accessed August 21, 2012.

32. Jansen KU, Shaw AR. Human papillomavirus vaccines and prevention of cervical cancer. *Annu Rev Med.* 2004;55:319–331.

33. FUTURE I/II Study Group. Four year efficacy of prophylactic human papillomavirus quadrivalent vaccine against low grade cervical, vulvar, and vaginal intraepithelial neoplasia and anogenital warts: randomised controlled trial. *BMJ.* 2010;340:c3493.

34. Centers for Disease Control and Prevention. Quadrivalent Human Papillomavirus Vaccine Recommendations of the Advisory Committee on Immunization Practices (ACIP) *MMWR Morb Mortal Wkly Rep.* 2007;56(RR-2).

35. Benítez-Bribiesca L. Ethical dilemmas and great expectations for human papilloma virus vaccination. *Arch Med Res.* 2009;40:499–502.

36. Balog JE. The moral justification for a compulsory human papillomavirus vaccination program. *Am J Public Health.* 2009;99:616–622.

37. Zimmerman RK. Ethical analysis of HPV vaccine policy options. *Vaccine.* 2006;24:4812–4820.

38. Mylonakis E, Paliou M, Hohmann EL et al. Listeriosis during pregnancy. a case series and review of 222 cases. *Medicine.* 2002;81:260–269.

39. Khuroo MS, Khuroo MS. Hepatitis E virus. *Curr Opin Infect Dis.* 2008;21:539–543.

40. Sharapov MB, Favorov MO, Yashina TL, Brown MS, Onischenko GG, Margolis HS, Chorba TL. Acute viral hepatitis morbidity and mortality associated with hepatitis E virus infection: Uzbekistan surveillance data. *BMC Infect Dis.* 2009;9:35.

41. Wells DL, Hopfensperger DJ, Arden NH, et al. Swine influenza virus infections. Transmission from ill pigs to humans at a Wisconsin agricultural fair and subsequent probable person-to-person transmission. *JAMA.* 1991;265:478–481.

42. Siston AM, Rasmussen SA, Honein MA, et al. Pandemic H1N1 Influenza in Pregnancy Working Group. Pandemic 2009 influenza A (H1N1) virus illness among pregnant women in the United States. *JAMA.* 2010;303:1517–1525.

43. Goldkind SF, Sahin L, Gallauresi B. Enrolling pregnant women in research—lessons from the H1N1 influenza pandemic. *N Engl J Med.* 2010;362:2241–2243.

44. Zetola NM, Bernstein KT, Wong E, et al. Exploring the relationship between sexually transmitted diseases and HIV acquisition by using different study designs. *J Acquir Immune Defic Syndr.* 2009:546–551.

45. Staras SA, Cook RL, Clark DB. Sexual partner characteristics and sexually transmitted diseases among adolescents and young adults. *Sex Transm Dis.* 2009;36:232–238.

46. Lee HC, Ko NY, Lee NY, et al. Trends in sexually transmitted diseases and risky behaviors among HIV-infected patients at an outpatient clinic in southern Taiwan. *Sex Transm Dis.* 2010;37:86–93.

47. Weinstock H, Berman S, Cates W, Jr. Sexually transmitted diseases among American youth: Incidence and prevalence estimates, 2000. *Perspect Sex Reprod Health.* 2004;36:6–10.

48. Kellogg N. The evaluation of sexual abuse in children. *Pediatrics.* 2005;116:506–512.

49. Berkoff MC, Zolotor AJ, Makoroff KL, et al. Has this prepubertal girl been sexually abused? *JAMA.* 2008;300:2779–2792.

50. Centers for Disease Control and Prevention. Vaccinia virus infection after sexual contact with a military smallpox vaccine—Washington, 2010. *MMWR Morb Mortal Wkly Rep.* 2010;59:773–775.

51. Ramos Jr AN, Matida LH, Saraceni V, et al. Control of mother-to-child transmission of infectious diseases in Brazil: progress in HIV/AIDS and failure in congenital syphilis. *Cad Saude Publica.* 2007;23:S370–S378.

52. Morse SS. Factors in the emergence of infectious diseases. *Emerg Infect Dis.* 1995;1:7–15.

53. Hahn BH, Shaw GM, De Cock KM, Sharp PM. AIDS as a zoonosis: scientific and public health implications. *Science.* 2000;287:607–614.

54. Wolfe ND, Daszak P, Kilpatrick AM, Burke DS. Bushmeat hunting, deforestation, and predicting zoonotic emergence. *Emerg Infect Dis.* 2005;11:1822–1827.

55. Myers G, MacInnes K, Myers L. Phylogenetic moments in the AIDS epidemic. In: Morse SS, ed. *Emerging Viruses.* New York and Oxford: Oxford Univ. Press; 1993:120–137.

56. Shilts R. *And the Band Played On.* New York: St. Martin's Press; 1987.

The Epidemiology of HIV/AIDS among American Women

Martha M. McKinney, PhD; Katherine M. Marconi, PhD, MS; and Lois J. Eldred, PA-C, MPH, DrPH

Introduction

Almost 280,000 women are estimated to be living with human immunodeficiency virus (HIV) infection in the United States.[1] In contrast to the early years of the epidemic when only homosexual men were thought to be at risk for this disease, women now account for 27% of annual new HIV infections and 25% of people living with HIV.[2]

As the U.S. HIV/AIDS (acquired immune deficiency syndrome) epidemic has evolved, the primary mode of transmission reported by women has shifted from injection drug use to high-risk heterosexual sex. HIV has spread disproportionately among racial/ethnic groups, with black and Hispanic women most seriously affected. In 2008, for example, black and Hispanic women accounted for an estimated 81% of adult/adolescent females diagnosed with HIV infection but only 25% of the female population ages 13 and older.[3] Across all racial/ethnic groups, HIV incidence rates are highest among women ages 30–39.[4]

This chapter examines HIV/AIDS among U.S. women from a public health perspective. After presenting a brief history of the early years of the epidemic, the chapter describes trends in HIV/AIDS incidence, prevalence, and mortality and the natural history of HIV infection in women. Additional sections discuss HIV risk factors and prevention strategies, trends in HIV testing and follow-up, and diagnosis and treatment issues. Finally, goals and challenges for the next decade are discussed.

Historical Background

Although sporadic case reports and other available data suggest that the current HIV/AIDS epidemic started in the mid- to late 1970s,[5] this disease went unrecognized in the public health arena until June 5, 1981 when the Centers for Disease Control and Prevention (CDC) reported five cases of *Pneumocystis carinii* pneumonia (PCP) in young men without any clinically apparent underlying immunodeficiency.[6] Noting that all of these men reported male-to-male sexual contact, CDC researchers hypothesized that "some aspect of a homosexual lifestyle or disease acquired through sexual contact" might predispose men to opportunistic infections.[6]

Table 13-1 tracks the evolution of the HIV/AIDS epidemic over the next 15 years. Initially, the CDC identified male injection drug users and men with one of the three "Hs"—homosexual orientation, Haitian origin, or hemophilia—as the groups at greatest risk for AIDS. By 1983, reports of serious opportunistic infections among women prompted the addition of female sexual partners of men with AIDS as a fifth risk group. Research by French virologists Françoise Barré-Sinoussi and Luc Montagnier and American virologist Robert Gallo led to the 1984 isolation of HIV as the infectious agent that causes AIDS.

People infected with HIV may remain symptom free for many years. AIDS develops in the later stages of HIV infection when the immune system has been severely damaged. Although the CDC first published a detailed AIDS surveillance case definition in 1986,[7] gender differences were not cited until 1992, when invasive cervical cancer was added as an AIDS-indicative condition.[8] In December 1995, the U.S. Food and Drug Administration approved saquinavir for use in treating advanced HIV infection. This antiretroviral drug introduced a new era of highly active antiretroviral therapy (HAART) designed to reduce viral replication by using different classes of antiretroviral agents to block the virus at each stage of its life cycle. Although there still is no cure for HIV disease, HAART has dramatically improved life expectancy for HIV-infected women and men.

HIV/AIDS Incidence and Prevalence in Women

Because many states and U.S. territories did not implement confidential name-based HIV reporting until 2008, AIDS incidence data provided the only means of assessing the impact of the epidemic. CDC researchers used back-calculation models based on AIDS incidence data and the probability distribution of the incubation period from HIV infection to AIDS diagnosis to analyze historical HIV incidence trends. However, these models provided no insights on current transmission patterns.[9] Following the introduction of antiretroviral therapies, back-calculation models based exclusively on incident AIDS cases were deemed invalid due to the difficulty of estimating the length of the incubation period at the population level.

Table 13-1

Highlights of the Pre-HAART era, 1981–1996

Date	Reported Event	Comment
1981	• 5 cases of *Pneumocystis carinii* pneumonia reported in homosexual men	Los Angeles, California
	• 26 additional cases of new immunodeficiency syndrome reported	California and New York
1982	• Cluster of immunodeficiency syndrome cases reported in California	First report that "infectious agents" might be sexually transmitted
	• Initial cases reported in people with hemophilia	
	• Term "acquired immune deficiency syndrome" used for first time (replacing "gay-related immune deficiency")	CDC identifies 4 risk factors: homosexuality, injection drug use, Haitian origin, hemophilia A
	• 5 cases in women reported, including 1 with only heterosexual exposure	
	• Initial vertically transmitted cases reported in 4 infants	
1983	• Drs. Françoise Barré-Sinoussi and Luc Montagnier isolate lymphadenopathy-associated virus, later to become known as human immunodeficiency virus or HIV	
	• CDC issues HIV prevention recommendations	Female sexual partners of men with AIDS added as a fifth risk group
1984	• Dr. Robert Gallo identifies HIV as the cause of AIDS	
	• CDC classifies AIDS as a "notifiable disease"	25 cases reported in first week
1985	• FDA licenses the first enzyme immunoassay to screen for HIV antibody	
	• U.S. Public Health Service issues first recommendations for preventing mother-to-child transmission of HIV	
1986	• CDC provides a surveillance case definition of AIDS	Updated in 1987 and 1993
	• Zidovudine, the first drug used to treat AIDS, begins clinical trials	
1987	• FDA approves zidovudine for clinical use	
1990	• First National Conference on Women and AIDS held in Boston	
1992	• FDA licenses first rapid HIV test	
1993	• CDC expands case definition of AIDS to include invasive cervical cancer and conditions prevalent among injection drug users	
	• Two major federally-funded research studies on women and HIV/AIDS begin: Women's Interagency HIV Study and HIV Epidemiology Study	
	• FDA approves female condom for sale in the United States	

1994	• A major clinical trial demonstrates that administering zidovudine to HIV-infected women and their newborns can substantial reduce perinatal transmission • U.S. Public Health Service recommends routine screening of pregnant women for HIV	CDC issues guidelines for using zidovudine to reduce perinatal transmission
1995	• FDA approves an oral HIV test, the first nonblood-based antibody test for HIV • FDA approves first protease inhibitor, saquinavir, ushering in a new era of highly active antiretroviral therapy	
1996	• FDA approves first nonnucleoside reverse transcriptase inhibitor, nevirapine • FDA approves viral load test to measure the level of HIV	

CDC = Centers for Disease Control and Prevention, FDA = Food and Drug Administration, HAART = highly active antiretroviral therapy, HIV = human immunodeficiency virus

Source: Data from Kaiser Family Foundation. The global HIV/AIDS epidemic: a timeline of key milestones. 2007. Available at http://www.kff.org/hivaids/timeline/hivtimeline.cfm. Accessed January 11, 2010; Sepkowitz KA. AIDS—the first 20 years. New Engl J Med 2001;344:1765.

In 2008, CDC researchers used 2006 case reports from 22 states that had implemented confidential name-based HIV reporting, combined with a laboratory assay—BED HIV-1—that could directly identify recent infections, to calculate more accurate U.S. incidence and prevalence estimates and to recalculate previous estimates. Their findings indicate that new HIV diagnoses have stabilized at about 55,000 infections per year; however, the female percentage has crept upward to 27%.[9] Women now account for one-quarter of the 1.1 million U.S. adults and adolescents living with diagnosed or undiagnosed HIV infection.[1] By comparison, the 15.7 million women living with HIV/AIDS worldwide comprise about half of the infected adult/adolescent population (UNAIDS and WHO, 2009).[10]

Table 13-2 shows the estimated number of women living with HIV/AIDS by year and transmission category in 37 states that have conducted confidential name-based HIV surveillance since at least 2005. Between 2005 and 2007, 70–73% of these women reported infection through high-risk heterosexual contact, and 26–28% reported injection drug use as the primary mode of transmission.

Table 13-2

Estimated numbers of adult/adolescent females living with a diagnosis of HIV infection by year and transmission category, 2005–2007—37 states with confidential name-based HIV infection reporting[a]

Transmission Category	2005	2006	2007
Injection drug use	40,082	40,245	40,197
High-risk heterosexual contact[b]	100,206	105,842	111,629
Other[c]	1,955	1,963	1,989
Subtotal[d]	142,242	148,051	153,814

Source: Adapted from Centers for Disease Control and Prevention. Table 15a. Persons living with a diagnosis of HIV infection, by year and selected characteristics, 2005–2007—37 states with confidential name-based HIV infection reporting. *HIV/AIDS Surveillance Report, 2008.* 2010;20:76. Available at http://www.cdc.gov/hiv/surveillance/resources/reports/2008report/pdf/2008SurveillanceReport.pdf. Accessed February 19, 2011.
[a]The data shown in this table include women with a diagnosis of HIV infection regardless of stage of disease at diagnosis. Estimated numbers were statistically adjusted to account for reporting delays and missing risk factor information but not for incomplete reporting.
[b]Heterosexual contact with a person known to have, or to be at high risk for, HIV infection.
[c]Includes hemophilia, blood transfusion, and risk factor not reported or identified.
[d]Because column totals for estimated numbers were calculated independently of the values for the subpopulations, the values in each column may not sum to the column total.

AIDS Trends

Figure 13-1 illustrates the rapid growth in female AIDS cases since 1985. Between 1985 and 2010, the female percentage of new adult and adolescent AIDS cases increased from 7% to 25%. AIDS incidence among women rose steadily through 1993, the year in which the AIDS definition was expanded to include invasive cervical cancer. Between 1993 and 1996, incidence leveled off at approximately 13,000 AIDS cases per year. Following the 1996 introduction of HAART, AIDS incidence declined to its current level of about 12,000 female cases per year.

Figure 13-2 illustrates the variations in AIDS rates among U.S. states and dependent areas in 2009. Although every state has reported some AIDS cases among women, the states and areas with the highest AIDS rates among women include District of Columbia, New York, U.S. Virgin Islands, Maryland, Puerto Rico, and Florida. Regionally, AIDS case rates are highest among women in the Northeast and the South.

Racial/Ethnic Differences in HIV/AIDS Rates

Since the beginning of the HIV/AIDS epidemic, black and Hispanic women have borne a disproportionate burden of this disease. Table 13-3 presents 2010 estimates of the number of women newly diagnosed with HIV and the diagnosis rates by race/ethnicity in 46 states that have conducted confidential name-based HIV surveillance since at least 2005. As in past years, black women accounted for more two-thirds of the HIV/AIDS cases. The estimated HIV/AIDS rate for black women (41.7 per 100,000) was 20 times higher than for white women (2.1 per 100,000). Although Hispanic women had fewer reported HIV/AIDS cases than white women, their HIV/AIDS rate (9.2 per 100,000) was almost four times higher.

Socioeconomic issues such as poverty, lack of health insurance coverage, limited access to health care and HIV prevention education may explain some racial/ethnic disparities in HIV/AIDS incidence.[11] Research studies indicate that black women are no more likely to have unprotected sex and multiple sexual partners or to abuse substances than women of other racial/ethnic groups.[12] However, some studies suggest that black women are more likely to have high-risk sexual partners.[12] For Hispanic women, language barriers and cultural factors such as *machismo*, which encourages male domination, and *marianismo*, which requires women to be submissive and obedient, may heighten risk for HIV by limiting their ability to negotiate safer sex.[13]

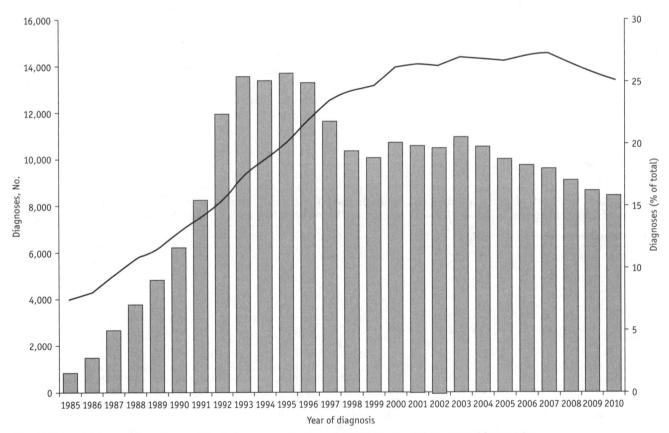

Note. All displayed data have been estimated. Estimated numbers resulted from statistical adjustment that accounted for reporting delays, but note for incomplete reporting.

Figure 13-1 AIDS diagnoses among adults and adolescent females, 1985–2010—United States and 6 dependent areas.

Reproduced from Centers for Disease Control and Prevention. AIDS Diagnoses among Adults and Adolescent Females, 1985–2010—United States and 6 Dependent Areas. Slide 10. Available at http://www.cdc.gov/hiv/topics/surveillance/resources/slides/women/index.htm

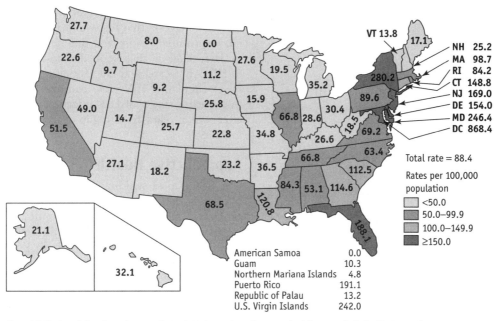

American Samoa 0.0
Guam 10.3
Northern Mariana Islands 4.8
Puerto Rico 191.1
Republic of Palau 13.2
U.S. Virgin Islands 242.0

Total rate = 88.4

Rates per 100,000 population
- <50.0
- 50.0–99.9
- 100.0–149.9
- ≥150.0

Note. All displayed data have been estimated. Estimated numbers resulted from statistical adjustment that accounted for reporting delays, but not for incomplete reporting. Rates are per 100,000 population.

Figure 13-2 Rates of adult and adolescent females living with an AIDS diagnosis, year–end 2009—United States and 6 dependent areas (N = 116,020).

Reproduced from Centers for Disease Control and Prevention. Rates of Adult and Adolescent Females Living with an AIDS Diagnosis, year–end 2009—United States and 6 Dependent Areas. Slide 17. Available at http://www.cdc.gov/hiv/topics/surveillance/resources/slides/women/index.htm

Table 13-3

Diagnoses of HIV infection among adult and adolescent females, by race/ethnicity, 2010–46 states[a]

Race/Ethnicity	Number	Rate
White, not Hispanic	1,733	2.1
Black/African American	6,268	41.7
Hispanic (any race)	1,533	9.2
Asian	134	2.5
Native Hawaiian/Other Pacific Islander	6	4.5
American Indian/Alaska Native	61	6.4
Multiple races	133	9.7
Total[b]	9,868	8.0

Reproduced from Centers for Disease Control and Prevention. Diagnoses of HIV Infection Among Adult and Adolescent Females, by Race Ethnicity, 2010–46 States. Slide 3. Available at http://www.cdc.gov/hiv/topics/surveillance/resources/slides/women/index.htm
[a]Data include people with a diagnosis of HIV infection regardless of stage of disease at diagnosis. Data are drawn from 46 states with confidential name-based HIV infection reporting since at least January 2005. All displayed data have been estimated. Estimated numbers resulted from statistical adjustment that accounted for reporting delays but not for incomplete reporting. Rates are per 100,000 population.
[b]Because column totals for estimated numbers were calculated independently of the values for the subpopulations, the values in each column may not sum to the column total.

Mortality Trends

In the post-HAART era, people with HIV/AIDS are living much longer, increasing the chances that more than 25% will die from other causes.[14] The Women's Interagency HIV Study (WIHS), a longitudinal, observational cohort study of HIV-infected women and demographically similar uninfected women, illustrates this trend.[15]

WIHS researchers tracked deaths among HIV-infected participants over 10 years to identify causes and predictors of mortality. Between 1998 and 2004, 47% of the 710 deaths with known causes were not related to any AIDS-defining condition. The most common non-AIDS causes of death were trauma or overdose, hepatitis C liver disease, cardiovascular disease, and non-AIDS malignancies.

Race/ethnicity	No.	Rate
American Indian/Alaska Native	26	2.8
Asian[a]	19	0.4
Black/African American	3,571	23.8
Hispanic/Latino[b]	754	4.5
Native Hawaiian/Other Pacific Islander	1	1.0
White	957	1.1
Multiple races	167	12.2
Total	**5,496**	**4.5**

Note. Data include persons with a diagnosis of HIV infection regardless of stage of disease at diagnosis. Deaths of persons with a diagnosis of HIV infection may be due to any cause. All displayed data have been statistically adjusted to account for reporting delays, but not for incomplete reporting. Rates are per 100,000 population.

[a]Includes Asian/Pacific Islander legacy cases.

[b]Hispanics/Latinos can be of any race.

Figure 13-3 Deaths of adults and adolescent females with a diagnosis of HIV infection, by race/ethnicity, 2009–46 states.

Source: Reproduced from Centers for Disease Control and Prevention. Deaths of adult and adolescent females with a diagnosis of HIV infection, by race/ethnicity, 2009—United States. Slide 8. Available at http://www.cdc.gov/hiv/topics/surveillance/resources/slides/women/index.htm.

In the United States, rates of death due to HIV disease have always been higher for men than for women. However, since 1987, the ratio of these rates has decreased from 10:1 to 3:1, and the female proportion of HIV-related deaths has increased from 10% to 28%.[16,17]

Although the HIV-related death rate among women has stabilized at about 4.5 deaths per 100,000 among all infected women, black women experience much higher annual death rates.[16] In 2009, for example, the age-adjusted average annual rate of HIV-related death among black women was about 23.8 deaths per 100,000.[18] This rate exceeded the rates reported for men and women of all race/ethnicities except black men. HIV-infected black women also have higher death rates due to any cause compared with women of other race/ethnicities (Figure 13-3).

Natural History

Research studies are beginning to shed light on gender-related differences in the natural history of HIV infection, but much remains to be learned. The increasing rate of new infections among women, along with advances in antiretroviral therapy and viral load measurement, provide an opportunity to investigate relationships between gender, disease progression, and response to treatment.

Disease Progression and Survival

Without treatment, an estimated 50–60% of HIV-infected individuals will develop an AIDS-defining condition in 10 years[19,20] and about 50% will die within 10 years of becoming infected.[21] Early in the HIV/AIDS epidemic, HIV-infected women appeared to experience more rapid progression of illness than men. However, more recent research suggests that disease progression rates are similar, with initially observed differences largely explained by later stage of disease at diagnosis, differential access to HIV/AIDS care, and later initiation of treatment.[22] The lower circulating HIV viral load observed among women in the early stages of HIV infection appears to dissipate after several years, resulting in similar rates of progression to AIDS.[23]

Reproductive Health

One of the most striking effects of antiretroviral therapy has been the sharp decline in mother-to-child transmission of HIV. HIV can be transmitted from mother to infant during pregnancy, labor, and delivery or postnatally through breastfeeding. Without prophylactic therapy, approximately 25% of infants born to HIV-infected women will become infected.[24]

Before the 1994 discovery that zidovudine administered to HIV-infected pregnant women and their newborns could significantly reduce perinatal HIV transmission, an estimated 15,000 children were born with HIV.[25] Increased rates of prenatal HIV screening, the timely administration of appropriate antiretroviral therapy during and after pregnancy, and/or prophylaxis during and after delivery have lowered the transmission rate to less than 2%.[26] Today, fewer than 200 HIV-infected infants are born in the United States each year.[27]

In the United States, approximately one in three HIV-infected women desire to bear children.[28] With antiretroviral therapy improving the health and longevity of HIV-infected women and greatly reducing the risk of perinatal HIV transmission, women are in a stronger position to make reproductive choices. Many therapeutic options exist for effectively managing HIV during pregnancy, with most antiretroviral regimens posing little risk to the fetus. Pregnancy seems to have little influence on the course of HIV infection. Although HIV-infected women experience a decrease in specific markers of immune system function during pregnancy, this can be partly explained by the dilutional effect of the increase in plasma volume during pregnancy and does not appear to have a clinically significant effect.[29]

Comorbidities

Clinical outcomes in the antiretroviral-therapy era are influenced by multiple factors, including comorbid conditions, aging, nonantiretroviral drug toxicity, and risk of comorbid behaviors.[30] It is often difficult to distinguish between HIV-related comorbidities and the long-term toxicities of antiretroviral therapy. Comorbidities also may interact with antiretroviral effects, as in the case of interaction of alcohol with antiretroviral-related liver toxicity. Some of the most common comorbidities observed in HIV-infected women are discussed next.

Viral Hepatitis
HIV-infected women are at risk for coinfection with hepatitis B (HBV) and/or hepatitis C (HCV) because these

blood-borne pathogens are transmitted through similar routes. HBV is most often transmitted through unprotected sexual intercourse or injection drug use. HCV is transmitted most efficiently through direct exposure to contaminated blood or blood products, most often through injection drug use. Both types of viral hepatitis significantly increase the risk of liver-related morbidity and mortality.

Although HBV can be prevented through vaccination, WIHS researchers found serological evidence of HBV infection in 43% of the HIV-infected women tested for this virus between 1994 and 1995.[31] During a later (2001–2002) WIHS enrollment period, the percentage of HIV-infected women testing positive for hepatitis B core antibody dropped to 19%.[32] Among women participating in the HIV Outpatient Study (HOPS), another long-term observational cohort study, the prevalence of chronic HBV infection increased from 3.3% to 5.1% between 1996 and 2007.[33]

Longitudinal analyses of WIHS and HOPS data suggest that the percentage of HIV-infected women with HCV coinfection may be declining. Over the two WIHS enrollment periods, about 35% of the HIV-infected women tested for HCV infection were seropositive.[34] HIV-infected women enrolled between 1994 and 1995 were three times more likely to have HCV than women enrolled between 2001 and 2002 (39% vs. 13%).[32] Among female HOPS participants, the prevalence of HCV decreased from 39% in 1996 to 27% in 2007.[35] Researchers attribute these declines to a shift from injection drug use to unprotected sex as the most common mode of HIV transmission.[32]

To date, research studies have not shown any association between HBV infection, progression to AIDS, or patients' viral or immunological responses to antiretroviral therapy.[36] Current public health guidelines recommend that HIV/HBV-coinfected patients be treated with antiviral agents active against both HIV and HBV.[37]

Coinfection with HIV and HCV accelerates progression to cirrhosis, decompensated liver disease, and hepatocellular carcinoma.[38] However, HCV does not appear to affect the progression of HIV disease or to compromise immunological or virological response to HAART.[39-41] Because current HCV therapies have significant toxicity and limited efficacy, clinical experts recommend treatment for HCV coinfection only when the risk of liver disease and the prospects for successful treatment outweigh the risk of therapy-induced adverse effects.[42]

Depression
Of the various psychiatric disorders associated with HIV/AIDS, substance use disorders and depression are the most common.[43] Although HIV-infected women are more likely to report depressive symptoms than men,[44] epidemiologic studies of major depression in HIV populations show similar prevalence ranges for women and men: 2%–18% and 4%–22% respectively.[45]

Research suggests that depression causes biologic changes in endocrine and immune function that accelerate the progression of HIV disease. Significant associations have been documented between depression and poorer virologic response, increased likelihood of immunologic failure, and incident AIDS-defining illnesses.[46] Both the WIHS and the HIV Epidemiologic Research Study found that women with chronic depressive symptoms were significantly more likely to die within the study period than women with intermittent or no depressive symptoms.[47,48] Other studies suggest that positive emotions and expectancy regarding health outcomes and the ability to find meaning in the illness experience have a protective effect against HIV-related mortality and immune decline and may even improve immune system functioning.[49,50]

Despite findings that depression can significantly reduce adherence to HAART regimens,[51] many HIV care providers do not routinely screen for depression.[52] Moreover, it is not always clear whether reported symptoms, such as fatigue, insomnia, and appetite loss, are caused by depression or HIV/AIDS itself. Treatment decisions are complicated by a paucity of research on antidepressant treatment in HIV-infected women and the potential for adverse drug interactions between antidepressants and antiretroviral medications. Studies suggest that HIV-infected women with high levels of depressive symptoms may be best served through comprehensive programs that integrate medical care with psychosocial interventions and antidepressant treatment.

Menopause and Aging Issues

With increasing life expectancy, more HIV-infected women are experiencing menopausal transition. The mean age at onset (47–48 years) is slightly lower than for uninfected women (49–51 years).[53,54] However, factors independently associated with early menopause, such as drug use, smoking, and low socioeconomic status, are common among HIV-infected women, making it difficult to assess the true impact of HIV.[55-57]

HIV-infected women tend to report more menopausal symptoms than uninfected women[58] even though no significant differences in estradiol and progesterone levels have been observed.[59] Results from a multisite prospective study of menopause suggest that economic hardship, unemployment, and lower socioeconomic status may confound the relationship between HIV and reported symptoms.[60]

It is well known that menopausal women experience an increase in total cholesterol once the protective effect of estrogen is lost. What is less clear is the extent of additive effects of HIV and menopause and the relative protective versus harmful effects of the new antiretroviral agents on bone mineral density, cardiovascular disease, and lipid abnormalities.

Osteoporosis
HIV-infected women increasingly are developing conditions usually seen only in aging adults. Several studies of women with normal body weight have documented lower bone mineral density among HIV-infected women, with one study reporting 10% incidence of osteoporosis among HIV-infected women as compared to 5% among uninfected women.[61] Neither the class nor duration of

antiretroviral therapy is predictive of decreased bone mineral density.[61,62] In one study, female participants showed no evidence of bone loss after initiation of antiretroviral therapy, suggesting that earlier use of antiretroviral therapy may have some protective effect.[63]

Cardiovascular Disease

Among women, age-related increases in cardiovascular morbidity and mortality begin after menopause, climbing precipitously over the ensuing decade until their risk equals that of men. HIV infection also accelerates cardiovascular risk. For example, in one study, the rate of myocardial infarction among HIV-infected women (12.71 per 1,000 person-years) was 2.6 times higher than the rate among uninfected women (4.88 per 1,000 person-years).[64]

Although some studies of HIV-infected patients show an increased risk of myocardial infarction following the initiation of antiretroviral therapy, new research indicates that this increased risk is partially due to genetic and lifestyle-related factors.[65] There is some evidence that the new antiretroviral agents may have a protective effect. For example, a study of 36,766 Veterans Administration patients (98% male) documented small decreases in the rates and hazards of cardiovascular and cerebrovascular events and a decreased hazard of death from any cause.[66] Whether postmenopausal HIV-infected women on antiretroviral therapy can achieve the same cardiovascular benefits is not yet known.

Lipid Abnormalities

Many HIV-infected women develop lipid abnormalities, such as hypertriglyceridemia (i.e., a condition of elevated cholesterol or triglyceride concentration in the blood), that increase their risk for cardiovascular disease. In a large study of untreated HIV-infected individuals, women had significantly higher levels of high-density lipoproteins and cholesterol than men.[67] Certain classes of antiretroviral agents also elevate lipids in the bloodstream, causing abnormalities in the adipose tissue that contains stored cellular fat.[68] In one multicenter study, 42% of HIV-infected women experienced adipose tissue alterations, as compared to 30% of men.[69] The gender-specific impact of newer antiretroviral agents on lipid levels and adipose tissue alterations is not yet known.

HIV Risk Factors and Prevention Strategies

Among U.S. women, the primary mode of HIV transmission is unprotected sexual intercourse with an already infected male. The CDC estimates that 72% of U.S. women living with HIV/AIDS acquired HIV through high-risk heterosexual sex, with an additional 26% acquiring HIV through injection drug use.[1] Although HIV can be acquired through mucous membrane exposure to vaginal secretions and menstrual blood, CDC has not yet received any confirmed cases of female-to-female transmission.[70]

HIV Risk Factors

Early Sexual Intercourse

An estimated 26–50% of U.S. residents infected through high-risk heterosexual sex contract HIV during their teens or early 20s.[71] As compared to young men, young women tend to have older sexual partners, putting them at risk for infection at an earlier age. Results from the 2002 National Survey of Family Growth, a nationally representative survey, indicate that women first engage in premarital sex at a median age of 17.2 years.[72] Thirteen percent of the women responding to this survey reported first having premarital sex by age 15, 54% by age 18, and 74% by age 20.

Sexually Transmitted Infections

Inflammatory and ulcerative infections greatly increase the likelihood of acquiring and transmitting HIV.[73] Sexually transmitted infections (STIs) make women more susceptible to HIV by creating breaks in the genital tract lining and increasing the number of CD4 cells in cervical secretions that can serve as targets for HIV. People coinfected with HIV and other STIs are more likely to shed HIV in their genital secretions, thereby heightening the risk of HIV transmission.[74] Because STIs are treatable, early detection and prompt treatment are critical for HIV prevention.

During 2009, women ages 15–24 accounted for the highest number of reported cases of chlamydia and gonorrhea.[75] Within this age category, women ages 15–19 had higher rates of reported chlamydia than women ages 20–24 (3,329.3 per 100,000 vs. 3,273.9 per 100,000). Women ages 15–19 also had higher gonorrhea rates (568.8 per 100,000 vs. 555.3 per 100,000). Between 2005 and 2009, the rate of primary and secondary syphilis among women ages 15–19 increased from 1.9 per 100,000 to 3.3 per 100,000. Among women ages 20–24, the rate increased from 3.0 per 100,000 to 5.6 per 100,000.

Over the years, minority women have experienced higher rates of sexually transmitted disease than white women. In 2009, for example, the rate of chlamydia among black women (2,096 per 100,000) was almost eight times higher than the rate among white women (270 per 100,000).[75] Higher chlamydia rates also were reported for American Indian/Alaska Native women (1,215 per 100,000) and Hispanic women (789 per 100,000).

More than one-quarter of U.S. women are infected with genital human papillomavirus (HPV), a major cause of neoplasias involving the female reproductive tract.[76] Although 90% of women with HPV infection naturally clear the virus within 2 years,[77] this percentage is lower among women with HIV.[78] HIV-infected women are at greater risk for HPV infection and for progression to HPV-related diseases, such as cervical intraepithelial neoplasia, the precursor to cervical cancer.[79-83] Two vaccines offer effective protection against the types of HPV that cause most cervical cancers. However, these vaccines are not recommended for women older than 26 years or for women previously infected with any strain of HPV.[84]

Among coinfected women, low CD4 count and high viral load are associated with a moderate increase in HPV persistence.[79] The impact of HIV-related antiretroviral therapy on HPV incidence and persistence remains unclear.[85] There is some evidence that HIV/HPV coinfection may hasten the progression of HIV (lower CD4 count and higher viral load), but this relationship also requires further investigation.[79]

Injection Drug Use

Although the percentage of U.S. women infected through injection drug use has declined since the early years of the HIV/AIDS epidemic, injecting drug users accounted for 14% of female incident HIV cases in 2007.[86] Female injection drug users tend to be diagnosed at a later stage of disease than heterosexually infected women, underscoring the critical need for outreach activities that integrate clean needle exchange with HIV prevention education and testing.

HIV Prevention Strategies

Over the next decade, the key HIV prevention challenges will be to reach diverse populations of high-risk women with age- and culturally-appropriate messages and to garner sufficient resources to support these interventions. As noted by the Joint United Nations Programme on HIV/AIDS, effective HIV prevention will require comprehensive and multimethod HIV interventions:

> Condoms are an essential part of combination prevention, which includes among other elements: access to information about HIV, access to treatment, harm reduction measures, waiting longer to become sexually active, being faithful, reducing multiple partners and concurrent relationships, male circumcision, ensuring human rights, and the reduction of stigma.[87]

Examples of effective HIV prevention programs targeted toward women, especially black women, can be found at the CDC's website on evidence-based HIV prevention interventions (http://www.cdc.gov/hiv/topics/research/prs/evidence-based-interventions.htm), the National Women's Health Information Center website (http://www.womenshealth.gov/hiv-aids/preventing-hiv-infection/), and the websites of AIDS-related organizations such as the National Minority AIDS Council (http://www.nmac.org). Organizations serving women, such as Planned Parenthood, typically integrate HIV prevention, testing, and counseling into their programs and offer HIV prevention education resources.

Over the past decade, HIV prevention programs have increasingly focused on "prevention with positives." The objective of these programs is to help HIV-infected individuals change behaviors that put their sex and/or needle-sharing partners at risk for infection. Studies indicate that the likelihood of unprotected sexual behavior is significantly higher among individuals who believe that HAART reduces the risk of HIV transmission during unprotected sex or who perceive HIV/AIDS as a less threatening disease because of HAART availability.[88] These beliefs may help explain why WIHS participants were more likely to report unprotected vaginal sex after HAART initiation.[89]

Prevention Funding

In fiscal year 2009, federal agencies distributed more than $3.1 billion for HIV prevention, treatment, and support services.[90] CDC's distribution of about half a billion dollars for HIV prevention activities accounted for only 17% of this amount.[91] Even with additional support from private foundations and state and local governments, total prevention expenditures were dwarfed by the amounts spent on HIV treatment and care.

HIV Prevention Research

Vaccines

Greater investments in HIV prevention, along with a reinvigorated portfolio of prevention interventions, should help reduce HIV incidence. However, an effective vaccine will be needed to completely eradicate the disease. Through clinical trials networks, such as the HIV Vaccine Trials Network and the U.S. Military HIV Research Program, a number of approaches to vaccination are in various stages of development. In the fall of 2009, researchers announced the first partially effective results from the RV144 Prime-Boost HIV Vaccine Clinical Trial in Thailand.[92] Preliminary results showed that an ALVAC-HIV primer vaccine followed by an AIDSVAX B/E booster reduced the risk of HIV infection by about 31%.

Microbicides

In addition to vaccines, researchers are investigating the safety and effectiveness of microbicides in reducing the risk of acquiring or transmitting HIV and other sexually transmitted diseases. Women are more likely than men to acquire HIV via sexual intercourse due to greater exposed surface area in the female genital tract. Yet, many women feel powerless to negotiate condom use. As a possible solution to this problem, a clinical trial conducted in South Africa between May 2007 and March 2010 assessed the effectiveness and safety of a vaginal tenofovir gel microbicide for HIV prevention.[93] Tenofovir gel reduced HIV acquisition by an estimated 39% overall and by 54% in women with high gel adherence. Once effective microbicides become more widely available, women will be able to apply them topically to the vagina without having to depend on their partners' cooperation.

Male Circumcision

Three clinical trials in Africa have documented a 50–60% reduction in HIV acquisition among men who are circumcised.[94-96] Although mass male circumcision may reduce women's risk of exposure to HIV at a population level, a protective effect for women has not been shown on an individual level. In Rakai, Uganda, for example, a 24-month study of serodiscordant couples found that circumcision of HIV-infected men did not reduce HIV transmission to female partners.[97] However, studies have demonstrated that male circumcision reduces the incidence and prevalence of high-risk HPV in female partners of circumcised men.[98,99]

Viral load suppression

Studies of serodiscordant heterosexual couples suggest that viral load suppression through antiretroviral therapy reduces the risk of HIV transmission.[100] Antiretroviral therapy holds considerable promise for slowing the transmission of HIV if prevention benefits are not offset by increases in risk behavior. Further research is needed to determine the extent to which virological suppression in the blood is associated with suppression in the genital fluids and to assess the applicability of these findings to other populations at risk for HIV.

HIV Testing and Follow-Up

Despite federal efforts to increase HIV screening, an estimated 53,200 women—19% of all U.S. women living with HIV—are unaware of their infection.[101] The high prevalence of undiagnosed HIV infection among U.S. women has enormous public health implications. First, women unaware of their infection are more likely to engage in high-risk activities that contribute to the spread of HIV. Second, women diagnosed with HIV late in the course of their infection often are too severely immunocompromised to benefit from antiretroviral therapy.

In 1985, the U.S. Food and Drug Administration licensed the first enzyme immunoassay (EIA) to screen for HIV antibody. Over the next 2 decades, public health guidelines recommended targeted testing of people with "high-risk" behaviors. In 2006, CDC sought to increase opportunities for early diagnosis by recommending that all patients aged 13–64 years be screened for HIV as part of routine clinical care. To simplify the screening process, CDC recommended that patients be informed orally or in writing that HIV testing would be performed unless they declined. This "opt-out" approach replaced earlier recommendations that patients receive pretest counseling and provide separate written consent.

Each year, the National Center for Health Statistics conducts a large-scale National Health Interview Survey (NHIS) of a statistically representative sample of U.S. adults aged 18 and older. Published results from these surveys indicate that, between 2002 and 2009, the percentage of women reporting at least one HIV test increased from 38% to 45%. As shown in Figure 13-4, the percentage of black women reporting at least one HIV test increased from 52% to 62% over this time period. Increases also were noted for Hispanic women (39% to 49%) and white women (35% to 41%). Despite these upward trends, testing rates remain suboptimal for women of all races and ethnicities.

Since the 1994 discovery that zidovudine could substantially reduce perinatal HIV transmission, the U.S. Public Health Service, the American College of Obstetricians and Gynecologists, and many other health professional organizations have recommended that HIV screening be included in the routine panel of prenatal tests. Although increasing numbers of pregnant women are being screened for HIV, national and state surveys indicate that this test has not yet become a routine part of prenatal care. Between 1995 and 2002, the percentage of pregnant women reporting an

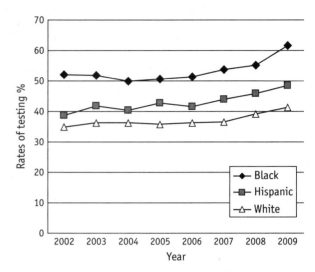

Figure 13-4 Age-adjusted percent distributions of human immunodeficiency virus testing status among women ≥ 18 years by race/ethnicity.

Source: Data from Table 41, Summary Health Statistics for U.S. Adults: National Health Interview Surveys, 2002–2009. http://www.cdc.gov/nchs/products/series.htm#sr10. Accessed January 14, 2011

HIV test in the past 12 months rose from 41% to 54%.[102,103] In the 2006 NHIS, 61% of pregnant women reported an HIV test in the past 12 months.[104] This percentage still is much lower than the ≥97% screening rates reported for other perinatally transmitted infectious diseases.[105] Data reported by 33 states with perinatal HIV-exposure reporting systems indicate that almost one-third of women giving birth to HIV-infected infants are not tested for HIV until after delivery.[106]

As noted earlier in this chapter, untreated individuals with HIV have a 2% probability of progressing to AIDS in the first 2 years following infection and a 50% probability at 10 years.[107] Thus, an AIDS diagnosis within 12 months of the initial HIV diagnosis suggests late testing for HIV infection. CDC's *HIV/AIDS Surveillance Reports* show that, between 2001 and 2006, the percentage of HIV-infected females (≥13 years) diagnosed with AIDS less than 12 months after the initial HIV diagnosis fluctuated between 32% and 36%. During 2007 and 2008, the percentages hovered between 30% and 31%.

Changes in HIV testing techniques and policies have reduced some barriers to HIV testing. Patients no longer have to wait a few days to 2 weeks to receive their test results. Rapid HIV tests yield results in 30 minutes or less, with sensitivities and specificities comparable to those of conventional EIAs. Universal HIV screening policies and the availability of new antiretroviral treatments have helped allay the fear and stigma associated with HIV testing. Although the opt-out approach is expected to increase HIV testing rates—especially among pregnant women—studies suggest that women who underestimate their risk for HIV infection may continue to decline testing.

The healthcare community has not yet reached consensus on whether clinicians should routinely screen female (or male) patients for HIV. Major medical associations have voiced strong support for routine testing. However,

Table 13-4

Centers for Disease Control and Prevention staging system for classifying Human Immunodeficiency Virus-infected adults

CD4 cell count, cells/mm3 (CD4 cell percentage)[a]	CDC Classification		
	A[b]	B[c]	C[d]
>500 (>29)	A1	B1	C1
200–500 (14–28)	A2	B2	C2
<200 (<14)	A3	B3	C3

Source: Data from Centers for Disease Control and Prevention. 1993 revised classification system for HIV infection and expanded surveillance case definition for AIDS among adolescents and adults. *MMWR* 1992;41:1–17. Available at http://www.cdc.gov/mmwr/preview/mmwrhtml/00018871.htm. Accessed January 24, 2010.

[a]The CD4 cell count and CD4 cell percentage provide a snapshot of the health of an individual's immune system. The more CD4 cells in circulation, the stronger the immune system. The CD4 percentage represents the percentage of all functional lymphocytes that are CD4 cells. By considering both CD4 cell count and CD4 cell percentage, clinicians and their patients can determine the best time to initiate HIV therapy.

[b]Asymptomatic, persistent generalized lymphadenopathy, or acute human immunodeficiency virus infection

[c]Symptomatic (not A or C)

[d]AIDS indicator condition

after reviewing available evidence on HIV screening effectiveness, the U.S. Preventive Services Task Force concluded that the benefits of screening people without risk factors were "too small relative to potential harms to justify a general recommendation."[108] Questions also have been raised about reimbursement for routine testing. Although CDC funds HIV testing in health departments and community-based settings, very few of these sites have adequate resources to conduct routine testing. Most private insurers and state Medicaid programs cover HIV testing only when known risk factors have been reported or clinical indications of infection are detected. Medicare reimbursement policies limit coverage to beneficiaries at increased risk for HIV infection.

As more women are screened for HIV, testing sites will be increasingly challenged to build internal capacity to provide HIV care and/or to develop effective referral systems. CDC researchers estimate that only 52% of newly diagnosed women are successfully linked to medical care within 12 months.[109] Studies indicate that the most effective strategies for transitioning HIV-infected clients from diagnosis to specialized HIV care include proactive case managers, intensive client contact, and client training on how to navigate the healthcare system.[110,111] The ability of testing sites to implement these strategies will depend upon the availability of HIV care providers, financial support for dedicated case managers, and the clinical staff's time and preparedness to counsel women about positive test results.

Diagnosis and Treatment

If left untreated, HIV leads to advanced immune suppression and AIDS. However, effective antiretroviral therapy has enabled acutely ill people diagnosed with AIDS to revert to a healthier state. To address this added complexity, CDC has developed a Clinical Staging System for HIV/AIDS that accounts for laboratory parameters of immunosuppression (e.g., CD4 cell count) and previous diagnosis of an HIV-related condition. As shown in Table 13-4, this staging system uses categories of disease (A, B, C) to further specify stages of disease.

For people with access to high-quality HIV/AIDS care and affordable medicine, HAART regimens have changed HIV from a universally fatal disease to a chronic disease. Entering into HIV treatment early in the course of disease decreases the risk for cardiovascular disease and AIDS-related cancers, lowers rates of treatment side effects and HIV drug resistance, and appears to extend longevity. In light of this evidence, the U.S. Department of Health and Human Services Panel on Antiretroviral Guidelines for Adults and Adolescents recommends that antiretroviral therapy be initiated in patients with a history of an AIDS-defining illness and/or CD4 counts ≤ 500 cells/mm^3.[37]

Studies of HIV-infected women suggest that the receipt of HAART is influenced by race/ethnicity, insurance status, and substance use behaviors.[112-114] A WIHS analysis of disparities in HAART use found that, in 2005, 29% of clinically eligible women were not on a HAART regimen.[114] Black women were twice as likely as white women to report nonuse, even after taking health insurance status into account. Regardless of race/ethnicity, uninsured women were two times more likely to report nonuse than women with Medicaid coverage. Surprisingly, women with private health insurance were less likely than Medicaid enrollees to report HAART use. The researchers hypothesized that higher copayments and deductibles or physicians with less HIV experience at their care sites might explain this finding. Women reporting moderate alcohol consumption were 1.72 times more likely to report nonuse than their nondrinking counterparts.

To date, no studies have found gender-based differences in clinical progression of HIV during long-term antiretroviral therapy.[115] However, gender-based differences in adverse reactions to antiretroviral therapy do exist. For example, nevirapine, an antiretroviral drug frequently used in the United States, and which serves as the backbone of treatment regimens in many developing countries, is associated with increased risk of liver toxicity in women.[116]

Gender Differences in Opportunistic Infections

The manifestation and frequency of opportunistic infections are similar among HIV-infected women and men with a few notable exceptions. Gynecological infections and cancers are a common manifestation of HIV-related immunosuppression in women. Kaposi's sarcoma, a cancer associated with HIV immunosuppression, occurs most frequently in men who have sex with men.

Adherence to Antiretroviral Therapy

Total adherence to the treatment regimen is needed for HAART to be most effective. Yet, most women and men find it difficult to maintain the strict adherence levels required. A prospective observational study of 161 HIV-infected women taking antiretroviral therapy found that adherence varied over time, decreasing from a mean of 64% in the first month of observation to 45% in month 6.[117] Virologic failure (defined as a viral load ≥500 RNA copies/ml) occurred in 71% of the women with ≤12% adherence and 43% of those with 13–44% adherence, as compared to only 17% of women with adherence ≥88%.

Adherence to antiretroviral therapy is influenced by multiple factors, including the complexity of the drug regimen, forgetting to take pills, depression, coinfections, treatment-related side effects, and the stigma associated with HIV/AIDS. Adherence also is inversely associated with the number of children living in the household, and the perceived level of difficulty in caring for them.[118] To effectively address these adherence barriers, high-quality HIV/AIDS care requires the incorporation of social and behavioral interventions. Methods of supporting adherence range from patient education, case management, and peer support to directly observed therapy and directly administered antiretroviral therapy.[119]

Summary

Although women constitute a minority of the U.S. population living with HIV/AIDS, their proportion has steadily increased since the early years of the epidemic. The growing numbers highlight the critical need for female-specific approaches to lowering HIV incidence, increasing HIV testing rates, and enhancing access to HIV/AIDS care. These new approaches must be driven by and targeted toward women at high risk for HIV infection, especially women from minority communities. Economic and social factors affecting HIV risk also influence access to treatment; these include poverty, unstable housing, single parenthood, and domestic violence, will need to be addressed. Moreover, women require reliable health insurance, HIV-knowledgeable clinicians who provide gynecological as well as general medical care, and affordable child care to fully engage in HIV/AIDS treatment. Addressing these issues will lay a strong foundation for women to benefit from future vaccines, microbicides, and treatments as they become available.

Discussion Questions

1. How many women are estimated to be living with HIV in the United States? What groups of women are most at risk for this disease?

2. What are the leading risk factors for HIV/AIDS among U.S. women? How have these risk factors changed over the course of the U.S. epidemic?

3. Among U.S. women, what are some of the most common morbidities associated with HIV/AIDS? How do these comorbidities affect HAART adherence and clinical outcomes?

4. How does pregnancy affect the course of HIV infection?

5. What are some examples of effective HIV prevention programs targeted toward women?

6. What areas of research may lead to new HIV prevention modalities?

7. What are the individual and public health benefits of early HIV detection?

8. What factors influence women's adherence to antiretroviral therapy?

References

1. Centers for Disease Control and Prevention. HIV prevalence estimates—United States, 2006. *MMWR Morb Mortal Wkly Rep.* 2008;57:1073–1076.

2. AIDS.gov. U.S. .statistics. 2011. http://aids.gov/hiv-aids-basics/hiv-aids-101/overview/statistics. Accessed February 25, 2011.

3. Centers for Disease Control and Prevention. Diagnoses of HIV infection among adult and adolescent females, by race/ethnicity, 2007–2010—46 states and 5 U.S. dependent areas. http://www.cdc.gov/hiv/topics/surveillance/resources/slides/women/slides/Women.pdf. Accessed February 25, 2011.

4. Centers for Disease Control and Prevention. Subpopulation estimates from the HIV incidence surveillance system—United States, 2006. *MMWR Morb Mortal Wkly Rep.* 2008;57:985–989.

5. Tatem AJ, Rogers DJ, Hay SI. Global transport networks and infectious disease spread. *Adv Parasitol.* 2006;62:293–343.

6. Centers for Disease Control and Prevention. Pneumocystis pneumonia—Los Angeles. *MMWR Morb Mortal Wkly Rep.* 1981;30:250–252.

7. Centers for Disease Control and Prevention. Current trends classification system for human t-lymphotropic virus type III/ lymphadenopathy-associated virus infections. *MMWR Morb Mortal Wkly Rep.* 1986;35:334–339.

8. Centers for Disease Control and Prevention. 1993 revised classification system for HIV infection and expanded surveillance case definition for AIDS among adolescents and adults. *MMWR Morb Mortal Wkly Rep.* 1992;41:1–17.

9. Hall HI, Song R, Rhodes P, et al. Estimation of HIV incidence in the United States. *JAMA.* 2008;300:520–529.

10. UNAIDS and World Health Organization. *2009 AIDS Epidemic Update.* Geneva, Switzerland: UNAIDS; December 2009. http://data.unaids.org/pub/Report/2009/JC1700_Epi_Update_2009_en.pdf. Accessed January 14, 2010.

11. Centers for Disease Control and Prevention. HIV among African Americans. 2010. http://www.cdc.gov/hiv/topics/aa/resources/factsheets/aa.htm. Accessed February 23, 2011.

12. Tillerson K. Explaining racial disparities in HIV/AIDS incidence among women in the U.S.: a systematic review. *Statist Med.* 2008;27:4132–4143.

13. Moreno CL. The relationship between culture, gender, structural factors, abuse, trauma, and HIV/AIDS for Latinas. *Qual Health Res.* 2007;17:340–352.

14. Centers for Disease Control and Prevention. Deaths due to HIV disease are not exactly the same as deaths of persons with AIDS. 2009. http://www.cdc.gov/hiv/topics/surveillance/resources/slides/mortality/slides/mortality3.pdf. Accessed February 22, 2011.

15. French, AL, Gawel, SH, Hershow, R, et al. Trends in mortality and causes of death among women with HIV in the United States: a ten-year study. *J Acquir Immune Defic Syndr.* 2009;51:399–406.

16. Centers for Disease Control and Prevention. Trends in annual age-adjusted rate of death due to HIV disease, by sex, United States, 1987–2008. 2009. http://www.cdc.gov/hiv/topics/surveillance/resources/slides/mortality/slides/mortality.pdf. Accessed February 22, 2011.

17. Centers for Disease Control and Prevention. Trends in the percentage distribution of deaths due to HIV disease, by sex, United States, 1987–2008. http://www.cdc.gov/hiv/topics/surveillance/resources/slides/mortality/slides/mortality.pdf. Accessed February 22, 2011.

18. Centers for Disease Control and Prevention. Age-adjusted average annual rate of death due to HIV disease by sex and race/ethnicity, United States, 2004–2008. Available at http://www.cdc.gov/hiv/topics/surveillance/resources/slides/mortality/slides/mortality.pdf. Accessed February 22, 2011.

19. Muñoz A, Wang MC, Bass S, et al. Acquired immunodeficiency syndrome (AIDS)—free time after human immunodeficiency virus type 1 (HIV-1) sero-conversion in homosexual men. *Am J Epidemiol.* 1989;130:530–539.

20. Rutherford GW, Lifson AR, Hessol NA, et al. Course of HIV-1 infection in a cohort of homosexual and bisexual men: an 11 year follow up study. *BMJ.* 1990;301:1183–1188.

21. Vella S, Giuliano M, Pezzotti P, et al. Survival of zidovudine-treated patients with AIDS compared with that of contemporary untreated patients. Italian Zidovudine Evaluation Group. *JAMA.* 1992;267:1232–1236.

22. Umeh OC, Currier JS. Sex differences in HIV: natural history, pharmacokinetics, and drug toxicity. *Curr Infect Dis Rep.* 2005;7:73–78.

23. Sterling TR, Vlahov D, Astemborski J, Hoover DR, Margolick JB, Quinn TC. Initial plasma HIV-1 RNA levels and progression of AIDS in women and men. *N Engl J Med.* 2001;344:720–725.

24. Connor EM, Sperling RS, Gelber R, et al. Reduction of maternal-infant transmission of human immunodeficiency virus type 1 with zidovudine treatment. *New Engl J Med.* 1994;331:1173–1180.

25. Centers for Disease Control and Prevention. Update: perinatally acquired HIV/AIDS—United States, 1997. *MMWR Morb Mortal Wkly Rep.* 1997; 46:1086–1092.

26. Mofenson LM. Advances in the prevention of vertical transmission of human immunodeficiency virus. *Semin Pediatr Infect Dis.* 2003;14:295–308.

27. Panel on Treatment of HIV-Infected Pregnant Women and Prevention of HIV Transmission. *Recommendations for Use of Antiretroviral Drugs in Pregnant HIV-1-Infected Women for Maternal Health and Interventions to Reduce Perinatal HIV Transmission in the United States.* May 24, 2010. http://www.aidsinfo.nih.gov/contentfiles/PerinatalGL.pdf. Accessed February 22, 2011.

28. Chen JL, Phillips KA, Kanouse DE, Collins RL, Miu A. Fertility desires and intentions of HIV-positive men and women. *Fam Plann Perspect.* 2001;33:144–152.

29. Anderson JR. HIV and reproduction. In: Anderson JR, ed. *A Guide to the Clinical Care of Women with HIV/AIDS. 2005 Edition.* Rockville, MD: HIV/AIDS Bureau, Health Resources and Services Administration; 2005: 241–330. http://hab.hrsa.gov/deliverhivaidscare/files/clinicalcareguide2005.pdf. Accessed February 23, 2011.

30. Justice AC. Prioritizing primary care in HIV: comorbidity, toxicity, and demography. *Top HIV Med.* 2007;14:159–163.

31. Tien PC, Kovacs A, Bacchetti P, et al. Association between syphilis, antibodies to herpes simplex virus type 2, and recreational drug use and hepatitis B virus infection in the Women's Interagency HIV Study. *Clin Infect Dis.* 2004; 39:1363–1370.

32. Bacon MC, von Wyl V, Alden C, et al. The Women's Interagency HIV Study: an observational cohort brings clinical sciences to the bench. *Clin Diagn Lab Immunol.* 2005;12:1013–1019.

33. Spradling PR, Richardson JT, Buchacz K, et al. Prevalence of chronic hepatitis B virus infection among patients in the HIV Outpatient Study, 1996–2007. *J Viral Hepat.* 2010;17:879–886.

34. Tsui J, Vittinghoff E, Anastos K, et al. Hepatitis C seropositivity and kidney function decline among women with HIV: data from the Women's Interagency HIV Study. *Am J Kidney Dis.* 2009;54:43–50.

35. Spradling PR, Richardson JT, Buchacz K, et al. Trends in hepatitis C virus infection among patients in the HIV Outpatient Study, 1996–2007. *J Acquir Immune Defic Syndr.* 2010;53:388–396.

36. Sulkowski MS. Viral hepatitis and HIV coinfection. *J Viral Hepat.* 2008;48:353–367.

37. Panel on Antiretroviral Guidelines for Adults and Adolescents. Guidelines for the use of antiretroviral agents in HIV-1-infected adults and adolescents. Department of Health and Human Services. January 10, 2011. http://www.aidsinfo.nih.gov/ContentFiles/AdultandAdolescentGL.pdf. Accessed January 18, 2011.

38. Koziel MJ, Peters MG. Viral hepatitis in HIV infection. *N Engl J Med.* 2007;356:1445–1454.

39. Al-Harthi L, Voris J, Du W, et al. Evaluating the impact of hepatitis C virus (HCV) on highly active antiretroviral therapy-mediated immune responses in HCV/HIV-coinfected women: role of HCV on expression of premed/memory t cells. *J Infect Dis.* 2006;193:1202–1210.

40. Hershow RC, O'Driscoll PT, Handelsman E, et al. Hepatitis C virus coinfection and HIV load, CD4+ cell percentage, and clinical progression to AIDS or death among HIV-infected women: Women and Infants Transmission Study. *Clin Infect Dis.* 2005;40:859–867.

41. Sullivan PS, Hanson DL, Teshale EH, Wotring LL, Brooks JT. Effect of hepatitis C infection on progression of HIV disease and early response to initial antiretroviral therapy. *AIDS.* 2006;20:1171–1179.

42. Sulkowski MS. Management of hepatic complications in HIV-infected persons. *J Infect Dis.* 2008;197:S279–293.

43. Jones DJ, Roberts GW. Substance abuse, HIV, and mental health issues: prevention and treatment challenges. In: Smith KY, Rawlings MK, Ojikutu B, Stone V, eds. *HIV/AIDS in U.S. Communities of Color.* New York: Springer; 2009:229.

44. Chander G, Himelhoch S, Moore RD. Substance abuse and psychiatric disorders in HIV-positive patients: epidemiology and impact on antiretroviral therapy. *Drugs.* 2006;66:769–789.

45. Benton TD. Depression and HIV/AIDS. *Curr Psychiatry Rep.* 2008;10: 280–285.

46. Anastos K, Schneider MF, Gange SJ, et al. The association of race, sociodemographic, and behavioral characteristics with response to highly active antiretroviral therapy in women. *J Acquir Immune Defic Syndr.* 2005;39:537–544.

47. Cook JA, Grey D, Burke J, et al. Depressive symptoms and AIDS-related mortality among a multisite cohort of HIV-positive women. *Am J Public Health.* 2004;94:1133–1140.

48. Ickovics JR, Hamburger ME, Vlahov D, et al. Mortality, CD4 cell count decline, and depressive symptoms among HIV-seropositive women: longitudinal analysis from the HIV Epidemiology Research Study. *JAMA.* 2001;285:1466–1474.

49. Cruess DG, Douglas SD, Petitto JM, et al. Association of resolution of major depression with increased natural killer cell activity among HIV-seropositive women. *Am J Psychiatry.* 2005;162:2125–2130.

50. Ickovics JR, Milan S, Boland R, Schoenbaum E, Schuman P, Vlahov D. Psychological resources protect health: 5-year survival and immune function among HIV-infected women from four U.S. cities. *AIDS.* 2006;20:1851–1860.

51. Horberg MA, Silverberg MJ, Hurley LB, et al. Effect of depression and selective serotonin reuptake inhibitor use on adherence to highly active antiretroviral therapy and on clinical outcomes in HIV-infected patients. *J Acquir Immune Defic Syndr.* 2008;47:384–390.

52. Rabkin JG. HIV and depression: 2008 review and update. *Curr HIV/AIDS Rep.* 2008;5:163–171.

53. Ortiz AP, Harlow SD, Sowers M, Nan B, Romaguera J. Age at natural menopause and factors associated with menopause state among Puerto Rican women aged 40–59 years, living in Puerto Rico. *Menopause.* 2006;13: 116–124.

54. Palmer JR, Rosenberg L, Wise LA, Horton NJ, Adams-Campbell LL. Onset of natural menopause in African American women. *Am J Public Health.* 2003;93:299–306.

55. McKinlay SM, Bifano NL, McKinlay JB. Smoking and age at menopause in women. *Ann Intern Med.* 1985;103:350–356.

56. Santoro N, Arnsten JH, Buono D, Howard AA, Schoenbaum EE. Impact of street drug use, HIV infection, and highly active antiretroviral therapy on reproductive hormones in middle-aged women. *J Womens Health.* 2005;14:898–905.

57. Schoenbaum EE, Hartel D, Lo Y, et al. HIV infection, drug use, and onset of natural menopause. *Clin Infect Dis.* 2005;41:1517–1524.

58. Miller SA, Santoro N, Lo Y, et al. Menopause symptoms in HIV-infected and drug-using women. *Menopause.* 2005;12:348–356.

59. Cu-Uvin S, Wright DJ, Anderson D, et al. Hormonal levels among HIV-1-seropositive women compared with high-risk HIV seronegative women during the menstrual cycle. Women's Health Study (WHS) 001 and WHS 001a study team. *J Womens Health Gend Based Med.* 2000;9:857–863.

60. Avis NE, Stellato R, Crawford S, et al. Is there a menopausal syndrome? Menopausal status and symptoms across racial/ethnic groups. *Soc Sci Med.* 2001;52:345–356.

61. Dolan SE, Huang JS, Killilea KM, Sullivan MP, Aliabadi N, Grinspoon S. Reduced bone density in HIV-infected women. *AIDS.* 2004;18:475–483.

62. Briot K, Kolta S, Flandre P, et al. Prospective one-year bone loss in treatment-naïve HIV+ men and women on single or multiple drug HIV therapies. *Bone.* 2011;48:1133–1139.

63. Amorosa V, Tebas P. Bone disease and HIV infection. *Clin Infect Dis.* 2006;42:108–114.

64. Triant VA, Lee H, Hadigan C, Grinspoon SK. Increased acute myocardial infarction rates and cardiovascular risk factors among patients with human immunodeficiency virus disease. *J Clin Endocrinol Metab.* 2007;92:2506–2512.

65. Rasmussen LD, Omland LH, Pedersen C, et al. Risk of myocardial infarction in parents of HIV-infected individuals: a population-based cohort study. *BMC Infect Dis.* 2010:14;10:169. http://www.biomedcentral.com/content/pdf/1471-2334-10-169.pdf. Accessed February 22, 2011.

66. Bozzette SA, Ake CF, Tam HK, Chang SW, Louis TA. Cardiovascular and cerebrovascular events in patients treated for human immunodeficiency virus infection. *N Engl J Med.* 2003;348:702–710.

67. El-Sadr WM, Mullin CM, Carr A, et al. Effects of HIV disease on lipid, glucose and insulin levels: results from a large antiretroviral naïve cohort. *HIV Med.* 2005;6:114–121.

68. Fontas E, van Leth F, Sabin CA, et al. Lipid profiles in patients receiving antiretroviral therapy: are different antiretroviral drugs associated with different lipid profiles? *J Infect Dis.* 2004;189:1056–1074.

69. Galli M, Veglia F, Angarano G, et al. Gender differences in antiretroviral drug-related adipose tissue alterations. Women are at higher risk than men and develop particular lipodystrophy patterns. *J Acquir Immune Defic Syndr.* 2003;34:58–61.

70. Centers for Disease Control and Prevention. HIV/AIDS among women who have sex with women. June 2006. http://www.cdc.gov/hiv/topics/women/resources/factsheets/wsw.htm. Accessed February 23, 2011.

71. Hader SL, Smith DK, Moore JS, Holmberg SD. HIV infection in women in the United States: status at the millennium. *JAMA*. 2001;285:1186–1192.

72. Finer LB. Trends in premarital sex in the United States, 1954-2003. *Public Health Rep*. 2007;122:73–78.

73. Risbud A, Chan-Tack K, Gadkari D, et al. The etiology of genital ulcer disease by multiplex polymerase chain reaction and relationship to HIV infection among patients attended sexually transmitted disease clinics in Pune, India. *Sex Transm Dis*. 1999;26:55–62.

74. Centers for Disease Control and Prevention. The role of STD detection and treatment in HIV prevention—CDC fact sheet. 2010. http://www.cdc.gov/std/hiv/STDFact-STD-HIV.htm. Accessed February 19, 2011.

75. Centers for Disease Control and Prevention. *Sexually Transmitted Disease Surveillance, 2009*. 2010. http://www.cdc.gov/std/stats09/toc.htm. Accessed February 22, 2011.

76. Dunne EF, Unger ER, Sternberg M, et al. Prevalence of HPV infection among females in the United States. *JAMA*. 2007;297:813–819.

77. Ho GYF, Bierman R, Beardsley L, Chang CJ, Burk RD. Natural history of cervicovaginal papillomavirus infection in young women. *N Engl J Med*. 1998;338:423–428.

78. Moscicki AB, Ellenberg JH, Farhat S, Xu J. Persistence of human papillomavirus infection in HIV-infected and -uninfected adolescent girls: risk factors and differences, by phylogenetic type. *J Infect Dis*. 2004;190:37–45.

79. Strickler HD, Burk RD, Fazzari M, et al. Natural history and possible reactivation of human papillomavirus in human immunodeficiency virus positive women. *J Natl Cancer Inst*. 2005;97:577–586.

80. Wright TC, Ellerbrock TV, Chiasson MA, et al. Cervical intraepithelial neoplasia in women infected with human immunodeficiency virus: prevalence, risk factors, and validity of Papanicolaou smears. New York Cervical Disease Study. *Obstet Gynecol*. 1994;84:591–597.

81. Massad LS, Riester KA, Anastos KM, et al. Prevalence and predictors of squamous cell abnormalities in Papanicolaou smears from women infected with HIV-1. *J Acquir Immune Defic Syndr*. 1999;21:33–41.

82. Massad LS, Ahdieh L, Benning L, et al. Evolution of cervical abnormalities among women with HIV-1: evidence from surveillance cytology in the Women's Interagency HIV Study. *J Acquir Immune Defic Syndr*. 2001;27:432–442.

83. Massad LS, Seaberg EC, Watts DH, et al. Low incidence of invasive cervical cancer among HIV-infected U.S. women in a prevention program. *AIDS*. 2004;18:109–113.

84. Immunization Action Coalition. Ask the experts: human papillomavirus (HPV). 2010. http://www.immunize.org/askexperts/experts_hpv.asp. Accessed February 23, 2011.

85. Shrestha S, Sudenga SL, Smith JS, Bachmann LH, Wilson CM, Kempf MC. The impact of highly active antiretroviral therapy on prevalence and incidence of cervical human papillomavirus infections in HIV-positive adolescents. *BMC Infect Dis*. 2010;10:295.

86. Centers for Disease Control and Prevention. *HIV/AIDS Surveillance Report, 2007*. 2009. http://www.cdc.gov/hiv/surveillance/resources/reports/2007report/table20.htm. Accessed February 23, 2011.

87. UNAIDS. UNAIDS promotes combination HIV prevention towards universal access goals. 2009. http://data.unaids.org/pub/PressStatement/2009/20090318_pressstatement_prevention_en.pdf. Accessed February 23, 2011.

88. Crepaz N, Hart TA, Marks G. Highly active antiretroviral therapy and sexual risk behavior: a meta-analytic review. *JAMA*. 2004;292:224–236.

89. Wilson TE, Gore ME, Greenblatt R, et al. Changes in sexual risk behavior among HIV-infected women after initiation of HAART. *Am J Public Health*. 2004;94:1141–1146.

90. Kaiser Family Foundation. Total HIV/AIDS federal funding, FY 2010 2010. http://www.statehealthfacts.org/comparetable.jsp?ind=528&cat=11. Accessed February 23, 2011.

91. Centers for Disease Control and Prevention. DHAP HIV funding awards by state and dependent area fiscal year 2009). April 2010. http://www.cdc.gov/hiv/topics/funding/state-awards/2009/index.htm. Accessed February 23, 2011.

92. Rerks-Ngarm S, Pitisuttithum P, Nitayaphan S, et al. Vaccination with ALVAC and AIDSVAX to prevent HIV-1 infection in Thailand. *N Engl J Med*. 2009;361:2209–2220.

93. Abdool Karim Q, Abdool Karim SS, Frohlich JA, et al. Effectiveness and safety of tenofovir gel, an antiretroviral microbicide, for the prevention of HIV infection in women. *Science*. 2010;329:1168–1174.

94. Auvert B, Taljaard D, Lagarde E, Sobngwi-Tambekou Sitta R, Puren A. Randomized, controlled intervention trial of male circumcision for reduction of HIV infection risk: the ANRS 1265 trial. *PLoS Med*. 2005;2:1112–1122.

95. Bailey RC, Moses S, Parker CB, et al. Male circumcision for HIV prevention in young men in Kisumu, Kenya: a randomised controlled trial. *Lancet*. 2007;369:643–656.

96. Gray RH, Kigozi G, Serwadda D, et al. Male circumcision for HIV prevention in men in Rakai, Uganda: a randomised trial. *Lancet*. 2007;369:657–666.

97. Wawer MJ, Makumbi F, Kigozi G, et al. Circumcision in HIV-infected men and its effect on HIV transmission to female partners in Rakai, Uganda: a randomised controlled trial. *Lancet*. 2009;374:229–237.

98. Wawer MJ, Tobian AA, Kigozi G, et al. Effect of circumcision of HIV-negative men on transmission of human papillomavirus to HIV-negative women: a randomised trial in Rakai, Uganda. *Lancet*. 2011;377:209–218.

99. Giuliano AR, Nyitray AG, Albero G. Male circumcision and HPV transmission to female partners. *Lancet*. 2011;377:183–184.

100. Spire B, de Zoysa I, Himmich H. HIV prevention: what have we learned from community experiences in concentrated epidemics? *J Int AIDS Soc*. 2008;11:5.

101. Campsmith M, Rhodes PH, Hall I, Green TA. Undiagnosed HIV prevalence among adults and adolescents in the United States at the end of 2006. *J Acquir Immune Defic Syndr*. 2010;53:619–624.

102. Lansky A, Jones JL, Frey RL, Lindegren ML. Trends in HIV testing among pregnant women: United States, 1994-1999. *Am J Public Health*. 2001;91:1291–1293.

103. Anderson JE, Sansom S. HIV testing in a national sample of pregnant U.S. women: who is not getting tested? *AIDS Care*. 2007;19:375–380.

104. Centers for Disease Control and Prevention. Persons tested for HIV—United States, 2006. *MMWR Morb Mortal Wkly Rep*. 2008;57:845–849.

105. Anderson JE, Sansom S. HIV testing among U.S. women during prenatal care: findings from the 2002 National Survey of Family Growth. *Matern Child Health J*. 2006;10:413–417.

106. Centers for Disease Control and Prevention. Reducing HIV transmission from mother-to-child: an opt-out approach to HIV screening. 2007. http://www.cdc.gov/hiv/topics/perinatal/resources/factsheets/opt-out.htm. Accessed February 23, 2011.

107. Centers for Disease Control and Prevention. Late HIV testing—34 states, 1996-2005. *MMWR Morb Mortal Wkly Rep*. 2009;58:661–665.

108. U.S. Preventive Services Task Force. Screening for HIV: recommendation statement. *Ann Intern Med*. 2005;143:32–37.

109. Centers for Disease Control and Prevention. Reported CD4+ T-lymphocyte results for adults and adolescents with HIV/AIDS—33 states, 2005. *HIV/AIDS Surveillance Supplemental Report* 2005;11:1–31. http://www.cdc.gov/hiv/surveillance/resources/reports/2005supp_vol11no2. Accessed February 23, 2011.

110. Liau A, Petters S, Crepaz N. A Systematic Review of U.S.-Based Interventions for Linking and Retaining HIV-Positive Persons in Medical Care. Atlanta, GA: Annual HIV Prevention Conference; August 23–26, 2009. http://www.2011nhpc.org/archivepdf/2009_NHPC_Abstract_Book_REV4_2011.pdf. Accessed August 21, 2012.

111. Craw JA, Gardner LI, Marks G, et al. Brief strengths-based case management promotes entry into HIV medical care. *J Acquir Immune Defic Syndr*. 2008;47:597–606.

112. Cook JA, Cohen MH, Grey D, et al. Use of highly active antiretroviral therapy in a cohort of HIV-seropositive women. *Am J Public Health*. 2002;92:82–87.

113. Cohen MH, Cook JA, Grey D, et al. Medically eligible women who do not use HAART: the importance of abuse, drug use, and race. *Am J Public Health*. 2004;94:1147–1151.

114. Lillie-Blanton M, Stone VE, Snow Jones A, et al. Association of race, substance abuse, and health insurance coverage with use of highly active antiretroviral therapy among HIV-infected women, 2005. *Am J Public Health*. 2010;100:1493–1499.

115. Nicastri E, Angeletti C, Palmisano L, et al. Gender differences in progression of HIV-1-infected individuals during long-term highly active antiretroviral therapy. *AIDS*. 2005;19:577–583.

116. Bartlett JG, Gallant JE. *Medical Management of HIV Infection*. Baltimore, MD: Johns Hopkins University Press; 2003.

117. Howard AA, Arnsten JH, Lo Y, et al. A prospective study of adherence and viral load in a large multi-center cohort of HIV-infected women. *AIDS*. 2002;16:2175–2182.

118. Merenstein D, Schneider MF, Cox C, et al. Association of child care burden and household composition with adherence to highly active antiretroviral therapy in the Women's Interagency HIV Study. *AIDS Patient Care STDS*. 2009;23:289–296.

119. Simoni JM, Amico KR, Pearson CR, Malow R. Strategies for promoting adherence to antiretroviral therapy: a review of the literature. *Curr Infect Dis Rep*. 2008;10:515–521.

Prevention of HIV/AIDS in Women

Zena Stein, MA, MB, BCh, Dr Med Sc (Hon) Witwatersrand, Dr Sc (Hon) Columbia University and Mervyn Susser, MB, BCh, Dr Med Sc (Hon) Witwatersrand, FRCP (Edinburgh), FRCP (London)

Introduction

This chapter outlines the ongoing search for preventing human immunodeficiency virus (HIV) infections in women, mainly women resident in the United States. Historically, in the developed world, both the recognition of the disease and the approaches to its avoidance in women were delayed by the initial understanding that only men were susceptible. We describe the evolution from this concept to an increasing awareness that women are not only at least as susceptible as men, but also that women with a sexually transmitted infection have their own specific needs. Development of this understanding and of the research and experience to provide them with protection are documented here, concluding with a critical summary of where we stand today.

However, as this is not a field that stands still, a timely update of government policy seems appropriate here. In July 2010 the United States issued the National HIV/AIDS Strategy for the United States.[1] This was the first statement in this country that served as a national plan. Regarding the themes developed in this chapter on prevention for women, this "strategy" document emphasizes the need for a combination of efforts in prevention, especially for those individuals and groups at high risk, as well as for the application of appropriate interventions for communities at high risk. It also demonstrated the very high relative risks for women of color in the United States, the concentration of at-risk women in geographic areas, and the need for attention to access for their care. Further actions regarding diagnosis and treatment are needed for women of color, to counter the high mortality among them for those infected with HIV.

The National Strategy also recommends increased emphasis on testing for seropositivity, an action not specifically developed elsewhere in this chapter. The purpose is to decrease the numbers of seropositive men and women in the community who are unaware of their HIV status. By identifying those who are seropositive before the typical symptoms develop, infected people could be connected sooner to clinical care. Provided adequate access is available, early connection to care and treatment would benefit them. From our perspective, adequate treatment would also reduce their infectivity. Moreover, it has been shown that knowledge of positive serostatus, even for the untreated, tends to reduce high-risk behavior. Hence, this strategy, involving behavioral, public health, and clinical actions, could contribute to prevention in women as well as in men.

Soon after the release of the National Strategy, the Office of AIDS Research (OAR) of the National Institutes of Health also published recommendations based on deliberations of the OAR Social and Behavioral Research Think Tank, which should be read alongside this chapter.[2] Similarly, the *Journal of Acquired Immune Deficiency Syndromes* (JAIDS) published a supplement in December 2010, also in some aspects supplementing this chapter.[3]

Historical Review

Initial understanding of the acquired immune deficiency syndrome (AIDS) epidemic arose from its manifest connection with men having sex with men.[4,5] Hence, "GRID" was the initial acronym assigned to gay-related-immunodeficiency-disease. At that time little thought was given to the susceptibility of women to this disease.[6] Indeed the neglect of sexually transmitted infections afflicting women goes back much further than the advent of this new plague. Thus, going by the earliest records we have, the condom in the late 18th century seemed to have been designed specifically to protect men from syphilis. During World War I, the use of condoms was emphasized for the soldiers on leave from the trenches. For sexually active women at that time, however, neither condoms nor the vaginal diaphragm were recommended even for sex workers, among whom sexually transmitted infections were a well-recognized occupational hazard. Indeed, women were typically seen as the vectors rather than the victims of sexually transmitted infections. For example, to support the assumed efficacy of the male condom, a trial to protect sailors on shore leave from contracting sexually transmitted infections is often quoted. Of course, such a trial says nothing about the protection needed for women.[7] In the United States late in the 20th century, the first women identified as HIV infected had acquired the disease from blood transfusions. Subsequent female victims were either injection drug users or the female partners of infected bisexual men. The numbers of U.S. women infected heterosexually grew slowly.[8,9] But as the epidemics in Africa, Haiti, and elsewhere were documented, women could no longer be ignored. Accordingly, the first injunction to women for self-protection was simple: "use a condom." It was actually some time into the epidemic before it dawned on policymakers that because women did not use male condoms, this was an unreal piece of advice: it is often socially impossible for a young woman to initiate condom use by the male partner. Even married women who propose condom use might seem to imply suspicion of their spouse's infidelities, or worse, might call up suspicion of extramarital encounters on their own part. Since the advent of hormonal contraceptives, moreover, in longstanding partnerships, resort to condom use primarily to prevent pregnancy is uncommon. As we discuss later, many women faced difficulties in introducing the condom into their encounters. From the start of the epidemic they have been made aware of their risks but not realistically of how to avoid them.[10]

Surprisingly, for many years even family planning clinics functioning almost exclusively for women failed to recognize that for women to sustain reproductive health required prevention both of sexually transmitted infections and unintended pregnancies. In part, this neglect may have been due to the advent and success of hormonal contraceptives, introduced in the 1960s. Revolutionary in its early years, the family planning movement had become conservative and long delayed the necessary efforts to attract and inform young unmarried women, as well as boys and men, of the advent of the new sex-associated hazard of HIV. For too long the need to emphasize the use of condoms as well as hormones (dual protection discussed later) found little support in the United States health services.[11]

In the face of the HIV epidemic, no professional group seized the initiative for protecting women. By contrast, women themselves, and the organizations in which their interests were dominant, as for instance the International Committee for Research on Women and the Population Council were quick to recognize the inadequacy of the advice to use a condom.[12]

Research in Prevention

In time the issue of prevention for women stimulated the growth of a major national and international research movement. Initially these investigators addressed three approaches to prevention. First was sexual abstinence, mainly directed in the United States at "delaying sexual debut" among adolescents. A second approach to women's self-protection aimed to create and provide a physical or chemical barrier against infection. A third approach seeks to promote behavioral change and self-protection among women by providing the knowledge, skills, and self-confidence needed to control their sexual encounters, for instance, by refusing to entertain sex without a condom. Behavioral skills would of course be needed both to sustain abstinence as well as to implement the wide use of whatever physical or chemical barriers become available. Subsequently, ideas for prevention expanded to include societal and service-based interventions.

Given this backdrop for the past 3 decades, by 2010 the HIV epidemic has spread unabated across the world. The full extent of the painful tragedy of the past 2 decades is hard to comprehend. In the recently liberated and democratized South Africa, for instance, a substantial proportion of a generation of young women has been infected, and many have died from the disease as noted in Figure 14-1.[13–15]

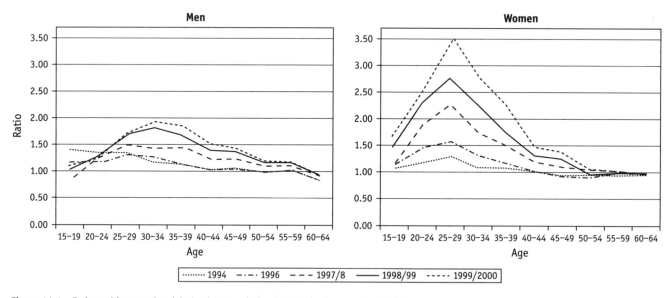

Figure 14-1 Estimated increase in adult death rates relative to 1985 death rates, South Africa.

In some ways, the movement to find new means of protection—essentially a research enterprise—took precedence over enhancing health education.[16] Even when the female condom was invented specifically to extend the options for women, little interest was expressed nor effort expended by U.S. public health clinics to promote its regular use. Nonetheless, it is encouraging that over the past 2 decades, and especially in 2010, both the search for physical and chemical barriers against the virus and the deployment of social and psychological modalities are at last showing progress. Meanwhile we await the anticipated advent of the "holy grail," an effective vaccine. In what follows, we summarize research efforts that have been undertaken and the present status of each.

Abstinence in Young People

A first approach was directed mainly toward deferring sexual encounters—"sexual debut"—until later ages among adolescents and young adults. This approach to prevention is often combined with a strong moralistic element that asserts the sinfulness of sex either before or outside marriage. Only stringent abstinence satisfies this approach. However, among young people "abstinence plus" is an alternative approach that aims to achieve the practical objectives of preventing both unwanted pregnancies and sexually transmitted infections, objectives that can be achieved without insisting absolutely on abstinence. Official U.S. policies often endorsed the moralistic position and invested in "abstinence only" programs, while omitting the education and encouragement to use the contraceptives and barriers integral to "abstinence plus."

Nonetheless, recent controlled trials among school children, which compare curricula for "abstinence only" with "abstinence plus" (namely, "comprehensive sex education") have been carefully evaluated. Although the latter programs emphasize abstinence as without question the safest behavior, they nonetheless subscribe to the use of condoms or other forms of contraception. Among such trials carefully assessed in a recent publication,[17] two-thirds of the comprehensive programs both delayed the onset of sexual activity and increased condom and contraceptive use among the young participants. By contrast, only three of nine "abstinence only" programs had any detectable effect on sexual behavior. One may conclude that in U.S. schools, the evidence supports the effectiveness of "abstinence plus" programs, but not of "abstinence only."

In the National Strategy for the United States, "abstinence" is barely mentioned. In the same year, in its Guide to Community Prevention Services,[18] the Center for Disease Control and Prevention (CDC)—unequivocally endorsed comprehensive approaches.

Physical Barriers

We turn next to a summary of those physical barriers that in the year 2010 seem to be firmly established, notwithstanding obstacles overcome in order to reach the tested and "evidence-based" status they now occupy.

The Male Condom

The oldest contraceptive device on record is the male condom. As described in the *Oxford Companion to the Body*, some very ancient specimens, made of a variety of materials, may have served magical rather than medical purposes, However, the Italian anatomist Gabrielo Fallopio, in an account published posthumously (he died in 1632) described a linen sheath to be fitted over the glans penis but under the foreskin, which he recommended as a protection against the "French disease" (syphilis: the name assigned to a lovelorn shepherd in a long poem by the 16th century physician and poet Fracastoro). Recently in England actual fragments of animal gut condoms were excavated from a 17th century manor, and in the 18th century both Casanova and James Boswell refer to such devices. Eventually, as noted previously, in World War I (1914–1918) rubber condoms were distributed to the British forces in France as protective against sexual transmission of infections. From the 1920s onward latex condoms began to play a part in contraception, as did also such contraceptive barriers for women as the diaphragm (known at that time as the "Dutch Cap").

With the advent of the HIV scourge in the early 1980s, it was taken for granted ("common sense")[14,19] that the male condom would be an effective barrier against whatever organism was responsible for transmission, as previously it had been shown to do for men with gonorrhea, and of course also against insemination. The conventional view was that the condom did not need further testing. Nevertheless, the reported success for contraception was only around 85%; failures could be attributed not only to "breakage or slippage" but also simply to the omission of use. For prevention of HIV, its effectiveness was established partly in the laboratory but later more convincingly by observations based on longitudinal studies of discordant couples (i.e., only one partner was infected).[20] The male condom was found to be protective if used in every sexual encounter or, at the least, in well over 90% of encounters, essentially a matter of all or none.

The Female Condom

The finding on the male condom was and is important. For one thing, at the time of this writing, we still do not have comparable data for protection conferred on either women or men by the female condom, the cervical cap, or the vaginal diaphragm.[21] Nevertheless, we do have evidence that, as a contraceptive, the female condom is at least as effective as the male condom (Figure 14-2).[22] Similarly, in trials where the female condom was introduced in a random fashion among the options for protection against infections, and at least some women substituted its use for the male condom, the rates of infection remained unchanged.[23] In a large observational study in public family planning clinics in Brazil, moreover, the introduction of the female condom reduced the reported rate of unprotected sex.[24] Appropriately, *Saving Lives Now*, a recent detailed comprehensive evaluation of the female condom, concludes emphatically that both male and female condoms should be made widely available.[25] The male

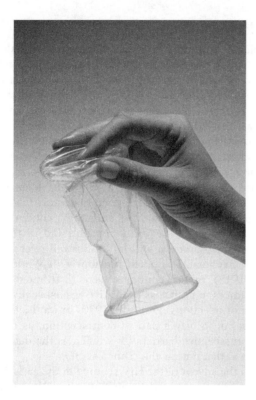

Figure 14-2A The female condom.

Source: © Jones & Bartlett Learning. Photographed by Kimberly Potvin.

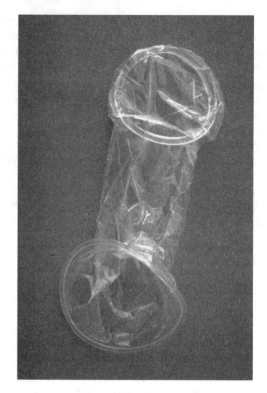

Figure 14-2B The female condom.

Source: © Photodisc.

condom on its own does not meet the needs of women. Resorting to common sense as previously we did for the male condom, since the female condom covers the vulva, vagina, and cervix and is also impervious to HIV in the laboratory, if it is used correctly it is in all probability protective. But it is even more important to recognize that, as with the male condom, safety is ensured only with correct use in every encounter: the appropriate slogan is that condoms on the shelf or in the pocket are not protective.

Returning to the female condom, much has been learned since it first became available for adoption and use among women. To begin with, it had to be understood and its application rendered familiar to both men and women. Surprisingly, in preparation for a sexual encounter few women actually saw or touched the male condom in its small neat package. With the female condom, however, women needed to become familiar and comfortable with the new device as indeed also did their male partners.

Essential to the dissemination of the female condom, in our view badly needed, is a trained and motivated public health workforce especially among those facilities serving women.[26] Although the female condom is more expensive than the male condom, price has probably not proved an insuperable obstacle to its uptake, because the usual providers are governments and donors rather than clients themselves. Indeed, if dissemination were wider, the price would be lower. Many men prefer their partner to take the initiative in prevention and in such partnerships female condoms work well.[27] They serve particularly well when the male partner is averse to the male condom. However,

were a woman to take the initiative in providing or insisting on the use of either a male or a female condom, it is patently far from a universal solution to the problem of prevention. Since the onset of the HIV epidemic the use of both male and female condoms has expanded sufficiently to halt the velocity of spread in some countries; still the incidence of new infections worldwide and among either sex has not ensured the decline of the epidemic.

This brings us to the heart of the problem. When couples known to be discordant for HIV are counseled together and agree to use condoms, the incidence of infection is less among them than among those not so counseled. Available barriers are not lacking so much as is the need for partner understanding, cooperation, and consensual behavior.[28] One might well argue that lack of such essential social and behavioral norms has enabled the HIV epidemic to break through all national and international boundaries. Sexual encounters take place at all times, among all kinds of people, and in many places. Unlike unwanted conceptions, transmission does not depend only on fertile periods. We belabor this point because over the last 2 decades, and still now, only modest success has attended the considerable effort concentrated on ensuring safe sex while the means to do so would seem to be readily at hand, namely, "use a condom."

It has become absolutely clear that women in relationships that involve intimacy, trust, coparenting, and economic dependence will be reluctant to use condoms. For all relationships, there will be some reluctance to use condoms: impediments regularly reported in field studies mention that condoms interrupt sexual encounters and reduce spontaneity. In addition, some couples believe the physical barrier impedes pleasure, whether this is real or imaginary. Still there remain the much more obstinate factors of relationships. An insightful study among sex-workers in Madagascar, for instance, exemplifies variation in condom nonuse by degree of fluidity in partnerships: here intimacy or trust is measured on a scale rather than by the more usual categories of partnerships as "stable" compared to "casual."[29] The evidence is compelling and confirmed universally, that the closer the couple, the greater the reluctance to use condoms.

Of course, many other women, single or married, have special needs or face particularly difficult circumstances, and it is almost axiomatic that social disadvantage accentuates the problems of self protection. Those with physical or mental disability come to mind, as do the very young and the very old, habitual users of drugs or alcohol, and those who for various reasons live impoverished and destitute. Commercial sex workers and women subject to intimate violence must also be included. Studies describing the daily lives of drug-using women illustrate the complex issues of self-protection they often face.[30] These considerations bolster the argument for providing protection that goes beyond the male or female condom alone.

Chemical Barriers

Vaginal Gels: The Microbicides

While we await the development of a vaccine or protective pill, a substance that a woman could use secretly and preferably apart from the moment of sexual intercourse (that is to say, "coitally independent") would be a boon for all women. This protective device could be a gel or a sponge that she would herself insert into her vagina. Undetectable by the partner through smell or taste or sensation and applied discreetly, what a relief! No arguments, no explanations. The protective device might also be a contraceptive but perhaps not always, because pregnancy may be desired. The hidden nature of the device was both trigger and challenge to the microbicide movement. Not that the element of secrecy would be endorsed by all men; some might well regard secrecy as deception.[31] But for women unable to engage in or even to contemplate the discourse among couples visualized for effective condom use, the concept of a "microbicide" is surely liberating.

Disregarded at first, the challenge, energized by women's movements everywhere, soon took hold and was in time recognized by private and eventually by government donors.[32] The pharmaceutical industry on the whole preferred not to push the issue, seeing its ultimate value among less developed countries where little profit might be made.

Controlled Trials

Trials involving human subjects were necessary for the development of a microbicide, even if the agent is active only against HIV and not against either sperm or other sexually transmitted infections. Preliminary evidence provided by laboratory animals would not suffice. Moreover, a necessary condition was that no risk of harm to the reproductive tract should attend microbicide use. Thus trials that aimed to reach many thousands of women first passed through a phase of testing to determine appropriate dosage, followed by a second and larger trial to ensure safety. Trials reaching a third phase without mishap were to provide the crucial evidence of effectiveness and hence were conducted among women evidently at "high" risk of infection, a group likely to provide the best opportunity to assess benefit. Even with all this, still the experiments faced unusual difficulties.[8,33]

Problems Facing Microbicide Trials

Intentionally, many participants were to be at high risk. This was requisite to achieving adequate numbers of newly infected women as participants in order to evaluate the success of the trials. Although regular use of the male condom by their partners was unlikely, an ethical commitment for investigators was always to counsel participating women to try to ensure condom use by their male partners. Of course, should such counseling prove effective, the trial could hardly succeed because the numbers of new infections would be insufficient. Then too, trials would have to randomize participants on the one hand to using the microbicide under test and on the other to using a supposedly inert substance as placebo. Such procedures require careful explanation to participants, few if any of whom will have had previous experience of such a concept. Moreover, the "inert" nature of the placebo would need to have been established beforehand as far as possible, apart from its performance during the trial. It was also preferable that women not become pregnant during the trial, because a test substance might possibly be toxic to an embryo. Finally, as with condom use, despite precautions, investigators would have no direct proof of correct and consistent use of either the microbicides under test or even of the placebo.

These are some among many difficulties faced in such trials. Indeed, the first completed trial was a serious setback when it not only proved ineffective but had possibly increased the risk of infection. Shortly thereafter, a second trial was abandoned as potentially also harmful. Yet a third trial was abandoned after failing to recruit sufficient numbers of infected women, whereas a fourth gave inconsistent results.

Preexposure Prophylaxis

Since 2007 this field has undergone serious reconsideration. The direction that further work in this field is likely to take deserves discussion. Arguing that some antiviral drugs deployed as therapeutic against AIDS are highly effective, could they also have a role in prevention?[34] Suffice it to say that, among health workers or others accidentally jabbed with infected needles or among victims of rape, the regular practice has been immediately to administer full treatment for a limited period of time. This approach (postexposure prophylaxis) has seemed to avert at least some infections that might otherwise have been expected. Other evidence of benefit has also accrued from cases of apparently infected newborn infants first treated postnatally. More important for persons at risk is a modified version of this approach (preexposure prophylaxis, or PrEP), which is to ingest antiretroviral drugs before exposure to the virus. In support of this approach, in which drugs are taken by the pregnant woman during pregnancy or intrapartum, is the undoubted protection provided to the infant.

Perhaps these drugs could also work as microbicides? At long last, in trials involving two different sites in South Africa one substance, comprising the antriretroviral drug Tenofovir 1% was shown to reduce the risk of infection as compared with the placebo.[35] This trial involved 880 participants over a period of up to 2 years and found a reduction in the incidence of new HIV infections that was modest but significant. Among women who used the microbicide as frequently as instructed, the protection was 54%. Since Tenofovir has already been used by millions of infected patients worldwide with very few adverse effects and is slow to induce resistance, there is much to believe that, as shown in the trial, it will prove acceptably safe as a microbicide. Unexpectedly, too, the incidence of herpes simplex virus 2 (HSV-2), a precursor of some cases of HIV, was halved. Moreover, important in terms of behavior, this gel was not used at the time of coitus, but at an estimated 12 hours before expected sexual encounters, as well as 12 hours later.

Widely recognized as a breakthrough, the next few years will be critical in raising the level of protection perhaps by the addition of other antiretroviral drugs to the gel, by varying the dose, or by substituting a cervical ring for the gel. These trials have together involved many investigators across the world and thousands of women, fortunately without harming them. At last, the hope of finding some preventive against infection appears to be realized.

The virus develops resistance against drugs used in treatments, however, and with prolonged use, some drugs manifest undesirable side effects. The drug Tenofovir described earlier as a microbicide, is relatively favorable in both these respects if taken before potential exposure.

A major trial of Truvada, a pill that combines two antiretroviral drugs—Tenofovir and Emtricitabine, was reported several months after the microbicide with Tenofovir was announced.[36] This trial tested the pill, taken daily, against a placebo, among 2,499 HIV negative men, mainly men who have sex with men, across six countries. The protective effect was similar to that for the microbicide: among all on the trial, the reduction in infections rate was 44%; among those apparently regular user, it was 73%, clearly statistically significant. Blood samples taken among men who did and did not become infected, confirmed this result beyond doubt: 95% protection.

Currently, these areas of study overlap with the application of vaginal microbicides.[37] Absorption into the body of Tenofovir, for instance, is more rapid via the reproductive tract than by mouth. Current experiments among women in communities of high prevalence are engaged in testing selected antiretroviral drugs, singly or in combination, both as microbicides applied to the vagina and by ingestion. At the time of writing, more trials are awaited.[38] They may well be in hand before an effective vaccine becomes available and, like a vaccine, these advances will protect men as well as women both directly and indirectly.

Behavioral Interventions

The year 2010 was certainly a watershed year for the prevention of HIV in women. We now have the promise of protection from microbicide use, as well, in all likelihood of a PrEP pill. Although a full range of choices will not be immediately available to the women who want or need them, we may assume some or all will in time enter the public health horizon in the United States. The National Strategy clearly recommends combinations of preventive actions.[1] However, it will still be in the hands of women whether or not they want to use some or any of these methods. The promise of protection will still ultimately depend on the social and behavior situations in which they are presented. Now, in addition to the evidence-based work presented later, fresh studies will be needed to measure the effects on women of these new methods, which so far provide only "partial protection": or alter risk reduction to favor "risk compensation." These will be new challenges for the future.[2] As always, we must start with what we do know.[39]

Hence, in addition to the above account of research aimed at developing, testing, and introducing physical and chemical barriers against HIV infection, we have still to consider studies aimed at behavior change. Given that condoms are effective barriers to sexually transmitted infections including HIV, researchers have recognized the major preventive potential of promoting incentives and action to sustaining consistent male or female condom use, both by women and by men.

Further preventive approaches would be to promote sustained abstinence among the young and thereby defer the age of sexual debut, to limit the number of partnerships, to limit unprotected sexual encounters to mutually monogamous partners, to avoid or at least reduce concurrent partnerships, to discourage violent behavior during sex, and to protect vulnerable groups, especially sex workers and users of drugs. The list is long and as already mentioned, behavior change in these situations will need to be considered with these and every other form of prevention, whether by education, use of barriers, PrEP or vaccines.

Attempts to create a theoretical model of individual behavior change that would meet the case for prevention of HIV have been many, some of which do share common elements.[40–42] A first step toward change calls for enhancing knowledge. In the face of the threat of HIV, sexually active persons need not only to recognize and sustain awareness of the risk of infection but also to acquire understanding of how the disease may spread and endanger themselves and others. Such understanding may not be readily internalized nor consistently applied. For women in particular, beyond cultivating awareness of potential risk, sexual activity calls for sustained appreciation of the difficulties of implementing such means of self-protection as are available against contracting the disease.

To ensure such self-protection is not simple. The earliest intervention studies learned that to face the new scourge, more is needed than simply acquiring a clear and "cognitive" understanding of what has to be done. An obvious requirement is that the means of protection, either with the male or female condom, must be on hand. Advice and practice are required in the use of the available means of self-protection. Also needed, more especially for a woman, is the cultivation of a degree of self-confidence sufficient to enable her to introduce and use a barrier: this may call for counseling to enhance self-awareness and the acquisition of the skills to render sexual encounters safe. The requisite knowledge and motivation should follow from all this, although successful execution is likely to depend heavily both on the circumstances and the nature of the partnership and also, in the same way as in all of these means, on the broader cultural background in which sexual engagement takes place.[14]

In the relatively new field of studies of HIV, in many countries and especially in the United States these theories and their variants have yielded nearly 2 decades of observation and experiment. Attempts to change behavior have been tested in many ways and in different settings: for instance, by mass education, videos in clinic rooms, recruitment and training of local leaders, and group workshops either in naturally occurring settings like classrooms and sports clubs or, more often, among specially constituted volunteer groups. Some few experiments have used one-on-one counseling.[42] More recently, interventions have taken advantage of the information technology now readily available to many.[2] Favorable results from many of these approaches have been followed by broader dissemination of particular interventions to other groups and other populations. In most cases, all these experiments have relied on reported behavior change (such as sustained abstinence, reduction in partner number, and fewer episodes of unprotected sex). These reports are important although many leave room for doubt about their validity. In very few cases (discussed later), could the response to an intervention be measured by a reduction in incidence either of HIV infection or even of other sexually transmitted infections. Moreover, the endpoints of observed or reported behavior have seldom been evaluated beyond a 6-month period.

Evidence and Methods

Fortunately, in a major contribution to rendering accessible the body of this now considerable literature on HIV, the CDC has collected, evaluated, and categorized so-called "evidence-based" intervention studies.[43] In what follows, we describe three such approaches in detail: one attempts to reach communities, a second selects and fol-

lows a specially constituted group of women, and a third is a study of individual one-on-one interactive counseling. All selected studies have been rigorously designed and implemented and appropriately analyzed.

Community-Wide Approach

We noted previously the recommendation contained in the National Strategy to identify communities at high risk of HIV and to devise appropriate strategies to meet their needs. Hence, we begin this section with a community-wide study known as "PROMISE" an acronym for "Peers reaching out and modeling intervention strategies for HIV/AIDS risk reduction in their community").[44] PROMISE, like each of the studies we discuss, begins by setting out its guiding theory. This study was in fact guided not by one but by three theoretical assumptions: first, people change behavior in a series of stages; second, reasoned action is guided by attitudes, beliefs, and the expectations of others; third, social cognitive theory, posits learning follows from observing the success of others practicing a new behavior. This very ambitious project was to operate in five U.S. cities and in each, to identify two communities, one subject to intervention and the other serving as untouched control. A team of advocates was dispatched to the intervention community to disseminate pamphlets with readings on HIV, supplies such as bleach to clean needles for use by injection drug users, and male condoms, for use by everyone. Over the 3 years of the study, interviews were conducted on 10 occasions with randomly chosen residents. These interviews reached over 15,000 persons in all.

Since the evaluation was based on the theory that behavior change occurs in phases, respondents were asked about the same issues at 10 successive interviews. For our specific purposes, four questions addressed condom use, specifically, the frequency, intended consistency and history of male condom use. Finally, each person was asked: Are you carrying a condom? Reported behavior at each phase could thus be categorized as indicating the intention or otherwise of the respondent to use a condom.

Comparisons of the data drawn from the many interviews conducted in the intervention and control communities enabled analysis of change over time. For instance, as to condom use in the intervention communities, the result was overwhelmingly favorable. In responding to the question "Are you carrying a condom," an affirmative response by the respondent was followed by the request to show one. From a baseline of 17.4% among intervention respondents, the rise to 30% at the end of the study is impressive, and the more so compared with virtually no change among controls viz. 18.5% at baseline and 18.9% at conclusion of the study (Figure 14-3). This highly original and intensive project of course posed many methodological challenges, not all of which could be completely resolved. Nevertheless, the innovative approach of the study is remarkable, in that promoting behavior change, reduced the risks for HIV with an apparently unique intervention, not yet repeated either within the United States nor elsewhere.

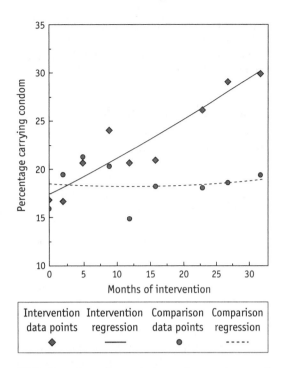

Figure 14-3 Percentage of respondents carrying a condom over time: CDC AIDS Community Demonstration Project, 1991–1994.

Source: Reproduced from Community-level HIV intervention in 5 cities: final outcome data from the CDC AIDS community demonstration projects. *Am J Public Health* 1999;89:336–345 with kind permission. © American Public Health Association.

Group-Based Studies

Another set of studies[45–47] exemplifies a design used more often in this field than any other. As a first example,[45] in 1992, African American women were recruited "on the street" in a San Francisco neighborhood that is home to many people of color who were mostly financially deprived, poorly educated, and among those American women at highest risk of HIV infection. Titled the SISTA project (Sisters Informing Sisters on topics concerning AIDS), it included an intervention delivered to one group over five sessions; a control group received only one session and intervention in a third group was deferred to the end of the study. Participating women were randomly assigned, each of whom responded to an interview at baseline, and to another at the end of the study, 3 months later. The key outcome sought was the reported consistency of male condom use.

The theory guiding this smaller scale and more modest study was also "social cognitive theory," similar in some ways to the "PROMISE" study described earlier. In the San Francisco study, however, a continuous relationship was sustained over 5 weeks in a weekly group meeting. Here gender and empowerment were taken to be central in guiding the development of social skills, ideas promoted in the steps outlined for each successive intervention session. At the outset, gender and pride were emphasized as positive attributes of African American women; a second session focused on education about the chances of HIV infection and the reduction of risk; a third session dealt with assertiveness; and a fourth with sexual self-control,

an aspect of the program explored in play acting set in typical scenarios. The fifth and last session rehearsed defensive action that could be used with noncompliant partners. For controls, a single session aimed to provide an overview of social cognitive skills.

This 3-month test of the intervention yielded a clear improvement in almost all the criteria of behavior change specified initially by the study. Reported male condom use doubled over time but only in the intervention group.[45]

A more elaborate and fully described intervention, conducted among 360 women attending family planning clinics in New York, is known as FIO (The Future is Ours).[46] This study compared the results in women assigned to one of three groups: one attended eight sessions of counseling, a second only four sessions, and a third group served as a "waiting control." Each counseling session, guided by a manual that set out each procedure, was described in detail. The underlying theory behind this work, like that described earlier, was designed specifically to meet the needs of women.[41] Evaluations and comparisons were carried out after 1 month and again after 12 months. The improvement in protective behavior during sexual encounters, accompanied by a marked decline in unprotected sex, reflected a significant advantage for the eight-session group on both follow-up occasions.

Individualized and Interactive Interventions

The individual one-on-one research, titled Project RESPECT, was developed by a large team of investigators, including several from the CDC, with additional advice and support from Martin Fishbein, a notable leader in formulating the theories of behavior change used in this and many other experiments.[39] The initial study for which Project RESPECT is best known covered some 5,000 men and women who were the clients of five clinics across the United States that provided treatment for sexually transmitted infections.[48] Those who agreed to participate were randomized into four groups, two of which followed the protocol-driven interactive procedure, and two of which were assigned only to the routine didactic counseling used in the clinics. Each counseling session lasted about 20 minutes. Counselors were carefully trained in the chosen approach and provided with a detailed procedural guide. The interactive procedure aimed essentially for counselor and client jointly to develop an intervention that would be practical and suitable for the client. In the event, when followed over a period of 12 months, those in the intervention program reported fewer episodes of unsafe sex; among the men but not the women, there were fewer reinfections of gonorrhea.

The CDC has since deepened its experience with both the two- and the four-session versions of the RESPECT approach.[43] Training manuals have been developed for counselors, and their applicability tested in a variety of circumstances, for instance as in HIV counseling and testing sites, as well as in less specialized clinics. Proponents claim that the two-session version, given no more than a quiet space for up to 20 minutes, can be used anywhere in a busy service setting. It can also be adapted to include other counseling purposes and integrated into the preventive program of other services. As one example, a small study in family planning clinics in New York City adapted the approach to introduce "dual protection (protection against unintended pregnancy and infections)," by a licensed practical nurse.[49,50]

Interventions among Seropositive People

In another set of evidence-based studies included in the CDC collection, researchers worked specifically with both women and men infected with HIV (The Healthy Living Project). The individualized interactive behavioral approach is similar to that in Project RESPECT, although the outcomes sought are more complex. The intervention involves a sequence of 15 sessions with study subjects, or alternatively, three series of five sessions, each first addressing the specific issue of safe sex and then maintenance of physical and mental health.[51]

Changes in the Wider Society

The Social Context: Public Health Structures and Services

In response to the recognized importance of the given social context in which the epidemic is rife, a broad array of interventions has been explored. Under the term "structural interventions," for instance, the course of public health action is located in contextual and environmental factors, rather than only or mainly with individual risk behaviors.[52] Such factors might operate at the highest level of government, as has been documented in Brazil[53] and as now appears to be taking place in South Africa.[54] Or, by contrast, they may operate at the level of a primary care facility or a hospital. Although changes like these can rarely be evaluated with the precision of "evidence-based" trials, either in terms of behavior change or incidence, still promising effects have been documented by observations, demonstration projects and on-the-ground reports.

Test and Treat: Models for Prevention

In 2008, WHO scientists proposed a theoretical approach toward reducing HIV prevalence and halting the epidemic; under this regime every adult would be tested annually for HIV, and any newly positive person would be immediately assigned to antiretroviral treatment.[55] If indeed such a program were to be implemented, undoubtedly the epidemic would decline to the benefit of both women and men. (It is well known that infected people who are under treatment are less likely to transmit the virus, because their viral load declines). Critics have questioned not only the feasibility of such a program, however, but also some assumptions of the proposed approach.[56] One critic suggests it would take 70 years to show an effective decline.[57] Nevertheless, preliminary efforts to implement the proposed intervention are ongoing, as indeed are widespread efforts to expand test-

ing in the community for one's serostatus. Reducing the numbers of infected people is a platform of prevention in itself, because it could start treatment earlier, and reduce transmission among them.

Male Circumcision

Male circumcision illustrates some of these possibilities. In 2007 in three separate and convincing experiments, carried out respectively in South Africa, Uganda, and Kenya, men were circumcised in excellent surgical sites.[58–60] In a subsequent follow up, the incidence of HIV infection was 60% lower than in an uncircumcised control group. The similarity of the findings in the three experiments is particularly impressive, even though there has been no similar trial in well-resourced countries. Were a populationwide policy of universal circumcision to be followed, the benefit for women is likely to depend on whether other risk reduction behavior such as condom use were to be unaffected by circumcision. Follow-up so far has been too brief to answer that question. Nonetheless, with all else remaining equal, the fewer the men infected, so too the fewer women would be infected, and would infect others.

Whether circumcision should be offered to all men, including those who are known to be HIV positive, is still in question. Since HIV-positive men will not themselves benefit directly from the procedure, which seems not to be protective against other sexually transmitted infections, it could be argued that including the procedure would unnecessarily raise costs. Moreover, troubling for women's health, if HIV-infected men undergo circumcision and engage in unprotected sex before the wound is healed (after some 6 weeks on average), the risk of transmission of HIV to partners is raised. On the other hand, larger numbers of uncircumcised men seem ready to undergo the procedure provided serostatus is not a condition for doing so. In some societies, moreover, stigma may attach to men not circumcised.

Other Societywide Interventions

Of course, any preventive approaches against HIV measures taken by the community (as illustrated with the PROMISE initiative), or that could reduce the incidence of infection as a vaccine or perhaps pre- or postexposure prophylaxis might accomplish, new infections among women would be reduced. Widespread treatment of those infected would have a similar effect among women as well as men. Since in general, public health preventive action tends to be more readily adopted by women than by men, the positive potential of such measures is likely to favor women. Among them, however, the poor and the uneducated are often the last to profit from public health preventive services.

Summary

A wholly effective vaccine against HIV would of course reduce the existing frequency and distribution of the disease, as in the differences between women and men, rich and poor, and wealthy and poor countries. Nothing so dramatic is yet on the horizon, but even at the time of writing in 2010, ongoing efforts toward prevention and treatment have advanced to the point of curbing the mass devastation initially wrought by the disease. At the same time, as yet neither in the United States nor globally is there room for complacency. Certainly, even in the United States today women are still in need both of protection from sexually transmitted diseases and of optimal care among those already infected. Under any circumstances, though most certainly among vulnerable groups, to neglect active intervention and the deployment of proven behavioral interventions is unjustifiable.[61]

In one U.S. example, an intervention was carried out among young low-income women attending family planning clinics, a group recognized as vulnerable to HIV infection.[62] At recruitment, many were users of condoms for contraception. All were instructed in the use of hormonal methods. These would prevent pregnancies, but of course would have no beneficial effect on the risk of sexually transmitted infection. On follow-up, almost all had adopted hormonal methods and discarded the use of condoms. This was clearly an unacceptable outcome. Counseling on the hazards of unprotected sex had been insufficiently emphasized, and certainly the implementation of an appropriate CDC preventive intervention like RESPECT had been neglected. Use of contraception and condoms to prevent both pregnancy and infection, known as dual protection, has to be the aim of counseling among groups of women likely to be at risk.[63,64]

Nor is optimal care widely provided for those women in the United States and elsewhere who are already seropositive for HIV, whether on active treatment or not. Although the recognized aim is so-called "normalization," this is seldom actively pursued in public services. As one example, among HIV-positive women conception and pregnancy should be seen as a possibility for those who desire it, but appropriate counseling and facilities are needed. Again, omission of such counseling is not an ethical option.[65] In short, despite 25 years of experience and research with extensive resources and despite considerable advances in knowledge, application of the knowledge we have deserves more intensive attention.

On a positive note, there has very recently been a flurry of activity in the United States to improve the situation, especially among groups who are at high risk. As described earlier, there is now a National HIV/AIDS strategy for the United States incorporated in several other documents, evidence of a renewed attempt to remedy some of the faults documented in recent publications.

Finally, a very important issue that has just reemerged in the scientific literature focuses even more attention on dual protection and the role of injectable hormones. In 1996, a challenging paper appeared in the journal *Nature*, demonstrating that in macaque monkeys, subcutaneous vaginal implants of progesterone (DMPA) greatly enhanced their susceptibility to SHIV, the equivalent to HIV in humans.[66] Although evidence of a similar effect of

progesterone in women exposed to HIV has been widely sought, results have been conflicting. As this chapter was going to press, a doubling of the HIV risk following the use of injectable hormones, either to the woman herself, or to her partner, has been published.[67]

Subject to intense evaluation, this study, based on some 3,000 discordant couples in seven African countries reopens a major controversy among public health planners. Contraception is on its own a profoundly important tool for women's health and especially for those residents in locations of high prevalence for HIV. How should we maximize prevention while facilitating contraception?[68]

Acknowledgment

The HIV Center for Clinical and Behavioral Studies, National Institute of Mental Health, P30 MH43520 (Anke A. Ehrhardt, PhD, Principal Investigator) has tendered generous support for this work We are grateful to Dr. Joanne Mantell and Dr. Ida Susser for careful and critical reading of this manuscript.

Discussion Questions

1. What are the benefits (a) for individuals and (b) for the community of early diagnosis of infection with HIV?
2. For scholars, policies of prevention have been distinguished as "abstinence" versus "abstinence plus." How do these two policies differ, and which do you favor?
3. What are your views about the female condom? Describe this device and who is likely to use it.

References

1. White House Office of National AIDS Policy. *National HIV/AIDS Strategy for the United States*. Washington, DC: The White House; July 13, 2010.
2. Office of AIDS Research, National Institutes of Health. Social and behavioral HIV prevention research Think Tank. September 26–28, 2010.
3. El-Sadr WM, Mayer KH, Adimora AA. The HIV epidemic in the United States: A time for action. *J AIDS*. 2010;55:S63.
4. Shilts R. *And the Band Played On: Politics, People, and the AIDS Epidemic*. New York: St. Martin's Press; 1987.
5. Bayer R, Oppenheimer GM. *AIDS Doctors: Voices from the Epidemic*. New York: Oxford University Press; 2000.
6. Flam R, Stein ZA. Behavior, infection and immune response: an epidemiological approach. In: Feldman DA, Johnson TM, eds. *The Social Dimension of AIDS: Methods and Theory*. New York: Praeger Press; 1986:61–76.
7. Cates W, Jr., Holmes KK. Condom efficacy against gonorrhea and nongonococcal urethritis (letter). *Am J Epidemiol*. 1996;143:843–844.
8. Susser M, Stein Z. Human immunodeficiency virus and the role of women: the new challenge. In: *Eras in Epidemiology: The Evolution of Ideas*. New York: Oxford University Press; 2009.
9. Centers for Disease Control and Prevention. Persons living with a diagnosis of HIV infection, by year and selected characteristics, 2005–2007—37 states with confidential name-based HIV infection reporting. *HIV/AIDS Surveillance Report, 2008*. 2010;20:76.
10. Stein ZA. HIV prevention: The need for methods women can use. *Am J Public Health*. 1990;80:460–462.
11. Cates W, Jr., Stone KM. Family planning, sexually transmitted diseases and contraceptive coice: a literature update part I. *Family Planning Perspective*. 1992;24:75–84.
12. Elias C, Heise L. Challenges for the development of female-controlled vaginal microbicides. *AIDS*. 1994;8:1–9.
13. Abdool Karim Q, Abdool Karim SS. South Africa: host to new and emerging epidemics. *Sex Transm Infec*. 1999;75:139–147.
14. Susser I. *AIDS, Sex and Culture: Global Politics and Survival in Southern Africa*. Chichester, England: Blackwell; 2009.
15. Dorrington R, Bourne D, Bradshaw D, Laubscher R, Timaeus IM. The impact of HIV/AIDS on adult mortality in South Africa. Medical Research Council Technical Report. September 2001.

16. Rosenfield A, Charo RA, Chavkin W. Moving forward on reproductive health. *N Engl J Med.* 2008;359:1869–1871.

17. Kirby DB. The impact of abstinence and comprehensive sex and STD/HIV education programs on adolescent sexual behavior. *Sex Res Social Policy.* 2008;5:18–27.

18. Collins C, Diallo DD. A prevention response that fits America's epidemics: Community perspectives on the status of HIV prevention in the United States. *J AIDS.* 2010;55:S148–S150.

19. Gramsci A. *Selections from the Prison Notebooks.* London: Lawrence and Wishart; 1971.

20. De Vincenzi I, for the European study Group on Heterosexual Transmission of HIV. A longitudinal study of human immunodeficiency virus transmission by heterosexual partners. *N Engl J Med.* 1994;331:341–346.

21. Alliance for Microbicide Development; Stone A., ed. Proceedings from Symposium on "Advancing Prevention Technologies for Sexual and Reproductive Health." September 2009.

22. Trussell J. Contraceptive efficacy of the Reality female condom. *Contraception.* 1998;58:147–148.

23. Latka M, Gollub E, French P, Stein Z. Male-condom and female-condom use among women after counseling in a risk-reduction hierarchy for STD prevention. *Sex Trans Dis.* 2000;27:431–437.

24. Barbosa RM, Kalckmann S, Berquo E, Stein Z. Notes on the female condom: experiences in Brazil. *Intl J STD AIDS.* 2007;18:261–266.

25. Center for Health and Gender Equity. *Saving Lives Now: Female Condoms and the Role of U.S. Foreign Aid.* Takoma Park, MD: Author; 2008.

26. Mantell JE, West B, Sue K, et al. Health care providers: A missing link in understanding acceptability of the female condom. *AIDS Educ Prev.* 2011;23:65–77.

27. Beksinska M, Smit J, Mabude Z, et al. Male partner involvement and assistance in female condom use. *Eur J Contracept Reprod Health Care.* 2008;13:400–403.

28. Mantell JE, Stein ZA, Susser I. Women in the time of AIDS: barriers, bargains, and benefits. *AIDS Educ Prev.* 2008;20:91–106.

29. Stoebenau K, Hindin MJ, Nathanson CA, et al. "... But then he became my *sipa*": the implications of relationship fluidity for condom use among women sex workers in Antananarivo, Madagascar. *Am J Public Health.* 2009;99: 811–819.

30. Gollub EL. A neglected population: drug-using women and women's methods of HIV/STI prevention. *AIDS Educ Prev.* 2008;20:107–120.

31. Mantell JE, Myer L, Carballo-Dieguez A, et al. Microbicide acceptability research: current approaches and future directions. *Soc Sci Med.* 2005;60:319–330.

32. Harrison PF, Lamphear TL. Microbicides. In Mayer KH, Pizer HF, eds. *The AIDS Pandemic: Impact on Science and Society.* San Diego, CA: Elsevier Academic Press; 2005:190–235.

33. Lagakos SW, Gable AR. Institute of Medicine Committee on Methodological Challenges in HIV Prevention Trials. *Methodological Challenges in Biomedical HIV Prevention Trials.* Washington, DC: National Academies Press; 2008.

34. Cohen MS, Gay C, Kashuba ADM, et al. Narrative review: Antiretroviral therapy to prevent the sexual transmission of HIV-1. *Ann Intern Med.* 2007; 146:591–601.

35. Abdool Karim Q, Abdool Karim SS, Frohlich JA, et al. Effectiveness and safety of Tenofovir gel, an antiretroviral microbicide, for the prevention of HIV infection in women. *Science.* 2010;329:1168–74.

36. Grant RM, Lama JR, Anderson PL, et al. Preexposure chemoprophylaxis for HIV prevention in men who have sex with men. *N Eng J Med.* 2010:363: 2587–2599.

37. AVAC Global Advocacy for AIDS Prevention. *A Cascade of Hope and Questions.* Vol. 2: Understanding the Results of CAPRISA 004. New York: Author; August 2010.

38. Kuhn L, Susser I, Stein Z. Can further placebo-controlled trials of antiretroviral drugs to prevent sexual transmission of HIV be justified? *Lancet* 2011;378:285–287.

39. Pequegnat W. AIDS behavioral prevention: unprecedented progress and emerging challenges. In Mayer KH, Pizer HF, eds. *The AIDS Epidemic: Impact on Science and Society.* San Diego, CA: Elsevier Academic Press; 2005: 236–260.

40. Fishbein M. *Theoretical Models of HIV Prevention, Abstract Book: Consensus Development Conference on Interventions to Prevent HIV Risk Behaviors.* Bethesda, MD: National Institutes of Health, 1997.

41. Fisher JD, Fisher WA. Changing AIDS-risk behavior. *Psychol Bull.* 1992;111:455–474.

42. Ehrhardt AA, Exner TM. Prevention of sexual risk behavior for HIV infection with women. *AIDS.* 2000;14:S53–S58.

43. Centers for Disease Control and Prevention. Diffusion of effective behavioral interventions (DEBI). 2009 Compendium of evidence-based HIV prevention interventions. http://www.cdc.gov/hiv/topics/research/prs/evidence-based-interventions.htm.

44. The CDC AIDS Community Demonstration Projects Research Group. Community-level HIV intervention in 5 cities: final outcome data from the CDC AIDS community demonstration projects. *Am J Public Health.* 1999;89:336–345.

45. DiClemente RJ, Wingood GM. A randomized controlled trial of an HIV sexual risk intervention for young African American women. *JAMA.* 1995;274:1271–1276.

46. Ehrhardt A, Exner TM, Hoffman S, et al. A gender-specific HIV/STD risk reduction intervention for women in a health care setting: short- and long-term results of a randomized clinical trial. *AIDS Care.* 2002;24:147–161.

47. Jemmott JB III, Jemmott LS. HIV risk-reduction behavioral interventions with heterosexual adolescents. *AIDS.* 2000;14:S40–S52.

48. Kamb ML, Fishbein M, Douglas JM, et al. Efficacy of risk-reduction counseling to prevent human immunodeficiency virus and sexually transmitted diseases. *JAMA.* 1998;280:1161–1167.

49. Exner TA, Mantell JE, Hoffman S, et al. Project REACH: A provider-delivered dual protection intervention for women using family planning services in New York City. *AIDS Care.* 2011;23:467–475.

50. Adams-Skinner J, Exner TM, Pili C, et al. The development and validation of a tool to assess nurse performance in dual protection counseling. *Patient Educ Couns.* 2008;76:265–271.

51. Healthy Living Project Team. Effects of a behavioral intervention to reduce risk of transmission among people living with HIV: The Healthy Living Project randomized controlled study. *J Acquir Immune Defic Syndr.* 2007;44: 213–221.

52. Blankenship KM, Friedman SR, Dworkin S, Mantell JE. Structural interventions: Concepts, challenges and opportunities for research. *J Urban Health.* 2006;83: 59–72.

53. Parker RG. Civil society, political mobilization, and the impact of HIV scale-up on health systems in Brazil. *JAIDS.* 2009;52:S49–51.

54. Chopra M, Lawn JE, Sanders D, et al. Lancet South Africa team. Achieving the health Millennium Development Goals for South Africa: challenges and priorities. *Lancet.* 2009;374:1023–1031.

55. Granich RM, Gibbs CF, Dye C, et al. Universal voluntary HIV testing with immediate antiretroviral therapy as a strategy for elimination of HIV transmission: a mathematical model. *Lancet.* 2009;373:48–57.

56. Dieffenbach CW, Fauci AS. Universal voluntary testing and treatment for prevention of HIV transmission. *JAMA.* 2009;301:2380–2382.

57. Wagner BG, Blower S. Voluntary universal testing and treatment is unlikely to lead to HIV elimination: a modeling analysis. *Nature Proceedings.* 2009; 3917:1.

58. Auvert B, Thljaard D, Lagrade E, et al. Randomized controlled intervention trial of male circumcision for reduction of HIV infection risk: the ANRS 1265 trial. *PLoS Med.* 2005;2:e298.

59. Gray RH, Kigozi G, Serwadda D, et al. Male circumcision for HIV prevention in men in Rakai, Uganda: a randomized trial. *Lancet.* 2007;369:657–666.

60. Bailey RC, Moses S, Parker CB, Agot K, et al. Male circumcision for HIV prevention in young men in Kisumu, Kenya: a randomized controlled trial. *Lancet.* 2007;369:643–656.

61. El-Sadr WM, Mayer KH, Hodder SL. AIDS in America—Forgotten but not gone. *N Engl J Med.* 2010;362:967–970.

62. Morroni C. *Condom and Dual Method Use among Young Minority Women Initiating Oral Contraception in the United States* [dissertation]. New York: Columbia University, Department of Epidemiology, Mailman School of Public Health; October 2007.

63. Cates W, Jr. Contraception, unintended pregnancies, and sexually transmitted diseases: why isn't a simple solution available? *Am J Epidemiol.* 1996;143:311–318.

64. Cates W, Jr., Steiner M. Dual protection against unintended pregnancy and sexually transmitted infections: what is the best contraceptive approach. *Sex Transm Dis.* 2002;29:168–174.

65. Mantell JE, Smit JA, Stein ZA. The right to choose parenthood among HIV-infected women and men. *J Public Health Policy.* 2009;30:367–378.

66. Marx PA, Spira AI, Gettie A, et al. Progesterone implants enhance SIV vaginal transmission and early virus load. *Nature Medicine.* 1996;2:1084–1089.

67. Heffron R, Donnell D, Rees H, et al. Use of hormonal contraceptives and risk of HIV-1 transmission: a prospective cohort study. *Lancet Infect Dis.* 2012;12:19–26. doi: 10.1016/S1473-3099(11)70247-X. Epub 2011 Oct 3.

68. Gollub E, Stein Z. Living with uncertainty: acting in the best interests of women. *Aids Res Treat* 2012;2012:524936.

Chronic Psychological and Psychosocial Conditions

Eating Disorders

Julia Sheehy, PhD

Dedicated to the memory of Melissa Rose Avrin 1989–2009

Melissa's Story

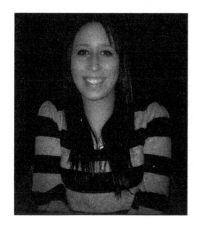

Source: Courtesy of Judy Avrin.

Melissa opened her college application essay with: "I was fourteen years old the first time I made myself throw up. If I had known that it was rapidly going to become my addiction, I would have never done it."

She was 13 and at sleep-away camp when she first became conscious of her body image after gaining some weight and beginning to menstruate. Her first eating disorder, chewing and spitting out food, escalated to binging and purging accompanied by constipation. She also started exercising compulsively and lost weight. Her doctors and her mother did not notice the subtle signs and symptoms of her developing eating disorder. Two days before her 16th birthday, Melissa was hospitalized and placed in an eating disorders program. During 2 weeks of aggressive inpatient therapy, she was stabilized medically. After leaving the hospital, she continued to be treated by a multidisciplinary team including a therapist, psychiatrist, and a nutritionist. While in treatment, Melissa continued to struggle with depression and symptoms of her eating disorder. Several years later she was hospitalized again for 4 weeks. Melissa appeared very motivated and eager to succeed in this new inpatient program. However, after leaving the hospital, she again experienced difficulties. While her parents and doctors were discussing the possible need for another hospitalization, Melissa died suddenly of a heart attack. She was 19 years old.

Someday Melissa, Inc. foundation is dedicated to promoting recognition and awareness of eating disorders and the importance of early treatment. http://www.somedaymelissa.com/

Introduction

Females account for the majority of the cases of anorexia and bulimia worldwide,[1–3] according to several estimates about 90%.[4–6] Girls and young women living in westernized cultures are the most susceptible.[7–10] The central features of these largely female disorders are disturbed body image, excessive dietary restraint and/or intake, and extreme means of manipulating their weight.

Binge eating disorder, in contrast, appears to affect males and females about equally according to data from the United States, Canada, and Australia.[11–14] Binge Eating Disorder is defined by excessive intake without accompanying compensatory behaviors (purging, restriction, and extreme exercise).

This chapter presents diagnostic categories and the prevalence and incidence of eating disorders. Risk factors, health consequences, and recovery and relapse rates are then reviewed. Prevention strategies and the effects of diagnostic globalization conclude the chapter.

Diagnosing Eating Disorders

The *Diagnostic and Statistical Manual of Mental Disorders*, Fourth Edition (DSM-IV)[7] provides a list of symptoms of anorexia nervosa. Symptoms include refusal to maintain a minimally healthy weight (specifically, ≤ 85% ideal body weight for height), intense fear of gaining weight, disturbed perceptions of weight and shape, overvaluation of weight and size on self-worth, denial of the seriousness of low weight, and amenorrhea. Two subtypes further define anorexia: restricting type in the absence of regular purging, and binge eating and purging type.

The DSM-IV provides a list of symptoms of bulimia, including episodes of binge eating (consuming larger amounts of food than most people would eat in discrete periods of time with loss of control over eating), recurring compensatory behaviors to compensate for binging, and overvaluation of weight and shape on self-worth. The criteria describe binging episodes and compensatory behaviors occurring at least twice weekly during a minimum of 3 months. Two subtypes further define bulimia: purging type involving regular self-induced vomiting or laxatives, diuretics, or enemas to compensate for binges in contrast to the nonpurging type relying on fasting or excessive exercise to compensate for excessive intake during binges.

Eating Disorder Not Otherwise Specified (EDNOS), a residual category, includes eating disorders that are variants of the more common disorders. For example, chewing and spitting out one's food and Binge Eating Disorder without compensatory behaviors is classified to the category of Eating Disorder Not Otherwise Specified in DSM-IV.

Eating disorder classifications are being actively debated and are likely to be modified in the next DSM,[15] scheduled for publication in 2013. Many people seeking treatment for an eating disorder, who experience functional impairment and psychological distress from their symptoms, do not meet criteria for either anorexia or bulimia and therefore are frequently assigned the diagnosis of Eating Disorder Not Otherwise Specified.[16–18] Many studies of eating disorders target individuals who meet criteria for anorexia or bulimia; therefore, those diagnosed with Eating Disorders Not Otherwise Specified are not included remaining an underresearched and poorly understood patient population. Patients classified with Eating Disorder Not Otherwise Specified often believe their diagnosis fails to capture the severity of their symptoms and suffering.[19]

Proposed changes in eating disorder classifications for the fifth edition of the DSM are listed on the American Psychiatric Association's DSM-5 Development website, at dsm5.org. In addition to eliminating the criterion of amenorrhea for anorexia, the task force proposes to reduce the required frequency of binging and purging from twice weekly for 3 months to once weekly for 3 months and to eliminate the subtypes of bulimia. Another modification proposed distinguishes Binge Eating Disorder from Eating Disorder Not Otherwise Specified basing the diagnosis on psychological features associated with binging behavior.

Prevalence and Incidence

Hoek and van Hoeken's 2003 review noted among young females an average prevalence rate of 0.3% for anorexia and 1% for bulimia.[16] The most recent studies reported slightly higher prevalence rates: 2.2% for anorexia[20] and 2.3% for bulimia.[21] Several studies that assessed partial-syndrome eating disorders indicated even higher prevalence rates: 3.7% for partial-syndrome anorexia and 5.4% for partial-syndrome bulimia.[22,23] Hoek and Hoeken concluded that the estimated prevalence rate for Binge Eating Disorder was 1% at a minimum.[16] A recent study on Eating Disorder Not Otherwise Specified found a prevalence rate of 2.37%.[24]

According to several long-term epidemiologic studies, the incidence of anorexia increased over the course of the 20th century until the 1970s, climbing most significantly from the 1950s to the 1970s when incidence stabilized. Rates were greatest for females between the ages of 15 and 19; this group accounted for about 40% of cases. These data were based on registered patients detected by healthcare practitioners.[16]

Although known cases of anorexia inarguably increased in the 1900s, the upward trend may have been due to improved understanding and detection of the disorder as well as greater treatment options.[16] A recent phone interview study conducted in Finland by clinicians trained in diagnosing eating disorders provided estimates for anorexia in the general population and reported substantially higher incidence rates than the studies limited to clinical samples.[20] Of the cases identified in this general population study, approximately half had been detected by healthcare practitioners.[20]

Scattered case histories describing overeating and vomiting date back centuries; however, reports early in the 20th century provided a few reports depicting bulimic behaviors as co-occurring with preoccupation with and intense fear of fatness. During the 1970s reports of this condition surged in the psychiatric literature creating the need for descriptive symptoms enabling the condition to be diagnosed and treated. Bulimia was defined by psychiatrist Gerald Russell in 1979[25] and included in the DSM in 1980.[26]

Several large-scale, long-term studies were then undertaken to assess the incidence of bulimia.[27,28] These studies found that rates increased sharply from 1980 to 1983, and from 1988 to 1993. Samples consisted of cases of bulimia that had been identified by healthcare practitioners, as documented in their medical records. Incidence rates were greatest for females between the ages of 20 and 24.[27]

A longitudinal study in Finland published in 2009 aimed to capture incidence rates of undetected as well as detected cases of bulimia in females by studying a nationwide, nonclinical sample.[21] Participants and their parents completed three follow-up questionnaires after baseline data collection at enrollment. As anticipated, incidence rates in the community sample were substantially higher than those found in the clinical sample, although accurate comparisons between the two are complicated by the studies' different assessment methods and targeted age groups. The community study also found that approximately one-third of the cases of bulimia had been detected by healthcare practitioners.

In DSM-IV, Binge Eating Disorder is included in the broad classification of Eating Disorder Not Otherwise Specified and is listed as a diagnosis "in need of further research."[7] Binge Eating Disorder affects 3.5% of females and 3% of males although believed to be prevalent among 30% of young people trying to lose weight.

Epidemiologic studies are believed to underestimate the actual numbers of people affected by eating disorders.[16] Although anorexia and bulimia have distinct definitions in the psychiatric nomenclature, psychological features intrinsic to the disorders including shame and denial continue to hinder accurate identification of cases. Shame and denial make it difficult for individuals to acknowledge the symptoms they are experiencing and to seek treatment. Some evidence suggests that eating disorders are underdiagnosed among some minorities. Preset concepts regarding diversity of populations who experience eating disorders may impede health professional from inquiring about symptoms and referring some groups for treatment affecting epidemiologic prevalence data.[29]

If the proposed diagnostic changes for the DSM-5 are implemented, prevalence and incidence rates of eating disorder diagnoses may not greatly change although redistribution is likely with higher rates of the formal categories of anorexia and bulimia and lower rates of Eating Disorders Not Otherwise Specified.

Risk Factors

Eating disorders grow out of a web of risk factors. Notably, being female is the single greatest risk factor for developing anorexia and bulimia,[30] with adolescent girls and young women particularly vulnerable.[16] In contrast, Binge Eating Disorder is equally likely to develop in males and females and may develop any time across the life span.[17,31]

Body dissatisfaction, defined as painfully negative appraisals of one's own body, has been suggested as a major risk factor in the development and maintenance of eating disorders. Body dissatisfaction is believed to stem from cultural pressures to conform to a narrow version of attractiveness that is impossible for most people to achieve.[32] Dieting, purging, and exercise are undertaken in an attempt to move one's body closer to the ideal.

Support for the role of cultural pressures in body dissatisfaction comes from a study conducted on the main island of Fiji. Fijian culture traditionally prized robust appetites and figures, and Fijian society had low rates of body dissatisfaction and eating disorders. After the arrival of western television shows, including *Xena: Warrior Princess* and *Beverly Hills 90210* in the 1990s, girls reported significant increases in body dissatisfaction and eating disorder symptoms. Many of the girls in the study explicitly said that they were striving to look like the characters they admired on television.[33]

Not only are females significantly more vulnerable to body dissatisfaction than males,[34] their body dissatisfaction is also unidirectional. In contrast to males who are dissatisfied with their bodies and are equally likely to want to be heavier or thinner,[35] females who are distressed about their bodies want only to be thinner. In a study reported in 2003, the prevalence of dieting was noted among 10-year-old girls and increased with age, as noted in Figure 15-1.

Although for decades eating disorders were assumed to affect white females primarily, the studies addressing ethnicity have not supported this assumption. Studies present a more complex linkage between ethnicity and types of eating pathology. Some evidence suggests that white females are more prone to restrictive and compensatory behaviors,[18] whereas binging has been shown consistently to cut across ethnicities.[13,36,37] Furthermore, among women with Binge Eating Disorder, black women report less psychological distress than white women.[38]

Differences within ethnic groups vary according to degree of exposure and acculturation to western ideals; the more individuals integrate into cultures that objectify females and prize thin bodies, the more likely they are to develop eating disorder symptoms.[8-10] Some women may be at greater risk including ballet dancers, gymnasts, wrestlers, models, or members of other subcultures that emphasize certain body sizes and shapes.[39]

Little is known about lesbianism and eating disorders. A nationwide study of eating behaviors of lesbians noted

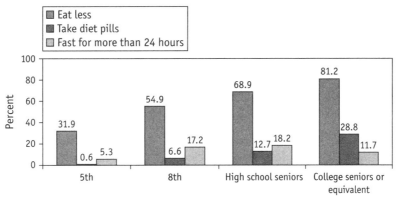

Figure 15-1 Dieting behaviors in the formative years

Source: Reproduced from The formative years: Pathways to substance abuse among girls and young women ages 8–22. New York: The National Center on Addiction and Substance Abuse (CASA) at Columbia University (2003).

overeating was much more common than undereating and vomiting in this population.[40] Another study reported lesbian college students indicated less body dissatisfaction and fewer eating disorder behaviors than heterosexual women, despite lesbians having significantly higher body mass index numbers than their counterparts.[41]

Researchers have investigated biologic risk factors associated with eating disorders, including genetic and neurobiologic. Family and twin studies have indicate that anorexia and bulimia aggregate in families. Relatives of individuals with a history of anorexia or bulimia are 10 times more likely to develop an eating disorder than those without an affected relative.[42] Twin studies indicate that heritability for anorexia ranges from 33%-85%, for bulimia 28%-83%, and for binge eating between 31% and 50%.[43]

Both anorexia and bulimia have also been associated with low levels of serotonin associated with acute phases of the disorders and following recovery. It is not yet clear, however, whether neurotransmitter abnormalities are causes or consequences of the disorders.[44] Most genetic studies of eating disorders have been conducted among women. Men may differ in their genetic vulnerability to eating disorders; more research is needed.

Childhood sexual abuse is a risk factor for the development of eating disorders, bulimia, and especially Binge Eating Disorder.[45,46] Although sexual abuse during childhood occurs among both genders,[47] female victims are more likely to internalize symptoms, such as suicidal thoughts and disordered eating. Male victims are more likely to develop externalizing symptoms, such as excessive drinking and delinquency.[48] Recent research also suggests that sexual abuse may be only one of many childhood traumas that predispose individuals to develop eating disorders later in life. Emotional and physical abuse, neglect, separation or loss, and major life changes may contribute to eating pathology.[49]

Personality factors associated with eating disorders include deficits in self-concept and perfectionism. Deficits in self-concept, i.e., feelings of ineffectiveness and low self-esteem, have been repeatedly associated with anorexia, bulimia, and Binge Eating Disorder.[50] However, such deficits predispose individuals to a broad range of psychopathology other than eating pathology specifically. Females score only slightly lower than males on global measures of self-esteem;[51] however, sources of self-esteem are known to vary by gender. For example, perceiving oneself as physically attractive is more strongly associated with female self-esteem,[52] suggesting that threats to self-esteem and consequent symptomatic expression may also vary by gender.

An ample body of evidence supports the association between perfectionism and eating disorders, even when varying measure have been used and different stages of the disorders have been assessed.[50] Although males and females are equally prone to perfectionism,[53] studies are needed to assess whether males and females manifest their perfectionism in different domains. Females may be more perfectionistic about their sources of self-esteem,

such as appearance, in extreme and maladaptive ways in the case of body dissatisfaction and eating disorders.

Over time researchers hope to understand the interconnection among various risk factors that collectively contribute to the development and maintenance of eating disorders.

Health Consequences

Eating disorders produce numerous medical risks, including fatality. At 5%, anorexia has been found to have the highest mortality rate of any psychiatric disorder.[54] Among the most severely ill who have been anorectic for 2 decades or more, the mortality rate is 20%.[55] The most common causes of death associated with anorexia are cardiac arrest and suicide. Less extreme but very serious medical consequences of anorexia include osteopenia and osteoporosis, stunted growth, cardiac dysfunction, seizures, and gastric problems.[1]

For decades, mortality associated with bulimia was considered "rare"[56] until a recent, large study noted a 3.9% mortality rate for bulimia, and even more surprisingly, 5.2% mortality rates for EDNOS.[57] Patients with Binge Eating Disorder were excluded from this study, meaning that EDNOS patients had subsyndrome anorexia or bulimia or variants of those disorders. Therefore, the findings indicate that mortality rates, including suicide, for all three categories of eating disorders may be "similar."[58]

A recent study by Miotto and Preti suggested that depression and aggressiveness accounted for the link between eating disorders and suicidal symptoms.[59] The authors noted that eating disorder pathology was not associated with elevated suicide risk, but depression and aggression induced these behaviors. The biologic impact of binging and purging negatively affects serotonin function and contributes to social withdrawal. Poor serotonin functioning and isolation raise depression and aggression, which may influence risk of suicide.

Bulimic behaviors can cause esophagus ruptures and cardiac dysfunction, as well as significant metabolic disturbances due to the purging behaviors and consequential depletion of needed electrolytes. Binge Eating Disorder, when associated with obesity (which it not always is), may result in high cholesterol, high blood pressure, and onset of diabetes.[1]

Eating disorders can also compromise reproduction, by way of amenorrhea and nutritional deficiencies. One small study conducted at an infertility clinic found active eating disorders among more than a third of the women undergoing ovulation induction.[60] Women with eating disorders who do become pregnant are at elevated risk for pre- and postnatal problems such as miscarriage, prematurity, and perinatal mortality.[61] Moreover, infants born at low weight are at greater risk for developing anorexia later in life.[62]

Most individuals with anorexia and bulimia do not seek out mental health treatment.[16] Medical providers, therefore, are in the primary position to detect eating disorders; clinicians may also be faced with management of medical conditions that accompany untreated psychiatric disorders when treating eating disordered patients.

Recovery and Relapse

The many outcome studies conducted on eating disorders are challenging to compare because of major differences including lack of consistent definitions of recovery (partial versus full), different sources for study populations (clinical versus community), and varied lengths of follow-up after initial diagnosis. Nevertheless, a recent comprehensive review of 26 studies published between 2004 and 2009 revealed course and outcome trends that can help inform treatment expectations and speculative prognoses.[63]

Anorexia is characterized by having substantial relapse rates, modest rates of full recovery, and the most protracted course of all the eating disorders.[63] Receiving inpatient treatment and struggling with severe and extended anorexia indicate poorer prognoses. Significant portions of individuals with anorexia also migrate into bulimia or the Eating Disorder Not Otherwise Specified category. Those who do fully recover from anorexia often continue to contend with persistent body dissatisfaction and psychosomatic symptoms.[20]

Bulimia is characterized by quicker rates of recovery and higher rates of both partial and full recovery than anorexia.[63] Severe comorbid psychopathology indicates a poorer prognosis, and those who remain ill for 5 years may be chronically affected. Significant portions of patients with bulimia also migrate into the Eating Disorder Not Otherwise Specified category. Many who do fully recover from bulimia experience ongoing problems with body image, self-esteem, anxiety, and psychosomatic symptoms.[21]

Preliminary research on Binge Eating Disorder and other Eating Disorder Not Otherwise Specified conditions suggest higher remission rates at 1-year follow-up than for anorexia and bulimia. Having few interpersonal supports may indicate poorer prognoses for these disorders. Those who have Binge Eating Disorder or Eating Disorders Not Otherwise Specified for 5 years may struggle with the disorder chronically.[63]

Prevention

Psychoeducation about eating disorders including information about behaviors and characteristics, health consequences and treatment, does not reliably reduce susceptibility to future eating pathology; in fact, pilot studies with school girls suggested that psychoeducation intensified the drive for thinness in some students.[64,65]

Successful eating disorder prevention programs do exist, however, and several are now considered empirically supported.[66] Effective prevention programs promote body acceptance and disrupt the internalization of thinness as ideal. When directed by professional staff, these programs produce the largest benefits if offered to high-risk, female-only groups whose participants are over the age of 15.[66]

Globalization of American Diagnoses

The DSM was created to provide clinicians and researchers with a common language for describing various mental illnesses. Diagnostic categories described in DSM have been developed by the American Psychiatric Association with significant collaboration of international experts. The categories and descriptions evolve with each DSM revision, as new research accumulates, clinical thinking and treatment approaches progress, and expressions of mental illness takes different forms.

Ethan Watters, a journalist who studies social trends, recently examined the influence of DSM categories and noted trends reflect symptomatic expression, especially as American diagnoses assume greater hegemony around the world. In a *New York Times Magazine*,[67] publication Watters cited an example from Dr. Sing Lee's work with anorectic patients in Hong Kong. Young women in Hong Kong suffered from the same behavioral symptoms as American anorectic patients; however, they complained of stomach bloating and digestion difficulties instead of fear of fatness and body dissatisfaction—their subjective symptoms differed. Dr. Lee has been researching culturally specific versions of anorexia.

In 1994, a Chinese girl died of complications due to anorexia on a crowded Hong Kong street. Her death garnered considerable media attention, and reporters employed the DSM's description of anorexia in an attempt to understand the girl's condition. Dr. Lee subsequently observed a sharp increase in the number of patients presenting with anorexia; moreover, his new patients were increasingly reporting fear of fatness. American anorexia had seemingly migrated into the Hong Kong psyche. As researchers and clinicians work to describe, measure, track, and treat eating disorders, these efforts may shape mental illness patterns of the future.

Summary

Anorexia and bulimia are primarily female disorders in contrast to Binge Eating Disorder, which appears to affect males and females about equally. Eating disorder diagnostic categories continue to be debated and may be revised for the next edition of the DSM, especially because a majority of eating disorder patients are assigned the diagnosis of eating disorder not otherwise specified. Eating disorders affect people of all ethnicities across the globe. However, relationships exist between prevalence rates and degree of exposure to western ideals, and between ethnicity and type of eating disorder. Anorexia, bulimia, and eating disorders not otherwise specified produce numerous medical consequences including reproductive problems and carry comparable mortality risks. Prevention research has indicated that psychoeducation may intensify preexisting restrictive tendencies in some individuals, although helpful prevention programs foster acceptance of various body types and question the idealization of thinness.

Discussion Questions

1. What are the types of eating disorders?
2. What impedes the accuracy of prevalence and incidence rates for eating disorders?
3. What are the known risk factors associated with anorexia and bulimia?
4. What are the health consequences associated with eating disorders?
5. What factors are known to be effective in eating disorder prevention?

References

1. American Psychiatric Association. Practice guideline for the treatment of patients with eating disorders (revision). *Am J Psychiatry.* 2000;157 (January suppl).
2. Hoek HW. Incidence, prevalence and mortality of anorexia and other eating disorders. *Curr Opin Psychiatry.* 2006;19:389–394.
3. Wittchen HU, Jacobi F. Size and burden of mental disorders in Europe—a critical review and appraisal of 27 studies. *Eur Neuropsychopharmacol.* 2005;15:357–376.
4. Anderson AE. Anorexia nervosa and bulimia nervosa in males. In: Garfinkle PE,. Gardner DM, eds. *Diagnostic Issues in Anorexia Nervosa and Bulimia Nervosa.* New York: Brunner/Mazel; 1998:166–207.
5. Hsu LKG. Epidemiology of the eating disorders. *Psychiatr Clin North Am.* 1996;19:681–700.
6. Whittchen HU, Nelson CB, Lachner G. Prevalence of mental disorders and psychosocial impairments in adolescents and young adults. *Psychol Med.* 1998;28:109–126.
7. *Diagnostic and Statistical Manual of Mental Disorders.* 4th ed. Washington DC: American Psychiatric Association; 1994.
8. Davis C, Katzman MA. Perfectionism as acculturation: psychological correlates of eating problems in Chinese male and female students living in the United States. *Int J Eat Disord.* 1999;25:65–70.
9. Gowen LK, Hayward C, Killen JD, et al. Acculturation and eating disorders: symptoms in adolescent girls. *J Res Adolesc.* 1999;9:67–83.
10. Gunewardene A, Huon GF, Zheng R. Exposure to westernization and dieting: a cross-cultural study. *Int J Eat Disord.* 2000;29:289–293.
11. Hay P. The epidemiology of eating disorder behaviors: an Australian community-based survey. *Int J Eat Disord.* 1998;23:371–382.
12. Lewinsohn PM, Seeley JR, Moerk KC, Striegel-Moore RH. Gender differences in eating disorder symptoms in young adults. *Int J Eat Disord.* 2002;32:426–440.
13. Reagan P, Hersch J. Influence of race, gender, and socioeconomic status on binge eating frequency in a population-based sample. *Int J Eat Disord.* 2005;38:252–256.
14. Woodside DB, Garfinkle PE, Lin E, et al. Comparisons of men with full or partial eating disorders, men without eating disorders, and women with eating disorders in the community. *Am J Psychiatry.* 2001;158:570–574.
15. Walsh T. Eating disorders in DSM-V: review of existing literature. *Int J Eat Disord.* 2009;42:579–580.
16. Hoek HW, van Hoeken D. Review of the prevalence and incidence of eating disorders. *Int J Eat Disord.* 2003;34:383–396.
17. Hudson JI, Hiripi E, Pope HG Jr, Kessler RC. The prevalence and correlates of eating disorders in the National Comorbidity Survey Replication. *Biol Psychiatry.* 2007;61:348–358.
18. Striegel-Moore RH, Franko DL, Thompson D, et al. An empirical study of the typology of bulimia nervosa and its spectrum variants. *Psychol Med.* 2005;35:1563–1572.
19. Ellin A. Narrowing an eating disorder. *The New York Times.* January 19, 2010.
20. Keski-Rahkonen A, Hoek H, Susser E, et al. Epidemiology and course of anorexia nervosa in the community. *Am J Psychiatry.* 2007;164:1259–1265.
21. Keski-Rahkonen A, Hoek HW, Linna, MS, et al. Incidence and outcomes of bulimia nervosa: a nationwide population-based study. *Psychol Med.* 2009;39:823–831.
22. Garfinkle PE, Lin E, Goering P, et al. Should amenorrhea be necessary for the diagnosis of anorexia nervosa. *Br J Psychiatry.* 1996;168:500–506.
23. Walters EE, Kendler KS. Anorexia nervosa and anorectic-like syndromes in a population-based female twin sample. *Am J Psychiatry.* 1995;152:64–71.
24. Machado P, Machado B, Goncalves S, Hoek H. The prevalence of eating disorders not otherwise specified. *Int J Eat Disord.* 2007;40:212–217.
25. Russell GFM. Bulimia nervosa: an ominous variant of anorexia nervosa. *Psychol Med.* 1979;9:429–448.
26. American Psychiatric Association. *Diagnostic and Statistical Manual of Mental Disorders.* 3rd ed. Washington DC: Author; 1980.
27. Soundy TJ, Lucas AR, Suman VJ, Melton LJ III. Bulimia nervosa in Rochester, Minnesota from 1980 to 1990. *Psychol Med.* 1995;25:1065–1071.
28. Turnbull S, Ward A, Treasure J, Jick, H, Derby L. The demand for eating disorder care: an epidemiological study using the General Practice Research database. *Br J Psychiatry.* 1996;169:705–712.
29. Becker A, Franko DL, Spek A, Herzog DB. Ethnicity and differential access to care for eating disorder symptoms. *Int J Eat Disord.* 2003;33:205–212.
30. Striegel-Moore RH, Bulik CM. Risk factors for eating disorders. *Am Psychologist.* 2007;62:181–198.
31. Kinzi JF, Traweger C, Trefalt E, et al. Binge eating disorder in males: a population-based investigation. *Eat Weight Disord.* 1999;4:169–174.
32. Paxton S. Body dissatisfaction and disordered eating. *J Psychosom Res.* 2002;53:961–962.
33. Becker AE. Television, disordered eating, and young women in Fiji: negotiating body image and identity during rapid social change. *Cult Med Psychiatry.* 2004;28:533–559.
34. Babio N, Arija V, Sancho C, Canals J. Factors associated with body dissatisfaction in non-clinical adolescents at risk of eating disorders. *J Public Health.* 2008;16:107–115.
35. Furnham A, Badmin N, Sneade I. Body image dissatisfaction: gender differences in eating attitudes, self-esteem, and reasons for exercise. *J Psychol.* 2002;136:581–596.
36. Hay P. The epidemiology of eating disorder behaviors: an Australian community-based survey. *Int J Eat Disord.* 1998;23:371–382.
37. Lewinsohn PM, Seeley JR, Moerk KC, Striegel-Moore R.H. Gender differences in eating disorder symptoms in young adults. *Int J Eat Disord.* 2002;32:426–440.
38. Pike KM, Dohm FA, Striegel-Moore RH, Wilfrey DE, Fairburn CG. A comparison of black women and white women with binge eating disorder. *Am J Psychiatry.* 2001;158:1455–1460.
39. Striegel-Moore RH. Risk factors for eating disorders. *Ann N Y Acad Sci.* 1997;817:98–109.
40. Bradford J, Ryan C, Rothblum ED. National Lesbian Health Care Survey: implications for mental health care. *J Consult Clin Psychol.* 1994;62:228–242.
41. Siever MD. Sexual orientation and gender as factors in socioculturally acquired vulnerability to body dissatisfaction and eating disorders. *J Consult Clin Psychol.* 1994;62:252–260.
42. Bulik CM. Exploring the gene-environment nexus in eating disorders. *J Psychiatry Neurosci.* 2005;30:335–339.
43. Bulik CM, Tozzi F. Genetics in eating disorders: state of the science. *CNS Spectrums.* 2004;9:511–515.
44. Kaye WH, Frank GK, Bailer UF, et al. Serotonin alterations in anorexia and bulimia nervosa: new insights from imaging studies. *Physiol Behav.* 2005;85:73–81.
45. De Groot J, Rodin GM. The relationship between eating disorders and childhood trauma. *Psychiatric Ann.* 1999;29:225–229.
46. Wonderlich SA, Brewerton TD, Jocic Z, et al. Relationship of childhood sexual abuse and eating disorders. *J Am Acad Child Adolesc Psychiatry.* 1997;36:1107–1115.
47. Banyard V, Williams L, Siegel J. Childhood sexual abuse: a gender perspective on context and consequences. *Child Maltreat.* 2004;9:223–238.
48. Chandy J, Blum R, Resnick M. Gender-specific outcomes for sexually abused adolescents. *Child Abuse Negl.* 1996;20:1219–1231.
49. Smyth JM, Heron KE, Wonderlich SA, Crosby RD, Thompson, KM. The influence of reported trauma and adverse events on eating disturbance in young adults. *Int J Eat Disord.* 2008;41:195–202.
50. Jacobi C, Hayward C, de Zwaan M, et al. Coming to terms with risk factors for eating disorders: application of risk terminology and suggestions for a general taxonomy. *Psychol Bull.* 2004;130:19–65.
51. Kling K, Hyde J, Showers C, Buswell B. Gender differences in self-esteem: a meta-analysis. *Psychol Bull.* 1999;125:470–500.
52. Andreja A. Gender differences in the structure of self-concept: are the self conceptions about physical attractiveness really more important for women's self-esteem? *Studia Psychol.* 2006;48:31–43.
53. Stoeber J, Stoeber F. Domains of perfectionism: prevalence and relationships with perfectionism, gender, age, and satisfaction with life. *Pers Individ Dif.* 2008;46:530–535.
54. Sullivan PF. Mortality in anorexia nervosa. *Am J Psychiatry.* 1995;152:1073–1074.
55. Theander S. Outcome and prognosis in anorexia nervosa and bulimia: some results of previous investigations, compared with those of a Swedish long-term study. *J Psychiatric Res.* 1985;19:493–508.
56. Garner DM, Garfinkel PE. *Handbook of Treatment for Eating Disorders.* 2nd ed. New York: Guilford Press; 1997.
57. Crow SJ, Peterson CB, Swanson SA, Raymond NC, Specker S, Eckert ED, et al. Increased mortality in bulimia nervosa and other eating disorders. *Am J Psychiatry.* 2009;166:1342–1346.
58. Kaye W. Eating disorders: hope despite mortal risk. *Am J Psychiatry.* 2009;166:1309–1311.
59. Miotto P, Preti A. Eating disorders and suicidal ideation: the mediating role of depression and aggressiveness. *Curr Opinion Psychiatry.* 2006;19:389–394.
60. Abraham S, Mira N, Llewellyn-Jones D. Should ovulation be induced in women recovering from an eating disorder or who are compulsive exercisers? *Fertil Steril.* 1990;53:566–568.
61. Key A, Mason H, Bolton J. Reproduction and eating disorders: a fruitless union. *Eur Eat Disord Rev.* 2000;8:98–107.

62. Cnattingius C, Hultman M, Dahl M, Sparen P. Very pre-term birth, birth trauma, and the risk of anorexia nervosa among girls. *Arch Gen Psychiatry.* 1999;56:634–638.

63. Keel P, Brown T. Update on course and outcome in eating disorder. *Int J Eat Disord.* 2010;43:195–204.

64. Carter JC, Stewart DA, Dunn VJ, Fairburn CG. Primary prevention of eating disorders: might it do more harm than good? *Int J Eat Disord.* 1997;22: 167–172.

65. Huon GF, Roncolato WG, et al. Prevention of diet-induced disorders: findings and implications of a pilot study. *Eating Disorders: J Treat Prev.* 1997;5: 280–293.

66. Stice E, Shaw H, Marti CN. A meta-analytic review of eating disorder prevention programs: encouraging findings. *Ann Rev Clin Psychol.* 2007;3:207–231.

67. Watters E. The Americanization of mental illness. *The New York Times Magazine.* January 10, 2010.

CHAPTER

16

Depression in Women

Daniel J. Pilowsky, MD, MPH and Katherine M. Keyes, PhD

Introduction

Major Depressive Disorder (MDD) affects an estimated 18.8 million Americans per year[1] and is among the leading causes of disability worldwide.[2] Women are more likely to be affected with depression than men, with sex ratios ranging from 1.5 to 3.1 across continents and cultures.[3] Over 30 years ago, Weissman and Klerman reviewed research dealing with gender differences in the prevalence of depression and concluded that depression was more prevalent in women than in men, both in clinical and community samples.[4] Until then some believed that the gender difference in the prevalence of depression was the result of differences in treatment-seeking behavior. Most individuals meeting criteria for MDD are not treated, and depressed men are less likely than their female counterparts to seek treatment. However, Weissman and Klerman found that depression was more prevalent in adult women not only in clinical samples but also in community surveys. Since then, the gender difference in the prevalence of depression has been one of the most consistent findings in psychiatric epidemiology, with researchers reporting these differences in a variety of samples.[5]

This chapter provides an overview of the depression diagnoses in the *Diagnostic and Statistical Manual of Mental Disorders*, currently in its fourth edition (DSM-IV[6]), describes prevalence estimates for MDD in the United States from major epidemiologic surveys, and discusses biologic and psychosocial risk factors for depression, with special emphasis on studies that examined risk factors that may have a dissimilar impact on men and women. We describe clinical presentations of depression related to the reproductive cycle, focusing on postpartum depression and premenstrual dysphoric disorder.

Diagnosing Major Depressive Disorder in the DSM-IV

The cardinal symptom of depression is persistent and impairing sadness. Because sadness is a universal and normative human experience, diagnostic criteria must quantify its magnitude and establish thresholds in order to ascertain who is clinically depressed—not simply sad.

Thus, we assume that everyone in the population has a value of depressed mood on an underlying continuum; once an individual passes beyond a certain threshold of depressed mood, we diagnose the individual as suffering from depression. An analogy can be made to high blood pressure diagnostics: although everyone has a blood pressure, we choose a clinical cut point beyond which individuals are considered to suffer from hypertension.

Neither sadness nor any of the other symptoms of depression can be measured using biologic or other classically objective measures. Thus, we resort to patients' reports and to our observations during the clinical interview to estimate the extent of each symptom and use a count of symptoms to establish a threshold. The DSM-IV provides a list of symptoms of major depressive episode (MDE) (see Table 16-1). Five or more of the symptoms shown in Table 16-1 must be present during the same 2-week period and at least one of the symptoms must be depressed mood or loss of interest or pleasure. As with most DSM-IV disorders the symptoms must cause clinically significant impairment or distress. A major depressive disorder is defined as having a single or multiple MDE episodes in individuals who have never met criteria for a bipolar disorder (also known as manic-depressive), while not meeting criteria for related disorders (e.g. schizoaffective disorder), as specified in DSM-IV.

MDD is not the only type of depression recognized by the DSM. A second type of depression, less severe but often chronic, is known as dysthymia. Dysthymia has a low prevalence in the population[7] and is characterized by depressed mood most of the day, for more days than not, for at least 2 years. A third situation arises when individuals become temporarily depressed following a stressful life event and the depression does not meet criteria for a specific psychiatric disorder. The DSM-IV provides two diagnoses, adjustment disorder "with depressed mood" and "with anxiety and depressed mood," that are applicable to this situation. Last, individuals who are sufficiently depressed to report impairment or distress but do not meet criteria for any of these other disorders, are diagnosed with "depressive disorder not otherwise specified." An example (given in DSM-IV) is an individual who has experienced four (rather than five) MDE symptoms

Table 16-1

DSM-IV criteria for Major Depressive Episode [6]

(A) Five (or more) of the following symptoms have been present during the same 2-week period and represent a change from previous functioning; at least one of the symptoms is either (1) depressed mood or (2) loss of interest or pleasure:

    (1) depressed mood most of the day, nearly every day, as indicated by either subjective report (e.g., feels sad or empty) or observation made by others (e.g., appears tearful). Note: In children and adolescents, can be irritable mood.

    (2) markedly diminished interest or pleasure in all, or almost all, activities most of the day, nearly every day (as indicated by either subjective account or observation made by others)

    (3) significant weight loss when not dieting or weight gain (e.g., a change of more than 5% of body weight in a month), or decrease or increase in appetite nearly every day. Note: In children, consider failure to make expected weight gains.

    (4) insomnia or hypersomnia nearly every day

    (5) psychomotor agitation or retardation nearly every day (observable by others, not merely subjective feelings or restlessness or being slowed down)

    (6) fatigue or loss of energy nearly every day

    (7) feelings of worthlessness or excessive or inappropriate guilt (which may be delusional) nearly every day (not merely self-reproach or guilt about being sick)

    (8) diminished ability to think or concentrate, or indecisiveness, nearly every day (either by subjective account or as observed by others)

    (9) recurrent thoughts of death (not just fear of dying), recurrent suicidal ideation without a specific plan, or a suicide attempt or a specific plan for committing suicide

(B) The symptoms do not meet criteria for a Mixed Episode.

(C) The symptoms cause clinically significant distress or impairment in social, occupational, or other important areas of functioning.

(D) The symptoms are not due to direct physiological effects of a substance (e.g., a drug of abuse, a medication) or a general medical condition (e.g., hypothyroidism).

(E) The symptoms are not better accounted for by Bereavement, i.e., after the loss of a loved one, the symptoms persist longer than 2 months or are characterized by marked functional impairment, morbid preoccupation with worthlessness, suicidal ideation, psychotic symptoms, or psychomotor retardation.

Source: Reproduced with permission from *Diagnostic and Statistical Manual of Mental Disorders*, 4th ed. Text Revision. Copyright © 2000. American Psychiatric Association.

for at least 2 weeks. When we use the term "depression" in this chapter we refer to any of the depressive disorders described here. However, when discussing the epidemiology of depression, we often refer to MDD, as this disorder has been the focus of most epidemiologic surveys.

Onset, Prevalence, and Trends in Depression Diagnoses from Major Epidemiologic Surveys

Onset of Depression and Gender Differences Through the Life Course

The median age of MDD onset is estimated to be at 30 years, dysthymia at 31, and any mood disorder at 30, but the range of MDD incidence varies throughout the life course.[8] Gender differences in the prevalence of MDD are not evident before puberty. The prevalence of MDD is very low before puberty and is either equally distributed in boys and girls, or slightly more prevalent in boys.[9] Figure 16-1 displays the age of depression onset for boys and girls in the Children in the Community Study, a longitudinal community sample in upstate New York.[9] After puberty preva-

lences of MDD diverge markedly by gender. By ages 12–15 girls are more likely to be depressed than boys. This pattern continues in adulthood, with women accounting for about two-thirds of prevalent cases.[4,10] Furthermore, the gender difference is also observed in studies that measure depressive symptoms rather than diagnoses.[11] In sum, the adult pattern of a higher prevalence of depression in women emerges in adolescence and continues in adulthood. A variety of theories have been proposed to explain this pattern, and they are discussed later in this chapter.

12-Month and Lifetime Prevalence of DSM-IV Major Depressive Disorder

Estimates of the incidence and prevalence of depressive disorders are best made from large, nationally representative surveys of the general population. In Table 16-2, we present estimates of the lifetime and 12-month (when available) prevalence of MDD in men and women. These estimates are based on large surveys in the United States since 1980. As shown in Table 16-2, they range from 2.6% for men in the Epidemiologic Catchment Area (ECA)[12] study to 22.9% for women in the National Comorbidity Survey Replication (NCSR).[13] Further, the ratio of

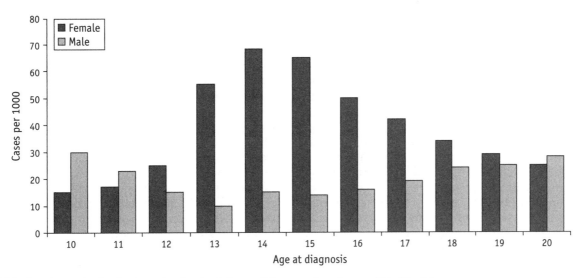

Figure 16-1 Prevalence rate of major depressive disorder during youth by age and gender, ages 10 to 20 years.

Source: Adapted from Cohen P, Cohen J, Kasen S, et al., An epidemiological study of disorders in late childhood and adolescence-I. Age- and gender-specific prevalence. J Child Psychol Psychiatry 1993;34:851-867.

Table 16-2

Lifetime and past-year prevalence of major depression by gender in large-scale epidemiologic surveys in the United States, 1980-2003

| Study | Years of data collection | Past 12-month | | | Lifetime | | | Reference |
		Women	Men	Women: men ratio	Women	Men	Women: men ratio	
U.S. ECA	1980-1985	2.7	1.2	2.3	7.0	2.6	2.7	[12]
NCS	1991-1992	12.9	7.7	1.6	21.3	12.7	1.7	[13]
NLAES	1991-1992	3.9	2.7	1.4	11.0	8.6	1.3	[14]
NESARC	2001-2002	6.9	3.6	1.9	17.1	9.0	1.9	[15]
NSAL: African American	2001-2003	n/a	n/a	n/a	13.1	7.0	1.9	[17]
NSAL: Caribbean Black	2001-2003	n/a	n/a	n/a	13.1	12.6	1.0	[17]
NSAL: White	2001-2003	n/a	n/a	n/a	19.5	16.2	1.2	[17]
WMH	2001-2003	10.2	6.2	1.6	22.9	15.1	1.5	[18]

n/a: past 12-month major depression estimates from the NSAL have not yet been published.

---

diagnosis between men and women ranges from 1 to 1 (virtually no difference in prevalence between men and women) for Caribbean Blacks in the National Survey of American Life (NSAL), to 2.7 to 1.0 for the Epidemiologic Catchment Area study.[17] Fewer studies have published prevalence of current depression by gender, but population estimates indicate a similar overrepresentation of women, with women to men ratios ranging from 1.4 to 1.0 in the National Longitudinal Alcohol Epidemiologic Survey (NLAES) survey[14] to 1.9 to 1.0 in the National

Epidemiologic Survey on Alcohol and Related Conditions (NESARC) survey.[15]

Temporal, Geographic, and Sociodemographic Trends in Depression Gender Differences

Epidemiologic evidence collected over the past 20 years indicates that major depression has been substantially increasing in recent birth cohorts in the United States.[16,17] The National Comorbidity Study Replication reported that the lifetime prevalence of major depression was 10.6% for individuals over the age of 60, compared to 19.8% for individuals ages 30–44 and 15.4% for individuals ages 18–29.[16] In addition, consistent evidence is emerging that the gender difference in depression is diminishing, both in the United States and worldwide,[18-20] especially in countries where traditional female roles have shifted over time (e.g., more women in the workforce), which suggests a strong psychosocial component to gender differences in depression. Hypotheses for the increase in prevalence among younger cohorts include artifacts of diagnosis such as the increased awareness of depression and its symptoms, and advances in pharmacotherapy and the consumer advertising that has accompanied these advances.[21] The increases also may be the result of increased exposure to or salience of stressful life events and other environmental risk factors.[22] The validity of these hypotheses remains open for debate.

Risk Factors for Depression

Depression is a complex disorder, and multiple factors likely contribute to elevated female risk. The body of research evaluating risk factors for depression in women is vast, and the reader is referred to several relevant publications.[23–25] In this chapter we focus on risk factors for depression that may contribute to the higher prevalence of depressive disorders in women compared to men: hormonal differences, stressful life events, genetic liability, and childhood anxiety disorders.

Hormone Differences Through the Life Course

Changes in mood associated with changes in sex hormone levels are often reported by women, for example, while using oral contraceptives or hormone replacement therapy,[26-27] during important developmental phases such as puberty and menopause, as well as during the luteal phase of the menstrual cycle and postpartum (reviewed in detail later). Thus, the association between hormones and depression status among women has been an area of empirical interest. Although this association seems intuitive to explain the sex difference in depression prevalence as hormones differ between men and women, the evidence for a role of hormones in the etiology of depression remains scant. We discuss the role of hormonal changes that may affect depression at various stages of women's lives here and describe the clinical presentation of premenstrual dysphoric disorder and postpartum depression in subsequent sections.

Adolescence

Because sex differences in the production of gonadal hormones emerge during puberty, it is reasonable to hypothesize that increasing levels of female sex hormones may play a causative role in sex differences in depression. Consistent with this hypothesis, Angold et al. demonstrated that the increased risk for depression in girls is better predicted by pubertal stage rather than chronological age.[28]

Other research, however, offers little empirical evidence to support a significant hormonal contribution to sex differences in depression.[29] Although early studies were plagued with methodologic issues (e.g., small sample sizes, unreliable measures of depression, indirect assessments of hormone levels), Brooks-Gunn and Warren[29] directly assessed hormone levels in 100 Caucasian girls and found psychosocial factors to be much stronger predictors of depression onset than hormone levels. Further, Hayward et al. reported that postmenarcheal differences between boys and girls on depressive scores were limited to Caucasian adolescents only.[30] These data suggest that psychosocial rather than biologic mechanisms may account for the sex difference. Further, Gilligan et al. assert that the onset of puberty corresponds to a developmental stage when societal expectations of young women change, with new pressures, both internal and societal, for thinness, beauty, and the adoption of feminine gender roles. Further, interpersonal conflicts arising from the struggle to conform to these roles may contribute to the emergence of gender differences in the prevalence of depression in adolescence.[31–33] Thus, many investigators currently conclude that the biologic hormone changes associated with puberty may not play a decisive role in female depression incidence.

Premenstrual Dysphoria

Women often experience sadness and irritability during the luteal phase of the menstrual cycle. Sadness and irritability that is clinically impairing has been defined in the DSM-IV as premenstrual dysphoric disorder (PMDD), and specific treatment recommendations have been proposed. The etiology of PMDD is unknown; little evidence has emerged of specific hormone imbalances among women with PMDD compared to those without.

Using data from a large community sample, Cohen at al. found that PMDD was strongly associated with previous history of depression and was also associated with low educational level, working outside the home, and current cigarette smoking.[34] There is abundant evidence that women with PMDD report more stressful life events and are more affected by stressors than women without PMDD.[35]

Postpartum

A majority of women experience some form of depressive symptoms following childbirth, thought to be caused by fluctuations in hormones such as estrogen and progesterone during this time.[36] The clinical presentation of postpartum depression is outlined later. Here we discuss the hypothesized increased risk for depression during the postpartum period. Whether postpartum women have an increased risk of MDD compared to similarly aged women not giving birth, however, is debatable. An early meta-analysis estimated that approximately 13% of women experience clinically significant MDD approximately 4 to 6 weeks after childbirth compared to 12% of women not giving birth.[37] Many of these studies were clinical samples of small size, however. More recent evidence suggests that the postpartum period does increase risk for depression.[38–40] For example, a nationally representative study of over 14,500 women reported that an increased risk for MDD persists for at least 1 year following childbirth.[38]

Menopause

The transition to menopause is associated with decreased levels of estrogen, which leads to a constellation of physical symptoms. Although it is a commonly held belief that menopause increases the risk for depressive symptoms, irritability, and major depressive disorder, empirical support for this belief is not consistent.[41] Studies using symptom scores and other nondiagnostic measures of depression have noted an association between mood and perimenopausal status (most often defined as the 1-year period prior to menopause when menopausal symptoms emerge),[42,43] but epidemiologic samples with diagnostic measures have raised doubts about this association in the general population.[44] There is overlap between the symptoms of menopause (e.g. irritability, insomnia, libido changes), as well as unique symptoms of menopause (e.g. vaginal dryness) and of depression (e.g. suicidal thoughts),[41] and this overlap contributes to the difficulty inherent in studying the relation between menopause and depression.

Psychosocial Factors

Stressful life events

Sex differences in depression are often attributed to gender differences in the experience of and response to stressful life events. Although studies have demonstrated that females and males experience the same number of stressful life events,[45,46] some investigators suggested that the stressful life events experienced by females are qualitatively different from those experienced by males. For example, interpersonal stress is associated with higher depressive symptoms compared to more general life stressors;[47] as women are more likely to report these types of stressors compared to men, the experience of these stressors may be one mediator of the gender difference. Other investigators posit that women are differentially sensitive to stressful life events. Maciejewski et al.[46] found that, compared to men, women are at three times greater risk for depression following a stressful event. Finally, Hammen[48] suggests that depressed women exhibit maladaptive traits that generate stressful life events (e.g., marital problems, job difficulties) and lock the women into cycles of chronic depression, thereby translating adolescent depression into a lifelong disability. However, Kessler refutes this hypothesis on methodologic grounds.[22] Because women with a history of depression, compared to those never depressed, are more likely to have experienced both stressful life events and prior depressive episodes, it is unclear whether stressful life events predict future depressive episodes independently of past depressive episodes.[22] Despite these methodologic concerns, the association between stressful life events and first onset depressive episodes remains a viable hypothesis.

Child sexual abuse (CSA) can be seen as a special class of stressful life events. CSA has been shown to predict psychopathology in adolescents and adults, most frequently depression.[49,50] Research suggests that females are more likely to experience CSA than males, and this differential exposure may partially explain the sex difference in adult depression rates.[51,52]

Gender Roles and Role Strain

Women tend to have greater responsibility for care giving compared to men, both with child and elder care.[53] Further, women tend to have larger social networks and stronger ties within those networks. In the "cost of caring" hypothesis, Kessler et al.[54] argue that women experience more psychological distress because of greater emotional involvement in the lives of those around them. Consistent with this hypothesis, married women have a higher prevalence of depression compared to never-married women.[55] Further, Nazroo et al.,[56] in a study of couples, reported that the increased risk of depression in women following a stressful life event was most marked when the event involved children, housing, and/or reproductive difficulties.

Genetic Liability and Familial Aggregation of Major Depression in Women

Many studies have shown that a family history of depression is a major risk factor for early-onset depression across both sexes. Having a depressed parent results in approximately a threefold increase in offspring depression,[57] and having two affected generations increases risk even further.[58] Broad heritability estimates range from 31–42%.[57] The preponderance of evidence, however, does not demonstrate sex differences in the heritability of depression; further, a large meta-analysis of twin studies consisting of more than 20,000 subjects found no consistent sex differences.[57]

Childhood Anxiety Disorders

Anxiety and depression are highly comorbid disorders.[59] In fact, many researchers posit that anxiety and depression may well be part of a single underlying disorder, which is both highly hereditable and more likely to occur in females. In studies of high-risk families, the offspring of depressed parents were shown to be at increased risk for both depression and anxiety.[60,61] Family studies have also shown significant genetic overlap for anxiety and depressive disorders in childhood.[62] In a longitudinal study of female twins, Silberg et al. modeled both common genetic and shared environmental pathways between childhood anxiety disorders and adolescent depression.[63]

Despite their common etiology, anxiety disorders can be distinguished from depressive disorders in the onset sequence. A body of research suggests that anxiety disorders usually precede depression, both in children of depressed parents and in samples not selected for parental depression,[64–66] and represent a risk for the subsequent onset of depressive disorders. In the Weissman et al. study of the offspring of depressed parents, an eightfold increase in risk of adolescent depression was found for children diagnosed with anxiety, and this risk was more pronounced in females.[61] Sex differences in anxiety are large and precede sex differences in depression; Lewinsohn et al. demonstrated that, by age 6 years, girls are twice as likely as boys to be diagnosed with an anxiety disorder.[67]

This body of literature has recently been challenged. Using prospective data from a longitudinal study of children in New Zealand, Moffit et al. have reported that depression precedes anxiety almost as often as anxiety precedes depression.[68] They suggested that the lifetime prevalence (i.e., estimates of the number of individuals who have had the disorder at any point in their life) of MDD and generalized anxiety disorder may have been underestimated in retrospective surveys. It is unclear, however, whether cultural differences between New Zealand and the United States might have contributed to discrepant findings.

Postpartum Depression

Childbirth is accompanied by major endocrine changes and is often experienced as a psychosocial stressor. There is a wide range of postpartum mood disturbances from mild manifestations (postpartum blues), to clinically significant depression (postpartum depression), and to a severe condition (postpartum psychosis) that has a very low prevalence.

The "blues" is a highly prevalent event (> 69%) considered a normal sequela of childbirth. It is often described as a mild and transient alteration of mood following delivery.[41] Postpartum depression (PPD) represents a clinically significant condition meeting criteria for a major depressive episode. The DSM-IV specifies a postpartum depression modifier applicable to major depressive episodes occurring within 4 weeks postpartum. Compared to controls, Cox and colleagues reported a threefold higher rate of onset of depression within 5 weeks of childbirth but no difference was found in the 6-month period following delivery between delivering mothers and controls (13.8% postnatal and 13.4% controls).[69] The onset of PPD characteristically takes place within the first four weeks postpartum, and the symptoms are similar to those observed in major depression not occurring during the postnatal period. Depressive symptoms and sequelae of childbirth often overlap (e.g., fatigue, alterations in sleep, and appetite changes). Furthermore, the anxiety associated with caring for a newborn may contribute to an overall sense of vulnerability. Therefore, a PPD diagnosis requires clinical acumen and knowledge of the physiologic concomitants of the normal postpartum period.

Risk factors for PPD include prior depressive episodes and multiple psychosocial factors, most prominently low social support, especially from the woman's partner.[37,70] Other factors include substance use and abuse,[71] past experiences of abuse,[71] lower socioeconomic status,[72] and stressful life events,[37] A frequently cited medical factor is obstetric complications.[72]

Depression is often diagnosed in the postpartum period, but clinical recognition after delivery does not necessarily imply a postnatal onset. Stowe et al. reported that whereas about two-thirds of women diagnosed with PPD had an early postpartum onset, over 10% had a prenatal onset, with the remaining women having a late postpartum onset.[73] These investigators concluded that the perinatal vulnerability to depression begins before delivery and extends beyond the early postpartum period (i.e., beyond 6 weeks postpartum).

Postpartum psychosis (PPP) is a severe mental illness and a psychiatric emergency due to the risk of suicide and the risk to the infant.[74] Fortunately, the incidence is very low, about one or two cases per 1,000 live births. The incidence of PPP is a lot higher, however, among women with history of a psychiatric hospitalization before delivery compared to those never admitted to a psychiatric hospital.[75] Obstetric variables are of minor importance.[76] The clinical implications are clear, i.e., women with a history of bipolar disorder or psychoses, and especially those hospitalized for these conditions, are at increased risk for PPP and should be carefully monitored during the postpartum period.

Premenstrual Dysphoric Disorder (PMDD)

PMDD is distinct from premenstrual syndrome (PMS), a common syndrome that includes a mix of psychiatric symptoms and vasomotor changes. The range of symptoms captured under the PMS banner is wide and includes mood fluctuations, anxiety, irritability, joint or muscle pain, and breast tenderness or bloating.[77] PMDD is considered by some a true mood disorder with symptoms that resemble the symptoms of major depression. In the DSM-IV, PMDD is classified under the rubric "depressive disorders not otherwise specified." About 3% to 6% of women meet criteria for PMDD.[41] A large study of a community-based sample of women aged 36–44 years found a prevalence of 6.4%[34] and reported several risk factors including current cigarette smoking (OR = 4.1, suggesting that PMDD was about four times more likely in women smoking cigarettes compared to those not smoking), and a history of major depression (OR = 3.6). The main difference between PMDD and MDD is that the depressive symptoms should be limited to the luteal phase (i.e., should precede menstruation) and should not represent an exacerbation of preexisting depression, anxiety, or personality disorder. In addition, they must be present in at least two consecutive menstrual cycles. A symptom-free period after menstruation helps distinguish PMDD from preexisting anxiety and mood disorders.[78]

Fertility and Depression

Although an association between depression and infertility has been documented, the causal direction of the association remains under debate as most studies have been either 1) cross-sectional assessments of psychiatric clinical samples, using number of children born as a proxy for fertility without controlling for potential confounders such as birth control usage,[79–81] or 2) cross-sectional assessments of infertility patients, including those engaged in vitro fertilization, using nondiagnostic symptom scales to assess depression and variable control groups.[82-86] Diagnostically reliable studies have shown that the prevalence of major depression is higher in women seeking care for infertility compared to women who do no,[87–89] but cross-sectional assessment again precludes firm conclusions about direction of effect. Thus, an association between infertility and depression exists, but it remains unclear whether 1) the presence of depression decreases the ability of conceive a child, 2) women who have problems conceiving are more likely to become depressed, and/or 3) a common antecedent cause such as hormone imbalance accounts for the relationship.

Summary

Boys and girls have a similar prevalence of depression before adolescence, when the adult pattern of a higher prevalence in women is established. There is no definitive explanation for the higher prevalence of depression in adult women, compared to adult men. Hormonal factors may play a role, but psychosocial factors may play an equal or greater role. The most consistent risk factor for postpartum depression is a prior episode of depression. Postpartum psychosis is a medical-psychiatric emergency and requires prompt intervention. Although menopause is believed to be associated with depression, studies in community samples have not shown a consistent association between menopause and the onset of depression.

Discussion Questions

1. What are the main differences between major depressive disorder and dysthymic disorder? Compare duration, severity of symptoms, and clinical presentation.
2. Compare the prevalence of major depression in boys and girls before and after puberty. What theories have been advanced to explain the change in prevalence that takes place in adolescence?
3. Compare and contrast postpartum depression and postpartum psychosis. Which one carries more risk?
4. What is the most consistently demonstrated risk factor for premenstrual dysphoria? What other factors may play a role?
5. Does an association between infertility and depression exist? Discuss the issues that have arisen regarding the direction of causality.

References

1. Robins LN, Regier DA. *Psychiatric Disorders in America: The Epidemiologic Catchment Area Study*. New York: The Free Press; 1990.
2. Murray CJ, Lopez AD. Alternative projections of mortality and disability by cause 1990-2020: Global Burden of Disease Study. *Lancet*. 1997;349:1498–1504.
3. Weissman MM, et al. Cross-national epidemiology of major depression and bipolar disorder. *JAMA*. 1996;276:293–299.
4. Weissman MM, Klerman GL. Sex differences and the epidemiology of depression. *Arch Gen Psychiatry*. 1977;34:98–111.
5. Hyde JS, Mezulis AH, Abramson LY. The ABCs of depression: integrating affective, biological, and cognitive models to explain the emergence of the gender difference in depression. *Psychol Rev*. 2008;115:291–313.
6. *Diagnostic and Statistical Manual of Mental Disorders*. 4th ed. Washington DC: American Psychiatric Association; 1994.
7. Weissman MM, et al. The epidemiology of dysthymia in five communities: rates, risks, comorbidity, and treatment. *Am J Psychiatry*. 1988;145: 815–819.
8. Kessler RC, et al. Lifetime prevalence and age-of-onset distributions of DSM-IV disorders in the National Comorbidity Survey Replication. *Arch Gen Psychiatry*. 2005;62:593–602.
9. Cohen P, Cohen J, Kasen S, et al. An epidemiological study of disorders in late childhood and adolescence-I. Age- and gender-specific prevalence. *J Child Psychol Psychiatry*. 1993;34:851–867.
10. Accortt EE, Freeman MP, Allen JJB. Women and major depressive disorder: clinical perspectives on causal pathways. *J Womens Health (Larchmt)*. 2008;17:1583–1590.
11. Allgood-Merten B, Lewinsohn PM, Hops H. Sex differences and adolescent depression. *J Abnorm Psychol*. 1990;99:55–63.
12. Weissman MM, Leaf PJ, Tischler GL, et al. Affective disorders in five United States communities. *Psychol Med*. 1988;18:141–53.
13. Kessler RC, McGonagle KA, Nelson CB, et al. Sex and depression in the National Comorbidity Survey I: Lifetime prevalence, chronicity and recurrence. *J Affect Discord*. 1993;29:85–96.
14. Grant BF, Harford TC. Comorbidity between DSM-IV alcohol use disorders and major depression: results of a national survey. *Drug Alcohol Depend*. 1995;39:197–206.
15. Hasin DS, et al. Epidemiology of major depressive disorder: results from the National Epidemiologic Survey on Alcoholism and Related Conditions.[see comment]. *Arch Gen Psychiatry*. 2005;62:1097–1106.
16. Kessler RC, Berglund P, Demler O, et al. Lifetime prevalence and age-of-onset distributions of DSM-IV disorders in the National Comorbidity Survey Replication. *Arch Gen Psychiatry*. 2005;62:593–602.
17. Williams DR, Gonzalez HM, Neighbors H, et al. Prevalence and distribution of major depressive disorder in African Americans, Caribbean blacks, and non-Hispanic whites: results from the National Survey of American Life. *Arch Gen Psychiatry*. 2007;64:305–315.
18. Seedat S, Scott KM, Angermeyer MC, et al. Cross-national associations between gender and mental disorders in the World Health Organization World Mental Health Surveys. *Arch Gen Psychiatry*. 2009;66:785–795.
19. Wickramaratne J, et al. Age, period and cohort effects on the risk of major depression: results from five United States communities. *J Clin Epidemiol*. 1989;42:333–343.
20. Joyce PR, et al. Birth cohort trends in major depression: increasing rates and earlier onset in New Zealand. *J Affect Disord*. 1990;18:83–89.
21. Olfson M, et al. National trends in the use of psychotropic medications by children. *J Am Acad Child Adolesc Psychiatry*. 2002;41:514–521.
22. Kessler RC. Epidemiology of women and depression. *J Affect Disord*. 2003;74:5–13.
23. Nolen-Hoeksema S, Larson J, Grayson C. Explaining the gender difference in depressive symptoms. *J Pers Soc Psychol*. 1999;77:1061–1072.
24. Barbee EL. African American women and depression: a review and critique of the literature. *Arch Psychiatr Nurs*. 1992;6:257–265.
25. Nolen-Hoeksema S, Girgus JS. The emergence of gender differences in depression during adolescence. *Psychol Bull*. 1994;115:424–443.
26. Yonkers KA Bradshaw KD. Hormone replacement and oral contraceptive therapy: do they induce or treat mood symptoms? In: Leibenluft E, ed. *Gender Differences in Mood and Anxiety Disorders: From Bench to Bedside*. Washington DC: American Psychiatric Press; 1999.
27. Yonkers KA, Bradshaw KD, Halbreich U. Oestrogens, progestins and mood. In: Steiner M, Yonkers KA, Eriksson E, eds. *Mood Disorders in Women*. London: Martin Dunitz; 2000:207–232.
28. Angold A, Costello EJ, Worthman CM. Puberty and depression: the roles of age, pubertal status and pubertal timing. *Psychol Med*. 1998;28:51–61.
29. Brooks-Gunn J, Warren MP. Biological and social contributions to negative affect in young adolescent girls. *Child Dev*. 1989;60:40–55.
30. Hayward C, et al. Ethnic differences in the association between pubertal status and symptoms of depression in adolescent girls. *J Adolesc Health*. 1999;25:143–149.
31. Gilligan C. *In a Different Voice: Psychological Theory and Women's Development*. Cambridge, MA: Harvard University Press; 1982.
32. Brown LM, Gilligan C. *Meeting at the Crossroads: Women's Psychology and Girls' Development*. Cambridge, MA: Harvard University Press; 1992.
33. Taylor JM, Gilligan C, Sullivan AM. *Between Voice and Silence: Women and Girls, Race and Relationship*. Cambridge, MA: Harvard University Press; 1995.
34. Cohen LS, et al. Prevalence and predictors of premenstrual dysphoric disorder (PMDD) in older premenopausal women. The Harvard Study of Moods and Cycles. *J Affect Disord*. 2002;70:125–132.
35. Fontana AM, Palfai TG. Psychosocial factors in premenstrual dysphoria: Stressors, appraisal, and coping processes. *J Psychosom Res*. 1994;38: 557–567.
36. Steiner M, Dunn E, Born L. Hormones and mood: From menarche to menopause and beyond. *J Affect Disord*. 2003;74:67–83.
37. O'Hara MW, Swain AM. Rates and risk of postpartum depression—A meta-analysis. *Int Rev Psychiatry*. 1996;8:37–54.

38. Vesga-López O, et al. Psychiatric disorders in pregnant and postpartum women in the United States. *Arch Gen Psychiatry*. 2008;65:805–815.

39. Eberhard-Gran M, et al. A comparison of anxiety and depressive symptomatology in postpartum and non-postpartum mothers. *Soc Psychiatry Psychiatr Epidemiol*. 2003;38:551–556.

40. Munk-Olsen T, et al. New parents and mental disorders: a population-based register study. *JAMA*. 2006;296:2582–2589.

41. Somerset W, et al. Depressive disorders in women: From menarche to beyond the menopause. In: Keyes CLM, Goodman SH, eds. *Women and Depression*. New York: Cambridge University Press; 2006:62–88.

42. Ballinger C. Psychiatric aspects of the menopause. *Br J Psychiatry*. 1990;156:773–787.

43. Collins A, Landgren BM. Reproductive health, use of estrogen and experience of symptoms in perimenopausal women: a population-based study. *Maturitas*. 1994;20:101–111.

44. Avis NE, et al. A longitudinal analysis of the association between menopause and depression. Results from the Massachusetts Women's Health Study. *Ann Epidemiol*. 1994;4:214–220.

45. Paykel ES, et al. Life events and social support in puerperal depression. *Br J Psychiatry*. 1980;136:339–346.

46. Maciejewski PK, Prigerson HG, Mazure CM. Sex differences in event-related risk for major depression. *Psychol Med*. 2001;31:593–604.

47. Rudolph KD, et al. Toward an interpersonal life-stress model of depression: the developmental context of stress generation. *Dev Psychopathol*. 2000;12:215–234.

48. Hammen C. Generation of stress in the course of unipolar depression. *J Abnorm Psychol*. 1991;100:555–561.

49. Dinwiddie S, et al. Early sexual abuse and lifetime psychopathology: a co-twin-control study. *Psychol Med*. 2000;30:41–52.

50. Kendler KS, Thornton LM, Prescott CA. Gender differences in the rates of exposure to stressful life events and sensitivity to their depressogenic effects. *Am J Psychiatry*. 2001;158:587–593.

51. Cutler SE, Nolen-Hoeksema S. Accounting for sex differences in depression through female victimization: Childhood sexual abuse. *Sex Roles*. 1991;24:452–438.

52. Whiffen VE, Clark SE. Does victimization account for sex differences in depressive symptoms? *Br J Clin Psychol*. 1997;36:185–193.

53. Sieber SD, Toward a theory of role accumulation. *Am Sociol Rev*. 1974; 39:567–578.

54. Kessler RC, Price RH, Wortman CB. Social factors in psychopathology: stress, social support, and coping processes. *Annu Rev Psychol*. 1985;36:531–572.

55. King CA, et al. Diagnosis and assessment of depression and suicidality using the NIMH Diagnostic Interview Schedule for Children (DISC-2.3). *J Abnorm Child Psych*. 1997;25:173–181.

56. Nazroo JY, Edwards AC, Brown GW. Gender differences in the onset of depression following a shared life event: a study of couples. *Psychol Med*. 1997;27:9–19.

57. Sullivan PF, Neale MC, Kendler KS. Genetic epidemiology of major depression: Review and meta-analysis. *Am J Psychiatry*. 2000;157;1552–1562.

58. Weissman MM, et al. Families at high and low risk for depression: a 3-generation study. *Arch Gen Psychiatry*. 2005;62:29–36.

59. Cloninger CR, Comorbidity of anxiety and depression. *J Clin Psychopharmacol*. 1990;10:43S–46S.

60. Weissman MM, et al. Incidence of psychiatric disorder in offspring at high and low risk for depression. *J Am Acad Child Adolesc Psychiatry*. 1992;31:640–648.

61. Weissman MM, et al. Offspring of depressed parents. 10 years later. [see comment]. *Arch Gen Psychiatry*. 1997;54:932–940.

62. Thapar A, McGuffin P. Anxiety and depressive symptoms in childhood: A genetic study of comorbidity. *J Child Psychol Psychiatry*. 1997;38(6):651–656.

63. Silberg J, et al. The influence of genetic factors and life stress on depression among adolescent girls. *Arch Gen Psychiatry*. 1999;56:225–32.

64. Weissman MM, et al. Families at high and low risk for depression: a 3-generation study. *Arch Gen Psychiatry*. 2005;62:29–36.

65. Kovacs M, et al. A controlled family history study of childhood-onset depressive disorder. *Arch Gen Psychiatry*. 1997;54:613–623.

66. Orvaschel H, Lewinsohn PM, Seeley JR. Continuity of psychopathology in a community sample of adolescents. *J Am Acad Child Adolesc Psychiatry*. 1995;34:1525–1535.

67. Lewinsohn PM, et al. Gender differences in anxiety disorders and anxiety symptoms in adolescents. *J Abnorm Psychol*. 1998;107:109–117.

68. Moffitt TE, et al. Depression and generalized anxiety disorder: cumulative and sequential comorbidity in a birth cohort followed prospectively to age 32 years. *Arch Gen Psychiatry*. 2007;64:651–660.

69. Cox JL, Murray D, Chapman G. A controlled study of the onset, duration and prevalence of postnatal depression. *Br J Psychiatry*. 1993;163:27–31.

70. Dennis C-L, Letourneau N. Global and relationship-specific perceptions of support and the development of postpartum depressive symptomatology. *Soc Psychiatry Psychiatr Epidemiol*. 2007;42:389–395.

71. Ross LE, Dennis C-L. The prevalence of postpartum depression among women with substance use, an abuse history, or chronic illness: A systematic review. *J Womens Health (Larchmt)*. 2009;18:475–486.

72. Campbell SB, Cohn JF. Prevalence and correlates of postpartum depression in first-time mothers. *J Abnorm Psychol*. 1991;100:594–599.

73. Stowe ZN, Hostetter AL, Newport DJ. The onset of postpartum depression: Implications for clinical screening in obstetrical and primary care. *Am J Obstet Gynecol*. 2005;192:522–526.

74. Tschinkel S, et al. Postpartum psychosis: Two cohorts compared, 1875–1924 and 1994–2005. *Psychol Med*. 2007;37:529–536.

75. Harlow BL, et al. Incidence of hospitalization for postpartum psychotic and bipolar episodes in women with and without prior prepregnancy or prenatal psychiatric hospitalizations. *Arch Gen Psychiatry*. 2007;64:42–48.

76. Nager A, et al. Obstetric complications and postpartum psychosis: a follow-up study of 1.1 million first-time mothers between 1975 and 2003 in Sweden. *Acta Psychiatr Scand*. 2008;117:12–19.

77. Johnson SR, McChesney C, Bean JA. Epidemiology of premenstrual symptoms in a nonclinical sample. I. Prevalence, natural history and help-seeking behavior. *J Reprod Med*. 1988;33:340–346.

78. Bhatia SC, Bhatia SK. Diagnosis and treatment of premenstrual dysphoric disorder. *Am Fam Physician*. 2002;66:1239–1248.

79. Jonsson SA. Marriage rate and fertility in cycloid psychosis: comparison with affective disorder, schizophrenia and the general population. *Eur Arch Psychiatry Clin Neurosci*. 1991;24:119–125.

80. Odegard O. Fertility of psychiatric first admissions in Norway 1936–1975. *Acta Psychiatr Scand*. 1980;62:212–220.

81. Calzeroni A, et al. Celibacy and fertility rates in patients with major affective disorders: the relevance of delusional symptoms and suicidal behaviour. *Acta Psychiatr Scan*. 1990;82:309–310.

82. Yong P, Martin C, Thong J. A comparison of psychological functioning in women at different stages of in vitro fertilization treatment using the mean affect adjective check list. *J Assist Reprod Genet*. 2000;17:553–556.

83. Beaurepaire J, et al. Psychosocial adjustment to infertility and its treatment: male and female responses at different stages of IVF/ET treatment. *J Psychosom Res*. 1994;38:229–240.

84. Kee BS, Jung BJ, Lee SH. A study on psychological strain in IVF patients. *J Assist Reprod Genet*. 2000;17:445–448.

85. Matsubayashi H, et al. Emotional distress of infertile women in Japan. *Hum Reprod*. 2001;16:966–969.

86. Domar AD, Zuttermeister PC, Friedman R. The psychological impact of infertility: a comparison with patients with other medical conditions. *J Psychosom Obstet Gynaecol*. 1993;14(suppl):45–52.

87. Chen TH, et al. Prevalence of depressive and anxiety disorders in an assisted reproductive technique clinic. *Hum Reprod*. 2004;19:2313–2318.

88. Downey J, et al. Mood disorders, psychiatric symptoms, and distress in women presenting for infertility evaluation. *Fertil Steril*. 1989;52:425–432.

89. Fassino S, et al. Anxiety, depression and anger suppression in infertile couples: a controlled study. *Hum Reprod*. 2002;17:2986–2994.

Bipolar Disorder

Elizabeth Saenger, PhD

Introduction

Bipolar Disorder, one of the most serious illnesses worldwide, is associated with functional impairment, comorbidity with psychiatric and nonpsychiatric illnesses, high use of health services, and suicide.[1] In the United States, it is less prevalent, but more persistent and impairing, than Major Depressive Disorder (MDD).[2] Women tend to experience serious forms and features of the illness far more often than men,[3] although both genders may have an age of onset in the teens or early 20s.[1]

This chapter describes the evolving concept of Bipolar Disorder (BP), and its problematic similarities and differences compared with recurrent MDD. Differences in BP by gender are addressed in terms of comorbidity and mortality. Finally, the chapter describes concerns unique to women with BP, including pregnancy, postpartum risks, and menopause.

Evolution of Bipolar Disorder as a Diagnosis

Bipolar Disorder has been evolving as a diagnosis since before the Christian era.[4] Until the mid-19th century, physicians and philosophers speculated about the causes, cures, and possible relationships between melancholia (a form of MDD) and mania (characterized then as persistent euphoria). Experts at that time concluded that the two extreme moods constituted parts of a single entity.[1] By the early 20th century, Emil Kraepelin, a German psychiatrist whom some regard as the founder of contemporary scientific psychiatry, developed a new classification of mental disorders. This paradigm-setting nosology (classification of illness) grouped hundreds of conditions identified in the 19th century according to Kraepelin's observations about their longitudinal course and *patterns* of symptoms (as opposed to merely the similarity of a few major symptoms). Kraepelin also differentiated between dementia praecox (schizophrenia) and a spectrum of conditions he called "manic-depressive illness"—a broad division that still shapes the development of contemporary research on mental illness, even as new findings in genetics challenge it.[5]

Kraepelin's classification, including his theoretically and clinically significant delineation of manic-depressive illness, had the advantage of being empirically based. It also had the disadvantage of relying on descriptions of symptoms, rather than their etiology, because he, like us, could not give a patient presenting with melancholia or mania a lab test to determine whether she had pathogens or genetic defects causing a disease or condition.

After Kraepelin, researchers around the world, especially in the United States, continued to create empirically based models of the illness. Often they divided the illness into categories, or subtypes, such as MDD and BP.[6] Many of these classifications, including the Diagnostic and Statistical Manuals developed by the American Psychiatric Association,[7] continued to regard the dysregulation of mood as a hallmark of the illness, although some researchers argue that other features, such as extremes in activity level,[8–10] may be more central.

The Diagnostic and Statistical Manual of Mental Disorders, Fourth Edition (DSM-IV)

Table 17-1 presents the latest divisions developed by the American Psychiatric Association[7] and widely used in the United States for research and insurance reimbursement. The most readily recognized form of mood disorders in this classification, Bipolar-I (BP-I), consists of at least one episode of either mania (a persistently elated or euphoric mood or an irritable mood), or mixed mania (manic and depressive features together), lasting for a week or longer. At least three or four of the following seven symptoms must always be present: decreased need for sleep, distractibility, exaggerated sense of self-importance, increase in goal-directed activity, a tendency to engage in pleasurable behaviors the person is likely to regret later, and an increase in the speed of talking (pressured speech) or thinking (racing thoughts). Racing thoughts, as opposed to pressured speech, must be self-reported. In severe cases, psychotic symptoms (hallucinations or delusions) may occur. BP-I typically includes depressive episodes, characterized by loss of interest in activities that used to be pleasurable; fatigue; feelings of worthlessness; disturbances of sleep or appetite; and inability to concentrate.

Table 17-1

Categories of key mood disorders in the *Diagnostic and Statistical Manual of Mental Disorders* (DSM-IV)

Criterion	MDD	BP-I	BP-II	Cyclothymic disorder	Bipolar disorder not otherwise specified
Manic or mixed episode (must last a week or more)	Absent	Present	Absent	Must not be present for the first two years	Absent
Major Depressive episode (must last two weeks or more)	Present	Optional	Present	No, but numerous periods with some of the symptoms	Absent
Hypomanic episode (must last four days or more)	Absent	Optional	Present	No, but numerous periods with some of the symptoms	Hypomanic episode(s) or relevant pattern of symptoms must be Present

Other forms of BP in the DSM-IV include Bipolar-II and Cyclothymic Disorder. Bipolar-II (BP-II) consists of one or more episodes of hypomania (a less extreme version of mania) lasting 4 days or longer and periods of major depression. BP-II is associated with major problems more often than BP-I, including a lower likelihood of returning to premorbid functioning, shorter periods of wellness, more impairment from depression, a greater likelihood of rapid cycling (four or more episodes of hypomania or depression in a year), and suicide.[11] Cyclothymic Disorder is a chronic condition characterized by at least 2 years of fluctuating highs and lows not severe enough to meet the criteria for an episode of mania or major depression.[7] In 15% to 50% of cases, Cyclothymic Disorder becomes BP-I or BP-II.[7] In clinic settings, Cyclothymic Disorder may be more common in women, although no gender difference appears in community samples.[7]

Women are more likely than men to have Bipolar-II (29% vs. 15%),[12] as well as more serious features of BP. Women are more vulnerable to mixed mania and to depressive episodes that are more frequent, more prolonged, and less effectively managed with medication.[13] Women are also more likely to have rapid cycling, which is less responsive to treatment and leads to worse outcomes.[1]

The Study of Bipolar Disorder

The investigation of BP requires an interdisciplinary team in which neuroscience plays an increasingly prominent role. For example, in response to the strong association of smoking with BP, reported by epidemiologists, geneticists created a model of gene–environment interaction of BP comorbid with nicotine addiction, suggesting it might be more difficult for a person with BP to stop smoking than for a person in the general population.[14] Geneticists also identified a gene region that may explain observations in other disciplines about disorders that are commonly comorbid with BP, including migraines, noting the success of some medications in reducing episodes of both problems.[15] In addition, the latest laboratory research on brain disorders lends credence to the idea that BP and recurrent MDD (but not single episodes it) are two sides of the same coin, because both appear to result from an abnormal functional organization of the same circuits.[16]

Epidemiological Sources of Data

Studies of BP in the United States generally estimate lifetime prevalence rates of about 1% to 2% in both women and men,[1] although these rates may be increasing.[10] Major epidemiologic studies include the small New Haven Survey of 1978, the first community survey to use standardized diagnostic criteria for mental health.[17] Three subsequent large-scale national surveys, the Epidemiological Catchment Area (ECA) study of 1980–1984,[18] the National Comorbidity Survey (NCS) of 1991–1992,[19] and the National Comorbidity Study Replication (NCS-R) of 2005,[20–21] found roughly similar results. Nevertheless, due to methodologic problems in collecting data, some experts estimate that 1 of 10 individuals in the community has the disorder, or is at risk for it.[22] Pharmaceutical companies selling drugs to treat BP promote even higher figures, such as "20%–30% of patients in the primary care setting."[23]

To reduce discrepancies, some prominent researchers have made adjustments in the way they count data. These modifications concern public health officials and insurance companies, because they underscore the impossibility of accurately determining the prevalence of BP today.[1]

Despite difficulties in estimating the prevalence of BP, evidence clearly indicates some relative risks among different groups. For example, successive cohorts born after 1935 are at increasing risk for mania.[1] In addition to youth, other variables associated with BP include being single or divorced and being homeless or incarcerated.[1] Variables that appear uncorrelated with BP include gender, race, and ethnicity (with the possible exception of lower rates among Asians); urban versus rural residence; and social class.[1]

Credibility Gaps in Prevalence Estimates

The many barriers to collecting accurate data describing BP include:

- low prevalence, which means that a large sample is needed for reasonable estimates
- high comorbidity with other psychiatric disorders sharing some of the symptoms, causing an interviewer to overlook bipolarity
- lack of reliability and equivalence of different interviewer instruments resulting in under- or overdiagnosis, complicating comparisons among studies[24-26]
- frequent use of trained nonclinician interviewers who achieve only modest interrater reliability compared with clinicians[1]
- failure to ask respondents about family history of mental illness even though the strongest predictor of BP is BP in first-degree relatives[1]
- absence of clinical consensus regarding definitions of BP[28-29]
- extrapolations necessary to estimate prevalence for a disorder that requires observation over time after initial onset due to symptoms resembling MDD[30]

In addition to methodologic problems that affect all epidemiologic research, studies of BP raise controversial questions of reliability and validity.[28-32] Recently, over an 8-year interval, outpatient visits for BP nearly doubled among adults, and increased fortyfold in children and adolescents.[32] This dramatic jump was not detected in community surveys.[32] These data highlight the need for clinically reliable studies to determine the incidence of BP, especially among children and adolescents. If the clinical diagnoses are accurate, pediatric BP would be an epidemic with huge public health implications. If the clinical diagnoses were *not accurate*, this would support the contention of leading researchers that some prominent psychiatrists encourage clinicians to diagnosis BP in an over-inclusive manner to increase the market for pharmaceutical products for children.[33]

Misdiagnosis

Prevalence estimates are also compromised by the widespread clinical confusion of BP with borderline personality disorder (BPD), which is characterized by pervasive instability in relationships, self-image, and mood. BPD is diagnosed three times more frequently in women than men, and is often comorbid with mood disorders.[7] BPD appears to be a risk factor for being diagnosed with BP,[35] and people with BPD were found to more frequently score BP-positive (vs. negative) on a simple, widely used screening test for BP.[35]

The misdiagnosis of BP as recurrent MDD has an even greater impact on prevalence estimates, because MDD is a common diagnosis given to women four times as often as men,[1] and among women especially, BP-II is commonly misdiagnosed as MDD.[28,36] Studies using methods ranging from insurance claims to patient medical records, and from surveys to interviews, find BP much more frequently diagnosed as MDD than vice versa.[28] This error is due partly to the ambiguous boundary between normal high spirits and hypomania, compared with the clear distinction between normal high spirits and mania. Consequently, women with BP-II may not recognize their hypomania as a problem.[1] Women with BP might also be more likely than men to be misdiagnosed with MDD because they are more likely to have a depression (vs. mania) for an initial episode.[1] Further, even when a BP diagnosis is rendered, the next professional involved in treatment may diagnose MDD, as happened to 27.5% of patients with new BP diagnoses, and 17.5% of those with older BP diagnoses, in two large samples.[37]

Misdiagnosis can have serious consequences for women with bipolar depression or recurrent MDD accompanied by the multiple risk factors for BP described later. A diagnosis of recurrent MDD often leads to taking antidepressants. In the short term, such drugs may precipitate manic episodes; in the long term, they may induce or intensify rapid cycling or worsen the course of the illness.[1,13,28]

In short, methodologic flaws in data collection make prevalence estimates of BP in women less credible, although these estimates do provide some useful data for comparisons among subgroups of the population.

Bipolar Disorder Not Otherwise Specified

Patients presenting with bipolar features that do not fit into defined categories, such as alternations between highs and lows of shorter duration or recurrent hypomanic episodes without any depression, are considered Bipolar Disorder Not Otherwise Specified (BPNOS) in the DSM-IV. Some experts speculate that the widely accepted prevalence estimates of BP are grossly underestimated[39] due to the inclusion of only BP-I, or only BP-I and BP-II, and the exclusion of Cyclothymic Disorder and BPNOS. Clinicians diagnose BPNOS when they are unsure about the specific BP diagnosis.

In many epidemiologic studies, women with repeated episodes of depression might be diagnosed with recurrent MDD even though mild hypomanic symptoms appeared during their illness. This diagnosis often occurs when hypomanic symptoms do not meet the minimum requirement of 4 days or the number and type of symptoms do not satisfy criteria for hypomania.

Interest in MDD with a trace of hypomania has recently increased in tabulations of BP by epidemiologists. As the last row in Table 17-2 shows, the American Psychiatric Association, in the next version of the *Diagnostic and Statistical Manual*, may redefine hypomania in terms of its duration or number of symptoms.[40]

Recent secondary analyses[39,41] of major epidemiologic studies indicate that lifetime prevalence estimates of BP increase significantly with the inclusion of BPNOS and that BPNOS is associated with substantial dysfunction. For example, the reanalysis of the NCS-R[41] defined BPNOS as "recurrent hypomania without a major depressive episode or with fewer symptoms than required for...hypomania." This reanalysis found that for women, the prevalence of BP-I was 1.1%, of BP-II 1.3%, and of BPNOS 2.1%.

A subsequent large-scale study in Munich[42] explored the idea that a more inclusive definition of BP would

Table 17-2

The evolving concept of Bipolar Disorder

Date	Diagnostic System	Conception of Bipolar Disorder
1952	DSM-I	Psychodynamic influence with disorders on a continuum of normal and abnormal; "manic-depressive reaction" and "psychotic depressive reaction" are subcategories of "affective reactions," viewed as one of four kinds of psychoses.
1968	DSM-II	Psychodynamic influence remains, with disorders on a continuum of normal and abnormal, but "manic-depressive reaction" becomes "manic-depressive illness," is separated from the psychosis category, and listed under major affective disorders.
1978	RDC (Research Diagnostic Criteria)	Research taxonomy designed by the National Institute of Mental Health to detect cases of psychiatric disorders, such as MDD, for epidemiologic and other investigations; high inter-rater reliability
1980	DSM-III	Based on the RDC; "bipolar disorder" replaces "manic depressive disorder" to emphasize mood polarity; bipolar disorder in a separate category from depression; high interrater reliability.
1987	DSM-III-R (DSM-III-Revised)	Bipolar disorders are subdivided into types, such as Bipolar Disorder-Manic and Bipolar Disorder-Mixed.
1994	DSM-IV	Bipolar II Disorder (BP-II) critically distinguished from Bipolar Disorder Not Otherwise Specified; includes operational definitions for rapid cycling and mixed episodes; excludes antidepressant-induced mood changes; distinguishes between having a single episode and more than one episode; adds an "atypical specifier" to major depressive episodes if there are symptoms, such as weight gain and excessive sleeping, which are more common in women.
Anticipated 2013	DSM-5	Depending on pending data analysis, may adjust 4-day duration criteria and number/type of symptoms criteria to qualify for hypomania; may include an anxiety dimension and a suicide assessment dimension for all mood disorders.

significantly increase prevalence estimates, especially among women. However, because the German and American healthcare systems differ, thus affecting the sampling procedure, these detailed and intriguing data might not generalize to the United States.

Bipolar Spectrum Disorder: A Paradigm for the Future?

The DSM-IV defines affective disorders using a categorical system classifying symptoms and diagnoses as present or absent. For example, if a woman has an episode of mania, she is diagnosed with BP-I. Leading experts, including the psychiatrist directing the development of DSM-5,[43] acknowledge this categorical model has been historically useful. However, the current categorical system does not accommodate comorbidity, suggesting to many researchers,[6,39,41] but not all,[10,44] that classifying sets of symptoms into discrete DSM categories does not accurately reflect reality.

How might a dimensional system differ from the categorical method used in the U.S.? In the extreme, such a classification might group Borderline Personality Disorder (BPD) with mood disorders. Both conditions are easily characterized along dimensions of affective instability, impulsivity, and chaotic relationships. From this vantage point, the temperamental terrain of the two disorders differs only in degree, with BPD characterized by nearly continuous emotional "mini-earthquakes" without full-scale earthquakes, and BP marked by periodic full-scale earthquakes without the constant backdrop of "mini-earthquakes."[45,46] Varied data support joining women from these two diagnostic categories in one classification given their similarities in responding to several medications that may improve or stabilize moods.[45,46] However, conceptualizing BPD in terms of the medical model, and treating the condition with drugs, rather than with the more psychodynamic framework currently applied, might have unintended consequences. The medical model blames women with personality disorders for their condition,[45] fostering professional hostility toward these patients.[47] Further, pharmaceutical treatment might marginalize the evidence-based psychotherapies that have been successful with BPD, including dialectical behavior therapy (DBT), which teaches patients specific skills, such as learning to tolerate stress and interact effectively with people.[48]

Most models focus narrowly on bipolar disorders and recurrent MDD. The key question is not whether someone has MDD or BP, but rather in what ways, and to what extent, an individual is at risk for a manic episode. Sufficient nonmanic risk factors for BP, even in the absence of ever having a hypomanic symptom, suggest she will become bipolar. Some experts recommend rating patients on the Bipolarity Index, which uses a continuum of bipolarity rather than a categorical diagnosis of BP or MDD.[6] This assessment tool organizes risk factors into five categories, each worth up to 20 points depending on the number of markers and the degree to which they predict BP. The categories, and strong predictors within them, include:

- Episode characteristics, such as psychosis or postpartum depression
- Age of onset, most tellingly illness beginning between the ages of 15 and 25
- Response to treatment: lack of response to three or more antidepressants, antidepressant-induced mania, or a positive response to mood stabilizers
- Family history, particularly the number of first-degree relatives with BP
- Course of illness, especially frequency of recurrence

The last predictor is important as single episodes of MDD have heterogeneous sources whereas recurrent MDD is a risk factor for BP. Therefore, recurrent MDD with additional nonmanic risk markers, but not single episodes, are considered part of the bipolar spectrum.[6] Consequently, a woman with repeated episodes of MDD beginning in her teens, who had postpartum depression and antidepressant-induced mania, and who has a mother and sister with BP, would fall within the bipolar spectrum even though her DSM diagnosis would be MDD because she would not meet the specific criteria for a hypomanic or manic episode shown in Table 17-3.

Advocates for retaining the DSM's categorical concept of BP see the bipolar spectrum as "bipolar imperialism,"[10] which goes beyond the data by including too many people originally diagnosed with other conditions. According to this view, the phenomenologic resemblances among mood disorders do not prove they are caused by a single pathological mechanism—an argument consonant with the genetic distinction between BP-I and BP-II.[10] Broadening the definition of BP risks "weakening or trivializing the core concept of bipolar disorder" and losing a "coherent, tractable phenotypic target for genetic, biologic, and experimental therapeutic studies."[44]

The use of a categorical (vs. dimensional or spectrum) system leads to the diagnosis of many women as entirely MDD when a broader approach would more precisely reflect clinical data recognizing degrees of bipolarity. The failure to check routinely for bipolarity leaves women at risk for the inappropriate treatment of bipolar depression as unipolar depression, or the misinterpretation of hypomania as joy postpartum.

Implications for Women

From the time Kraepelin developed the concept of manic-depression until its recent reincarnation as the bipolar spectrum, research on BP focused on BP-I as the epitome of the disorder, obscuring variants of manic-depression that occur more frequently and more seriously in women. Thus BP-I is referred to as the "classic" type of BP and the mania that defines it is the "standard" for the disorder.[28] However, both BP-II and MDD with traces of bipolarity, which disproportionately strike women, are associated with great impairment including higher risk of suicide than BP-I.[1] Consequently, the DSM-IV has classified manic-depressive illness into categories that do not acknowledge the degrees of bipolarity that cloud the

Table 17-3
Defining symptoms of hypomanic or manic episode
The DSM-IV requires a cluster of four or five of these characteristics for a diagnosis of hypomania (if they last together for at least 4 days), or mania (if they persist for 7 or more days):   • A euphoric, expansive, or irritable mood (the primary symptom)   • Exaggerated self-esteem or self-worth   • Decreased need for sleep   • Pressure to talk or more talkativeness than normal   • An absence of a logical connection between one idea and the next, or the feeling that thoughts are racing   • Difficulty focusing   • Increased activity, either in term of an abundance of goals and projects, or agitation   • Extensive involvement in pleasurable activities, such as spontaneous sexual affairs, irrational buying sprees, unnecessary world travel, or patently unsound business ventures, with harmful consequences   To meet DSM criteria, symptoms must: • Affect functioning (for hypomania) or impair functioning (for mania)   • Be noticeable by others   • Occur for a reason other than the administration of antidepressants and other treatment; alcohol or drugs; and other medical conditions   • Exist without a simultaneous episode of major depression

gravity of mood disorders among women, especially those with BP-II. In addition, the dichotomous partitioning of the bipolar spectrum into BP and MDD may inadvertently contribute to the high prevalence of iatrogenic antidepressant treatment for many women whose MDD has bipolar features. This problem might be exacerbated if, as two studies suggest, antidepressants are more likely to precipitate both mania and rapid cycling in women (vs. men) with bipolar depression.[1]

Comorbidity

Psychiatric Comorbidity

BP is characterized by pervasive psychiatric comorbidity, and bipolarity has even been called "a marker for comorbidity."[49] A secondary analysis of the NCS-R[41] indicated almost all people with BP had at least one lifetime psychiatric comorbidity. Three or more lifetime comorbidities were reported by 86% of people with BP-I, 86% with BP-II, and 57% with BPNOS. Anxiety disorders, especially panic attacks, impulse control disorders, and substance use disorders were most common. Such large-scale comorbidity both (1) suggests BP is associated with dysfunction in multiple regulatory systems, thus warranting investigation[41] and (2) complicates treatment, since comorbidity is correlated with a more severe course of illness, including more recurrent depression, and a higher rate of suicidality.[50]

From a clinical perspective, the most significant comorbidity for women with BP is alcohol addiction. The rate of problem drinking in the general population is much higher in men than women. Consequently, although having BP significantly raises the risk of alcohol use, women (OR = 7.35, 95% CI = 3.32 – 16.26) are far more vulnerable than men (OR = 2.77, 95% CI = 1.59 – 4.81).[51] Comorbidity with such disorders seriously worsens the course of BP, resulting in higher rates of mixed mania, rapid cycling, exacerbated symptoms of mania and depression, and increases in aggressiveness and suicidality.[52] Comorbid alcohol disorders may also reduce response to lithium during mania and decrease treatment adherence.[52] In addition, comorbid substance abuse is a risk factor for arrest, especially in women.[53]

Do women with BP drink to self-medicate? In one sample, people with BP used drugs to reduce feelings of depression (87%) or racing thoughts (58%). At least one symptom was relieved, 67% reported.[54] However, other studies found the two disorders share common mechanisms, such as impulsivity and excessive attraction to rewarding stimuli; drinking may simply be a manifestation of those mechanisms.[1,52] Some authorities have concluded a subgroup of people with BP use alcohol to self-medicate; others do not consider the self-medication hypothesis resolved.[1,52]

Although comorbid alcohol abuse worsens bipolar symptoms, smoking may have the opposite effect.[55] During mania, smoking may reduce auditory overstimulation. In addition, smoking cessation may increase the risk of depression among women with BP. Therefore, it seems logical to infer that starting to smoke, or continuing to smoke, may lower the probability of depression in these patients.

Medical Comorbidity

A population-based study found women with BP consistently more likely than controls (41% vs. 12%) to have medical comorbidities including asthma, renal failure, and acquired immune deficiency syndrome (AIDS).[56] Substantially elevated adjusted odds ratios for many debilitating conditions spanned cardiovascular, neurologic, pulmonary, endocrine, gastrointestinal, and all other organ systems. Consequently, healthcare costs for people with BP are four times higher than for age- and gender-matched controls.[56]

Some comorbidity is related to the interaction of BP and gender. Migraine headaches are more common in people with BP than the general population (25% vs 10%), and among women with BP (35%) than their male counterparts (15%).[57] Thyroid disease affected 27% of women with BP compared with 6% of men—four times greater than in the general population.[58] Hypothyroidism and subclinical hypothyroidism have been linked to depressive episodes, and some researchers find that treating these conditions improves the response to antidepressants, especially in women.[1]

Neuropsychologic Comorbidity

BP is associated with a broad range of neuropsychologic deficits in all phases of the disorder. Language and reasoning, and a few other aspects of intelligence relying on premorbid functioning, including memory of past events, are exceptions.[1] Attention appears to be a key problem, and impairment in this area presumably limits learning, memory, and visuospatial skills.[1] The severity of the course of illness, including features such as psychosis and rapid cycling, exacerbates cognitive deficits, and the effects of medications may be mixed. In addition, many deficits develop independent of episodes, and may even predate them.[1]

Mortality

General medical conditions and suicide are the two leading causes of death among people with BP. A recent meta-analysis[59] of 17 studies on bipolar spectrum disorders concluded that most excess mortality in BP is secondary to comorbidity with general medical conditions. As in the population at large, cardiovascular disease is the leading killer of women with a history of BP.[59] Cardiovascular problems are related to metabolic abnormalities, especially obesity, which is more prevalent among women with BP than female controls.[60]

Data from a prospective study noted women with BP-I have more hypertension and abdominal obesity, and are at a higher risk for future weight gain, diabetes, and cardiovascular disease.[61] Further, elevated body mass index is associated with a poorer prognosis, including more episodes and greater disability.[62]

Suicide

Available data on suicide in BP are fragmentary and unlinked, in part because few studies look specifically at BP apart from mood disorders as a whole,[63] and because early, often-cited studies sampled severely ill patients and excluded outpatients.[1] Nevertheless, experts agree people with BP are far more likely than the general population to die from suicide. Recent meta-analyses estimate that suicide may be up to 22 times more common among people with BP.[64] In the general population, women are three times as likely as men to attempt suicide, but four times as many men succeed.[1] Among people with BP, however, women are as likely or more likely to succeed as men.[1]

Risk factors for suicidal acts differ by gender. A prospective two-year study[65] of MDD and BP patients at high risk of suicide found each prior attempt increased the chance of future attempts sixfold for women compared with threefold for men. Additional risk factors for women were suicidal ideation and prior attempts using methods likely to be effective, such as shooting oneself or jumping off a bridge, rather than less effective methods, such as overdosing. Hostility, subjective depressive symptoms, fewer reasons for living, cigarette smoking, and comorbid borderline personality disorder were also risk factors for women.

Three powerful risk factors for suicide, shown in Figure 17-1, are features of BP more common in women, including depression, mixed episodes (episodes with depressive and manic symptoms), and rapid cycling (four or more episodes per year).[1] Treatment with the mood stabilizer lithium did not prevent suicide attempts, but reduced success rates far more than any other medication.[66,67]

Box 17-1 Patient with Bipolar Disorder

Melody O'Hara,* age 47, experienced her first serious episode of depression at 13, when she felt abandoned after her mother's death and father's remarriage. She began cycling between mania and depression, with multiple mixed episodes, as depicted at the far left and far right of the mood chart.

Melody suffered another major loss in her 20s when she was forced to relinquish custody of her twins after she left them alone overnight during a manic episode. Her children's absence gnawed at her and often made her feel suicidal.

Because of her frequent changes in residence and failure to return phone calls, Melody lost touch with many friends. When hypomanic, however, she indulged her passion for baking and invited people to her home for a feast. Her specialty was making cakes with creative and humorous decorations—a talent that provided a meager income.

After being hospitalized for depression, Melody began attending a weekly support group for people with bipolar disorder. The group helped her feel less alone although she still became highly anxious when manic or depressed. She felt calmer after having unprotected sex with strangers.

Despite the metabolic problems medications caused, Melody conscientiously began taking three prescribed drugs to control her disorder. Nevertheless, her rapid cycling continues, and her illness remains a defining, and often incapacitating, feature of her life.

*Identifying details have been changed to protect this woman's privacy.

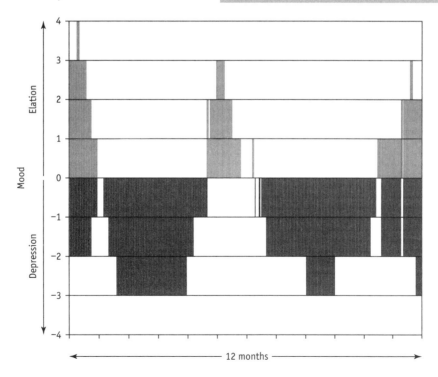

Figure 17-1 This mood chart presents a year in the life of a woman with severe bipolar disorder and three risk factors for suicide which appear more frequently in women: rapid cycling, long periods of depression, and mixed episodes. In mixed episodes, shown at the far left and far right. Depressive symptoms and hypomanic or manic symptoms occur at the same time.

Source: Adapted from the Bipolar Collaborative Network.

Meta-analysis showed that on lithium maintenance, risks for all suicidal acts/100 person years were reduced by 67% for BP-I and 82% for BP-II.[68]

Treatment and Prevention

The usual management of BP disorder involves medications, particularly mood stabilizers, antipsychotics, and antidepressants in addition to psychosocial treatment and support groups. Early adequate treatment is necessary not only to reduce symptoms in a given episode, but to avoid changing the brain in ways believed to increase risk of both future episodes—a phenomenon known as "kindling"—and treatment resistance (limitations on a person's ability to respond favorably to medication).[69]

"Mood stabilizer," a designation the Food and Drug Administration (FDA) does not define,[1] usually refers to drugs taken as maintenance medications to reduce the chances of relapses. Drugs widely prescribed as mood stabilizers include lithium as well as several anticonvulsants, primarily divalproex (valproate, valproic acid), carbamazepine, and lamotrigine.[70,71] Only lithium—and recently, to a lesser extent, the antipsychotic quetiapine—have demonstrated efficacy in reducing the likelihood of both manic and depressive episodes.[71] As noted earlier, lithium also decreases rates of suicide and attempted suicide.[66-68] Consequently, despite its many side effects, lithium remains the first-line agent for adults,[71] including the elderly.[72]

Antipsychotics work quickly to eliminate hallucinations and delusions,[1] but frequently have unpleasant or dangerous side effects. Older antipsychotics typically produce sedation[1] and rarely cause tardive dyskinesia (disfiguring, jerky, involuntary movements), a side effect more frequently affecting people with mood disorders,[71] particularly women.[73] Newer, so-called second-generation, antipsychotics, are less likely to cause movement disorders, but they create rapid weight gain and other, well-documented, adverse metabolic results.[74]

Antidepressants are still widely prescribed, even though they create serious risks and have not been approved by the FDA for monotherapy in BP.[71] Two 2010 meta-analyses concluded antidepressants are poorly tolerated and not very effective for patients with BP.[75,76] A third recent meta-analysis[38] found that antidepressants used for 6 months or more in randomized, controlled trials reduced the risk of new depression by 27%, but increased the odds of new mania by 72%—a danger to which women may be particularly vulnerable.[77] Women with rapid cycling are especially susceptible to the destabilizing effects of antidepressants; the discontinuation of these drugs consistently appears to be the best treatment for rapid cycling, even though it runs counter to the tendency of many physicians to prescribe, rather than stop, medication.[78]

In general, women are more likely to be prescribed antidepressants and combinations of drugs (polypharmacy), such as two or more antidepressants or combinations of antidepressants and antipsychotics.[79-81] However, it is difficult to interpret studies of these drugs as few people with BP are included even when sample sizes are large.[80]

Despite the risks of antidepressants in BP and limited evidence for efficacy of some combinations, polypharmacy is increasing, with the accompanying risks of more side effects and potential for drug–drug interactions.[81] Further, the frequent treatment of major mental illness with expensive, on-patent medications[82] often supplants psychosocial treatments.[83] As Thomas R. Insel, MD, director of the National Institute of Mental Health observed, "aside from the evident success of marketing … specific medications, what is perhaps most worrisome is the relative neglect of effective non-pharmacological interventions … for mood and anxiety disorders."[84]

Effective treatments for bipolar depression[85] other than medication include:

- psychoeducation as a first-line treatment or a component of other therapies
- cognitive behavior therapy, to help clients change the distorted thinking that contributes to depression, and to improve problem-solving abilities
- family-focused therapy to improve the system of which the client is a part, and to reduce the expressed negative emotion and stress that contribute to relapse
- interpersonal therapy and interpersonal-social rhythm therapy to help clients improve relationships and develop regular sleeping habits, because disruption in sleeping patterns can precipitate episodes, as well as being a symptom of mania and hypomania

Other successful treatments for bipolar depression include light therapy, particularly in seasonal and chronic cases, and adjustments in sleep. These measures strengthen circadian rhythms, the disruption of which is associated with dysfunction in moods.[86] For severe cases not responsive to medication, electroconvulsive therapy (ECT) is a first-line choice, and has a response rate of 65% to 85%.[71] Vagus nerve stimulation and transcranial magnetic stimulation are newer options for treatment-resistant depression.[1]

To reduce the chances of an episode, people with BP can identify and avoid likely triggers, particularly loss of sleep, and develop good support systems to reduce the impact of stress in their lives.[88] In contrast to the population at large, women with BP find marriage a buffer from stress, lowering risk of depression.[89]

Sometimes people with BP can also learn to recognize precursors[90] in time to seek clinical care and inquire about recovery-oriented services. Such care includes treatment plans tailored to patient goals, increasing the likelihood of adherence. Professionals can collaborate with patients to identify underlying issues for nonadherence, and customize evidence-based interventions to address them.[91] A growing body of research supports the value of patient-provider partnering, patient satisfaction with care, and patient education. These shared responsibilities have been associated with patient hope and self-efficacy with better outcomes than the more traditional evaluations of symptom reduction and relapse prevention.[92]

More appropriate prescribing would also improve treatment outcomes. Many psychiatrists ranging from 20.6%

in community mental health centers to 38.9% in private practice do not use practice guidelines at all.[93] Consequently, it is not surprising that the NCS-R reported most patients were not taking appropriate medication, particularly if they were seeing general practitioners rather than psychiatrists. However, it is not known the extent to which this failure reflects patient noncompliance or inadequate prescribing.[41]

Bipolar Disorder across a Woman's Reproductive Lifespan

BP usually begins in the late teens to early 20s—the early reproductive years—creating innumerable clinical complications related to the hypothalamic-pituitary-gonadal (HPG) axis.[60]

Menstrual and metabolic dysfunction often occur in women both before and after the development of BP,[60] including risk of polycystic ovary syndrome (PCOS), a common reproductive and metabolic disorder that raises the risk for coronary artery disease and type 2 diabetes.[60] PCOS also affects women's reproductive functioning, because it is characterized by hyperandrogenism, anovulation, infertility, and recurrent miscarriages.[60] Some medications prescribed for BP exacerbate these problems. A randomized trial showed that 21% of women on divalproex, compared with 7% on placebo, gained 5% of their body weight in a year.[60] Antipsychotics, especially the newer medications, often cause serious metabolic problems including weight gain.[74] Older antipsychotics and the newer antipsychotic risperidone interfere with the menstrual cycle, reducing fertility and increasing the risk of osteoporosis.[94]

Attention to contraception may be particularly relevant for women with BP for three reasons. First, one of the symptoms of mania and hypomania is excessive involvement in pleasurable activities, including "sexual indiscretions," possibly resulting in an unplanned pregnancy. Second, the hormones in oral contraceptives may help stabilize a woman's emotional state.[95] The larger mood fluctuations experienced by women may correlate with cyclical hormones of the menstrual cycle,[96] although consistent relationships among depression, mania, and phases of the menstrual cycle have not been demonstrated.[97] Third, medications for BP may decrease the effectiveness of oral contraceptives, and oral contraceptives may alter effect of BP medications.[98] There have been no reports of drug–drug interactions between oral contraceptives and both atypical antipsychotics and some mood stabilizers, although research on these possible dangers is limited.[98]

Pregnancy

Prenatal counseling should present the risks associated with pregnancy, including genetic transmission of susceptibility to BP.[95] These risks include the substantial dangers to fetal development caused by some medications; some are known to be teratogenic, including spina bifida. Risk may be reduced by folate supplementation beginning before conception; vitamin K during pregnancy and regular exercise have also been recommended.[99] Discontinuing medication to reduce the chances of teratogenesis doubles the risk of episodes and increases the amount of time spent ill fivefold.[99] More such episodes (47%) occur in the first trimester than the second (32%) or third (19%).[99]

Additional issues associated with pregnancy include physiological changes that influence drug metabolizing and renal clearance rates, altering the effect of antidepressants as well as some mood stabilizers.[95] Consequently, prenatal recommendations include frequent blood tests for medication levels in the pregnant woman,[95] as well as specific screening for abnormal fetal development specific to the medication being used: e.g., for lithium, an ultrasound and echocardiogram for cardiac malformation at 16–18 weeks.[100] Women on lithium also need monthly monitoring of electrolytes and thyroid functioning.[95]

Because untreated maternal depression is associated with postpartum depression in mothers, and lethargy, irritability, and low birth weight in infants, treatment is increasingly recommended.[101] Pregnant women with depression, not necessarily bipolar depression, appear to benefit most from interpersonal therapy; cognitive therapy; a form of acupuncture designed to alleviate depression; and (albeit with less rigorous data) massage.[101] For more serious depressions, especially those with psychotic or suicidal features, ECT may be considered in lieu of medications.[95] Although ECT is not a first-line treatment under other circumstances, when appropriate precautions are taken, ECT is allegedly safe for women during pregnancy, and has not been known to harm the fetus.[95]

Mood stabilizers increase various risks to the fetus at different stages of pregnancy. Divalproex is particularly dangerous during the first trimester and may cause major congenital malformations (6.2%–20.3%) depending on the dose—more than lamotrigine (1.0%–5.6%) and carbamazepine (2.2%–7.9%).[99] In utero exposure to divalproex, compared with other mood stabilizers, is also associated with far more neurobehavioral deficits for babies, including developmental delays (25%–71%) and decreases in verbal IQ (22%–30%), often necessitating special education.[99] Lithium, if taken during the first trimester, increases the incidence of a congenital heart defect by a factor of one to eight.[99] If taken during the second or third trimester, lithium can cause premature delivery, thyroid abnormality, and excess fluid in the amniotic sac. Other problems include "floppy baby syndrome" (abnormal limpness) and decreased Apgar scores.[99] Overall, exposure to lithium is associated with major congenital malformations in 4.05–12.0% of fetuses.[99] All other mood stabilizers are also associated with varied risks.[1]

Less is known about the problems posed by other medications for BP. Nevertheless, antidepressants, benzodiazepines (antianxiety agents), older antipsychotics, and newer antipsychotics (except clozapine) all have demonstrated an adverse effect on the fetus in animal studies and/or human beings.[1] Clozapine appears safer although the fetus, just like an adult patient, must be monitored for agranulocytosis, a potentially fatal increase in white blood cells.[95] For all the foregoing medications, using as small a dose as possible, taking a single medication, and monitoring results are recommended.[95]

Given the foregoing information about complications of pregnancy unique to women with BP, it may be understandable that in one study, 37% of such women decided not to pursue pregnancy when provided with accurate information about their treatment options.[102] Due to the threat of teratogenesis, the first impulse of a woman with BP and an unplanned pregnancy might be to stop taking medication immediately. However, this course of action is problematic, because abruptly discontinuing many psychotropic drugs, particularly after chronic use, could precipitate relapse.[101,104] In addition, by the time a woman realizes she is pregnant, drugs have already had the opportunity to compromise the health of the fetus. Consequently, several studies have concluded that the benefit of discontinuing mood stabilizers would be limited and the risk of relapse is substantial. Among women followed in a prospective study,[105] relapse rates doubled if mood stabilizers were used at the time of conception and throughout pregnancy. Further, the time to the first recurrence of an episode was four times shorter, and the proportion of time spent ill during pregnancy was five times greater, among those who discontinued medication.[105] Although the risk of relapse from discontinuing medication is greater than the probability of teratogenesis, women's perception of risk from a "man-made" cause, and their attitudes towards therapeutic abortion, may cause some women to forgo treatment.[106]

Pregnancy itself may exacerbate the risk of depression, hypomania, and mania.[95] However, some reports, and a study of women with BP-I who were responsive to lithium before pregnancy, suggest that pregnancy may decrease the chances of an episode among women who are not on medication.[107]

Postpartum

After delivery, 20%–50% of women with BP[108] (vs. 10–15% of women in the general population)[107] experience postpartum depression,[109] and 20%–30% have postpartum psychosis.[110] Postpartum depression, and especially postpartum psychosis, increase the short-term risk of suicide and infanticide.[111,112] In untreated postpartum psychosis, the risk of the latter is as high as 4% in the general population.[113] Consequently, treatment, including medication, psychotherapy, and/or ECT, are recommended. Interpersonal psychotherapy treatment (ITP) is particularly appropriate in helping women cope with role changes and relationships accompanying parturition.[114] ECT is also effective and leads to faster and more complete remission among women with postpartum psychosis than those with psychosis unrelated to childbearing.[114] Longitudinal data show that most women with BP and postpartum psychosis have a good prognosis and fare far better than women with psychotic episodes not triggered by sudden hormonal shifts.[114]

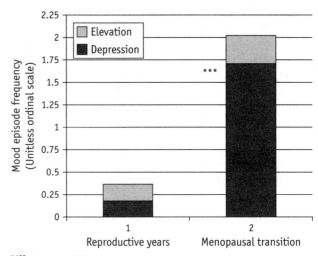

Figure 17-2 Mood episode frequency before and during menopause transition of 27 women with Bipolar Disorder.

Source: Reproduced from Marsh WK, Templeton A, Ketter TA, Rasgon NL. Increased frequency of depressive episodes during the menopausal transition in women with bipolar disorder: preliminary report. J Psychiatr Res. 2008;42:247–251. ©Elsevier 2008.

Breastfeeding complicates the clinical picture due to sleep loss, and may precipitate mania or postpartum psychosis.[114] In addition, breastfeeding is sometimes contraindicated for mothers taking BP medication,[95] as these drugs would be secreted in breast milk.[1] Because infants do not have developed livers and kidneys, these drugs may affect neurodevelopment.[106] If a mother must nurse while taking medication, it is advisable to divide daily doses to reduce peak serum concentrations,[114] taking drugs just after breastfeeding or right before the neonate is scheduled to sleep.[95]

Perimenopause and Menopause

Few data exist on BP in older women, compared with those of reproductive age. Nevertheless, it is clear that perimenopause is associated with an increase in depressive episodes compared with younger women (30–40 years old).[115] In one study of the menopausal transition, 68% of women with BP had at least one depressive episode during an average of 17 months.[116] Perimenopause and menopause are associated with an increase in episodes of depression, agitated depression, and psychosis.[108]

Additional concerns of older women with BP suggest increased need for monitoring. For example, it seems probable that when anticonvulsant medications are used long term, older women with BP might require more bone mineral density (BMD) screenings because some of these drugs exacerbate the bone loss. This change peaks at menopause and makes women more vulnerable to fractures.[117]

Future Directions

Increasing knowledge of disturbances underlying the many comorbidities of BP suggests the condition is more than a psychiatric illness. Consequently, a new paradigm views

BP as a combination of four core dysfunctions: abnormal emotional reactivity or instability; problems with circadian rhythms; cognitive impairment; and a collection of co-occurring medical problems, such as obesity, with far-reaching consequences.[118] This vision of BP might encourage patients, providers, and policymakers to address risks that typically accompany the mood disorder.[118] For example, women with BP have more abdominal fat than obese controls, which increases cardiovascular disease; this fat releases substances that increase the severity of depression.[119] Psychiatrists and allied health professionals would treat BP more effectively by using weight management strategies as well as medication and psychosocial care.

Comparisons of BP in the United States vs. Europe might also yield useful hypotheses and information. BP has a more serious course in the United States, where patients are more likely to have earlier age at diagnosis, greater likelihood of a positive family history of the disorder, comorbid anxiety, substance abuse, and/or rapid cycling.[120] American patients are more often treated with valproate and atypical antipsychotics, whereas those in Europe much more frequently receive lithium and typical antipsychotics with better long-term outcomes than people in the United States who received the same drugs.[120]

Summary

Bipolar Disorder is one of the most serious illnesses worldwide due to the functional impairment and high use of health services. Until recently, the prevalence of BP was estimated at 1% to 2% in women and men. Lately many authorities argue that in both epidemiologic studies and clinical practice most cases of BP are not recognized, especially in women. Instead, Major Depressive Disorder is often overdiagnosed at the expense of BP and Bipolar Disorder Not Otherwise Specified. BP is highly comorbid with other psychiatric disorders and has been regarded as a marker for comorbidity. By far the most clinically harmful comorbidity for women is alcohol dependence; BP raises a woman's chance of having an alcohol use disorder more than sevenfold.

Women with BP are 20 times more likely to die from suicide than women in the general population, but the main sources of premature mortality in this illness are general medical illnesses, particularly cardiovascular disease. Dysfunction in the hypothalamic-pituitary-gonadal (HPG) axis is associated with cardiovascular disease, as well as reproductive and metabolic irregularities. These abnormalities put women with BP at risk of obesity, PCOS, postpartum psychosis, and other difficulties across the life span. Unfortunately, medications commonly used to treat BP exacerbate these problems, pose serious teratogenic risks, and, in the case of antidepressants, worsen the course of the illness.

Discussion Questions

1. What is BP, and how does it differ in men and women?
2. Why it is hard to estimate the prevalence of BP, especially the prevalence of BP in women? How does our classification system contribute to this problem?

3. What is the most serious psychiatric comorbidity for women with BP? Why?
4. What are the two biggest causes of premature mortality in women with BP? Why?
5. How does BP affect women across the life span? In particular, how might BP affect contraception, pregnancy, postpartum issues, and menopause?

References

1. Goodwin F, Jamison K. *Manic-Depressive Illness: Bipolar Disorders and Recurrent Depression*. New York: Oxford University Press; 2007.
2. Kessler RC, Merikangas KR, Wang PS. Prevalence, comorbidity, and service utilization for mood disorders in the United States at the beginning of the twenty-first century. *Annu Rev Clin Psychol*. 2007;3:137–158.
3. Ketter TA. Diagnostic features, prevalence, and impact of bipolar disorder. *J Clin Psychiatry*. 2010;71:e14.
4. Pies R. The historical roots of the "bipolar spectrum": did Aristotle anticipate Kraepelin's broad concept of manic-depression? *J Affect Disord*. 2007; 100:7–11.
5. Craddock N, Owen MJ. The Kraepelinian dichotomy—going, going…but still not gone. *Br J Psychiatry*. 2010;196:92–95.
6. Phelps J, Angst J, Katzow J, Sadler J. Validity and utility of bipolar spectrum models. *Bipolar Disord*. 2008;10:179–193.
7. *Diagnostic and Statistical Manual of Mental Disorders*. 4th ed. Washington DC: American Psychiatric Association; 1994:317–391, 650–654.
8. Vieta E, Suppes T. Bipolar II disorder: arguments for and against a distinct diagnostic entity *Bipolar Disord*. 2008;10:163–178.
9. Akiskal HS. Searching for behavioral indicators of bipolar II in patients presenting with major depressive episodes: the "red sign," the "rule of three" and other biographic signs of temperamental extravagance, activation and hypomania. *J Affect Disord*. 2005;84:279–290.
10. Paris J. The bipolar spectrum: a critical perspective. *Har Rev Psychiatry* 2009;17:206–213.
11. Novick DM, Swartz HA, Frank E. Suicide attempts in bipolar I and bipolar II disorder: a review and meta-analysis of the evidence. *Bipolar Disord*. 2010;12:1–9.
12. Baldassano CF, Marangell LB, Gyulai L, et al. Gender differences in bipolar disorder: retrospective data from the first 500 STEP-BP participants. *Bipolar Disord*. 2005;7:465–470.
13. Ghaemi SN. Treatment of rapid-cycling bipolar disorder: are antidepressants mood destabilizers? *Am J Psychiatry*. 2008;165:300–302.
14. McEachin RC, Saccone NL, Saccone SF, et al. Modeling complex genetic and environmental influences on comorbid bipolar disorder. *BMC Med Genet*. 2010;11:14.
15. Oedegaard KJ, Greenwood TA, Johansson S, et al. A genome-wide association study of bipolar disorder and comorbid migraine. *Genes Brain Behav*. 2010;9:673–680.
16. Ongür D, Lundy M, Greenhouse I, et al. Default mode network abnormalities in bipolar disorder and schizophrenia. *Psychiatry Res*. 2010;183:59–68.
17. Weissman MM, Myers JK. Epidemiology of mental disorders: emerging trends in the United States. *Arch Gen Psychiatry*. 1978;35:1304–1311.
18. Regier DA, Meyers JM, Kramer M, et al. The NIMH Epidemiologic Catchment Area Program. *Arch Gen Psychiatry*. 1984;41:934–941.
19. Kessler RC, McGonagle KA, et al. Lifetime and 12-month prevalence of DSM-III-R psychiatric disorders in the United States: results from the National Comorbidity Study. *Arch Gen Psychiatry*. 1994;51:8–19.
20. Kessler RC, Berglund P, Demler O, et al. Lifetime prevalence and age-of-onset distributions of DSM-IV disorders in the National Comorbidity Survey Replication. *Arch Gen Psychiatry*. 2005;62:593–602.
21. Kessler RC, Chiu WT, Demler O, Walters EE. Prevalence, severity, and comorbidity of 12-month DSM-IV Disorders in the National Comorbidity Survey Replication. *Arch Gen Psychiatry*. 2005;62:617–627.
22. Akiskal HS. The emergence of the bipolar spectrum: Validation along clinical-epidemiologic and familial-genetic lines. *Psychopharm Bull*. 2007;40:99–115.
23. CME Institute, JCP E-lert: Recognizing Bipolar Disorder. *Prim Care Companion J Clin Psychiatry*. 2010;12(suppl 1).
24. Helzer JE, Robins LN, McEvoy LT, et al. A comparison of clinical and Diagnostic Interview Schedule diagnoses. *Arch Gen Psychiatry*. 1985;42:657–666.
25. Carta MG, Hardoy MC, Fryers T. Commentary: Are structured interviews truly able to detect and diagnose Bipolar II disorders in epidemiological studies? The king is still nude! *Clin Pract Epidemiol Ment Health*. 2008;4:28–31.
26. Narrow WE, Rae, DS, Robins LN, Regier DA. Revised prevalence estimates of mental disorders in the United States: Using a clinical significance criterion to reconcile surveys' estimates. *Arch Gen Psychiatry*. 2002;59:115–123.
27. Barnett JH, Smoller JW. The genetics of bipolar disorder. *Neuroscience*. 2009;164:331–343.
28. Ghaemi SN, Ko JY, Goodwin FK. "Cade's Disease" and beyond: misdiagnosis, antidepressant use, and a proposed definition for bipolar spectrum disorder. *Can J Psychiatry*. 2002;47:125–134.

29. Carta MG, Angst J. Epidemiological and clinical aspects of bipolar disorders: controversies or a common need to redefine the aims and methodological aspects of surveys. *Clin Pract Epidemiol Ment Health.* 2005;1:1–4

30. Bebbington P, Ramana R. The epidemiology of bipolar affective disorder. *Soc Psychiatry Psychiatr Epidemiol.* 1995;30:279–292.

31. Parens E, Johnston J. Controversies concerning the diagnosis and treatment of bipolar disorder in children. *Child Adolesc Psychiatry Ment Health* 2010;4:9:1–14.

32. Moreno C, Laje G, Blanco C, et al. M. National trends in the outpatient diagnosis and treatment of bipolar disorder in youth. *Arch Gen Psychiatry.* 2007;64:1032–1039.

33. Frances A. Psychiatric diagnosis gone wild: the "epidemic" of childhood bipolar disorder. *Psychiatr Times.* April 8, 2010. http://www.psychiatrictimes.com/display/article/10168/1551005. Accessed February 7, 2011.

34. Zimmerman M, Galione JN, Ruggero CJ, et al. Screening for bipolar disorder and finding borderline personality disorder. *J Clin Psychiatry.* 2010;71:1212–1217.

35. Ruggero CJ, Zimmerman M, Chelminski I, Young D. Borderline personality disorder and the misdiagnosis of bipolar disorder. *J Psychiatr Res.* 2010;44:405–408.

36. Awad AG, Rajagopalan K, Bolge SC, McDonnell DD. Quality of life among bipolar disorder patients misdiagnosed with major depressive disorder. *Prim Care Companion J Clin Psychiatry.* 2007;9:195–202.

37. Stensland MD, Schultz JF, Frytak JR. Depression diagnoses following the identification of bipolar disorder: costly incongruent diagnoses. *BMC Psychiatry.* 2010;10:39–47.

38. Ghaemi SN, Wingo AP, Filkowski MA, Baldessarini RJ. Long-term antidepressant treatment in bipolar disorder: meta-analyses of benefits and risks. *Acta Psychiatr Scand.* 2008;118:347–356.

39. Judd LL, Akiskal HS. The prevalence and disability of bipolar spectrum disorders in the US population: re-analysis of the ECA database taking into account subthreshold cases. *J Affect Disord.* 2003;73:123–131.

40. American Psychological Association DSM-V Task Force. Hypomanic episode: proposed revision. Updated May 21, 2010. http://www.dsm5.org/ProposedRevisions/Pages/proposedrevision.aspx?rid=426. Accessed January 17, 2011.

41. Merikangas KR, Akiskal HS, Angst J, et al. Lifetime and 12-month prevalence of bipolar spectrum disorder in the National Comorbidity Survey Replication. *Arch Gen Psychiatry.* 2007;64:543–552.

42. Zimmermann P, Brückl T, Nocon A, et al. Heterogeneity of DSM-IV major depressive disorder as a consequence of subthreshold bipolarity. *Arch Gen Psychiatry.* 2009;66:1341–1352.

43. Regier DA, Narrow WE, Kuhl E, Kupfer DJ. The conceptual development of DSM-V. *Am J Psychiatry.* 2009;166:645–650.

44. Baldessarini RJ. A plea for the integrity of the bipolar disorder concept. *Bipolar Disord.* 2000;2:3–7.

45. Akiskal HS. The temperamental borders of affective disorders. *Acta Psychiatr Scand.* 1994;89(suppl 379):32–37.

46. Henry C, Mitropoulou V, New AS, et al. Affective instability and impulsivity in borderline personality and bipolar II disorders: similarities and differences. *J Psychiatr Res.* 2001;35:307–312.

47. Bodner E, Cohen-Fridel S, Iancu I. Staff attitudes toward patients with borderline personality disorder. *Compr Psychiatry.* 2011;52:548–555.

48. Weinberg I, Ronningstam E, Goldblatt MJ, et al. Common factors in empirically supported treatments of borderline personality disorder. *Curr Psychiatry Res.* 2011;13:60–68.

49. McElroy, SL. Diagnosing and treating comorbid (complicated) bipolar disorder. *J Clin Psychiatry* 2004;65(15 suppl):35–44.

50. Baldassano CF. Illness course, comorbidity, gender, and suicidality in patients with bipolar disorder. *J Clin Psychiatry.* 2006;67:8–11.

51. Frye MA, Altshuler LA, McElroy SL, et al. Gender differences in prevalence, risk, and clinical correlates of alcoholism comorbidity in bipolar disorder. *Am J Psychiatry.* 2003;160:883–889.

52. Swan AC. The strong relationship between bipolar and substance-use disorder. *Ann NY Acad Sci.* 2010;1187:276–293.

53. McDermott BE, Quanbeck CD, Frye MA. Comorbid substance use disorder in women with bipolar disorder associated with criminal arrest *Bipolar Disord.* 2007;9:536–540.

54. Weiss RD, Kolodziej M, Griffin ML, et al. Substance use and perceived symptom improvement among patients with bipolar disorder and substance dependence *J Affect Disord.* 2004;79:279–283.

55. Leonard S, Adler LE, Benhammou K, et al. Smoking and mental illness. *Pharmacol Biochem Behav.* 2001;70:561–570.

56. Carney CP, Jones LE. Medical comorbidity in women and men with bipolar disorders: A population-based controlled study. *Psychosom Med.* 2006;68:684–691.

57. McIntyre RS, Konarski JZ, Wilkinds K, et al. The prevalence and impact of migraine headache in bipolar disorder: results from the Canadian Community Health Survey. *Headache.* 2006;46:973–982.

58. Baldassano CF, Marangell LB, Gyulai L, et al. Gender differences in bipolar disorder: retrospective data from the first 500 STEP-BD participants. *Bipolar Disord.* 2005;7:465–470.

59. Roshanaei-Moghaddam B, Katon W. Premature mortality from general medical illness among persons with bipolar disorder: A review. *Psychiatric Serv.* 2009;2:147–156.

60. Kenna HA, Jiang B, Rasgon NL. Reproductive and metabolic abnormalities associated with bipolar disorder and its treatment. *Harv Rev Psychiatry.* 2009;17:138–146.

61. Fleet-Michaliszyn SB, Soreca I, Otto AD, et al. A prospective observational study of obesity, body composition, and insulin resistance in 18 women with bipolar disorder and 17 matched control subjects. *J Clin Psychiatry.* 2008;69:1892–1900.

62. Calkin C, van de Velde C, Ruzickova M, et al. Can body mass index help predict outcome in patients with bipolar disorder? *Bipolar Disord.* 2009;11:650–656.

63. Goldsmith KS, Pellmar TC, Kleinman AM, Bunney WE, eds. *Reducing Suicide: A National Imperative.* Washington, DC: Institute of Medicine of the National Academies Press; 2002. http://www.nap.edu/catalog.php?record_id=10398. Accessed January 2011.

64. Tondo L, Isacsson G, Baldessarini RJ. Suicide behavior in bipolar disorder: risk and prevention. *CNS Drugs* 2003;17:491–511.

65. Oquendo MA, Bongiovi-Garcia ME, Galfavy H, et al. Sex differences in clinical predictors of suicidal acts after major depression: a prospective study. *Am J Psychiatry.* 2007;164:134–141.

66. Baldessarini RJ, Tondo L, Hennen, J. Treating the suicidal patient with bipolar disorder. Reducing suicide risk with lithium. *Ann N Y Acad Sci.* 2001;932:24–38.

67. Dunner DL. Correlates of suicidal behavior and lithium treatment in bipolar disorder. *J Clin Psychiatry.* 2004;65(suppl 10):5–10.

68. Baldessarini RJ, Tondo L, Hennen J. Lithium treatment and suicide risk in major affective disorders: update and new findings. *J Clin Psychiatry.* 2003;64(suppl 5):44–52.

69. Post RM. Mechanisms of illness progression in the recurrent affective disorders. *Neurotox Res.* 2010;18:256–271.

70. Van Lieshout RJ, MacQueen GM. Efficacy and acceptability of mood stabilisers in the treatment of acute bipolar depression: systematic review. *Br J Psychiatry.* 2010;196:266–273.

71. Ansari A, Osser DN. The psychopharmacology algorithm project at the Harvard South Shore Program: an update on bipolar depression. *Harv Rev Psychiatry.* 2010;18:36–55.

72. Shulman KI. Lithium for older adults with bipolar disorder: should it still be considered a first-line agent? *Drugs Aging.* 2010;27:607–615.

73. Schwartz T, Raza S. Aripiprazole (Abilify) and tardive dyskinesia. *P&T.* 2008;33:32–34.

74. Maayan L, Correll CU. Management of antipsychotic-related weight gain. *Expert Rev Neurother.* 2010;10:1175–1200.

75. Correa R, Akiskal H, Gilmer W, et al. Is unrecognized bipolar disorder a frequent contributor to apparent treatment resistant depression? *J Affect Disord.* 2010;127:10–18.

76. Ghaemi SN, Ostacher MM, El-Mallakh RS, et al. Antidepressant discontinuation in bipolar depression: a Systematic Treatment Enhancement Program for Bipolar Disorder (STEP-BD) randomized clinical trial of long-term effectiveness and safety. *J Clin Psychiatry.* 2010;71:372–380.

77. Burt VK, Rasgon N. Special considerations in treating bipolar disorder in women. *Bipolar Disord.* 2004;6:2–13.

78. Ghaemi SN. Treatment of rapid-cycling bipolar disorder: Are antidepressants mood destabilizers? *Am J Psychiatry.* 2008;165:300–302.

79. Marcus SC, Olfson M. National trends in the treatment for depression from 1998 to 2007. *Arch Gen Psychiatry.* 2010;67:1265–1273.

80. Mojtabai R. Increase in antidepressant medication in the US adult population between 1990 and 2003. *Psychother Psychosom.* 2008;77:83–92.

81. Mojtabai R, Olfson M. National trends in psychotropic medication polypharmacy in office-based psychiatry. *Arch Gen Psychiatry.* 2010;67:26–36.

82. Frank RG, Conti RM, Goldman HH. Mental health policy and psychotropic drugs. *Milbank Q.* 2005;83:271–298.

83. Mojtabai R, Olfson M. National trends in psychotherapy by office-based psychiatrists. *Arch Gen Psychiatry* 2008;65:962–970.

84. Insel TR. Psychiatrists' relationships with pharmaceutical companies: part of the problem or part of the solution? *JAMA.* 2010;303:1192–1193.

85. Vieta E, Pacchiarotti I, Valenti M, et al. A critical update on psychological interventions for bipolar disorders. *Curr Psychiatry Rep.* 2009;11:494–502.

86. Wirtz-Justice A, Benedetti F, Terman M. *Chronotherapeutics for Affective Disorders: A Clinician's Manual for Light and Wake Therapy.* New York: Karger; 2009.

87. Dell'Osso B, Mundo E, D'Urso N, et al. Augmentative repetitive navigated transcranial magnetic stimulation (rTMS) in drug-resistant bipolar depression. *Bipolar Disord.* 2009;11:76–81.

88. Suto M, Murray G, Hale S, et al. What works for people with bipolar disorder? Tips from the experts. *J Affective Disord.* 2010;124:76–84.

89. Lieberman DZ, Massey SH, Goodwin FK. The role of gender in single vs married individuals with bipolar disorder. *Compr Psychiatry.* 2010;51:380–385.

90. Goossens PJ, Kupka RW, Beentjes TA, van Achterberg T. Recognising prodromes of manic or depressive recurrence in outpatients with bipolar disorder: a cross-sectional study. *Int J Nurs Stud.* 2010;47:1201–1207.

91. Velligan DI, Weiden PJ, Sajatovic M, et al. Assessment of adherence problems in patients with serious and persistent mental illness: recommendations from the expert consensus guidelines. *J Psychiatr Pract.* 2010;16:34–45.

92. Morris CD, Miklowitz DJ, Wisniewski SR, et al. Care satisfaction, hope, and life functioning among adults with bipolar disorder: data from the first 1000 participants in the Systematic Treatment Enhancement Program. *Compr Psychiatry*. 2005;46:98–104.

93. Perlis RH. Use of treatment guidelines in clinical decision making in bipolar disorder: a pilot survey of clinicians. *Curr Med Res Opin*. 2007;23: 467–475.

94. Joffe H. Reproductive biology and psychotropic treatments in premenopausal women with bipolar disorder. *J Clin Psychiatry*. 2007;68(suppl 9);10–15.

95. Rasgon NL, Zappert, LN. Special considerations for women with bipolar disorder. In: Bowden C, Calabrese J, Ketter T, eds. *Advances in the Treatment of Bipolar Disorder*. vol 24. Washington, DC, American Psychiatric Publishing; 2005:211–241.

96. Rasgon N, Bauer M, Grof P, et al. Sex-specific mood changes by patients with bipolar disorder. *J Psychiatric Res*. 2005;39:77–83.

97. Shivakumar G, Bernstein IH, Suppes T, et al. Are bipolar mood symptoms affected by the phase of the menstrual cycle? *J Womens Health*. 2008;17: 473–478.

98. Marangell LB. Current issues: women and bipolar disorder. *Dialogues Clin Neurosci*. 2008;10:229–238.

99. Nguyen HT, Sharma V, McIntyre RS. Teratogenesis associated with antibipolar agents. *Adv Ther*. 2009;26:281–294.

100. Cohen LS, Wang B, Nonacs R, et al. Treatment of mood disorders during pregnancy and the postpartum. *Psychiatr Clin N Am*. 2010;33:273–293.

101. Harvard Medical School. Alternatives to antidepressants during pregnancy. *Harv Ment Health Lett*. 2010;27:4–5.

102. Viguera AC, Cohen LS, Bouffard S, et al. Reproductive decisions by women with bipolar disorder after pregnancy psychiatric consultation. *Am J Psychiatry*. 2002;159:2102–2104.

103. Howland RH. Potential adverse effects of discontinuing psychotropic drugs—part 1. *J Psychosoc Nurs Ment Health Serv*. 2010;48:11–14.

104. Howland RH. Potential adverse effects of discontinuing psychotropic drugs—part 2. *J Psychosoc Nurs Ment Health Serv*. 2010;48:9–12.

105. Viguera AC, Whitfield T, Baldessarini RJ, et al. Risk of recurrence in women with bipolar disorder during pregnancy: prospective study of mood stabilizer discontinuation *Am J Psychiatry*. 2007;164:1817–1824.

106. Dodd S, Berk M. The safety of medications for the treatment of bipolar disorder during pregnancy and the puerperium. *Curr Drug Saf*. 2006;1:25–33.

107. Grof P, Robbins W, Alda M, et al. Protective effect of pregnancy in women with lithium-responsive bipolar disorder. *J Affect Disord*. 2000;61:31–39.

108. Sit D. Women and bipolar disorder across the life span. *JAMA*. 2004;59: 91–100.

109. Garcia KS, Flynn P, Pierce, KJ, Caudle M. Repetitive transcranial magnetic stimulation treats postpartum depression. *Brain Stimul*. 2010;3:36–41.

110. Freeman MP, Smith KW, Freeman SA, et al. The impact of reproductive events on the course of bipolar disorder in women. *J Clin Psych*. 2002;63:284–287.

111. Jones I, Craddock N. Familiality of the puerperal trigger in bipolar disorder: results of a family study. *Am J Psychiatry*. 2001;158:913–917.

112. Kelly E, Sharma V. Diagnosis and treatment of postpartum bipolar depression. *Expert Rev Neurother*. 2010;7:1045–1051.

113. Spinelli M. Maternal infanticide associated with mental illness: Prevention and the promise of saved lives. *Amn J Psychiatry*. 2004;161:1548–1557.

114. Sit D, Rothschil AJ, Wisner KL. A review of postpartum psychosis. *J Womens Health*. 2006;15:352–368.

115. Marsh WK, Ketter TA, Rasgon NL. Increased depressive symptoms in menopausal age women with bipolar disorder: age and gender comparison. *J Psychiatr Res*. 2009;43:798–802.

116. Marsh WK, Templeton A, Ketter TA, Rasgon NL. Increased frequency of depressive episodes during the menopausal transition in women with bipolar disorder: preliminary report. *J Psychiatr Res*. 2008;42:247–251.

117. Pack AM, Walczak TS. Bone health in women with epilepsy: clinical features and potential mechanisms. In: Gidal BE, Harden CL, eds. *Epilepsy in Women: The Scientific Basis for Clinical Management*. Boston: Elsevier; 2008. *International Review of Neurobiology*; vol 83.

118. Leboyer M, Kupfer DJ. Bipolar disorder: new perspectives in health care and prevention. *J Clin Psychiatry*. 2010;71:1689–1695.

119. Kemp DE, Gao K, Chan PK, et al. Medical comorbidity in bipolar disorder: relationship between illnesses of the endocrine/metabolic system and treatment outcome. *Bipolar Disord*. 2010;12:404–413.

120. Post R. More early onsets and difficult courses of bipolar illness occur in the US than in the Netherlands and Germany. *Bipolar Network News*. 2010;14:1, 5.

Posttraumatic Stress Disorder in Women

Eun Jung Suh, PhD and Clara Li, MA

Introduction

Posttraumatic Stress Disorder (PTSD) is an anxiety disorder that may occur after learning of or personally experiencing a traumatic event, estimated to affect approximately 8% of American adults.[1] PTSD is the most common type of anxiety disorder among women in the United States[2] occurring more frequently among women than men,[3] and females have a greater risk for developing PTSD than males following exposure to a traumatic event.[4]

Definition of PTSD

According to the American Psychiatric Association,[1] the essential features of PTSD noted in Table 18-1 include development of symptoms following exposure to a

Table 18-1

DSM-IV Checklist for PTSD

(A) A traumatic event is characterized by both of the following:
- A death, serious injury, or threat to the physical integrity of self or others
- Intense fear, helplessness, or horror

(B) Reexperienced symptoms with at least one of the following:
- Recurrent recollections of the trauma
- Recurrent dreams of the trauma
- Recurrent flashbacks of the trauma
- Psychologically distressed at stimuli resembling the trauma
- Physiologically aroused to stimuli resembling the trauma

(C) Avoidance symptoms, absent before the trauma, with at least three of the following:
- Avoiding thoughts, feelings, or conversations associated with the trauma
- Avoiding activities, places, or people associated with the trauma
- Unable to remember important aspects of the trauma
- Feeling detached from others
- Having restricted affect or emotions
- Having a sense of a foreshortened future

(D) Physical symptoms, absent before the trauma, with at least two of the following:
- Insomnia
- Irritability
- Difficulty concentrating
- Hypervigilance
- Easily startled

(E) Duration of the symptoms in Criteria B, C, and D lasts more than 1 month.

(F) Symptoms cause significant impairments in at least one of the following areas:
- Emotional distress
- Impairment of social, occupational, or other aspects of functioning.

Source: Data from American Psychiatric Association. (2000). *Diagnostic and statistical manual of mental disorders DSM-IV-TR*. Arlington, VA: American Psychiatric Publishing, Inc.

traumatic event involving death, serious injury, or a threat to the physical integrity of others or oneself (Criterion A). Among traumatized individuals, their responses to the stressful event must involve intense fear, feeling of helplessness, or horror (among children, the response has to involve disorganized or agitated behavior). Other symptoms following the exposure to the traumatic event include persistent reexperiencing of the trauma (Criterion B), persistent avoidance of stimuli relating to the trauma and persistent experience of numbing (Criterion C), as well as persistent symptoms of anxiety or increased physical arousal that were absent prior to the trauma (Criterion D). These symptoms must be present for more than 1 month (Criterion E) and induce clinically significant distress or impairment in functioning (Criterion F).

Epidemiology of PTSD in Women

Some researchers attributed differences in rates of PTSD by gender to differences in traumatic experiences,[2] post-trauma social support,[5] and bias in sample selection.[6] However, other studies have shown that gender differences remained significant even after controlling for potential confounders such as numbers and types of traumatic events,[2,7] cultural background,[8] diversity of study populations, and methods of assessment.[9] An early empirical study showed that women and men differed in frequency of PTSD, in which nearly 31% of females were shown to develop PTSD after being exposed to a trauma as opposed to 19% of males.[10] A subsequent epidemiologic survey in the general population also reported that PTSD was almost twice as prevalent in females as males.[2] Similar results have been replicated by a number of other recent epidemiologic studies.[11,12] In contrast, several early clinical studies did not find evidence for gender differences in the rate of PTSD;[13,14] however, these data were either collected from an extremely small sample[13] or lacked standard assessments of PTSD.[13,14] A review of recent American studies of PTSD by gender is presented in Table 18-2.

Traumatized women with a diagnosis of PTSD are at increased risk for both psychiatric disorders[25] and health-related problems.[26] PTSD is linked to poor self-reported physical health and greater use of medical services.[27] Pregnant women with PTSD were more likely to display comorbid depression and anxiety than those without PTSD.[28] Experience of a potentially traumatic event was consistently identified as a contributor to smoking behavior,[29-31] and individuals with PTSD were more likely to be smokers than those without PTSD.[32] In addition to increased smoking, experience of potentially traumatic events and diagnosis of PTSD were also associated with increased nonmedical use of prescription drugs both in adults[33] and adolescents.[34] Traumatic exposure may also result in cognitive impairment as individuals with PTSD often exhibited difficulties in neurocognitive tasks.[35]

Gender Differences in PTSD

Given the significant health impact of PTSD, a need exists to understand why women are at greater risk than men for the disorder and to further investigate women's vulnerability to PTSD. In this chapter, we explore several plausible explanations, including gender differences in (1) types of trauma, (2) feelings of betrayal, (3) social roles, (4) social supports, (5) interpersonal relationships, (6) cognitive appraisals, (7) acute stress responses, (8) acute dissociative reactions, (9) child sexual abuse, (10) genes, (11) hormonal environment, (12) neurotransmitter systems, (13) intelligence quotient, and (14) verbal memory. Methodologically, the present chapter describes (15) types of sample, (16) forms of assessment, and (17) definitions of trauma as important contributing factors for the gender disparity in the rate of PTSD.

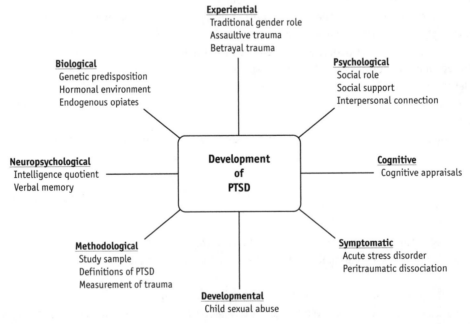

Figure 18-1 Risk factors for the development of PTSD.

Table 18-2

Lifetime prevalence of PTSD by gender in epidemiologic surveys, United States

Study	Sample size	Sample description	Lifetime prevalence		References
			Females [%]	Males [%]	
Helzer et al., 1987	2,493	General population	1.3	0.5	[15]
Breslau et al., 1991	1,007	Urban population of young adults aged between 21 and 30 years	30.7	14.0	[16]
Kessler et al., 1995	5,877	National noninstitutionalized civilian respondents aged 15 to 54 years	10.4	5.0	[17]
Singer et al., 1995	1,265	Six public school students (in Cleveland, Ohio, Denver, Colorado, and Northeast Ohio) aged between 14 and 19 years	16.2	7	[18]
Boney-McCoy & Finkelhor, 1995	2,000	National telephone sample of youths aged between 10 and 16 years	15.3	5.9	[19]
Harrison et al., 1997	122,824	Minnesota public school students aged between 12 and 18 years	8.0	2.2	[20]
Breslau et al., 1998	2,181	Community samples in the Detroit area aged between 18 and 45 years	18.3	10.2	[21]
Kessler et al., 1999	2,181	National sample aged between 18 and 45	20.4	8.1	[22]
Breslau et al., 2004	1,698	Public school students in mid-Atlantic city with an average age of 21 years	7.9	6.3	[23]
Kessler et al., 2005	9,282	National face-to-face sample aged 18 years and older	9.7	3.6	[24]

Known and Suspected Risk Factors

Experiential Factors

Differences in Traumatic Experiences

Even though men were found to be more inclined than women to report a traumatic event,[9] women were hypothesized to experience more traumatic events that have greater potential for developing PTSD,[2] such as sexual assaults.[9,36] Indeed, data suggest that nonsexual assaults are more commonly experienced by men,[16] and interpersonal forms of assault are more commonly experienced by women.[2] However, women still have higher rates of PTSD than men following exposure to the same type of trauma.[37] Data from a community-based random digit dialed survey conducted in Detroit, Michigan, in 1996 among a representative sample of 2,181 women and men ages 18 to 45 provided gender specific conditional risks of PTSD among those exposed to traumatic events (Table 18-3). Ever experiencing a traumatic event was more frequently reported by women (92.2%) than men (87.1%). The conditional risk of PTSD with any trauma was 13% among women and 6.2% among men ($P < .001$).[38]

Experiences of Betrayal Trauma

According to the Betrayal Trauma Theory,[39] greater experiences of betrayal are observed among women relative to men following traumatic events. Women are more likely than men to be violated by one of their caregivers or acquaintance.[39] These survivors' thoughts, perceptions, and interpretations of situations are greatly influenced by feelings of betrayal.[39] In addition, memory loss of traumatic events frequently occurs among victims whose caregivers are the perpetrators of their trauma.[40] Although this theory appears to explain why there are gender differences in symptoms of PTSD, specifically in memory loss,[8] it was noted that greater rates of

Table 18-3

Conditional risk of PTSD among respondents exposed to specific traumas by gender[38]

Type of Trauma	Females [%]	Males [%]
Assaultive violence	35.7	6.0
Rape	49.0	--
Sexual assault other than rape	24.4	15.7
Mugged/ threatened with a weapon	17.5	2.4
Badly beaten	56.2	6.4
Serious car accident	3.6	1.6
Other injury or shocking event	5.4	6.6
Learning of trauma to others	3.2	1.4
Unexpected death or relative or friend	16.2	12.6
Any trauma	13.0	6.2

Source: Adapted from Breslau, N. The epidemiology of trauma, PTSD, and other posttrauma disorders. *Trauma Violence Abuse.* 2009;10:198–211.

PTSD were consistently found in women regardless of the type of trauma experienced.[16] Accordingly, it is unlikely that the feelings of betrayal are the primary reason for such gender disparity in the rates of PTSD.[8]

Psychosocial Factors

Social Roles

In explaining the phenomenon where gender was considered a risk factor for PTSD, some researchers proposed a close association between female social roles and high levels of negative stressors.[41] Gender differences in expression of emotion can be observed as early as infancy when girls are often taught to show and share their emotions to others in contrast to boys who are often taught to suppress and hide their emotions.[42] There is evidence suggesting that females' social roles are likely to expose them to higher levels of negative support[43] and emotional distress[44] in comparison to men. The culturally sanctioned roles of women as mothers[45] as well as their caregiving responsibilities[6] were hypothesized as contributors to the gender difference in PTSD owing to an increased level of distress associated with disruption at home. Both culturally and socially, women have often been labeled as "cold" if they do not cry for their loss of a child; they are called "sluts" if they engage in copulation within days of a rape.[8] Other socially constructed stressors, such as male domination and social insinuations of reporting traumatic events were also recognized as contributors to the differential rate

of PTSD between the two genders.[8] The traditional sex role of men being valiant seems to have prevented them from reporting sexual traumas[9] and describing situations as stressful[46,47] to interviewers. Even though social roles appeared to have great influence on the answering styles and levels of distress by gender, the question regarding how the social experiences of being men or women influence their responses to traumatic events remains unknown.[8]

Social Support

It was hypothesized that social support was the mediator in the relationship between gender and psychological distress,[43] and there is strong empirical support for this hypothesis.[41] Theoretically, female emotional health is closely related to other individuals, given their propensity toward the desire to form bonding relationships.[48] Consistent with the theory, a significant relationship between perceived social support and PTSD symptoms was found only among women.[41] In addition, when a relationship between negative support and PTSD symptoms was identified, such associations were observed in females but not in males.[41] Furthermore, although lack of social support was seen as a significant predictor for PTSD in both genders,[49] women appeared to receive lower levels and less benefit of social support relative to men following traumatic events.[41] In a civilian population, for instance, female victims of violent crime were more likely than males to report negative responses from family and friends.[41] Recent data suggest that PTSD may be related to marital status, in which prevalence of PTSD is significantly higher among unmarried adults (i.e., separated, divorced, or widowed) relative to those who are married.[50] Considering marital status as an indication of social support, the results are in accordance with previous findings regarding the importance of social support roles on PTSD rate.[50] Future research is needed to investigate the impact of gender roles on social support following traumatic events.[8]

Interpersonal Relationships

According to attachment theories, all humans need social connections in addition to food, clothing, and shelter.[51] Although an individual's fulfillment is largely dependent on interpersonal connection and relationships,[51] men and women have different ways of defining such fulfillment.[8] Self-fulfillment among women is defined by their ability to create and maintain relationships,[52] whereas self-fulfillment for men is highly related to societal and cultural prescriptions of masculinity.[53] Accordingly, compared with men, women have been described as being more compassionate,[54] more invested in relationships,[8] and emotionally more sensitive to the needs of others.[55] Considering women's greater connection with family and close friends, some researchers posited that disasters in home and community would have a greater impact on women than on men.[56] Similarly, learning of a trauma experienced by children or significant others may also elevate the level of distress in women compared to men because of their close personal relationships.[6] Nevertheless, there is a paucity of empirical research that has investigated the relationship between an individual's attachment to others and the development of PTSD.[8]

Cognitive Factors

Subjective Experience of Traumatic Events

Gender differences in cognitive appraisal have been recognized since the 1980s. Research among high school seniors indicated that females were more likely than males to report major life events and school-related stressors affected their locus of control.[57] It was suggested that such self appraisals are closely related to a higher rate of mental disorders in women,[58] especially stress-related disorders.[59] Some researchers have proposed that gender disparities in response to traumas[60] as well as the prevalence of PTSD[61] were byproducts of the gender differences in cognitive appraisal. Women were significantly more inclined than men to pick up on threat signals,[62] perceive the world as dangerous,[63] describe a situation as a threat,[46] blame themselves for the trauma, and perceive themselves negatively.[9] These findings were thought to be consistent with greater reports of PTSD and poorer prognosis of the disease among women.[16] Nevertheless, these findings do not provide information regarding how or why gender-specific differences in their cognitive interpretations develop.

Symptomatic Factors

Acute Stress Responses

Acute stress response is an individual's initial reaction in response to traumatic events.[61] A diagnosis of Acute Stress Disorder (ASD) in women appeared to be a stronger predictor of PTSD relative to men.[64] A higher percentage of females with ASD (93%) subsequently developed PTSD within 6 months of a traumatic event compared with 57% of similarly affected men.[64] Consequently, women are believed to have their own specific acute stress response that increases their vulnerability to the development of PTSD than men.[64] Although the diagnosis of ASD better predicted the presence of PTSD in females, such diagnosis was a greater predictor in the absence of PTSD among men.[64] The gender differences in the relationship between ASD and PTSD were hypothesized to result from greater prevalence of dissociation in females.[64] However, it remains unclear why women and men display such diverse initial reactions in response to trauma.

Peritraumatic Dissociation

Peritraumatic dissociation is a limited or distorted awareness during and shortly after the traumatic events.[61] An early meta-analysis of PTSD identified peritraumatic psychological processes as the strongest predictor for the disease.[65] Given that women with PTSD exhibited a greater degree of peritraumatic dissociation than men,[66] the greater rate of PTSD among women was thought to be related to their unique dissociative responses.[64] Conversely, another study failed to replicate the gender differences in prevalence of peritraumatic dissociation and suggested that PTSD was not a unique consequence of peritraumatic dissociation.[67] However, the research was limited to single-source information and retrospective reporting,[67] in which traumatic memories tended to be distorted and repressed by the survivors.[68] Accordingly, there was a call for conceptualizing a wider range of peritrauma-related symptoms in future PTSD studies.[67]

Developmental Factors

Child Sexual Abuse

Child sexual abuse was highly associated with etiology[18] and prognosis of mental health.[69] There is evidence suggesting that the prevalence of child sexual abuse differed by gender with 13–16% in males[70] and 15–33% in females.[71] Even though child sexual abuse psychologically affects both boys and girls, female victims with severe abuse reported more trauma symptoms than the male victims.[72] In addition, there were gender differences in their postabuse coping strategies.[73] Male sexual abuse survivors were more inclined than females to act out aggressively and engage in externalizing behavior after abuse,[74] whereas female sexual abuse victims were more likely to display internalizing behavior[9] and avoidance coping.[73] Such gender differences in coping strategies were identified as signficant predictors for both posttraumatic morbidity[75] and PTSD severity.[76]

Biologic Factors

Genetic Predisposition

The greater susceptibility to stress among women has been largely ascribed to biologic differences[77] in which women may be genetically more predisposed to PTSD compared with men.[8] An early twin study showed that genetic factors explained approximately 30% of the variance in PTSD symptoms, and such results remained strong even after controlling for differences in trauma exposure between the twins.[78] There is recent evidence suggesting that genetic factors accounted for greater variance in PTSD relative to individual-specific environmental factors.[79] Literature showed that individuals with certain premorbid personality characteristics, such as neuroticism,[80] and preexisting mood disorders, including depression and anxiety,[81] had increased risk for PTSD. In addition, having a family history of mood disorders was also thought to be evidence of a genetic susceptibility factor for PTSD.[82] Another more recent twin study has indicated that genetic factors can alter the risk of exposure to certain types of traumatic experiences, in which monozygotic twins exhibited greater correlations than dizygotic twins for assaultive trauma but not nonassaultive trauma.[83] Some researchers attributed the development of PTSD to dysregulation of the hypothalamic-pituitary-adrenal (HPA) axis,[84] which is a major stress response system that closely interacts with immune function.[85] Some researchers have hypothesized that exposure to a traumatic experience could alter gene expression and consequently cause failure in the immune system that regulates the HPA axis.[86] Further research is needed to investigate the relationship between genetic factors and gender differences in PTSD.

Hormonal Differences

The brain's hormonal environment during adulthood is considered an essential element in understanding gender differences in psychopathology.[87] Studies indicate that the hormonal environment is undifferentiated between males and females until the development of testes and the production of androgens. Before such hormonal maturation, boys are more vulnerable to psychological disturbances than girls.[87] Following menarche, hormones fluctuate across the menstrual cycle and reproductive stage,[87] increasing susceptibility of females to certain psychiatric disorders.[88] Consequently, the menstrual cycle and reproductive system are considered two primary factors contributing to gender differences in PTSD incidence patterns.[8] Given that women report premenstrual and postpartum-induced anxiety and panic states, hormonal fluctuations appear to be a good explanation for the phenomenon.[87] Indeed, a majority of neurotransmitters germane to PTSD are highly alterable by female sex hormones.[89] Female hormones, estrogens in particular, are thought to increase vulnerability to the development of PTSD among women compared with men following traumatic events regardless of the nature of the trauma.[87] Nevertheless, there are no empirical data linking hormone changes associated with the menstrual cycle and/or the reproductive system with the stress response system.[60]

Neurotransmitter Systems

Neurotransmitter systems may play an essential role in understanding the development and causes of PTSD.[90] Evidence from animal studies suggests that stressful events are associated with a depletion of dopamine and serotonin,[91] leading to release of endogenous opiates to alleviate levels of anxiety.[89] Since women have fluctuating levels of endogenous opiates during their menstrual cycle,[92] they may experience higher risks than men for developing anxiety-related disorders or PTSD. The relationship between PTSD symptoms and levels of endogenous opiates remains unclear.[93] Despite the increasing evidence suggesting a neurological perspective to explain PTSD, there is a lack of information regarding gender differences in neural responses to traumatic imagery.

Cerebral Blood Flow

Medial prefrontal structural abnormalities were evident in individuals with PTSD.[94] The medial prefrontal cortex of the brain is an important area for processing stress responses. PTSD patients exhibit marked increases in blood flow to medial prefrontal cortex relative to control groups.[95] Similarily, patients with PTSD exhibited increased brain activations in the medial frontal gyrus during a dissociative state.[96] In contrast, another study found decreased cerebral blood flow in the medial frontal cortex of both male and female Vietnam veterans with PTSD.[97] Additional studies are needed in order to confirm the effect of PTSD and gender on the responsivity of the medial frontal cortex.

Neuropsychological Factors

Intelligence Quotient (IQ)

As early as the 1990s, a low full-scale IQ was perceived as a risk factor for more severe PTSD symptoms.[98] Examining pretrauma IQ scores, a number of studies concluded that a low IQ score predisposed the development of PTSD,[98,99] whereas a high verbal IQ score appeared to protect against the mental disorder.[100] However, veterans with PTSD were not significantly different from control subjects in their performance on general intellectual functioning.[102] Similarly, there was no association between IQ subtests and trauma symptoms in female survivors of childhood abuse.[103,104] Other studies of traumatized children, adolescents, and adults also found no association.[101] There is insufficient evidence to support the theoretical proposition that IQ is an explanation for the greater rate of PTSD in women relative to men.

Verbal Memory

Verbal memory impairments were consistently exhibited among PTSD patients.[105,106] Studies on both traumatized adults and adolescents provided support for the relationship between PTSD and deficits in verbal memory functions.[107] Although alcohol misuse, depression, lower IQ, and attention deficits were identified as contributors to verbal memory impairments, the relationship between such problems and PTSD remained significant even after adjusting for comorbidity, attention problems, and intellectual functioning.[108] Although some researchers considered verbal memory deficits a risk factor for PTSD, others perceived verbal memory as a predictor of treatment outcomes for Cognitive Behavioral Therapy (CBT).[109] Relative to those with an intact verbal memory, PTSD patients with a poor verbal memory showed less progression with CBT.[109] Although most research indicates women are more proficient than men in verbal memory tasks,[110] few studies have investigated how verbal memory may be related to gender difference in the rate of PTSD.

Methodologic Factors

Types of sample

Although men appeared to have higher risks of traumatic experiences than women in studies using adult samples,[111] such findings appeared to be the opposite in research among adolescents.[9] Questions remain regarding the interaction of gender and age in the development of PTSD as age of participants may contribute to observed gender differences.[9] In addition, studies of gender effects on PTSD among participants in a randomly selected epidemiologic sample may yield different results than response from a convenience sample, such as college students,[9] because (1) abused victims were more likely to drop out of college[94] and (2) females were more likely than males to have been sexually abused.[71] Furthermore, sites of recruitment were also considered important in studying the gender effect on PTSD.[6] Postdisaster experiences of women were likely to be more severe in developing countries compared with those in developed countries where resources were more available and gender roles were less delineated for women.[6]

Form of Measurement

Although a number of studies used semistructured interviews as assessment tools for studies of traumatic experiences and PTSD, others relied on self-report questionaires.[9]

Such methodologic differences were hypothesized to contribute to gender effects of PTSD as men are less likely than women to report their emotional disturbances and sexual traumatic events during an interview.[9] Some investigators have suggested that anonymously completed questionnaires may result in more accurate responses from men relative to interviews due to the social pressure to act in their more traditional role of being invulnerable.[9] In addition, studies of gender in relation to PTSD appeared to yield different results depending on whether traumas were assessed over the individuals' entire life span or a discrete interval of time, in which the latter tended to yield an insignificant gender effect.[9] Despite having this methodologic bias, issues regarding instrumentation have not yet been investigated in empirical studies.[8]

Definitions of PTSD

Another essential element in understanding gender effects on PTSD was the diverse definitions of trauma and criteria for a diagnosis.[9] A shift in diagnostic criteria of PTSD occurred since the 1980s according to the third edition of the *Diagnostic and Statistical Manual of Mental Disorders* (DSM) when traumatic events were simply defined by the nature of the events themselves. In the fourth edition,[1] nevertheless, two additional criteria (A) were added in which the nature of trauma and the individual's peritraumatic response were more well defined and specific than in the previous edition. In criterion A, traumatic events were defined as: a death, serious injury, or threat to the physical integrity of self or others. The second component required a response of intense fear, helplessness, or horror. The definition change increased the diagnosis of PTSD among women when both criteria were applied.[9] These findings have provided signficant implications for the use of epidemiologic instruments and potential differences in documenting symptom differences between men and women.

Summary

Despite robust findings demonstrating gender disproportion in the rate of PTSD, the reasons why such gender differences exist have remained unclear. Based on current literature, no definitive explanation has been developed for the greater frequency of PTSD among women than men. Additional research is required to understand the relationship of higher rates of PTSD among women, including further exploration of biologic and psychosocial factors as well as consideration of methodologic issues.

Discussion Questions

1. Which psychosocial factor is perceived to have a mediating effect in the relationship between gender and psychological distress? What is the theory supporting the mediating effect?
2. Does a diagnosis of Acute Stress Disorder (ASD) predict the development of PTSD? Explain how such a diagnosis predicts the prevalence of PTSD among men compared with women.

3. Do gender differences in postabuse coping strategies exist? Describe how male and female sexual abuse survivors differ in coping with their sexual trauma.
4. Which three methodologic factors are used in this chapter to explain the gender disparity in the prevalence of PTSD? Describe how these factors contribute to gender differences in PTSD rates.

References

1. *Diagnostic and Statistical Manual of Mental Disorders*. 4th ed. Washington DC: American Psychiatric Association; 1994.
2. Kessler RC, Sonnega A, Bromet E, et al. Posttraumatic stress disorder in the national comorbidity survey. *Arch. Gen. Psychiatry.* 1995;52:1048–1060.
3. Blanchard E B. Who develops PTSD from motor vehicle accident? *Behav Res Therapy.* 1996;34:1–10.
4. Kimerling R, Ouimette PC, Weitlauf J. Gender issues in PTSD. In: Friedman MJ, Keane TM, Resick PA, eds. *PTSD: Science and Practice—A Comprehensive Handbook.* New York: Guilford Press; 2005.
5. Ozer EJ, Best SR, Lipsey TL, Weiss DS. Predictors of posttraumatic stress disorder and symptoms in adults: A meta-analysis. *Psychol Bull.* 2003;129:52–73.
6. Kimerling R, Mack K, Alvarez J. Women and disaster. In: Neria Y, Galea S, Norris F, eds. *Mental Health and Disasters.* New York: Cambridge University Press; 2009:203–217.
7. Breslau ND. Sex differences in posttraumatic stress disorder. *Arch Gen Psychiatry.* 1997;54:1044–1048.
8. Simmons CA. Speculation as to why women "get" PTSD more often than men. *Women Ther.* 2007;30(1):85–98.
9. Tolin DF, Foa EB. Sex differences in trauma and posttraumatic stress disorder: a quantitative review of 25 years of research. *Psychological Trauma: Theory, Research, Practice, and Policy.* 2008;S(1):37–85.
10. Helzer JE, Robins LN, McEvoy L. Post-traumatic stress disorder in the general population. *N Engl J Med.* 1987;317:1630–1634.
11. Breslau N, Anthony JC. Gender differences in the sensitivity to posttraumatic stress disorder: an epidemiological study of urban young adults. *J Abnormal Psychol.* 2007;116:607–611.
12. Breslau ND. Gender differences in trauma and posttraumatic stress disorder. *J Gend Specif Med.* 2002;5:34–40.
13. Koltek MWT. The prevalence of posttraumatic stress disorder in an adolescent inpatient unit. *Can J Psychiatry.* 1998;43:64–68.
14. Davidson JSR. Traumatic experiences in psychiatric outpatients. *J Trauma Stress.* 1990;3:459–475.
15. Helzer, JE, Robins LN, McEvoy L. Post-traumatic stress disorder in the general population. *N Engl J Med.* 1987;317:1630–1643.
16. Breslau N, Davis GC, Andreski P, Peterson EL. Traumatic events and posttraumatic stress disorder in an urban population of young adults. *Arch Gen Psychiatry.* 1991;48:216–222.
17. Kessler RC, Sonnega A, Bromet E, Hughes M, Nelson CB. Posttraumatic stress disorder in the National Comorbidity Survey. *Arch Gen Psychiatry.* 1995;52:1048–1060.
18. Singer MI, Anglin TM, Song L, Lunghofer L. Adolescents' exposure to violence and associated symptoms of psychological trauma. *JAMA.* 1995;273:477–482.
19. Boney-McCoy S, Finkelhor D. Psychosocial sequelae of violent victimization in a national youth sample. *J Consult Clin Psychol.* 1995;63:726–736.
20. Harrison PA, Fulkerson JA, Beebe TJ. Multiple substance use among adolescent physical and sexual abuse victims. *Child Abuse Negl.* 1997;21:529–539.
21. Breslau N, Kessler RC, Chilcoat HD, et al. Trauma and posttraumatic stress disorder in the community: the 1996 Detroit Area Survey of Trauma. *Arch Gen Psychiatry.* 1998;55:626–632.
22. Kessler RC, Sonnega A, Bromet E, et al. PTSD in the National Comorbidity Survey. *Arch Gen Psychiatry.* 1995;52:1048–1060.
23. Breslau N, Wilcox HC, Storr CL, et al. Trauma exposure and posttraumatic stress disorder: a study of youths in urban America. *J Urban Health.* 2004;81:530–544.
24. Kessler RC, Chiu WT, Demler, O, et al. Prevalence, severity, and comorbidity of 12-month DSM-IV disorders in the National Comorbidity Survey Replication. *Arch Gen Psychiatry.* 2005;62:617–27.
25. Breslau N, Davis GC, Peterson EL, Schultz LR. A second look at comorbidity in victims of trauma: the posttraumatic stress disorder-major depression connection. *Biol Psychiatry.* 2000;48:902–909.
26. Simpson TL. Women's treatment utilization and its relationship to childhood sexual abuse history and lifetime PTSD. *Subst Abus.* 2002;23:17–30.
27. Schnurr. P.P., Jankowski, M.K. Physical health and post-traumatic stress disorder: review and synthesis. *Semin Clin Neuropsychiatry.* 1999;4:295–304.
28. Seng JS, Low LK, Sperlich M, et al. Prevalence, trauma history, and risk for posttraumatic stress disorder among nulliparous women in maternity care. *Obstet Gynecol.* 2009;114:839–47.

29. Amstadter AB, Nugent NR, Koenen KC, et al. Association between COMT, PTSD, and increased smoking following hurricane exposure in an epidmiologic sample. *Psychiatry*. 2009;72:360-9.

30. Joseph S, Yule W, Williams R, Hodgkinson P. Increased substance use in survivors of the Herald of Free Enterprise disaster. *Br J Med Psychology*. 1993;66:185–191.

31. Parslow R, Jorm AF. Tobacco use after experiencing a major natural disaster: analysis of a longitudinal study of 2063 young adults. *Addiction*. 2006;101:1044–1050.

32. Op Den Velde W, Aarts PG, Falger PR, et al. Alcohol use, cigarette consumption and chronic post-traumatic stress disorder. *Alcohol Alcohol*. 2002;37:355–361.

33. McCauley JL, Amstadter A, Danielson CK, et al. Mental health and rape history in relation to nonmedical use of prescription drugs in a national sample of women. *Addict Behav*. 2009;34:641–648.

34. McCauley JL, Danielson CK, Amstadter AB, et al. The role of traumatic event history in non-medical use of prescription drugs among a nationally representative sample of US adolescents. *J Child Psychol Psychiatric*. 2010;51:84–93.

35. Gilbertson M, Paulus L, Williston S, et al. Neurocognitive function in monozygotic twins discordant for combat exposure: Relationship to post-traumatic stress disorder. *J Abnorm Psychol*. 2006;115:484–495.

36. Kessler RC, Sonnega A, Bromet E, et al. Epidemiologic risk factors for trauma and PTSD. In: Yehuda R, ed. *Risk Factors for Posttraumatic Stress Disorder*. Washington, DC, American Psychiatric Press; 1999:23–59.

37. Shore JH, Tatum EL, Vollmer WM. Psychiatric reactions to disaster: the Mount St. Helens experience. *Am J Psychiatry* 1986;143:590–595, 76–83.

38. Breslau N. The epidemiology of trauma, PTSD, and other post trauma disorders. *Trauma Violence Abuse*. 2009;10:198–211.

39. DePrince AP. Intersection of gender and betrayal in trauma. In: Kimerling R, Ouimette P, Wolfe J, eds. *Gender and PTSD*. New York, Guilford Press; 2002:98–116.

40. Freyd JJ. *Betrayal Trauma: The Logic of Forgetting Childhood Abuse*. Cambridge, MA: Harvard University Press; 1996.

41. Andrews CR. Social support and PTSD victims of violent crime. *Traumatic Stress*. 2003;16:421–427.

42. Worell J, Johnson DM. Feminist approaches to psychotherapy. In: Worell J, ed. *Encyclopedia of Women and Gender*. New York: Academic Press; 2001: 425–437.

43. Turner H. Gender and social support: taking the bad with the good. *Sex Roles*. 1994;30:521–541.

44. Kaniasty KF. Social support and victims of crime: matching event, support, and outcome. *Am J Comm Psychol*. 1992;20:211–241.

45. Yuksel S. Collusion and denial of childhood sexual trauma in traditional societies. In: Shalev AY, Yehuda R, McFarlane AC, eds. *International Handbook of Human Response to Trauma*. New York: Plenum/Kluwer; 2000: 153–161.

46. Eisler RM. Masculine gender role stress. Scale development and component factors in the appraisal of stressful situations. *Behav Modif*. 1987;11: 123–136.

47. Timmer, SG. Life stress, helplessness, and the use of alcohol and drugs to cope: an analysis of national survey data. In: Shiffman S, Wills TA, eds. *Coping and Substance Use*. New York: Academic Press; 1985:171–198.

48. Kessler RC, McLeod JD. Sex differences in vulnerability to undersirable life events. *Am Soc Review*. 1984;49:620–631.

49. King DW. Posttraumatic stress disorder in a national sample of female and male Vietnam veterans: risk factors, war-zone stressors and resilience-recovery variables. *J Abnorm Psychol*. 1999;108:164–170.

50. Weissman MM, Neria Y, Das A, et al. Gender differences in posttraumatic stress disorder among primary care patients after the World Trade Center attack of September 11, 2001. *Gend Med*. 2005;2:76–86.

51. Bowlby J. *Loss, Sadness, and Depression*. New York: Basic Books; 1980. *Attachment and Loss*; vol. 3.

52. Miller JB. *Toward a New Psychology of Women*. 2nd ed. Boston: Beacon Press; 1976.

53. Pleck JH. The gender role strain paradigm: an update. In: Levant RF, Pollack WF, eds. *A New Psychology of Men*. New York: Basic Books; 1995:11–32.

54. Hoffman ML. Sex differences in empathy and related behaviors. *Psychol Bull*. 1977;54:712–722.

55. Hall JA. Gender effects in decoding nonverbal cues. *Psychol Bull*. 1978;85:845–857.

56. Morrow BH, Enarson E. Hurricane Andrew through women's eyes: issues and recommendations. *Int J Mass Emergencies Disasters*. 1996;14:5–22.

57. Cole T, Sapp GL. Stress, locus of control, and achievement of high school seniors. *Psychol Rep*. 1988;63:355–359.

58. van Nieuwenhuizen C. Sekseverschillen in het omgaan met stress. Een overzicht van recente literatuur [Sex differences in coping with stress. A review of recent literature.]. *Gedrag & Gezondheid*. 1994;22:55–68.

59. Norris FH. 60,000 disaster victims speak: part I. An empirical review of the empirical literature.1981–2001. *Psychiatry*. 2002;65:207–239.

60. Rasmusson AM. Gender issues in the neurobiology of PTSD. In: Kimerling R, Ouimette P, Wolfe J, eds. *Gender and PTSD*. New York: Guilford Press; 2002:76–97.

61. Olff M, Langeland W, Draijer N, Gersons BP. Gender differences in post-traumatic stress disorder. *Psychol Bull*. 2007;133:183–204.

62. Kemp AH. Gender differences in the cortical electrophysiological processing of visual emotional stimuli. *NeuroImage*. 2004;21:632–646.

63. Kimerling R, Ouimette P, Wolfe J, eds. *Gender and PTSD*. New York: Guilford Press; 2002.

64. Bryant RA. Gender differences in the relationship between acute stress disorder and posttraumatic stress disorder following motor vehicle accidents. *Aust N Z J Psychiatry*. 2003;37:226–229.

65. Ozer EJ. Predictors of posttraumatic stress disorder and symptoms in adults: a meta-analysis. *Psychol Bull*. 2003;129:52–73.

66. Fullerton CS. Gender differences in posttraumatic stress disorder after motor vehicle accidents. *Am J Psychiatry*. 2005;158:1486–1491.

67. Raija-Leena Punamäki IH. The role of peritraumatic dissociation and gender in the association between trauma and mental health in a Palestinian community sample. *Am J Psychiatry*. 2005;162:545–551.

68. van der Kolk BA, BJ. The psychobiology of traumatic memory: clinical implications of neuroimaging studies. *Ann NY Acad Sci*. 1997;821:99–113.

69. Banyard VL. Characteristics of child sexual abuse as correlates of women's adjustment: A prospective study. *J Marriage Family*. 1996;58:853–865.

70. Polusny MA. Long-term correlates of child sexual abuse: theory and review of the empirical literature. *Appl Prev Psychol*. 1995;4:143–166.

71. Kendall-Tackett KA. Impact of sexual abuse on children: a review and synthesis of recent empirical findings. *Psychol Bull*. 1993;113;164–180.

72. Ketring SA. Perpetrator-victim relationship: long-term effects of sexual abuse for men and women. *Am J Fam Ther*. 1999;27:109–120.

73. Ullman SE. Gender differences in social reactions to abuse disclosures, post-abuse coping, and PTSD of child sexual abuse survivors. *Child Abuse Neglect*. 2005;29:767–782.

74. Gomes-Schwartz BH. *Child Sexual Abuse: The Initial Effects*. Newbury Park, CA: Sage; 1990.

75. Chang CM, Connor KM, Davidson JRR, Jeffries K, Lai TJ. Posttraumatic distress and coping strategies among rescue workers after an earthquake. *J Nervous Mental Dis*. 2003;191:391–398.

76. Bryant RA. Coping style and post-traumatic stress disorder following severe traumatic brain injury. *Brain Injury*. 2000;14:175–180.

77. Young EA. Sex differences and the HPA axis: implications for psychiatric disease. *J Gender Specific Med*. 1998;1:21–27.

78. True WR, Rice J, Eisen SA, Heath AC, Goldberg J, Lyons MJ, Nowak J. A twin study of genetic and environmental contributions to liability for posttraumatic stress symptoms. *Arch Gen Psychiatry*. 1993;50:257–264.

79. Sartor CE, McCutcheon VV, Pommer, NE, et al. Common genetic and environmental contributions to post-traumatic stress disorder and alcohol dependence in young women. *Psychol Med*. 2010;8:1–9.

80. Brewin CR, Andrews B, Valentine JD. Meta-analysis of risk factors for post-traumatic stress disorder in trauma-exposed adults. *J Consult Clin Psychol*. 2000;68:748–766.

81. Davidson JRT, Swartz M, Storck M, Krishnan KRR, Hammett E. A diagnostic and familial study of posttraumatic stress disorder. *Am J Psychiatry*. 1985;142:90–93.

82. Comings DE, Muhleman D, Gysin R. Dopamine DRD2 gene and susceptibility to posttraumatic stress disorder: a study and replication. *Biol Psychiatry*. 1996;40:368–372.

83. Stein MB, Jang KL, Taylor S, et al. Genetic and environmental influences on trauma exposure and posttraumatic stress disorder symptoms: a twin study. *Am J Psychiatry*. 2002;159:1675–1681.

84. Yehuda R, LeDoux J. Response variation following trauma: a translational neuroscience approach to understanding PTSD. *Neuron*. 2007;56:19–32.

85. Wong CM. Post-traumatic stress disorder: advances in psychoneuroimmunology. *Psychiatr Clin North Am*. 2002;25:369–383.

86. Uddin M, Aiello AE, Wildman DE, et al. Epigenetic and immune function profiles associated with posttraumatic stress disorder. *Proc Natl Acad Sci U S A*. 2009;107:9470–9475.

87. Seeman MV. Psychopathology in women and men: focus on female hormones. *Am J Psychiatry*. 1997;154:1641–1647.

88. Earls F. Sex differences in psychiatric disorders: origins and developmental influences. *Psychiatr Dev*. 1987;1:1–23.

89. Vasterling JJ, Brewin CR, eds. *Neuropsychology of PTSD: Biological, Cognitive, and Clinical Perspectives*. New York: Guilford Press; 2005.

90. Charney DS, Deutch AY, Krystal JH, Southwick SM, Davis M. Psychobiologic mechanisms of posttraumatic stress disorder. *Arch Gen Psychiatry*. 1993;50:294–305.

91. Van der Kolk BA, Greenberg M, Boyd H, Krystal J. Inescapable shock, neurotransmitters, and addiction to trauma: toward a psychobiology of post-traumatic stress. *Biol Psychiatry*. 1985;20:314–325.

92. Chuong CJ, Coulam CB, Kao PC, Bergstralh EJ, Go VL. Neuropeptide levels in premenstrual syndrome. *Fertil Steril*. 1985;44:760–763.

93. Yonkers KA, Gurguis G. Gender differences in the prevalence and expression of anxiety disorder. In: Seeman, MV, ed. *Gender and Psychopathology*. New York, American Psychiatric Publishing, Inc; 1995:113–130.

94. Rauch SL, Shin LM, Segal E, et al. Selectively reduced regional cortical volumes in post-traumatic stress disorder. *Neuroreport*. 2003;14: 913–916.

95. Zubieta JK, Chinitz JA, Lombardi U, Fig LM, Cameron OG, Liberzon I. Medial frontal cortex involvement in PTSD symptoms: a SPECT study. *J Psychiatr Res*. 1999;33:259–264.

96. Laniusa RA. Brain activation during script-driven imagery induced dissociative responses in PTSD: a functional magnetic resonance imaging investigation. *Biol Psychiatry*. 2002;52:305–311.

97. Shin LM. Regional cerebral blood flow in the amygdala and medial prefrontal cortex during traumatic imagery in male and female Vietnam veterans with PTSD. *Arch Gen Psychiatry*. 2004;61:168–176.

98. Gurvits T, Gilbertson MW, Lasko NB, et al. Neurologic soft signs in chronic posttraumatic stress disorder. *Arch Gen Psychiatry*. 2000;57:181–186.

99. Macklin ML, Metzger LJ, Litz BT, et al. Lower precombat intelligence is a risk factor for posttraumatic stress disorder. *J Consult Clin Psychol*. 1998;66:323–326.

100. Vasterling JJ, Brailey K, Constans JI, Borges A. Assessment of intellectual resources in Gulf War veterans: relationship to PTSD. *Assessment*. 1997;4:51–59.

101. Saltzman KM, Weems CF, Carrion VG. IQ and posttraumatic stress symptoms in children exposed to interpersonal violence. *Child Psychiatry Hum Dev*. 2006;36:261–274.

102. Bremner JD, Scott TM, Delaney RC, et al. Deficits in short-term memory in posttraumatic stress disorder. *Am J Psychiatry*. 1993;150:1015–1019.

103. Bremner JD, Randall P, Scott TM, et al. Deficits in short-term memory in adult survivors of childhood abuse. *Psychiatry Res*. 1995;59:97–107.

104. Stein MB, Hanna C, Vaerum V, Koverola C. Memory functioning in adult women traumatized by childhood sexual abuse. *J Trauma Stress*. 1999;12:527–534.

105. Vasterling JJ, Duke LM, Brailey K, et al. Attention, learning, and memory performances and intellectual resources in Vietnam veterans: PTSD and no disorder comparisons. *Neuropsychology*. 2002;16:5–14.

106. Bremner J, Vermetten E, Afzal N, Vythilingam M. Deficits in verbal declarative memory function in women with childhood sexual abuse-related posttraumatic stress disorder. *J Nerv Mental Dis*. 2004;192:643–649.

107. Acosta E. Memory functions in adolescents with posttraumatic stress disorder. *Dissertation Abstracts International: Section B: Sciences and Engineering*. 2000:61:3267.

108. Gilbertson MW, Gurvits TV, Lasko NB, et al. Multivariate assessment of explicit memory function in combat veterans with posttraumatic stress disorder. *J Trauma Stress*. 2001;14:413–432.

109. Wild J, Gur R. Verbal memory and treatment response in post-traumatic stress disorder. *Br J Psychiatry*. 2008;193:254–255.

110. Kemenoff LA, Lengenfelder J, Kramer JH, Delis DC. Gender differences in vulnerability to interference using the California verbal learning Test-II. 2000. *Arch Clin Neuropsychol*. 15;8:682–683.

111. Cuffe SP. Prevalence of PTSD in a community sample of older adolescents. *J Am Acad Child Adolesc Psychiatry*. 1998;37:147–154.

112. American Psychiatric Association. *Diagnostic and Statistical Manual of Mental Disorders*. 3rd ed. Washington, DC: Author; 1980.

113. American Psychiatric Association. *Diagnostic and Statistical Manual of Mental Disorders*. 3rd ed., rev. Washington, DC: Author; 1987.

Substance Use Disorders*

Susan E. Foster, MSW and Linda Richter, PhD

Introduction

Substance use disorders are chronic diseases affecting 17.1 million girls and women in the United States today.[1] Despite a substantial body of science demonstrating that these conditions can be prevented and treated effectively, services to address these disorders remain largely divorced from medical practice; those providing such services lack the knowledge and capacity to provide health care, and healthcare professionals are poorly trained in prevention, diagnosis, and treatment of substance use disorders.[2] The result is that the conditions too often go unrecognized and untreated and result in unnecessary pain and suffering and costly consequences to society.

Addiction is the primary preventable contributor to some of the most common causes of death among women, including heart disease and cancer, and it is an aggravating factor for many other ailments including respiratory disease, infertility, pregnancy complications, depression, anxiety, and eating disorders. Risky substance use and untreated addiction also drive homicides, accidents, suicides, child abuse and neglect, sexual assaults, domestic violence, unplanned pregnancies, sexually transmitted diseases, academic failure, lost productivity, unemployment, poverty, and homelessness.[3] Girls and women have different motivations than men for using addictive substances, progress from substance use to addiction at lower levels of use and more quickly, and suffer the consequences sooner and more intensely. Despite these facts, gender differences rarely are taken into account in prevention and treatment.

This discussion draws from more than 10 years of research on women and substance use at the National Center on Addiction and Substance Abuse (CASA) at Columbia University, much of which was included in CASA's 2006 book, *Women under the Influence*, published by the Johns Hopkins University Press.

What Are Substance Use Disorders?

A substance use disorder is a chronic brain disease that can result from repeated use of tobacco, alcohol, controlled prescription medications, and illicit drugs. It involves structural and functional changes in the brain manifested by physical, psychological, and behavioral symptoms including compulsive drug seeking and use despite adverse health and social consequences.[4] Substance use disorders frequently co-occur with other physical and mental health problems.[5] They are considered developmental disorders because they typically emerge in childhood or adolescence—a time when the developing brain is most vulnerable to substance use.[6] Subclinical manifestations involving underage substance use or adult risky or excessive use are the precursors of addiction.

Substance use disorders can be treated effectively with a host of evidence-based pharmacologic and behavioral interventions and, like other chronic diseases, they can be managed effectively;[7] subclinical manifestations can be prevented and reduced by implementing public health-based approaches to disease prevention.[8]

How Many Women Have Substance Use Disorders and Who Gets Treated?

In 2008, 13.3% of females ages 12 and older (17.1 million) who were current users of tobacco, alcohol, and illicit or controlled prescription drugs had a substance use disorder; they met clinical diagnostic criteria for alcohol abuse/dependence or drug abuse/dependence in the past 12 months or nicotine dependence in the past 30 days (compared to 18.4% of males). Figure 19-1 indicates that young adult women ages 18 to 25 were the most likely to have a substance use disorder (22.5%), followed by 26- to 34-year-olds (18.4%), those 35 years and older (11.4%), and girls ages 12 to 17 (7.0%).

*Portions of this chapter based on material from *Women under the Influence* by the National Center on Addiction and Substance Abuse at Columbia University. Published by the Johns Hopkins University Press. Funded by the Bristol-Myers Squibb Foundation.

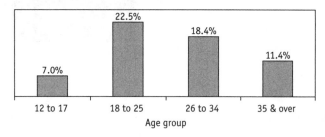

Figure 19-1 Prevalence of substance use disorders among girls and women (nicotine, alcohol or other drugs) by age group.

Source: Reproduced from The National Center on Addiction and Substance Abuse (CASA) at Columbia University. CASA analysis of data from 2008 National Survey on Drug Use and Health. New York: The National Center on Addiction and Substance Abuse (CASA) at Columbia University; 2010.

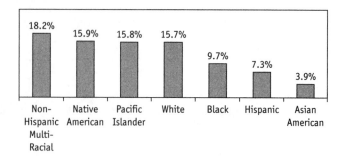

Figure 19-2 Prevalence of substance use disorders among girls and women by race/ethnicity.

Source: Reproduced from The National Center on Addiction and Substance Abuse (CASA) at Columbia University. CASA analysis of data from 2008 National Survey on Drug Use and Health. New York: The National Center on Addiction and Substance Abuse (CASA) at Columbia University; 2010.

Race/ethnicity prevalence of substance use disorders are noted in Figure 19-2. Women who identified as non-Hispanic multiracial were most likely to have a substance use disorder (18.2%), followed by Native American women (15.9%), Pacific Islander women (15.8%), and white women (15.7%). Black women had lower rates of substance use disorders (9.7%) followed by Hispanic women (7.3%) and Asian American women (3.9%). Another 19.6% of girls and women, although not meeting clinical criteria for a substance use disorder, engaged in risky use of these substances in a manner that threatened public health and safety (i.e., risky use includes underage drinking, adult drinking in excess of the U.S. Department of Agriculture (USDA) dietary guidelines, illicit drug use and misuse of controlled prescription drugs that do not meet clinical diagnostic criteria). In 2008, only 4.9% of current female users with an alcohol or other drug use disorder (6.4% of men) received any treatment in the past year in a professional setting (comparable treatment data are not available for those receiving treatment for nicotine dependence, so those whose only addiction was to nicotine were excluded from this analysis).[1]

Do Addictive Substances Affect Women Differently from Men?

Despite smoking cigarettes with lower nicotine levels, smoking fewer cigarettes, and inhaling less deeply than men, women are just as likely as men, on average, to become addicted to nicotine.[9] Smoking half a pack of cigarettes a day increases the risk of nicotine dependence in women to a greater extent than it does in men.[10] This gender difference can be seen at an early age: girls report more symptoms of nicotine dependence than boys at the same levels of use and became dependent in a shorter amount of time than boys.[11]

The physiologic impairments from alcohol, including the development of alcohol use disorders, occur among women at an earlier stage of drinking than men and after having consumed less alcohol.[12] Women metabolize alcohol less efficiently: they have decreased activity of the enzyme alcohol dehydrogenase, which breaks down alcohol in the liver and stomach keeping it from entering

the bloodstream and, because women's bodies contain less water and more fatty tissue than men of similar sizes, they maintain higher concentrations of alcohol in their blood.[13] As a result, women get intoxicated faster and have worse hangovers even when drinking the same amount as men; generally, one alcoholic drink for a woman has the same impact as two drinks for a man.[14] Women also become dependent on marijuana, heroin, cocaine, and certain psychoactive prescription drugs more easily than men.[15]

Pathways to Substance Use Disorders among Women

Females often have different reasons than males for initiating substance use; for example, they are more likely than males to smoke, drink, or use other drugs to lose weight, relieve stress, improve their mood, reduce inhibitions, and self-medicate anxiety, depression, and the negative feelings associated with physical and sexual trauma.[16] Girls are more responsive to the influence of substance-using peers and family members than are boys[17] and are targeted more frequently in media messages that make substance use appear sexy or glamorous.[16] Many factors contribute to a person's susceptibility to the use of addictive substances and to the likelihood that such use will progress to a clinical disorder.

Genetic and Biologic Factors

Whether a girl or woman begins to smoke, drink alcohol, or use other drugs is determined primarily by environmental influences; however, genetic and biologic factors determine whether such use will develop into a disorder.[18] Underage initiation of substance use is a particular concern. Key areas of the brain that control functions linked to substance use—decision making, judgment, impulse control, emotion, and memory—continue to develop both structurally and functionally throughout childhood and into early adulthood. These brain functions remain highly vulnerable to the influences of addictive substances and may be altered permanently by early substance use.[6]

Girls with earlier than average physical and sexual maturation are at increased risk of engaging in substance use at younger ages, more frequently, and in greater quantities than their peers who mature later.[19] Women with a family history of alcohol use disorders show greater physical tolerance for alcohol[20] and react in ways that reflect heightened risks for heavy drinking, have more intense alcohol craving, and more likely to develop future alcohol problems.[21] Physical tolerance for alcohol and other drugs declines with age because of slower metabolism and other age-related physiologic changes.[22] As a result, what might have been safe levels of alcohol use in earlier adulthood can be quite harmful and addictive in older age.[22]

Personal Factors

Teenage girls with low self-confidence are at twice the risk of substance use as those with higher self-confidence.[23] A key component of self-image for girls and women is body image; those who engage in unhealthy dieting behaviors may use addictive substances to self-medicate negative feelings or to aid in their efforts to lose weight.[24] Stress also increases risk and girls and women are more likely than boys and men to respond to stress with substance use.[25] Women experience physical and sexual abuse, the pressures of caring for relatives, depression, and anxiety more often than males and are likelier to self-medicate the negative feelings associated with these problems by turning to substance use;[26] this increases their risk of developing substance use disorders later in life.[27]

Environmental Factors

Parents are the strongest influence on children's decisions regarding whether or not to engage in substance use[28] and girls appear to be more responsive than boys to such parental influences.[16] Children of parents who engage in unhealthy substance use, who have permissive attitudes about substance use, or who are uninvolved or disengaged in their children's lives are at considerably increased risk for smoking, drinking, and using other drugs.[29] Peers also strongly influence the substance use attitudes and behaviors of girls.[30] When several of a girl's closest friends smoke or drink, she is more than seven times likelier to drink alcohol (compared to three times among boys).[31]

Neighborhoods, schools, and communities that are supportive, provide positive role models, hold high expectations for achievement, and encourage youth participation tend to protect against substance use,[32] whereas those that tolerate substance use or in which addictive substances are easily available increase risk.[33] Although such substances generally are more readily available to boys than girls,[34] once presented with the opportunity, equal numbers of males and females engage in substance use.[35]

The tobacco and alcohol industries have a long history of marketing to women, profiting from their desire to appear sophisticated, fun-loving, sexy, and thin.[16] More recently, direct-to-consumer advertisements for prescription drugs including sleep aids and attention boosters help to create a climate where there is a pill for every ill; excessive use of these medications increase the chances of drug dependence and addiction in women.[36]

Life Transitions and Late Onset Triggers that Increase Risk

As girls and women make key life transitions, they face significant changes in their physical and social environments, some of which heighten their risk of substance use.[37] During the transition to adolescence, girls begin to shift their focus from their parents to peers and popular culture—contexts often rife with temptations to smoke, drink, or use other drugs. Upon entering college, young women may take advantage of their new independence or respond to increased stress by engaging in substance use. After college or when entering the workforce, young women are faced with the stress of finding a job and developing a balance between career and family goals; these pressures can precipitate a desire to alleviate the stress via substance use.[38] Women experiencing the stresses of adulthood—marriage, pregnancy, child rearing, financial concerns, divorce, empty nest, retirement, declining health, or family illness or death—might turn to addictive substances for escape or comfort.[39] Some older women, whose physical or mental ailments are treated with potentially addictive prescription drugs, might misuse these drugs, become dependent on them, and ultimately develop a substance use disorder.[40]

Morbidity, Comorbidity, and Mortality Related to Substance Use Disorders in Women

Substance use disorders are causal factors in more than 70 known diseases requiring hospitalization.[41] In women, these disorders also frequently co-occur with depression, anxiety, schizophrenia, and eating disorders.[42] Nearly 2 million adult women in the United States have both a serious mental illness and an alcohol or other drug use disorder.[43]

Substance use during pregnancy increases the risk of miscarriages, stillbirths, premature births, low birth weight, congenital defects, and neonatal death; it also hikes the odds of mental retardation, poor cognitive skills, and conduct disorders among prenatally exposed children.[44] The most visible result of drinking during pregnancy is fetal alcohol spectrum disorder, characterized by growth deficiency, facial malformations, retardation, and other cognitive deficiencies.[45]

Approximately 400,000 preventable and premature deaths occur each year in the United States as a result of tobacco use.[46] Smoking shortens the life span of women to a greater extent than men (a loss of 15 vs. 13 years)[47] and almost half the women who smoke ultimately will die from smoking-related diseases.[48] Women are more susceptible than men to tobacco carcinogens.[49] Among women, smoking is related to cancer of the lung, larynx, oral cavity, esophagus, breast, bladder, pancreas, stomach, cervix, and ovaries;[50] doubles the risk of stroke;[51] increases the risk of death from respiratory disease tenfold; and increases the risk of menstrual problems.[52] Female smokers, on average, demonstrate lung damage and develop lung cancer at a younger age and at lower levels of tobacco use than men.[53] Smoking also increases a woman's chance of having and dying from a heart attack,[54] particularly if she uses oral contraceptives;[55] nearly 40% of teenage girls who use oral contraceptives also smoke.[56]

Women with alcohol use disorders are more likely than men to suffer from alcohol-related suicide, accidents, heart disease and other circulatory system disorders, cirrhosis of the liver, and hepatitis, and tend to develop these problems sooner and at lower levels of drinking.[57] Women also are more susceptible than men to alcohol-induced impairments in learning, memory, abstract thinking, problem solving, perception, and motor skills[58] and demonstrate memory loss and cognitive deterioration after fewer years of drinking than men.[59]

The misuse of illicit and certain psychoactive prescription drugs contributes to depression and is associated strongly with suicide.[60] It also is a key risk factor for burns, trauma, acquired immune deficiency syndrome (AIDS), sexually transmitted diseases, heart disease, stroke, hepatitis A, B, and C, and pregnancy-related complications including spontaneous abortion.[61] Teenage girls are more than twice as likely as boys to be admitted to a hospital for acute drug intoxication.[62]

Prevention

As with other chronic conditions, preventing the development of substance use disorders is a public health issue, which involves educating the population about the disease, its risk factors, and opportunities for prevention. Support is often needed to translate the knowledge gained into practice. In the case of preventing addictive disorders, it is critical that girls and women receive support from people close to them who understand the gender differences that influence risk.

The best window of opportunity for prevention is during childhood, when efforts should focus on reducing experimentation, increasing knowledge, developing healthy attitudes and beliefs about substance use, and helping girls navigate messages from peers and the media about the benefits of smoking, drinking, and using other drugs. Parents have the strongest influence—for better or worse—over their daughters' substance-related attitudes and behaviors.[16] Other key sources of influence include physicians, teachers, clergy, and community leaders. Because substance use disorders do develop among adult women, it is important to identify signs of risk—including a family history of substance use disorders, a history of abuse and violence, depression, anxiety, and eating disorders—and to help women get the care and support they need for these problems as well.[63] Although any encounters frequented by women offer opportunities for prevention and early intervention, including healthcare professionals' offices, educational settings, churches, support groups, and domestic violence or homeless shelters, those offering services require specialized training to enhance their potential success in preventing substance use disorders.

Tax and regulatory policies also are effective prevention strategies. Increasing taxes on cigarettes and alcohol has been strongly associated with lower levels of use,[64] particularly among young people and pregnant women.[65] Comprehensive tobacco control programs involving increased cigarette taxes, indoor smoking bans, and increased access to cessation treatment are associated with significant reductions in smoking, particularly among pregnant women.[66] Limiting the density of alcohol retail outlets, prohibiting low-price alcohol promotions such as "ladies' nights," banning alcohol advertising on college campuses or youth-oriented magazines, and ensuring consistent enforcement of alcohol policies are effective in reducing underage and excessive drinking.[67]

Early Diagnosis and Treatment for Women

An enormous body of evidence demonstrates that the most cost-effective approach to interrupt the progression of substance use to addiction is via regular screenings and brief interventions.[68] For women with consistent access to health care, physicians and other health professionals are in an ideal position to educate girls and women about the risks of substance use, screen for signs of risk, intervene early with those who have of a problem, and refer those in need to treatment. Screenings and brief interventions have been demonstrated to be effective in many settings ranging from colleges and universities to trauma centers.[68] Yet existing screening and assessment tools for substance-related problems tend to focus on issues that are more relevant to men—such as work related problems rather than domestic violence or family conflict—and measures of substance use frequency and quantity rarely are sensitive to gender differences in metabolism and other relevant physiologic factors. As such, it is critical that screening and assessment tools, as well as treatment protocols, be tailored to women.

If screening suggests the existence of a substance use disorder, comprehensive assessment in a medical setting must be done to determine the nature and severity of the disorder and the existence of any co-occurring health problems that also require treatment.[69] As with other chronic health conditions, the standard medical practice should be to screen, diagnose, and treat or refer for specialty care. Science-based, effective treatment approaches include psychosocial interventions, which attempt to modify patients' substance-related attitudes and behaviors, enhance coping skills, and help patients control cravings, avoid substance use triggers, and deal effectively with lapses,[70] and pharmacological interventions, which aim to inhibit substance use and its associated cravings, lessen the effects of addictive substances once they are taken, and prevent relapse.[71] Used together, these therapies enhance treatment efficacy.[72]

Disease Management and Recovery Supports

Because addiction is a chronic disease prone to relapse, long-term management is required; this includes comprehensive medical and behavioral health care and a range

Table 19-1

Evidence-based therapies to treat addiction

Behavioral Therapies

> Motivational interviewing
> Motivational Enhancement Therapy
> Cognitive Behavioral Therapy
> The Community Reinforcement Approach
> Contingency management
> Couples/family therapy
> Multisystemic therapy
> Therapeutic Community

Pharmacologic Therapies

Smoking Cessation

> Nicotine Replacement Therapy
> Antidepressant medication
> Varenicline
> Clonidine

Alcohol

> Disulfiram
> Naltrexone
> Acamprosate
> Anticonvulsants

Cocaine

> Disulfiram
> Modafinil

Marijuana

> Rimonabant
> Oral Tetrahydrocannabinol

Opioids

> Methadone
> Buprenorphine
> Naltrexone

of recovery supports by nonmedical professionals and paraprofessionals.[73] Many with substance use disorders also benefit from mutual support programs.[74] Nonmedical professionals and motivated and experienced nonprofessionals can provide social support, encourage patients to adhere to their treatment regimens, and help patients maintain key lifestyle changes that reduce the risk of relapse.[75]

Barriers to Early Intervention and Treatment for Women

Women are less likely than men to seek help, be diagnosed with a substance use problem, receive treatment or have treatment options tailored to their needs, and they are more likely than men to face barriers to accessing treatment[76] including lack of recognition of the disease by patient[77] and fear of professional help to address the problem.[78] Other barriers to treatment include lifestyle constraints such as lack of time or competing responsibilities,[77] lack of child care,[79] insufficient financial resources (insurance coverage) to pay for treatment,[80] inadequate social support,[77] and lack of information regarding where to turn for help.[80] In addition to these formidable personal barriers, there are institutionalized barriers to treatment access that require large-scale policy changes to overcome.

Stigma, Discrimination, and Public Misconceptions of Addiction

Misunderstanding of the disease of addiction has led to stigma and discrimination, which prevent people from receiving high-quality care.[81] Untreated addiction too frequently results in criminal activity, fueling public perceptions of addicted individuals as criminals.[82] Stigma and discrimination can be particularly problematic for women who are pregnant or postpartum and who may be wary of the involvement of child protective services should they seek treatment.[83] Institutional discrimination limits insurance coverage of addiction screening and treatment. Underlying the stigma and consequent discrimination associated with addiction is the misunderstanding of addiction as a moral failing rather than a chronic relapsing disease.

Lack of Training of Healthcare Professionals

The extent and quality of healthcare professionals' training in the signs and symptoms of addiction and their treatment are inexcusably deficient.[84] There are no national standards of education, training, practice, or accountability for general healthcare providers who typically are the first to encounter patients in need of help, and the standards for those in the addiction treatment profession are inadequate as well. In addition, many addiction treatment providers are not clinicians and therefore incapable of assessing and treating co-occurring health disorders and uable to prescribe pharmacological therapies. Thus, very few people receive care that is consistent with scientific knowledge.[2]

Fewer than 30% of girls say their doctors discuss smoking, drinking, or drug use with them.[85] More than 90% of primary care physicians screen their teen patients for high blood pressure more frequently than for smoking or drug use.[86] Less than 1% of primary care physicians consider a substance use disorder diagnosis when presented with the early symptoms of alcohol or prescription drug misuse in an older woman.[87] Further more, when physicians do screen for these conditions, they rarely provide guidance or follow-up care.[88]

Status of the Research

Although there has been considerable progress since the 1970s, the failure to include women in most studies of substance use and addiction has drastically limited knowledge of effective prevention and treatment options for women. The few published studies that included women focused less on the effects of substance use on the participants than on their children.[89] Most researchers who included women in their samples either combined the results with those of men, assumed the results to be opposite those of men, or simply excluded reporting the data on women.[90] More recently, government-funded studies have been required to include women in research samples, which should enhance the quality of future research providing greater knowledge of substance use disorders in women.[91]

Changing Policy and Practice

To reduce the prevalence of substance use disorders among women, the population must be educated to understand the chronic nature of addiction, learn about common risk factors and consequences of misuse among women and effects on their children, understand that these disorders can be prevented and treated, and know where to seek help. Prevention and treatment services should address problems related to substance use including risky sex, physical and sexual abuse, eating disorders, depression, anxiety, and other physical and mental health problems.[16]

Opportunities for Prevention among Girls and Women

The effective prevention of substance use disorders among girls and women requires a comprehensive, long-term approach that starts in childhood and addresses all the areas of influence on a girl's or woman's life that can increase risk. These include influences from parents, peers, schools, communities, and the media. Interventions for girls and young women should address parent–child communication and parental monitoring of children's behaviors, social norms regarding substance use, coping and social skills, and media influences on substance use. Interventions for adult women should address risks associated with women's substance use disorders such as domestic violence, eating disorders, depression and anxiety, and work- and family-related stress, as well as the risks of substance use during pregnancy.[89] Policy interventions that involve increased taxes, smoking bans, and regulation of tobacco and alcohol marketing and Internet sales of tobacco, alcohol, and prescription drug products can have an enormous impact on women's substance use.[92]

Improving Early Intervention, Treatment, and Disease Management for Girls and Women

Medical schools, licensing boards, public and private insurers, physicians, and other healthcare providers must work together to ensure that physicians are well trained to diagnose addictive disorders in general and among women in particular, that they make screening a priority, and that they either can treat and manage the disorder themselves or refer patients to effective specialty treatment and disease

management.[93] Policymakers should require adherence to appropriate science-based standards for all those providing addiction treatment, including tailoring programs to address the unique needs of girls and women.[94] Treatment programs should accommodate the transportation and childcare needs of parenting women and include a family component to ensure social support and boost the odds of treatment adherence and relapse prevention. And much like other chronic diseases, treating substance use disorders requires a long-term care approach focused on recovery management. Although symptoms may recur as they do with other chronic diseases, this does not necessarily indicate a failure in treatment. Effective chronic disease management for addiction requires medical management, aftercare services, and long-term recovery support.[95] Parents, other family members, teachers, coaches, clergy, and other community leaders should be aware of signs of trouble and how to get help.

Insurance Coverage

Despite significant gains in reducing the treatment gap resulting from the recent passage of parity for mental health and addiction coverage included in the Patient Protection and Affordable Care Act of 2010,[96] loopholes remain allowing insurance plans to avoid paying for high-quality treatment. Efforts must be made to remove the loopholes in coverage and ensure that all girls and women can access affordable and effective preventive services and treatment.

Shifting Public Investments

Federal, state, and local governments in the United States spend more than $467 billion each year on substance misuse and addiction. Of each dollar federal and state governments spend, 95.6 cents pays for the consequences of our failure to prevent and treat the problem and less than 2 cents goes to prevention.[97] Shifting public investment to prevention, early intervention, treatment, disease management, and research can have a profound effect on reducing the costs of substance use disorders to women, families, and the public. Doing so is not only sound economic policy; it is a moral responsibility and good medicine.

Summary

Addressing the full spectrum of substance use problems for women—from experimentation to risky or excessive use to clinical dependence—requires fundamental changes in the way the public views these problems and the way the healthcare profession, government, and other service providers respond to them. To reduce substance use disorders in girls and women, we have to address not only the unique motivations for use, consequences of use, barriers to treatment, and treatment needs, but also ensure that the public is educated about this disease. Prevention and treatment providers must be well trained to administer gender-sensitive services including screening, intervention and treatment with costs covered by public and/or private insurance. Unless we commit our nation to making drastic but feasible changes in policy and practice, addiction will continue to be the number one preventable public health problem in the United States and the destructive, intergenerational cycle of addiction and relapse will continue to devastate women, families and communities and waste scarce government resources.

Discussion Questions

1. What factors are associated with greater vulnerability of girls and women to substance use compared to boys and men?
2. How could healthcare providers in clinical medicine and dentistry provide advice about substance use?
3. What are the best opportunities for education and prevention of substance use?
4. How have public programs influenced access to substance use by young girls and women?

References

1. National Center on Addiction and Substance Abuse at Columbia University. *CASA Analysis of Data from 2007 National Survey on Drug Use and Health.* New York: National Center on Addiction and Substance Abuse (CASA) at Columbia University; 2009.
2. Institute of Medicine. *Improving the Quality of Health Care for Mental and Substance-use Conditions: Quality Chasm Series.* Washington, DC: Institute of Medicine; 2005.
3. McLellan AT, Lewis DC, O'Brien CP, Kleber HD. Drug dependence, a chronic medical illness: implications for treatment, insurance, and outcomes evaluation. *JAMA.* 2007;284:1689–1695.
4. *Diagnostic and Statistical Manual of Mental Disorders.* 4th ed. Washington DC: American Psychiatric Association; 1994.
5. Epstein J, Barker P, Vorburger M, Murtha C. *Serious Mental Illness and Its Co-occurrence with Substance Use Disorders, 2002.* Rockville, MD: U.S. Department of Health and Human Services, Substance Abuse and Mental Health Services Administration, Office of Applied Studies; 2004.
6. National Institute on Drug Abuse. Addiction: *Drugs, Brains, and Behavior: The Science of Addiction.* Bethesda, MD: U.S. Department of Health and Human Services, National Institutes of Health, National Institute on Drug Abuse; 2008. http://www.drugabuse.gov/scienceofaddiction/scioffaddiction.pdf. Accessed October 28, 2009.
7. Erickson CK. *The Science of Addiction.* New York: WW Norton & Company; 2007.
8. Bodenheimer TS, Grumbach K. *Understanding Health Policy: A Clinical Approach.* 5th ed. Atlanta, GA: Centers for Disease Control and Prevention; 2009.
9. Perkins KA. Sex differences in nicotine versus nonnicotine reinforcement as determinants of tobacco smoking. *Exp Clin Psychopharmacol.* 1996;4:166–177.
10. Kandel DB, Chen K. Extent of smoking and nicotine dependence in the United States: 1991–1993. *Nicotine Tob Res.* 2000;2:263–274.
11. DiFranza JR, Savageau JA, Rigotti NA, et al. Development of symptoms of tobacco dependence in youths: 30 month follow up data from the DANDY study. *Tob Control.* 2002;11:228–235.
12. Fuchs CS, Stampfer MJ, Colditz GA, et al. Alcohol consumption and mortality among women. *N Engl J Med.* 1995; 332:1245–1250.
13. Hill SY, Smith TR. Evidence for genetic mediation of alcoholism in women. *J Subst Abuse.* 1991;3:159–174.
14. Ely M, Hardy R, Longford NT, Wadsworth MEJ. Gender differences in the relationship between alcohol consumption and drink problems are largely accounted for by body water. *Alcohol Alcohol.* 1999;34:894–902.
15. National Institute on Drug Abuse. *NIDA Research Report: Prescription Drugs: Abuse and Addiction.* Bethesda, MD: U.S. Department of Health and Human Services, National Institutes of Health, National Institute on Drug Abuse; 2001. NIH publication 05–4881.
16. National Center on Addiction and Substance Abuse at Columbia University. *The Formative Years: Pathways to Substance Abuse Among Girls and Young Women Ages 8–22.* New York: National Center on Addiction and Substance Abuse at Columbia University; 2003.
17. Block J, Block JH, Keyes S. Longitudinally foretelling drug usage in adolescence: early childhood personality and environmental precursors. *Child Dev.* 1988;59:336–355.
18. Han C, McGue MK, Iacono WG. Lifetime tobacco, alcohol and other substance use in adolescent Minnesota twins: univariate and multivariate behavioral genetic analyses. *Addiction.* 1999;94:981–993.
19. Bauman KE, Foshee VA, Koch GG, Haley NJ, Downtown MI. Testosterone and cigarette smoking in early adolescence. *J Behav Med.* 1989;12:425–433.
20. Schuckit MA, Smith TL, Kalmijn J, Tsuang J, Hesselbrock V, Bucholz K. Response to alcohol in daughters of alcoholics: a pilot study and a comparison with sons of alcoholics. *Alcohol Alcohol.* 2000;35:242–248.
21. Lundahl LH, Lukas SE. The impact of familial alcoholism on alcohol reactivity in female social drinkers. *Exp Clin Psychopharmacol.* 2001;9:101–109.
22. Atkinson RM, Ganzini L, Bernstein MJ. Alcohol and substance-use disorders in the elderly. In: Birren JE, Sloane RB, Cohen GD, eds. *Handbook of Mental Health and Aging.* New York: Academic Press; 1992:516–555.
23. Ludwig KB, Pittman JF. Adolescent prosocial values and self-efficacy in relation to delinquency, risky sexual behavior, and drug use. *Youth Soc.* 1999;30:461–482.
24. National Center on Addiction and Substance Abuse at Columbia University. *Food for Thought: Substance Abuse and Eating Disorders.* New York: National Center on Addiction and Substance Abuse at Columbia University; 2003.
25. Byrne D, Byrne A, Reinhart M. Personality, stress and the decision to commence cigarette smoking in adolescence. *J Psychosom Res.* 1995;39:53–62.
26. Flanigan BJ, Potrykus PA, Marti D. Alcohol and marijuana use among female adolescent incest victims. *Alcohol Treat Q.* 1988;5:231–248.
27. Brennan PL, Moos RH, Kim JY. Gender differences in the individual characteristics and life contexts of late-middle-aged and older problem drinkers. *Addiction.* 1993;88:781–790.
28. Johnson PB, Johnson HL. Reaffirming the power of parental influence on adolescent smoking and drinking decisions. *Adolesc Family Health.* 2000;1:37–43.
29. Adlaf EM, Ivis FJ. Structure and relations: the influence of familial factors on adolescent substance use and delinquency. *J Child Adolesc Subst Abuse.* 1996;5:1–19.
30. Barber JG, Bolitho F, Bertrand LD. Intrapersonal versus peer group predictors of adolescent drug use. *Child Youth Serv Rev.* 1999;21:565–579.
31. Simons-Morton B, Haynie DL, Crump AD, Saylor KE. Peer and parent influences on smoking and drinking among early adolescents. *Health Educ Behav.* 2001;28:95–107.
32. Bernard, B. *Fostering Resiliency in Kids: Protective Factors in Family, School, and Community.* Portland, OR: Northwest Regional Educational Laboratory; 1991.
33. Allison KW, Crawford I, Leone PE, et al. Adolescent substance use: preliminary examinations of school and neighborhood context. *Am J Community Psychol.* 1999;27:111–141.
34. Crum RM, Lillie-Blanton M, Anthony JC. Neighborhood environment and opportunity to use cocaine and other drugs in late childhood and early adolescence. *Drug Alcohol Depend.* 1996;43:155–161.
35. Van Etten ML, Neumark YD, Anthony JC. Male-female differences in the earliest stages of drug involvement. *Addiction.* 1999;94:1413–1419.
36. National Center on Addiction and Substance Abuse at Columbia University. *Under the Counter: The Diversion and Abuse of Controlled and Prescription Drugs in the U.S.* New York: National Center on Addiction and Substance Abuse at Columbia University; 2005.
37. Cullen KW, Koehly LA, Anderson C, et al. Gender differences in chronic disease risk behaviors through the transition out of high school. *Am J Prev Med.* 1999;17:1–7.
38. Golombek H, Marton P, Stein B, Korenblum M. A study of disturbed and non-disturbed adolescents: Tte Toronto Adolescent Longitudinal Study. *Can J Psychiatry.* 1986;31:532–535.
39. Brennan PL, Moos RH. Late-life drinking behavior: The influence of personal characteristics, life context and treatment. *Alcohol Health Res World.* 1996;20:197–204.
40. Jinks MJ, Raschko RR. A profile of alcohol and prescription drug abuse in a high-risk community-based elderly population. *Ann Pharmacother* 1990; 24:971–975.
41. National Center on Addiction and Substance Abuse at Columbia University. *The Cost of Substance Abuse to America's Health Care System: Report 1, Medicaid Hospital Costs.* New York: National Center on Addiction and Substance Abuse at Columbia University; 1993.
42. Patton GC, Coffey C, Carlin JB, Degenhardt L, Lynskey M, Hall W. Cannabis use and mental health in young people: Cohort study. *BMJ.* 2002;325:1195–1198.
43. Substance Abuse and Mental Health Services Administration, Office of Applied Studies. *Women with Co-occurring Serious Mental Illness and a Substance Use Disorder: The NSDUH Report.* Rockville, MD: U.S. Department of Health and Human Services; 2004.
44. Brady JP, Posner, M, Lang, C, Rosati MJ. *Risk and Reality: The Implications of Prenatal Exposure to Alcohol and Other Drugs.* Washington, DC: U.S. Department of Education, Office of Educational Research and Improvement; 1994.
45. Weinberg NZ. Cognitive and behavioral deficits associated with parent alcohol use. *J Am Acad Child Adolesc Psychiatry.* 1997;36:1177–1186.
46. Centers for Disease Control and Prevention. Health effects of cigarette smoking. 2009. http://www.cdc.gov/tobacco/data_statistics/fact_sheets/health_effects/effects_cig_smoking/. Accessed October 20, 2009.
47. Centers for Disease Control and Prevention. Annual smoking-attributable mortality, years of potential life lost, and economic costs—United States, 1995–1999. 2002. http://www.cdc.gov/mmwr/preview/mmwrhtml/mm5114a2.htm. Accessed October 28, 2009.

48. Husten CG, Chrisman JH, Reddy MN. Trends and effects of cigarette smoking among girls and women in the United States, 1965–1993. *J Am Med Womens Assoc.* 1996;51:11–18.

49. International Early Lung Cancer Action Program Investigators, Henschke CI, Yip R, Miettinen OS. Women's susceptibility to tobacco carcinogens and survival after diagnosis of lung cancer. *JAMA* 2006;296:180–184.

50. Terry PD, Miller AB, Rohan TE. Cigarette smoking and breast cancer risk: a long latency period? *Int J Cancer.* 2002;100;723–728.

51. Aronow WS, Ahn C, Gutstein H. Risk factors for new atherothrombotic brain infarction in 664 older men and 1,488 older women. *Am J Cardiol* 1996; 77:1381–1383.

52. Office of the Surgeon General. *Women and Smoking: A Report of the Surgeon General* Washington, DC: U.S. Government Printing Office; 2001. GPO item 0483-L-06.

53. Science Daily. Women more vulnerable to tobacco carcinogens, new results show. 2009. http://www.sciencedaily.com/releases/2009/05/090503082340.htm. Accessed October 29, 2009.

54. Willett WC. Green A, Stampfer MJ. Relative and absolute excess risks of coronary heart disease among women who smoke cigarettes. *N Engl J Med* 1987;317: 1303–1309.

55. Rosenberg L, Kaufman DW, Helmrich MS, et al. Myocardial infarction and cigarette smoking in women younger than 50 years of age. *JAMA* 1985;253:2965–2969.

56. Paulus D, Saint-Remy A, Jeanjean M. Oral contraception and cardiovascular risk factors during adolescence. *Contraception.* 2000;62:113–116.

57. U.S. Department of Health and Human Services. *Alcohol and Health: Tenth Special Report to the U.S. Congress.* Washington, DC: U.S. Department of Health and Human Services; 2000.

58. Hommer DW, Momenan R, Kaiser E, Rawlings RR. Evidence for a gender-related effect of alcoholism on brain volumes. *Am J Psychiatry* 2001; 158:198–204.

59. Nixon SJ. Cognitive deficits in alcoholic women. *Alcohol Health Res World.* 1994;18:228–232.

60. American Academy of Pediatrics, Committee on Adolescents. Suicide and suicide attempts in adolescents. *Pediatrics.* 2000;105:871–874.

61. National Center on Addiction and Substance Abuse at Columbia University. *The Costs of Substance Abuse to America's Health Care System: Report 1, Medicaid Hospital Costs.* New York: National Center on Addiction and Substance Abuse at Columbia University; 1993.

62. Gauvin F, Bailey B, Bratton SL. Hospitalizations for pediatric intoxication in Washington State, 1987–1997. *Arch Pediatr Adolesc Med.* 2001;155: 1105–1110.

63. National Center on Addiction and Substance Abuse at Columbia University. *Substance Abuse and the American Woman.* New York: National Center on Addiction and Substance Abuse at Columbia University; 1996.

64. Grossman M, Sindelar JL, Mullahy J, Anderson R. Policy watch: alcohol and cigarette taxes. *J Econ Perspect.* 1993;7:211–222.

65. Ringel JS, Evans WN. Cigarette taxes and smoking during pregnancy. *Am J Public Health.* 2001;91:1851–1856.

66. Stein CR, Ellis JA, Savitz, DA, Vichinsky L, Perl SB. Decline in smoking during pregnancy in New York City, 1995–2005. *Public Health Rep.* 2009;124:841–849.

67. National Center on Addiction and Substance Abuse at Columbia University. *Wasting the Best and the Brightest: Substance Abuse at America's Colleges and Universities.* New York: National Center on Addiction and Substance Abuse at Columbia University; 2007.

68. Substance Abuse and Mental Health Services Administration, Center for Substance Abuse Treatment. Screening, brief intervention, and referral to treatment: Frequently asked questions for the public. http://www.samhsa.gov/prevention/SBIRT/index.aspx. Accessed August 29, 2012.

69. American Society of Addiction Medicine. Public policy statement on screening for addiction in primary care settings. 1997. http://www.asam.org/advocacy/find-a-policy-statement/view-policy-statement/public-policy-statements/2011/12/16/screening-for-addiction-in-primary-care-settings. Accessed August 29, 2012.

70. Carroll KM. Relapse prevention as a psychosocial treatment: a review of controlled clinical trials. *Exp Clin Psychopharmacol.* 1996;4:46–54.

71. Suh JJ, Pettinati HM, Kampman KM, O'Brien CP. The status of disulfiram: a half of a century later. *J Clin Psychopharmacol.* 2006;26:290–302.

72. Center on Substance Abuse Treatment. *Enhancing Motivation for Change in Substance Abuse Treatment.* Rockville, MD: Substance Abuse and Mental Health Services Administration; 1999. Treatment Improvement Protocol (TIP) Series 35.

73. Master RJ, Eng C. Integrating acute and long-term care for high-cost populations. *Health Aff.* 2001;20:161–172.

74. McKellar J, Stewart E, Humphreys K. Alcoholics Anonymous involvement and positive alcohol-related outcomes: cause, consequence, or just a correlate? A prospective 2-year study of 2,319 alcohol-dependent men. *J Consult Clin Psychol.* 2003;71:302–308.

75. United Nations International Drug Control Programme. *Contemporary Drug Abuse Treatment: A Review of the Evidence Base.* New York: United Nations Office on Drugs and Crime; 2002.

76. Bertakis KD, Azari R, Helms J, et al. Gender differences in the utilization of health care services. *J Fam Pract.* 2000;49:147–152.

77. Rapp RC, Xu J, Carr CA, et al. Treatment barriers identified by substance abusers assessed at a centralized intake unit. *J Subst Abuse Treat.* 2006;30:227–235.

78. Tsogia D, Copello A, Orford J. Entering treatment for substance misuse: a review of the literature. *J Mental Health.* 2001;10:481–499.

79. Ashley OS, Marsden ME, Brady TM. Effectiveness of substance abuse treatment programming for women: A review. *Am J Drug Alcohol Abuse.* 2003;29:19–53.

80. Battjes RJ, Onken LS, Delany PJ. Drug abuse treatment entry and engagement: report of a meeting on treatment readiness. *J Clin Psychol* 1999; 55:643–57.

81. McLellan AT, Meyers K. Contemporary addiction treatment: a review of systems problems for adults and adolescents. *Biol Psychiatry.* 2004;56:764–770.

82. National Center on Addiction and Substance Abuse at Columbia University. *Behind Bars: Substance Abuse and America's Prison Population.* New York: National Center on Addiction and Substance Abuse at Columbia University; 1998.

83. Appel PW, Ellison AA, Jansky HK, Oldak R. Barriers to enrollment in drug abuse treatment and suggestions for reducing them: opinions of drug injecting street outreach clients and other system stakeholders. *Am J Drug Alcohol Abuse.* 2004;30:129–153.

84. Miller NS, Sheppard LM, Colenda CC, Magen J. Why physicians are unprepared to treat patients who have alcohol- and drug-related disorders. *Acad Med.* 2001;7:410–418.

85. Sarigiani PA, Ryan L, Petersen AC. Prevention of high-risk behaviors in adolescent women. *J Adolesc Health.* 1999;25:109–119.

86. Ellen JM, Franzgrote M, Irwin CE, Millstein SG. Primary care physicians' screening of adolescent patients: a survey of California physicians. *J Adolesc Health.* 1998;22:433–438.

87. National Center on Addiction and Substance Abuse at Columbia University. *Under the Rug: Substance Abuse and the Mature Woman.* New York: National Center on Addiction and Substance Abuse at Columbia University; 1998.

88. Bernstein LR, Folkman S, Lazarus RS. Characterization of the use and misuse of medications by an elderly, ambulatory population. *Med Care.* 1989;27:654–663.

89. Wetherington, CL, Roman AB. Drug addiction research and the health of women. 1998. http://archives.drugabuse.gov/WHGD/DARHW-Download2.html. Accessed August 29, 2012.

90. Reed BG. Developing women-sensitive drug dependence treatment services: why so difficult? *J Psychoactive Drugs* 1987;19:151–163

91. Office of Research on Women's Health. Inclusion of women and minorities in clinical research. 2012. http://orwh.od.nih.gov/research/inclusion/index.asp. Accessed August 29, 2012.

92. Foster SE, Vaughan RD, Foster WH, Califano JA. Alcohol consumption and expenditures for underage drinking and adult excessive drinking. *JAMA.* 2003;289:989–995.

93. National Center on Addiction and Substance Abuse at Columbia University. *Missed Opportunity: National Survey of Primary Care Physicians and Patients on Substance Abuse.* New York: National Center on Addiction and Substance Abuse at Columbia University; 2000.

94. Ellis RA, O'Hara M, Sowers, KM. Profile-based intervention: developing gender-sensitive treatment for adolescent substance abusers. *Res Soc Work Pract.* 2000;10:327–347.

95. Wagner EH, Austin BT, Davis C, et al. Improving chronic illness care: translating evidence into action. Interventions that encourage people to acquire self-management skills are essential in chronic illness care. *Health Aff.* 2001;20:64–78.

96. U.S. Congress. H. 1424: The Emergency Economic Stabilization Act of 2008. 2008. http://thomas.loc.gov. Accessed October 29, 2009.

97. National Center on Addiction and Substance Abuse at Columbia University. *Shoveling Up II: The Impact of Substance Abuse on Federal, State and Local Budgets.* New York: National Center on Addiction and Substance Abuse at Columbia University; 2009.

Intimate Partner Violence and Women's Health in the USA

Leslie L. Davidson, MD, MSc and Cynthia Golembeski, MPH

Introduction

Intimate partner violence (IPV) seriously compromises the short- and long-term health and well-being of women who experience it, of those who perpetrate it, and of children who witness it. Although violence against women has gained increasing recognition as a human rights issue, IPV often remains hidden, stigmatized, underrecognized, and underreported.[1] Studies incorporating diverse population samples, definitions, and research methods have found 25% to 54% of women reporting lifetime exposure to IPV.[2,3]

This chapter focuses on health conditions associated with IPV and addresses definitional challenges that complicate understanding the epidemiology of IPV. A detailed review of the costs to individuals and to society are beyond the scope of this chapter but estimates of the costs of intimate partner rape, physical assault, and stalking exceed $5.8 billion annually, nearly $4.1 billion of which is for direct medical and mental health services. The total costs of IPV also include almost $1 billion in lost productivity from paid work and household chores for those experiencing nonfatal IPV and a similar dollar figure in lost lifetime earnings of IPV homicide victims.[4–6] Cost aside, IPV is one of the most prevalent health-related conditions suffered by women significantly affecting women's survival and well-being, including physical, mental, and reproductive health. IPV cuts across all social, racial, ethnic, religious groups and educational and economic strata.

Historical Perspective

In 1871, Alabama was the first state to rescind men's right to beat their wives but it took close to 100 years before spousal assault and "domestic" violence came to be identified as a critical social issue. As recently as a few decades ago, violence against women in the home was largely regarded as a private family matter.[7] Initially advocates just identified "battered" women, somewhat mirroring the concurrent efforts regarding "battered" children. In 1975, Gelles and Straus[8] conducted the first nationally representative family violence survey that included the dimension of spousal abuse, and other research examined the social construction of *patriarchal* violence as a "private" event.[7–9] Due to advocacy efforts, social norms began to shift; in 1985 the Surgeon General's office convened a workshop on violence and public health declaring that "domestic violence" was the biggest public health crisis of the decade. Increasing media coverage contributed to shifting social norms towards the perception of partner violence as unacceptable.

In the United States these shifts culminated in the passage of the Violence Against Women Act of 1994.[10] This act provided $1.6 billion to enhance investigation and prosecution of violent crimes perpetrated against women, imposed automatic and mandatory restitution on those convicted, and allowed civil redress in cases prosecutors chose to leave unprosecuted. It also provided the Office on Violence Against Women with authority to develop federal policy around issues relating to intimate partner violence and sexual violence.[11]

In 1999, the Centers for Disease Control and Prevention (CDC) suggested dropping the word "domestic" from the term and using "intimate partner" instead to more accurately describe the vulnerable population and to differentiate partner violence from other forms of family violence, such as child maltreatment and elder abuse. Practitioners, academics, and both governmental and nongovernmental organizations, such as the World Health Organization (WHO), CDC, and the Family Violence Prevention Fund (FVPF), define IPV as consisting of violent or coercive behaviors (including threats), which may be physical, sexual, emotional and/or controlling, committed by a current or former intimate partner. IPV may vary in both frequency and severity of impact and occurs in one or more of the following several forms:[12,13]

- **Physical abuse**: Acts such as slapping, hitting, punching, kicking, pushing, assaults with a weapon, choking, and homicide
- **Sexual abuse**: Forced or unwanted intercourse or participation in other sexual acts and/or sexual coercion
- **Psychological or emotional abuse**: Behaviors that undermine the emotional well-being of the person, including threats of physical or sexual abuse, intimidation, property destruction, humiliation, neglect, threats to remove or harm children, pets, etc.

• **Various controlling behaviors**: Behaviors that may include separating a person from family or friends, monitoring their movements (i.e., surveillance, stalking, checking email or phone records), and undermining economic security (i.e., preventing employment, confiscation of earnings, restricting access to financial resources, etc.)

IPV is thus a constellation of coercive behaviors with the goal of gaining power and control over an intimate partner.[14] Research evidence supports the centrality of control within this constellation: the presence of a highly controlling partner is associated with higher risk of injury or death to the other partner.[15]

IPV is found across all cultural and racial groups, social classes, genders, and age groups. In the lives of society's more vulnerable, IPV is associated with numerous other health and social problems, such as substance use, housing insecurity, and family fragmentation[16,17] often concentrated among the poor and marginalized members of the society such as immigrants. Poverty in association with IPV poses challenges to victims related to work, training, education, and efforts toward establishing economic independence. Vulnerable populations, migrants, immigrants, women living with a disability, and those serving in or involved with a partner in the military are at higher risk.[3,7,16] Within these groups adolescents and young adult women are at highest risk of partner violence.[18]

Although men and women both perpetrate physical or psychological violent *behavior* against their partners with similar frequency, the majority of cases of IPV with a serious *impact* are perpetrated against women.[3,19] Women are much more likely to suffer sexual violence as well as physical, psychological, and emotional *harm*, including depression and posttraumatic stress disorder (PTSD), in comparison to men.[19] Female victims of IPV experience greater levels of fear than male victims.[3,13,20] Compared to men, women are twice as likely to sustain an injury and over seven times more likely to report being beaten, choked, or restrained.[3] CDC survey data indicated the prevalence of women having experienced coercive sex or physical violence in the preceding year was 1.4% and 23.6% over the lifetime, twice that reported by men. National Violence Against Women Survey (NVAWS) findings are similar except that they note lifetime prevalence for men was even lower than the CDC study, one-third the frequency reported by women.[21] Prevalence rates of IPV involving same-sex female partners range from 17% to 52% similar to IPV rates related to women in heterosexual relationships.[22]

Beginning with Straus and Gelles researchers increasingly recognized the occurrence of perpetration of physical violence by both partners within a relationship, which may be described as mutual, reciprocal, or symmetrical violence.[4] A large national survey (N = 11,370) found that half of the violent relationships included perpetration by both partners, which was associated with greater injury than unidirectional violence, regardless of the perpetrator's gender.[23] The apparent gender symmetry of the occurrence of violent or coercive behavior within partner relationships contrasted with clear evidence of the imbalance of significant harm to women challenged the research findings of epidemiologists and social scientists. In the last decade, researchers have worked to reconcile the contradiction through better defining different types of partner violence. Johnson proposed a model that distinguished between typologies based on the level of control driving the violent behavior within the couple:[14]

1. **Intimate terrorism** constitutes violence "embedded in a general pattern of controlling behaviors, indicating that the perpetrator is attempting to exert general control over his partner." This type of violence perpetrated by a very controlling partner has also been referred to as "patriarchal terrorism," "coercive controlling violence," or "coercive control."[24] In these situations, it is primarily the male who perpetrates.

2. **Violent resistance** is a violent yet noncontrolling response to intimate terrorism initiated by a violent and controlling abusive partner.

3. **Situational couple violence** or "common couple violence," which may be the most prevalent type, "does not involve any attempt on the part of either partner to gain control over the relationship." Such violence may be situationally provoked, chronic, or severe, yet does not reflect "relationship-wide evidence of an attempt to exert general control over one's partner." The impact of this type of violence is less severe than that of intimate terrorism. This is the more common typology.

4. **Mutual violent control** consists of both persons being violent and very controlling and is rare.

In applying these subgroups in a reanalysis of data from a previous study.[14] Johnson found that intimate terrorism is almost exclusively perpetrated by men whereas *situational couple violence* is likely to involve males and females to an equal extent. Using these same subtypes, Johnson and Leone analyzed the NVAWS data and found systematic differences in the frequency, chronicity, severity of impact, and loss of work time between intimate terrorism and situational violence.[14]

Screening, Surveillance, and Measurement

How one defines and measures IPV affects estimates of incidence and prevalence rates, patterns and associations, demographic differences, and health consequences, which in turn will affect clinical and policy decisions. Valid, reliable measures are emerging for screening and clinical assessment as well as research. The strengths, limitations, and weaknesses of various measures have been documented recently by the CDC.[25] Debate continues on the appropriateness of screening for IVP universally within healthcare settings. On the one hand, the WHO conditions for screening are not met;[26,27] in particular, there is insufficient evidence about effective interventions for victims of IPV following a positive screen.[28] On the other hand, a consistent majority of women of all ages and nationalities support healthcare screening.[29,30] Within a healthcare setting, asking about the occurrence of partner violence fits within the routine social history alongside other health risks such as smoking or alcohol abuse. Excluding routine questions about partner violence in health encounters because it does not meet screening criteria does women a disservice.

IPV rates vary widely by data source with estimates given for 1-year prevalence and/or lifetime prevalence rates. Incidence rates are rarely given. These may reflect ongoing, intermittent, or previous experiences related to IPV.[31] The prevalence of IPV depends on the definitions and measures applied, the interviewer and the setting, and assurance of anonymity or confidentiality. For instance, variations in the definition of IPV may influence the reported levels of severity among the respondents studied. Variability of the time frame in which violence is measured may challenge comparisons given the lack of reliability of some data on the extent and nature of IPV. In addition, methodology issues including small or inappropriate samples, a lack of controlled analysis and adjustment for confounders, and inconsistent measurements or definitions complicate analyses. The combination of these issues impedes fruitful comparisons needed for meaningfully understanding the health effects of IPV. Moreover, data collection and analysis may be hindered by the influence of social and cultural norms in determining what constitutes violence, discrepancies in reporting, particular framings of questions, limited access to target populations, and whether the responses are restricted to the current relationship.[3]

Data Sources

Despite a rapid rise in the number of IPV publications, the lack of regular, ongoing surveillance and use of uniform definitions and survey methods across states has hindered efforts to 1) establish robust national estimates of the prevalence of IPV, 2) to study risk, and 3) to evaluate IPV prevention or intervention programs.[21] Social surveys, hospital and medical reports, and official reports, such as death certificates, medical examiners' records, and police and judiciary records, constitute the three main data sources on IPV. Cross-sectional population-based surveys offer the most complete data on the prevalence of IPV, particularly because clinical samples may not be representative of the population and are prone to selection biases.

Records-based research often focuses on a single traumatic event that garners attention of the health or justice systems, yet victimization histories often include multiple events and violent precursors to the given offense. These depend on the appropriate questions being asked and documented in the record. In addition, emergency department records, a frequent source for studies, may document the injury as intentional but often fail to document the relationship between victim and perpetrator, leading to an undercount of IPV occurrence. Emergency records also focus primarily on *physical* harm, only one dimension of IPV, capture cases of greater severity, and measure only acute, not long-term impact. Legal data focus on perpetration, are subject to selection bias, and may not specify well the impact of the initial injury itself.

National Data Sources

Routinely collected national data sources useful in establishing estimates of *fatal* IPV include the Federal Bureau of Investigation's (FBI's) Uniform Crime Reports-Supplemental Homicide Reports (UCR-SHR) based on crime reports, the CDC's National Vital Statistics System (NVSS) obtained from death certificates, and the National Violence Death Reporting System (NVDRS) drawing on death certificates and crime and coroner reports.

Representative data sources regarding *nonfatal* IPV exist and include the FBI's National Incidence-Based Reporting System, the CDC and National Institute of Justice's National Violence Against Women Survey, the Bureau of Justice Statistics' National Crime Victimization Survey (NCVS), the CDC and National Center for Health Statistics' National Hospital Ambulatory Medical Care Survey, the National Electronic Injury Surveillance System, and the Behavioral Risk Factor Surveillance System (BRFSS) on the CDC website.[32] The 1996 NVAWS is the largest-scale IPV specific prevalence study. In 2005, the first-ever IPV module within the CDC's BRFSS telephone survey was administered to over 70,000 respondents in 18 states; one in four women reported lifetime experience of at least one form of physical or sexual IPV victimization during their lifetime.[21]

Limiting the research focus to severe forms of violence tends to highlight gender differences, whereas including minor forms tends to increase gender symmetry. In addition, population-based studies reveal higher rates of IPV as well as more gender symmetry than crime-based or health based studies, which is likely a consequence of the sample and of the severity of the violence. Consequently, national crime surveys may underestimate IPV prevalence.[21,33] In addition, much of our present knowledge is primarily derived from studies of main effects models, which largely focus on the impact of one type of violence on the individual without incorporating analysis of the interactions between different types of abuse or multiple experiences of abuse.[14,34]

Underreporting

The National Center for Injury Prevention and Control estimated in 2003 only 20% of IPV cases are reported.[1] Many reasons have been found to explain the underreporting of IPV, including fear for personal safety due to retribution, shame, self-blame for victimization, fear of being blamed, fear of negative outcomes following disclosure, such as financial insecurity, loss of family stability such as removal of children, or an end to the relationship.[13,35,36] Anonymous or confidential surveys consistently find higher rates than research based on disclosure or justice data.

Some research suggests women of color may face stigma due to perceptions of IPV in their respective communities and to the omission of people of color from public health messages and campaigns Bent-Goodley[36] suggests stereotypes and labeling combined with cultural and language barriers may particularly interfere with women of color's abilities to receive appropriate IPV related care and services, especially in light of negative experiences with health care and formal service systems.[29,37] In addition, discriminatory treatment, such as greater dual arrests, likelihood of prosecution, and a higher degree of child removals when IPV is involved in regards to people of color may compromise help-seeking behavior.[36] These systematic variations in the willingness of respondents to disclose experiences of IPV may bias research in examining disparities in occurrence by race or ethnic group.

Role of Health Care Providers in Documenting IPV

Despite clear policies by the majority of professional organizations, healthcare providers frequently fail to either screen or conduct case finding during health-related visits despite the availability of simple evaluated screening instruments.[25] Reasons for this failure include limited education or training in relation to IPV, feelings of not being adequately qualified, a lack of referral resources, language and cultural barriers, fear of being incorrect, a lack of privacy, and concerns regarding an additional workload.[38,39] Women report negative experiences with health professionals, which include a tendency for professionals to ignore the signs of abuse or their lack of support even if caregivers do acknowledge IPV. The meta-analysis of 25 qualitative studies by Feder et al. concludes that perceptions of appropriateness of the response partly depend on the context of the medical consultation, capability and desire of professionals to address IPV, and the relationship between the woman and the healthcare professional.[40] Although the majority of women in all studies confirm they do not mind being asked about or explicitly screened for IPV, confidentiality as well as a relationship of trust is imperative for disclosure, which is often facilitated by continuity of care.[30,41] Women need nonjudgmental, nondirective, and individually tailored responses from healthcare professionals that acknowledge the complexity of IPV.[40] This has consequences for studying the epidemiology of IPV as well as for improving the care of women facing IPV. This failure will contribute to underreporting the occurrence of IPV, because many studies rely on clinical samples.

Risk Factors

Because longitudinal studies of IPV are rare, it is difficult to disentangle risks for IPV from consequences of IPV. IPV victimization is characterized by multilevel and multifactorial causes, including individual, dyadic, family, community, and societal determinants, though most research focuses on the individual victim or perpetrator.[42] Because partner violence involves a couple, a comprehensive investigation of risks for IPV should include factors associated with the dyad, the couple. Few studies do and the epidemiology of IPV perpetration is beyond the scope of this chapter.

Individual factors associated with an increased risk of IPV victimization include past history of child abuse; witnessing parental IPV; IPV perpetrated by a prior partner; prior injury or verbal abuse by the current partner; youth; lack of health insurance or receipt of medical assistance; mental health risks including anxiety, depression, or history of suicide attempts; and victim and/or partner use of drugs or alcohol and pregnancy.[3,43]

Intergenerational Transfer of Violence

Cross-sectional and longitudinal studies associate childhood exposure to IPV with both later victimization and perpetration of dating and marital aggression.[44,45] For instance, analysis of the Adverse Childhood Experiences (ACE) study data concludes that among those who have grown up with a battered mother and experienced childhood sexual and physical abuse, the risk of IPV victimization and perpetration increases 3.5 times for women and 3.8 times for men. Multiple studies indicate that approximately 20–25% of children report witnessing IPV incidents involving their parents, which places them at greater risk of developing behavioral, social, emotional, cognitive, attitudinal, and long-term problems.[46,47] Problems of IPV and child abuse and neglect within families are interconnected.[2,45,48] Despite evidence for the intergenerational transfer of IPV, no prospective studies have investigated the mechanisms by which it occurs.[13] Experience of IPV may significantly contribute to increased risk for child maltreatment by the IPV victim, perhaps mediated by maternal stress, depression, and unwanted or unintended pregnancy, all of which are associated with both child maltreatment and IPV victimization.[49,50]

Socioeconomic Risks

Women who experience IPV are at an increased risk of experiencing unemployment, health problems, and housing instability[17,51] which could put them at increased risk of IPV or may result from the IPV itself or both. Steady employment may be affected by stress and injury, contacts with the criminal justice system, or other negative consequences of IPV. Family separation, resulting in income reduction, combined with limited access to other important resources such as affordable housing may also prolong the experience of IPV (and thus increase prevalence) by inhibiting women from leaving violent relationships or disclosing information regarding IPV. This would result in an increased prevalence rate of IPV particularly in poorer women since women with more economic or social resources would not be so constrained.

Race

The role of race in relation to IPV is contested and several factors including reporting bias may play a role. Studies suggest higher reporting rates of IPV incidents by medical providers, police, and other professionals for African Americans than for whites.[36] This is corroborated by the National Violence Against Women Survey.[3] In a large, multicenter study reviewing emergency department records, Dearwater et al. did not find a higher prevalence of African Americans among those who experienced partner violence than those who presented with other problems.[52] Differences in education and income have been put forward as explanation for previous assumptions of IPV being associated with race factors.[53] To date, definitive studies have not been published.

Immigration Status

A review of Asian immigrants by Lee and Hadeed[54] found no increase in national rates contrasting to an increase found in local studies and surmised that there may have been underreporting in the national studies. They also found that changes in status may aggravate risk of violence. Similarly, Klevans[55] reviewed research on prevalence in Latinos and did not find an increase once confounders had been adjusted for. However, Frye et al.[56] found that foreign birth was the most powerful risk factor for femicide in an urban neighborhood study. The National Violence Against Women study suggests that IPV *incidence* is no higher among immigrant women, explaining that that IPV *prevalence* is increased by their relative inability to leave the relationship because of language barriers, social isolation, lack of access to equitable jobs, tenuous legal status, and fear of contact with government authorities. Moreover, immigration status may additionally be used as a tool of control, which may influence a woman's ability to seek help.[57]

Homelessness

Rates of severe IPV are extremely high among homeless women with serious mental illness. However, homelessness may also be a result of IPV: one study found that over 30% of women in homeless shelters are there in direct response to abusive relationships.[58] In a study involving 99 episodically homeless women with mental illness, 70% had been physically assaulted, 30% had been sexually assaulted by a partner, 87% had experienced physical abuse in adulthood, and 76% had experienced sexual abuse in adulthood.[59]

Substance Use

Many studies note a link between substance abuse and IPV, yet further investigation regarding the strength and direction of substance use association with IPV is necessary. A meta-analysis by Black et al.[60] examining alcohol use or excessive drinking as a risk factor for partner violence found a significant association, with correlation coefficients ranging from $r = 0.21$ to $r = 0.57$. Regardless of conflicting perspectives regarding the causal role of alcohol, evidence suggests women who live with heavy drinkers face a much higher risk of physical partner violence and that men who have been drinking inflict more serious violence at the time of assault. Moreover, the clinic-based family study conducted by Coker et al.[61] determined that women who reported that both they and their partner had a drug and alcohol problem were at increased risk for sexual, physical, or psychological IPV. Case control studies involving female emergency department patients indicate problem drinking and drug use were significantly associated with risk of IPV injury.[62,63] Similarly, Caetano et al.'s analysis of 1995 national study data reveals that 30%

to 40% of the men and 27% to 34% of the women who perpetrated violence against their partners were drinking at the time.[64]

Alcohol use is highly correlated with IPV, yet may be both a direct cause and a result of partner violence.[65] Researchers suggest cognitively mediated effects of alcohol may operate as a situational factor, increasing the likelihood of violence by reducing inhibitions, clouding judgment, and impairing an individual's ability to interpret clues.[66] The meta-analytic review by Foran and O'Leary[67] demonstrates that alcohol plays a role in IPV yet it is neither a sufficient or necessary factor. Despite the absence of establishing the precise etiologic role of alcohol in the occurrence of IPV, empirical evidence suggests alcohol use often precedes or accompanies acts of mental aggression for both victims and perpetrators.[68]

Relationship/Dyadic Characteristics

Dyadic models of couples aggression may better elucidate the etiology and developmental course of violence within relationships.[69] The dyadic context in which men perpetrate IPV against women includes relationship features, stress between partners, individual characteristics, and communication styles. At an interpersonal level, the most consistent marker for IPV is relationship conflict or discord. Other salient relationship factors associated with IPV include male dominance within the family unit and poor family functioning.[70] Status inconsistency, whereby the female partner occupies a higher educational, professional, and/or income status than her male partner, has been identified as a risk factor for IPV in both civilian and active duty military populations.[3]

Neighborhood Effects

The limited research on neighborhood effects and the risk of IPV suggest low neighborhood socioeconomic position and high levels of neighborhood mobility are associated with higher risk of partner violence.[62,71] High levels of collective efficacy in a neighborhood have been identified as protective factors against partner violence.[72] However, to date only a narrow range of neighborhood characteristics has been examined in relation to IPV, which coincides with a lack of comprehensive understanding of how neighborhoods affect the risk of partner violence.[73,74]

Resilience/Protective Factors

Little is known about what enables women to avoid or leave abusive partners or what makes certain women resilient in the face of partner violence, because most of the research focuses on deficits and risk factors.[13] The research that has been done finds social support a central protective factor. It has been identified as a key factor in assisting women both to avoid and to escape IPV.[75,76] Social support has also been found to diminish negative mental health outcomes and to predict lower levels of violence with the exception of women victims of the most profound IPV.[77] Coker et al.[78] conclude in their cross-sectional study that stronger social support was associated with better physical and mental health status among women currently experiencing IPV and suggest that such support is a key factor in improved coping with IPV. In women leaving IPV shelters, employment and social support predicted lower rates of IPV 1 year later.[79] A recent Cochrane Review finds initial evidence that intensive advocacy and provision of services for victims may be more effective in ensuring their long-term safety than treatment programs for perpetrators.[80]

Prevention

World Health Organization guidelines[81] suggest IPV may be significantly reduced through "well-planned and multi-sector strategies that tackle multiple causes using frameworks such as the public health approach," whereas costly policing and correctional approaches result in minimal returns. The Institute of Medicine (IOM), addressing the role of health professionals and systems, supports a multifaceted, systems change approach to IPV service implementation, which generally consists of a supportive environment, identification of IPV and appropriate referrals, on-site healthcare services, community resource linkages, and appropriate leadership and oversight.[82]

Public health researchers have often approached IPV using a surveillance framework, in which the goal is to quantify, monitor, and reduce risk factors that negatively affect population health.[83] In the last decade, they have adopted a multilevel socioecological model. Primary prevention has consisted of risk reduction seeking to prevent the initial occurrence of IPV through early education, changing sex role-stereotyped attitudes and behaviors. More recently the focus has been on changing social norms and on working to achieve gender equality in terms of power differentials between men and women.[84] There is broader understanding of the need to break the intergenerational cycle of violence through early intervention targeting children who witness or experience violence.[85] Secondary prevention now includes multisectoral identification of women at risk with appropriate evaluated interventions, such as advocacy.[80] A socioecological model presupposes intervention acting on multiple levels.[86]

Intervention for Women Experiencing IPV

Rigorous evidence on interventions that have lasting effects in reducing IPV levels is beginning to emerge and supports the use of advocacy, social support, and early intervention strategies along with programs designed to decrease the proximal influences of environmental stressors and interpersonal conflict that may precipitate IPV. The Nurse Family Partnership, evaluated through randomized controlled trials, found that low-income women who had received nurse visits before and after birth reported decreased IPV.[35,87]

A recent Cochrane review found modest evidence for a protective effect of advocacy-based interventions to support women disclosing IPV in health or social service settings.[80] The strongest initial evidence for advocacy interventions came from a randomized controlled trial

of community-based advocacy support for women in shelters provided evidence that advocacy interventions could offer effective secondary prevention for women experiencing severe abuse.[88] A follow-up study explored the mechanisms by which the intervention worked, finding that the initial advocacy assisted women to access needed resources and to increase social support, increasing overall quality of life, which then seemed to serve as a protective factor.[79] Though health and social systems may be prime candidates for intervention programs, such programs must ensure approaches to minimize differences in access to and use of care by vulnerable groups. Bent-Goodley[36,89,90] documents how women of color often first seek out services via informal providers, such as faith-based communities and friends, as opposed to resorting to mental health, criminal justice, or health professionals as a primary alternative.

The increase in the number of interactions with healthcare providers during pregnancy provides opportunities for intervention with women who may otherwise be isolated from health care.[91] The increasing availability of orders of protection and better trained policing may also offer promising avenues for intervention that are largely unevaluated.

Health Consequences of IPV

The WHO world report on violence and health[86] identifies various IPV outcomes found to be highly correlated with the experience of IPV by women:

- **Physical**: abdominal and thoracic injuries, bruises and welts, chronic pain, disability, fibromyalgia, fractures, gastrointestinal disorders, irritable bowel syndrome, lacerations and abrasions, ocular damage, decreased physical function.
- **Psychological and behavioral**: alcohol and drug misuse, depression, anxiety, eating and sleeping disorders, feelings of shame and guilt, phobias and panic disorders, physical inactivity, poor self-esteem, posttraumatic stress disorder, psychosomatic disorders, smoking, suicidal behavior and self-harm, unsafe sexual behaviors.
- **Sexual and reproductive**: Gynecological disorders, infertility, pelvic inflammatory disease, pregnancy complication, sexual dysfunction, unwanted pregnancy, unsafe abortion, sexually transmitted infections including human immune deficiency virus (HIV).
- **Fatal health consequences**: AIDS-related mortality, maternal mortality, homicide, suicide.

The high prevalence rates of IPV among women seeking medical care have been captured by numerous studies both for injury-related and noninjury-related visits. Both clinical and population-based studies demonstrate women who have experienced IPV are at increased risk of emergency visits and hospitalization for health conditions not directly connected to injury—somatic complaints, obstetric complications, and psychiatric diagnoses.[92] Although injuries from IPV are not the sole reason that abused women present to the emergency department (ED), evidence suggests that women experiencing IPV often visit the ED with noninjury complaints and then later return to the ED with IPV-related injuries.[93]

Physical impacts of IPV are often dose-dependent such that as either duration or severity of IPV increases, so too does outcome severity, including fractures, head trauma, disfiguring, and death.[61,94,95] Moreover, the influence of different types and multiple episodes of abuse can persist long after the abuse itself has stopped.[95,96] Women who have experienced IPV are also more likely to perceive their overall health as poor.[97,98] Studies demonstrate that women who have experienced physical or sexual abuse experience ill health more frequently than other women, particularly in regard to physical functioning, psychological well-being, and the adoption of further risk behaviors, including smoking, physical inactivity, and alcohol and drug use.[95,96,99,100] In addition, women involved in violent relationships have faced restriction in accessing services, public life, and emotional support from friends[70] resulting in failure to address health problems with effective intervention.

Injury Resulting from IPV

IPV is one of the primary causes of nonfatal injuries to women, characterized in particular by injuries to the face, neck, upper torso, breast, and abdomen.[29] Women seeking medical attention for head, neck, and facial injuries are 7.5 times more likely to be victims of IPV than women with injuries limited to other locations.[101] A 2000 review[102] estimates that half of all acute injuries and one in five of injuries in women acutely requiring surgery were the result of IPV. A national population-based study found that 40% of the almost 5 million sexual and physical IPV assaults perpetrated against women annually result in an injury.[15]

Case Fatality and IPV Injury

Campbell et al.[15] identify nine near-lethal incidents for every IPV femicide (gunshot or stab wound to head, neck or torso; choking or immersion in water to the point of unconsciousness; severe head injuries with a blunt object weapon). Campbell et al. suggest the risk factors for near-lethal IPV incidents against women were substantially the same as for femicide (including approximately 75% with prior IPV experience).

Intimate Partner Homicide

Due to varying definitions, health and justice department systems report somewhat different estimates for the proportion of men and of women killed by an intimate partner, but in both systems, far higher proportions of murders in women are caused by an intimate partner. In 2000, three times as many women as men were reported murdered by an intimate partner according to Bureau of Justice Statistics. In addition, they report that 30% of all murders of women are caused by an intimate partner compared to only 5% of murders of men.[103,104] Based on state- and national-level health data, 40%–50% of all female

homicides were committed by a male intimate partner.[15] Data from 13 states participating in the National Violent Death Reporting System found that 77.2% of all intimate partner homicide victims in 2003 were women.[21]

Among states participating in the NVDRS, 20% of homicides were directly associated with intimate partner conflict and among cases of homicide followed by a suicide, 58% of the victims were a current or former partner of the perpetrator. In these cases, 92% of the perpetrators were male and 75% of the victims were female.[105,106] Lee et al.[107] note the IPV homicide rate for African American women is more than twice that observed for white women, despite little difference between white women and African American women in lifetime incidence of IPV.

In an 11-city case control study, 70% of the male perpetrators were using drugs and/or alcohol at the time of the homicide incident.[108] Other identified risk factors associated with intimate partner femicide include perpetrator's unemployment status, avoidance of arrest for IPV, access to a firearm, previous threat with a weapon, victim's child by another man, estrangement particularly from a controlling partner, a highly controlling partner, attempted strangulation, along with prior physical violence against the victim serving as a primary risk factor.[15,108] Firearms were the major weapon used in intimate partner homicides from 1981 to 1998.[109] Other significant bivariate-level risks include stalking, forced sex, and abuse during pregnancy.[15,108,110] In addition, never having lived together, as well as prior IPV arrest, were associated with lower risks of homicide.

Research evidence offers potential for intervention to prevent femicide. Campbell et al.[15] demonstrate that the greatest risk factor for intimate partner homicide, regardless of the gender of the victim (65–70% of cases where the female is killed; 75% of the cases where the male partner is killed), is prior IPV perpetrated against the female partner. In addition, various studies suggest that approximately 40% of female intimate partner homicide victims had been in contact with the healthcare system within 1 or 2 years of their death.[43,111] The majority of victims or perpetrators (up to 83% of the cases) or both had contact with criminal justice, victim assistance, and/or healthcare agencies in the year prior to the homicide, which indicates opportunities for intervention.[15]

Reproductive and Sexual Health

Both physical and sexual IPV are associated with a range of adverse sexual or reproductive outcomes including sexual risk-taking behaviors. Concepts of reproductive choice, including factors such as consent, timing, type of sexual activity, pregnancy and disease prophylaxis, condom use, and pregnancy retention, are often highly restricted within the context of an abusive relationship, which may lead to unintended pregnancies associated with serious risks to maternal, perinatal, and infant health.[50] For instance, women experiencing IPV may be less likely to negotiate using condoms for fear of greater abuse or subject to birth control obstruction, placing them in a position of enhanced risk for contracting HIV and other sexually transmitted infections (STIs).[112–114] Furthermore, women who are HIV positive and experiencing IPV may face barriers to health care and be less likely to adhere to antiretroviral medication regimes.[115,116]

Sexual Abuse

Sexual abuse frequently involves physical abuse or the threat of physical abuse. Sexual and physical violence combined have been found to be more detrimental to physical and emotional health than experiencing physical violence alone.[61,117] Coker's systematic literature review offers strong evidence that physical IPV is consistently associated with sexual risk taking, inconsistent condom use, partner nonmonogamy, having an unplanned pregnancy or induced abortion, having a STI, and other sexual or reproductive dysfunction.[118] Coercing and controlling female partners through force or fear to engage in risky behaviors, including illicit drug use and sex work, may substantially increase risk for HIV and other threats to well-being, including incarceration.[113]

HIV, STIs, and IPV

Partner violence puts women at risk of HIV, particularly through inconsistent condom use.[119] In turn, HIV infection puts women at higher risk of IPV. Gielen et al.[113] conclude HIV-positive women may be at risk for elevation in IPV when their HIV status is disclosed. Rates of lifetime physical or sexual IPV were nearly equivalent between HIV-positive and HIV-negative women and across seven cross-sectional and longitudinal studies comparing HIV-negative and HIV-positive samples. Moreover, studies find higher severity and greater frequency of IPV among HIV-positive women in comparison to HIV-negative women, findings consistent with Wyatt et al.[112] that noted HIV-positive women report more severe trauma histories.

Pregnancy and IPV

In addition to unwanted pregnancy, an outcome of physical and sexual IPV, a pregnancy often precipitates physical abuse.[50] Though prevalence estimates for IPV during pregnancy vary, pregnancy is generally acknowledged to be a time of increased risk for IPV. In a review, Gazmararian et al.[91] identified substantial variation in IPV occurrence during pregnancy though the majority were in the range of 4% to 8%, consistent with findings from U.S. statewide surveys. According to Saltzman et al.,[120] 50–70% of women who experienced IPV prior to pregnancy experience it again during pregnancy. Approximately 14% report a first incident of abuse during a pregnancy.[121]

Characteristics that increase the likelihood of IPV during pregnancy include being less than 20 years old, having less than a high school education, economic difficulties, use of alcohol, tobacco or other drugs, prior STIs, unmarried status, current or prior unintended pregnancy and/or termination, interpregnancy interval of less than 24 months, and history of suicidal ideation, depression, or other psychiatric illness.[91,122]

IPV during pregnancy is a significant health concern with harms extending beyond the victim and implications from preconception through the postpartum period.[91] Women living in Seattle who experienced IPV during pregnancy that was reported to the police had a higher rate of antenatal hospitalization compared to women without such a report who had a singleton or a fetal death during the same time period.[123] Janssen et al.[124] report on the impact of exposure to physical intimate partner violence during pregnancy in almost 5,000 Vancouver women. They found a substantial and significant increase in antepartum hemorrhage (OR = 3.79), intrauterine growth restriction (OR = 3.0), and perinatal death (OR = 8.0). If a woman feared her partner but did not receive physical violence, there was no association with adverse pregnancy outcomes. Findings from numerous other studies indicate that women who experience IPV during pregnancy frequently have delayed prenatal care, show a substantial increase in their own prenatal and perinatal health conditions (including infection, high blood pressure, uterine rupture, and a higher incidence of fetal injury), experience more premature birth, and have babies with lower birth weight and increased need for intensive care and other healthcare service needs after birth.[29,37] Moreover, IPV during pregnancy has been identified as a specific time-related risk factor for femicide.[15] Chang et al.[110] found homicide, which accounts for over 31% of maternal injury deaths, to be the leading cause of traumatic death for pregnant and recently pregnant women in the United States from 1991 to 1999.

Mental Health Outcomes

IPV has also been associated with a wide range of adverse mental health conditions often involving high-risk behavior in addition to the direct risk of injury and death. Mental health conditions include depression and posttraumatic stress disorder, drug use, and suicide.[29,94,117,125] Because few studies are longitudinal, few can clarify the interrelationships, chronicity, or sequence of evolution. Bonomi et al.[94] and Plichta[37] draw attention to the lack of studies simultaneously focusing on or disentangling relationships between the nature of IPV exposure and women's health, differential healthcare use, and co-occurrence of risk behaviors. Uncertainty remains as to whether these health problems result from or increase risk for IPV.

IPV is strongly associated with an increase in the development of a mental health condition and with an exacerbation of an existing one. As in the case of alcohol and substance abuse, the direction of effect may be dual in that the experience of IPV may lead to a mental health condition such as depression whereas an existing mental illness may increase vulnerability to IPV. A meta-analysis of mental illness among women who had experienced IPV conducted in 1999 found three to five times the risk of depression, suicidal ideation or attempts, posttraumatic stress disorder (PTSD), and substance use in comparison to those who have not experienced IPV.[126] Many other mental health conditions such as anxiety, low self-esteem, eating disorders, sleep disorders, personality disorders, and nonaffective psychosis have also been associated with exposure to IPV.[61,127,128] Differences in risk of depression have been linked to severity and chronicity of abuse, co-occurrence of IPV types or extent of violence experienced, and the presence or absence of social support and safety options.[13,19,29,76,117] Numerous studies report the co-occurrence of IPV, HIV risk, and substance use and underscore the significance of such comorbidity in women's lives, particularly those comprising most highly vulnerable subgroups.[113] Major depression is often comorbid with PTSD in women experiencing IPV.[117] Multiple experiences of victimization throughout adulthood and childhood, especially among women experiencing current IPV with previous experience of childhood sexual abuse, have been found to be associated with a higher prevalence of PTSD.

Areas for Future Research

Research in IPV prevention and intervention is a clear priority for future investigations and is now a priority for the CDC, the National Institutes of Health, and the National Institute of Justice as well as for major advocacy organizations. The National Academy reported on some recommendations in 2004.[129] Priorities for research include the study of strategies on how to shift social norms that tolerate or accept IPV and on better understanding how IPV occurrence is determined in part by the socioecological context.

Multilevel studies that take account of the socioecological model proposed by Heise[42] and replicated in the *World Report on Violence and Health*[86] published by WHO (Figure 20-1) will be essential in moving toward effective prevention. Jewkes suggests primary prevention strategies addressing IPV by targeting poverty, reducing alcohol consumption, and improving the status of women[130] consistent with these recommendations. Cunradi[68] suggests that public health approaches to changing the availability of alcohol through policy interventions may be a fruitful approach to prevention. Also important is the implementation of longitudinal approaches to better understand how relationship violence develops across the life span and across generations. Longitudinal research is essential in understanding the complex temporal relationships between IPV and other health problems. Improving the quality of IPV information in routinely collected data including guidelines for definitions and opportunities for linkage is essential.

During the last decade substantial progress has been achieved in understanding differential patterns of IPV, distinguishing situational couple violence from "intimate

terrorism" and making better sense of what appeared to be decades of conflicting research findings and subsequent differential interpretation. Epidemiologists need to investigate the development and consequences of these different typologies to lay the groundwork for public health strategies to prevent the prevalent, harmful, and intergenerational consequences of IPV.

Summary

A high percentage of American women experience intimate partner violence at some point across their life course, resulting in lasting physical and psychological damage at great cost to their families, communities, and society. Although women in all cultural and racial groups have been at risk of violence within family settings, among disadvantaged members of society the prevalence of intimate partner violence is greater, often occurring at younger ages and with greater frequency. However, researchers have difficulty obtaining accurate measures of IPV due to study factors such as: identification of appropriate study populations, differing definitions of abuse, and varying lengths of exposure to abuse. In addition, study participants may limit responses to questionnaires or interviews due to a desire for confidentiality. Women experiencing IPV are more vulnerable to acquiring sexually transmitted infections and pregnancies; therefore, healthcare providers are valuable contributors to detection of IPV. During routine examination clinicians may observe evidence of physical or sexual abuse and through nonjudgmental questioning may identify patients' experiences of psychological or emotional abuse requiring referral to appropriate treatment. Because of the personal and societal burden created by IPV, the World Health Organization and the Institute of Medicine, as well as other agencies have advocated a multidimensional approach to prevention though coordinated efforts within communities, states and by the federal government to reduce levels of poverty, mental illness and substance abuse that are major contributors to intimate partner violence.

Discussion Questions

1. What interventions to prevent partner violence might be developed as a result of a public health approach rather than a clinical approach?
2. How does Johnson's typology of different forms of couples violence assist in explaining the differences in prevalence found when considering severity of impact compared to occurrence of behaviors?
3. Discuss the debate on whether healthcare professionals should screen all women for partner violence. How do you balance the views and wishes of women against the WHO guidelines for screening?
4. How would prospective longitudinal studies help untangle the co-occurrence of violence, depression, and substance use?
5. Might partner violence have an impact on longer term chronic illness such as cardiovascular disease? What might be the mechanism? How would you study this?

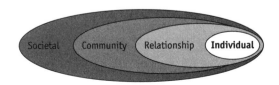

Figure 20-1 Socio-ecological model for understanding violence.

Source: Reproduced from Krug EG et al., eds. World report on violence and health, Geneva: World Health Organization, 2002.

References

1. National Center for Injury Prevention and Control. *Costs of Intimate Partner Violence against Women in the United States.* Atlanta: Centers for Disease Control and Prevention; 2003.

2. Thompson RS, Bonomi AE, Anderson M, et al. Intimate partner violence: prevalence, types, and chronicity in adult women. *Am J Prev Med.* 2006; 30:447–457.

3. Tjaden P, Thoennes N. *Full Report of the Prevalence, Incidence, and Consequences of Violence against Women: Findings from the National Violence against Women Survey: Research Report.* Rockville, MD: National Institute of Justice, Centers for Disease Control; 2000.

4. Whitaker DJ, Halleyesus T, Swahn M, Saltzman LS. Differences in frequency of violence and reported injury between relationships with reciprocal and nonreciprocal intimate partner violence. *Am J Public Health.* 2007;97: 941–947.

5. Gerberding J. National Center for Injury Prevention and Control. *Costs of Intimate Partner Violence Against Women in the United States.* Atlanta, GA: Centers for Disease Control and Prevention; 2003.

6. Corso PS, Mercy JA, Simon TR, et al. Medical costs and productivity losses due to interpersonal and self-directed violence in the United States. *Am J Prev Med.* 2007;32:474–482.

7. Campbell JC, Moracco KE, Saltzman LE. Future directions for violence against women and reproductive health: science, prevention, and action. *Matern Child Health J.* 2000;4:149–154.

8. Gelles R, Straus M. *Intimate Violence: The Causes and Consequences of Abuse in the American Family.* New York: Simon and Schuster; 1988.

9. Stark E, Flitcraft A, Frazier W. Medicine and patriarchal violence: the social construction of a "private" event. *Int J Health Serv.* 1979;9:461–493.

10. Factsheet: The Violence Against Women Act. http://www.whitehouse.gov/sites/default/files/docs/vawa_factsheet.pdf. Accessed November, 2012.

11. Office of Violence Against Women: United States Department of Justice. http://www.ovw.usdoj.gov/index.html. Accessed November 2012.

12. Saltzman LE, Fanslow JL, McMahon PM, Shelley GA. *Intimate Partner Violence Surveillance: Uniform Definitions and Recommended Data Elements, ver. 1.0.* Atlanta, GA: U.S. Department of Health and Human Services, Public Health Service, Centers for Disease Control and Prevention; 2002.

13. Bogat GA, Levendosky AA, von Eye A. The future of research on intimate partner violence: person-oriented and variable-oriented perspectives. *Am J Community Psychol.* 2005;36:49–70.

14. Johnson MP. Conflict and control: gender symmetry and asymmetry in domestic violence. *Violence against Women.* 2006;12:1003–1018.

15. Campbell JC, Glass N, Sharps PW, et al. Intimate partner homicide: review and implications of research and policy. *Trauma, Violence Abuse.* 2007;8: 246–269.

16. Lown EA, Schmidt LA, Wiley J. Interpersonal violence among women seeking welfare: unraveling lives. *Am J Public Health.* 2006;96:1409–1415.

17. Pavao J, Alvarez J, Baumrind N, et al. Intimate partner violence and housing instability. *Am J Prev Med.* 2007;32:143–146.

18. Bureau of Justice Statistics Special Report, *Intimate Partner Violence and Age of Victim,* 1993–99. Washington, DC: U.S. Department of Justice; 2001.

19. Cascardi M, Langhinrichsen J, Vivian D. Marital aggression: Impact, injury, and health correlates for husbands and wives. *Arch Inter Med.* 1992;152:1178–1184.

20. Brush LD. Violent acts and injurious outcomes in married couples: methodological issues in the national survey of families and households. *Gender and Society.* 1990;4:56–67.

21. Breiding MJ, Black MC, Ryan GW. Prevalence and risk factors of intimate partner violence in eighteen U.S. states/territories, 2005. *Am J Prev Med.* 2008;34:112–118.

22. Freedner N, Freed LH, Yang YW, Austin SB. Dating violence among gay, lesbian, and bisexual adolescents: results from a community survey. *J Adolesc Health.* 2002;31:469–474.

23. Graham-Kevan N, Archer J. Intimate terrorism and common couple violence: a test of Johnson's predictions in four British samples. *J Interpers Violence.* 2003;18:1247–1270.

24. Stark E. *Coercive Control: How Men Entrap Women in Personal Life.* New York: Oxford University Press; 2007.

25. Thompson MP, Basile KC, Hertz MF, Sitterle D. *Measuring Intimate Partner Violence Victimization and Perpetration: A Compendium of Assessment Tools.* Atlanta, GA: Centers for Disease Control and Prevention, National Center for Injury Prevention and Control; 2006.

26. MacMillan HL, Wathen CN, Jamieson E, et al. Violence Against Women Research Group. Screening for intimate partner violence in health care settings: a randomized trial. *JAMA.* 2009;302:493–501.

27. Ramsay J, Richardson J, Carter YH, et al. Should health professionals screen women for domestic violence? *BMJ.* 2002;325:314–319.

28. Wathen CN, MacMillan HL. Interventions for violence against women: scientific review. *JAMA.* 2003;289:589–600.

29. Campbell JC. Health consequences of intimate partner violence. *Lancet.* 2002;359(9314):1331–1336.

30. Zeitler MS, Paine AD, Breitbart V, et al. Attitudes about intimate partner violence screening among an ethnically diverse sample of young women. *J Adolesc Health.* 2006;39:119.1–8.

31. Saltzman LE, Houry D. Prevalence of nonfatal and fatal intimate partner violence in the United States. In: Mitchell C, Anglin D, eds. *Intimate Partner Violence: A Health-Based Perspective,* New York: Oxford University Press; 2009:31–38.

32. Centers for Disease Control and Prevention. Intimate partner violence: data sources. http://www.cdc.gov/ViolencePrevention/intimatepartnerviolence/datasources.html. Accessed May 1, 2011.

33. Bachman RA. Comparison of annual incidence rates and contextual characteristics of intimate-partner violence against women from the National Crime Victimization Survey (NCVS) and the National Violence against Women Survey (NVAWS). *Violence Against Women.* 2000;6:839–867.

34. Williams LM. Understanding child abuse and violence against women: a life course perspective. *J Interpers Violence.* 2003;18:441–451.

35. Marks JS, Cassidy EF. Does a failure to count mean that it fails to count? Addressing intimate partner violence. *Am J Prev Med.* 2006;30:530–531.

36. Bent-Goodley TB. Health disparities and violence against women: why and how cultural and societal influences matter. *Trauma Violence Abuse.* 2007;8:90–104.

37. Plichta SB. Intimate partner violence and physical health consequences: policy and practice implications. *J Interpers Violence.* 2004;19:1296–1323.

38. Sugg NK, Inui T. Primary care physicians' response to domestic violence: opening Pandora's box. *JAMA.* 1992;267:3157–3160.

39. Easteal PW, Easteal S. Attitudes and practices of doctors toward spouse assault victims: an Australian study. *Violence Victims.* 1992;7: 217–228.

40. Feder GS, Hutson M, Ramsay J, Taket AR. Women exposed to intimate partner violence: expectations and experiences when they encounter health care professionals: a meta-analysis of qualitative studies. *Arch Intern Med.* 2006;166:22–37.

41. Davidson LL, Grisso JA, Garcia-Moreno C, et al. Training programs for healthcare professionals in domestic violence. *J Womens Health Gend Based Med.* 2001;10:953–969.

42. Heise LL. Violence against women: an integrated, ecological framework. *Violence against Women.* 1998;4:262–290.

43. Crandall ML, Nathens AB, Kernic MA, et al. Predicting future injury among women in abusive relationships. *J Trauma.* 2004;56:906–912.

44. Ehrensaft MK, Cohen P, Brown J, et al. Intergenerational transmission of partner violence: a 20-year prospective study. *J Consulting Clin Psychol.* 2003;71:741–753.

45. Bensley L, Van Eenwyk J, Wynkoop Simmons K. Childhood family violence history and women's risk for intimate partner violence and poor health. *Am J Prev Med.* 2003;25:38–44.

46. McCloskey LA, Walker M. Posttraumatic stress in children exposed to family violence and single-event trauma. *J Am Acad Child Adolesc Psychiatry.* 2000;39:108–115.

47. Dube SR, Anda RF, Felitti VJ, et al. Exposure to abuse, neglect and household dysfunction among adults who witnessed intimate partner violence as children: implications for health and social services. *Violence Victims.* 2002;17:3–17.

48. Widom CS. Does violence beget violence? A critical examination of the literature. *Psychol Bull.* 1989;106:3–28.

49. Taylor CA, Guterman NB, Lee SJ, Rathouz PJ. Intimate partner violence, maternal stress, nativity, and risk for maternal maltreatment of young children. *Am J Public Health.* 2009;99:175–183.

50. Pallitto CC, Campbell JC, O'Campo P. Is intimate partner violence associated with unintended pregnancy? A review of the literature. *Trauma, Violence Abuse.* 2005;6:217–235.

51. Lloyd S, Taluc N. The effects of male violence on female employment. *Violence against Women.* 1999;5:370–392.

52. Dearwater SR, Coben JH, Campbell JC, et al. Prevalence of intimate partner abuse in women treated at community hospital emergency departments. *JAMA.* 1998;280:433–438.

53. Hastings JE, Hamberger LK. Sociodemographic predictors of violence. *Psychiatr Clin North Am.* 1997;20:323–335.

54. Lee Y-S, Hadeed L. Intimate partner violence among Asian immigrant communities: health/mental health consequences, help-seeking behaviors and service utilization. *Trauma, Violence Abuse.* 2009;10:143–170.

55. Klevans J. An overview of intimate partner violence among Latinos. *Violence against Women.* 2007;13:111–122.

56. Frye V, Galea S, Tracy M, et al. The role of neighborhood environment and risk of intimate partner femicide in a large urban area. *Am J Public Health.* 2008;98:1473–1479.

57. Orloff L, Kaguyutan JV. Offering a helping hand: legal protections for battered immigrant women, a history of legislative responses. *Am Univ J Gender, Social Policy and the Law.* 2002;10:95–183.

58. Bassuk EL, Rosenberg L. Why does family homelessness occur? A case-control study. *Am J Public Health* 1988;78:783–788.

59. Goodman LA, Dutton MA, Harris M. Episodically homeless women with serious mental illness: prevalence of physical and sexual assault. *Am J Orthopsychiatry.* 1995;65:468–478.

60. Black M, Breiding M. Adverse health conditions and health risk behaviors associated with intimate partner violence—United States, 2005. *MMWR Morb Mortal Wkly Rep.* 2008;57:113–117.

61. Coker AL, Smith PH, Bethea L, et al. Physical health consequences of physical and psychological intimate partner violence. *Arch Fam Med*. 2000;9: 451–457.

62. Grisso JA, Schwarz DF, Hirschinger N, et al. Violent injuries among women in an urban area. *N Engl J Med*. 1999;341:1899–1905.

63. Kyriacou DN, Anglin D, Taliaferro E, et al. Risk factors for injury to women from domestic violence. *N Engl J Med*. 1999;341:1892–1898.

64. Caetano R, Schafer J, Cunradi CB. Alcohol-related intimate partner violence among white, black, and Hispanic couples in the United States. *Alcohol Res Health*. 2001;25:58–65.

65. Kantor GK, Straus MA. Substance abuse as a precipitant of wife abuse victimizations. *Am J Drug Alcohol Abuse*. 1989;15:173–189.

66. Flanzer JP. Alcohol and other drugs are key causal agents of violence. In: Gelles RJ, Loseke DL, eds. *CurrentCcontroversies on Family Violence*. Newbury Park, CA: Sage; 1993:171–181.

67. Foran HM, O'Leary KD. Alcohol and intimate partner violence: a meta-analytic review. *Clin Psychol Rev*. 2008;28:1222–1234.

68. Cunradi CB. Neighborhoods, alcohol outlets and intimate partner violence: addressing research gaps in explanatory mechanisms. *Int J Environ Res Public Health*. 2010;7:799–813.

69. Capaldi DM, Kim HK. Typological approaches to violence in couples: a critique and alternative conceptual approach. *Clin Psychol Rev*. 2007;27: 253–265.

70. Heise LL, Garcia Moreno C. Violence by intimate partners. In: *World Report on Violence and Health*. Geneva, Switzerland: World Health Organization; 2002:87–121.

71. Cunradi CB, Caetano R, Clark C, Schafer J. Neighborhood poverty as a predictor of intimate partner violence among White, Black, and Hispanic couples in the United States: a multilevel analysis. *Ann Epidemiol*. 2000;10: 297–308.

72. Browning CR. The span of collective efficacy: extending social disorganization theory to partner violence. *J Marriage Fam*. 2002;64:833–850.

73. O'Campo P. Invited commentary: Advancing theory and methods for multilevel models of residential neighborhoods and health. *Am J Epidemiol*. 2003;157:9–13.

74. O'Campo P, Burke J, Peak GL, et al. Uncovering neighbourhood influences on intimate partner violence using concept mapping. *J Epidemiol Community Health*. 2005;59:603–608.

75. Goodman LA, Dutton MA, Vankos N, Weinfurt K. Women's resources and use of strategies as risk and protective factors for re-abuse over time. *Violence Against Women*. 2005;11:311–336.

76. Campbell JC, Rose LE, Kub J. The role of social support and family relationships in women's responses to battering. *Health Care Women Int*. 2000;21:27–39.

77. Carlson BE, McNutt LA, Choi DY, Rose IM. Intimate partner abuse and mental health: the role of social support and other protective factors. *Violence Against Women*. 2002;8:720–745.

78. Coker AL, Smith PH, Thompson, MP, et al. Social support protects against the negative effects of partner violence on mental health. *J Womens Health Gend Based Med*. 2002;11:465–476.

79. Bybee DI, Sullivan CM. The process through which an advocacy intervention resulted in positive change for battered women over time. *Am J Community Psychol*. 2002;30:103–132.

80. Ramsay J, Carter Y, Davidson LL, et al. Advocacy interventions to reduce or eliminate violence and promote the physical and psychosocial well-being of women who experience intimate partner abuse. *Cochrane Database Syst Rev*. 2009;3. CD005043.

81. World Health Organization. *Preventing Violence: A Guide to Implementing the Recommendations of the World Report on Violence and Health*. Geneva, Switzerland: World Health Organization; 2004.

82. Institute of Medicine. *Confronting Chronic Neglect: The Education and Training of Health Professionals on Family Violence*. Washington, DC: National Academy Press; 2001.

83. Saltzman LE. Issues related to defining and measuring violence against women: response to Kilpatrick. *J Interpers Violence*. 2004;19:1235–1243.

84. Rice J. Preface. In: *Annals of the New York Academy of Sciences*, 1087 (Violence and Exploitation against Women and Girls). New York: New York Academy of Sciences; 2006:xi–xv.

85. Garcia-Moreno C, Jansen HA, Ellsberg M, et al. Public health: violence against women. *Science*. 2005;310(5752):1282–1283.

86. Krug EG. World Health Organization. *World Report on Violence and Health*. Geneva: World Health Organization; 2002.

87. Olds DL, Robinson J, O'Brien R, et al. Home visiting by paraprofessional and by nurse: a randomized-controlled trial. *Pediatrics*. 2004;110:486–496.

88. Sullivan CM, Bybee DI. Reducing violence using community-based advocacy for women with abusive partners. *J Consult Clin Psychol*. 1999;67:43–53.

89. Bent-Goodley TB. Perceptions of domestic violence: a dialogue with African American women. *Health Soc Work*. 2004;29:307–316.

90. Bent-Goodley TB. Domestic violence and kinship care: connecting policy with practice. *J Health Soc Policy*. 2006;22:65–83.

91. Gazmararian JA, Petersen R, Spitz AM, et al. Violence and reproductive health: current knowledge and future research directions. *Matern Child Health J*. 2000;4:79–84.

92. Kernic MA, Wolf ME, Holt VL. Rates and relative risk of hospital admission among women in violent intimate partner relationships. *Am J Public Health*. 2000;90:1416–1420.

93. Muelleman RL, Liewer JD. How often do women in the emergency department without intimate violence injuries return with such injuries? *Acad Emerg Med*. 1998;5:982–985.

94. Bonomi AE, Thompson RS, Anderson M, et al. Intimate partner violence and women's physical, mental, and social functioning. *Am J Prev Med*. 2006;30:458–466.

95. Koss MP, Woodruff WJ, Koss PG. Criminal victimization among primary care medical patients: prevalence, incidence, and physician usage. *Behav Sci Law*. 1991;9:85–96.

96. Felitti VJ, Anda RF, Nordenberg D, et al. Relationship of childhood abuse and household dysfunction to many of the leading causes of death in adults. The Adverse Childhood Experiences (ACE) Study. *Am J Prev Med*. 1998;14:245–258.

97. Lown EA, Vega WA. Intimate partner violence and health: self-assessed health, chronic health, and somatic symptoms among Mexican American women. *Psychosom Med*. 2001;63:352–360.

98. Resnick HS, Acierno R, Kilpatrick DG. Health Impact of interpersonal violence. 2: Medical and mental health outcomes. *Behav Med*. 1997;23:65–78.

99. Golding JM. Sexual assault history and limitation in physical functioning in two population samples. *Res Nurs Health*. 1996;19:33–44.

100. Dickinson LM, deGruy FV 3rd, Dickinson WP, Candib LM. Health-related quality of life and symptom profiles of female survivors of sexual abuse. *Arch Fam Med*. 1999;8:35–43.

101. Perciaccante VJ, Ochs HA, Dodson TB. Head, neck, and facial injuries as markers of domestic violence in women. *J Oral Maxillofac Surg*. 1999;57: 760–763.

102. Guth AA, Pachter L. Domestic violence and the trauma surgeon. *Am J Surgery*. 2000;179:134–140.

103. Bureau of Justice Statistics. *Intimate partner violence, 1993–2001*. Washington, DC: U.S. Department of Justice; 2003. Crime Data Brief NCJ 197838.

104. Bureau of Justice Statistics. *Intimate partner violence in the US, 1993–2004*. Washington, DC: U.S. Department of Justice; 2006.

105. Karch DL, Lubell KM, Friday J, et al. Surveillance for violent deaths—National Violent Death Reporting System, 16 states, 2005. *MMWR Morb Mortal Wkly Rep*. 2008;57(SS03):11–43,45.

106. Bossarte RM, Simon TR, Barker L. Characteristics of homicide followed by suicide incidents in multiple states, 2003–04. *Inj Prev*. 2006;12(suppl 2): ii33–ii38.

107. Lee RK, Thompson VL, Mechanic MB. Intimate partner violence and women of color: a call for innovations. *Am J Public Health*. 2002;92:530–534.

108. Campbell JC, Webster D, Koziol-McLain J, et al. Risk factors for femicide in abusive relationship: results from a multisite case controls study. *Am J Public Health*. 2003;93:1089–1097.

109. Sorenson SB, Wiebe DJ. Weapons in the lives of battered women. *Am J Public Health*. 2004;94:1412–1417.

110. Chang J, Berg CJ, Saltzman LE, Herndon J. Homicide: a leading cause of injury deaths among pregnant and postpartum women in the United States, 1991–1999. *Am J Public Health*. 2005;95:471–477.

111. Sharps PW, Koziol-McLain J, Campbell J, et al. Health care providers' missed opportunities for preventing femicide. *Prev Med*. 2001;33:373–380.

112. Wyatt GE, Myers HF, Williams JK. Does a history of trauma contribute to HIV risk for women of color? Implications for prevention and policy. *Am J Public Health*. 2002;92:660–665.

113. Gielen AC, Ghandour RM, Burke JG, et al. HIV/AIDS and intimate partner violence: intersecting women's health issues in the United States. *Trauma Violence Abuse*. 2007;8:178–198.

114. Wingood GM, DiClemente RJ, Harrington KF, et al. Efficacy of an HIV prevention program among female adolescents experiences gender-based violence. *Am J Public Health*. 2006;96:1085–1090.

115. Lichtenstein B. Domestic violence in barriers to health care for HIV-positive women. *AIDS Patient Care STDS*. 2006;20:122–132.

116. Beadnell B, Baker S, Knox K, et al. The influence of psychosocial difficulties on women's attrition in an HIV/STD prevention program. *AIDS Care*. 2003;15:807–820.

117. Dutton MA, Green BL, Kaltman SI, et al. Intimate partner violence, PTSD, and adverse health outcomes. *J Interpers Violence*. 2006;21:955–968.

118. Coker AL. Does physical intimate partner violence affect sexual health? A systematic review. *Trauma Violence Abuse*. 2007;8:149–177.

119. Frye V, Ompad D, Chan C. Intimate partner violence perpetration and condom use-related factors: associations with heterosexual men's consistent condom use. *AIDS Behav*. 2011;15:153–162.

120. Saltzman LE, Johnson CH, Gilbert BC, Goodwin MM. Physical abuse around the time of pregnancy: an examination of prevalence and risk factors in 16 states. *Matern Child Health J*. 2003;7:31–34.

121. Jasinski JL. Pregnancy and domestic violence. *Trauma Violence Abuse*. 2004;5: 47–64.

122. Bohn DK, Tebben JG, Campbell JC. Influences of income, education, age, and ethnicity on physical abuse before and during pregnancy. *J Obstet Gynecol Neonatal Nurs*. 2004;33:561–571.

123. Lipsky S, Holt VL, Easterling TR, Critchlow CW. Police-reported intimate partner violence during pregnancy and the risk of antenatal hospitalization. *Matern Child Health J*. 2004;8:55–63.

124. Janssen PA, Holt VL, Sugg NK, et al. Intimate partner violence and adverse pregnancy outcomes: a population-based study. *Am J Obstet Gynecol*. 2003;188:1341–1347.

125. Zlotnick C, Johnson DM, Kohn R. Intimate partner violence and long-term psychosocial functioning in a national sample of American women. *J Interpers Violence*. 2006;21:262–275.

126. Golding JM. Intimate partner violence as a risk factor for mental disorders: a meta-analysis. *J Family Violence*. 1999;14:99–132.

127. Danielson KK, Moffitt TE, Caspi A, Silva PA. Comorbidity between abuse of an adult and DSM-III-R disorders: evidence from an epidemiological study. *Am J Psychiatry*. 1998;155:131–133.

128. Plichta SB. Interactions between victims of intimate partner violence against women and the health care system: policy and practice implications. *Trauma Violence Abuse*. 2007;8:226–239.

129. Kruttschnitt C, McLaughlin BL, Petrie CV. *Advancing the Federal Research Agenda on Violence against Women*, Washington, DC: National Academies Press; 2004.

130. Jewkes R. Intimate partner violence: causes and prevention. *Lancet*. 2002;359(9315):1423–1429.

Endocrine and Autoimmune Conditions

Asthma

Judith S. Jacobson, DrPH, MBA

Introduction and Natural History

Asthma is a chronic (intermittent, persistent) condition in which the bronchi (airways) tend to become constricted, inflamed, and filled with mucus in response to allergens or other stimuli. Such exacerbations or attacks vary in frequency and resolve spontaneously, but may cause dyspnea (shortness of breath), wheezing (whistling sounds in the chest during breathing), and chest tightness. Even in the absence of an exacerbation, asthmatics may have persistent symptoms, such as frequent coughing as if to clear the throat, nighttime coughing, dyspnea in response to exertion, and chest tightness.

Asthma is highly variable in severity; among some individuals, symptoms are mild or occur only in the presence of specific triggers that can readily be avoided. Among other patients, the condition can be disabling or even fatal, sometimes with little or no warning. The condition also varies in age of onset, from infancy to old age. Many children who have asthma symptoms in the first year or two of life are symptom-free when they grow older. However, repeated exacerbations can contribute to lung remodeling and long-term deterioration of lung function.

Extrinsic or atopic (allergic) asthma is often considered a different phenotype from intrinsic asthma, in which exacerbations are not associated with exposure to particular allergens or allergy seasons but to airborne chemical pollutants and irritants, such as paint fumes, or cold air, physical exertion (including hearty laughter),[1] respiratory infections, or even psychological factors, such as anxiety. About 70% of asthmatics have allergies.[2] However, many people with atopic asthma also develop exacerbations due to cold air and other factors considered triggers for intrinsic asthma.

Adult onset asthma may be related to occupational exposures or to catastrophic events, such as the September 11, 2001 attack on the World Trade Center; the high volume of combustion products clearly played a causal role in the development of asthma among many individuals who worked at Ground Zero in the weeks and months after the September 11 attack.[3]

For many years, asthma was thought to be a relatively rare disease and one that mainly affected the affluent. However, during the past 40 years, the prevalence of the condition has risen markedly worldwide. Increasingly, in developed countries, it affects residents of low-income urban communities. In the United States, prevalence increased by 75% from 1980 to 1994.[4] The annual economic cost of asthma is estimated at $19.7 billion.[5] In 2003, the condition accounted for 12.8 million missed school days among children aged 5–17 years and about 10.1 million missed work days among adults aged 18 and over.[6] In 2005, asthma accounted for 3,384 deaths.[7] More than 18 million adults in the United States suffer from asthma. Current asthma prevalence (a doctor's diagnosis of asthma plus symptoms in the past year) is 8.2% overall, 6.0% among males and 10.3% among females.[8] However, among children, asthma is more prevalent among males than females (Figure 21-1).

Among the elderly, asthma is often underdiagnosed.[9] Seniors with asthma often have less lung compliance and respiratory muscle strength; less of a sensation of air hunger and bronchoconstriction; less energy expenditure; and more progressive, irreversible, and severe disease than younger patients. Mortality data are ambiguous, but some data suggest that asthma mortality is higher among individuals aged 65 and over than in younger age groups. Seniors also may have comorbid conditions, such as cardiac disease, that complicate treatment. Whether asthma in the elderly who have late-onset disease differs from that in individuals who had developed the condition at younger ages is unknown; no cohort studies specifically focusing on elderly people with asthma have been published.

Asthma as a Women's Health Issue

Among infants, the male/female ratio of wheeze (asthma cannot be definitively diagnosed in small children) prevalence is high; the gender difference is often attributed to slower fetal lung maturation[10] and higher rates of preterm birth among males.[11] However, during puberty, boys outstrip girls in thoracic growth rates, and their lung capacity continues to grow until later ages. Older adolescent boys generally have 25% greater lung function than girls of equal height.[12,13] Those patterns may help to account for the gender crossover of asthma that occurs in adolescence although the male/female ratio decreases throughout most

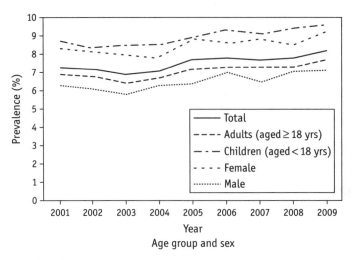

Figure 21-1 Asthma prevalence by age and gender.

Source: Reproduced from Zahran HS, Bailey C, Garbe P. Vital signs: Asthma prevalence, disease characteristics, and self-management education—United States, 2001–2009. Morbidity Mortality Weekly Report. 2011;60:547–552. http://www.cdc.gov/mmwr/preview/mmwrhtml/mm6017a4.htm

of the life span for reasons that are not well understood. Some evidence suggests that postmenopausal women are less likely to have asthma than younger women or men of comparable age.[14] However, as they age, women increasingly outnumber men; hence adult asthma is predominantly a disease of older women.[15]

Incidence

Asthma incidence is difficult to measure because it is not a reportable disease and no asthma registries exist. A diagnosis of asthma involves identification of episodic symptoms, such as wheezing, cough, shortness of breath, and chest tightness. The frequency of bronchial hyperresponsiveness and airflow obstruction fluctuates over time.[16] Spirometry is used to determine the adverse effects of challenge with methacholine (a mild lung irritant), cold air, or physical exertion on lung function and the ability of a bronchodilator to reverse those effects.

In population surveys asking about asthma, respondents are not always asked if they have had a doctor's diagnosis. A recent analysis of asthma incidence in the United States used data from the National Health Interview Survey (NHIS), relying on self-report from respondents who also provided information on other members of the household. To ascertain asthma status, respondents were asked: "During the past 12 months, did anyone in the family have asthma?" Respondents who answered *Yes* were then asked which family member and "When was the asthma first noticed?" Based on responses to those questions, incidence rates increased from 5.7 to 10.1 per 1,000 among children and from 1.2 to 4.0 per 1,000 among adults between 1980 and 1996.[17] Among adults, a gender crossover was observed; in 1982, the incidence rate was 4.8 per 1,000 among males and 2.2 per 1,000 among females, but by 1992 the rate was 3.7 per 1,000 among males and 6.2 per 1,000 among females. The change in female rates was statistically significant only among women. Incidence also increased more rapidly among nonwhites than whites (Figure 21-2).

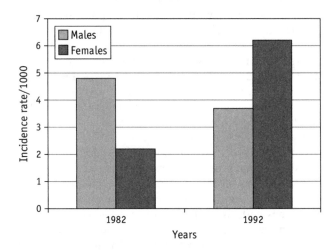

Figure 21-2 Gender crossover in asthma incidence rates.

Source: Reproduced from National Health Interview Survey, National Center for Health Statistics, Centers for Disease Control and Prevention.

Spectrum of Research

In response to the overall rising asthma prevalence and incidence rates, often described as an asthma epidemic, research is increasingly addressing the causes of asthma and assessing the potential epidemic levels including the relationship between asthma and gender. A number of studies have documented the age/gender crossover in asthma. Research has confirmed that asthmatic episodes may be affected by the menstrual cycle, pregnancy, and menopause but has not identified the mechanisms underlying the associations. Research is also addressing the relationship between allergy and reproductive hormones. Studies of common risk factors, both genetic and environmental, are increasingly considering differences by gender. Asthma among the elderly received little attention from investigators until recently, but the need for studies of the 65 and older age group is beginning to be recognized. Psychosocial factors, such as anxiety and domestic partner violence, are also beginning to be addressed. Differences by gender in disease severity, in the relationship between disease severity and standard measures of lung function, and in treatment response are also being acknowledged.

Risk Factors and Gender

A number of risk factors, some of them gender-related, are associated with asthma (Table 21-1).

Genetic/Familial Factors

Among the strongest risk factors for asthma is having a first-degree relative with asthma or atopy (the tendency to develop allergy symptoms and/or elevated immunoglobulin E (IgE) on exposure to common allergens). Several gene mutations or polymorphisms have been associated with asthma, some with age of onset or severity,[18] and a few specifically with gender differences in asthma. For example, in one of the few genetic studies stratified by gender, a polymorphism of the cytotoxic T lymphocyte-associated 4 receptor (CTLA-4) genotype was associated with cord blood and serum IgE, but only in females.[19,20] Estrogen receptor alpha gene polymorphisms have also been associated with bronchial hyperreactivity, particularly among females.[21] Genes have also been found to be associated with response to asthma therapy.[22] Researchers are exploring gender differences in phenotype and patterns of maternal and paternal inheritance. Some have found stronger associations of children's risk with maternal than paternal asthma, but whether that difference is due to children's environmental exposures being more like those of their mothers than of their fathers, to the greater availability of information about mothers' asthma and atopy status (in part because adult males may not recall their early childhood asthma), or to true differences in genetic inheritance patterns is not clear. Genetic risk is unlikely to account for the asthma epidemic or increasing incidence among women observed in recent decades.

Table 21-1

Asthma Risk Factors and Gender

Risk factor	Direction and gender relevance
Family history	Maternal asthma more associated with risk than paternal asthma
Genetic mutations/polymorphisms	Some associations with gender-specific risk
Ethnicity/immigration	Higher prevalence among blacks and Puerto Ricans Little gender stratification
Respiratory infections	Associated with early childhood asthma, especially in males Asthma trigger in adults
Smoking	Maternal smoking affects boys more than girls
Breastfeeding	Some evidence of benefit for breastfed children of both genders
Diet	Some evidence of benefit from Mediterranean diet Maternal diet may affect offspring's asthma risk No evidence of gender difference
Obesity	Obesity more associated with asthma in women than in men
Allergens	Allergens are asthma triggers in atopic patients; little evidence of gender difference in effects
Occupational exposures	Some evidence that workplace exposures to allergens and irritants affect women more than men; increase asthma risk in offspring
Reproductive/hormonal factors in females	
Menarche/puberty	Associated with increased asthma risk
Menstrual cycle	Exacerbations more common in luteal than follicular phase
Pregnancy/oral contraceptives	Associated with both risk and remission
Menopause	Associated with remission or reduced risk
Hormone replacement therapy	Associated with increased asthma risk
Psychosocial factors	Anxiety/depression associated with increased risk Partner violence associated with increased risk
Hygiene hypothesis	No evidence of gender difference

Ethnicity/Immigration/Socioeconomic Status

In the United States, asthma is notably more prevalent among African Americans and some Hispanic subgroups than among whites and Asians, and among those living in low-income urban neighborhoods than among those living in suburban or rural areas. Our recent studies of preschool-age children in New York City have found prevalence highest among children of Puerto Rican background and lowest in those of Mexican origin.[23] However, in international studies, asthma prevalence is highest in New Zealand, Britain, and the United States and lowest in the poorest countries of Africa and Latin America. In samples of 1,000 children each from 22 industrialized and developing countries collected for the International Study of Asthma and Allergies in Childhood (ISAAC) found the prevalence of wheeze attributable to skin prick test reactivity (a marker of atopy) strongly associated with gross national income, a measure of economic development.[24]

Several studies have confirmed low prevalence among Mexicans but increasing prevalence among Mexican Americans following immigration to the United States. The growth of minority and immigrant communities in U.S. inner cities in the last few decades of the 20th century is thought to have contributed to the asthma epidemic. The high prevalence of asthma in those communities is often attributed to poor housing conditions and proximity to sources of air pollution. Minority and immigrant women and children may be more exposed to those adverse environmental conditions, especially indoor air pollution, than men, who generally spend more time outdoors. Men are also more geographically and socially mobile due to work or cultural factors. The hygiene hypothesis (discussed later) suggests that lack of exposure to infectious agents may contribute to asthma risk. However, among Mexico- and U.S.-born children of Mexican-born parents living in Chicago, asthma was strongly associated with being born in the United States or immigrating at a young age with longer residence after controlling for other recognized risk factors, including exposure to animals or pets, history of infections, acetaminophen use, and antibiotic use in infancy.

Respiratory Infections

Asthma/wheeze in early childhood is strongly associated with a history of respiratory infections, including both viruses and ear infections, in early infancy.[26–28] Boys appear to be more susceptible to such infections than girls, but that difference in susceptibility may reflect the same developmental factors that account for boys' higher rates of asthma or may be on the causal pathway leading to early childhood asthma. Girls who have virus-associated wheezing in childhood are more likely than boys to develop severe asthma or, after an asthma-free period in later childhood and adolescence, to experience recurrence in adulthood.[29]

Airborne Pollutants, Smoking, and Environmental Tobacco Smoke

The rising prevalence rate of asthma during the 20th century may reflect changing patterns of smoking among women, which increased significantly when women joined the workforce during World War II. Among children exposed to maternal smoking *in utero*, boys showed larger deficits in lung function than girls at ages 7–19 years.[30] However, the effect of paternal smoking on children's lung function did not differ by the gender of the child.[31] Adolescent boys who smoke are more likely to wheeze than girls who smoke, perhaps because girls with labile airways are less likely to smoke than boys.[32] Other airborne pollutants, such as nitrogen dioxide and sulfur dioxide, have been associated with asthma exacerbations and emergency department admissions.

Breastfeeding

Children who have been breastfed are thought to have a lower risk for asthma than other children, but the data are equivocal. Studies differ in recording of breastfeeding history; some count children who were ever breastfed, however briefly, as exposed, while others include only children who were breastfed exclusively for at least 6 months. Some studies have found that the benefit accrues only to offspring of nonasthmatic or nonatopic mothers; others find the reverse. One hypothesis is that the benefit of breastfeeding lies in the passive immunity it confers, protecting the child from respiratory infections, during the high-risk months of infancy. However, if respiratory infection mediates that benefit, controlling for it may bias the effect of breastfeeding toward the null. There is little evidence that the benefits of breastfeeding differ between male and female offspring.[33]

Diet

A variety of dietary factors have been studied as possibly contributing to asthma prevention or control.[34] The evidence for a benefit of dietary antioxidants or antioxidant vitamin supplements has been considered strong enough to justify further research, including studies of the relationship between maternal diet during pregnancy and asthma in offspring,[35] but does not warrant recommendations for supplementation at this time. Vitamin D has been found to offer some protection against asthma and asthma severity.[36,37] The Mediterranean dietary pattern (high in fruits, vegetables, and fish and low in meat and saturated fats) has also shown a benefit in some but not all studies.[38] Gender differences in diet or in benefit from dietary components have not been studied.

Obesity

The asthma epidemic has developed concurrently with the current epidemic of obesity; these two major public health issues have similar geographical, socioeconomic, and racial distribution.[39] Studies have found that obesity is associated with asthma[40] and with asthma hospitalization[41] more in women than in men. In our New York City study of preschool children, an association of asthma/wheeze with overweight was driven by girls, not because girls were more likely than boys to be overweight but because a few very lean boys, but no very lean girls, were asthmatic.[23] A similar J-shaped association of asthma with body size has been observed among adult males.[42] A study of asthmatic adolescents noted a strong association between obesity and asthma-related hospitalizations as well as missed school days among boys more than among girls.[43] Further evidence for the association comes from findings that weight loss predicted improvement in asthma outcomes.[44]

Allergens

Allergy/atopy is strongly associated with asthma, and many asthma exacerbations are triggered by allergen exposure. However, contrary to widespread belief, it is not clear that allergen exposure actually induces the development of asthma.[45] Both indoor allergens (e.g., dust mite, cockroach, and mouse allergens) and seasonal plant allergens (e.g., ragweed) have been associated with asthma exacerbations. In a German birth cohort, atopy was not associated with asthma symptoms until age 5.[46] Our New York data identified differences in levels of specific IgE among preschool boys and girls, which may reflect differences in patterns of active play by gender.[47] Allergic and nonallergic rhinitis are strongly associated with asthma, as are allergen exposure[48] and allergic sensitization as measured by IgE,[49] but the pathways through which exposure to an allergenic substance may affect asthma status and the role of gender in these processes are poorly understood.

Occupational Exposures

About 10–15% of new-onset adult asthma is thought to be related to occupational exposure.[50] Many blue-collar and agricultural occupations[51] as well as pink-collar occupations[52] have been linked to asthma. Although efforts are being made to promote workplace safety, new materials are constantly being introduced; their safety in an industrial setting is often assumed in the absence of evidence of harm. Increasing incidence and prevalence of asthma among women have occurred as more women work outside the home. Some evidence suggests that women may be more likely than men to develop asthma in response to such exposures.[53] However, women, especially those employed in home cleaning,[54] are also exposed to allergens and irritants at home.[55] A diagnosis of asthma or asthma exacerbation linked to workplace exposures may lead to income loss and emotional distress.[56] In addition, both mothers' and fathers' workplace exposures have been linked to asthma in their offspring.[57]

Reproductive Events/Sex Hormones

Early puberty has been associated with asthma persistence, even when body size is taken into account.[58] New-onset of asthma after puberty has been linked to early menarche.[59] Among cycling women with asthma, more than 50% experienced increased symptoms and were more dependent on medications during the luteal phase than the follicular phase of the cycle.[60] Among female athletes with mild atopic asthma, menstrual cycle phase was found to affect the severity of exercise-induced bronchoconstriction.[61] Use of oral contraceptives has been associated with asthma risk among women who have no history of asthma and with remission of symptoms among women with such

a history.[59] Use of hormone replacement therapy increased the risk of asthma among nonobese women.[62]

Asthma is one of the most common diseases complicating pregnancy. Some data had suggested that the gender of the fetus might affect the risk of asthma exacerbations during pregnancy, but a large cohort study found no statistically significant effects of fetal gender.[63] A review concluded that the worsening of asthma during pregnancy cannot be attributed to either asthma or pregnancy but to a complex combination of factors and events.[64] Fear of the adverse effects of medication can result in undertreatment of asthma during pregnancy, which has been recognized as a problem for emergency departments.[65]

Women with poorly controlled asthma and those who were hospitalized for asthma during pregnancy have been found to have a higher risk of preterm birth than those whose asthma was well controlled.[66] An observational study found that offspring of women who used montelukast (a widely used controller or maintenance treatment for asthma) had lower birth weights and shorter gestation than offspring of women who did not, but did not differ in risk for malformations.[67] However, the investigators concluded that the indications for medication use, rather than the medication itself, may have accounted for the differences in pregnancy outcomes. Another study found that personal smoking but not environmental tobacco smoke exposure among pregnant women with asthma was associated with number of symptomatic days, number of nights with sleep disturbance due to symptoms, and with low birth weight of the offspring. Maternal smoking,[68] diet, and infections during pregnancy have also been associated with asthma in offspring.[69] Even maternal anxiety during pregnancy has been found to predict children's asthma.[70] Apart from effects on offspring, the association of reproductive events with asthma risk and severity clearly points to a relationship between sex hormones and asthma and to a need for research on that relationship and its possible relevance to asthma treatment.

Psychosocial Factors/Stress/Domestic Partner Violence

A number of studies have found associations between adverse emotional states and asthma. Anxiety and depression have been linked to asthma in young adults.[71] In a nationwide sample of adults who underwent spirometry, those with impaired lung function were more likely than others to have mental health problems; females in the sample were less likely than males to have impaired lung function.[72] In a birth cohort of children of asthmatic mothers, both child psychological risk and maternal depression were predictive of asthma at ages 6–8 years.[73] Children living in dilapidated homes and whose mothers were experiencing chronic intimate partner violence had more than four times the risk of children without those exposures or with only one of active asthma at age 36 months.[74]

The Hygiene Hypothesis

One of the most important theories proposed to account for the asthma epidemic in industrialized countries is the hygiene hypothesis, which suggests that infants who are excessively sheltered from the immune stimulation afforded by exposure to infectious agents are more susceptible. Many bacteria and parasites elicit an immune response that down-regulates the inappropriate reaction to allergy and other autoimmune diseases. Children in large families have been found to have fewer allergies and eczema than children without siblings.[75] Infants on farms where mothers milked the cows and brought the baby into the barn regularly were less likely to develop asthma than other children.[76] Children who lived with dogs or cats[77] or entered day care in their first year[78] also had lower risk of asthma/allergy in later childhood. Although women are in general more susceptible than men to autoimmune diseases, the relationship of the hygiene hypothesis to this gender difference has not been studied.

Issues in Asthma Diagnosis

Among patients with respiratory symptoms, making a diagnosis of asthma requires a detailed clinical history and lung function testing. The measurement most often used to assess pulmonary airflow obstruction is forced expiratory volume in one second (FEV_1). However, FEV_1 is not diagnostic assessment because it does not correspond well to symptoms and exacerbations, particularly in women.[79] Making the diagnosis requires ruling out viral infections, smoker's cough, chronic obstructive pulmonary disease (COPD), emphysema, vocal cord dysfunction, and gastroesophageal reflux.

Treatment and Therapeutic Interventions

The National Asthma Education and Prevention Program (NAEPP)[80] and the Global Initiative for Asthma (GINA)[81] provide similar guidelines for treatment of men and women with asthma. The goal of treatment is to alleviate persistent wheezing, cough, shortness of breath, and chest tightness, and to prevent exacerbations. Specific allergens and irritants that trigger exacerbations should be identified and avoided. Obviously, patients should avoid smoking and being exposed to secondhand smoke.

Controller Medications

Most people with asthma should use a controller medication, usually an inhaled corticosteroid such as fluticasone or budesonide, on a daily basis. Controller medications prevent airway inflammation. Long-term use of inhaled corticosteroids does not carry the risk of side effects that are associated with oral steroids. Some patients may also use long-acting beta-2 agonists (LABAs), such as salmeterol and formoterol. Patients who derive little benefit from corticosteroids should use leukotriene modifiers, such as montelukast and zileutron.

Rescue Medications

To keep on hand for exacerbations, patients should also have a rescue or quick-relief medication, such as albuterol (a short-term beta-2 agonist) or ipatropium. Rescue medications are bronchodilators; they relax the airway muscles to open the airway, making it easier to breathe. Rescue medications should not be used regularly; most patients who use them frequently probably should have their controller medication dosage increased instead. Exacerbations are best prevented than treated; evidence increasingly suggests that exacerbations predict lung function decline and airway remodeling and obstruction.[82] However, athletes and others with asthma who are subject to exercise-induced exacerbations are encouraged to use rescue medication just prior to exercising. Such use can prevent the exacerbation and enable patients to adhere to a good exercise program, which can maintain fitness and prevent obesity.

Immunotherapy

Patients whose asthma is triggered by specific allergens, such as pet or seasonal plant allergens, may also be treated with immunotherapy, a series of injections of the allergen at very low doses to induce desensitization. However, immunotherapy is not as effective for allergic asthma as it is for allergic rhinitis.

Treatment Issues

Unfortunately, undertreatment and poor adherence to treatment, especially to controller treatment, are common. Many patients dislike or cannot afford to take a controller medication daily. Many are fearful of the side effects of long-term use. Patients who have an inhaled corticosteroid prescription filled often use their inhalers incorrectly or not at all. A study of patients seen in an emergency department (ED) for an asthma exacerbation found that few subsequently received controller medications and that continuity of care between the ED and the primary care physician was poor.[83] In a survey of 1,006 asthma patients in Detroit, factors associated with nonadherence were nonwhite race, female gender, low income, and difficulty affording medication; when medication-related beliefs were taken into account, the association with race was no longer statistically significant.[84] Education is often invoked as the solution to the problems of nonadherence and treatment errors, as for similar problems in other chronic diseases, but more user-friendly and affordable treatments and preventive measures are also needed.

Research is in progress on asthma vaccines based on infectious agents and parasites common in settings where asthma is rare. Hormonal factors and immune system modulators are also being explored as treatment or preventive agents.

Summary

Asthma is a chronic (intermittent, persistent) condition in which the bronchi (airways) become constricted, inflamed, and filled with mucus in response to allergens or other stimuli. The condition varies in severity; among some individuals, symptoms are mild or occur only in the presence of specific triggers that can be readily avoided. Among other patients, asthma can be disabling or even fatal, sometimes with little or no warning. The condition also varies in age of onset, from infancy to old age. Many children who have asthma symptoms in the first year or two of life are symptom free when they grow older.

Asthma is more prevalent among males than females before puberty but more prevalent among females in adulthood. The age/gender crossover suggests that hormonal factors may play a role in the development and persistence of asthma, but the specific mechanisms are unknown.

Diagnosis is somewhat more challenging in women than in men because the standard lung function tests appear to be less informative among women. Asthma incidence and prevalence have increased dramatically in the past 4 decades, especially in industrialized countries and among women and children.

Among the strongest risk factors for asthma is having a first-degree relative with asthma or atopy. Several gene mutations or polymorphisms have been associated with asthma, but genetics and family history do not account for the recent asthma epidemic. In the United States ethnicity is strongly associated with asthma; prevalence is highest among blacks and Puerto Ricans and lowest among Asians and Mexicans. Asthma/wheeze in early childhood is strongly associated with a history of respiratory infections in early infancy, including both colds and ear infections. However, increasing evidence suggests that early exposure to infectious agents or a dirty environment may be protective against asthma in the long term, supporting the so-called hygiene hypothesis. Smoking and environmental smoke exposure have also been associated with asthma. Many asthma exacerbations are triggered by allergen exposure, but contrary to widespread belief, it is not clear that allergen exposure actually induces the development of asthma. Being breastfed as an infant appears to be protective, as does a diet high in fruit, vegetables, and fish and low in meats and saturated fats. Obesity is a strong risk factor, especially among women. Occupational exposures to lung irritants have been associated with the development of asthma among both workers and their offspring. Among women, reproductive and hormonal events, including menarche, pregnancy, and menopause, have been associated with new-onset asthma and remission. Psychological stress has also been associated with asthma.

For most patients, asthma treatment involves both a daily controller medication and a rescue medication for use during exacerbations. Immunotherapy may also be helpful. However, nonadherence is a pervasive problem associated with gender and affordability of medication. New simpler and more affordable treatment and preventive measures are needed.

Discussion Questions

Introduction and Natural History

1. What is asthma? What is the difference between extrinsic and intrinsic asthma?
2. What is the evidence for an asthma epidemic? What groups are most affected?
3. Is asthma a women's health issue? Why or why not?

Incidence

1. How are asthma incidence rates ascertained in population surveys? What are the strengths and limitations of that approach?

Spectrum of Research

1. Of the various avenues of research described, which do you think has the most potential value? Why? How would you approach it?

Risk Factors and Gender

1. What bearing, if any, do familial or genetic factors have on the recent increase in asthma prevalence?
2. What clues might immigrant studies yield regarding asthma etiology?
3. What is the hygiene hypothesis? What are the arguments for and against it?
4. Why does the association of asthma with obesity appear to be stronger in females than males?

Treatment and Therapeutic Interventions

1. What is the difference between controller and rescue medications?
2. Why is adherence to asthma treatment poor?

References

1. Liangas G, Yates DH, Wu D, et al. Laughter-associated asthma. *J Asthma*. 2004;41:217–221.
2. World Health Organization. *Global Surveillance, Prevention and Control of Chronic Respiratory Diseases: A Comprehensive Approach*. Geneva, Switzerland: Author; 2007.
3. Brackbill RM, Hadler JL, DiGrande L, et al. Asthma and posttraumatic stress symptoms 5 to 6 years following exposure to the World Trade Center terrorist attack. *JAMA*. 2009;302:502–516.
4. Centers for Disease Control. Surveillance for asthma—United States, 1960–1995. *MMWR Morb Mortal Wkly Rep*. 1998;47(SS-1).
5. American Lung Association. Epidemiology & Statistics Unit, Research and Program Services. *Trends in Asthma Morbidity and Mortality*. Washington, DC: Author; 2007.
6. Akinbami, L. Asthma prevalence, health care use and mortality: United States 2003–05. Atlanta, GA: Centers for Disease Control and Prevention, National Center for Health Statistics; 2006.
7. Kung HC, Hoyert DL, Xu JQ, Murphy SL. *Deaths: Final Data for 2005*. Hyattsville, MD: National Center for Health Statistics; 2008. National Vital Statistics Reports; vol 56 no 10.
8. New York State Department of Health. Adult Asthma Prevalence in the United States and New York State—2006 Behavioral Risk Factor Survey Statistics. http://www.health.state.ny.us/statistics/ny_asthma/asthmaprevalence06.htm. Accessed January 2, 2010.
9. Stupka E, DeShazo R. Asthma in seniors: part 1. Evidence for underdiagnosis, undertreatment, and increasing morbidity and mortality. *Am J Med*. 2009;122:6–11.
10. Hepper PG, Shannon EA, Dornan JC. Sex differences in fetal mouth movements. *Lancet*. 1997;350:1820.
11. Ingemarsson I. Gender aspects of preterm birth. *BJOG*. 2003;110(suppl 20): 34–38.
12. DeGroodt EG, van Pelt W, Borsboom GJ, et al. Growth of lung and thorax dimensions during the pubertal growth spurt. *Eur Respir J*. 1988;1:102–108.
13. Nève V, Girard F, Flahault A, Boulé M. Lung and thorax development during adolescence: relationship with pubertal status. *Eur Respir J*. 2002;20:1292–1298.
14. Troisi RJ, Speizer FE, Willett WC, et al. Menopause, postmenopausal estrogen preparations, and the risk of adult-onset asthma. A prospective cohort study. *Am J Resp Crit Care Med*. 1995;152:1183–1188.
15. Postma DS. Gender differences in asthma development and progression. *Gender Med*. 2007;4:S133–S146.
16. Holgate ST. Has the time come to rethink the pathogenesis of asthma? *Curr Opin Allergy Clin Immunol*. 2010;10:48–53.
17. Rudd RA, Moorman JE. Asthma incidence: data from the National Health Incidence Survey, 1980–1996. *J Asthma*. 2007;44:65–70.
18. Sleiman PM, Flory J, Imielinski M, et al. Variants of DENND1B Associated with Asthma in Children. *N Engl J Med*. 2010;362:36–44. Erratum in: *N Engl J Med*. 2010;363:994.

19. Chang JC, Liu CA, Chuang H, et al. Gender-limited association of cytotoxic T-lymphocyte antigen-4 (CTLA-4) polymorphism with cord blood IgE levels. *Pediatr Allergy Immunol.* 2004;15:506–512.

20. Yang KD, Liu CA, Chang JC, et al. Polymorphism of the immune-braking gene CTLA-4 (+49) involved in gender discrepancy of serum total IgE levels and allergic diseases. *Clin Exp Allergy.* 2004;34:32–37.

21. Dijkstra A, Howard TD, Vonk JM, et al. Estrogen receptor 1 polymorphisms are associated with airway hyper-responsiveness and lung function decline, particularly in female subjects with asthma. *J Allergy Clin Immunol.* 2006;117:604–611.

22. Finkelstein Y, Bournissen FG, Hutson JR, Shannon M. Polymorphism of the ADRB2 gene and response to inhaled beta-agonists in children with asthma: a meta-analysis. *J Asthma.* 2009;46:900–905.

23. Jacobson JS, Mellins RB, Garfinkel R, et al. Asthma, body mass, gender, and Hispanic national origin among 517 preschool children in New York City. *Allergy.* 2008;63:87–94.

24. Weinmayr G, Weiland SK, Björkstén B, et al. ISAAC Phase Two Study Group. Atopic sensitization and the international variation of asthma symptom prevalence in children. *Am J Respir Crit Care Med.* 2007;176:565–574.

25. Eldeirawi K, McConnell R, Furner S, et al. Associations of doctor-diagnosed asthma with immigration status, age at immigration, and length of residence in the United States in a sample of Mexican American School Children in Chicago. *J Asthma.* 2009;46:796–802.

26. Jackson DJ, Gangnon RE, Evans MD, et al. Wheezing rhinovirus illnesses in early life predict asthma development in high risk children. *Am J Resp Crit Care Med.* 2008;178:667–672.

27. Jacobson JS, Goldstein IF, Canfield SM, et al. Early respiratory infections and asthma among New York City Head Start children. *J Asthma.* 2008;45:301–8.

28. Wu P, Dupont WD, Griffin MR, et al. Evidence of a causal role of winter virus infection during infancy in early childhood asthma. *Am J Resp Crit Care Med.* 2008;178:1123–1129.

29. Bush A, Menzies-Gow A. Phenotypic differences between pediatric and adult asthma. *Proc Am Thoracic Soc.* 2009;6:712–719.

30. Li YF, Gilliland FD, Berhane K, et al. Effects of in utero and environmental tobacco smoke exposure on lung function in boys and girls with and without asthma. *Am J Respir Crit Care Med.* 2000;162:2097–2104.

31. Venners SA, Wang X, Chen C, et al. Exposure-response relationship between paternal smoking and children's pulmonary function. *Am J Resp Crit Care Med.* 2001;164:973–976. (Correction in *Am J Resp Crit Care Med.* 2002;166:775.)

32. Rasmussen F, Siersted HC, Lambrechtsen J, et al. Impact of airway lability, atopy, and tobacco smoking on the development of asthma-like symptoms in asymptomatic teenagers. *Chest.* 2000;117:1330–1335.

33. Scholtens S, Wijga AH, Brunekreef B, et al. Breast feeding, parental allergy and asthma in children followed for 8 years. The PIAMA birth cohort study. *Thorax.* 2009;64:604–609.

34. Devereux G. Session 1: Allergic disease Nutrition as a potential determinant of asthma. *Proc Nutr Soc.* 2009;69:1–10.

35. Allan K, Kelly FJ, Devereux G. Antioxidants and allergic disease: a case of too little or too much? *Clin Exp Allergy.* 2010;40:370–380.

36. Hughes DA, Norton R. Vitamin D and respiratory health. *Clin Exp Immunol.* 2009;158:20–25.

37. Litonjua AA. Childhood asthma may be a consequence of vitamin D deficiency. *Curr Opin Allergy Clin Immunol.* 2009;9:202–207.

38. Chatzi L, Kogevinas M. Prenatal and childhood Mediterranean diet and the development of asthma and allergies in children. *Public Health Nutr.* 2009;12:1629–1634.

39. Lucas SR, Platts-Mills TA. Paediatric asthma and obesity. *Paediatr Respir Rev.* 2006;7:33–38.

40. Camargo CA Jr, Weiss ST, Zhang S, et al. Prospective study of body mass index, weight change, and risk of adult-onset asthma in women. *Arch Intern Med.* 1999;159:2582–2588.

41. Lin RY, Lee GB. The gender disparity in adult asthma hospitalizations dynamically relates to age. *J Asthma.* 2008;45:931–935.

42. Litonjua AA, Sparrow D, Celedon JC, et al. Association of body mass index with the development of methacholine airway hyper-responsiveness in men: the Normative Aging Study. *Thorax.* 2002;57:581–585.

43. Joseph CL, Havstad SL, Ownby DR, et al. Gender differences in the association of overweight and asthma morbidity among urban adolescents with asthma. *Pediatr Allergy Immunol.* 2009;20:362–369.

44. Eneli IU, Skybo T, Camargo CA Jr. Weight loss and asthma: a systematic review. *Thorax.* 2008;63:671–676.

45. Pearce N, Pekkanen J, Beasley R. How much asthma is really attributable to atopy? *Thorax.* 1999;54:268–272.

46. Illi S, von Mutius E, Lau S, et al. Multicentre Allergy Study (MAS) group. Perennial allergen sensitization early in life and chronic asthma in children: a birth cohort study. *Lancet.* 2006;368:763–770.

47. Canfield SM, Jacobson JS, Perzanowski MS, et al. Total and specific IgE associations between New York City Head Start children and their parents. *J Allergy Clin Immunol.* 2008;121:1422–1427.

48. Gent JF, Belanger K, Triche EW, et al. Association of pediatric asthma severity with exposure to common household dust allergens. *Environ Res.* 2009;109:768–774.

49. Rotsides DZ, Goldstein IF, Canfield SM, et al. Asthma, allergy, and IgE levels in NYC Head Start children. *Respir Med.* 2010;104:345–355.

50. Stenton SC. Occupational and environmental lung disease: occupation asthma. *Chron Respir Dis.* 2010;35–46.

51. Cherry N, Beach J, Burstyn I, et al. Data linkage to estimate the extent and distribution of occupational disease: new onset adult asthma in Alberta, Canada. *Am J Ind Med.* 2009;52:831–840.

52. Reutman SR, Rohs AM, Clark JC, et al. Respiratory health assessment of nail technicians: Symptoms, lung function, and airway inflammation. *Am J Ind Med.* 2009;52:868–875.

53. Tarlo SM, Malo JL; Third Jack Pepys Workshop on Asthma in the Workplace Participants. An official ATS proceedings: asthma in the workplace: the Third Jack Pepys Workshop on Asthma in the Workplace: answered and unanswered questions. *Proc Am Thorac Soc.* 2009;6:339–349.

54. Medina-Ramón M, Zock JP, Kogevinas M, et al. Asthma symptoms in women employed in domestic cleaning: a community based study. *Thorax.* 2003;58:950–954.

55. Bernstein JA, Brandt D, Rezvani M, et al. Evaluation of cleaning activities on respiratory symptoms in asthmatic female homemakers. *Ann Allergy Asthma Immunol.* 2009;102:41–46.

56. Yacoub MR, Lavoie K, Lacoste G, et al. Assessment of impairment/disability due to occupational asthma through a multidimensional approach. *Eur Respir J.* 2007;29:889–896.

57. Tagiyeva N, Devereux G, Semple S, et al. Parental occupation is a risk factor for childhood wheeze and asthma. *Eur Respir J.* 2009;35:987–993.

58. Guerra S, Wright AL, Morgan WJ, et al. Persistence of asthma symptoms during adolescence: role of obesity and age at the onset of puberty. *Am J Respir Crit Care Med.* 2004;170:78–85.

59. Salam MT, Wenten M, Gilliland FD. Endogenous and exogenous sex steroid hormones and asthma and wheeze in young women. *J Allergy Clin Immunol.* 2006;11:1001–1007.

60. Murphy VE, Gibson PG. Premenstrual asthma: prevalence, cycle-to-cycle variability and relationship to oral contraceptive use and menstrual symptoms. *J Asthma.* 2008;45:696–704.

61. Stanford KI, Mickleborough TD, Ray S, et al. Influence of menstrual cycle phase on pulmonary function in asthmatic athletes. *Eur J Appl Physiol.* 2006;96:703–710.

62. Gómez Real F, Svanes C, Björnsson EH, et al. Hormone replacement therapy, body mass index and asthma in perimenopausal women: a cross sectional survey. *Thorax.* 2006;61:34–40.

63. Firoozi F, Ducharme FM, Lemière C, et al. Effect of fetal gender on maternal asthma exacerbations in pregnant asthmatic women. *Respir Med.* 2009;103:144–151.

64. Clifton V. Maternal asthma during pregnancy and fetal outcomes: potential mechanisms and possible solutions. *Curr Opin Allergy Clin Immunol.* 2006;6:307–311.

65. Gluck JC. The change of asthma course during pregnancy. *Clin Rev Allergy Immunol.* 2004;26:171–180.

66. Bakhireva LN, Schatz M, Jones KL, Chambers CD; Organization of Teratology Information Specialists Collaborative Research Group. Asthma control during pregnancy and the risk of preterm delivery or impaired fetal growth. *Ann Allergy Asthma Immunol.* 2008;101:137–143.

67. Sarkar M, Koren G, Kalra S, et al. Montelukast use during pregnancy: a multicentre, prospective, comparative study of infant outcomes. *Eur J Clin Pharmacol.* 2009;65:1259–1264.

68. Lannerö E, Wickman M, Pershagen G, Nordvall L. Maternal smoking during pregnancy increases the risk of recurrent wheezing during the first years of life (BAMSE). *Respir Res.* 2006;7:3.

69. Kumar R. Prenatal factors and the development of asthma. *Curr Opin Pediatr.* 2008;20:682–687.

70. Cookson H, Granell R, Joinson C, et al. Mothers' anxiety during pregnancy is associated with asthma in their children. *J Allergy Clin Immunol.* 2009;123:847–853.e11.

71. Goodwin RD, Fergusson DM, Horwood LJ. Asthma and depressive and anxiety disorders among young persons in the community. *Psychol Med.* 2004;34:1465–1474.

72. Goodwin RD, Chuang S, Simuro N, et al. Association between lung function and mental health problems among adults in the United States: findings from the First National Health and Nutrition Examination Survey. *Am J Epidemiol.* 2007;165:383–388.

73. Klinnert MD, Nelson HS, Price MR, et al. Onset and persistence of childhood asthma: predictors from infancy. *Pediatrics.* 2001;108:E69.

74. Franco Suglia S, Duarte CS, Sandel MT, Wright RJ. Social and environmental stressors in the home and childhood asthma. *J Epidemiol Community Health.* 2010;64:636–642.

75. Strachan DP. Hay fever, hygiene, and household size. *BMJ.* 1989;299:1259–1260.

76. Douwes J, Cheng S, Travier N, et al. Farm exposure in utero may protect against asthma, hay fever and eczema. *Eur Respir J.* 2008;32:603–611.

77. Ownby DR, Johnson CC. Does exposure to dogs and cats in the first year of life influence the development of allergic sensitization? *Curr Opin Allergy Clin Immunol.* 2003;3:517–522.

78. Ball TM, Castro-Rodriguez JA, Griffith KA, et al. Siblings, day-care attendance, and the risk of asthma and wheezing during childhood. *N Engl J Med.* 2000;343:538–543.

79. Godfrey JR. Toward optimal health: Sally Wenzel, MD discusses the need for better asthma management in women. *J Womens Health.* 2006;15:230–233.

80. National Heart, Lung, and Blood Institute. National Asthma Education and Prevention Program. *Expert Panel Report 3. Guidelines for the Diagnosis and Management of Asthma. Full Report 2007.* Bethesda, MD: U.S. Department of Health and Human Services; 2007. http://www.nhlbi.nih.gov/guidelines/asthma/asthgdln.pdf. Accessed January 2, 2010.

81. Bateman ED, Hurd SS, Barnes PJ, et al. Global strategy for asthma management and prevention: GINA executive summary. *Eur Respir J* 2008;31:143–178. http://www.ncbi.nlm.nih.gov/pubmed/18166595

82. Bai TR. Evidence for airway remodeling in chronic asthma. *Curr Opin Allergy Clin Immunol.* 2010;10:82–86.

83. Cydulka RK, Tamayo-Sarver JH, Wolf C, et al. Inadequate follow-up controller medications among patients with asthma who visit the emergency department. *Ann Emerg Med.* 2005;46:316–322.

84. Wells K, Pladevall M, Peterson EL, et al. Race-ethnic differences in factors associated with inhaled steroid adherence among adults with asthma. *Am J Respir Crit Care Med.* 2008;178:1194–1201.

Multiple Sclerosis

William A. Sheremata, MD

Introduction

Multiple sclerosis (MS) is a uniquely human nervous system disorder affecting young women more than twice as often as men.[1,2] It is the most common neurologic disorder of young adults and is the most frequent cause of chronic disability in this population.[2,3] Commonly referred to as "MS," the illness is characterized by recurrent attacks of nervous system impairment (*relapses*) that occur unpredictably and vary greatly in character, severity, and their propensity to remit (*relapsing-remitting*). Clinical manifestations of MS reflect involvement of different parts of the brain and spinal cord by an inflammatory demyelinating disease process, generally accepted to be autoimmune (Figure 22-1.).

Brain lesions termed plaques may occur without any detectable focal neurologic manifestations (Figures 22-2 and 22-3.). Traditionally, the diagnosis of MS is made by a neurologist determining that the disease is "disseminated both in space and in time." That means the plaques are scattered through the nervous system and have occurred at least two times.

The clinical manifestations of MS are as varied as those in the entire range of neurologic illness. In many patients MS may be readily diagnosed at its onset by an experienced neurologist.[1,2] However, its recognition in some patients may be challenging for the physician and frustrating for the patient. A common and easily recognized symptom is loss of vision due to optic neuritis and is the initial problem

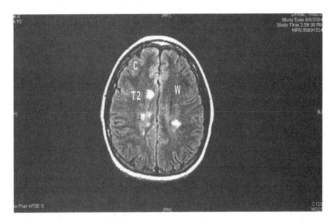

Figure 22-2 MRI of the brain.

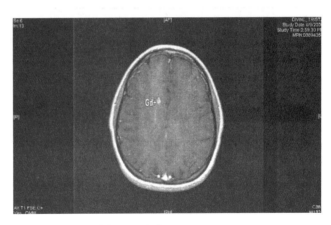

Figure 22-3 MRI of the same brain.

in 15–20% of cases. Inflammation in the affected optic nerve is typically associated with loss of vision and pain in the eye due to inflammation in the optic nerve. Recovery typically occurs within days to weeks and often seems complete, though varying degrees of visual impairment may remain. Of all the initial attacks of MS, almost half are associated with difficulty in walking.[2–5] Gait problems are related to plaques in a number of different areas within the brain or spinal cord. As with optic neuritis, gait disturbance often appears evanescent. However, the experienced neurologist is able to detect some residual impairment. Relapses average 0.7 annually in untreated women.[4]

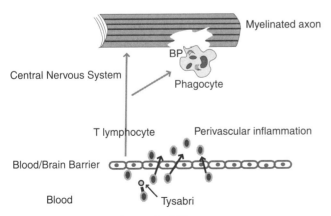

Figure 22-1 Immunopathogenesis of MS.

MS patients often appear normal for many years despite having had past attacks. McAlpine described a variety of types of clinical progression in graphical form that give a better idea of the clinical types of illness (Figure 22-4.).

A minority of patients will have "benign" illness with no limitation of function evident for protracted periods of time. Once gait is clearly altered following recovery from an attack, increasing neurologic deficits can be predicted.[3] Reports not based on natural history studies, suggest that a cane may be necessary within a couple of years or so; and use of a walker or wheelchair may become necessary soon after. However, natural history studies in Canada, France, and Minnesota suggest a better prognosis.[3–6] The unpredictability of MS contributes significantly to anxiety and depression as accompaniments to other clinical manifestations. Emotional symptoms may dominate the clinical picture and lead to diagnostic difficulty.

Progressive illness may begin at any time for reasons unknown.[1,2,5–8] *Secondary progressive MS*—the most common type—is identified by the appearance of clinically worsening neurologic findings occurring between, or in the absence of, exacerbations. The proportion of untreated patients developing such illness has variably been estimated to be between 50–70% of patients. Fortunately, clinical trials conducted in the last 15 years have clearly demonstrated a reduction of the risk of both relapses and progression of disability with active treatment.

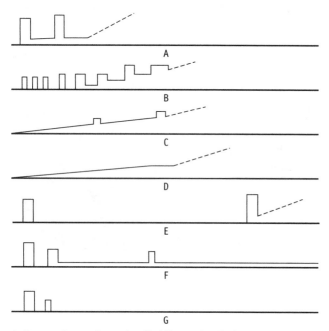

A. Severe relapses, increasing disability, and early death. B. Many short attacks, tending to increase in duration and severity. C. Slow progression from onset, superimposed relapses, and increasing disability. D. Slow progression from onset without relapses. E. Abrupt onset with good remission followed by long latent phase. F. Relapses of diminishing frequency and severity, slight residual disability only. G. Abrupt onset, few if any relapses after first year, no residual disability.

Figure 22-4 Clinical course of MS.

Reproduced from McAlpine, D., Compston, N.D., and Acheson, E.D.: *Multiple Sclerosis: A reappraisal.* Ed. 2, p. 32. Churchill Livingston, London. © Elsevier 1998.

Primary progressive MS, illness not associated with relapses and remissions, occurs in approximately 15% of MS patients.[9] This illness often has an insidious onset as a slowly progressive gait disorder appearing in midlife. It is slightly more common in men and is twice as common in Irish and European Jewish (Ashkenazi) populations.

Relapsing-progressive MS is a less common illness where remission may be associated with limited or no recovery. Often, in such patients the severity and propensity to relapse and acquire disability may be established at its very outset. Weinschenker and colleagues in 1989 published a natural history study indicating 50% of untreated patients with three exacerbations in their first year of illness were wheelchair bound within 5 years of onset.[5] More aggressive illness of this nature is seen more often in African American patients. Aggressive immunosuppressive treatment, first used in Europe over a half century ago, has markedly improved the outcome for such patients.

Sources of Data: Spectrum of Research Addressing the Topic

Epidemiologic research has contributed substantially to the understanding of MS. Alter presented a number of important epidemiologic observations on MS in Minnesota and in Israel.[7] Subsequently, Kurtzke in a 1980 review of a series of important studies of U.S. veterans reported that temperate latitudes were associated with a greater risk for MS.[8] Paty, in establishing an MS database in London, Ontario 35 years ago, provided the foundation for a series of valuable population-based reports on the natural history of MS. Using this database, Weinschenker and coworkers have generated several papers on the natural history.[5,9,10] Ebers, now at Oxford (England), and others have continued their studies.[9,10] Mayr et al. in 2003 published newer observations on the Olmsted County, Minnesota, population.[6] Several important reports on the natural history of MS have also come from a Lyon, France database.[3,4]

Genetic Research

Hauser, working with an International MS Consortium based at University of California, San Francisco, Harvard, Massachusetts Institute of Technology, Duke University, and the University of Miami in the United States, as well as several other international centers, have contributed several definitive reports on genetic risks in MS.[11,12] Autoimmune diseases, including MS, are now recognized to have a complex polygenic background. The majority of the genes contributing to the risk of MS are located in a large genomic region—the Major Histocompatibility Complex (MHC) locus at chromosome 6p21 (Figure 22-5). A few other genes with important roles in immune function, including IL-2 (T-cell growth factor) and IL-2 receptor genes are located elsewhere.[11,12] This productive collaboration is continuing to define gene function and correlate findings with human disease phenotypes. This work is being done in parallel with research into the functional immunology of these genes.

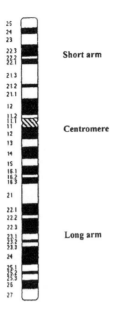

Figure 22-5 Drawing of chromosome 6 from the Human Genome Project. Courtesy of the National Library of Medicine.

Neurovirology

In the last half century many viruses have been implicated as potential causes of MS but most have subsequently been discarded. At present, the Epstein-Barr virus (EBV) and herpes simplex-6 viruses (HSV-6) are the major focus of this research.[12] Molecular mimicry, the immune recognition of viral gene products as structural myelin proteins, has become a major research focus.

Incidence and Prevalence Rates

MS is a disease typically found in persons of European origin.[1,2,7–10] It is rare in Africa and in Asia, as well in persons originating from those geographic areas.[7,8] Kurtzke, in his 1980 review, reported high frequency rates, rates over 30/100,000, occur in white populations between 65° and 45° North latitude (southern Canada and northern United States).[8] Similar high rates occur in New Zealand and southern Australia. He reported that low prevalence rates (less than 5/100,000) occurred in Asia and Africa except for one area, South Africa. Migration from a high-incidence area in Europe to South Africa at age 15 or less reduced a high risk of MS and vice versa. Migration after that age had no effect on the risk of MS. A similar phenomenon was observed in populations moving to and from Israel and in the male veteran population migrating within the United States. Male African Americans had approximately half of the risk of MS compared with white Americans. Very few cases were diagnosed among Native Americans and Asians.

Mayr et al. recently reported updated prevalence and incidence rates for whites with MS in Olmsted County, Minnesota.[6] This study probably represents the most complete case ascertainment of any population in the United States. The residents are well educated and receive excellent medical care and the county has many neurologists familiar with MS. Repeated study of the Olmsted population has contributed to excellent ascertainment with a reported raw prevalence of MS of 177/100,000 and a raw annual incidence rate of 7.5/100,000 as of last data tabulation in December 2000. The investigators concluded that after age and sex adjustment, these prevalence and incidence rates have been stable for over 20 years. Rates reported appear high compared with those from 20 centers in United States and Europe.

Reported incidence rates for MS varied from 0.86 in Romania to "10.1–12.2" in southeastern Scotland. Other reports show that low prevalence rates in Sardinia and Palermo, Sicily, rose substantially when Northern European trained neurologists returned to those areas. Madrid is now listed as a "high-incidence area" with clinicians now in residence who are skilled at diagnosis of multiple sclerosis. A recent study based on electronic death certificates from all 50 states and the District of Columbia was undertaken to estimate the U.S. MS mortality rate; MS was a contributing cause on 0.2% death certificates (approximately 45,000 deaths) between 1990 and 2001and the death rate increased from 1.2 to 1.6 deaths per 100,000 population during these years.[13]

The geographic distribution noting MS was uncommon in the southern states based on the earlier Kurtzke data. The first neurologist (Peritz Scheinberg), arrived in Florida in 1953 but was drafted into the military. Returning 2 years later, he began a department of neurology at the University of Miami, the first medical school in Florida. An incomplete 1983 Florida state MS survey yielded a prevalence of nearly 80/100,000; just 6 years after, the first MS center was established in Florida. In 1985, Sheremata (with Poskanzer and Roman) reported on an MS "cluster" in Key West, Florida—the southernmost city in the United States. The raw prevalence rate was 145/100,000 among the resident population. Although half of the 30,000 residents of the island were of African ancestry, no MS cases were found within that group. Illness among whites born or raised in Key West prior to adolescence did not differ in character from those who moved there from other parts of the United States. It seems clear that the true incidence and prevalence of MS cannot be ascertained without community awareness of the condition diagnosed by trained neurologists in collaboration with well-designed repeated population studies.

Mean Ages at Diagnosis and Changes over Time

The median age of MS onset in Olmsted County was 35.4 years (range 17.3–59.6) in women and 37.2 years in men (range 16.7–67). Median time from onset of symptoms to diagnosis was 2 years. This contrasts with Alter's earlier finding in Minnesota that the median age of onset of relapsing-remitting in women with MS was 24 years of age. Mean age of onset of MS in the Faroe Islands, where an epidemic of MS occurred, was between 23.07 and 26.85 years of age for women and men, respectively.[7,14] Median age of onset in Lyon, France was 30 years. Populations in England have been reported to be older at onset. The reasons for the later onset of symptoms reported by Mayr and coworkers in the Olmsted population are unexplained. Although there is a perception that the incidence and prevalence of MS is increasing,[13] the Olmsted study[6] appears to refute this, attributing the changes to more complete case ascertainment.

Pittock et al. reported the outcome of a group of untreated patients in Olmsted County examined at intervals over 10 years. There was "no significant increase in disability" over a 10-year period; however, 30% of the patients required ambulatory assistance by the end of the study.[15] Gait abnormality at onset, onset of progressive disease, and longer duration of disease were risk factors for disability. The French natural history study from Lyon showed that patients took an average of 11.4 years to reach an expanded disability status scale (EDSS) score of 4 (obvious gait difficulty); 23.1 years to reach an EDSS of 6 (use of one cane needed); and 33.1 years to reach an EDSS of 7 (a walker required to walk 20 feet).[3] The "favorable" prognosis for the French cohort of MS patients in Lyon was questioned as being too optimistic by some academics when published in 1980. Differences may be explained, at least in part, by the referral patterns to American academic centers versus experience with a population study. The 2004 Olmsted County experience is therefore more similar to that in Lyon.[15]

In an Arizona study, a number of factors were found to affect relapse rates in MS.[16] Infection, electric shock, pregnancy, and spinal anesthetics tended to increase MS relapse rate, whereas surgery, not associated with spinal anesthetics, and trauma did not. Clearly, pregnancy and infection are contributing factors in the French studies.[3,4] There are no known factors that influence the development of secondary progressive or primary progressive MS.

Emotional Stress

Cosgrove's initial observations (personal communication) at McGill showed "major life stress" had a significant negative impact on MS. Such stress was temporally associated with onset of MS and an increased risk of relapse. Subsequent controlled studies were performed by Grant (with Brown and coworkers at the National Hospital at Queen Square, London, England) and reported in 1989.[17] Findings showed a highly significantly greater occurrence of severe threat, but not minor stress, in MS patients compared with controls. In MS, there was a proximate relation between severe threat and the risk onset and of MS relapse. Mohr and coworkers in 2000 documented that major life stress and "hassles" resulted in an increased numbers of plaques in brain magnetic resonance imaging (MRI) studies, the primary outcome measure.[18]

Pregnancy

Confavreaux reported that women in Lyon, France had a relapse frequency of 0.7 attacks per year.[4] Pregnancy resulted in a slight initial increase in relapses in the first trimester of pregnancy, followed by a marked drop in the second trimester. The relapse rate increased toward the end of the third trimester and peaked in the first

6 months after delivery; during which time the rate was three times higher than the baseline rate. Following this 6-month postpartum period, the relapse rate dropped, but remained double the baseline rate for the next 30 months, (the duration of the period of observation). These findings are in agreement with earlier observations by Alter in Minnesota.[7]

Morbidity and Mortality

Morbidity in MS is measured by the Kurtzke expanded disability status scale, which was initially designed for epidemiologic studies in 1984 and is now universally used for assessment of outcomes in therapeutic trials. The scale has a ranges from 0 to 10; "0" represents the presence of neither symptoms nor abnormalities on examination; "4" generally is associated with mild but definite gait abnormality, "6" the use of one cane; "8" the use of a wheelchair, and "10" death. The reproducibility of the scale is good, particularly in the range of 4–10. Descriptions of morbidity are ordinarily in terms of time to reach an end point. Averages of disability points are not informative or statistically valid.

Mortality rates provided by early studies are difficult to interpret. Redelings et al. have recently reported the age-adjusted MS mortality rate from 1990–2001 was 1.44 deaths per 100,000 population in the United States.[13] The report also concludes that the mortality rates increased throughout the study period. There is a minimal shortening of life expectancy in MS, documented in the Canadian actuarial study.[19] MS is not a reportable disease, and until recently, recognition of illness (and hence case ascertainment) was low. In the past, when post mortem examinations were common, many cases were identified only then. In many communities in the United States, consultant neurologists and MRI equipment are now available, resulting in greater frequency and accuracy of the diagnosis of MS. The conclusion that mortality rates were increasing from 1990 to 2001 in the United States[13] contrasts with the observations in Olmsted County, Minnesota[6] where there were no increases in incidence and prevalence rates over a longer period of time.[6]

The Olmsted County, Canadian, and French natural history studies probably represent some of the best available data in more modern times. The outcomes measured are consistent and verifiable. Assessments of the impact of drugs on the natural history will require long periods of observation, but the available short-term observations are encouraging. Acceptance of the greater impact of instituting therapy at the very outset of disease, and recognizing the futility of delaying treatment until advanced disability prevails, will improve the outlook for new patients.

Detection Methods and Screening Patterns

MS in its typical presentations is recognized by physicians regardless of their training, although the diagnosis is accepted only when made by a neurologist. However, most general physicians and internists will recognize the neurologic nature of the patient's complaints. The investigation may be initiated by ordering imaging studies of the brain and spinal cord and even a cerebrospinal fluid examination, but insurance companies may impede this effort. Despite this, a woman's complaints of heat intolerance, fatigue, and/or tingling of her extremities, which are indeed highly suggestive of MS to the experienced specialist, may not arouse concern in some busy physicians. The common response is that these symptoms reflect an emotional problem, which is more likely if anxiety or depression is prominent.

Diagnosis of Multiple Sclerosis

Diagnostic criteria were originally developed to select a more homogeneous cohort of patients for studies. Many patients with the illness did not meet the original 1963 *Schumacher criteria*. The 1983 *Poser criteria* included laboratory support including MRI evoked response testing and cerebrospinal fluid (CSF) examination for the first time. The more recent *MacDonald criteria*[20] are accepted for referral of patient for early treatment based on studies that have shown substantially better outcomes, regardless of specific medications. These criteria allow the identification of "clinically isolated syndromes" (optic neuritis, and brain stem or acute myelitis) with very high (> 80%) probability of a subsequent diagnosis of clinically definite MS (one or more additional attacks within 2 years). Imaging provides the additional evidence required to establish the presence of dissemination of lesions both in time and space, without requiring a second clinical attack for diagnosis. Early diagnosis of MS and earlier introduction of treatment predicts a superior outcome.

Imaging (MRI) studies have become especially helpful in establishing the diagnosis earlier than previously possible. This is important, as early institution of treatment is especially effective in preventing both relapses and disease progression. However, MRI studies performed early in the illness may not detect the typical changes in brain or spinal cord. Twenty-five years ago, we reported that within 3 years of their initial symptoms, only half of patients with clinically definite MS had the anticipated MRI brain lesions. However, of those with no brain lesions, half had spinal cord lesions. Neuroimaging has improved but a proportion of patients with MS do not have detectable brain MRI lesions visible early in their illness. New imaging techniques have revealed the presence of cortical brain lesions that are not evident in conventional studies early in MS. It has been established recently that by pathological examination these cortical lesions may precede the appearance of white matter lesions at the outset of MS.

Recognized and Suspected Risk Factors
Genetic Risk for MS

Alter recognized that a family history of MS conferred an increased risk of the disease developing in blood relatives.[7] Within three generations, the risk is 10 times higher on average than among individuals without a family history. However, the risk of a child born to a mother with MS is

increased by 20–40 times. Virtually all large centers have found that 20% of MS patients will have a family history of illness. This is true in the Cuban population and other ethnic populations in South Florida.

In 1972 Jersild first reported a genetic association of genes within the major histocompatibility locus (MHC) with a risk of MS.[21] Since that early report it is now clearly established that HLA DR2 (DR1*1501 specifically) is twice as common in MS compared with the general population. It is half as common in African Americans and is uncommon in Africa. The gene also confers a higher risk of MS and greater disease severity. Presence of the gene is also associated with higher levels of antibody to EBV. Patients with high levels of antibody and that possess DR1*1501 have a markedly increased risk of MS.[20] Many other genes with polymorphisms located on the short arm of chromosome 6p21 are associated with a risk of MS (Figure 22-5). The concept of each of several genes making a small additive contribution to a risk of MS has been proposed.[11,21]

Environmental Risks Associated with MS

Environmental risk factors have been recently been reviewed by Ascherio and Munger.[22,23] MS is an illness of Europeans and their descendants living in the north temperate latitudes, and to a more limited extent in the south temperate latitudes. The U.S. veterans studies reported by Kurtzke appear to show a striking latitudinal MS distribution.[8] Migration studies of veterans have also shown that prepubertal migration from the southern low-risk area of the United States to a higher-risk northern area results in an increased risk. However, these observations have been challenged by Ebers who, using the Veterans Administration data, showed that those with Scandinavian surnames had the same MS risk regardless of whether they lived in the north or in the south. In the history of migration to the new world, in reality it appears that most migrants have immigrated to areas of the world more similar to their homelands. Despite this, other migration studies have shown that prepubertal migration from a low-risk area of the world to a high-risk area (such as moving from South Africa to Holland) results in a higher risk of MS. The opposite is also true. These observations imply an infectious risk for MS. These interpretations have been supported by the Faroe Island epidemic of MS.

The Faroe Islands is a Danish administered territory comprised of a Celtic population genetically similar to northern and western Scotland and Iceland. Health care was provided by physicians from Denmark who were familiar with MS but who had not documented a single case on the islands prior to 1943. British troops (very young men) occupied the islands in 1941, and this historical fact was followed by an epidemic of MS.[8,14] Sixteen MS patients were diagnosed in the first wave of cases, beginning 2 years after the arrival of the British. Studies showed that these troops were camped in the areas where pubertal Faroese resided in 1941 and who subsequently developed MS. A second wave occurred in persons who were in Denmark for the duration of World War II and who later returned to the islands. A third wave of MS occurred in persons who had been in contact with the original MS Faroese population. Kurtzke has interpreted these findings, and complementary observations in Iceland, as providing strong support for the conclusion that an infectious environmental factor contributes to the risk for MS.[14] Many different viruses have been suspected to play a role in MS. Because the British soldiers took their dogs to the Faroe Islands, canine distemper, which is related to human measles virus, was investigated but eventually discarded as a candidate virus. Measles and related viruses were also extensively investigated. Retroviruses, especially HTLV-I, which can cause nervous system disease somewhat resembling MS, were also investigated extensively.

Urban dwellers have a higher risk of MS, suggesting a probable increased risk of exposure to a causative agent. As well, a higher socioeconomic status is also associated with an increased risk of MS. Independent of the first hypothesis, it has been proposed that this may be related to delayed exposure to a common infectious agent. An age-dependent altered immune response is hypothesized to occur, such as occurs with infectious mononucleosis. In infectious mononucleosis, disease results from an active immune response to Epstein-Barr virus infection from adolescence to college age, whereas infection earlier or later in life does not.[22] At present, there is an accumulating literature implicating EBV and another closely related herpes virus; herpes simplex-6 (HSV6). An antibody to an EBV polymerase gene product has been shown to cross-react with a structural myelin protein (myelin basic protein) capable of inducing experimental demyelinating disease in rodents.[24,25] This is an example of molecular mimicry. A more recent publication[26] has shown that a specific Epstein Barr nuclear antigen-IgG antibody (but not a neutralizing antibody to EBV) rises with exacerbations proportional to the volume of brain affected in MS attacks. Other work has shown that HSV6, like EBV, infects lymphocytes but EBV also infects oligodendrocytes (the myelin producing cells in the nervous system) in MS patients compared with brain specimens for cases without MS. This is an important area for additional research.

Vitamin D and Risk of MS

Vitamin D deficiency has been associated with risk of MS.[27,28] Geographic areas with limited sunlight, at least for parts of the years, correspond to the areas reported to have the highest risk for MS, as proposed by Kurtzke. The large Harvard Nurses' Health Study (NHS) and Nurses' Health Study II (NHS II) were established in 1976 and 1989 respectively and provided 92,253 women for analysis. A higher risk for MS was documented when vitamin D3 serum levels were low (less than 100 nmol/L) and small supplemental doses of vitamin D (300 IU daily) reduced the risk of MS by 40%. Preliminary studies in Canada suggest that women, but not men, may receive greater benefit from vitamin D replacement (2,000 IU daily). The reasons for the apparent sex difference are speculative, and the findings must be replicated by additional studies. The risk of excessive absorption and high calcium serum levels that may lead to kidney stone formation is a concern. The

NHS studies have also documented a doubling of the risk for MS in smokers and a similar increased risk of disability in women who continue to smoke.[29]

Effect of Pregnancy on MS

Based on the observations that pregnancy reduces the risk of relapse in MS interest in the possible role of estrogens has arisen. MRI studies have provided preliminary evidence that relatively high doses of estrogen may reduce the risk of new disease activity. Despite the inherent risks of such an approach, the role of estrogens as a possible therapy for MS is now being actively investigated for women.

Treatment and Therapeutic Interventions

Treatment of MS falls into three categories: symptomatic treatment, management of acute relapses, and treatment aimed at reducing the risk of relapses and neurologic disability.

Symptomatic Treatment

In the past and to the present, symptomatic treatment of anxiety, depression, fatigue, sleep disorders, spasticity, paroxysmal disorders, pain, and a host of other problems complicating MS have been important aspects of the medical management. Most MS patients are anxious about their future, which is often unfounded as pessimistic perceptions fuel these concerns. Young adults are also more likely to react emotionally to the clinical reality of MS. Their emotional response to the common occurrence of headaches may occasionally be interpreted as their principal problem whereas specific aspects of MS may be ignored, consequently delaying diagnosis and treatment. These issues are not addressed here except to mention an important group of commonly unrecognized or misdiagnosed complications of MS. Ordinarily, symptoms are not considered to be related to MS if they do not last more than 24 hours.

Paroxysmal disorders, composed of a group of unusual recurrent manifestations, typically last seconds to minutes and occur almost exclusively in MS. These include paroxysmal dystonia (parosyxmal tonic spasms), paroxysmal akinesia, paroxysmal choreoathetosis, paroxysmal dysarthria, and brief pains, such as trigeminal neuralgia. They may occur in isolation or in concert with other manifestations of MS. The most commonly occurring is *paroxysmal dystonia*, which, along with other paroxysmal problems, is often misinterpreted as evidence of a conversion reaction, especially when this occurs early in the clinical course. The increased muscle tone is a strange transient, but recurring, alteration of limb posture which may affect one, two, or all the limbs although rarely involving the entire trunk. Severe dystonia may be associated with severe pain lasting minutes to hours.

Paroxysmal dystonia and other paroxysmal disorders are usually attributed (perhaps incorrectly) to crosstalk between demyelinated axons in the spinal cord or brain stem. Psychiatric care does not help the affected individuals but small doses of anticonvulsants (i.e., carbamazepine) prescribed for a few months are usually very effective. Over the years, many unfortunate patients have received inappropriately high doses of psychotropic medications prescribed for months, without benefit.

Management of Acute Relapses

If a patient becomes incapacitated, medication may be appropriate to shorten more severe attacks although recovery will occur to the same degree with or without treatment. Adrenocorticotrophic hormone or ACTH (ACTHAR® Gel), also called corticotrophin, is the only validated Food and Drug Administration (FDA) approved treatment for relapses of MS. Most neurologists, however, prescribe either oral or high-dose intravenous steroids (methylprednisolone, Medrol®) for exacerbations of MS. Some neurologists prescribe them chronically although there is no scientific basis for this practice. In addition, there are many potential side effects.

Glucocorticoids "steroids" do reduce fatigue and often induce a sense of well-being but their many side effects do not justify their use for those reasons alone. The national optic neuritis study sponsored by the National Institutes of Health documented faster recovery from attacks of optic neuritis after the use of high-dose intravenous (IV) methylprednisolone. In contrast, oral steroids did not shorten the attacks but actually doubled the risk of relapse of optic neuritis as compared with oral placebo. There is often a rapid response to either drug in patients with acute, severe relapses, but there are no adequate comparison studies of IV methylprednisolone with ACTH or compared with higher doses of oral steroids. Side effects of steroids include an increased risk of viral, bacterial, yeast, fungal, and parasitic infestations. Infections include progressive multifocal leukoencephalopathy (PML) due to John Cunningham virus infection of the brain. Other complications of steroids include psychiatric problems, cataracts, osteoporosis, and ischemic necrosis of hips and other joints. Steroids, including methylprednisolone, induce programmed cell death (apoptosis), not only in lymphocytes but in neurons in the brain and the retina. In contrast, studies performed more than 3 decades ago have shown the corticotrophin has a powerful neuroprotective effect. This is yet another reason for supporting use of ACTH.

Treatment Aimed at Reducing the Risk of Relapses and Neurologic Disability

Treatments demonstrated to prevent attacks and reduce the risk of disability that have been approved for use include three forms of interferon-beta (Betaseron®, Avonex®, and Rebif®) and glatiramer acetate (Copaxone®). They are sometimes referred to as the "ABC" first wave of injectable drug products that have been modestly effective, especially if initiated at the onset of MS. They reduce the risk of attacks by approximately 30%, but when used early, they are about 50% more effective. The reduction in the risk of progression appears to be between 35–40%. Natalizumab (Tysabri®) an IV drug that has been more recently approved, appears to be about twice as effective as the first wave drugs in preventing relapses and in preventing disease progression. However, there is a risk associated with the use of Tysabri® of 1/1,000 developing PML, a serious and often fatal brain infection.

The first of a third wave of oral products, Fingolimod (Gilenya®), was approved September 22, 2010. After 1 year in a drug comparison study, it was 50% more effective than interferon-beta 1a (Avonex®) in reducing relapses. In a second study, Fingolimod was 54% more effective than placebo after 2 years in reducing relapses. Fingolimod and another drug, cladribine, have reported effectiveness approaching that of Tysabri® in reducing relapses but with important side effects including an increased risk of viral infections. Cladribine was not approved in 2011 "pending further safety-benefit analysis." Other oral products as well as two intravenous drugs are currently under investigation. A concern is that oral drugs are more convenient but decreased compliance outside of studies is a reality. The interferon-beta injectable drugs produce a variable local reaction as well as a "flulike" systemic reaction. Nonsteroidal anti-inflammatory drugs are quite effective in minimizing the systemic reaction, which includes an anxiety-like reaction with respiratory distress and rapid heart rate.

Prevention, Control, and Adherence Patterns

As the first decade of the 21st century has passed, research has not yet identified a means for preventing MS. Not quite a century ago, Roy Swank while training at Cambridge in England studied the relationship between diet and the risk of MS, based on his observation that a coastal Norwegian diet appeared to be protective.[30] He concluded that animal fat consumption increased both serum lipids and the risk of MS. He showed for the first time that a low animal fat diet reduced serum lipids and also appeared to reduce the risk of MS relapse. He published a series of long term follow-up papers reporting favorable outcomes in a Montreal cohort of MS patients who had been followed for up to 40 years. Others reported a reduction in relapses with similar dietary management in controlled trials. Although Swank proposed that a low animal fat diet supplemented with cod liver oil would decrease the risk of MS,[31] no population studies have been undertaken as yet.

Vitamin D Deficiency

Vitamin D deficiency has emerged as relevant to the risk of MS and as an opportunity to easily control an important environmental factor. Recommended doses of vitamin D have recently been revised upward from 300 IU to 800–900 IU daily, based on the recognition that average serum vitamin D levels that had been accepted as normal were actually low. Work at the Harvard School of Public Health has implicated values below 100 nmol/L are a risk for MS, which may be greater in women. Preliminary treatment trials have shown that women benefit from aggressive supplementation.

Smoking

Smoking has been documented to double the risk of MS and also to double the risk of disability in studies.[27,28] Cigarette smoking is also known to increase symptoms in MS. It is obvious that this unhealthy habit has an important but remediable impact on MS. There is no reason to expect risks of relapse or disability to differ with use of marijuana because smoke activates immune responses in the lungs, which is hypothesized to be the mechanism leading to disease activation.

Relapse Prevention

Relapse prevention (control) has been the primary goal of the initial trials of therapeutic of interferon-beta-1b (Betaseron®) and other agents for MS. The reduction of the risk of disability first demonstrated for interferon-beta-1a (Avonex®) has been accepted as a more important longer term goal. However, therapeutic trials still focus on relapse prevention, which is easier to document. An important issue in connection with treatment in any illness is compliance with treatment. In MS centers where education of the patient is emphasized and the patient's trust is gained, compliance with injectable treatment is 70% or greater. In community neurologists' offices the compliance rates are substantially lower, averaging about 20%. A common misperception among patients and professionals is that patients' disabilities are likely to be reduced by the ABC and other drugs. Although disability may occasionally be reduced in some individuals, improvement rarely occurs. Patients must be guided to accept the reality of their illness and any residual disability or they may be become disillusioned and stop therapy inappropriately.

Summary

Multiple sclerosis is the most common neurologic disease and cause of disability in young adults, primarily those of European descent. This inflammatory, demyelinating, autoimmune disorder primarily affects the brain and spinal cord, but visual problems are common. Despite a risk of progressive disability, life expectancy is minimally reduced in untreated patients. Prevalence rates appear to be increasing nationally although population-based studies in Olmsted County, Minnesota, have not shown this. This county is the most intensively and repeatedly studied population in the United States and has the highest reported MS incidence and prevalence rates. Diagnosis of MS has been greatly facilitated by incorporating MRI and analyses of spinal fluid among diagnostic criteria. These criteria have led to earlier initiation of standard treatment producing superior long-term control.

The most common difficulties encountered in MS involve vision, ability to walk, and control of bladder and bowel. Impaired cognition as well as anxiety and depression occur with some frequency. Standard treatments (Avonex®, Betaseron®, Copaxone®, and Rebif®) are modestly effective, especially when introduced early in the illness. More aggressive treatments are available (Cytoxan, Novantrone, Tysabri®) but their use is associated with not only greater potential benefit but more potential harm. Of the new highly effective oral agents, Fingolimod is the only approved agent but others are likely to be approved in the U.S. by the FDA and in other countries.

Infectious factors in genetically primed hosts are hypothesized to be important in MS but a specific infectious etiology has not been identified. Genetic factors contribute to the risk of MS as the disease occurs among blood relatives. Research has strongly implicated smoking as a risk for developing MS and for increasing disability. Vitamin D deficiency has also been convincingly demonstrated to be a risk factor that appears to be greater in women who alone appear to benefit by treatment with high doses (2,000 IU daily). As more neurologists with expertise in MS are trained, more complete case ascertainment is anticipated as in Olmsted County and the rate will appear to rise throughout the United States in genetically predisposed individuals.

Discussion Questions

1. What factors predispose to MS? Discuss factors that predispose to relapses in MS.
2. Why might women be predisposed to MS?
3. Why might the incidence and prevalence rates for MS be higher in Minnesota? What factors might be implicated?
4. Do you think that data from mortality rates recorded for MS are useful? Discuss the strengths and weaknesses of using mortality rates for studying MS.
5. Discuss molecular mimicry in relationship to immune responses and its potential relevance to MS.

References

1. McAlpine D, Compston ND, and Acheson ED. *Multiple Sclerosis: A reappraisal.* Ed. 2. London. Churchill Livingston, Copyright Elsevier 1998, p32.
2. Noseworthy JH, Luccinetti C, Rodriguez M, Weinschenker BG. Multiple sclerosis. *N Engl J Med.* 2000;343:938–952.
3. Confavreux C, Vukusic S, Moreau T, Adeline P. Relapses and progression of disability in multiple sclerosis. *N Engl J Med.* 2000;343:1430–1438.
4. Confavreux C, Hutchinson M, Hours MM, et al. Rate of pregnancy-related relapse in multiple sclerosis. *N Engl J Med.* 1998;339:285–291.
5. Weinschenker BG, Bass B, Rice GPA, et al. The natural history of multiple sclerosis: a geographically based study. 1. Clinical course and disability. *Brain.* 1989;112:133–146.
6. Mayr WT, Pittock SJ, McClelland RL, et al. Incidence and prevalence of multiple sclerosis in Olmsted County, Minnesota. *Neurology.* 2003;61:1373–1377.
7. Alter M., Kurtzke JF. *The Epidemiology of Multiple Sclerosis.* Springfield, IL: Thomas; 1968.
8. Kurtzke JF. Epidemiological contributions in multiple sclerosis: an overview. *Neurology.* 1980;30:61–79.
9. Cotttrel DA, Kremenchutzky M, Rice GPA. The natural history of multiple sclerosis: a geographically based study. 5: the clinical features and natural history of primary progressive multiple sclerosis. *Brain.* 1999;122:641–647.
10. Ebers GC, Koopman WJ, Hader W, et al. The natural history of multiple sclerosis: a geographically based study. 8: familial multiple sclerosis. *Brain.* 2000;123;631–640.
11. Sawyer S, Ban M, Maraniah M., et al. A high-density screen for linkage in multiple sclerosis. *Am J Hum Genet.* 2005;77:454–467.
12. The International Multiple Sclerosis Consortium. Risk alleles for multiple sclerosis identified by a genomewide study. *N Engl J Med.* 2007;357:1–12.
13. Redelings MD, McCoy L, Sorvillo F. Multiple sclerosis mortality and patterns of comorbidity in the United States from 1990 to 2001. *Neuroepidemiology.* 2006;26:102–107.
14. Kurtzke JF. Epidemiologic evidence for multiple sclerosis as an infection. *Clin Microbiol Rev.* 1993;6:382–427.
15. Pittock SJ, Mayr WT, McClelland RI, et al. Change in MS-related disability in a population-based cohort. A 10-year follow-up study. *Neurology.* 2004;62:51–59.

16. Bamford CR, Sibley WA, Thies C, et al. Trauma as an etiologic and aggravating factor in multiple sclerosis *Neurology.* 1981;31:1229–1234.

17. Grant I, Brown GW, Harris T, et al. Severely threatening events and marked life difficulties preceding onset or exacerbation of multiple sclerosis. *J Neurol Neurosurg Psychiatr.* 1989;52:8–13.

18. Mohr DC, Goodkin DE, Bacchetti P, et al. Psychological stress and the subsequent appearance of new brain MRI lesions in MS. *Neurology.* 2000;55:55–61.

19. Sadovnik AD, Ebers GC, Wilson RW, Paty DW. Life expectancy in patients attending multiple sclerosis clinics. *Neurology.* 1992;42:991–994.

20. McDonald WI, Compston A, Edan G, et al. Recommended diagnostic criteria for multiple sclerosis: guidelines from the International Panel on the Diagnosis of Multiple Sclerosis. *Ann Neurol.* 2001;50:121–127.

21. Jersild C, Fog T. HLA antigens and multiple scleroses. *Lancet.* 1972;1240–1241.

22. Ascherio A, Munger KL. Environmental risk factors in multiple sclerosis. Part I: the role of infection. *Ann Neurol.* 2007;61:288–299.

23. Ascherio A, Munger KL. Environmental risk factors in multiple sclerosis. Part II: noninfectious factors. *Ann Neurol.* 2007;61:504–515.

24. Olson JK, Croxford J, Calenoff MA, et al. A virus-induced molecular mimicry model of multiple sclerosis. *J Clin Invest.* 2001;108:311–318.

25. Wekerle H, Hohlfeld R. Molecular mimicry in multiple sclerosis. *N Engl J Med.* 2003;349:185–186.

26. Farrell RA, Wall GR, Clark DA, et al. Humoral immune response to EBV in multiple sclerosis is associated with disease activity on MRI. *Neurology.* 2009;73:32–38.

27. Munger KL, Zhang SM, O'Reilly E, et al. Vitamin D intake and incidence of multiple sclerosis. *Neurology.* 2004;62:60–65.

28. Munger K, Levin LL, Hollis BW, et al. Serum 25-hydroxyvitamin D levels and risk of multiple sclerosis. *JAMA.* 2006;296:2832–2838.

29. Hernan MA, Olek MJ, Ascherio A. Cigarette smoking and incidence of multiple sclerosis. *Am J Epidemiol.* 2001;154:69–74.

30. Swank RL, Lerstad O, Stroom A, Backer J. Multiple sclerosis in rural Norway. Its geographic and occupational incidence in relation to nutrition. *N Engl J Med.* 1952;246:722–728.

31. Swank RL, Dugan BB. *The Multiple Sclerosis Diet Book.* New York: Random House; 1987.

Systemic Lupus Erythematosus

Archana Vasudevan, MD and Ellen M. Ginzler, MD, MPH

A Typical Lupus Patient named Cora

At age 9, Cora began to feel sick as the new school year began. When she turned 10 years old, Cora began to have severe fatigue, a facial rash, and joint pains, and was found to be severely anemic. She was diagnosed with systemic lupus erythematosus (SLE) and treated with prednisone and hydroxychloroquine. Her SLE was well controlled on low-dose prednisone until she was a teenager, when she developed a flare of her rash and arthritis. Early in her 20s, Cora developed a seizure disorder and lupus nephritis, which were treated with mycophenolate mofetil, prednisone, and hydroxychloroquine. During the course of her disease, Cora also developed severe osteoporosis with multiple vertebral compression fractures and macular toxicity from antimalarial medications. Her SLE remains active with cutaneous flares. She continues to be treated with mycophenolate mofetil and low-dose prednisone for lupus. Cora is now treated with bisphosphonates for osteoporosis. Her growth was impaired by the medications and chronic illness. She finished high school and college but had to drop out of graduate school because of her illness. Now in her 30s, Cora is thinking about her chances of having a family and children.

Introduction

Systemic lupus erythematosus (SLE) is an autoimmune condition that may affect almost any organ in the body. The Centers for Disease Control and Prevention (CDC) website states that 322,000 to over 1 million people have been affected by lupus in the United States.[1,2] However, the actual incidence and prevalence of lupus is probably much higher, as these numbers do not include patients with overlapping features of other autoimmune conditions such as scleroderma or Sjögren's syndrome. Furthermore, patients with incomplete expression of the disease based on the American College of Rheumatology (ACR) criteria for diagnosis (Table 23-1) and undiagnosed patients are not included.[3] Moreover, with the SLE classification criteria being revised, the incidence and prevalence may change again.

Ninety percent of lupus patients are women who are diagnosed most frequently with symptoms during their reproductive years between ages 20 and 39.[4,5] This gender predilection may be explained by genetic abnormalities in some studies. Men with an extra X chromosome, i.e., Klinefelter's syndrome, (47, XXY), have been found to have the same risk for developing lupus as women (46, XX).[6] Abnormal DNA methylation that can activate or inactivate genes involved in regulation of the immune system on the X chromosome have been described in women with lupus.[7] Cytokines—proteins involved in cellular signaling—known to be pathogenetic in SLE such as interferons are produced in much higher quantities by lymphocytes in women.[8]

People belonging to minority populations—blacks, Asians, and Hispanics—are affected much more often and have more severe disease than Caucasians.[9–11] The manifestations also differ between various ethnic groups, with renal problems developing during the course of the disease among 30–50% of African-Americans compared with 13% of Caucasian patients.[10–12] A study conducted in Sweden indicated risk of lupus among immigrants tends to parallel the risk of developing lupus in the country of origin.[13]

Recent studies indicate an improvement in survival of lupus patients from less than 50% alive 5 years after diagnosis in 1955 to over 85% at 10 years,[14] although lupus patients still face a 1.5- to 5-fold greater risk of mortality compared to the general population.[15] In earlier decades, mortality was related to progressive organ failure; however, with the introduction of immunosuppressive agents including steroids, newer antihypertensives, dialysis, and renal transplantation, the causes of death shifted to include complications resulting from treatment such as infections and accelerated atherosclerosis.[15] Despite improvements in overall survival, a large international cohort study of more than 9,500 SLE patients provided the standardized mortality rate (SMR, the ratio of observed number of deaths to the expected number of deaths among women of the same age and calendar-year cohort) of 2.2 for the United States although the rate was significantly greater among African Americans with an SMR of 2.6 [95% CI = 2.3–2.9] than Caucasians, SMR = 1.4 [95% CI = 1.2–1.7].[16]

Table 23-1

The 1997 American College of Rheumatology (ACR) Revised Criteria for the Classification of Systemic Lupus Erythematosus (SLE)

1. Malar rash—Fixed malar erythema, flat or raised

2. Discoid rash—Erythematous raised patches with keratotic scaling and follicular plugging; atrophic scarring may occur

3. Photosensitivity—Skin rash as an unusual reaction to sunlight, by patient history or physician observation

4. Oral ulcers—Oral or nasopharyngeal ulcers, usually painless, observed by physician

5. Arthritis—Nonerosive arthritis involving two or more peripheral joints, characterized by tenderness, swelling, or effusion

6. Serositis—Pleuritis (convincing history of pleuritic pain or rub heard by physician or evidence of pleural effusion) OR pericarditis (documented by ECG, rub, or evidence of pericardial effusion)

7. Renal disorder—Persistent proteinuria (> 0.5 g/d or $> 3+$) OR cellular casts of any type

8. Neurologic disorder—Seizures (in the absence of other causes) OR psychosis (in the absence of other causes)

9. Hematologic disorder—Hemolytic anemia OR leukopenia ($< 4,000$/mL on two or more occasions) OR lymphopenia ($< 1,500$/mL on two or more occasions) OR thrombocytopenia ($< 100,000$/mL in the absence of offending drugs)

10. Immunologic disorder—Antidouble-stranded DNA OR anti-Sm OR positive finding of antiphospholipid antibodies based on (1) an abnormal serum level of immunoglobulin G (IgG) or M (IgM) anticardiolipin antibodies, (2) a positive test result for lupus anticoagulant using a standard method, or (3) a false-positive serologic test for syphilis known to be positive for at least 6 months and confirmed by *Treponema pallidum* immobilization or fluorescent treponemal antibody absorption test

11. Antinuclear antibody—An abnormal titer of antinuclear antibody (ANA) by immunofluorescence or an equivalent assay at any time and in the absence of drugs known to be associated with "drug-induced lupus syndrome"

Diagnosis of SLE for inclusion in clinical trials requires 4 of 11 criteria.

Sources: Data from Tan EM, Cohen AS, Fries JF, et al. The 1982 revised criteria for the classification of systemic lupus erythematosus. *Arthritis Rheum.* 1982; 25:1271–1277.
Hochberg MC. Updating the American College of Rheumatology revised criteria for the classification of systemic lupus erythematosus. *Arthritis Rheum.* 1997; 40:1725.

Pathophysiology of SLE

Lupus is an autoimmune disease with a complex interplay of genetic and environmental factors playing a role in its pathophysiology. A susceptible person with multiple SLE predisposing genes may experience an environmental trigger such as an infection or radiation. This second trigger may set into motion events that occur in the immune system of the genetically susceptible patient. The damage to the various tissues by lupus is mediated by both the innate and adaptive components of the immune system. Although some cells—antigen presenting cells, B and T helper cells—may be overactive, others such as the regulatory cells may be underfunctioning. Antigens that are normally immunologically sequestered may be exposed to lymphocytes and antigen presenting cells. These cells, due to loss of tolerance and decreased apoptosis, undergo abnormal, prolonged activation resulting in inflammatory response.[17]

Clinical Manifestations and Complications of SLE

Lupus may affect almost any organ in the body and with varying degrees of severity. Accrual of clinical and serologic criteria for diagnosis may take months to years from the time of onset of symptoms.[18,19] Many patients present with nonspecific symptoms such as fatigue, anorexia, alopecia, headaches, Raynaud's phenomenon, and myalgias before being diagnosed with SLE.[19]

Of all the clinical manifestations of lupus, cutaneous and musculoskeletal are the most common including malar rash on the face (Figure 23-1) and hands crippled with arthritis (Figure 23-2).[17] These can decrease the quality of life due to disability and cosmetic effects. However, renal and central nervous system manifestations cause more morbidity. Lupus nephritis has been classified into six categories as listed in Table 23-2. The glomerular capillaries in lupus nephritis are damaged by deposition of immune complexes (antigen-antibody complexes, complement components, and immunoglobulins) resulting in various clinical features—hematuria, pyuria, cellular casts, hypertension, and proteinuria. Thromboses within these renal blood vessels due to the presence of antiphospholipid antibodies causing microangiopathy can present similarly.[20]

In addition to the clinical features of SLE itself, healthcare providers also have to be vigilant about the complications of the disease and its treatment. Accelerated atherosclerosis has been well documented in women with SLE and even in the pediatric age group.[15,21] The relative risk of atherosclerosis in women with SLE under the

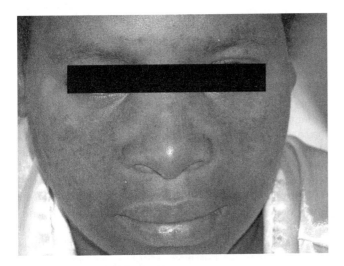

Figure 23-1 Malar facial rash of lupus.

Courtesy of Archana Vasudeva and Ellen M. Ginzler

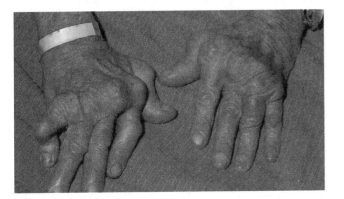

Figure 23-2 Crippling arthritis of lupus.

Source: Courtesy of Leonard V. Crowley, MD, Century College.

age of 45 is five times that of the general population.[22] The traditional risk factors for coronary atherosclerosis such as hyperlipidemia, hypertension, diabetes, metabolic syndrome, smoking, and postmenopausal status are accentuated in SLE patients, contributing to this higher risk. Furthermore, certain nontraditional cardiovascular risk factors—nephrotic syndrome, body mass index, and low physical activity, which result more from fatigue, arthralgias/arthritis and myalgia than active lupus—increase within the first 3 years of SLE diagnosis. A multivariate analysis of all the traditional and nontraditional cardiovascular risk factors has found SLE itself to be an additional risk factor. Some of these factors such as morbid obesity, smoking, and sedentary lifestyle are significantly higher in African Americans with SLE.[15,23]

Osteoporosis prevalence is also increased in SLE patients, which may result from treatment with steroids. African American, Hispanic, and Asian populations with SLE have also been found to have a lower bone mineral density (BMD) than Caucasian populations.[24–26] Similarly patients with juvenile onset of the disease have lower BMD then age-matched populations.[27] However, a third of SLE patients with vertebral and nonvertebral fractures may have a normal bone mineral density.[28]

Table 23-2

Abbreviated International Society of Nephrology/Renal Pathology Society Classification of Lupus Nephritis (2003)

Class I	Minimal lupus nephritis
Class II	Proliferative lupus nephritis
Class III	Focal lupus nephritis
Class IV	Diffuse segmental (IV-S) or global (IV-G) lupus nephritis
Class V	Membranous lupus nephritis
Class VI	Advanced sclerosing lupus nephritis

Source: Data from Weening JJ, D'Agati VD, Schwartz MM, et al. on behalf of the International Society of Nephrology and Renal Pathology Society Working Group on the Classification of Lupus Nephritis. The classification of glomerulonephritis in systemic lupus erythematosus revisited. *J Am Soc Nephrol.* 2004; 15:241–250.

Age-appropriate screening for malignancies is absolutely essential as SLE patients treated with immunosuppressive agents are at increased risk. Pap smears are recommended annually and should be enforced as the risk of cervical dysplasia is increased in SLE patients treated with immunosuppressive agents.[29]

Agents Used in the Treatment of SLE and Their Complications

The main goal of treatment has been to prevent or reduce damage to organs. Steroids, cyclophosphamide, azathioprine, mycophenolate mofetil, methotrexate, leflunomide, and cyclosporine A are all used in the treatment of lupus as immunosuppressive agents.[30] Steroids are the first line of therapy. Other immunosuppressive medications are used to prevent disease exacerbations and as steroid-sparing drugs to avoid the long-term side effects such as osteoporosis, diabetes, and avascular necrosis. Alkylating agents like cyclophosphamide have serious side effects of infertility, infections, cancers, and bone marrow suppression, which have to be weighed against the benefits for individual cases.

Newer medications such as mycophenolate mofetil have better side effect profiles with equal efficacy, which make them more attractive for both physicians and patients. Other medications such as dapsone, colchicine, intravenous immunoglobulin, and thalidomide have been used for certain manifestations of SLE. Biologics—medications prepared by using DNA recombinant technology—have been aimed at controlling abnormal cytokines or cells that are shown to be pathogenic in SLE. Examples include rituximab (targets B cells), belimumab (targets cytokine—B lymphocyte stimulator) and abatacept (targets the T cell costimulatory pathway). Most of these therapeutic agents are commercially available but used "off label" for SLE.

Antimalarials—hydroxychloroquine—were initially used for controlling skin rashes and arthritis. Recent research has shown such widespread survival and response advantages for antimalarials with such small risk of retinal toxicity that they are now prescribed for most patients with SLE. Medications for other indications are commonly prescribed in the treatment regimens by rheumatologists. Antihypertensives such as angiotensin receptor blockers and angiotensin converting enzyme inhibitors are used to control proteinuria in patients with lupus nephritis. Other antihypertensives such as calcium channel blockers are used for Raynaud's and pulmonary hypertension management. Bisphosphonates are prescribed for prophylaxis as well as treatment of glucocorticoid-induced osteoporosis. Prophylaxis for osteoporosis and monitoring with biennial bone mineral densities should be done for most patients unless the patient has chronic renal failure or is in the pediatric age group. Though the role of BMD testing in predicting fractures in SLE patients is not comparable to other populations, it does identify the majority of patients at risk.

Close monitoring and management of patients by rheumatologists is required as patients with quiescent disease may require tapering of steroids, initiation of steroid-sparing agents or prophylactic treatment. Some care may be adequately provided by primary care physicians but most primary care providers are not comfortable making changes to treatment regimens or with routine monitoring of patients with SLE.[31]

Several indicators have been developed for monitoring disease activity such as SLEDAI (Systemic Lupus Erythematosus Disease Activity Index) and BILAG (British Isles Lupus Assessment Group).[32–34] These descriptive criteria have been revised several times to more accurately capture minor changes in disease activity. SLICC/DI (Systemic Lupus Erythematosus International Collaborating Clinics Damage Index) has been developed to assess the damage due to SLE, its treatment and the consequences of prolonged survival of these patients.[35] Data indicate that lupus patients with more damage earlier in the course of their disease experience higher mortality rates.

Lupus at Each Stage of Life

Adolescence

About 15% of lupus patients have disease onset before age 16, when lupus tends to be more severe than in adults. Adolescents also have more persistently active disease that, when treated with immunosuppressive medications, may result in delayed growth and pubertal development.[36] As with other chronic illnesses during adolescence, lupus also leads to altered mood and cognitive dysfunction. However, distinguishing neuropsychiatric SLE (NP-SLE) from primary mood disorders is essential as both may have their onset in this age group.[37]

Damage accrual is more rapid among teenage patients than adults, especially within the first 6 months of disease onset and tends to increase with younger age at onset, persistently active disease and recurrent infections.[38,39] Although cosmetic effects of medications should be considered at every life stage, peer pressure and the desire to "fit in" may lead to decreased compliance with treatment regimens, particularly among adolescents.

Reproductive

The burden of the disease is highest in the reproductive age group. Although mortality rates have been reduced, a third of the deaths from lupus continue to occur among patients aged 15 to 44. Women in this group also have higher prevalence of mood and anxiety disorders.[40] Patients without active neuropsychiatric SLE (NP-SLE) may also have decreased attention, memory, and reasoning abilities.[41] Emotional distress is accentuated by increased prevalence of impaired sexual function due to increased fatigue, bodyaches, and depression.[42]

Contraceptive use is recommended for all women in this age group, especially in the presence of active disease or while receiving most immunosuppressive agents. Low estrogen oral contraceptives are prescribed for stable lupus patients if they do not have antiphospholipid antibody syndrome. Contraceptive methods such as intrauterine devices have increased incidence of infections in SLE and progesterone only oral contraceptives lead to accelerated bone loss and, therefore, are usually not recommended.[43]

Despite misconceptions among patients with SLE, fertility rates are normal with a pregnancy rate of 2–2.4 per person, with lower rates seen mainly in patients with lupus nephritis (1.9 versus 2.5, $P = 0.01$).[44] Ovarian function is retained among younger patients even while being treated with cyclophosphamide. Lupus patients often experience difficulty with childcare involving lifting, carrying, and bathing young children.[45] Women who develop lupus later in life have usually experienced worse pregnancy outcomes prior to being diagnosed with the disease compared to other healthy women.[46] These adverse pregnancy outcomes may result from the appearance of autoantibodies in their serum long before the clinical manifestations of SLE.[47,48] However, prepregnancy counseling, better treatment options, closer monitoring, and joint management by obstetricians, perinatalogists, cardiologists, and rheumatologists have led to improved pregnancy outcomes with fewer flares during pregnancy and postpartum. Among women with active lupus, approximately 50% flare during pregnancy and a significant proportion have poor fetal outcomes. Outcomes are even better when the disease is quiescent before conception with disease flares occurring in only 8% during pregnancy and 10% of these women experience fetal loss.[49,50] The main risk factors for poor pregnancy outcomes are proteinuria, antiphospholipid antibody syndrome (APS), thrombocytopenia, and hypertension.[51] Hypertensive complications occur in 10–20% of women with SLE especially with a history of lupus nephritis. There is also an increased incidence of preeclampsia toxemia.[49,50] A useful resource for providers and patients alike is the ACR website at http://www.rheumatology.org/practice/clinical/patients/diseases_and_conditions/pregnancy.asp.

A small number of newborns to mothers with anti-SSA/Ro or anti-SSB/La antibodies may develop skin, blood, liver, and heart abnormalities. Together these conditions are termed neonatal lupus syndrome, which parallels the presence of maternal autoantibodies until the sixth to eighth month of life. However, congenital heart block that occurs in utero to the developing fetal heart tissue is irreversible and carries very high morbidity and mortality risk.

Women with these autoantibodies require fetal echocardiograms performed weekly from week 16 to monitor high-risk fetuses.[17] If the fetuses show signs of cardiac involvement (bradycardia, heart blocks, heart failure) or hydrops, then the mothers may be treated with oral dexamethasone or apheresis to remove maternal antibodies from circulation and prevent progression of fetal cardiac disease. However, these treatments are of limited value in preventing progression of heart block in affected fetuses. Children born with first- or second-degree heart blocks may progress to third degree after birth and require pacemakers for survival. Once the cardiac conduction system is scarred by the auto-antibodies, the heart block is irreversible.[52]

Older Years

A study in Sweden noted menopause occurred earlier among lupus patients (44.9 years vs. 46.8 years) and the use of hormone replacement therapy for symptoms also started earlier than in healthy women.[44] The gender disparity usually seen in lupus is less pronounced in this older population. Compared to younger women at initial presentation of lupus, the 5- and 10-year survival rates of patients diagnosed after the age of 50 are lower due to comorbidities associated with aging common in the general population. The diagnosis may be missed due to a higher frequency of nonspecific symptoms that are common to other diseases. Older age at SLE onset is characterized by slower disease progression involving organ systems and lower prevalence of the more severe manifestations of SLE such as lupus nephritis and neuropsychiatric lupus and higher incidence of serositis, interstitial lung disease and Sjögren's syndrome.[53,54]

Key Points

Minorities Have Higher Prevalence of SLE

The LUpus in MInorities: NAture vs. nurture (LUMINA) study was started in 1994 to identify the differences between three racial/ethnic groups—African American, Hispanic, and Caucasian populations. Some manifestations of SLE are more common in certain groups such as myocarditis, which was seen in 60% of African American patients with SLE whereas it was seen only in 1.9% of Hispanic patients in the study.[55] Among African Americans receiving renal transplantation for end-stage renal disease secondary to lupus nephritis, the risk of recurrent lupus nephritis in their posttransplant kidneys is higher than for others.[56] Damage index scores increase more rapidly in Hispanic populations with SLE than Caucasian or African American populations.[57] Older age and greater lupus activity were associated with this increase in damage along with ethnicity and lower household incomes.[58]

Quality of Life (QoL)

Review of multiple studies has demonstrated that even though the health-related quality of life (HRQoL) is reduced in SLE patients, it appears to correlate more with the age of the patient than disease activity.[59] The QoL also depends on a Hassles index, which measures minor stressors that everyone encounters in daily life. SLE patients with higher Hassles index and renal involvement have lower QoL.[60,61]

Work Disability

Three-quarters of SLE patients have problems with hand function and about 42% are unable to perform their daily activities.[62] Disability earlier in the course of the disease is determined by higher disease activity at diagnosis, higher physical demands of the job, and lower educational level. Patients from a lower socioeconomic status, as measured by educational level and occupational prestige are more likely to become disabled as well.[58,63] However, when applying for Social Security benefits, SLE patients have been reported to be less successful in obtaining benefits, as their medical records may not accurately document their functional disability.[64] Survival is also lower in SLE patients who have household incomes below $25,000 per year (70% vs. 86%) than those with higher incomes.[65] An important point of note is that in 2004, more women live under the poverty line than men.[66]

Social Support

Married women or women with a live-in partner scored higher in their physical function than single women. Family size is, however, smaller than in controls. The patient's culture appears to be a better predictor of family size with patients belonging to ethnic minority populations having larger families than whites. The effect of social support on disease activity also appears to differ according to the patient's culture. Social support appeared to benefit the patient's physical functioning more for those patients with social, economic, and health advantages.[42,67]

Health Insurance

Uninsured patients had far fewer visits to healthcare providers than patients with Medicaid. Medicaid patients had to travel longer distances to see their rheumatologists. These patients had more emergency room visits and were often required to see their primary care physician before being referred to a rheumatologist.[68] Ethnic and income differences also appear to predict the type and use of insurance. African American patients were less likely to be privately insured and more likely to have no insurance.[68] Hispanic populations appear to underuse their Medicaid and Medicare coverage compared to other populations including their prescription programs, hospitalizations, or outpatient follow-ups.[69,70] Poor prognosis in patients with SLE has not been shown to be related to underuse or noncompliance with medication use or limited access to medical care. However, the improved survival rates of SLE patients with introduction of steroids, newer antihypertensive medications, renal dialysis, and transplantation does suggest that lack of treatment with newly available prescribed medications would result in diminished survival rates reported prior to the 1950s when 50% of patients died within 4 years of diagnosis of SLE.[71]

Key Research Studies

Only two medications, corticosteroids and hydroxychloroquine, are approved by the Food and Drug Administration (FDA) for the treatment of SLE, although in the last 2 decades there have been an increasing number of clinical trials for SLE, with over 200 trials listed on www.clinicaltrials.gov in September 2009. These include both interventional and noninterventional clinical trials for treatment and prevention of SLE, its complications, and comorbidities. Some biologic agents, such as abatacept and rituximab, have failed to show superiority over placebo on a background of currently available disease-modifying antirheumatic drugs, whereas others, such as the monoclonal antibody to CD40 ligand, had side effects that resulted in the trials being terminated early.[30,72]

Some of the key studies of importance have been the following:

1. Mycophenolate mofetil (Cellcept®) was shown in clinical trials for lupus nephritis to be as effective if not superior to intravenous cyclophosphamide with higher rates of partial and complete remission and fewer complications.[73–75]
2. Oral contraceptives were shown not to lead to lupus flares in patients with stable disease.[76]
3. Hydroxychloroquine (Plaquenil®) was shown to give an advantage in response to treatment and in survival in SLE patients and to reduce flares in pregnant women.[77]
4. Belimumab (Benlysta) has shown efficacy in patients with serologically active disease along with standard of care therapy in phase II and III trials.[78]

Unanswered Questions

The risks of treating pediatric patients with the same medications as adults with SLE need to be studied. An example as mentioned in the clinical vignette of the young girl with a long history of SLE. The effects of bisphosphonates prescribed for osteoporosis prophylaxis in pediatric and reproductive age group on "normal" bone growth have not been demonstrated.

1. Not many interventional and noninterventional clinical trials are designed for juvenile SLE patients.
2. Persistently active disease has never been targeted in trials, even though this is the more common state of disease activity in SLE patients.
3. Multiple registries have been established to study the natural history of SLE and its complications, but the need to study the effect of ethnic admixture on the risk of SLE still exists.

Summary

SLE is a prototype of chronic autoimmune diseases that is characterized by relapses and remissions. Although the disease may affect any age group, women in the reproductive age group are the most affected. Multidisciplinary management of pregnant women with lupus has shown improved outcomes in recent years with better treatment options. However, there is no effective prophylaxis or treatment for fetuses or neonates at risk for or with cardiac involvement. In conclusion, considerable clinical and basic science research in the last few decades has been translated into significant improvement in the management of lupus with improved morbidity and mortality. Many unanswered questions remain to be the focus of research in the coming years.

Discussion Questions

1. How would you compare the problems that women with SLE face with that of women afflicted with diabetes mellitus, as both involve multiple systems?
2. What factors should you take into consideration when a woman with SLE is planning a pregnancy?
3. Describe areas not studied or other unanswered questions in research in SLE.
4. What factors determine prognosis in SLE patients?
5. What are the different comorbidities to be considered in the three age groups—adolescence, reproductive age group, and postmenopausal age groups?

References

1. Office of Minority Health and Disparities. Eliminate disparities in lupus. http://www.cdc.gov/omhd/amh/factsheets/lupus.htm#8.
2. Helmick CG, Felson DT, Lawrence RC, et al. National Arthritis Data Workgroup. Estimates of the prevalence of arthritis and other rheumatic conditions in the United States: part 1. *Arthritis Rheum.* 2008;58:15–25.
3. Hochberg MC. Updating the American College of Rheumatology revised criteria for the classification of systemic lupus erythematosus. *Arthritis Rheum.* 1997;40:1725.
4. Office of Women's Health. Could I have lupus? http://www.womenshealth.gov/about-us/government-in-action/couldihavelupus.cfm. Accessed August 26, 2012.
5. McCarty DJ, Manzi S, Medsger TA, et al. Incidence of systemic lupus erythematosus. Race and gender differences. *Arthritis Rheum.* 1995;38(9):1260–1270.
6. Scofield RH, Bruner GR, Namjou B, et al. Klinefelter's Syndrome (47,XXY) in male systemic lupus erythematosus patients support for the notion of a gene-dose effect from the X chromosome. *Arthritis Rheum.* 2008;58:2511–2517.
7. Lu Q, Wu A, Tesmer L, et al. Demethylation of CD40LG on the inactive X in T cells from women with lupus. *J Immunol.* 2007;179:6352–6358.
8. Berghofer B, Frommer T, Haley G, et al. TLR7 ligands induce higher IFN-α production in females. *J Immunol.* 2006;177:2088–2096.
9. Lau CS, Yin G, Mok MY. Ethnic and geographical differences in systemic lupus erythematosus: an overview. *Lupus.* 2006;15:715–719.
10. Kumar K, Chambers S, Gordon C. Challenges of ethnicity in SLE. *Best Pract Res Clin Rheumatol.* 2009;23:549–561.
11. Cooper GS, Parks CG, Treadwell EL, et al. Differences by race, sex and age in the clinical and immunologic features of recently diagnosed systemic lupus erythematosus patients in the southeastern United States. *Lupus.* 2002;11:161–167.
12. Bastian HM, Roseman JM, McGwin G, et al for the LUMINA study group. Systemic lupus erythematosus in three ethnic groups. XII. Risk factors for lupus nephritis after diagnosis. *Lupus.* 2002;11:152–160.
13. Li X, Sundquist J, Sundquist K. Risks of rheumatic diseases in first- and second-generation immigrants in Sweden. A nationwide followup study. *Arthritis Rheum.* 2009;60:1588–1596.
14. Pistiner M, Wallace DJ, Nessim S, et al. Lupus erythematosus in 1980s: a survey of 570 patients. *Semin Arthritis Rheum.* 1991;21:55–64.
15. Borchers AT, Keen CL, Shoenfeld Y, Gershwin ME. Surviving the butterfly and the wolf: mortality trends in systemic lupus erythematosus. *Autoimmun Rev.* 2004;3:423–453.
16. Bernatsky S, Boivin JF, Joseph L, et al. Mortality in systemic lupus erythematosus. *Arthritis Rheum.* 2006;54:2550–2557.
17. Wallace DJ, Hahn BH, eds. *Dubois' Lupus Erythematosus.* 7th ed. Philadelphia: Lippincott Williams & Wilkins; 2007: 47–53, 639–646, 1059–1080.
18. Arbuckle MR, McClain MT, Rubertone MV, et al. Development of autoantibodies before the clinical onset of systemic lupus erythematosus. *N Engl J Med.* 2003;349:1526–33.
19. Heinlen LD, McClain MT, Merrill J, et al. Clinical criteria for systemic lupus erythematosus precede diagnosis, and associated autoantibodies are present before clinical symptoms. *Arthritis Rheum.* 2007;56:2344–2351.

20. Seshan SV, Jennette C. Renal disease in systemic lupus erythematosus with emphasis on classification of lupus glomerulonephritis. Advances and implications. *Arch Pathol Lab Med.* 2009;133:233–248.

21. Schanberg LE, Sandborg C. Dyslipoproteinemia and premature atherosclerosis in pediatric systemic lupus erythematosus. *Curr Rheumatol Rep.* 2004;6:425–433.

22. Hahn BH. Systemic lupus erythematosus and accelerated atherosclerosis. *N Engl J Med.* 2003;349:2379–2380.

23. Petri M. Detection of coronary artery disease and the role of traditional risk factors in the Hopkins Lupus Cohort. *Lupus.* 2000;9:170–175.

24. Lee C, Almagor O, Dunlop DD, et al. Association between African American race/ethnicity and low bone mineral density in women with systemic lupus erythematosus. *Arthritis Rheum.* 2007;57:585–592.

25. Mok CC, Mak A, Ma KM. Bone mineral density in postmenopausal Chinese patients with systemic lupus erythematosus. *Lupus.* 2005;14:106–112.

26. Mendoza-Pinto C, García-Carrasco M, Sandoval-Cruz H, et al. Risks factors for low bone mineral density in pre-menopausal Mexican women with systemic lupus erythematosus. *Clin Rheumatol.* 2009;28(1):65–70.

27. Lilleby V. Bone status in juvenile systemic lupus erythematosus. *Lupus.* 2007;16:580–586.

28. Li EK, Tam LS, Griffith JF, et al. High prevalence of asymptomatic vertebral fractures in Chinese women with systemic lupus erythematosus. *J Rheumatol.* 2009;36:1646–1652.

29. Bernatsky S, Ramsey-Goldman R, Clarke AE. Malignancy in systemic lupus erythematosus: what have we learned? *Best Pract Res Clin Rheumatol.* 2009;23:539–547.

30. Vasudevan AR, Ginzler EM. Established and novel treatments for lupus. *J Musculoskel Med.* 2009;26:291–300.

31. Urowitz MB, Kagal A, Rahman P, Gladman DD. Role of specialty care in the management of patients with systemic lupus erythematosus. *J Rheumatol.* 2002;29:1207–1210.

32. Bombardier C, Gladman DD, Urowitz MB, et al. Derivation of the SLEDAI. A disease activity index for lupus patients. The Committee on Prognosis Studies in SLE. *Arthritis Rheum.* 1992;35:630–640.

33. Symmons DP, Coppock JS, Bacon PA, et al. Development and assessment of a computerised index of clinical disease activity in systemic lupus erythematosus. Members of the British Isles Lupus Assessment Group (BILAG). *Q J Med.* 1988;69:927–937.

34. Isenberg DA, Rahman A, Allen E, et al. BILAG 2004: development and initial validation of an updated version of the British Isles Lupus Assessment Group's disease activity index for patients with systemic lupus erythematosus. *Rheumatology.* 2004;44:902–906.

35. Gladman DD, Urowitz MB. The SLICC/ACR damage index: progress report and experience in the field. *Lupus.* 1999;8:632–637.

36. Beresford MW, Davidson JE. Adolescent development and SLE. *Best Pract Res Clin Rheumatol.* 2006;20:353–368.

37. Klein-Gitelman M, Brunner HI. The impact and implications of neuropsychiatric systemic lupus erythematosus in adolescents. *Curr Rheumatol Rep.* 2009;11:212–217.

38. Descloux E, Durieu I, Cochat P, et al. Influence of age at disease onset in the outcome of paediatric systemic lupus erythematosus. *Rheumatology.* 2009;48:779–784.

39. Lee PPW, Lee TL, Ho MHK, et al. Recurrent major infections in juvenile-onset systemic lupus erythematosus—a close link with long-term disease damage. *Rheumatology.* 2007;46:1290–1296.

40. Bachen EA, Chesney MA, Criswell LA. Prevalence of mood and anxiety disorders in women with systemic lupus erythematosus. *Arthritis Rheum.* 2009;61:822–829.

41. Kozora E, Arcineigas DB, Filley CM, et al. Cognitive and neurologic status in patients with systemic lupus erythematosus without major neuropsychiatric syndromes. *Arthritis Rheum.* 2008;59:1639–1646.

42. Vinet E, Pineau C, Gordon C, et al. Systemic lupus erythematosus in women: impact on family size. *Arthritis Rheum.* 2008;59:1656–1660.

43. Culwell K, Curtis K, del Carmen Cravioto M. Safety of contraceptive method use among women with systemic lupus erythematosus: a systematic review. *Obstet Gynecol.* 2009;114:341–353.

44. Ekblom-Kullberg S, Kautiainen H, Alha P, Helve T, Leirisalo-Repo M, Julkunen H. Reproductive health in women with systemic lupus erythematosus compared to population controls. *Scand J Rheumatol.* 2009:1–6

45. Ostensen M, Rugelsjoen A. Problem areas of the rheumatic mother. *Am J Reprod Immunol.* 1992;28:254–255.

46. Dhar JP, Essenmacher LM, Ager JW, Sokol RJ. Pregnancy outcomes before and after a diagnosis of systemic lupus erythematosus. *Amer J Obstet Gynecol.* 2005;193:1444–1455.

47. Arbuckle MR, McClain MT, Rubertone MV, et al. Development of autoantibodies before the clinical onset of systemic lupus erythematosus. *N Engl J Med.* 2003;349:1526–1533.

48. Heinlen LD, McClain MT, Merrill J, et al. Clinical criteria for systemic lupus erythematosus precede diagnosis, and associated autoantibodies are present before clinical symptoms. *Arthritis Rheum.* 2007;56:2344–2351.

49. Yuen SY, Krizova A, Ouimet JM, Pope JE. Pregnancy outcome in systemic lupus erythematosus (SLE) is improving: results from a case control study and literature review. *Open Rheumatol J.* 2008;2:89–98.

50. Dhar JP, Sokol RJ. Lupus and pregnancy: complex yet manageable. *Clin Med Res.* 2006;4:310–321.

51. Clowse ME, Magder LS, Witter F, Petri M. Early risk factors for pregnancy loss in lupus. *Obstet Gynecol.* 2006;107:293–299.

52. Buyon JP, Clancy RM, Friedman DM. Cardiac manifestations of neonatal lupus erythematosus: guidelines to management, integrating clues from the bench and bedside. *Nat Clin Pract Rheumatol.* 2009;5:139–148.

53. Boddaert J, Huang DLT, Amoura Z, Wechsler B, Godeau P, Piette JC. Late-onset systemic lupus erythematosus. A personal series of 47 patients and pooled analysis of 714 cases in the literature. *Medicine.* 2004;83:348–359.

54. Rovensky J, Tuchynova A. Systemic lupus erythematosus in the elderly. *Autoimmun Rev.* 2008;7:235–239.

55. Aptel M, McGwin G, Vila LM, et al for the LUMINA Study Group. Associated factors and impact of myocarditis in patients with SLE from LUMINA, a multiethnic US cohort. *Rheumatology.* 2008;47:362–367.

56. Burgos PI, Perkins EL, Pons-Estel GJ, et al. Risk factors and impact of recurrent lupus nephritis in patients with systemic lupus erythematosus undergoing renal transplantation. Data from a single US institution. *Arthritis Rheum.* 2009;60:2757–2766.

57. Alarcón GS, McGwin G Jr, Bartolucci AA, et al. Systemic lupus erythematosus in three ethnic groups. IX. Differences in damage accrual. *Arthritis Rheum.* 2001;44:2797–2806.

58. Demas KL, Costenbader KH. Disparities in lupus care and outcomes. *Curr Opin Rheumatol.* 2009;21:102–109.

59. McElhone K, Abbott J, The LS. A review of health related quality of life in systemic lupus erythematosus. *Lupus.* 2006;15:633–643.

60. Da Costa D, Dobkin PL, Pinard L, et al. The role of stress in functional disability among women with systemic lupus erythematosus: a prospective study. *Arthritis Care Res.* 1999;12:112–119.

61. Appenzeller S, Clarke AE, Panopalis P, et al. The relationship between renal activity and quality of life in systemic lupus erythematosus. *J Rheumatol.* 2009;36:947–952.

62. Johnsson PM, Sandqvist G, Bengtsson A, Noveda O. Hand function and performance of daily activities in systemic lupus erythematosus. *Arthritis Care Res.* 2008;59:1432–1438.

63. Partridge AJ, Karlson EW, Daltroy LH, et al. Risk factors for early work disability in systemic lupus erythematosus. Results from a multicenter study. *Arthritis Rheum.* 1997;40:2199–2206.

64. Liang MH, Daltroy LH, Larson MG, et al. Evaluation of social security disability among claimants with rheumatic disease. *Ann Int Med.* 1991;115:26–31.

65. Kasitanon N, Magder LS, Petri M. Predictors of survival in systemic lupus erythematosus. *Medicine (Baltimore).* 2006;85:147–156.

66. Legal Momentum. *Reading between the Lines: Women's Poverty in the United States, 2010.* New York: Author; 2010. http://www.legalmomentum.org/our-work/women-and-poverty/resources--publications/reading-between-the-lines.pdf. Accessed August 26, 2012.

67. Bae SC, Hashimoto H, Karlson EW, et al. Variable effects of social support by race, economic status, and disease activity in systemic lupus erythematosus. *J Rheumatol.* 2001;28:1245–1251.

68. Waters TM, Chang RW, Worsdall E, Ramsey-Goldman R. Ethnicity and access to care in systemic lupus erythematosus. *Arthritis Care Res.* 1996;9:492–500.

69. Gillis JZ, Yazdany J, Trupin L, Julian L, et al. Medicaid and access to care among persons with systemic lupus erythematosus. *Arthritis Care Res.* 2007;57:601–607.

70. Nichol MB, Shi S, Knight TK, Wallace DJ, Weisman MH. Eligibility, utilization, and costs in a California Medicaid lupus population. *Arthritis Rheum.* 2004;51:996–1003.

71. Chambers SA, Rahman A, Isenberg DA. Editorial. Treatment adherence and outcome in systemic lupus erythematosus. *Rheumatology (Oxford).* 2007;46:895–898.

72. Merrill J, Neuwelt C, Wallace D, et al. Efficacy and safety of rituximab in patients with moderately to severely active systemic lupus erythematosus (SLE): results from the randomized, double-blind phase II/III study EXPLORER. *American College of Rheumatology National Meeting.* 2008; Abstract L12.

73. Chan TM, Li FK, Tang CS, et al. Efficacy of mycophenolate mofetil in patients with diffuse proliferative lupus nephritis. Hong Kong-Guangzhou Nephrology Study Group. *N Engl J Med.* 2000;343:1156–1162.

74. Ginzler EM, Dooley MA, Aranow C, et al. Mycophenolate mofetil or intravenous cyclophosphamide for lupus nephritis. *N Engl J Med.* 2005;353:2219–2228.

75. Chan TM, Tse KC, Tang CS, et al. Hong Kong Nephrology Study Group. Long-term study of mycophenolate mofetil as continuous induction and maintenance treatment for diffuse proliferative lupus nephritis. *J Am Soc Nephrol.* 2005;16:1076–1084.

76. Petri M, Kim MY, Kalunian KC, et al for the OC-SELENA Trial. Combined oral contraceptives in women with systemic lupus erythematosus. *N Engl J Med* 2005;353:2550–2558.

77. Ruiz-Irastorza G, Ramos-Casals M, Brito-Zeron P, Khamashta MA. Clinical efficacy and side effects of antimalarials in systemic lupus erythematosus: a systematic review. *Ann Rheum Dis.* 2010;69:20–28.

78. Wallace DJ, Stohl W, Furie RA, et al. A phase II, randomized, double-blind, placebo-controlled, dose-ranging study of belimumab in patients with active systemic lupus erythematosus. *Arthritis Rheum.* 2009;61:1168–1178.

Diabetes Across the Stages of a Woman's Life*

Julie C. Will, PhD, MPH; Gloria L. A. Beckles, MD, MSc; and Michelle D. Owens-Gary, PhD

Introduction and Natural History

Definition and Description of Diabetes

Diabetes mellitus, referred to as "diabetes," is a group of metabolic diseases characterized by hyperglycemia that results from defects in insulin secretion, insulin action, or both.[1] In the United States the majority of cases of diabetes are classified as type 1 or type 2, accounting for 5–10% and 90–95% of cases, respectively.

Type 1 diabetes, formerly called insulin-dependent diabetes, results from an absolute deficiency of insulin secretion that is caused by destruction of the pancreatic beta cells by the body's immune system. The onset of type 1 diabetes occurs most commonly in childhood and young adulthood.

Type 2 diabetes, formerly called noninsulin-dependent diabetes, results from a combination of resistance to insulin action and inadequate insulin secretion. Onset of type 2 diabetes is typically diagnosed at older ages, but recently, although still rare, type 2 diabetes has been more frequently diagnosed among children and adolescents.[2]

A third type of diabetes is gestational diabetes (GDM), which is defined as glucose intolerance with onset or first recognition during pregnancy.[3]

Diabetes is a major public health problem in the United States, exerting a considerable and costly burden on society and individuals.[4,5] It is the principal cause of new cases of end-stage renal disease, blindness among adults of working age, and nontraumatic lower extremity amputation. In addition, mortality from cardiovascular disease is two- to fourfold higher among people with diabetes.[6] In 2007, the estimated total societal cost of diabetes was about $174 billion (in 2007 dollars), with direct healthcare costs estimated at about $117 billion and indirect costs (lost productivity) at $58 billion.[7] In one study that examined age and gender as related to total medical costs (outpatient care, inpatient care, medications and medical supplies), the financial burden increased with age in both men and women with diabetes. Women, however, spent more than men, with the greatest disparity (US$1,345) occurring in young adulthood (ages 19–34 years).[8]

Diabetes as a Woman's Health Issue

In 1985, the Public Health Service Task Force on Women's Health Issues published a set of five criteria that were developed to evaluate woman's health issues associated with specific conditions.[9] The criteria required that the problem, condition, or disease must be unique, more prevalent (i.e., disparities in burden are evident), more serious among women, or some subgroup of women, and the risk factors or interventions must differ for women or some subgroup of women. By these criteria, and as illustrated throughout this chapter, diabetes is a major woman's health issue.

General Prevalence, Incidence, Trends

Currently, as reflected in Figure 24-2, no major incidence difference of diabetes has been noted by gender for several decades.[10,11] For both men and women, age-adjusted

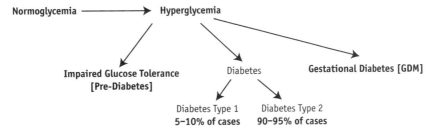

Figure 24-1 Spectrum of Diabetes.

*This chapter is in the public domain and may be reproduced freely with proper citation.

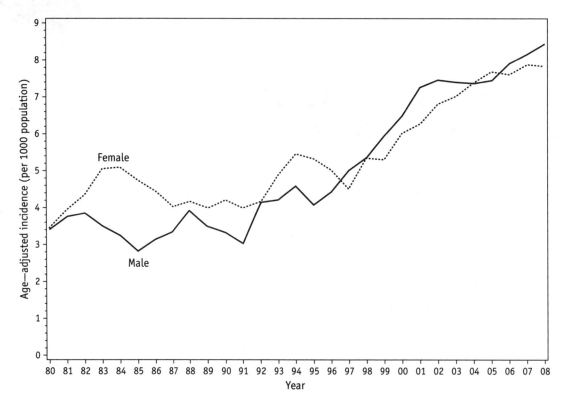

Figure 24-2 Age-adjusted incidence of diagnosed diabetes, aged 18–79 Years, by gender, United States, 1980–2008.

Source: Reproduced from Centers for Disease Control and Prevention (CDC), National Center for Health Statistics, Division of Health Interview Statistics, data from the National Health Interview Survey. http://www.cdc.gov/diabetes/statistics/incidence/fig4.htm

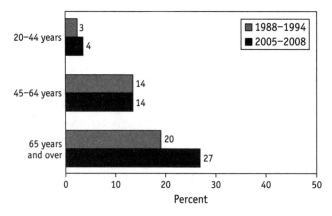

Figure 24-3 Increased incidence of diabetes mellitus by age group, United States.

Source: Reproduced from CDC/NCHS, Health, United States, 2010, Figure 5. Data from the National Health and Nutrition Examination Survey. http://www.cdc.gov/nchs/data/hus/hus10.pdf#fig05

incidence of diagnosed diabetes was more than two times higher in 2008 than in 1980, with most of the increase occurring in the latter half of the time period. In 2008, the age-adjusted incidence was similar among men and women (8.4 vs 7.8 per 1,000). Because of the female advantage in longevity, the number of women diagnosed with diabetes in the middle and older years based on current prevalence patterns and increases noted in the past 2 decades in Figure 24-3, the number of women affected is projected to exceed that of their male counterparts through to 2050.[12,13]

Also, across all life stages, diabetes is two to four times more prevalent among women in the high-risk nonwhite racial/ethnic subgroups of African American, Mexican American, American Indian, and Alaska Native, and some Asian women than among non-Hispanic white women.[2,14,15] Furthermore, although the prevalence of diabetes has increased steadily in all subgroups of women since the early 1990s, the rate of increase has been projected to be steepest in these nonwhite racial/ethnic populations.[10,12,13] Although diabetes is a major risk factor for coronary heart disease in both sexes, diabetes has a more powerful effect on the occurrence of fatal and nonfatal coronary heart disease among women than men.[16] Furthermore, when measured in relation to in-hospital and 5-year survival after myocardial infarction, prognosis is worse for women than men.[17]

Risk factors for type 2 diabetes are the same in both sexes but many of the major risk factors are more prevalent in women. Women are more likely than men to be older, to report a family history of diabetes, to be poorly educated, or to live in low-income households.[18,19] Beginning in adolescence, women are also more likely than men to be obese and physically inactive and less likely to engage in regular leisure-time physical activity.[20,21] Compared to non-Hispanic white women, these characteristics are at least twice as common among women of African American, Mexican American, American Indian, Alaska Native, or Asian American origins.[18–21]

Spectrum of Research Addressing the Problem

Key Research Advances in the Past 20 Years

There have been major breakthroughs in diabetes research that have enabled clinicians to move from "believing" that certain strategies are effective to "knowing" that specific strategies, if applied with fidelity, are effective. The key research advances are: 1) type 2 diabetes can be prevented or delayed through multicomponent lifestyle interventions,[22] 2) microvascular complications of type 1 and type 2 diabetes can prevented or delayed through improved glycemic control,[23] and 3) in certain subsets of the population with diabetes, there is some promise that the macrovascular complications of type 1 and type 2 diabetes can be prevented or delayed through improved glycemic control.[23]

Prevention of Type 2 Diabetes

Multicomponent lifestyle interventions that successfully increase physical activity and improve diet (and, it is hoped, improve body weight and other anthropometric measurements) reduce the risk of diabetes in persons at high risk (i.e., those with impaired glucose tolerance) by about 40% compared to persons who receive a less-intensive comparison intervention.[22] It is unclear, however, whether physical activity or diet alone delays the onset of diabetes. Studies of the individual components of a multicomponent intervention have not generally yielded strong evidence showing that a single component is as effective as the multicomponent intervention.[22,24,25] Multicomponent interventions have also been shown to have long-term effects—lowering the incidence of diabetes for up to 20 years.[26]

Successfully delaying or preventing type 2 diabetes appears to apply equally to men and women. For example, in the Diabetes Prevention Program (DPP) study,[27] women who received the lifestyle intervention saw a decrease in incidence of diabetes by 54% compared to women who received the control condition. For men, the decrease was

65%; however, this decrease was not statistically different from the decrease of 54% for women. Results also appear to apply to women with gestational diabetes [GDM] who have a 71% higher rate of diabetes after pregnancy than women who do not develop GDM. In the DPP,[28] those with a history of GDM who were treated by lifestyle interventions showed a 50% decrease in diabetes incidence compared to those who did not receive such treatment.

Prevention of Microvascular Complications

For persons with either type 1 or type 2 diabetes, the benefits of intensive control of blood sugar (i.e., glycemic control) on microvascular and neuropathic complications have become well established during the past 20 years.[23] The benefits are apparent for both men and women. Physicians recommend that patients routinely monitor their blood glucose levels to ensure that they generally remain below a certain level (as measured by glycated hemoglobin or A1C). Even lower targets for glycemic control have been established for women with GDM and for women with pre-existing type 1 or type 2 diabetes who become pregnant.[23]

Prevention of Macrovascular Complications

Diabetes dramatically closes the gap in deaths from heart disease and stroke between men and women.[29] Evidence that intensive glycemic control provides protection against heart disease and stroke is still unclear due to conflicting study results.[23] In fact, some studies have indicated that cardiovascular disease deaths increased in the group with tighter glycemic control; others have found that certain subgroups of the diabetes population appear to benefit from lower levels of blood sugar. Some researchers have hypothesized that intensive glycemic control early after diabetes development may have a critical impact on prevention of diabetes complications, although intensive control at a later stage of diabetes may not be as effective.[30] Regardless of whether an individual can prevent or delay heart disease and stroke by achieving tight glycemic control, it is essential that they control the risk factors for heart disease and stroke such as high blood pressure, abnormal lipids, and tobacco use.[23]

Impact of Diabetes across the Life Stages

Diabetes has been recognized as an important women's health issue; research advances have improved the lives of the increasing number of women with diabetes or who are at increased risk of developing diabetes. This section highlights those conditions or risk factors that contribute to our understanding of diabetes as a women's health issue through their uniqueness, higher prevalence, or seriousness. In addition, this section provides illustrations of how recent research has improved the lives of women. Conditions and intervention strategies will be illustrated across four life stages: older youth, women of reproductive age, midlife women, and older women. Such an approach highlights the richness of women's lives and the unique struggles they face to achieve maximum health and the highest quality of life.

Older Youth

Racial/Ethnic Disparities in the Burden of Disease

During the past 20 years, a number of epidemiologic studies have examined the prevalence and incidence of diabetes in youth.[31] This section, however, draws mainly on the SEARCH for Diabetes in Youth Study, a population-based study conducted in the United States in multiple centers to gather detailed information on diabetes status and other health conditions for youth aged 10–19 at baseline (2001).[2]

In this study, these same youth were followed during 2002–2005 to detect incident cases of diabetes and to collect other relevant health information. Focusing on the SEARCH for Diabetes in Youth Study and on youth aged 10–19 at diagnosis (referred to as older youth throughout the remainder of this section) allows for an important discussion of the emergence of type 2 diabetes in older youth, a relatively new and potentially reversible public health phenomenon. Also, SEARCH allows an examination of differences by racial/ethnic groups in the prevalence and incidence of type 1 and type 2 diabetes (Table 24-1 and Table 24-2).[32,36]

In the past, the primary form of diabetes among older youth of all racial/ethnic groups was type 1 diabetes mellitus. Non-Hispanic whites, both females and males, continue to have the highest prevalence of type 1 diabetes

---

Table 24-1

Prevalence and Incidence Rates of Type 1 Diabetes Mellitus among Youth Diagnosed at 10–19 Years of Age, by Racial/Ethnic Group and Gender, SEARCH for Diabetes in Youth Study, 2001–2005

Burden	Non-Hispanic White	African American	Hispanic	Asian/Pacific Islander	Navajo
Prevalence (per 1,000)					
Female	2.85 (2.71–3.00)	2.17 (1.90–2.49)	1.58 (1.39–1.79)	0.91 (0.73–1.14)	0.24 (0.11–0.52)
Male	2.92 (2.78–3.07)	1.91 (1.66–2.21)	1.59 (1.41–1.80)	0.64 (0.49–0.83)	0.32 (0.16–0.62)
Incidence (per 100,000)					
Female	19.70 (18.20–21.30)	18.20 (15.40–21.50)	11.80 (9.60–14.50)	7.50 (5.20–10.07)	2.97 (1.01–8.74)
Male	25.30 (23.60–27.10)	13.20 (10.90–16.10)	15.80 (13.20–18.80)	7.40 (5.20–10.60)	2.97 (1.01–8.74)

Source: Data from the SEARCH for Diabetes in Youth Study. Diabetes Care 2009; 32(Supplement 2): S102-S147

Table 24-2

Prevalence and Incidence Rates of Type 2 Diabetes Mellitus in Youth Diagnosed at 10–19 Years of Age, by Racial/Ethnic Group and Gender, SEARCH for Diabetes in Youth Study, 2001–2005

Burden	Non-Hispanic White	African American	Hispanic	Asian/Pacific Islander	Navajo
Prevalence (per 1,000)					
Female	0.22 (0.18–0.26)	1.47 (1.24–1.73)	0.52 (0.42–0.65)	0.54 (0.40–0.73)	1.67 (1.23–2.25)
Male	0.15 (0.12–0.19)	0.67 (0.53–0.86)	0.40 (0.32–0.51)	0.50 (0.37–0.68)	1.23 (0.86–1.74)
Incidence (per 100,000)					
Female	3.90 (3.30–4.70)	25.10 (21.80–29.00)	13.80 (11.40–16.70)	13.50 (10.40–17.60)	33.70 (24.12–47.08)
Male	3.40 (2.90–4.10)	13.00 (10.60–15.80)	9.40 (7.50–11.80)	10.70 (8.0–14.40)	21.79 (14.39–33.00)

Source: Data from the SEARCH for Diabetes in Youth Study. Diabetes Care 2009; 32(Supplement 2): S102-S147.

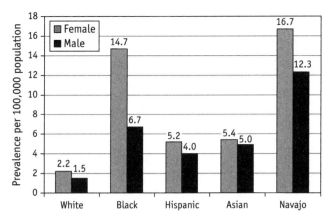

Figure 24-4 Prevalence of type 2 diabetes mellitus among youth aged 10-19 years, by racial/ethnic group and gender, SEARCH for Diabetes in Youth Study, 2001-2005.

Source: Data from the SEARCH for Diabetes in Youth Study. Diabetes Care 2009; 32(Supplement 2): S102–S147.

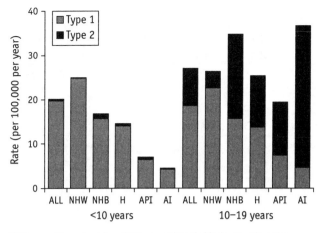

NHW = non-Hispanic whites; NHB = non-Hispanic blacks; H = Hispanics; API = Asians/Pacific Islanders; AI = American Indians

Figure 24-5 Rate of new cases of type 1 and type 2 diabetes among youth aged <20 years, by race/ethnicity, 2002–2005.

Source: Data from the SEARCH for Diabetes in Youth Study. Diabetes Care 2009; 32(Supplement 2): S102–S147.

in this group in the United States (females, 2.85/1,000; males, 2.92/1,000).[32] The widest gap in prevalence occurs between Navajo youth (females, .24/1,000; males, .32/1,000) and non-Hispanic white youth where there is an approximately 10-fold difference in the prevalence rates of type 1 diabetes (Table 24-1).[32,36] In contrast to racial/ethnic differences in rates of type 1 diabetes, there appears to be little differences in rates within racial/ethnic groups by gender.

Type 2 diabetes appears to be an emerging problem among older youth, especially among Navajo boys (1.23/1,000) and girls (1.67/1000), and among African American girls (1.47/1,000). Comparing prevalence rates of type 1 and type 2 diabetes mellitus diagnosed in 2001, the percentage of all cases that were diagnosed as type 2 diabetes mellitus was 87% for Navajo girls, 79% for Navajo boys, 44% for Asian/Pacific Islander boys, and 40% for African American girls (percentages derived from Tables 24-1 and 24-2). Asian/Pacific Islander boys, however, have relatively low prevalence rates for both type 1 (0.64/1,000) and type 2 (0.50/1,000) diabetes.

The incidence of diabetes from 2002–2005, both type 1 and type 2, among older youth also varies by race and ethnicity. For type 1 diabetes, the highest incidence rates of females were among Non-Hispanic Whites (25.3/100,000) and African Americans (18.2/100,000) (Table 24-1). For males, it was highest in the non-Hispanic white group (25.3/100,000). Both male and female Navajo youth had very low incidence rates of type 1 diabetes. For type 2, however, the incidence for female Navajo youth was 33.7/100,000 (the highest incidence rate for any group for either type of diabetes) and for male Navajo youth it was 21.8/100,000. African American females, in addition to their high incidence rates for type 1 diabetes, also had a high incidence rate of type 2 diabetes (25.1/100,000).

Figure 24-5 presents newly diagnosed cases of type 1 and type 2 diabetes for males and females combined by two age groups: younger than age 10 and 10–19 years as recorded in the SEARCH study. When the incidence rates

for type 1 and type 2 are combined (43.3/100,000), older African American girls are the unfortunate leaders in developing new cases of diabetes, regardless of type. Thus, it is especially important to understand why older girls from minority populations are bearing an increased burden of early chronic disease and the implications of this for their futures.

Extended Disparities Resulting in Serious and Long-Term Consequences

Development of type 2 diabetes in adolescents may have a cascading effect leading to the development of other chronic diseases at an earlier age than usually seen in the population. For example, results from multiple studies have found that the risk of developing an abnormal lipid condition in adulthood was significantly higher in adolescents with borderline- and high-risk levels of all lipoprotein variables compared with those with normal levels for all lipoprotein variables.[37] Consequently, if cardiovascular disease risk factors and hyperglycemia are left untreated, one may see earlier development of heart attacks and stroke among youth with earlier onset type 2 diabetes.

The SEARCH study found that a relatively high proportion of youth with type 2 diabetes have elevated blood pressure (from 15% to 28% varying by racial/ethnic group) and abnormal lipid profiles; at least 50% have high low-density lipoprotein (LDL) in all groups except the Navajo; however, three-quarters of the Navajo youth were found to have high triglycerides (Table 24-3). Furthermore, these youth are also at risk for the early development of microvascular complications due to poor control of blood glucose levels[23] as assessed by the A1C test, which provides a long-term assessment of blood sugar control. With A1C equal to or greater than 9.5%, poor control and higher risk of complications was noted among 43% Navajo; 28% Hispanic; 27% Asian;

Table 24-3

Characteristics of Youth with Type 2 Diabetes Mellitus, by Racial/Ethnic Group, SEARCH for Diabetes in Youth Study Results

% (95% CI)		Non-Hispanic White n = 115^	African American N = 212^	Hispanic n = 127^	Asian only n = 45^	Navajo n = 66^
Obese						
	Male	77.1 (65.2, 89.0)	85.5 (76.1, 94.8)	67.4 (53.8, 80.9)	78.6 (57.1, 100)	69.2 (51.5, 87.0)
	Female	80.7 (70.5, 90.9)	80.3 (73.4, 87.2)	76.7 (67.0, 86.4)	64.7 (42.0, 87.4)	66.7 (51.3, 82.1)
	Total	79 (71.3, 86.8)	81.9 (76.3, 87.5)	73.1 (65.1, 81.1)	71 (55.0, 86.9)	67.7 (56.1, 79.4)
No diabetes medications		5.6 (1.2, 9.9)	9.1 (5.1, 13.1)	11.8 (5.8, 17.9)	14.3 (2.7, 25.9)	15.1 (5.5, 24.7)
Family history of diabetes		77.9 (70.2, 85.5)	92.3 (88.7, 95.9)	84.8 (78.5, 91.1)	64.9 (49.5, 80.2)	92.2 (85.6, 98.8)
Poor glycemic control (A1c ≥ 9.5%)		12.3 (6.0, 18.5)	22.3 (16.1, 28.5)	28.1 (19.8, 36.3)	26.9 (9.9, 44.0)	43.3 (30.8, 55.9)
Elevated blood pressure*		16 (9.1, 23.0)	23.4 (17.3, 29.5)	20.8 (13.6, 28.1)	27.6 (11.3, 43.9)	14.5 (5.7, 23.3)
High triglycerides (≥ 110 mg/dl)		59.4 (49.8, 69.0)	34.6 (27.2, 42.0)	67.7 (58.5, 76.9)	40 (20.8, 59.2)	73.7 (62.3, 85.1)
High TG adjusted for duration†		59.6 (49.9, 68.5)	36.1 (29.2, 43.5)	67.9 (58.7, 75.9)	42.4 (25.3, 61.7)	72.6 (59.3, 82.7)
Low HDL cholesterol (≤ 40 mg/dl)		63.2 (54.0, 72.4)	36 (28.9, 43.2)	53.6 (44.3, 62.8)	42.3 (23.3, 61.3)	44.1 (31.4, 56.7)
Low HDL adjusted for duration†		61.1 (51.2, 70.1)	35.4 (28.5, 42.9)	52.8 (43.4, 62.0)	39.8 (23.1, 59.2)	51.1 (37.6, 64.3)
High LDL cholesterol (≥ 100 mg/dl)		51.5 (41.7, 61.2)	61 (53.4, 68.6)	56.6 (46.8, 66.3)	60 (40.8, 79.2)	45.6 (32.7, 58.5)
High LDL adjusted for duration†		53.5 (43.8, 62.9)	61.0 (53.5, 68.1)	58.2 (48.7, 67.1)	64.0 (44.4, 79.8)	38.5 (26.5, 52.1)

*Elevated blood pressure defined as measured blood pressure (SBP or DBP) ≥ age, gender, and height-specific 95th percentile
† Adjusted using logistic regression for diabetes duration and racial/ethnic category
^Denominators for cells may vary slightly due to missing data

Source: Data from the SEARCH for Diabetes in Youth Study. Diabetes Care 2009; 32(Supplement 2): S102–S147.

22% African American; and 12% non-Hispanic white patients. One prospective study in Sweden of diabetes patients diagnosed between the ages of 15 and 34 found that nephropathy can occur during the first 10 years after diabetes diagnosis for selected patients.[38] Risk factors for such early development include poor glycemic control, high blood pressure, and type 2 diabetes (as opposed to type 1 diabetes).[38]

Applying Research Results for Type 2 Diabetes Prevention

Because the chances of developing type 2 diabetes increase with high body mass index (BMI), weight gain, centralized fat, and high waist-to-hip ratio,[31] trends in obesity among adolescents may project future increases in type 2 diabetes. In the United States, the prevalence of overweight among children increased between 1980 and 2004, and the heaviest children were getting heavier.[39] Although additional years of data are needed, there is some evidence that these trends are beginning to level off.[39] Globally, however, the prevalence of childhood overweight has been increasing in many countries throughout the world, especially in relation to high-income and urban areas of developing countries.[40] Consequently, overweight youth around the world will likely experience higher rates of type 2 diabetes than seen in previous decades.

Large randomized controlled trials of strategies to prevent or delay diabetes have been conducted in adults and not in youth; however, these trials found that lifestyle interventions (including weight loss, healthier eating, and increased physical activity) prevent or delay type 2 diabetes in persons at high risk.[23] Because these results were found to apply to all participants regardless of racial/ethnic group, gender, or age, there is reason to believe that diabetes can also be prevented or delayed in youth. In a recent review of obesity prevention programs aimed at children and adolescents,[41] evidence suggested that current programs lead to short-term improvements in a variety of outcomes. However, to have maximum impact, the authors concluded that population health approaches need to be strengthened and added to the large number of one-on-one weight loss programs that currently exist.

Women of Reproductive Age

Gestational Diabetes Mellitus

GDM affects approximately 5% of all pregnancies, or more than 200,000 American women annually.[42,43] GDM, a public health concern, is associated with various adverse outcomes for the baby and the mother, including increased infant birth weight, birth trauma, hypoglycemia, and an increased risk for preeclampsia.[44–46] GDM also increases the chances that a woman will require a cesarean delivery. Infants of high birth weight are at increased risk of becoming obese during childhood or adolescence, which then increases their risk for later development of type 2 diabetes.

Although GDM usually ends after delivery, up to one-third of women will have developed type 2 diabetes when screened postpartum; non-white and Hispanic women with a history of GDM are particularly vulnerable.[42] Yet, not all women who had GDM during pregnancy necessarily develop diabetes mellitus. GDM presents an opportunity for early detection and the development of interventions to prevent or delay the development of type 2 diabetes.[45]

Applying Research Results for Diabetes Prevention in Women of Reproductive Age

Lifestyle Intervention and/or Medication for Women with GDM

The Diabetes Prevention Program (DPP), discussed in an earlier section, is a major study showing that type 2 diabetes is preventable in women with a history of GDM through modest weight loss associated with dietary changes and increased physical activity or treatment with the oral diabetes drug metformin (Glucophage).[47,48] Over 2,000 women included in the DPP study were asked about their history of GDM;[28,49] 350 women reported having a history of GDM. All participants were randomly assigned to one of three arms: a standard lifestyle intervention with placebo, metformin therapy, or to an intensive lifestyle intervention. Women with a history of GDM who received the standard lifestyle intervention and placebo had a 71% higher incidence of diabetes than did women with no history of GDM. However, women with a history of GDM who received either the intensive lifestyle intervention or metformin had a 50% reduction in the incidence of diabetes.[28,49]

Prevention through Preconception Care

Preconception and interconception care include a "set of interventions that aim to identify and modify biomedical, behavioral, and social risks to a woman's health or pregnancy outcome through prevention and management."[50] All women of reproductive age should receive such care before becoming pregnant as well as between pregnancies.[50] An important aspect of such care is to encourage women to adopt behaviors such as healthy eating and physical activity that should lower their risk of developing GDM and type 2 diabetes.[50,51]

Several barriers exist in ensuring preconception or interception care including: 1) primary care practices that do not have or use established guidelines for providing such care, 2) flawed systems for identifying women who are at risk of developing GDM or type 2 diabetes, 3) ineffective reminder systems to ensure postpartum follow-up care,[42,43] and 4) limited access to care because of financial and social factors such as no health insurance,[52,53] no child care, lack of affordable transportation, and geographic isolation.

Diabetes in the Middle Years

Diabetes as a Risk Factor for Other Diseases

Cardiovascular Disease

Historically, coronary heart disease (CHD) was identified as "a man's disease."[54,55] Heart disease is now recognized as the number one cause of death for women over age 65 in the United States.[56,57] Among midlife women (aged 40–59 years), cardiovascular disease (CVD) is equally prevalent in men and women. At age 80 years and older, however, CVD is more prevalent in women than in men.[58]

Diabetes is an important risk factor for coronary heart disease; women with diabetes have greater relative risks for heart disease than men with diabetes[16,57,59,60] and greater risk of developing heart disease and stroke than women without diabetes.[29] In addition, women with diabetes who develop CHD are more likely than men to experience adverse outcomes. For example, after having a myocardial infarction, mortality is greater for women with diabetes compared to their male counterparts.[55,59,61–62]

Depression

Depression is a common and serious medical condition that can affect the way women think and feel as well as their ability to function and cope with life's demands.[63] Research has noted an association between diabetes and depression;[64,65] females with diabetes are almost twice as likely as men with diabetes to develop depression.[54] An estimated 10–25% of women will experience depression at some point in their lifetime.[66]

Depression often contributes to poor glucose control as well as difficulty in following and maintaining a treatment plan. Depression may affect day-to-day functioning for women with diabetes as some depressed women may adopt unhealthy behaviors, such as being physically inactive or eating an unhealthy diet. When depression remains untreated, people with diabetes are at increased risk for complications such as heart disease, blindness, amputations, stroke, and kidney disease.[67,68] In addition, untreated depression may result in a decreased quality of life, increased healthcare usage with higher costs, as well as an increased risk of mortality.[67,68]

Underuse of Public Health Interventions

Cancer Screenings

Diabetes increases the risk of breast, colorectal, and uterine cancer.[69–71] Although the U.S. Preventive Services Task Force recommends mammograms every 1–2 years for women age 50 and older, some women fail to receive routine screening.[72,73] Even with more healthcare visits, women with diabetes are even less likely than women without diabetes to receive a mammogram according to these guidelines.[74] Diabetes care is often complex and may result in other healthcare recommendations being neglected.[74]

Immunizations

Immunizations are important for people with diabetes who are more susceptible to a number of viral conditions and complications.[75] The Advisory Committee on Immunization Practices recommends women with diabetes to be immunized against influenza annually[75] and to be immunized against pneumococcal infection once with additional vaccination for those age 65 years of age and older.[75] Among women with diabetes, less than half (47.9% for influenza and 46.7% for pneumococcal) reported ever having receiving the appropriate vaccinations.[76]

Applying Research Results on Prevention of Macrovascular Complications

Evidence that intensive glycemic control provides protection against heart disease and stroke is still unclear due to conflicting study results.[23] Despite the ability to prevent or delay heart disease and stroke by achieving tight glycemic control, it is essential that women control the risk factors for heart disease and stroke such as high blood pressure, abnormal lipids, and tobacco use.[23]

The Older Years

Longer Life Span and Diabetes Risk

Diabetes is well known to accelerate the aging process resulting in discordance between biologic and chronologic age.[77] The changing demography of the U.S. population is characterized by the "feminization of old age," a phenomenon in which women outnumber men markedly in the older years. For example, in 2008, there were 136 women aged 65 years and older and 207 women aged 85 years and older for every 100 men of comparable age.[78] Between 2010 and 2050, the number of women 65 years and older is projected to increase more than twofold to 48.6 million and the number aged 85 years and older to increase threefold to 11.6 million.[78]

National data show that, in the mid-2000s, more than one in three women 60 years and older had impaired fasting glucose;[14] among women 65–74 years of age, 7 out of 10 were overweight or obese (BMI $\geq$ 25 kg/m²), nearly 2 out of 5 were obese (BMI $\geq$ 30 kg/m²); about half (49.0%) were inactive and only 1 in 4 reported regular leisure-time activity.[20] The relationship of these risk factors to development of diabetes among older adults appears to be strong and more pronounced among women than men.[27,79,80] The combination of increasing numbers of older women with high prevalence of risk factors for diabetes portend a growing burden of diabetes among older women.

The prevalence of diagnosed and undiagnosed diabetes increases with age such that estimates for women 60 years and older are more than five to seven times higher than for women aged 20–39.[14] During 1999–2002 the prevalence of diagnosed diabetes among women 60 years and older was 14.4% and 4.9% were found to have undiagnosed diabetes. However, rates were considerably higher for non-Hispanic black women and Mexican American women with 24.7% diagnosed and 7.6% undiagnosed compared with non-Hispanic white women (12.3%, 4.7%).[14] These estimates reflect the growing burden of diabetes among older adults in the United States. Data from national longitudinal analysis of Medicare claims indicate prevalence increased by 62% and incidence by 23% between 1994 and 2003.[81] Data on incidence of diabetes among older women are sparse. National data based on self-reported diagnosis in the past year show that among women aged 65–79 years incidence was 11.0 per 1,000 in 2007.[82] Studies of selected populations suggest that the increasing trends in prevalence are being driven in turn by increasing rates of obesity.[81,83,84]

Diabetes is among the major causes of death among women 65 years and older in the United States.[85] When listed as underlying cause of death, diabetes ranked seventh overall, fifth for white women and fourth for women in all nonwhite racial/ethnic groups. Vital statistics underestimate the health impact of diabetes, which is underreported on U.S. death certificates, listed on 2 of 5 death certificates and as the underlying cause of death on only 1 of 10 death certificates of decedents with diabetes.[86,87] Many epidemiologic studies have established diabetes as a major risk factor for mortality and cardiovascular (primarily heart disease and stroke) and microvascular complications (retinopathy, nephropathy, neuropathy). Recent evidence indicates that the excess mortality and cardiovascular risk attributed to diabetes among older adults is lower than the twofold excess generally reported.[88,89]

Complicated Aging for Women with Diabetes

In addition to the traditional vascular complications of diabetes, evidence is accumulating that suggests a causal relation between diabetes and a variety of conditions or geriatric syndromes that occur among older adults are multifactorial in cause and often contribute to functional decline.[90] Because there is lack of consensus about the definition of a geriatric syndrome, the data presented are for conditions on which there is consensus: cognitive decline, dementia, recurrent falls, and incontinence. Figure 24-6 presents the risk of these conditions among older women.[90]

Cognitive Decline and Dementia

Several prospective population-based studies of older adults revealed that diabetes is a significant risk factor for incidence of cognitive impairment and acceleration of cognitive decline.[91,92] The relationship did not differ between men and women but, in both sexes, cognitive decline worsened with increasing duration of diabetes.[91] In addition, meta-analyses showed that the overall relative risk (RR) of developing dementia for persons with diabetes compared to those without diabetes was 1.47 (95% CI = 1.25–1.73), for Alzheimer's disease 1.39 (95% CI = 1.16–1.66), and for vascular dementia 2.38 (95% CI = 1.79–3.18).[91]

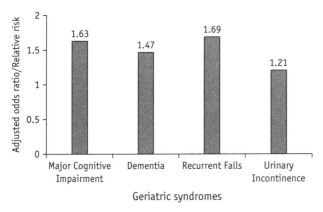

Figure 24-6 Association of diabetes mellitus with geriatric syndromes among older women.

Source: Data from Hanlon JT, Landerman LR, Fillenbaum GG, Studenski S. Falls in African American and white Community-dwelling elderly residents. J Gerontr A Biol Sci Med Sci 2002;57:M473–M478.; Lifford KL, Curhan GC, Hu FB, et al. Type 2 diabetes mellitus and risk of developing urinary incontinence. J Am Geriatr Soc 2005;53:1851–1857.; Jackson SL, Scholes D, Boyko EJ, et al. Urinary incontinence and diabetes in postmenopausal women. Diabetes Care 2005;28:1730–1738.

Recurrent Falls

Diabetes is also associated with incidence and frequency of falls among older adults.[91,93–96] One study of 9,249 older women showed that during 7.2 years of follow-up, incident falls increased with age and women with diabetes had higher age-specific rates than women without diabetes.[96] In this study, females with diabetes experienced increased risk of falling more than once a year compared to those without diabetes: age-adjusted odds ratios were 1.69 (95% CI = 1.37–2.07) for women who did not use insulin and 2.78 (95% CI = 1.82–4.24) for insulin users.

Urinary Incontinence

Urinary incontinence (UI) imposes a considerable individual and societal burden in the United States, affecting an estimated 17% to 49% of women aged 60 years and older, and accounting for direct medical costs of US$19.5 to US$26 billion annually.[97,98] Population-based studies show significantly higher odds of UI among women with diabetes compared to those without diabetes, even after multivariate adjustment.[79,97–99] The only prospective study, the Nurses' Health Study, conducted when participants were 50–75 years of age noted the incidence of UI was significantly higher among women with diabetes compared to women without diabetes, with the strength of the association increasing with increasing severity of incontinence.[97] Multivariate-adjusted relative risks ranged from 1.21 (95% CI = 1.02–1.43) to 1.97 (95% CI = 1.24–3.12). Studies also showed that risk increased with duration and indicators of severity of diabetes, such as insulin use and evidence of micro-vascular disease.[79,80,97–99]

Limited Research on Older Women with Diabetes

Although research has shown that older women are a high-risk group for diabetes and that diabetes is a more powerful predictor of fatal and nonfatal cardiovascular disease among women than men,[16,100] studies of older adults seldom present findings stratified by sex.

Recommendations and Future Directions

To improve the future of women with diabetes or at risk of diabetes, the following recommendations are provided:

1. Continue research into the prevention of heart disease and stroke for people (in all life stages) with diabetes to resolve the potential preventive role of intensive glycemic control.
2. Continue surveillance on the potential epidemic of type 2 diabetes in youth.
3. Remove racial/ethnic, age, and gender disparities in the implementation of evidence-based programs to prevent diabetes and its complications; strengthen approaches to include population as well as individual strategies.
4. Strengthen systems to ensure greater access to care preconception, interconception, and postpartum.
5. Educate healthcare providers regarding national recommendations for preventive care for women with diabetes or at risk for diabetes.

6. Create a sense of public health urgency around the issue of women and heart disease and emphasize the critical role of diabetes as a modifiable risk factor for heart disease and stroke.
7. Improve surveillance on women and diabetes, especially in the older age groups.

Summary

Diabetes is a chronic illness that requires continual medical care and patient self-management to prevent acute and long-term complications. Incidence has been steadily rising during the past 2 decades among males and females. Patterns of disease onset and prevalence vary by race/ethnicity and among older populations by gender. Race/ethnicity differences were also evident among the youth included in the SEARCH study; differences were noted by incidence and prevalence of types 1 and 2 diabetes. Gestational diabetes occurs to some susceptible women complicating approximately 5% of pregnancies and increasing the subsequent risk of diabetes mellitus. Interventions developed through the Diabetes Prevention Program successfully lowered the risk of diabetes postpartum and among other high-risk populations. Diabetes is a major risk factor for cardiovascular disease; therefore, reducing or delaying the onset of diabetes also reduces or delays the onset of heart disease and stroke. Older women with diabetes are at increased risk of geriatric syndromes including cognitive impairment, repeated falling, and urinary incontinence. Efforts to reduce the rate of obesity and increase physical activity are primary behavioral changes that may reduce the risk of diabetes and its complications among the aging American population.

Discussion Questions

1. How does the incidence of diabetes differ among women compared to men? By race/ethnicity? By age? How do these estimates affect risks of other chronic diseases?
2. Do types 1 and 2 diabetes have the same risk factors? What other type of diabetes is of major concern? Do preventive interventions prevent or delay all types of diabetes?
3. How does access to health care affect the incidence and prevalence of diabetes?
4. Are death certificates used to estimate diabetes mortality? Are the estimates valid? If not, why not?
5. How does diabetes affect older women?

References

1. American Diabetes Association. Diagnosis and classification of diabetes mellitus. *Diabetes Care.* 2009;32(suppl 1):S62–S67.
2. Mayer-Davis EJ, Bell RA, Dabelea D, et al. SEARCH for Diabetes in Youth Study Group. The many faces of diabetes in American youth: type 1 and type 2 diabetes in five race and ethnic populations: The SEARCH for Diabetes in Youth Study. *Diabetes Care.* 2009;32(suppl 2): S99–S101.
3. Metzger BE, Buchanan TA, Coustan DR, De Leiva A, Dunger DB, Hadden DR, et al. Summary and Recommendations of the Fifth International Workshop-Conference on Gestational Diabetes Mellitus. *Diabetes Care.* 2007;30(suppl 2): S251–S260.
4. Vinicor F. Is diabetes a public-health disorder? *Diabetes Care.* 1994;17(suppl 1): 22–27.
5. Narayan KM, Gregg EW, Fagot-Campagna A, et al. Diabetes—a common, growing, serious, costly, and potentially preventable public health problem. *Diabetes Res Clin Pract.* 2000;50(suppl 2):S77–S84.
6. Centers for Disease Control and Prevention. National Diabetes Surveillance. Age-adjusted percentage of civilian, noninstitutionalized population with diagnosed diabetes, by race and sex, United States, 1980–2010. http://www.cdc.gov/diabetes/statistics/prev/national/figraceethsex.htm.
7. American Diabetes Association. Economic cost of diabetes. *Diabetes Care.* 2008;31:1–20.
8. Zhang P, Imai K. The relationship between age and healthcare expenditure among persons with diabetes mellitus. *Expert Opin Pharmacother.* 2007;8:49–57. doi:10.1517/14656566.8.1.49.
9. U.S. Public Health Service. *Women's Health: Report of the Public Health Service Task Force on Women's Health Issues.* Vol. 1. Washington, DC: U.S. Department of Health and Human Services; 1985.
10. Cowie CC, Williams DE, Rust KF, et al. Full accounting of diabetes and pre-diabetes in the U.S. population in 1988–1994 and 2005–2006. *Diabetes Care.* 2009;32:287–294.
11. Geiss LS, Pan L, Cadwell B, et al. Changes in incidence of diabetes in U.S. adults, 1997–2003. *Am J Prev Med.* 2006;30(5):371–377.
12. Boyle JP, Honeycutt AA, Narayan KMV, Hoerger TJ, et al. Projection of diabetes burden through 2050. *Diabetes Care.* 2001;24:1936–1940.
13. Wild S, Roglic G, Green A, et al. Global prevalence of diabetes: Estimates for the year 2000 and projections for 2030. *Diabetes Care.* 2004;27:1047–1053.
14. Cowie CC, Rust KF, Byrd-Holt DD, et al. Prevalence of diabetes and impaired fasting glucose in adults in the U.S. population. *Diabetes Care.* 2006;29:1263–1268.
15. CDC. Diagnosed diabetes among American Indians and Alaska Natives aged < 35 years—United States, 1994–2004. *MMWR Morb Mortal Wkly Rep.* 2006;55:1201–1203.
16. Huxley R, Barzi F, Woodward M. Excess risk of fatal coronary heart disease associated with diabetes in men and women: meta-analysis of 37 prospective cohort studies. *BMJ.* 2006:332(7533):73–78. doi:10.1136/bmj.38678.389583.7C.
17. Crowley A, Menon V, Lessard D, et al. Sex differences in survival after acute myocardial infarction in patients with diabetes mellitus (Worcester Heart Attack Study). *Am Heart J.* 2003;146:824–831.
18. Annis AM, Caulder MS, Cook ML, Duquette D. Family history, diabetes, and other demographic and risk factors among participants of the National Health and Nutrition Examination Survey 1999–2002. *Prev Chronic Dis.* 2005;Apr, 2(2):1–12. Epub 2005 Mar 15. Available from http://www.cdc.gov/pcd/issues/2005/apr/04_0131.htm. Accessed June 4, 2009.
19. Beckles GLA, Thompson-Reid PE. Socioeconomic status of women with diabetes—United States, 2000. *MMWR Morb Mortal Wkly Rep.* 2002;51(7): 147–148, 159.
20. National Center for Health Statistics. *Health, United States, 2008.* With Chartbook. Hyattsville, MD: Author; 2009. http://www.cdc.gov/nchs/data/hus/hus08.pdf. Accessed, June 3, 2009.
21. Centers for Disease Control and Prevention. Youth Risk Behavior Surveillance—United States, 2007. Surveillance Summaries. June 6, 2008. *MMWR Morb Mortal Wkly Rep.* 2008;57(SS–4).
22. Orozco LJ, Buchleitner AM, Gimenez-Perez G, et al. Exercise or exercise and diet for preventing type 2 diabetes mellitus. *Cochrane Database Syst Rev.* 2008; Issue 3. Art. No.:CD003054. DOI: 10.1002/14651858.CD003054.pub3.
23. American Diabetes Association. Standards of medical care in diabetes-2009. *Diabetes Care* 2009;32(suppl 1):S13–S61.
24. Nield L, Summerbell CD, Hooper L, et al. Dietary advice for the prevention of type 2 diabetes mellitus in adults. *Cochrane Database Syst Rev.* 2008; Issue 3. Art. No:CD005102. DOI: 10.1002/14651858.CD005102.pub2.
25. Norris SL, Zhang X, Avenell A, et al. Long-term non-pharmacological weight loss interventions for adults with pre-diabetes. *Cochrane Database Syst Rev.* 2005; Issue 2. Art. No.:CD005270. DOI: 10.1002/14651858.CD005270.
26. Li G, Zhang P, Wang J, et al. The long-term effect of lifestyle interventions to prevent diabetes in the China Da Qing Diabetes Prevention Study: a 20-year follow-up study. *Lancet.* 2008;371:1783–1789.
27. Diabetes Prevention Program Research Group. Reduction in the incidence of type 2 diabetes with lifestyle intervention or metformin. *N Engl J Med.* 2002;346:393–403.
28. Ratner RE, Costas AC, Boyd EM, et al. Prevention of diabetes in women with a history of gestational diabetes: effects of metformin and lifestyle interventions. *J Clin Endocrinol Metab.* 2008;93:4774–4779.
29. Barrett-Connor E, Giardina EV, Gitt AK, et al. Women and heart disease: the role of diabetes and hyperglycemia. *Arch Intern Med.* 2004;164:934–942.
30. Soldatos F, Cooper ME. Does intensive glycemic control for type 2 diabetes mellitus have long-term benefits for cardiovascular disease risk? *Nat Clin Pract Endocrinol Metab.* 2009;5(3):138–9. EPub 2009 Feb 3.
31. Nadeau K, Dabelea D. Epidemiology of type 2 diabetes in children and adolescents. *Endocr Res.* 2008;33:35–58.
32. Bell RA, Mayer-Davis EJ, Beyer J, et al. SEARCH for Diabetes in Youth Study Group. Diabetes in Non-Hispanic White Youth: Prevalence, incidence, and clinical characteristics: the SEARCH for Diabetes in Youth Study. *Diabetes Care.* 2009;32(suppl 2):S102–S111.

33. Mayer-Davis EJ, Beyer J, Bell RA, et al. SEARCH for Diabetes in Youth Study Group. Diabetes in African American youth: Prevalence, incidence, and clinical characteristics: the SEARCH for Diabetes in Youth Study. *Diabetes Care.* 2009;32(suppl 2):S112–S122.

34. Lawrence JM, Mayer-Davis EJ, Reynolds K, et al. SEARCH for Diabetes in Youth Study Group. Diabetes in Hispanic American youth: Prevalence, incidence, demographics, and clinical characteristics: the SEARCH for Diabetes in Youth Study. *Diabetes Care.* 2009;32(suppl 2):S123–S132.

35. Liu LL, Yi JP, Beyer J, et al. SEARCH for Diabetes in Youth Study Group. Type 1 and Type 2 diabetes in Asian and Pacific Islander U.S. youth: the SEARCH for Diabetes in Youth Study. *Diabetes Care.* 2009;32(suppl 2): S133–S140.

36. Dabelea D, DeGroat J, Sorrelman C, et al. SEARCH for Diabetes in Youth Study Group. Diabetes in Navajo youth: Prevalence, incidence, and clinical characteristics: the SEARCH for Diabetes in Youth Study. *Diabetes Care.* 2009;32(suppl 2):S141–S147.

37. Magnussen CG, Raitakari OT, Thomson R, et al. Utility of currently recommended pediatric dyslipidemia classifications in predicting dyslipidemia in adulthood: evidence from the Childhood Determinants of Adult Health (CDAH) Study, Cardiovascular Risk in Young Finns Study, and Bogalusa Heart Study. *Circulation.* 2008;117:32–42.

38. Svensson M, Sundkvist G, Arnqvist HJ, et al. Signs of nephropathy may occur early in young adults with diabetes despite modern diabetes management: results from the nationwide population-based Diabetes Incidence Study in Sweden (DISS). *Diabetes Care.* 2003;26(10):2903–2909.

39. Ogden CL, Carroll MD, Flegal KM. High body mass index for age among US children and adolescents, 2003–2006. *JAMA.* 2008;299(20):2401–2405.

40. Wang Y, Lobstein T. Worldwide trends in childhood overweight and obesity. *Int J Pediatric Obesity.* 2006;1:11–25.

41. Flynn MAT, McNeil DA, Maloff B, et al. Reducing obesity and related chronic disease risk in children and youth: a synthesis of evidence with "best practice" recommendations. *Obes Rev.* 2006;7(suppl 1):7–66.

42. England LJ, Dietz PM, Njoroge T, et al. Preventing type 2 diabetes: public health implications for women with a history of gestational diabetes. *Am J Obstet Gynecol.* 2009:200:365.e1–365.e8.

43. Kim C, Tabaei BP, Burke R, et al. Missed opportunities for type 2 diabetes mellitus screening among women with a history of gestational diabetes. *Am J Public Health.* 2006;96:1643–1648.

44. Mullholland C, Njoroge T, Mersereau P, Williams J. Comparison guidelines available in the United States for diagnosis and management of diabetes before, during, and after pregnancy. *J Womens Health.* 2007;16:790–801.

45. Kapustin JF. Postpartum management for gestational diabetes mellitus: policy and practice implications. *J Am Acad Nurse Practitioners.* 2008;20:547–554.

46. Santos-Ayarzagoitia M, Salinas-Martinez AM, Villarreal-Perez JZ. Gestational diabetes: Validity of ADA and WHO diagnostic criteria using NDGG as the reference test. *Diabetes Res Clin Pract.* 2006;74:322.

47. Knowler WC, Barrett-Connor E, Fowler SE, et al. Reduction in the incidence of type 2 diabetes with lifestyle intervention or metformin. *N Engl J Med.* 2002;346:393–403.

48. National Diabetes Information Clearinghouse. Diabetes Prevention Program. http://diabetes.niddk.nih.gov/dm/pubs/preventionprogram/. Accessed July 3, 2009.

49. Bentley-Lewis R, Levkoff S, Stuebe A, Seely EW. Gestational diabetes mellitus: postpartum opportunities for the diagnosis and prevention of type 2 diabetes mellitus. *Nat Clin Pract Endocrinol Metab.* 2008;4:552–555.

50. Posner SF, Johnson K, Parker C, Atrash H, Biermann J. The national summit on preconception care: a summary of concepts and recommendations. *Matern Child Health J.* 2006;10(5 suppl):S197–S205.

51. Owens, MD, Kieffer E, Chowdhury FC. Preconception care and women with or at risk for diabetes: implications for community intervention. *Matern Child Health J.* 2006;10(5 Suppl):S137–S141.

52. Korenbrot CC, Steinberg A, Bender C, Newberry S. Preconception care: a systematic review. *Matern Child Health J.* 2002;6:75–88.

53. Bernasko J. Contemporary management of type 1 diabetes mellitus in pregnancy. *Obstet Gynecol Surv.* 2004;59:628–636.

54. Killien M, Bigby JA, Champion V, et al. Involving minority and underrepresented women in clinical trials: The National Centers of Excellence in Women's Health. *J Womens Health Gend Based Med.* 2000;9:1061–1070.

55. Sowers JR. Diabetes mellitus and cardiovascular disease in women. *Arch Intern Med.* 1998;158:617–621.

56. World Health Statistics Annual Report. *Vital Statistics and Cause of Death.* Geneva, Switzerland: World Health Organization; 1990.

57. Mankad R, Best PJ. Cardiovascular disease in older women: a challenge in diagnosis and treatment. *Womens Health.* 2008;4:449–464.

58. Lloyd-Jones D, Adams R, Carnethon M, et al. Heart disease and stroke statistics—2009 update: a report from the American Heart Association Statistics Committee and Stroke Statistics Subcommittee. *Circulation.* 2009;119: 480–486.

59. Koerbel G, Korytkowski M. Coronary heart disease in women with diabetes. *Diabetes Spectr.* 2003;16:148–153.

60. Hu G, Jousilahti P, Qizo Q, et al. The gender-specific impact of diabetes and myocardial infarction at baseline and during follow-up on mortality from all-causes and coronary heart disease. *J Am Coll Cardiol.* 2005;45:1413–1418.

61. Galcera-Tomas, Melgarejo-Moreno A, Garcia-Alberola A, et al. Prognostic significance of diabetes in acute myocardial infarction. Are the differences linked to female gender? *Int J Cardiol.* 1999;69:289–298.

62. Preis SR, Hwang S, Coady S, et al. Trends in all-cause and cardiovascular disease mortality among women and men with and without diabetes mellitus in the Framingham Heart Study, 1950–2005. *Circulation.* 2009;119:1728–1735.

63. American Psychiatric Association. *Diagnostic and Statistical Manual of Mental Disorders.* 4th ed., text rev. Washington, DC: American Psychiatric Association; 2000.

64. Knol MJ, Twisk JWR, Beekman ATF, et al. Depression as a risk factor for the onset of type 2 diabetes mellitus: a meta-analysis. *Diabetologia.* 2006;49: 837–845.

65. Anderson RJ, Clouse RE, Freeland KE, Lustman PJ. The prevalence of comorbid depression in adults with diabetes. *Diabetes Care.* 2001;24:1069–1078.

66. National Institute of Mental Health. (2011). Depression (NIH Publication No. 11–3561).Washington, DC: U.S. Department of Health and Human Services.

67. Lustman PJ, Clouse RE. Depression in diabetic patients: The relationship between mood and glycemic control. *J Diabetes Complications.* 2005;19:113–122.

68. Zhang X, Norris SL, Gregg EW, et al. Depressive symptoms and mortality among persons with and without diabetes. *Am J Epidemiol.* 2005;161:652–660.

69. Larsson SC, Mantzoros CS, Wolk A. Diabetes mellitus and risk of breast cancer: a meta-analysis. *Intl J Cancer.* 2007;121:856–862.

70. Friberg E, Mantzoros CS, Wolk A. Diabetes and risk of endometrial cancer: a population-based prospective cohort study. *Cancer Epidemiol Biomarkers Prev.* 2007;16:276–280.

71. Larsson SC, Orsini N, Wolk A. Diabetes mellitus and risk of colorectal cancer: a meta-analysis. *J Natl Cancer Inst.* 2005;97:1679–1687.

72. U.S. Preventive Service Task Force. Screening for breast cancer, recommendations, and rationale. *Ann Intern Med.* 2002;137:344–346.

73. Hsia J, Kemper E, Kiefe C, et al. The importance of health insurance as a determinant of cancer screening: evidence from the women's health initiative. *Prev Med.* 2000;31:261–270.

74. Lipscome LL, Hux JE, Booth GL. Reduced screening mammography among women with diagnosed diabetes. *Arch Intern Med.* 2005;165:2090–2095.

75. Recommendations and Reports: Prevention and control of influenza. *MMWR Morb Mortal Wkly Rep.* 2007;56:1–54.

76. Owens MD, Beckles GLA, Ho KK, et al. Women with diagnosed diabetes across the life stages: underuse of recommended preventive care services. *J Womens Health.* 2008;17:1–9.

77. Morley JE. Diabetes and aging: epidemiologic overview. *Clin Geriatr Med.* 2008;24:395–405.

78. U.S. Census Bureau. Table 2. Annual estimates of the resident population by sex and selected age groups for the United States: April 1, 2000 to July 1, 2008 (NC-EST2008–02).

79. Crandall J, Schade D, Ma Y, et al. The influence of age on the effects of lifestyle modification and metformin in prevention of diabetes. *J Gerontology A Biol Sci Med Sci.* 2006;61A:1075–1081.

80. Mozaffarian D, Kamineni A, Carnethon M, et al. Lifestyle risk factors and new-onset diabetes mellitus in older adults. The Cardiovascular Health Study. *Arch Intern Med.* 2009;169:798–807.

81. Sloan FA, Bethel A, Ruiz Jr D, et al. The growing burden of diabetes mellitus in the US elderly population. *Arch Intern Med.* 2008;168:192–199.

82. Centers for Disease Control and Prevention. Incidence of diagnosed diabetes per 1,000 population aged 18–79 years, by sex and age, United States, 1997–2007. http://www.cdc.gov/diabetes/statistics/incidence/fig4.htm. Accessed, July 2009.

83. Leibson CL, O'Brien PC, Atkinson E, et al Relative contributions of incidence and survival to increasing prevalence of adult-onset diabetes mellitus: a population-based study. *Am J Epidemiol.* 1997;146:12–22.

84. Gregg EW, Cheng YJ, Narayan V, et al. The relative contributions of different levels of overweight and obesity to the increased prevalence of diabetes in the United States: 1976–2004. *Prev Med.* 2007;45:348–352.

85. Centers for Disease Control and Prevention. Leading causes of death in females, United States, 2004. http://www.cdc.gov/women/lcod/. Accessed July 2009.

86. Will JC, Vinicor F, Stevenson J. Recording of diabetes on death certificates: has it improved? *J Clin Epidemiol.* 2001;54:239–244.

87. McEwen LN, Kim C, Haan M, et al. Diabetes reporting as a cause of death. *Diabetes Care.* 2006;29:247–253. E-pub DOI:10.2337/dc07–0238.

88. CDC. Major cardiovascular disease (CVD) during 1997–1999 and major CVD hospital discharge rates in 1997 among women with diabetes in the United States. *MMWR Morb Mortal Wkly Rep.*2001;50:948–954.

89. Bethel MA, Sloan FA, Belsky D, Feinglos MN. Longitudinal incidence and prevalence of adverse outcomes of diabetes mellitus in elderly patients. *Arch Intern Med.* 2007;167:921–927.

90. Cigolle CT, Langa KM, Kabeto MU, et al. Geriatric conditions and disability: the Health and Retirement Study. *Ann Intern Med.* 2007;147:156–164.

91. Lu F-P, Lin K-P, Kuo H-K. Diabetes and the risk of multi-system aging phenotypes: a systematic review and meta-analysis. *PloS ONE.* 2009;4:e4144. doi:10.1371.

92. Okereke OI, Kang JH, Cook NR, et al. Type 2 diabetes mellitus and cognitive decline in two large cohorts of community-dwelling older adults. *J Am Geriatr Soc.* 2008:56:1028–1036.

93. Hanlon JT, Landerman LR, Fillenbaum GG, Studenski S. Falls in African American and White community-dwelling elderly residents. *J Gerontol A Biol Sci Med Sci.* 2002;57:M473–M47.

94. Reyes-Ortiz CA, Snih SA, Loera J, et al Risk factors for falling in older Mexican Americans. *Ethnic Dis.* 2004;14:417–422.

95. Lee PG, Cigolle C, Blaum C. The co-occurrence of chronic diseases and geriatric syndromes: the Health and Retirement Study. *J Am Geriatr Soc.* 2009;57:511–516.

96. Schwartz AV, Hiller TA, Sellmeyer DE, et al. Older women with diabetes have a higher risk of falls. *Diabetes Care.* 2002;25:1749–1754.

97. Jackson RA, Vittinghoff E, Kanaya AM, et al. Urinary incontinence in elderly women: findings from the Health, Aging, and Body Composition Study. *Obstet Gynecol.* 2004;104:301–307.

98. Lifford KL, Curhan GC, Hu FB, et al. Type 2 diabetes mellitus and risk of developing urinary incontinence. *J Am Geriatr Soc.* 2005;53:1851–1857.

99. Jackson SL, Scholes D, Boyko EJ, et al Urinary incontinence and diabetes in postmenopausal women. *Diabetes Care.* 2005;28:1730–1738.

100. Pearte CA, Furberg CD, O'Meara ES, et al. Characteristics and baseline clinical predictors of future fatal versus nonfatal coronary heart disease events in older adults. The Cardiovascular Health Study. *Circulation.* 2006;113:2177–2185.

Diabetes Treatment Success Stories

Adolescent Years

© Galina Barskaya/ShutterStock, Inc.

Linda is a 14-year-old athlete who enjoys playing tennis with her siblings and on the varsity team at school. Like most teenagers with diabetes, Linda has type 1 diabetes. She was diagnosed with diabetes when she was 14 months old. Being diagnosed at such a young age, meant that Linda's parents, who did not have a family history of diabetes prior to Linda's diagnosis, had to learn quickly what diabetes is and how to keep it under control. Linda's mom admits that initially it was hard to know what to do for a 14-month- old with diabetes. But with a lot of guidance, education, and support from healthcare professionals, Linda's parents learned how to prepare healthy foods and to teach Linda about her diabetes as she got older. Aside from her insulin pump, Linda is now your average teenage girl. Linda says that as long as she stays physically active, watches what she eats, and maintains good control of her blood sugar, she can live a normal life.

Reproductive Years

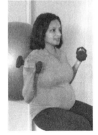

© leezsnow/iStockphoto.com

When Melinda was 26 years old, she got some surprising news from her OB-GYN. She was told that she had gestational diabetes, diabetes that occurs or is first recognized in pregnancy. Because Melinda has gestational diabetes, she must carefully monitor her blood sugar levels, develop a plan for maintaining regular physical activity, and modify her diet. Melinda learned that she now has a lifelong risk of developing type 2, but if she maintains her healthy lifestyle after the baby is born, she can reduce this risk. By losing weight after the baby is born and starting a regular exercise program, many people are able to get their blood sugar levels back to normal, delaying the onset of diabetes or even preventing it altogether.

Middle Years

© Comstock Images/Thinkstock

Veronica is a 51-year-old registered nurse and diabetes educator, who was diagnosed with type 2 diabetes in her mid 20s. She admits how challenging it was to accept the diagnosis of diabetes and to actually begin changing her lifestyle. Veronica says that she found it difficult to manage her diabetes while focusing on her career and starting a family. As a diabetes educator, she knew all of the things she should have been doing—exercising several times a week, changing her diet—but it took her some time to figure out how to fit it all into her busy schedule. This is very common for women in the middle years, who find themselves balancing careers with the needs of dependent children and aging parents. What turned Veronica around and on a healthy path was that she had a strong support system that included her family and friends, especially her friends with diabetes. They all work together to keep each other motivated. Veronica now runs a support group of her own and she also visits local churches and neighborhoods to offer information about diabetes.

Older Years

© wavebreakmedia/ShutterStock, Inc.

Eva, who is now 65 years old, has had type 2 diabetes since she was 29 years old. She says that managing diabetes in the older years can be tough because older people often have special challenges that other age groups may not readily have to deal with, like arthritis, depression, and memory loss. Older people facing these challenges may have trouble remembering to take their medications or follow their diet restrictions. Eva says that having friends and family members who check in on her and who buy her nutritious groceries has helped her tremendously. She says that there have been several times when she has felt so depressed that, although she knew needed to eat healthfully and exercise, she could not get the energy to get out of bed. Having people to talk with in a support group and family members who come to visit have all given Eva a new outlook on her life with diabetes. She admits that it is tough being alone trying to manage diabetes by herself. As a support group leader now, she gets strength from others in the group as they share their common stories and successes with managing diabetes.

Malignancies

Lung Cancer

Yuan-Chin Amy Lee, PhD and Zuo-Feng Zhang, MD, PhD

Introduction

Lung cancer is a malignant disease with abnormal lung cells, characterized by uncontrollable and unlimited growth. As classified by conventional microscopy, over 90% of all lung cancer patients fall into the four major histological types: squamous cell carcinoma (SCC), large cell carcinoma (LC), adenocarcinoma (AC), and small cell carcinoma (SC).[1] Clinically, lung cancer can be further classified into two groups according to its cell types: non-small cell lung cancer (NSCLC), including SCC, AC, and LC, and small cell lung cancer (SCLC, or oat cell cancer).

Lung cancer holds a distinguished position among malignancies with the second highest incidence rate but the highest mortality rate among all forms of cancer in the United States. In addition, the treatment of lung cancer has not advanced significantly over the last few decades. As a result, understanding the etiology, early detection, and prognosis of lung cancer is critical for identifying means of prevention to reduce incidence and improve prognosis.

Lung cancer among women is a serious public health issue as studies have shown that the proportion of never smokers and of adenocarcinoma are greater among female cases of lung cancer than male cases. Furthermore, over the past 2 decades the incidence of lung cancer among males has decreased, in contrast to no observed decline among women until the first dip was noted in 2010. In this chapter, we first provide an overview of lung cancer statistics, discuss general epidemiologic factors, focus on specific characteristics of lung cancer in women, and briefly describe the current diagnosis and treatment of lung cancer.

Descriptive Epidemiology of Lung Cancer

In the United States, lung cancer incidence ranks second to prostate cancer among men (116,470 new cases, 14% of all male cancers) and second to breast cancer among women (109,690 new cases, 14% of all female cancers), whereas estimated lung cancer mortality ranks number one in males (87,750 deaths, 29%) and females (72,590 deaths, 26%).[2] Compared to the death rate caused by other cancers, among women lung cancer is far more lethal than other malignancies as noted in Figure 25-1[2]

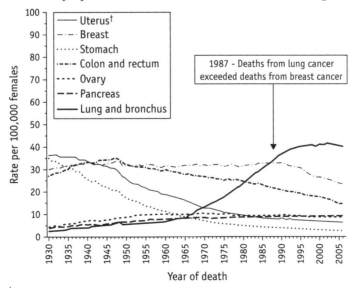

Figure 25-1 Age-adjusted cancer death rates, females by cancer site, 1930–2006.

Source: Reproduced from Cancer Facts & Figures 2010, Jemal A, Siegel R, Xu J, Ward E. Cancer Statistics, 2010. CA: Cancer J Clin 2010;60:277–300.

Deaths due to lung cancer among women exceed the number dying of both breast and colon cancer.

Since 1984, the mortality rate among males has been decreasing in contrast to the steady increasing rate noted among females since 1930 until the slight downturn recently reported by the American Cancer Society (Figure 25-2). Among females lung cancer deaths steadily increased between 1975 and 2000 when rates became stable (Figure 25-2).[2,3] Historical differences in cigarette smoking between men and women have contributed to the lag in the gender specific temporal trend of lung cancer deaths. The peak year of cigarette smoking in women was approximately 20 years later than that in men. The evident consequence of cigarette smoking is the greater mortality among women from lung rather than breast cancer beginning in 1987.[4] However, the trend for women has remained level at the peak rates for about 10 years rather than decreasing as observed among men (Figures 25-2 and 25-3). This observation reflects the sharper decline of male smoking.[5] In general, female lung cancer patients tend to be younger, are more likely to be never smokers, have higher incidence of adenocarcinoma, and generally have better survival than male patients.[6]

During the last 2 decades, the proportion of histological types has been changing; squamous.cell carcinoma, formerly the predominant type, has decreased and adenocarcinoma has increased in both men and women.[7] The increasing adenocarcinoma incidence may be attributable to changes in cigarette composition and/or the use of filters,[8] which may have resulted in deeper inhalation by the smokers for deeper penetration of lung carcinogens.

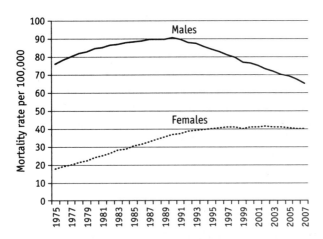

Figure 25-2 Lung cancer age-adjusted mortality rates per 100,000 in the US from 1975 to 2007 by gender.

Source: Data from Howlader N, Noone AM, Krapcho M, Neyman N, Aminou R, Waldron W, Altekruse SF, Kosary CL, Ruhl J, Tatalovich Z, Cho H, Mariotto A, Eisner MP, Lewis DR, Chen HS, Feuer EJ, Cronin KA (eds). SEER Cancer Statistics Review, 1975-2009 (Vintage 2009 Populations), National Cancer Institute. Bethesda, MD, http://seer.cancer.gov/csr/1975_2009_pops09/, based on November 2011 SEER data submission, posted to the SEER web site, April 2012.

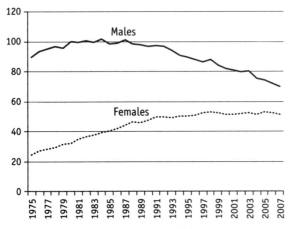

Figure 25-3 Lung cancer age-adjusted incidence rates per 100,000 in the US from 1975 to 2007 by gender.

Source: Data from Howlader N, Noone AM, Krapcho M, Neyman N, Aminou R, Waldron W, Altekruse SF, Kosary CL, Ruhl J, Tatalovich Z, Cho H, Mariotto A, Eisner MP, Lewis DR, Chen HS, Feuer EJ, Cronin KA (eds). SEER Cancer Statistics Review, 1975-2009 (Vintage 2009 Populations), National Cancer Institute. Bethesda, MD, http://seer.cancer.gov/csr/1975_2009_pops09/, based on November 2011 SEER data submission, posted to the SEER web site, April 2012.

Risk and Protective Factors among Women

Active Smoking

The increase and decline in cigarette sales were parallel to that of lung cancer deaths with an approximate 20-year gap (Figure 25-4).[9] Cigarette smoking has been established as the most important risk factor for lung cancer, including all major histological types, although the association is stronger for squamous cell carcinoma than adenocarcinoma.[10] Approximately 75%–80% of lung cancer deaths in women and 90% in men in the United States each year are estimated to be caused by active smoking.[11] The International Agency for Research on Cancer (IARC)[12] has identified 81 carcinogens in mainstream cigarette smoke to have sufficient evidence for carcinogenicity in humans or laboratory animals.[13] Duration of smoking has the strongest impact on lung cancer risk among smokers.[14] Lung carcinogens include polycyclic aromatic hydrocarbons such as benzo(a) pyrene and N-nitrosamines such as nicotine-derived nitrosamine ketone. Active tobacco smoking has been established as the strongest risk factor for lung cancer with an average risk ratio of 10.[15]

There has been a fair amount of controversy over whether female smokers are at a higher risk of lung cancer than male smokers with a similar level of exposure to tobacco smoke. Several case-control and prospective studies reported women are more susceptible to tobacco carcinogens than men.[16] On the other hand, cohort studies have reported similar relative risks for lung cancer among men and women.[16] Most recently, Patel et al. concluded that lung cancer risks among men and women are similar at given levels of smoking.[16]

Although active smoking is the primary cause of lung cancer, worldwide about 25% of cases among women occur among never smokers.[17] In the United States, an estimated 19% of female lung cancer cases are diagnosed among never smokers in contrast to 7% of male cases among never smokers.[16,18]

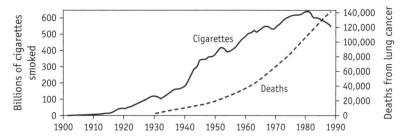

Figure 25-4 The trend of cigarette consumption and the number of lung cancer deaths in the United States, 1900–1990.

Source: Reproduced from U.S. Department of Agriculture, National Center for Health Statistics in Smoking, Tobacco, and Cancer Program 1985–1989 Status Report, NIH publication No. 90-3107.

When lung cancer cases among never smokers are considered separately, the disease ranks as the seventh most common cause of cancer deaths worldwide.[17] Several environmental, genetic, and reproductive factors have been studied as potential risk/protective factors for lung cancer in women.

Involuntary Smoking

Involuntary exposure to smoke has been investigated as a potential determinant for lung cancer development among never smokers. A review on the genotoxicity of involuntary smoking noted a biologically plausible association between tobacco smoking and smoking-related cancers in the population exposed to cigarette smoke.[19] Involuntary smoking includes exposure to mainstream smoke (approximately 20%) and the more concentrated sidestream smoke (about 80%), which has higher levels of some carcinogens such as benzo(a)pyrene, nitrosamine, and polonium than the mainstream.[20]

An IARC monograph review concluded that involuntary exposure to smoking is carcinogenic to humans[12] with a 20% increase in risk for females and 30% for males who were never active smokers. Although the study showed a smaller risk increase for women compared to men, the percentage of never smokers in women (19%) who have lung cancer is higher than that for men (7%). This observation also implies the existence of other important risk factors specific to lung cancer in women such as air pollution and hormonal factors discussed later. The evidence of an involuntary smoking effect has been observed for exposures at home and at work, but limited research has addressed exposure to tobacco smoke during childhood.[21] A pooled analysis from two case-control studies reported a consistent dose response with duration of exposure for all types of lung cancer.[22] In a recent unpublished pooled analysis with the largest sample size from the International Lung Cancer Consortium, Lee et al. observed an OR of approximately 1.38 (95% CI = 1.18−1.50) with ever exposure to involuntary smoking for both male and female nonsmokers and an even stronger association (OR~1.77, 95% CI = 1.42–2.20) for small cell lung cancer.[23] A modest association was observed when the residual confounding from active tobacco smoking was ruled out.

Air Pollution

In addition to involuntary smoking, exposure to air pollution may contribute to the development of lung cancer. Several studies in the United States reported an association between long-term exposure to particulate air pollution and lung cancer mortality.[24–26] The evidence was prominent with fine particulate material < 2.5µ (PM$_{2.5}$, RR = 1.14, 95% CI = 1.04−1.23 with a 10 µg/m^3 change) after appropriate adjustment by confounders.[26] The exposure response relationship strengthened the causal relationship.[26] However, the impact of air pollution has not been reported by gender.

Indoor Air Pollution

Smoke produced by burning domestic fuel such as coal, wood, and biomass for cooking and heating has been associated with lung cancer.[27] However, Straif et al. of IARC classified biomass use (primarily wood) as a Group 2A carcinogen because there was limited epidemiological evidence.[28] A recent pooled analysis in the International Lung Cancer Consortium by Hosgood et al. observed that predominant coal use was associated with an increased risk of lung cancer compared to nonsolid fuel use (OR = 1.15, 95% CI = 1.02−1.30), when the studies in North America and Europe were included.[29] In the same study, predominant wood use was associated with increased lung cancer risk (OR = 1.34, 95% CI = 1.18−1.52) when compared to nonsolid fuel use.[29] Similar associations were observed for men, women, and never smokers. Wood use among never-smoking women was associated with an increased risk of lung cancer (OR = 1.66, 95% CI = 1.21−2.24).[29]

Indoor Exposure to Radon

Radon, a well-established respiratory carcinogen, is a problem not only for underground miners but also for the general population.[30] The biologic mechanism by which radon initiates lung tissue is through alpha-particle emissions from inhaled radon progeny.[31] A pooled analysis of seven case-control studies in North America reported residential radon is associated with a 10% increase of lung cancer risk among never smokers.[32] Indoor radon is among the leading causes of lung cancer among never smokers.[30] As women are more likely to be never smokers and spend more time at home, the impact of indoor radon may play a more significant role in lung cancer development in women.

Family History of Cancer

As with other malignancies, a familial predisposition to lung cancer has been reported, with an early age at diagnosis supporting the hypothesis of inherited susceptibility.[33] A family history of lung cancer among first-degree relatives has been associated with an approximate two- to fivefold greater risk, particularly of early onset at ages less than 46 years noted by some researchers or younger than age 55 by other investigators.[34,35] One multi-center case-control study also found a family history of gastric cancer associated with a twofold increased risk of non-small cell lung cancer before age 55, which increased to threefold elevated risk at older age.[35] Studies suggest estrogen-related genes may be the link between a maternal history of breast cancer and high lung cancer risk.[35] Two international studies of female lung cancer showed similar results of a twofold increased risk associated with family history,[36,37] potentially associated with genetic factors, shared environmental/lifestyle factors, or gene–environment interactions.

Genetic Factors

The relationship between family history of cancer and lung cancer development implies an underlying genetic susceptibility. The frequency of mutations of epidermal growth factor receptor (EGFR) is higher among nonsmoking women and East Asian ethnic groups.[38] EGFR mutations are observed in 20% of female and in 9% of male lung cancer cases.[38] Lower frequency of Kras (v-Ki-ras2 Kirsten rat sarcoma viral oncogene) and tumor protein p53 (TP53) mutations is reported in lung tumors of never smokers than malignancies of smokers.[39] Female smokers have increased expression of CYP1A1 in lung tissue compared to male smokers, possibly resulting from induction by hormones, particularly estrogen.[40] A recent study examined the patterns of oncogenic and molecular signaling pathway activation and NSCLC survival and demonstrated different genomic profiles between men and women.[41] Tumor characteristics varied by gender: high-risk female patients showed increased invasiveness and activation of signal transducer and activator of transcription 3 (STAT3) in contrast to high-risk male patients whose tumors exhibited increased activation of the STAT3, tumor necrosis factor, EGFR, and wound healing.[41] Recent genomewide association studies have identified three chromosomal regions at 15q25, 5p15, and 6p21 associated with lung cancer.[42–45] Furthermore, lung cancer risk was increased more than fivefold among women with a family history of lung cancer and two copies of the risk alleles rs8034191 or rs105130 located in 15q24-25.1.[46] The single-nucleotide polymorphism (SNP) of the human telomerase reverse transcriptase (TERT) gene, rs2736100, was specifically associated with women, nonsmokers and adenocarcinoma in a large-scale replication study.[47]

Hormonal Factors

The gender-specific variation in expression of lung cancer-related genes may be associated with estrogen level differences. In addition, estrogen and progesterone receptors are expressed in the normal lung and in lung cancer cell lines. Formation of DNA adducts and activation of growth factors may be the mechanism explaining estrogen's effect on lung cancer development.[48] Furthermore, a recent study on second primary cancer following a first primary lung cancer reported an association with breast cancer, suggesting the role of hormones in lung cancer development.[49] The evidence for hormonal factors affecting lung cancer risk has been controversial. Early age at menopause ($\leq$ 40 years old) was inversely associated with lung adenocarcinoma risk with an OR of 0.3 (95% CI = 0.1−0.8); use of estrogen-replacement therapy was positively associated with lung adenocarcinoma risk, OR = 1.7 (95% CI = 1.0−2.5).[50] However, Blackman et al. did not observe an association with estrogen-replacement therapy,[51] in contrast to Schabath et al., who reported a 34% decreased lung cancer risk associated with hormone use.[52] A recent review of studies published between January 1966 and July 2008 indicated an approximate 76% increase of adenocarcinoma among ever users of hormone therapy among nonsmoking women.[53] In a randomized trial in the Women's Health Initiative, hormone-replacement therapy was not associated with increased lung cancer risk but higher mortality among women diagnosed with nonsmall cell lung cancer.[54] A prospectively followed cohort of peri- and postmenopausal women revealed the use of estrogen plus progestin increased lung cancer risk with a dose-response relationship; use of the combined therapy for ten years or longer was associated with a 50% greater lung cancer risk.[55]

Another publication from the Women's Health Initiative indicated bilateral oophorectomy was associated with higher risk of lung cancer (HR = 1.26, 95% CI = 1.02−1.56) and higher mortality due to lung cancer (HR = 1.31, 95% CI = 1.02−1.68).[56] Schwartz et al. demonstrated postmenopausal hormone use was associated with a decreased risk of estrogen receptor alpha (ER-α) and/or beta (ER-β) positive non-small cell lung cancer.[57] Therefore, individual ER status may modify the influence of hormone use on lung cancer development and may have contributed to the inconclusive studies of hormonal factors and lung cancer risk. In addition, the possible 2- to 3-decade lag time from hormonal exposures to lung cancer development may require longer duration of follow-up than studies have considered.[8]

Infection

Infection may be associated with lung cancer development via an inflammatory pathway. Chronic obstructive pulmonary disease (COPD) is an independent risk factor for lung cancer and has been found to coexist in 40% to 60% of lung cancer cases. Compared to smokers with normal lung function, smokers with COPD are two to six times more likely to develop lung cancer.[58]

HPV

Human papillomavirus (HPV) infection is an established risk factor for cervical cancer and has been suggested to be an important risk factor for lung cancer. Both HPV oncoproteins and E6 and E7 transcripts have been observed in lung tissue.[59] A Taiwanese study showed the presence of HPV DNA (types 16 and 18, which are classified as the most carcinogenic HPV types in humans[60]) in the cancer cells of never-smoking female lung cancer cases.[61] Several studies have reported the absence or low frequency of HPV infection in lung cancer cells[62,63] although others have observed higher frequencies (25.6−78.3) in Japan, Northern Iran, Finland, and Norway.[64–67] The mean prevalence of HPV in lung cancer was 24.5%; the average frequency was 17% in Europe, 15% in North America, and 35.7% in Asia.[68] A recent study of stage 1 lung cancer patients in Taiwan demonstrated high expression of HPV-16 and -18 among nonsmoking women with adenocarcinoma.[69] The results of *p53* mutations in female lung cancer patients suggested that HPV infection might be associated with lung cancer development via a HPV E6-dependent *p53* degradation pathway[70] The association between HPV infection and lung cancer seems dependent on geographic location, race, or host genetic susceptibility.[61] The HPV vaccine may play a role in the protection of women from lung cancer potentially lowering risk.

Dietary Factors

The results of studies assessing dietary factors and lung cancer risk have been inconsistent except for the protective effect of high consumption of fresh vegetables and fruits, which has been challenged by the results of a recent prospective study conducted among older Americans.[71] Wright et al. did not demonstrate a protective relationship between total fruit and vegetable consumption and lung cancer risk for either men or women. However, inverse associations with higher intake of some botanical groups, including Rosaceae (apples, peaches, nectarines, plums, pears, and strawberries), Convolvulaceae (sweet potatoes and yams), and Umbelliferae (carrots), were reported for lung cancer risk in men, but not in women.[71] Such gender differences may be due to the potential influence of estrogen or hormonally-related factors in women or superior and more accurate dietary recall by women.

The results from randomized trials indicated supplemental beta-carotene at high doses increased lung cancer risk among current smokers.[72,73] Such observations may be explained by the dose of purified beta-carotene, which is much greater than levels from normal dietary consumption, resulting in the loss of the anticancer action of fresh produce.[74] A recent systematic review of selective high-quality studies reported no compelling evidence that higher consumption of fruit and vegetables or serum concentrations of individual carotenoids decreases lung cancer risk.[74] On the other hand, an inverse association between total carotenoids and lung cancer risk was observed although study results may be explained by other exposures such as confounding due to healthier lifestyle, smoking history or use of carotenoid measurements as a proxy for estimated consumption of fruit and vegetables. Further investigation on dietary factors is necessary

in larger prospective studies in order to minimize residual confounding.

Occupational Factors

No female-specific estimates have been published indicating occupational carcinogens and lung cancer; the small number of exposed cases resulted in unstable estimates.[75] Considering men and women together, occupational exposure to carcinogens plays an important role in the development of lung cancer. Worldwide estimates for 2000 indicated 10% of lung cancer deaths in men and 5% in women were attributable to occupational exposures to lung carcinogens including arsenic, asbestos, beryllium, cadmium, chromium, diesel fumes, nickel, and silica.[76–78] An alternative study design is required to accurately assess the impact of work related exposures to lung cancer among women.

Lung Cancer Following Radiotherapy for Breast Cancer

Although associated with a small attributable fraction, radiotherapy has been suggested as a primary cause of lung cancer in women treated for breast cancer. Such an association has been reported from randomized trials and cancer registry-based studies.[79] High-dose radiotherapy was associated with an increased risk for second cancers in exposed tissues of the lungs, esophagus, pleura, bone, and soft tissue (RR = 1.45, 95% CI = 1.33−1.58).[79]

Screening Methods

No standardized population-based screening method has been established for lung cancer due to the lack of cancer-specific symptoms indicative of early stage disease although early diagnosis in stage 1 is associated with 5-year survival of 65–75%.[80] Since annual chest x-ray (CXR) did not reduce mortality compared to cases diagnosed after symptoms developed among nonscreened patients, routine CXR was discontinued.[81] Several studies have shown that screening with Computed Tomography (CT)[54] detects 58–93% of lung cancers at stage 1, approximately four times better than with CXR.[80] A recent randomized controlled trial to compare three annual screenings by either low-dose CT or single-view CXR enrolled more than 50,000 current or former smokers (including 20,000 women) from 33 U.S. medical centers. Results reported in 2011 after more than 5 years of follow-up revealed lung cancer mortality was reduced by 20% among those screened by CT.[80] However, low-dose CT screening was associated with a high rate of false positive findings which required invasive lung biopsies to rule out cancer. Although this trial provided significant evidence of improved survival, many questions remain to be addressed before public policy recommendations can be established. The investigators warned that survival benefits must be weighed against the recognized harms including the potential for overdiagnosis. The high costs of mass screening must also include the clinical costs of the essential pathologic evaluation of detected lesions.[80] The research team has encouraged development of additional early detection modalities including molecular markers in blood, sputum, and urine as a means of selecting patients at highest risk who might benefit the most from low-dose CT screening.[80]

Diagnostic Procedures, Pathologic Criteria and Staging

The tumor, node, metastasis (TNM) classification for NSCLC was adopted in 1974[82] and has been improved to involve imaging and tissue acquisition.[80] Although the increasing use of imaging has enabled earlier detection,[83] histologic confirmation is essential after positive imaging and before clinical decisions regarding treatment options.[84] Minimally invasive techniques such as endobronchial ultrasound-guided fine-needle aspiration (EBUS-FNA) are methods being studied for staging of lung cancer.[85–86] Several metagene models with gene and micro RNA signatures have been identified to assist in prognosis predictions of stage 1 lung cancer.[80] However, these techniques still need to be refined in order to improve the precision in diagnosis prior to clinical treatment decisions.

Treatment

To date surgery is considered the best option for lung cancer patients, particularly those with localized early-stage NSCLC. Treatment decisions for early-stage lung cancer vary by gender[87] with women more likely to have surgery than men. Men are more likely to receive radiotherapy then women.[87] However, such treatment differences do not fully explain the better survival of women.[88–90] For patients with advanced disease, platinum-based chemotherapy options, including paclitaxel, docetaxel, vinorelbine, or gemcitabine, all provide similar survival benefits compared to best supportive care.[91] Better treatment approaches are needed to improve survival of patients with advanced NSCLC. Several other treatment options are based on targeted inhibition of vascular endothelial growth factor (VEGF) or inhibition of epidermal growth factor receptor. The former includes bevacizumab, whereas the latter includes gefitinib and erlotinib. As mentioned earlier, female lung cancer patients are more likely to have EGFR mutations than male patients, and response to treatment by gefitinib and erlotinib is observed particularly in women, Japanese people, nonsmokers, and patients with adenocarcinoma.[92] Therefore, it is essential to define treatment options based on clinical features of the tumor and patient characteristics.

Summary

Lung cancer is the number one cause of cancer death for both women and men worldwide. Active tobacco smoking is considered the major cause of lung cancer although variation in susceptibility to tobacco smoke by gender has been suggested but the evidence seems equivocal. Risk factors other than active smoking include involuntary exposure to tobacco smoke with an approximate 20–30% increase in lung cancer risk. In addition, residential exposure to radon is associated with a 10% increased risk among never smokers. The impact of occupational exposure to lung carcinogens needs to be studied among more females from diverse worksites to identify specific adverse exposures and to provide adequate power for stable estimates. The family history association with lung cancer risk implies genetic susceptibility in association with environmental exposures. Similarly, hormonal factors such as postmenopausal hormonal therapy have been studied with inconsistent results, possibly due to the receptor status of tumor tissue. Future studies with comprehensive consideration of hormone-related factors are necessary to elucidate the impact of various exposures on lung cancer development among women. In addition to environmental, occupational, and genetic factors, infections with HPV may influence lung cancer risk. Improved and effective early detection modalities with minimal false positive results may enable diagnosis at more treatable stages leading to improved survival. In addition, patient characteristics such as EGFR mutations may assist in treatment decisions to improve survival. Cancer mortality rates will decline as detection and treatment of lung cancer improves for women and men.

Discussion Questions

1. What is the number one cause of cancer death in women?
2. What is the main cause of lung cancer development in both genders? Explain the concept of attributable fraction and discuss the attributable fraction of this risk factor?
3. Are women more susceptible to tobacco smoking exposure than men? What approach would you consider to elucidate such a potential variation/similarity?
4. Which histological subtype of lung cancer is more common among women than men? What are possible explanations?
5. What are possible mechanisms underlying the relationship between reproductive factors and lung cancer risk?
6. Which factors should be considered when decisions on treatment options need to be made?

References

1. Janssen-Heijnen ML, Coebergh JW. Trends in incidence and prognosis of the histological subtypes of lung cancer in North America, Australia, New Zealand and Europe. *Lung Cancer.* 2001;31:123–137.
2. Siegel R, Naishadham MA, Jemal A Cancer Statistics, 2012. *CA Cancer J Clin.* 2012;62:10–29.
3. Fast Stats: An interactive tool for access to SEER cancer statistics. Bethesda, MD: Surveillance Research Program. National Cancer Institute; 2010.
4. Devesa SS, Blot WJ, Stone BJ, et al. Recent cancer trends in the United States. *J Natl Cancer Inst.* 1995;87:175–182.
5. Wang H, Preston SH. Forecasting United States mortality using cohort smoking histories. *Proc Natl Acad Sci U S A.* 2009;106:393–398.
6. Harichand-Herdt S, Ramalingam SS. Gender-associated differences in lung cancer: clinical characteristics and treatment outcomes in women. *Semin Oncol.* 2009;36:572–580.
7. Travis WD, Lubin J, Ries L, Devesa S. United States lung carcinoma incidence trends: declining for most histologic types among males, increasing among females. *Cancer.* 1996;77:2464–2470.

8. Egleston BL, Meireles SI, Flieder DB, Clapper ML. Population-based trends in lung cancer incidence in women. *Semin Oncol.* 2009;36:506–515.

9. National Institutes of Health. *Smoking, Tobacco and Cancer Program 1985-1989 Status Report.* Bethesda, MD: National Cancer Institute, National Institutes of Health; 1990. NIH publication 90–3107.

10. Khuder SA. Effect of cigarette smoking on major histological types of lung cancer: a meta-analysis. *Lung Cancer.* 2001;31:139–148.

11. Hecht SS. Tobacco smoke carcinogens and lung cancer. *J Natl Cancer Inst.* 1999;91:1194–1210.

12. IARC Working Group on the Evaluation of Carcinogenic Risks to Humans. Tobacco smoke and involuntary smoking. *IARC Monogr Eval Carcinog Risks Hum.* 2004;83:1–1438.

13. Smith CJ, Perfetti TA, Garg R, Hansch C. IARC carcinogens reported in cigarette mainstream smoke and their calculated log P values. *Food Chem Toxicol.* 2003;41:807–817.

14. Doll R, Peto R, Boreham J, Sutherland I. Mortality in relation to smoking: 50 years' observations on male British doctors. *BMJ.* 2004;328:1519.

15. Vineis P, Alavanja M, Buffler P, et al. Tobacco and cancer: recent epidemiological evidence. *J Natl Cancer Inst.* 2004;96:99–106.

16. Patel JD. Lung cancer: a biologically different disease in women? *Womens Health (Lond Engl).* 2009;5:685–691.

17. Parkin DM, Bray F, Ferlay J, Pisani P. Global cancer statistics, 2002. *CA Cancer J Clin.* 2005;55:74–108.

18. Wakelee HA, Chang ET, Gomez SL, et al. Lung cancer incidence in never smokers. *J Clin Oncol.* 2007;25:472–478.

19. Husgafvel-Pursiainen K. Genotoxicity of environmental tobacco smoke: a review. *Mutat Res.* 2004;567:427–45.

20. Lam WK. Lung cancer in Asian women—the environment and genes. *Respirology.* 2005;10:408–417.

21. Boffetta P, Tredaniel J, Greco A. Risk of childhood cancer and adult lung cancer after childhood exposure to passive smoke: a meta-analysis. *Environ Health Perspect.* 2000;108:73–82.

22. Brennan P, Buffler PA, Reynolds P, et al. Secondhand smoke exposure in adulthood and risk of lung cancer among never smokers: a pooled analysis of two large studies. *Int J Cancer.* 2004;109:125–131.

23. Lee Y-CA, Hung R, Boffetta P, et al. A pooled analysis on the associations between involuntary smoking and lung cancer risk by histological types. [Unpublished]

24. Dockery DW, Pope CA, 3rd, Xu X, et al. An association between air pollution and mortality in six U.S. cities. *N Engl J Med.* 1993;329:1753–1759.

25. Pope CA, 3rd, Thun MJ, Namboodiri MM, et al. Particulate air pollution as a predictor of mortality in a prospective study of US adults. *Am J Respir Crit Care Med.* 1995;151:669–674.

26. Pope CA, 3rd, Burnett RT, Thun MJ, et al. Lung cancer, cardiopulmonary mortality, and long-term exposure to fine particulate air pollution. *JAMA.* 2002;287:1132–1141.

27. Hosgood HD, 3rd, Chapman R, Shen M, et al. Portable stove use is associated with lower lung cancer mortality risk in lifetime smoky coal users. *Br J Cancer.* 2008;99:1934–1939.

28. Straif K, Baan R, Grosse Y, et al. Carcinogenicity of household solid fuel combustion and of high-temperature frying. *Lancet Oncol.* 2006;7:977–978.

29. Hosgood HD, Paolo B, Greenland S, et al. In-home coal and wood use and lung cancer risk: a pooled-analysis of the International Lung Cancer Consortium. [Unpublished]

30. Samet JM, Avila-Tang E, Boffetta P, et al. Lung cancer in never smokers: clinical epidemiology and environmental risk factors. *Clin Cancer Res.* 2009;15:5626–5645.

31. Committee on Health Risks of Exposure to Radon (BEIR VI), National Research Council. *Health Effects of Exposure to Radon. BEIR IV.* Washington, DC: National Academy Press; 1999.

32. Krewski D, Lubin JH, Zielinski JM, et al. Residential radon and risk of lung cancer: a combined analysis of 7 North American case-control studies. *Epidemiology.* 2005;16:137–145.

33. Li X, Hemminki K. Familial and second lung cancers: a nation-wide epidemiologic study from Sweden. *Lung Cancer.* 2003;39:255–263.

34. Gao Y, Goldstein AM, Consonni D, et al. Family history of cancer and nonmalignant lung diseases as risk factors for lung cancer. *Int J Cancer.* 2009;125:146–152.

35. Cassidy A, Balsan J, Vesin A, et al. Cancer diagnosis in first-degree relatives and non-small cell lung cancer risk: results from a multi-centre case-control study in Europe. *Eur J Cancer.* 2009;45:3047–3053.

36. Rachtan J, Sokolowski A, Niepsuj S, et al. Familial lung cancer risk among women in Poland. *Lung Cancer.* 2009;65:138–143.

37. Wang XR, Yu IT, Chiu YL, et al. Previous pulmonary disease and family cancer history increase the risk of lung cancer among Hong Kong women. *Cancer Causes Control.* 2009;20:757–763.

38. Planchard D, Loriot Y, Goubar A, et al. Differential expression of biomarkers in men and women. *Semin Oncol.* 2009;36:553–565.

39. Sun S, Schiller JH, Gazdar AF. Lung cancer in never smokers—a different disease. *Nat Rev Cancer.* 2007;7:778–790.

40. Mollerup S, Ryberg D, Hewer A, et al. Sex differences in lung CYP1A1 expression and DNA adduct levels among lung cancer patients. *Cancer Res.* 1999;59:3317–3320.

41. Mostertz W, Stevenson M, Acharya C, et al. Age- and sex-specific genomic profiles in non-small cell lung cancer. *JAMA.* 2010;303:535–543.

42. Hung RJ, McKay JD, Gaborieau V, et al. A susceptibility locus for lung cancer maps to nicotinic acetylcholine receptor subunit genes on 15q25. *Nature.* 2008;452:633–637.

43. Amos CI, Wu X, Broderick P, et al. Genome-wide association scan of tag SNPs identifies a susceptibility locus for lung cancer at 15q25.1. *Nat Genet.* 2008;40:616–622.

44. Thorgeirsson TE, Geller F, Sulem P, et al. A variant associated with nicotine dependence, lung cancer and peripheral arterial disease. *Nature.* 2008;452:638–642.

45. McKay JD, Hung RJ, Gaborieau V, et al. Lung cancer susceptibility locus at 5p15.33. *Nat Genet.* 2008;40:1404–1406.

46. Liu P, Vikis HG, Wang D, et al. Familial aggregation of common sequence variants on 15q24-25.1 in lung cancer. *J Natl Cancer Inst.* 2008;100:1326–1330.

47. Truong T, Hung RJ, Amos CI, et al. Replication of lung cancer susceptibility loci at chromosomes 15q25, 5p15, and 6p21: a pooled analysis from the International Lung Cancer Consortium. *J Natl Cancer Inst.* 2010;102:959–971.

48. Thomas L, Doyle LA, Edelman MJ. Lung cancer in women: emerging differences in epidemiology, biology, and therapy. *Chest.* 2005;128:370–381.

49. Chuang SC, Scelo G, Lee YC, et al. Risks of second primary cancer among patients with major histological types of lung cancers in both men and women. *Br J Cancer.* 2010;102:1190–1195.

50. Taioli E, Wynder EL. Re: Endocrine factors and adenocarcinoma of the lung in women. *J Natl Cancer Inst.* 1994;86:869–870.

51. Blackman JA, Coogan PF, Rosenberg L, et al. Estrogen replacement therapy and risk of lung cancer. *Pharmacoepidemiol Drug Saf.* 2002;11:561–567.

52. Schabath MB, Wu X, Vassilopoulou-Sellin R, et al. Hormone replacement therapy and lung cancer risk: a case-control analysis. *Clin Cancer Res.* 2004;10:113–123.

53. Greiser CM, Greiser EM, Doren M. Menopausal hormone therapy and risk of lung cancer—Systematic review and meta-analysis. *Maturitas.* 2010;65:198–204.

54. Chlebowski RT, Schwartz AG, Wakelee H, et al. Oestrogen plus progestin and lung cancer in postmenopausal women (Women's Health Initiative trial): a post-hoc analysis of a randomised controlled trial. *Lancet.* 2009;374:1243–1251.

55. Slatore CG, Chien JW, Au DH, et al. Lung cancer and hormone replacement therapy: association in the vitamins and lifestyle study. *J Clin Oncol.* 2010;28:1540–1546.

56. Parker WH, Jacoby V, Shoupe D, Rocca W. Effect of bilateral oophorectomy on women's long-term health. *Womens Health (Lond Engl).* 2009;5:565–576.

57. Schwartz AG, Wenzlaff AS, Prysak GM, et al. Reproductive factors, hormone use, estrogen receptor expression and risk of non small-cell lung cancer in women. *J Clin Oncol.* 2007;25:5785–5792.

58. Young RP, Hopkins RJ, Hay BA, et al. A gene-based risk score for lung cancer susceptibility in smokers and ex-smokers. *Postgrad Med J.* 2009;85:515–524.

59. Giuliani L, Favalli C, Syrjanen K, Ciotti M. Human papillomavirus infections in lung cancer. Detection of E6 and E7 transcripts and review of the literature. *Anticancer Res.* 2007;27:2697–2704.

60. Cogliano V, Baan R, Straif K, et al. Carcinogenicity of human papillomaviruses. *Lancet Oncol* 2005;6:204

61. Cheng YW, Chiou HL, Sheu GT, et al. The association of human papillomavirus 16/18 infection with lung cancer among nonsmoking Taiwanese women. *Cancer Res.* 2001;61:2799–2803.

62. Clavel CE, Nawrocki B, Bosseaux B, et al. Detection of human papillomavirus DNA in bronchopulmonary carcinomas by hybrid capture II: a study of 185 tumors. *Cancer.* 2000;88:1347–1352.

63. Coissard CJ, Besson G, Polette MC, et al. Prevalence of human papillomaviruses in lung carcinomas: a study of 218 cases. *Mod Pathol.* 2005;18:1606–1609.

64. Tsuhako K, Nakazato I, Hirayasu T, et al. Human papillomavirus DNA in adenosquamous carcinoma of the lung. *J Clin Pathol.* 1998;51:741–749.

65. Nadji SA, Mokhtari-Azad T, Mahmoodi M, et al. Relationship between lung cancer and human papillomavirus in north of Iran, Mazandaran province. *Cancer Lett.* 2007;248:41–46.

66. Soini Y, Nuorva K, Kamel D, et al. Presence of human papillomavirus DNA and abnormal p53 protein accumulation in lung carcinoma. *Thorax.* 1996;51:887–93.

67. Hirayasu T, Iwamasa T, Kamada Y, et al. Human papillomavirus DNA in squamous cell carcinoma of the lung. *J Clin Pathol.* 1996;49:810–817.

68. Klein F, Amin Kotb WF, Petersen I. Incidence of human papilloma virus in lung cancer. *Lung Cancer.* 2009;65:13–18.

69. Hsu LH, Chu NM, Liu CC, et al. Sex-associated differences in non-small cell lung cancer in the new era: is gender an independent prognostic factor? *Lung Cancer.* 2009;66:262–267.

70. Cheng YW, Wu MF, Wang J, et al. Human papillomavirus 16/18 E6 oncoprotein is expressed in lung cancer and related with p53 inactivation. *Cancer Res.* 2007;67:10686–10693.

71. Wright ME, Park Y, Subar AF, et al. Intakes of fruit, vegetables, and specific botanical groups in relation to lung cancer risk in the NIH-AARP Diet and Health Study. *Am J Epidemiol.* 2008;168:1024–1034.

72. Albanes D, Heinonen OP, Taylor PR, et al. Alpha-tocopherol and beta-carotene supplements and lung cancer incidence in the alpha-tocopherol, beta-carotene cancer prevention study: effects of base-line characteristics and study compliance. *J Natl Cancer Inst.* 1996;88:1560–1570.

73. Mayne ST, Handelman GJ, Beecher G. Beta-carotene and lung cancer promotion in heavy smokers—a plausible relationship? *J Natl Cancer Inst.* 1996;88:1513–1515.

74. Gallicchio L, Boyd K, Matanoski G, et al. Carotenoids and the risk of developing lung cancer: a systematic review. *Am J Clin Nutr.* 2008;88:372–383.

75. De Matteis S, Consonni D, Bertazzi PA. Exposure to occupational carcinogens and lung cancer risk. Evolution of epidemiological estimates of attributable fraction. *Acta Biomed.* 2008;79(suppl 1):34–42.

76. Driscoll T, Nelson DI, Steenland K, et al. The global burden of disease due to occupational carcinogens. *Am J Ind Med.* 2005;48:419–431.

77. Fingerhut M, Nelson DI, Driscoll T, et al. The contribution of occupational risks to the global burden of disease: summary and next steps. *Med Lav.* 2006;97:313–321.

78. Nelson DI, Concha-Barrientos M, Driscoll T, et al. The global burden of selected occupational diseases and injury risks: methodology and summary. *Am J Ind Med.* 2005;48:400–418.

79. Berrington de Gonzalez A, Curtis RE, Gilbert E, et al. Second solid cancers after radiotherapy for breast cancer in SEER cancer registries. *Br J Cancer.* 2010;102:220–226.

80. The National Lung Screening Trial Research Team. Reduced lung-cancer mortality with low-dose computed tomographic screening. *N Engl J Med* 2011;365:395–409.

81. Bach PB, Niewoehner DE, Black WC. Screening for lung cancer: the guidelines. *Chest.* 2003;123:83S–88S.

82. International Union against Cancer. *TNM Classification of Malignant Tumours.* 2nd ed. Geneva, Switzerland: UICC; 1974

83. van Tinteren H, Hoekstra OS, Smit EF, et al. Effectiveness of positron emission tomography in the preoperative assessment of patients with suspected non-small-cell lung cancer: the PLUS multicentre randomised trial. *Lancet.* 2002;359:1388–1393.

84. Silvestri GA, Gould MK, Margolis ML, et al. Noninvasive staging of non-small cell lung cancer: ACCP evidenced-based clinical practice guidelines. 2nd ed. *Chest.* 2007;132:178S–201S.

85. Gomez M, Silvestri GA. Endobronchial ultrasound for the diagnosis and staging of lung cancer. *Proc Am Thorac Soc.* 2009;6:180–186.

86. Wallace MB, Pascual JM, Raimondo M, et al. Minimally invasive endoscopic staging of suspected lung cancer. *JAMA.* 2008;299:540–546.

87. Belani CP, Marts S, Schiller J, Socinski MA. Women and lung cancer: epidemiology, tumor biology, and emerging trends in clinical research. *Lung Cancer.* 2007;55:15–23.

88. Fu JB, Kau TY, Severson RK, Kalemkerian GP. Lung cancer in women: analysis of the national Surveillance, Epidemiology, and End Results database. *Chest.* 2005;127:768–77.

89. Moore R, Doherty D, Chamberlain R, Khuri F. Sex differences in survival in non-small cell lung cancer patients 1974-1998. *Acta Oncol.* 2004;43:57–64.

90. Batevik R, Grong K, Segadal L, Stangeland L. The female gender has a positive effect on survival independent of background life expectancy following surgical resection of primary non-small cell lung cancer: a study of absolute and relative survival over 15 years. *Lung Cancer.* 2005;47:173–181.

91. Chemotherapy in non-small cell lung cancer: a meta-analysis using updated data on individual patients from 52 randomised clinical trials. Non-small Cell Lung Cancer Collaborative Group. *BMJ.* 1995;311:899–909.

92. Siegel-Lakhai WS, Beijnen JH, Schellens JH. Current knowledge and future directions of the selective epidermal growth factor receptor inhibitors erlotinib (Tarceva) and gefitinib (Iressa). *Oncologist.* 2005;10:579–589.

Breast Cancer

Ruby T. Senie, PhD

Dedicated to the memory of Sharon Brous 1956–1991

Sharon's Story

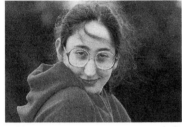

Source: Courtesy of Joan Brous.

Sharon was destined to be a film star from her early acting days in high school and college. Sharon's career was developing at ABC television where she contributed to special programs and docudramas until she was selected by Woody Allen for *Stardust Memories*. As her face filled the movie screen, her film career was launched. But Sharon was born during the era of diethylstilbestrol (DES), prescribed during pregnancy specifically for women who had experienced a miscarriage. Research has now linked Sharon's exposure in utero with her breast cancer, diagnosed when she was 30 years old. A recent publication documented additional health problems diagnosed among exposed mothers and their daughters as they grow older. Although Sharon was advised of her gynecologic abnormalities and potential vaginal cancer risk, physicians were not yet aware of increased breast cancer among DES-exposed women. When Sharon's grandmother, age 75, and a paternal aunt, age 65, developed breast cancer, the family was alerted to the disease. Sharon, on self-exam, found a lump in her breast. Although she had surgery to remove the cancer, the disease defied chemotherapy treatment. Sharon was 35 years old when she died; DES exposure may have compounded risk associated with her family history.

Introduction

Breast cancer is the most frequently diagnosed malignancy and second leading cause of cancer death among American women; the American Cancer Society (ACS) has estimated one in eight women will be diagnosed with invasive breast cancer by age 85. Current data from the Surveillance Epidemiology and End Results (SEER) program of the National Cancer Institute (NCI) indicate 2.6 million American women have a personal history of the disease. Primary, secondary, and tertiary prevention opportunities have been defined during the past several decades to address the public health burden of breast cancer. In the United States incidence and mortality rates are strongly influenced by screening practices, personal behaviors, and improved treatment options. Extensive research over several decades among diverse populations has identified numerous reproductive and environmental factors that

affect risk although their combined effects are limited compared with a positive family history especially with recognized inherited susceptibility. However, the recently recognized BRCA1, BRCA2, and other susceptibility genes account for only a small percentage of breast cancer, and many "environmental" factors also have a genetic origin. Therefore, researchers are now focused on more prevalent low-penetrance genetic markers associated with more modest levels of risk that may account for a greater proportion of disease in the general population. Gene–environment interactions are of major interest as some women may be more genetically susceptible to adverse effects of specific exposures such as hormone therapy. This chapter provides an overview of the extensive breast cancer literature noting the importance of timing of exposures at different ages and including some controversial aspects of the benefits and risks of early detection.

Incidence and Mortality Trends

The ACS estimated 226,870 women with invasive breast cancer and 63,300 cases of in situ disease would be diagnosed in 2012 and 39,920 would die of the disease.[1] Breast cancer also occurs in men with a ratio of 1 male case per 100 female cases; an estimated 2,190 men would be diagnosed and 410 would die of the disease in 2012.[1] Using SEER data to study breast cancer incidence trends, the ACS plotted increases noted during three time intervals between 1975 and 2002,[2] rates increased approximately 8.5% per year between ages of menarche and menopause before slowing to 2.5% increase among older women.[3] These data translate to diagnosis of 1 woman in 207 before age 40, rising to 1 in 27 between ages 40 and 59 and 1 in 15 among older women.[4] The ACS's frequently quoted "one in eight" estimate refers to risk across a full life span to age 85.

Figure 26-1 notes the long recognized age-related crossover of incidence rates among black women (15.5/100,000) compared with white women (13.1/100,000) between ages 40 and 45 that reverse at older ages.[2,5] The decline of breast cancer incidence rates after age 75 in the two later timeframes, 1985–1989 and 1998–2002, may be associated with age-related lower endogenous hormone levels, presence of comorbid chronic conditions, and reduced screening frequency.

Between 1975 and 2002 (Figure 26-2) screening mammography became widely accepted, increasing detection of invasive and duct carcinoma in situ (DCIS) breast cancer among women ages 50 and older whereas rates among younger women remained stable.[4] Since 2002 declining rates have been associated with the abrupt cessation of hormonal therapy (HT) among postmenopausal women following publication of the Women's Health Initiative (WHI) trial discussed later in this chapter.[6,7] Some researchers suspected reduced mammography screening may have contributed to reduced incidence[8] although declines also occurred among screened women who discontinued hormone use.[9]

Mortality Trends

Researchers have noted a continuing paradox: increased frequency of screening has raised incidence rates but mortality rates remained relatively stable until the slight decline noted in 1990, which was associated with more effective combined multimodality treatment and earlier diagnosis.[10] However, survival disparities remain evident, which Albano et al. suggested were due to less access to health care, high prevalence of comorbid conditions, adverse personal behaviors (smoking and obesity), and treatment options limited by the high costs of oncology drugs.[11–13]

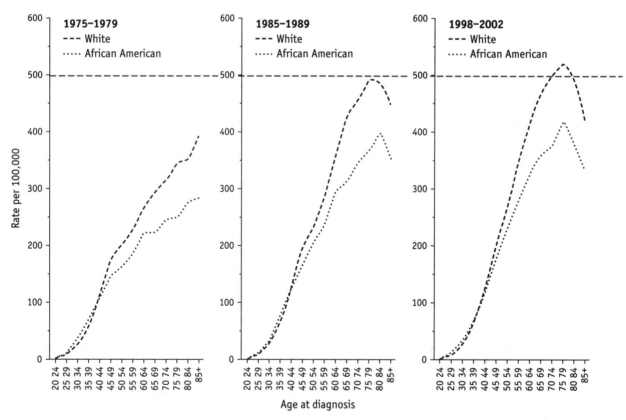

Figure 26-1 Increasing age-specific breast cancer incidence among white and black women during three time intervals [SEER Data].

Source: Reproduced from Smigal C, Jemel A, Ward E, et al. Trends in breast cancer by race and ethnicity: Update 2006. *CA Cancer J Clin* 2006; 56:168–183. Figure 3.

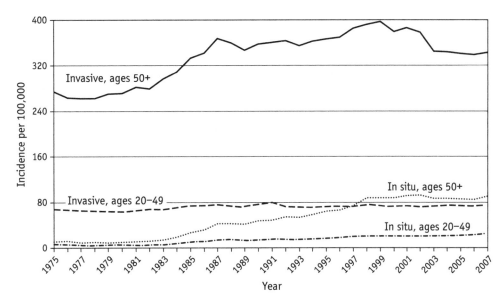

Figure 26-2 In situ and invasive breast cancer incidence rates by age group and year.

Data from SEER Cancer Statistics Review, 1975–2007, National Cancer Institute, National Center for Health Statistics, Centers for Disease Control and Prevention. Age-adjusted to the 2000 U.S. Standard Population.

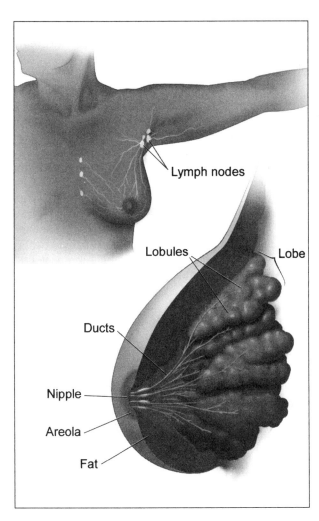

Figure 26-3 Internal structures of the mammary gland and ducts.

Source: Courtesy of the National Cancer Institute. Art by Don Bliss.

Biology of Breast Cancer

Breast Structure and Tissue Susceptibility

Breast tissue contains stromal and epithelial components that evolve over the life course from minimal development in utero and during childhood, development during puberty, full tissue differentiation during pregnancy, and regression after menopause.[14] The rudimentary ducts that develop during fetal growth are stimulated by maternal hormones. After birth, little change occurs in breast tissue until puberty. Cyclical hormones of each menstrual cycle cause breast cell proliferation and regression, while lobules expand slowly between puberty and first pregnancy, preparing for lactation.[15] Milk, produced by secretory epithelial cells lining the alveoli, flows through branching ducts to the nipple (Figure 26-3).

Benign Breast Conditions

Some women experience clinically detectable breast tissue changes stimulated by cyclical hormones; these palpable lesions cause concern and often lead to biopsy. Dupont and Page identified a spectrum of benign conditions identified in breast tissue obtained from biopsies (Figure 26-4).[16] The normal duct lined with a single layer of cells may develop hyperplasia (excessive growth) that undergoes transformation to atypical ductal hyperplasia, abnormal cells, on the path to duct carcinoma in situ. Benign tumors are generally circumscribed, slow growing, composed of well-differentiated cells that do not invade adjacent tissue. In the breast these nonproliferative lesions include cysts that rarely progress to cancer. In contrast, risk is elevated 1.5 to 2 times following diagnosis of proliferative lesions characterized by excess growth of normal appearing cells (hyperplasia without atypia), and three to five times after diagnosis of ductal or lobular

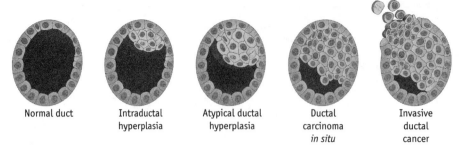

Figure 26-4 Breast cancer development–from normal duct to benign lesions and subsequent invasive ductal cancer.

Source: Adapted from the National Cancer Institute.

proliferation with atypia, abnormal nuclei in misshaped cells. Ten to 20 years after a biopsy indicated atypical ductal hyperplasia, cancer was diagnosed in 30% to 50% of the patients[17] including participants in the Breast Cancer Detection Demonstration Project (BCDDP) described later in this chapter; during follow-up of 15 to 20 years women were at increased risk of invasive cancer (RR = 3.0) following a diagnosis of hyperplasia with atypia.[18]

Malignant Transformation

A critical first step in cancer development is malignant transformation of a normal cell beginning with damaged DNA (Figure 26-5). Normal functioning tumor suppressor genes in the cell nucleus control repair of damaged DNA that may occur during cell division induced by normal aging, radiation, or other environmental exposures. If the protective genes are damaged or mutated, a normal cell may be transformed. When initiated cells survive and begin unrestrained growth, environmental promoting factors may enable transformed cells to proliferate, forming in situ or invasive breast cancer.[19] Approximately 90% of breast cancers originate in ducts and lobules (Figure 26-3). Before pregnancy, the DNA of breast cells is susceptible to damage; after a term pregnancy and breastfeeding the cells are fully differentiated, which lowers but does not eliminate risk of DNA damage.[15]

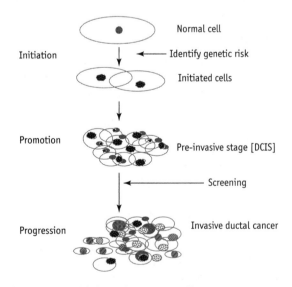

Figure 26-5 Initiation and progression of breast cancer.

Localized, preinvasive cancer cells that proliferate may disseminate from ducts to regional lymph nodes (Figure 26-3) in the glandular tissue of either breast[20] although the left breast is more frequently affected.[21] Genetic changes that permit cancer to develop and spread may be inherited, acquired through spontaneous mutations, or induced by environmental carcinogens.[22]

Invasive and In Situ Histology

Progression of cancer from in situ to invasive stage (Figure 26-4 and Figure 26-5) may be influenced by differing epidemiologic risk and prognostic factors discussed in this chapter. In situ disease was rarely diagnosed before 1980, but incidence increased 200% between 1987 and 2001[23] in parallel with enhanced mammographic detection.[24] Among the estimated 63,300 in situ cancers, 85% are ductal (ductal carcinoma in situ or DCIS) and 15% occur in lobules (lobular carcinoma in situ or LCIS). Tumors classified as DCIS exhibit diverse prognostic characteristics ranging from low-grade lesions that are unlikely to progress to high-grade lesions that more frequently become invasive cancers.[23] Although studies indicate progression from DCIS to invasive cancer may evolve over decades, DCIS is often aggressively treated.[23] Figure 26-6 presents the change in frequency of mammography and DCIS between 1987 and 2004.[24] Recent SEER data indicate 25% of breast cancer cases are classified as DCIS; incidence has increased from 5.8 per 100,000 women in 1975 to 32.5 per 100,000 in 2004 in parallel with increased mammography screening as noted in Figure 26-6. In contrast to DCIS, the incidence of invasive breast cancer has remained stable at a considerably higher rate of 123 per 100,000.

Tumor Histology and Tumor Markers

Breast cancer is a heterogeneous disease with distinctively different subtypes reflecting genetic patterns detectable by tumor tissue staining, an essential component for clinical decisions regarding appropriate treatment. Pathologically defined breast cancer may reflect differing pathways to tumor development as research has identified differing risk factors among patients with lobular, ductal, medullary, and mucinous invasive tumors. Of more than 27,300 invasive breast cancers diagnosed in the British Million Women Study, 65% were ductal, 12% lobular, 4% tubular

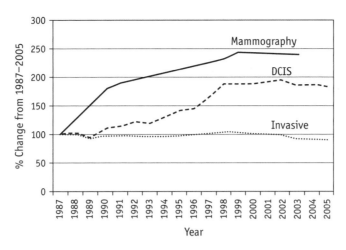

Figure 26-6 Percent change in DCIS, invasive breast cancer, and mammography, 1987–2005, United States.

Source: Reproduced from Virnig BA, Shamliyan T, Tuttle TM, et al. Diagnosis and management of Ductal Carcinoma in Situ (DCIS), Evidence Reports/Technology Assessments, No.185, Rockville (MD): Agency for Healthcare Research and Quality (US) 2009 Sep. www.ncbi.nlm.nih.gov/books/NBK32570/#ch3.s1

cancer, 3% medullary, and 1% mucinous.[25] An earlier American case series treated at one cancer center revealed similar histologic distributions with 66% ductal and 7% lobular but included more medullary (9%) cases.[26]

Microarray technology has provided new methods of classifying invasive breast cancer.[27] Paraffin sections of tumor tissue can be immunostained to identify distinct molecular subtypes: luminal A and B, the Her-2/neu, and a group defined as basal-type cancers. Some recognized breast cancer risk factors differed among the histologic subgroups, suggesting tumor development by differing biologic mechanisms.

Estrogen and Progesterone Receptors

Breast tissue and other hormone dependent tissues vary in their sensitivity to endogenous and exogenous hormones, which interact through estrogen (ER) and progesterone (PR) receptors located within the cells. Because tumors vary by receptor status, the influence of hormone exposure on risk and prognosis also varies.[28] Most luminal A tumors are ER-positive and, therefore, strongly hormone dependent.[27] Approximately 80% of invasive breast cancers are receptor positive, especially when diagnosed among older women. ER-negative breast tumors are more frequent among young, premenopausal women and among African American patients more than white women.[5] ER-positive tumors tend to be well differentiated, more responsive to hormonal or antiestrogen therapy improving prognosis. Reproductive risk factors such as age at menarche, parity, and body mass index have been more strongly associated with ER- and PR-positive than ER-and PR-negative tumors.[14]

Human Epidermal Growth Factor Receptor (HER2/neu)

Another tumor marker more frequently diagnosed among young breast cancer patients with aggressive disease is HER2/neu, a protooncogene that is identified in

approximately 20% of invasive breast cancers.[29] Among patients with lymph node involvement, HER2 gene was an indicator of poor prognosis until the drug herceptin was developed. When this targeted treatment was combined with chemotherapy, survival significantly improved.

Triple-Negative Tumors (TNBC)

Triple-negative breast cancers, defined as ER-negative, PR-negative and HER2-negative, account for 10% to 25% of invasive disease.[29] Rates for triple-negative breast cancer per 10,000 women were 2.44 for non-Hispanic white and 4.57 for African American women. These tumors tend to be more aggressive and fewer treatment options have been defined; therefore, triple-negative disease is characterized by poor survival compared with receptor positive and HER2/neu positive cancers.[30] In contrast, rates of receptor-positive disease were 23.3/10,000 among non-Hispanic white women and 14.2/10,000 among African Americans.[30]

Recent technologic advances have enabled extensive molecular characterization of breast tumors. Enhanced technology targeted to distinctive tumor markers is expected to increase treatment options. Ultimately, the more aggressive disease diagnosed at young ages among some American women will be more readily controlled with the expectation of reducing survival disparities by race/ethnicity.

Early Detection and Screening Modalities

Although early detection modalities have been promoted for more than 50 years, controversy continues to surround the use of available procedures and equipment as new technology has increased options. Persistent debates continue regarding age at first screening, frequency of repeated screening, age to discontinue screening, and the combinations of modalities to be used. The recently revised recommendations of the United States Preventive

Services Task Force (USPSTF), based on extensive accumulated scientific findings, were disputed by many clinicians and patients.[31] Studies indicated most women consider cancer screening a valuable component of their health care. Enthusiasm is not reduced by risk of a false positive test or the possibility of unnecessary treatment.[32] This section describes past and current early detection modalities conducted within the US.

Mammography

In 1963 clinicians and researchers, seeking to lower breast cancer mortality, developed a randomized controlled trial within the Health Insurance Plan (HIP) of New York, providers of insurance for city employees. The study, using the best equipment available in the 1960s, provided the first evidence of an estimated 30% reduction in mortality associated with annual mammography and clinical breast examination (CBE) followed by prompt treatment. The control group received comparable cancer treatment after symptoms were detected.[33]

American clinicians and researchers were convinced by the HIP results. Rather than conducting additional research, a national screening program, Breast Cancer Detection Demonstration Project (BCDDP), was launched in 1973 by the ACS collaborating with the National Cancer Institute. The goal of the BCDDP was to determine if the HIP results could be replicated in community-based screening centers across the United States.[34] More than 270,000 self-selected American women enrolled in BCDDP to receive free mammography. Because the program was not a randomized trial, many researchers questioned the value of the project, the usefulness of any generated data, and characteristics of the self-selected participants.[35] Among issues raised were the potential for harm from radiation and the possibility of overdiagnosis among patients treated by mastectomy for very early disease. These concerns forced improved film quality, which required lower radiation exposure for clear images. To address the potential for overdiagnosis, a panel of four expert breast pathologists was requested to review thousands of histologic slides submitted by all 29 participating screening centers. Cancer was confirmed in all but 48 cases; the physician of each patient was advised by BCDDP administration of the potential erroneous diagnosis.[35]

Most American health insurance plans eventually covered the cost of annual mammography and expenses related to subsequent clinical care. To address documented disparities in mortality by race/ethnicity and socioeconomic status that were potentially associated with late stage disease, the Congressional Caucus for Women's Issues initiated the Women's Health Equity Act in 1990 providing funds for the National Breast and Cervical Cancer Early Detection Program to provide screening and diagnostic services for low-income, uninsured women.[36]

Screening centers had operated without oversight or assurance of high quality films until the Mammography Quality Assurance Act of 1992 established federal standards and required accreditation.[1] The quality standards were developed initially for the federal program but subsequently all screening centers were required to comply. Federal standards and insurance coverage increased acceptance of routine screening by an increasing percentage of American women especially after referral by primary care physicians. Breast cancer incidence continued to rise as mammography screening increased although mortality remained unchanged. Hundreds of studies assessed personal, psychological, and cultural factors associated with screening frequency. Interventions to improve compliance were developed and studied. Some researchers were surprised to learn that most women were not deterred from subsequent screening after a false positive mammogram.[32]

Table 26-1 presents data from the National Health Interview Survey (NHIS) of 2008 indicating percentages of women reporting annual or biannual mammography by age, race/ethnicity, education, and health insurance status.[1] Although the recommendations of ACS for annual mammography from age 40 to elder years were considered the standard of care, some American professional organizations and many Europeans health departments advised first screening at age 50.[37,38] Over several decades proposed changes in age at initiation of mammography have met with public indignation[32] although radiologists were the most critical of the USPSTF recommendations of 1997 and 2002.[38]

Esserman et al. noted the media contributed to the strong response from the public by focusing each October on the benefits of screening while rarely mentioning limitations or potential harms.[39] Among young women with dense breast tissue stimulated by cyclical hormones, high mammographic density may impede tumor detection while exposing the breast to radiation.[40] Some clinicians have recommended premenopausal women schedule screening during the follicular phase of the menstrual cycle to obtain better images when hormonal stimulation is lower and breast tissue is less dense.[41,42]

Baines found higher frequency of falsely negative mammograms occurred during the luteal compared to the follicular phase of the menstrual cycle.[43] Excessive radiation exposure precluded repeat mammography to document image differences by menstrual cycle phase; however, magnetic resonance imaging (MRI) has confirmed that breast tissue density responds to cyclical hormones.[44] Using sequential MRI, several research groups have noted increased water retention and fibroglandular volume associated with progesterone elevations during the luteal phase.[45] Screening centers could enhance optimum images of premenopausal patients and reduce false negative screens by considering cycle phase when scheduling mammography.[46]

Recently, American and international investigators have questioned potential overdiagnosis which was defined on an NCI website as "screening that identifies clinically insignificant cancers" on an NCI website,[4] suggesting some detectable cancers may not progress during an individual's lifetime.[39] To confirm this possibility, Welch and Black reviewed seven published autopsy studies including more than 1,000 women of varying ages who died with no history of breast cancer. DCIS or

Table 26-1

Mammography among women ages 40 and older, United States, 2008

Characteristic	% Mammogram ≤ 12 months	% Mammogram ≤ 24 months
Age		
40–49	47.3	61.5
50–64	58.6	74.2
65+	53.2	65.4
Race/Ethnicity		
Hispanic	46.8	61.5
White [non-Hispanic]	54.2	68.0
African American	52.2	67.7
Asian American	52.2	65.1
Education		
≤ 12 years	49.2	64.3
13–15	55.2	69.1
16 +	64.5	77.9
Health Insurance		
No	26.0	35.6
Yes	56.2	70.5

Source: American Cancer Society, Surveillance Research 2011; National Health Interview Survey Public Use Data File 2008, National Center for Health Statistics, Centers for Disease Control and Prevention, 2009.

small invasive cancers were pathologically identified in each series ranging from 5% to 25%.[47] These authors suggested lack of agreement among pathologists may have contributed to potential overdiagnosis. Several studies found expert breast pathologists disagreed when asked to distinguish benign lesions and noninvasive malignant tissue,[48] potentially increasing the incidence of DCIS. A statewide New Hampshire study of 35 practicing pathologists each reviewed slides from 30 breast cases; high Kappa agreement (kappa coefficient = 0.95) was found when classifying tissue as benign or malignant but the score was considerably lower when noninvasive malignant samples were compared with benign lesions (kappa coefficient = 0.59); therefore, clinicians often seek additional pathologic review of the tissue.[49]

Differing interpretations of mammograms may also have an impact on the diagnosis of benign versus malignant findings. Significant differences in classification of abnormalities and clinical recommendations by 10 board-certified radiologists were documented when each reviewed the same 150 randomly selected mammograms from cancer patients and women without cancer.[50] Therefore, diversity of interpretation by radiologists and pathologists may significantly affect breast cancer incidence, treatment recommendations, and patients' quality of life.[51]

The 2009 updated USPSTF evidence-based recommendation against routine screening before age 50 or after age 75 for women at average risk,[31] was strongly opposed by women, clinicians, and advocacy groups who consider screening a basic "human right."[52] Regardless of age, USPSTF advised biannual mammography would provide equal benefit as annual screening with lower risks.[24,31,53] Data presented in Table 26-1 indicate many women have recently reported biannual rather than annual screening. Therefore, clinical concerns regarding decreased compliance with annual screening in response to the USPSTF changes may be unfounded as less frequent screening has already been reported by many women.[8]

Computer-Enhanced Mammography

Studies using the computer-aided detection (CAD) software, developed to improve the sensitivity of mammograms, revealed detection by a single radiologist plus CAD was comparable to detection recorded independently by two radiologists reviewing the same mammograms.[54] However, Fenton et al. assessed a screened population before and after CAD software was added and found CAD increased detection of DCIS, decreased specificity (true negative screening), and minimally improved sensitivity (true positive test).[55] Berry noted CAD use increased from 40% to 75% of screening centers since its introduction in 2007 although limited scientific research supported its use.[56] The CAD system is included in new digital mammography equipment and Medicare covers the additional charge ($16.50 as of 2010). Berry expressed concern that radiologists may rely on CAD even though the readings may not be accurate but may provide defense in medical malpractice suits.[56]

Ultrasound

Sonograms produced by high-frequency sound waves can distinguish solid tumors from fluid-filled breast cysts and may detect tumors missed by mammography, especially in dense breasts.[37] Ultrasound alone identified 25% of nonpalpable invasive cancers with mean size of 1.4 cm in a large series of screened women, many of whom had scar tissue from prior benign biopsies. To avoid additional exposure to radiation but provide additional screening, sonograms are frequently scheduled between routine mammography.[37]

Magnetic Resonance Imaging

Breast magnetic resonance imaging is increasingly used to assess breast tissue before surgery, especially to detect multicentric cancer cells scattered in the breast and to screen the opposite breast.[23] Although a study of mutation carriers did not identify any significantly increased risk associated with radiation exposure from repeated mammography,[57] ACS guidelines in 2007 encouraged greater use of MRI to avoid frequent mammography among women at high risk due to one of the following: a *BRCA* mutation or extensive family history, prior radiation therapy to the upper body before age 30, or projected lifetime risk of 20% to 25% based on the Gail model discussed later in this chapter.[58,59]

Palpation

For much of the 20th century breast cancer was diagnosed when tumors were large and adjacent lymph nodes contained cancer cells. The stage at diagnosis declined when women were encouraged by surgeons[60] and ACS advertisements to seek medical care immediately upon discovering a breast lump.[35] In 1974, breast cancer became the focus of women's fears when Betty Ford, wife of President Ford, was diagnosed with breast cancer, and Margaretta (Happy) Rockefeller, wife of Vice President Rockefeller, discovered the lump in her breast after hearing of Mrs. Ford's experience.[51] Following the extensive media coverage, many movie stars and other famous women spoke publically about their personal breast cancer experiences, which stimulated activists to launch campaigns demanding more funding for research.[35] The ACS began promotion of breast self-examination (BSE), providing instruction booklets and training programs;[35] research documented earlier stage disease associated with routine BSE[61,62] and lower mortality rates,[63] especially after BSE instruction.[64]

Before promotion of BSE and mammography, clinical breast examination (CBE) was the primary diagnostic modality; systematic palpation remains an important component of diagnosis for women with breast symptoms.[58] A literature review by Barton et al. indicated CBE detected between 3% and 45% of cancers missed by mammography in screening trials;[65] however, few clinicians use standardized procedures described in detail by Saslow et al.[58] including adequate time to systematically palpate all breast tissue. More than 70% of women report receiving a CBE during routine clinical care; therefore, inefficient clinical palpation may provide false reassurance and may result in missed cancer detection.[37,55] Clinical breast examination by skilled nurse examiners contributed significantly to disease detection in Canadian screening trials. However, comparable training and systematic procedures essential for controlled trials are rare among community-based healthcare providers.[64]

Women have been pressured by ACS, their doctors, and the press to receive routine screening although an estimated 20% of tumors are missed and ultimately detected as interval cancers by women themselves or clinicians.[51] The 2009 USPSTF screening guidelines advised doctors *not* to teach breast self-examination (BSE) and women were informed BSE was no longer encouraged as a monthly health practice.[31] This major health behavior change resulted from findings of a BSE education trial among randomized factories in China; breast cancer mortality did not differ by group assignment, and more benign biopsies were performed among those receiving BSE education.[66] Regardless of these study findings and USPSTF recommendations, genetic counselors continue to encourage monthly BSE in addition to routine CBE, MRI, and sonograms for women with a family history, genetic susceptibility, or a prior benign biopsy. A letter to the *New York Times* in response to the media report of the USPSTF 2009 advisory discouraging BSE expressed the concern of a patient who detected her "interval" cancer.[67]

LETTER; Breast Screening: Making Sense of the New Advice

New York, Nov. 17, 2009
To the Editor:
Five years ago, I had a mammogram revealing no abnormalities in the breast. Three months later, I found a lump through self-examination. The tumor was fast-growing, invasive and estrogen-receptor negative, one of the most aggressive kinds of breast cancer tumors.

Yes, the mammogram missed my tumor. And without self-examination, I would be dead by now. So maybe mammograms are not always infallible. But who decided that self-examination, a free and thoroughly noninvasive cancer-detection method, should be eliminated? Where is the logic in that decision?
Marilyn Hillman
New York, Nov. 18, 2009

Courtesy of Marilyn Hillman.

Breast Cancer among Men

Compared with women, male breast cancer is extremely rare, with less than 1 case per 100,000 American men. It is often diagnosed at advanced stages with positive axillary lymph nodes. Male breast tissue is composed of rudimentary ducts surrounded by stroma and adipose and subcutaneous tissue. Studies of tumor receptor status by gender noted more ER-positive tumors (87%) among men than women (55%).[68] The histology of male tumors is most frequently invasive ductal with DCIS occasionally detected, generally occurring at older ages by self-detection of a painless thickening or lump. Family history is reported by 15% to 20% of male cases, in contrast to 7% of men without personal history of breast cancer.[69] Male patients diagnosed before age 60 frequently have an affected relative who was diagnosed before age 45, suggesting inherited susceptibility. Risk was sixfold higher among men with an affected male relative and twofold higher with an affected female relative.[70] Gender-specific risk factors include Klinefelder's syndrome (XXY males),[71] history of gynecomastia,[68] and occupational exposures.[70] Breast cancer survival 10 years after diagnosis was comparable for men and women from hospital series and SEER data; 16% of female and male breast cancer patients died of the disease between 1975 and 2007.[68,69,72]

Breast Cancer Risk Factors among Women

Studies have repeatedly identified exposure of breast tissue to estrogen as a major aspect of known and suspected risk factors including early menarche, late menopause, first birth after age 30, and being overweight or obese after menopause. Many personal behaviors influence the levels of circulating hormones that vary during a woman's life course. Current research indicates 40% to 50% of cancer development may be attributable to personal differences in reproductive decisions, physical activity, alcohol consumption, and/or dietary patterns. However, having an affected relative is the strongest risk factor especially in families with inherited susceptibility. Table 26-2 lists many of the known and suspected factors that are continually being studied in different populations revealing differing levels of increased or decreased risk; these among others are briefly addressed in this section.

Age and Race/Ethnicity

As presented in Figure 26-1, breast cancer risk varies considerably by age and race. Among American women, incidence in 2010 was 123 cases per 100,000 females, higher among white (126.5/100,000) than black (118.3/100,000), Asian/Pacific Islander (90/100,00), or Hispanic (86/100,00) women.[1] Several breast cancer risk factors noted in the following sections differed by race including average age at menarche, age at first birth, intervals between births, total parity, age at and type of menopause. Some of these factors are believed to influence the incidence crossover pictured in Figure 26-1 with African American women at higher risk before age 45 than white women.[73]

International incidence comparisons reveal similar frequencies of breast cancer in northern Europe, Great Britain, Israel, and the United States with lower rates among women living in Asian and developing countries. However, breast cancer incidence doubled in Japan during the last few decades of the 20th century potentially associated with American influences during U.S. occupation following World War II. American breast cancer rates differ by migration status and country of origin. Research has indicated cultural or environmental factors shared by migrants from low incidence countries retain lower breast cancer risk if migration occurred after adolescence or at older ages. But migrants arriving before puberty from low incidence countries tend to have breast cancer rates similar to American-born women.[74] These patterns were significant predictors among the growing population of Hispanic women included in a population-based statewide case-control study in California. Lower breast cancer incidence was correlated with shorter residence in the United States and older ages at migration.[75] Compared with U.S.-born postmenopausal women, foreign-born Hispanic women retained their lower breast cancer risk even after 40 years with an OR = 0.66.[75] Increasing incidence rates among subsequent generations of immigrants from various low-risk countries may reflect changing reproductive patterns, increasing obesity, postmenopausal HT use, and acceptance of routine mammographic screening.

Family History

Although international incidence patterns and migration studies implicated environmental and cultural influences, researchers have known for more than a century that some families are at greater breast cancer risk than others. More than 4 decades ago, Lynch et al. collected extensive family histories from patients and identified hereditary syndromes characterized by young ages at diagnosis, high incidence of bilateral disease, cancer of other organs, and vertical transmission through several generations.[76] Although genetic risk was suspected, technology had not yet advanced to enable determination of specific genes associated with disease patterns in these families.

In 1980, the Centers for Disease Control and Prevention (CDC) launched a major population-based case-control study, the Cancer and Steroid Hormone Study (CASH), to assess the role of oral contraceptives in cancer development. Data collection included extensive family history that confirmed the reports of Lynch et al. indicating multiple cases of breast and other cancers in some families in contrast to others without any or only one affected relative. Thompson analyzed the spectrum of risk among first-degree relatives, number of affected

Table 26-2	
Factors known or suspected to be associated with breast cancer risk	
Increasing age	Body mass index
Genetic susceptibility	Alcohol intake/diet
Family history of breast or ovarian cancer	Aspirin, NSAIDS, other medications
Mammographic density	
Race/ethnicity	Screening history
Socioeconomic status	Prior benign breast surgery
Reproductive history	Smoking history
	Physical activity
Oral contraceptive use	Environmental carcinogens
Breastfeeding	Radiation exposure
Menopausal status	Mammary tumor virus
Postmenopausal hormone use	Diethylstilbestrol (DES) exposure

relatives, and ages at diagnosis (Table 26-3).[77] Risk was higher among relatives of women diagnosed before age 45. Segregation analyses of family pedigrees suggested inherited susceptibility, including male breast cancer and paternal relatives.[77] Although most epidemiologic studies include family history, the extent of affected relatives has often been more limited than in the CASH project and too frequently cancer history among paternal relatives is not considered.[77]

A collaborative reanalysis of individual data from 52 epidemiological studies confirmed these findings; breast cancer risk increased with number of first-degree affected relatives (Table 26-4),[78] similar findings to the CASH analyses.[77] Among 20-year-old women with two affected relatives, the probability of being diagnosed by age 70 was 21%. However, both studies indicate most relatives of affected women will *not* develop the disease in their lifetime; in addition, most women diagnosed with breast cancer do not have an affected relative.[78]

Risch noted that familial aggregation was a necessary aspect of inherited risk but was not sufficient to confirm genetic susceptibility. Therefore, he compared cancer incidence of monozygotic and same-sex dizygotic twins to differentiate genetic and nongenetic lifestyle contributors to familial risk. Estimates from these analyses suggested heritable factors account for 27% or more of familial aggregation.[79] Yasul et al. created a Family History Score from data collected in a large population-based case-control breast cancer study enabling assessment of effect modifications by environmental risk factors. The authors noted that familial disease may not be inherited but instead may reflect modifiable shared environmental and cultural patterns that may provide avenues for disease prevention.[80]

Genetic Susceptibility

BRCA1 and BRCA2

Technologic advances enabled high-throughput genotyping, which accelerated genetic analyses of high-risk families leading to identification of two susceptibility genes, *BRCA1* and *BRCA2* associated with a major proportion of inherited breast and ovarian cancer. *BRCA1*, located on chromosome 17, was identified in 1994,[81] and in 1995

Table 26-3

Spectrum of breast cancer risk among female relatives of breast cancer cases and control subjects, ages 20–44 & 45–54, Cancer and Steroid Hormone Study

Breast Cancer in Female Relative	Odds Ratio (95% Confidence Interval)
Ages 20–44 at diagnosis	
No affected relatives	1.00 [referent]
Mother affected	3.11 [2.33–4.17]
Sister affected	3.10 [1.82–5.30]
Mother or sister < 45 yr	3.54 [2.29–5.49]
Ages 45–54 at diagnosis	
No affected relatives	1.00 [referent]
Mother affected	1.88 [1.49–2.36]
Sister affected	2.20 [1.60–3.07]
Mother or sister < 45 yr	2.80 [1.92–4.08]

Source: Adapted from Thompson WD. Genetic epidemiology of breast cancer. *Cancer*. 1994;74:279–287.

Table 26-4

Breast cancer risk associated with number of affected first-degree relatives

Number of First-Degree Relatives with Breast Cancer	Risk Ratio (95% Confidence Interval)
None	1.00 [0.97–1.03]
One	1.80 [1.70–1.91]
Two	2.93 [2.37–3.63]
Three or more	3.90 [2.03–7.49]

Reproduced from Familial breast cancer: collaborative reanalysis of individual data from 52 epidemiological studies including 58,209 women with breast cancer and 101,986 without the disease. *The Lancet* 2001;358:1389–1399 with permission from Elsevier.

BRCA2 was identified on chromosome 13.[82] Genetic susceptibility increases risk of premenopausal, bilateral breast cancer and 64% of carriers are at risk for a second breast primary by age 70 (Figure 26-7). Approximately 5% to 10% of all breast cancer cases and 20 to 25% of familial breast cancer is associated with *BRCA1* or *BRCA2*. These genes have also been linked to 11–15% of ovarian cancer cases. *BRCA2* was found to be more strongly associated with male breast cancer than *BRCA1*.[83] Normal functioning *BRCA* genes suppress malignant transformation by repairing damages to DNA that may have occurred during cell division.[84] Identification of *BRCA* susceptibility genes included potential paternal transmission; male carriers were found to be at risk of breast, prostate, and other cancers.

More than 5,000 different mutations of *BRCA* genes have been identified each with varying ability to impede DNA repair, permit uncontrolled cell proliferation, and enable cancer development. A meta-analysis of 22 studies including 500 women unselected for family history indicated cumulative breast cancer risk by age 70 was 65% among *BRCA1* carriers compared with 45% among *BRCA2* carriers; risks were higher among more recent birth cohorts than women born before 1940.[85] Some female mutation carriers develop breast cancer, others ovarian cancer, some are diagnosed with both malignancies, although some mutation carriers remain free of cancer.

Statistical models developed by Berry, Parmigiani, and others predicted *BRCA* mutation status based on family pedigree data from three generations including gender, cancer status, age at each cancer diagnosis, site of cancer, current age, and age at death. The models guided genetic counselors' recommendations for *BRCA* testing and options for prevention.[86] The initial BRCAPRO model predicted only *BRCA1* carriers but was amended after *BRCA2* was identified and penetrance data was available including the higher carrier probability among Ashkenazi families[87] and among women of diverse race/ethnic heritages.[88] Claus et al. used CASH data to determine that family history remained a risk factor among noncarrier families depending upon number of first- and second-degree affected relatives; relative risks ranging from 1.5 to 2.5 were assumed to be influenced by shared environmental exposures including economic status, health behaviors, and additional susceptibility genes yet to be identified.[89] However, relatives negative for the family-specific mutation were not found to be at higher risk; the incidence of disease among these relatives was comparable to women in the general population based on age, race, and geographic setting.[90,91]

Data from Myriad Genetics in Figure 26-7 notes women with either *BRCA* mutation have an 87% likelihood of breast cancer by age 70, 44% risk of ovarian cancer, and a 90% risk of either cancer by age 80.[92] In addition, not all mutations of a gene have equal impact on cancer risk. In some small families with few female relatives a young breast cancer patient may test positive for a *BRCA* mutation in contrast to other affected relatives who may be *BRCA* negative (Table 26-5).[92]

High-risk family registries supported by federal funding enabled research to assess family prevalence patterns such as the composite pedigree of three generation (Figure 26-8) created to present features of inherited disease. This hypothetical family demonstrates inheritance of a specific *BRCA2* mutation by one of two brothers from their mother who had been diagnosed with bilateral breast cancer at ages 59 and 60 followed by ovarian cancer at age 82, a strong indicator of genetic susceptibility. To further breast cancer research, affected and unaffected members of high-risk families donate blood or saliva samples for genetic analyses. The hypothetical pedigree notes the mother's carrier status could not be determined as she died at age 83 before testing was available. However, her son was found to have inherited the *BRCA2* mutation after his diagnosis of breast cancer at age 74. His wife, whose parents had no cancer history, developed sporadic breast cancer at age 70 and was negative for both *BRCA1* and *BRCA2*. Their son was tested and found to be mutation negative. One daughter, who was diagnosed with breast cancer at age 39, died at age 42 before genetic testing was available but is assumed to have been a mutation carrier. Her sister was tested and found to have inherited the father's *BRCA* mutation. After she was diagnosed with a benign breast tumor, she elected to have prophylactic mastectomies to reduce her risk of developing breast cancer. An increasing number of women are choosing preventive surgery, procedures that significantly reduce cancer risk. Klitzman, in his recent book, presented the diverse responses he heard during interviews with women about their genetic testing experiences and their decisions regarding preventive modalities.[93]

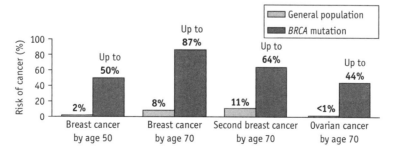

Figure 26-7 Risk of breast cancer and ovarian cancer among women with a *BRCA* mutation compared to women without a *BRCA* mutation.

Source: Courtesy of Myriad Genetics Laboratories, Inc. Mutation Prevalence Tables. http://www.myriadpro.com/bracanalysis-prevalence-tables. Last updated Feb. 2010.

Table 26-5

Factors suspected of influencing cancer diagnosis in high-risk families

(a) Inheritance of family-specific mutation of susceptibility gene

(b) Inheritance of low-penetrance genes affecting responses to environmental exposures; gene–environment interactions

(c) Inheritance of mutation of susceptibility gene and low penetrance genes; gene–gene interactions

(d) Penetrance of inherited mutation may vary by differing adult lifestyles including reproductive decisions, hormone use, body mass index

(e) Shared early life exposures in utero, during breastfeeding, and early childhood

(f) Common home environment during youth: nutritional patterns, physical exercise, parental smoking, drinking habits, access to health care

(g) Shared cultural factors influencing education goals, reproductive decisions, hormone use

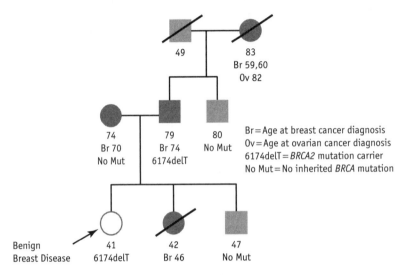

Br = Age at breast cancer diagnosis
Ov = Age at ovarian cancer diagnosis
6174delT = *BRCA2* mutation carrier
No Mut = No inherited *BRCA* mutation

Figure 26-8 Pedigree of family with male breast cancer carrying a *BRCA2* mutation.

A review by Giordano et al. indicated men were at higher breast cancer risk if they carried a mutation of *BRCA2* rather than *BRCA1*.[69] Multiple case breast cancer families with at least one male affected have a 60% to 76% risk of carrying a *BRCA2* mutation. Although men may be concerned for their mother, sisters, or daughters who are found to have a *BRCA* mutation, they often do not recognize their own risk of disease from a family-specific mutation.[69]

The proportion of breast cancer due to mutations in *BRCA1* or *BRCA2* varies considerably among the populations studied, although *BRCA1* mutations are more frequent than *BRCA2* with an overall ratio being 2:1. Families participating in registries have provided essential personal and cancer history information as well as biosamples to enable mutation testing for research.[94] Study populations of Ashkenazi Jews revealed three "founder" mutations (*BRCA1* (185delAG, 5382insC) and *BRCA2* (6174delT)) that account for 30% of diagnosed breast cancer,[83] raising the risk of the disease to 12% in this ethnic group.[95–97] Few studies have estimated prevalence of *BRCA* mutations in the U.S. general population, although among 2,500 population-based breast and ovarian cancer cases reported to SEER in California the prevalence of *BRCA1* mutation carriers was 0.24% (95% CI = 0.15–0.39%) among non-Hispanic white breast cancer patients in contrast to 1.2% (95% CI = 0.5–2.6%) among Ashkenazi patients.[98]

In addition to the 20% to 25% of familial risk associated with mutations of *BRCA* genes, an addition 5% to 6% of familial disease has been linked to uncommon moderate penetrance variants and common low penetrance polymorphism. Among these genetic markers are three that are more frequently studied: *TP5*, *ATM*, and *CHEK2*. Germline mutations in tumor protein p53 (*TP53*) increase risk of diverse cancers associated with Li-Fraumeni Syndrome, including HER-2 breast cancer diagnosed at young ages.[99] Female relatives who may have inherited one mutated copy of *ATM* have an estimated twofold increased risk of breast cancer (RR = 2.37, 95% CI = 1.51–3.78) similar to the risk associated with a mutation of *CHEK2*, another gene known to block DNA repair.[100,101]

Genetic testing of *BRCA1* and *BRCA2*, initially offered only through academic settings, has become widely available, especially after approval for Medicaid and Medicare coverage for testing and genetic counseling. Knowledge of inherited susceptibility is now an accepted component of clinical care and is considered essential for guiding treatment decisions of newly diagnosed patients.[102] As genetic counseling with testing has informed family members of their genetic status,[103] mutation carriers have sought clinical guidance and emotional support to address their inherited susceptibility. Facing Our Risk of Cancer Empowered (FORCE) is a nonprofit organization with professional direction providing online education, in-person support group meetings, and an annual conference for researchers to share their latest findings with FORCE coordinators and all interested members of the wider community (www.facingourrisk.org).[104] At a 2012 FORCE meeting in New York City, 12 women with an inherited *BRCA* mutation spoke of their physical and emotional responses to testing decisions, prophylactic surgeries, and use of reproductive technology to obtain preimplantation genetic testing as a component of in vitro fertilization.[105]

Genomewide Association Studies

Recently, genomewide association studies (GWAS) have been focused on identifying lower penetrance polymorphisms that may collectively interact with environmental factors to influence breast tumor development. The earliest studies of single nucleotide polymorphisms (SNPs) focused on genes affecting hormone metabolism, oxidative stress, and other known pathways associated with malignant transformation. Technologic advances have increased the mapping of genetic variation; with the growing number of SNPs studied, the need for specialized statistical methods was recognized. Researchers are now conducting pooled analyses of independent GWAS studies to achieve greater study power with larger, more diverse populations. In one study, GWAS identified markers among African American women,[106] although traditional reproductive factors were more predictive than the low-penetrance genes found in another GWAS study of white women.[107] Gene–environment interaction studies are now the focus of many large collaborative investigations of breast cancer etiology.

Early Life Exposures

Although breast cancer was believed to develop over decades, many epidemiologists questioned the hypothesis of Trichopoulos published in 1990 suggesting prenatal exposures might influence breast cancer risk in adulthood.[108] However, the concept of adverse in utero exposures resulting in disease years later was documented by Herbst et al., who reported vaginal cancer diagnosed in young women exposed prenatally to diethylstilbestrol (DES), a potent synthetic estrogen. DES had been prescribed early in pregnancy, often at high doses, to prevent repeated miscarriage.[109] Clinical trials indicating the drug caused increased rather than decreased rates of miscarriage were ignored. Between the 1940s and 1970 DES was given to more than 2.5 million American women,[110] a drug Lynch and Reich termed the first transplacental carcinogen identified in humans.[111] DES was associated with a 35% increased risk of breast cancer among mothers more than 30 years after initially exposure.[112] Recent reports estimated an almost twofold increased breast

cancer risk among exposed daughters, primarily diagnosed after age 40.[113] DES has also been associated with gynecological abnormalities impeding pregnancy which also increases breast cancer risk. To monitor long-term health risks the NCI created the DES Combined Cohort Follow-up Study; a recent publication documented "high lifetime risk of a broad spectrum of adverse health outcomes" including breast cancer (HR = 1.82, 95% CI = 1.04–3.18).[110] Adverse effects of DES have been greater among the daughters exposed in utero than among their mothers, documenting the adverse impact of environmental exposures during fetal development.

The changing breast cancer incidence patterns by birth cohorts noted in Figure 26-1 may reflect life-course events such as earlier age at puberty, later age at first birth, initiation and duration of breastfeeding, hormone use, personal health behaviors, etc. In a review by Xue and Michels intrauterine exposures modestly increased risk among offspring of older parents although risk was lower among twins and daughters whose mothers experienced preeclampsia (RR = 0.48, CI = 0.30–0.78).[114] Breast cancer risk was associated with greater height reached at an early age[115] and higher birth weight.[116] which was also found in studies among Asian-American women.[117] The positive association of birth weight and breast cancer risk suggested to some investigators that heavier female offspring may have larger mammary glands with greater number of breast cells subsequently susceptible to DNA damage.[118] Breast cancer risk was also associated with nutrition levels during childhood and adolescence as reflected among women with anorexia nervosa who were 50% less likely to develop the disease.[119]

Environmental exposures at young ages may augment inherited risk as found among women exposed during infancy or at young ages to radiation, which raised breast cancer risk 15 to 20 years later and remained elevated for more than 50 years.[120] Recent gene–environment studies have reported higher risk among *BRCA* mutation carriers born after 1940 compared with carriers born before World War II. Changes that may contribute to the differences include greater use of medical X-rays, delayed childbearing, greater availability of nutritional resources, access to new medications developed for the military, etc.[121]

Reproductive History

Figure 26-9 notes the potential exposures with influences on breast tissue that may occur during a longer interval between menarche and first birth. Until first birth, breast cells remain susceptible to environmental exposures that may result in DNA damage during menstrual cycle-related cell divisions.[5,116] Longer intervals between menarche and first birth delay the protective effect of maximum differentiation of breast tissue.[15] Researchers have long recognized the combined protection provided by late menarche, early first birth, and high parity associated with fewer ovulatory cycles during reproductive years. These factors lower exposure of breast tissue to hormonal stimulation. Risk was reduced 23% when menarche occurred at age 16 or older compared with age 12 or

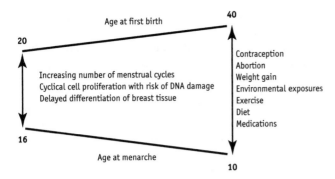

Figure 26-9 Potential decisions affecting breast cancer risk between menarche and first birth.

younger.[122] Ecologic studies support these associations; in countries with lower breast cancer rates, menarche occurs later followed by higher parity, and fewer regularly spaced cycles.[123] Hispanic women in the United States who have more children and earlier ages at first birth similarly experience less breast cancer. Changing childbearing practices closely paralleled regional differences in breast cancer rates in America before screening influenced incidence patterns.[124]

Parity has a dual effect on breast cancer risk. Before age 40 a transient two- to threefold increased risk occurs for about 10 years after each term birth compared with nulliparous women (Figure 26-10) but after age 40 early first births were protective.[125–127] Pathak suggested the pregnancy-related increased risk reflected stimulation of "initiated cells" by the hormonal milieu of pregnancy. Subsequently, breast cancer risk reduction follows a term pregnancy as breast cells are more fully differentiated especially after breastfeeding.[126] Pathak also suggested the short-term postpartum risk increase might be associated with the crossover of breast cancer incidence noted among African Americans in Figure 26-1.[126] Supporting this suggestion are data from the Women's Contraceptive and Reproductive Experiences (CARE) study that reported significant race-specific differences in the percentage of first births

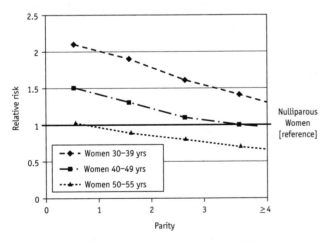

Figure 26-10 Age-specific risk by parity relative to nulliparous women.

Source: Data from Lambe M, Hsieh CC, Trichopoulos D, et al. Transient increase in the risk of breast cancer after giving birth. *N Engl J Med* 1994;331:5–9.

before age 20: 34% of black compared with 11.5% of white women,[128] suggesting early parity may have contributed to lower rates of postmenopausal disease among blacks while increasing their risk before ages 45.[129]

Pathologic comparisons of breast tissue from parous and nulliparous women obtained following mammary gland reduction surgery revealed pregnancy-induced differences in DNA repair and transcription regulation.[130] Colditz et al. noted premenopausal breast cancer increased 1.7% for each year between menarche and first pregnancy; closer spacing of births lowered risk.[3] The CARE study indicated that the risk was reduced for parous compared to nulliparous women although risk increased among women with longer delay between menarche and first birth; the interval was an independent risk factor specifically for ER-positive tumors.[128] Among women aged 50 to 79 participating in the WHI, estrogen-receptor-positive breast cancer risk was more frequently diagnosed among nulliparous than parous women (HR = 1.35, 95% CI = 1.20–1.52) in contrast to risks of triple-negative tumors, which were associated with higher parity.[30] Although preeclampsia is hazardous to pregnant women and the developing fetus, breast cancer risk is lower among parous women after multiple episodes of preeclampsia.[131]

The relationship of reproductive history to risk among *BRCA* mutation carriers was similar to women unselected for inherited susceptibility; Andrieu et al. reported each birth reduced risk among mutation carriers by 14% but only after age 40.[132] These authors found early age at first birth protective for *BRCA1* carriers but increased risk of *BRCA2* carriers.[92,132] To assess a potential transient effect of childbirth, 1,260 matched case-control sets of mutation carriers were studied; a nonsignificant increased risk within 2 years of childbirth was evident only among *BRCA2* carriers; *BRCA1* carriers were at lower risk, suggesting genetic differences in tissue responsiveness to hormonal stimulation.[133]

Breastfeeding

Breastfeeding has become more culturally acceptable and convenient especially for employed women who benefitted from legal requirements of employers to allocate private settings for expressing milk during the work day. Health benefits for mother and child have been recognized including enhanced bonding, optimum nutrition for the newborn, and lower breast cancer risk for mothers after prolonged breastfeeding. A biologic mechanism associated with lactation suggests estrogen levels of breast fluid are reduced and prolactin levels are elevated to stimulate breastmilk production.[134] Newcomb et al. found longer duration of lactation provided reduced risk of premenopausal breast cancer compared with parous women who did not breastfeed (RR = 0.78, 95% CI = 0.66–0.91); however, postmenopausal women did not share this benefit.[135] International data from more than 50,000 breast cancer cases and 95,000 controls reported a 4.3% risk reduction for each 12 months of breastfeeding.[136] Extended breastfeeding is known to induce protective biologic changes in breast tissue, delay resumption of regular ovulatory cycles, and depress estrogen levels in breast fluid.[134,135] *BRCA1* carriers were less likely to develop breast cancer after breastfeeding for 12 months or longer than parous women who did not breastfeed (OR = 0.55, 95% CI = 0.38–0.80) although no protection was evident among women with a *BRCA2* mutation.[134] Interestingly, being breastfed by a mother who developed breast cancer did not increase risk among her daughters years later.[137]

Abortion and Miscarriage

Several studies conducted among differing populations have suggested spontaneous and induced abortions may have a modest impact on breast cancer risk[138–140] before a first birth and among nulliparous women.[141] Although self-reported history may be biased by the legality of abortion and social acceptability, recent data from 16 countries and more than 50 investigations indicated interrupted pregnancy, spontaneous or induced, had no adverse impact on breast cancer risk. [142] A recent report from the prospective California Teachers Study confirmed these findings.[143] Among women with an inherited susceptibility, interrupted pregnancy did not increase breast cancer risk; however, Friedman et al. found risk reduced among *BRCA2* mutation carriers following repeated therapeutic abortion (OR = 0.36; 95% CI = 0.16−0.83) with no effect among *BRCA1* carriers.[92]

Weight Gain and Body Size

Body mass index (BMI) and weight gain cause subclinical inflammation in adipose tissue, increasing breast cancer risk differently among pre- and postmenopausal women. BMI of 30 or greater, classified as obese, compared to women with BMI of 25 or less, was associated with a twofold higher risk only among postmenopausal women in most epidemiologic studies. Huang et al. attributed 30% of postmenopausal breast cancer to weight gain, hormone use, or their combined effect.[144] Among nurses followed prospectively, weight gain of 20 kg or more between ages 18 and adulthood was associated with a twofold increased risk of postmenopausal breast cancer compared with women whose weight remained stable.[144] The biologic explanation for the association of weight gain and increased risk suggests breast tissue is stimulated by aromatization of androstenedione to estrogen in adipose tissue after menopause in the absence of ovarian hormones.[145] Recent research correlated breast cancer risk with the severity of breast inflammation, level of obesity, and elevated aromatase expression.[146]

In contrast to risk associated with obesity in postmenopausal women, Kelsey and Bernstein noted excess weight among premenopausal women was protective ranging from RR = 0.7 to 0.9 due to anovulatory cycles and lower endogenous estrogen levels.[145] John et al. found higher body mass (BMI ≥ 30 vs. < 25) reduced risk only of ER- and PR-positive premenopausal breast cancer (OR = 0.42, 95% CI = 0.29–0.61).[147] Several studies have noted taller premenopausal women are at increased risk (OR = 1.77, 95% CI = 1.23–2.53) suggesting early nutrition may have enhanced childhood growth

rates.[147] Among premenopausal women in the Nurses' Health Study II, body fatness recalled over several childhood and adolescent ages was inversely related to breast cancer; the most overweight women during childhood compared with the leanest were more protected (RR = 0.48).[148] However, research is needed to clarify the transition between the benefits associated with obesity at premenopausal ages and the adverse effects of excess weight after menopause.

Endogenous Hormones

Reproductive and body mass characteristics affect breast cancer risk by influencing levels of endogenous estrogen and progesterone exposure of breast tissue.[149] Observing lower risk associated with either premenopausal oophorectomy or administration of an antiestrogen led to several hypotheses associated with exposure to endogenous hormones.[145] Epidemiology studies of risk factors noted increased risk for ER-positive tumors among postmenopausal women with higher serum levels of estradiol and testosterone;[150] similar findings from the Nurses' Health Study indicated a two- to threefold increased risk of ER-positive and PR-positive breast cancer associated with the highest compared to lowest levels of testosterone and estradiol.[151]

Prospectively collected biosamples from WHI participants indicated higher prediagnostic serum levels of testosterone and estradiol were predictive of increased risk of ER-positive breast cancer.[6] Circulating estrogens were lower among postmenopausal women reporting moderate physical activity compared to sedentary women.[152] Lower circulating hormone levels among Asian women were linked to their lower risks of developing breast cancer although the biologic mechanisms for the findings have not been explained. Progesterone levels are also important as greater cell division occurs in breast tissue during the luteal phase of the menstrual cycles of premenopausal women.[153]

Oral Contraceptives (OCs)

When introduced in 1960 oral contraceptives contained large doses of estrogen and progestin. Some women and clinicians questioned the potential adverse effects of these medications on risk of breast cancer as high parity was believed protective against the disease. Since OCs were first marketed, many epidemiologic investigations have been conducted to address potential risks and benefits. The CASH Study, mentioned previously, was a large national population-based case-control study conducted by CDC; after extensive assessment of OC use in the 1980s, no adverse effect on risk of breast cancer was noted (RR = 1.0, 95% CI = 0.9–1.1).[154] Numerous additional case-control and cohort studies supported these findings in addition to revealing a strong protective role against ovarian and uterine cancer.[155] Recent formulations have lower hormonal dosages that balance contraceptive efficacy with minimal side effects and no increased risk of breast cancer.[156]

Studies of oral contraceptives are complicated by varying patterns of use (before and/or between pregnancies), recency and duration of use, changing dosages of estrogen and progestin, and interactions with potential confounders including family history and body size. A meta-analysis joined data from 54 international studies and reported a slightly increased risk of breast cancer among women with recent OC use (RR = 1.07, 95% CI = 1.03–1.10).[157] Risk was higher while women were using OCs (RR = 1.24, CI = 1.16–1.32), especially before age 25, and risk remained elevated for about 5 years before diminishing after use was discontinued.[157] However, breast cancers diagnosed among OC users were less clinically advanced than breast tumors in women not using OCs potentially associated with greater access to medical care required for OC prescriptions or influenced by OC control of ovulation. The results of international studies are influenced by the wide variety of OCs that may have differing effects on breast tissue.

Reports in 2002 from the CARE study conducted by CDC provided assessment of OCs currently approved for sale in the United States. Among the large population of women ages 35 to 64, no adverse effect was observed among current or former OC users compared with never users regardless of family history or genetic risk.[158] More than 75% of cases and controls had used combination OCs and many began use before age 20. These results were reassuring given the size of the study, the racial mix (25% black or Hispanic), and the high proportion of women ever using these preparations.[159] A new analysis from CARE assessed the many different formulations of OCs used and found no adverse effect associated with any combined OC preparation.[156] Among women with inherited susceptibility, breast cancer risk was not associated with OC use for 1 year although after 5 or more years a modest increase was noted only among BRCA2 mutation carriers.[160] Differences by specific gene, BRCA1 versus BRCA2, have been noted in other risk factor studies.

Infertility

Infertility, due to a variety of causes including low endogenous hormonal levels, has been associated with lower breast cancer risk. Women with an ovulatory disorder experience fewer cyclical hormone cycles reducing cancer risk.[161] Infertile participants in the Nurses' Health Study II were at diminished breast cancer risk (HR = 0.75, 95% CI = 0.59–0.96) compared with women who had no difficulty conceiving and risk was lowest after ovulation-induction therapy.[161] Clinical records of women who sought infertility treatment in Seattle between 1974 and 1986 were linked to SEER cancer files; cancer risk was similar to the general population although fewer infertile women developed breast cancer after clomiphene treatment compared women who had not used the medication.[162] In contrast, Brinton et al. reported a 30% increased risk of invasive breast cancer 20 years after clomiphene treatment among women evaluated for infertility between 1965 and 1988, suggesting the need for long-term monitoring to adequately assess risk.[163]

Venn et al. studied cancer risks among women who registered with an Australian in vitro fertilization (IVF) clinic and found comparable breast cancer rates to the general population although more cases than expected were diagnosed within the year after IVF. The authors suggested fertility drugs used for superovulation may have promoted preexisting cancer cells similar to the transient increased risk after term pregnancy.[164] Cancer risk among women in Sweden was increased before IVF but reduced after IVF with the strongest effect among those with multiple birth deliveries (OR = 0.33, 95% CI = 0.18–0.61) compared with women having single births (OR = 0.86, 95% CI = 0.68–1.08).[165] Assisted reproductive technologies have enabled increased frequency of multiple births, which have long been associated with reduced breast cancer risk. Preeclampsia, another factor associated with reduced breast cancer risk, often occurs in IVF pregnancies.[165]

Menopausal Transition

Breast cancer rates increases rapidly until about age 50 when incidence slows during the menopausal transition.[166] Risk is significantly reduced when natural menopause occurs before age 40. The combined effects of later age at menarche, earlier age at menopause, and higher parity diminish total number of ovulatory cycles, thus reducing exposure of breast tissue to cyclical endogenous estrogens. Studies indicate natural menopause at age 55 or older is associated with a twofold greater breast cancer risk compared with menopause at age 45.[167] However, bilateral oophorectomy at ages 40–45 provided a 45% risk reduction,[122] also found among women with a BRCA mutation.[168] Protection was greater after abrupt cessation of hormones compared with slower declines following natural menopause.[169] Data from the Nurses' Health Study noted hysterectomy with bilateral oophorectomy significantly lowered risk compared with women who retained their ovaries (HR = 0.75, 95% CI = 0.68–0.84) especially if surgery occurred before age 45 (HR = 0.62, 95% CI = 0.53–0.74).[170] Subsequent studies have indicated hormone use delayed the protective effect of bilateral oophorectomy.[153] African American women experience earlier natural and surgical menopause compared to white or Hispanic women, potentially contributing to their lower risk of postmenopausal breast cancer evident in Figure 26-1.[171,172]

Menopausal Hormone Therapy

Estrogen, introduced in the 1930s, was prescribed for many clinical conditions including menopausal symptoms until 1975 when increased endometrial cancer necessitated the addition of progestin. During recent decades 20% to 30% of American women were prescribed estrogen or combined therapy in response to reports of health benefits, including reduced risks of heart disease, stroke, and hip fracture while only slightly affecting risk of breast cancer.[173] Authors of a meta-analysis published in 1992 suggested hormonal therapy should be prescribed following hysterectomy and after diagnosis of heart disease, although they acknowledged their recommendations were based on potentially biased observational data.[173] Many studies published in the 1990s suggested hormone use would improve quality of life for postmenopausal women.[174] Other researchers encouraged assessment of person-specific benefits and risks in relation to family history of heart disease, breast cancer, and personal health status.[175] Several investigators found healthier women were more frequently prescribed HT than women with comorbid conditions, biasing study findings of some investigations, including the observational component of the WHI noted later.[176]

Most case-control and cohort studies reported increased breast cancer incidence among women using HT although the magnitude of risk was considered low compared to the protective role against heart disease. However, HT for 5 years or longer elevated breast cancer risk (RR = 1.35, 95% CI = 1.21–1.49) in the collaborative analyses of 51 international studies[177] and among American women in the BCDDP cohort reported by Schairer et al. who found the impact of estrogen alone (RR = 1.2) was less than combined therapy (RR = 1.4), which increased risk 8% per year of use.[178] A Los Angeles County population-based case-control study noted an adverse effect of 10 years of combined therapy (OR = 1.5) compared with no increased risk for estrogen alone.[179] The authors related the elevated risk of combined therapy to the known higher mitotic activity of breast tissue stimulated by progesterone during the luteal phase of the menstrual cycle.[180]

Additional studies reported HT increased risk although regional differences were evident. A population-based case-control study in three states reported use of estrogen alone for 5 or more years raised risk by 2% per year compared with 4% associated with combined therapy.[181] Higher risk levels were associated with longer term use of HT (OR = 3.93, 1.4–10.8) among cases compared with controls from two counties on Long Island, New York.[182] In addition, women ages 50–79 enrolled in a California-based screening program who had used HT for 5 years or longer were at 46% increased risk although shorter use had no adverse effect; the researchers suggested hormone-associated mammographic density may have delayed tumor detection.[183]

The two randomized controlled trials (RCTs) of the WHI were expected to clarify the benefits and risks of HT among healthy postmenopausal women ages 50 to 79. Criteria at enrollment included normal mammograms and clinical breast exams to ensure no detectable breast cancer was present before randomization. The trial of combined therapy, conjugated equine estrogens (0.625 mg) plus medroxyprogesterone acetate (2.5 mg) versus placebo, was stopped prematurely because "…health risks were shown to exceed the benefits" (pp. 573); these included increased cardiovascular disease and more cases of breast cancer diagnosed at advanced stages among treated than control women (HR = 1.26, 95% CI = 1.02–1.55).[184] Although the study results shocked the public and many of their physicians, in her book published in 1997 Dr. Susan Love was critical of prescribing habits and warned women to make informed choices about hormone therapy.[185] She was heavily criticized for scaring women about increased risk of breast cancer. When her beliefs were supported

by the WHI RCT results, she simply stated "… medical practice, as it often does, got ahead of the science" (pp. 2).[186] Interestingly, initiation of combined therapy was often associated with breast tenderness and greater mammographic density than estrogen alone.[187,188] In addition, the WHI data indicated randomization to estrogen plus progestin was associated with increased frequency of abnormal mammograms resulting in higher rates of breast biopsies, suggesting HT may have impeded disease detection.[184,189]

The observational component of the WHI provided evidence of significant differences between women clinically prescribed HT and nonusers supporting the prior biased results from some observational studies. HT use was reported more frequently by white, young, highly educated, more physically active women, with lower BMI and lower estimated breast cancer risk based on the Gail-model (discussed later in Table 26-6); however, their actual risk of disease was nearly twofold greater compared with nonusers.[184]

When the WHI trial of combined therapy was terminated, each WHI participant received a letter noting the RCT results. The public response to these findings was reflected in the reported 43% decline in hormone use among American women and a parallel decline in breast cancer incidence in 2003.[7] Some investigators suggested reduced screening explained the lower incidence rate although several studies conducted among screening registry participants limited this alternative explanation. Figure 26-6 notes invasive breast cancer rates remained relatively stable between 1987 and 2005 whereas mammography and in situ disease increased significantly. As both in situ and invasive ER-positive breast cancer declined among screened women after the WHI report, risk reduction was related to change in hormone use.[190] The California Teachers' Study noted 50% reduction in hormone use (estrogen or estrogen plus progestin) between enrollment in 1995–1996 and 2005–2006 at the most recent follow-up questionnaire, which was paralleled by a 45% reduction in ER-positive breast cancer.[192] In the San Francisco region a sharp decrease in HT use and breast cancer occurred beginning in 2002.[191]

Mammographic Density

With increasing use of mammography for early detection, Wolfe et al. identified four mammographic patterns that were predictive of cancer development.[193] Subsequently, the patterns were correlated with mammographic density, which has been more readily and consistently measured. Risk of disease was fourfold greater among women with both extensive patterning and density,[193] a component of the Breast Imaging Reporting and Data System (BI-RADS) designed by the American College of Radiology to standardize mammography reports by radiologists.[194] To assess the link between density and risk, total breast area and the dense component were measured on baseline mammograms of cases and controls enrolled in the BCDDP; cases had significantly greater density up to 5 years before breast cancer diagnosis compared to controls.[195] Byrne et al. identified density as an independent risk factor with greater magnitude than family history, age at first birth, or history of benign breast biopsy.[195]

A computer-assisted method enabling more standardized measurement of density was developed by Byng et al. and applied to digitized mammograms to calculate percent density from total breast area and area of dense tissue (Figure 26-11).[196] Known breast cancer risk factors including age, parity, and BMI were four to five times greater among women with 75% density compared with little or no density, indicating that mammographic density is one of the strongest recognized breast cancer risk factors.[197] A study of paired twins noted hereditary factors contribute to percentage of density with heritability ranging from 60% to 75%. Measurements were twice as strongly correlated among monozygotic twins than dizygotic twins.[198] GWAS has identified genes potentially influencing both breast tissue density and breast cancer risk.[199] Having both a family history and density of 75% or greater was associated with an RR = 5.43 for breast cancer among participants in the Canadian screening trial. Density assessed by a radiologist using the BI-RADS system indicated on mammography reports was closely correlated with measures obtained from the computer-assisted program.[200]

Among premenopausal women cyclical hormones complicated measurements of breast tissue density, which change with phases of each menstrual cycle. During the menopausal transition density generally declines as endogenous hormone levels diminish; however, density remains high among women using estrogen/progestin combined therapy.[201] Data from the WHI indicated hormone use significantly increased density among women aged 60–79 lasting for 2 years or longer after treatment was terminated.[202] Other data noted density declined when HT use ended or chemopreventive medication was used.[203] Density was studied in a collaborative multiethnic population in relation to breast cancer risk factors; no

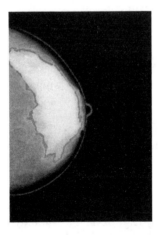

Figure 26-11 Digitized mammogram and computer-assisted measurement of density.

Source: Method: Byng JW, Boyd NF, Fishell E, et al. The quantitative analysis of mammographic densities. *Phys Med Biol* 1994;39:1629–1638; film created for research at Mailman School of Public Health.

differences by race/ethnicity were found but age and BMI were both inversely associated with density.[204] Moderate drinking compared with no alcohol intake was also linked to higher density.[205] Pike suggested mammographic density should be considered a modifiable intermediate marker of breast cancer risk as reduced density followed tamoxifen treatment, an antiestrogenic agent prescribed for women at high risk.[166]

Radiation Exposure

Ionizing radiation increased risk of breast cancer years after an intense single exposure[206] or following repeated diagnostic or therapeutic low-level exposures among women with scoliosis,[207] tuberculosis,[208] postpartum mastitis,[209] or Hodgkin's disease.[210] Thirty years after the atomic bomb, survivors had significantly higher breast cancer risk although their ages at diagnosis resembled onset in the general female population.[206,211] Studies of radiation indicated the dose was often less predictive of cancer development than age at exposure.[212] Between 1926 and 1957 some female infants were radiated for an enlarged thymus; threefold elevated breast cancer risk was found 35 years later[214] and remained evident for more than 55 years after initial treatment.[120]

The magnitude of adverse effect of radiation was greater than risks associated with reproductive history or other recognized risk factors.[214] Adams et al. concluded that breast tissue is most susceptible to malignant transformation when ductal cells are actively developing during puberty and first pregnancy[120] with risk almost sixfold greater following radiation at young ages.[210] Women treated with radiation for Hodgkin's disease before age 21 were at almost 20% increased risk of breast cancer during 30 years of follow-up; risk increased as age at treatment decreased.[210] Breast cancer developed in 35% of Hodgkin's disease patients treated with radiation before age 17 and one of eight treated before age 40, a rate comparable to risk in the general female population living to age 85.[215]

Among high-risk families enrolled in the Breast Cancer Family Registry, risk was increased by radiation treatment received for a prior cancer (OR = 3.55) or diagnostic X-rays for tuberculosis (OR = 2.49) or pneumonia (OR = 2.19).[216] Diagnostic chest X-rays also increased breast cancer risk among 1,601 *BRCA1/2* carriers in an international cohort; risk was highest among women exposed to radiation before age 20 who were born after 1949 (HR = 4.64, 95% CI = 2.2–10.9).[132]

Women have been assured that radiation exposure from mammography is limited and benefits out weight any risks;[1] however, ACS has recently recommended greater reliance on MRI and ultrasound for young women from high-risk families who need repeated screening.[58] Radiation exposure during diagnostic procedures is often essential although ultrasound, MRI, and other scanning modalities are frequent alternatives. However, concerns remain regarding low dose radiation exposures for clinical care, security procedures, and in other settings.[217]

Alcohol Consumption

Moderate levels of alcohol drinking have been associated with increased inflammation and altered hormone levels by stimulating estrogen conversion in fat tissue.[19] Studies conducted among diverse populations have assessed alcohol consumed daily or weekly and types of beverage: wine, beer, or liquor. Among participants in the National Health and Nutrition Examination Survey (NHANES) I follow-up study a dose response was noted; increased breast cancer risk among drinkers compared with nondrinkers was observed ranging from RR = 1.4 to 1.6.[218] Longnecker et al. found dose response effects of lifetime alcohol intake; risk associated with one drink per day before age 30 was lower than among older women rising from RR of 1.09 to 1.21 in contrast with RR = 2.3 after three or more drinks per day.[219] Data from the California Teachers Study also revealed increased risk associated with two or more drinks per day only among postmenopausal women, especially in combination with HT use.[220] The CARE study of CDC reported elevated risk among women ages 50–64 who indicated seven or more alcoholic drinks per week.[221] Although consumption of hard liquor increased breast cancer risk among postmenopausal women in a large population-based case-control study, exclusively drinking of either red or white wine did not have an adverse effect.[222]

Among Kaiser Permanente subscribers, alcohol drinking was associated with risk of ER-positive tumors rising from a nonsignificant 1.08 for one drink per day to RR = 1.21 (95% CI = 1.05–1.4) for one to two drinks daily and RR = 1.38 (95% CI = 1.13–1.68) for three or more drinks per day.[223] Risk of lobular cancer was increased almost twofold compared with 1.2 for ductal cancer, specifically for ER-positive tumors, in a Washington State study.[224] Regardless of number of drinks per week, moderate alcohol consumption did not affect risk of postmenopausal DCIS in the WHI suggesting alcohol increased proliferation of cancer cells destined to progress to invasive disease.[225] Some research suggested high intake of folic acid mitigated risk associated with alcohol intake although folic acid had no influence on risk among the nondrinkers.[226] The relationship between alcohol and breast cancer risk should be balanced by reports of healthy aging among women with moderate alcohol consumption.[227]

Cigarette Smoking

Tobacco smoke is a known strong carcinogen in many organs systems. Research has indicated carcinogens from tobacco smoke enter the circulation and are stored in breast adipose tissue where tobacco-specific DNA adducts have been detected. Aspirated nipple fluid also contained chemicals from cigarette smoking.[228] Smokers were found to have lower urinary estrogen levels[229] and earlier age at natural menopause, two factors associated with lower breast cancer risk.[230] In 1996, Ambrosone et al. reported N-Acetyltransferase 2 (NAT2), a metabolizing enzyme, was found to regulate detoxification and/or activation of aromatic amines in tobacco smoke influencing breast cancer risk among smokers.[231] In a meta-analysis smoking was an independent risk factor regardless of menopausal

status although among postmenopausal women with the variant of NAT2 slow clearance of aromatic amines increased breast cancer risk.[231]

Most epidemiologic studies assess risk of smoking based on interview data without benefit of biospecimens to confirm smoking status or identify enzyme activity. Among smokers enrolled in the Canadian National Breast Screening Study (NBSS) breast cancer risk was 16% higher compared to nonsmokers. Young age at initiating smoking raised the relative risk (RR = 1.50, 95% CI = 1.19–1.89).[228] Breast cancer incidence was also greater among current smokers than nonsmokers in the California Teachers Study.[232] In addition, nonsmokers living with a smoking spouse were at twofold higher risk and both active and passive smoking were linked to detection of ER-positive tumors in a large case-control study.[233] Others also noted increased ER-positive tumors among long-term smokers who began smoking at young ages, especially before first-term pregnancy.[234]

Women younger than age 50 with a BRCA mutation who smoked were at twofold greater breast cancer risk than nonsmokers in a nested case-control study among members of a family registry.[235] Another study of more than 2,500 matched pairs of BRCA mutation carriers reported past smoking of at least six pack years was associated with breast cancer only among BRCA1 mutation carriers (OR = 1.27, 95% CI = 1.06–1.50).[236]

Nonsteroidal Anti-Inflammatory Drugs (NSAIDS)

Epidemiologic studies have suggested nonsteroidal anti-inflammatory drugs (NSAIDS) including aspirin may lower breast cancer risk, as previously found for colon cancer. A follow-up study of NHANES I participants who reported aspirin use in the month before interview revealed reduced risk (RR = 0.72, 95% CI = 0.52–1.00) especially among women younger than age 50.[237] The small sample size and limited exposure information were questioned by Egan et al. who found no protective effect of long-term aspirin use among nurses[238] and only ibuprofen use reduced breast cancer in the WHI observational study.[239] However, a population-based case-control study reported reduced risk of ER-positive breast cancer among women using aspirin or other NSAID at least once per week for at least 6 months (OR = 0.80) and the protection was stronger among more frequent users.[240]

Data from the California Teachers Study indicated increased ER/PR negative breast cancer (RR = 1.81, 95% CI = 1.12–2.92) associated with long-term daily users of ibuprofen or aspirin in addition to a nonsignificant lower risk of ER/PR positive tumors (RR = 0.80, 95% CI = 0.62–1.03).[241] Neither NSAIDs nor aspirin alone provided protection in the national ACS cohort[242] and limited reductions of ER-positive in situ tumors were found among American Association of Retired Persons (AARP) study participants.[243] However, a meta-analysis of data from 38 international epidemiologic studies reported an overall breast cancer reduction (RR = 0.88, 95% CI = 0.84–0.93) following any NSAID use regardless of dose or duration of use.[244] The prospective Iowa Women's

Health Study indicated aspirin use lowered risk by 20% among postmenopausal women regardless of ER or PR tumor status, suggesting lower risk may be due to reduced inflammation.[245] A modest inverse association between total NSAIDs use and serum levels of estradiol and the ratio of estradiol to testosterone were reported from the Nurses' Health Study, suggesting a potential hormonal role.[246] NSAIDs may provide a modest reduction in breast cancer although the potential adverse risks of gastrointestinal bleeding may limit benefit for some women.

Physical Exercise

Risk reduction associated with physical activity was welcome guidance as few readily modifiable lifestyle factors have been identified. Although exercise across the life span is encouraged for women, the strongest protective aspect for breast cancer has been related to exercise-induced delayed puberty and irregular menstrual cycles which lower endogenous estrogen stimulation of breast tissue.[247] Vigorous, routine exercise such as ballet dancing, swimming, and gymnastics initiated at young ages before puberty caused more anovulatory cycles among postmenarcheal high school girls who reported 2 or more hours per week of swimming, jogging, or tennis playing.[123] Strenuous athletic training was also associated with secondary amenorrhea and luteal phase deficiency of progesterone.[248]

Compared with college athletes, alumni who had not been involved with sports were at significantly increased risk of breast cancer (RR = 1.86) more than 30 years after graduation[249] and risk differences remained during 15 additional years of follow-up.[250] Among adult women age 40 or younger, 4 or more hours per week of physical activity significantly lowered risk of breast cancer (OR = 0.42, 95% CI = 0.27–0.64) compared with similarly aged inactive women; the relationship was strongest among parous women.[251] Similarly, parous premenopausal nurses followed prospectively were at 20% lower breast cancer risk if they had engaged in physical activity during youth and adult years compared with less active nulliparous women.[252]

Exercise was also associated with enhanced immune function, which impedes cancer initiation and promotion. In their review of epidemiologic studies linking physical activity to reduced breast cancer risk, Gammon et al. reported benefit for physically active pre- and postmenopausal women who maintained a healthy body size, had lower serum hormone levels, and enhanced immune function.[152] A recent intensive 12-month exercise program requiring about 5 hours per week successfully lowered reproductive hormone levels among 320 postmenopausal women aged 50–74,[253] although questions about the effect on breast cancer risk remained to be determined.[254] Rundle noted that studies need to identify biomarkers that might indicate the beneficial mechanisms of routine physical exercise; he suggested understanding the biology of these mechanisms could provide targets for lifestyle or pharmaceutical interventions.[255]

Diet

The role of diet in the etiology of breast cancer has been extensively studied but remains controversial. International breast cancer rates have suggested diet may contribute to differing risk patterns given lower incidence among women in Asian and developing countries than in western nations. Recent increased incidence has been documented in some countries following cultural changes including a greater variety of available foods. For example, Japan experienced dramatic dietary changes after U.S. occupation following World War II with increased breast cancer mortality related to consumption of foods high in fat and animal protein and less fiber than traditional diets.[256] Breast cancer patterns in Japan now resemble the increased incidence found among offspring of Japanese-American immigrants but not the immigrants themselves whose risk remained lower. This pattern suggests adverse effects of western diets have occurred at young ages among Japanese women.

Early ecologic studies linked national per capita fat consumption with breast cancer incidence and mortality patterns although no data was available to control for other known and suspected risk factors.[14] The WHI Dietary Modification trial reported breast cancer risk was not significantly influenced by the low-fat intervention compared to control status (usual diet) during 8 years of follow-up among more than 48,000 randomized women. However, 15% less disease was diagnosed among women who were more adherent to the assigned dietary pattern.[257] Some argued the trial was too short to produce major changes. Other researchers suggested preventive aspects of diet may be evident only when initiated at young ages.

High fiber consumption, which inhibits reabsorption of estrogens in the intestines, was proposed to be similarly protective in humans as found in mice.[258] However, prospective studies have not supported the fiber concept.[226] Frequent consumption of meat, particularly when well done with high levels of heterocyclic amines, has been associated with increased risk. Inconsistent results have been reported from studies assessing intake of retinol, cruciferous vegetables, and soy. Diet remains a field of intense epidemiologic research based primarily on food frequency questionnaire data that may not adequately enable classification of study participants by their diversity of nutrient intake.

Vitamin D Exposure

Ecologic studies suggested a potential protective role of vitamin D and lower rates of breast cancer incidence and mortality in southern latitudes compared with northern U.S. states implying greater exposure to sunlight enhanced natural production of vitamin D.[259,260] Some researchers suggested the protective effect resulted from vitamin D binding to receptors in breast tissue stimulating cellular differentiation.[261] John et al. analyzed follow-up data from NHANES I and reported 25%–65% risk reduction among long-term residents of southern states with high solar exposure who also reported higher consumption of foods containing vitamin D or used vitamin D supplements.[261]

Recent studies based on measured serum concentrations of 1,25-(OH)$_2$D (25-OHD) indicated higher vitamin D levels inhibited cell proliferation and increased apoptosis of normal and malignant cells.[262] Plasma levels of 25-OHD above 40 ng/mL were associated with significantly reduced breast cancer among postmenopausal women (OR = 0.56, 95% CI = 0.41−0.78).[262] Similar findings from the Nurses' Health Study were limited to women aged 60 or older.[263] Garland et al. also reported a strong dose response as women with lowest blood levels of 25-OHD had the highest risk of breast cancer.[264]

In contrast to these reports, invasive breast cancer was not diminished among women randomized in the WHI trial to calcium and vitamin D supplements compared with placebo. Among trial participants circulating 25-hydroxyvitamin D levels were not associated with breast cancer diagnois.[265] However, a 4-year placebo-controlled RCT of calcium alone (1400–1500 mg) or calcium with vitamin D reported 60% reduction in overall cancer incidence when combined treatment was compared to placebo among women aged 55 and older. The authors noted the importance of higher vitamin D dose, 400–500 mg greater than the WHI RCT, for cancer prevention.[266] Mortality from any cause was modestly reduced in a meta-analysis of nine RCTs of vitamin D supplementation with doses ranging from 300 to 2,000 IU/day.[267] A meta-analysis of data from observational studies indicated the association of breast cancer risk with vitamin D supplementation differed by study design: a protective effect (summary RR = 0.83) was noted when cases and controls were compared but analyses of data from the more reliable prospective studies indicated vitamin D had no significant effect (summary RR = 0.97).[268]

Environmental Exposures

As originally suggested by Trichopoulos, Fenton et al. suggested environmental exposures could significantly alter breast tissue during vulnerable periods of prenatal and neonatal development.[269] Potential adverse effects of estrogen-disrupting chemicals at younger ages may increase malignant transformation of dividing mammary cells. Hormonal exposures at older ages may promote tumor proliferation of previously transformed cells (Figure 26-5).[270] Some synthetic chemicals suspected of being carcinogenic, including those classified as phthalates and endocrine disruptors, may stimulate early breast development, accelerate onset of puberty, and result in epigenetic changes potentially increasing risk of cancer at adult ages.

To assess adult levels of environmental risk factors, several large case-control and cohort studies were conducted. Among long-term residents of Long Island participating in a case-control study, self-reported ever use of pesticides (within the home and garden) was associated with a modestly elevated breast cancer risk (OR = 1.39, 95% CI = 1.15–1.68) although no dose response relationship was detected.[271] Serum levels from this case-control study failed to identify or confirm a relationship between breast cancer and past exposures to organochlorine compounds such as DDT that are now banned.[272] Few environmental contaminants have been linked to breast cancer partially due to inadequate measures of exposure.[273] New technology will enhance detection of potential environmental contaminants in future studies.

Viral Etiology

The mammary tumor virus (MMTV), first recognized by Bittner in the milk of mice at high risk of mammary cancer, was associated with earlier tumor development among offspring exposed to MMTV compared with offspring not exposed to the virus.[274] Recently several investigators, searching for a comparable human virus, have reported evidence of MMTV-like genetic sequences in some human breast cancers from female and male patients but very rarely in normal tissue.[275] A research team has recently identified the complete structure of a retrovirus in human breast cancer that shares 85%–95% of the MMTV characteristics and has been designated as human mammary tumor virus (HMTV).[276] One study identified the same MMTV-like DNA sequences in the breast cancer tissue of a family triad: mother, father, and daughter who had been living together for decades in the same house. The authors noted viral particle sequences were of mouse origin and could have resulted from a common exposure in the home.[277] A more recent report from Australian researchers identified MMTV-like gene sequences in 5% of breastmilk samples from healthy lactating women that could potentially be transmitted to offspring.[278]

Recent studies have also considered a potential role of human papillomavirus (HPV) in breast cancer etiology although no consistent findings have been reported. Among a series of 54 frozen breast cancer tissue samples from Australia, HPV-18 was detected by polymerase chain reaction (PCR) in 50% although Antonsson et al. indicated their research could not determine if the HPV was associated with infection.[279] Lower prevalence of HPV was reported from an American study of 70 samples (8.6%) representing a more diverse patient population.[280] As this brief report noted, interest in a viral etiology, and the associated potential development of a preventive vaccine, has been discussed for many years; meaningful results may not be achieved for decades although recent technological advances may accelerate the pace.

Predictive Models

To identify women at elevated risk who might benefit from chemopreventive agents, Gail and colleagues developed a multivariate statistical model using data from women screened annually in the BCDDP to combine estimate individual risk levels during 10, 20, or 30 years of follow-up (Table 26-6). The model computes an absolute risk: "the chance that a woman of a specific age with specific risk factors will develop breast cancer in a specific interval of time."[59] A minimal Gail risk score (1.66% risk within 5 years) was established for participation of healthy women in the Breast Cancer Prevention Trials. The original model was modified to specifically predict invasive disease with separate estimates for white and black women[281,282] as well as Asian women[283] which have been consistently validated in cohort[284] and case-control study populations.[285] Women, their physicians, genetic counselors, and others may obtain personalized estimates of risk to guide screening frequencies, preventive modalities, and surgical options.[59] Because many women overestimate their personal risk of breast cancer, the model may provide reassurance although some overestimates have been reported among women who receive less than annual screening.[282] Some researchers have suggested predictive models risk estimates that are comparable to mammographic density using BI-RADS methodology adjusted for age and race.[286]

Bilateral Breast Cancer

Among the estimated 2 million U.S. breast cancer survivors, approximately 5%–10% have had a second primary in the opposite breast. Simultaneous bilateral disease was diagnosed in 1% to 2% of cases and 12% to 15% following diagnostic bilateral biopsies.[145] Incidence of second primary cancers has recently increased as improved adjuvant treatment, chemotherapy and radiation therapy, have prolonged survival.[287] Kuian et al. used SEER data assess frequency of bilateral disease and reported a tenfold risk of a second ER-negative breast cancer after an ER-negative first primary especially among young patients.[288] Another analysis of SEER data indicated second primaries were more frequent after menopause among black compared with white breast cancer patients, which may have been associated with their greater frequency of ER-negative tumors.[289] Among newly diagnosed patients with no palpable lesion and negative contralateral mammogram, MRI has identified second primaries in 3% of cases, although a false-positive rate of 10% led to additional contralateral breast biopsies.[290]

Lobular cancer is more frequently multicentric and often bilateral compared with ductal tumors; therefore, some surgeons have screened and/or biopsied the contralateral breast of patients with lobular lesions to rule out a second breast cancer.[26] The histology of the first primary and treatment with radiation therapy were associated with cancer in the opposite breast in the Women's Environmental Cancer and Radiation Epidemiology Study (WECARE).[291] Radiation-induced contralateral breast cancer was associated with higher radiation dose and age less than 40 at time of initial treatment[287] but risk was reduced by adjuvant chemotherapy.[292] Among Hodgkin's patients treated with radiation, bilateral breast cancer was fourfold greater than matched breast cancer cases with no prior cancer.[293] New technologies enabling targeted therapy may lower risk of radiation-induced bilateral disease.

As noted in Figure 26-7, inherited susceptibility significantly increases the likelihood of contralateral breast cancer compared to patients without a BRCA mutation. Cumulative risk at 10 years was greater among carriers of BRCA1 (4.5 times increased) than women with a BRCA2 mutation (3.4 times increased).[294] Bilaterality was reduced by chemotherapy, tamoxifen therapy or bilateral oophorectomy, especially among premenopausal patients.[295] An additional genetic marker, a variant of the ATM gene, was identified in the WECARE study. Patients with the variant treated with radiation therapy were at greater risk of bilateral disease than breast cancer patients who carried the wild type ATM and did not receive radiotherapy.[291]

Table 26-7 provides a summary of scientifically assessed major risk factors associated with breast cancer. Studies currently being conducted focus on gene–environment interactions; others use mammographic density as an intermediate marker to assess the degree of potential reduction that may be achieved through health behaviors such as weight loss, increased exercise, and routine NSAID use. GWAS studies are addressing genetic associations of lower magnitude that may affect risk of disease in the general population and some research is assessing epigenetic influences on risk across the life span.

Breast Cancer Treatment

Surgery

Radical mastectomy, a life-prolonging procedure when introduced in 1890, remained the standard of care until the 1980s, causing considerable physical and psychological morbidity for many women.[296] With increased awareness, emphasis on earlier stage at diagnosis, and pressure by affected women, treatment standards began to change after the publication in 1985 of the clinical trial revealing equal survival for patients treated by mastectomy or breast

Table 26-6	
Breast cancer risk factors included in the Gail Model[59]	
Current Age	Number of benign breast biopsies
Race	Diagnosis of atypical hyperplasia
Age at menarche	Number of affected first-degree relatives
Age at first birth/nulliparous	[mother, sisters, daughters]

Data from Gail MH, Brinton LA, Byer DP, et al. Projecting individualized probabilities of developing breast cancer for white females who are examined annually. *J Natl Cancer Inst.* 1989;81:1879–1886.

conserving surgery (lumpectomy) followed by adjuvant radiation. Treatment by conservative surgery grew from 25% in 1990, when a National Institutes of Health consensus conference concluded lumpectomy was appropriate for women with stage I or II breast cancer, to 80% by 2005.[296] Since early research indicated 30% of patients treated by lumpectomy might experience recurrence, radiation therapy to remaining breast tissue was considered essential.[20] However, detection of diffuse microcalcifications following improved mammography and MRI has increased diagnosis of multicentric DCIS, raising the frequency of clinical recommendations for mastectomy rather than conservative surgery,[23] especially among young women with risk of contralateral breast cancer estimated to reach 11% after 20 years follow-up.[297] Among almost 1,000 DCIS cases, Dick et al. reported recurrent disease at 5 years was lowest following mastectomy, highest among patients treated by lumpectomy alone, and intermediate for DCIS cases with radiation therapy after lumpectomy.[298] Detection of multicentric DCIS by MRI following mammography has increased the frequency of mastectomy by almost 200% between 1998 and 2005 including prophylactic mastectomy of the opposite breast with many women requesting immediate reconstruction of both breasts.[297] Prophylactic mastectomy has been shown to nearly eliminate risk of subsequent malignancy.[299]

Chemotherapy and Hormonal Therapy

Before technology enabled determination of tumor receptor status, Beatson in 1896 reported regression of breast cancer following bilateral oophorectomy among young patients with advancing disease.[300] Surgical menopause became a standard treatment for premenopausal patients until the late 1970s when various chemotherapy agents caused permanent or temporary ovarian failure, reducing ovarian estrogen levels and lowering risk of recurrent disease.[301,302] Although bilateral oophorectomy is still considered a treatment option,[303] most women with positive axillary lymph nodes and others at increased risk of disease progression receive chemotherapy. Among older premenopausal women, chemotherapy-induced amenorrhea has been associated with reduced risk of recurrent disease, which some clinicians consider comparable to surgical ovarian ablation.[302] Younger premenopausal women may retain or regain their fertility after chemotherapy, presenting the option of subsequent pregnancy. Histologic tumor grade, a measure of tissue differentiation, is another criterion guiding treatment decisions; less well differentiated tumors require more aggressive therapy.[7]

Tamoxifen, a synthetic antiestrogen known as a selective estrogen receptor modulator (SERM) was introduced 30 years ago and has effectively reduced risk of recurrent and contralateral disease for women with ER-positive

Table 26-7

Major factors associated with increased breast cancer risk

Risk Factor	Relative Risk
BRCA1 or *BRCA2* mutation	10.0–32.0
Family history of breast cancer (in the absence of a known mutation, risk varies by age at diagnosis)	
1 first-degree relative: mother, sister, or daughter	1.5–2.0
2 first-degree relatives	3.0
3 or more first-degree relatives	4.0
1 second-degree relative: grandmother, aunt, cousin	1.2–1.5
Radiation therapy to the chest before age 30	7.0–17.0
Mammographic density >75%	4.0–5.0
Benign breast surgery (atypia with hyperplasia or LCIS)	4.0
Hormonal exposures	
Late age first birth (> 35 yrs) or nulliparity	1.2–1.7
Early menarche (< 12 yrs), late menopause (> 55 yrs)	1.2–1.3
Combined estrogen/progestin hormone therapy (use > 10 yrs)	1.5
Postmenopausal overweight or obesity	1.2–1.9
Alcohol consumption (2 drinks or more per day)	1.2
Smoking (> 6 pack years)	1.3–1.5
Lack of physical activity	1.1–1.8

Adapted from Warner E. Breast cancer screening. *N Engl J Med*. 2011;365:1025–1032.

breast cancer.[304] This medication provides no benefit for women with ER-negative breast cancer.[305] A meta-analysis of 55 international studies documented 50% reduced recurrence of ER-positive disease and contralateral breast cancer after 5 years of adjuvant tamoxifen.[306] Similarly, a meta-analysis of 20 international RCTs indicated breast cancer mortality was reduced more than 30% over 15 years of follow-up.[307]

Among several unpleasant side effects, tamoxifen has been associated with two potentially lethal conditions, endometrial cancer and thromboembolic disease.[308] Endometrial cancer among postmenopausal breast cancer patients treated with tamoxifen was associated by Bernstein et al. with prediagnosis obesity and hormone use.[309] These adverse side effects led to testing of a second SERM, raloxifene, which also provided long-term reduced risk of recurrent disease without the threat of endometrial cancer. Recently, both medications were studied as chemoprevention agents for healthy women.[310]

Radiation Therapy

In past decades, treatment of advanced breast cancer often included radiotherapy following radical mastectomy. As screening coupled with greater awareness of palpable tumors led to earlier stage at diagnosis, more limited surgery became acceptable when coupled with adjuvant radiation therapy to potentially eliminate cancer cells in retained breast tissue.[311] Subsequently, pooled data from several trials indicated risk of recurrent disease after lumpectomy was 7% with and 26% without adjuvant radiotherapy, although differences were attenuated in women aged 70 and older.[312] Therefore, after conservative surgery, radiation therapy to retained breast tissue became the standard of care to avoid subsequent cancer. However, patients and clinicians have questioned the need for radiotherapy for older patients, as treatment only with tamoxifen may adequately prevent further disease. A clinical trial conducted among newly diagnosed women age 70 or older with stage I estrogen-positive breast cancer who were randomized after lumpectomy (partial mastectomy or wide local excision) to 6 weeks of radiation or not; women in both groups were prescribed 20 mg tamoxifen daily.[313] Tumor size was restricted to 2 cm and axillary lymph node dissection was discouraged. Among the 600 patients enrolled between 1994 and 1999, radiation reduced risk of recurrent disease in the treated breast by 3% but survival did not differ when the two groups were compared. Therefore, tamoxifen only after breast conserving surgery has been recommended for elderly patients.[313]

Lymphedema

Among the 2 million American women who have a personal history of breast cancer, approximately 10% develop lymphedema and related unpleasant arm sensations; approximately 200,000 survivors are estimated to cope daily with physical discomforts and emotional reminders of breast cancer treatment. Lymphedema is interstitial fluid collection caused by disruption of lymph circulation. Among patients followed for 20 years after mastectomy at one cancer center, almost 30% had measurable arm swelling.[314] Onset of lymphedema generally occurred within 2 or 3 years of axillary lymph node surgery, often associated with weight gain or following injury or infection in the affected arm.[314,315] Another prospective study reported 8% of breast cancer patients experienced arm swelling and 37% arm discomforts without measurable swelling. These symptoms were associated with obesity, more extensive axillary surgery, higher number of nodes removed, and/or adjuvant radiation.[316] Other investigators also noted obesity raised the risk of lymphedema threefold.[317] Decongestive lymphatic therapy[318] is one of few treatment options to reduce arm swelling. An alternative treatment was suggested in a recent report that noted 30% reduction of lymphedema after 4 weeks of acupuncture.[319] The new surgical technique, sentinel lymph node biopsy using mapping of lymphatic drainage to enable node sampling, has reduced lymphedema to 3% in a series of more 900 breast cancer patients compared with 27% of patients with axillary dissection followed for 5 years after initial diagnosis.[320]

Reconstruction

Many women, disturbed by their altered body image following mastectomy, have opted for breast reconstruction for cosmetic and psychological benefits. Reconstruction may be accomplished by either a breast implant or autologous transfer of tissue from a distant site to the chest.[321] Autologous reconstruction requires more extensive surgery than a breast implant containing either saline or silicone gel. Owing to feared systemic disease following rupture of silicone implants, the Food and Drug Administration (FDA) banned their use until research identified the very limited adverse effects to very few of the millions of women with implants. However, the FDA approval is accompanied by a warning label noting implants may cause localized complications potentially requiring additional surgery or removal.

Studies of reconstruction among patients in four counties of southern California indicated that access to reconstruction was limited by cost to breast cancer patients with personal funds or variable coverage by health insurance.[322] Kruper et al. noted reconstruction was twice as frequent after diagnosis of DCIS than invasive disease, especially among younger, non-Hispanic white patients treated at teaching hospitals.[322] Although breast conserving surgery is offered for DCIS detected by mammography, women have been increasingly selecting mastectomy followed by reconstruction.[297] The passage of the Women's Health and Cancer Rights Act (WHRCA) in 1998 required health insurance plans to pay for reconstruction.[323]

Prognostic Factors

Tumor size and lymph node status, criteria for staging, remain primary factors predicting risk of recurrence and long-term survival. As suggested by the findings from the HIP study previously discussed, early detection followed promptly by surgery resulted in lower mortality among screened women compared with controls regardless of race/ethnicity or economic status.[324] Therefore, recognized breast cancer survival disparities were partially associated with delayed diagnosis and inadequate treatment.

Beginning in 1990, national data indicated declining mortality as use of early detection modalities increased and use of adjuvant therapy was expanded. To address the continuing higher mortality among black compared with white women, Congress passed the Breast and Cervical Cancer Mortality Prevention Act enabling CDC to create the National Breast and Cervical Cancer Early Detection Program providing mammography for poor women lacking health insurance.[325] Recent national survey data indicate screening is now comparable among race/ethnic groups (Table 26-1), although SEER data continue to reveal survival disparities. Data collected prospectively in Connecticut by Jones et al. suggested African American women received inadequate communication regarding mammography results that may have delayed clinical care.[326] Other factors appear to influence poor survival including young age at diagnosis, ER-negative tumor status, overexpression of HER2, and higher proliferation rates among African American women. However, stage-for-stage comparisons with white patients identified higher prevalence of some comorbid conditions significantly contributed to survival differences.[327] Researchers have suggested disparities among Hispanic women may also result from language barriers delaying diagnosis after suspicious mammography.[328]

Although adjuvant chemotherapy has significantly improved prognosis, Devitt noted long ago that patients of the same age with comparable tumor size and nodal status may experience very different outcomes.[20] Multimodality treatment may improve population-based survival rates but person-specific factors also influence prognosis including behaviors prior to and following diagnosis, treatment compliance, and socioeconomic status.[20]

Compliance with prescribed treatment has a significant impact on risk of recurrence. Adjuvant chemotherapy significantly reduced mortality but only when full treatment was administered as planned. Budman et al. noted patients receiving less than 85% of prescribed dosages experienced mortality rates comparable to untreated patients.[329] When adjuvant hormonal therapy prescribed for ER-positive postmenopausal patients was not received for the full 5 years, 26% increased risk of death was noted.[12] Factors leading to discontinued treatment included side effects, comorbid conditions, psychological problems, and high cost of drugs, among others.[330] Research using SEER data indicated that race/ethnicity disparities may be due to inadequate health insurance, which limited access to complete, effective, and high-cost adjuvant therapy,[12,330] as well as comorbid conditions including obesity-related chronic conditions that influenced treatment options.[331]

Personal behaviors including smoking were associated with higher mortality in a prospective study by the ACS; fatal breast cancer was more prevalent among smokers (RR = 1.26, 95% CI = 1.05–1.50) and was positively associated with increasing number of cigarettes and years of smoking.[332] These findings agreed with Scanlon et al. who reported smokers were at greater risk of lung metastases compared with nonsmoking breast cancer patients (RR = 3.73, 95% CI = 1.6–8.9).[333] Among smokers who developed breast cancer and were treated with radiation, Neugut et al. found a synergistic effect with a 33-fold increased risk of lung cancer in the radiation-exposed lung, in contrast to a two- to threefold elevated risk of radiation-induced lung cancer in nonsmokers.[13]

Most studies of prognostic factors reported overweight and obesity (BMI < 30 kg/m[2]) were associated with recurrent disease and diminished survival.[334,335] The presumed biologic mechanisms included higher circulating estrogens associated with excess adipose tissue and stimulation of proliferating breast cancer cells from insulin-like growth factors associated with visceral obesity.[336] Obese women were 34% more likely to have died of disease 15 years after participation in the CASH study[337] in addition to the more recent CARE study;[338] black women were more likely to be obese at diagnosis although death from obesity-related comorbid conditions may have preceded development of metastatic breast cancer in obese patients.[338] Obese women are often diagnosed with more advanced disease potentially due to less frequent mammography, greater difficultly receiving adequate screening, or inadequate communication regarding screening results.[326,336]

Weight gain of 5–20 lbs often occurs postdiagnosis while patients are receiving adjuvant chemotherapy.[335] Data from the combined Life after Cancer Epidemiology (LACE) Study and the Women's Healthy Eating and Living (WHEL) Study followed more than 3,000 patients and found no adverse effect of treatment-related weight gain,[336] although weight control may reduce morbidity and mortality due to other chronic conditions associated with aging.[335] Dietary patterns emphasizing consumption of fruit, vegetables, whole grains, and low-fat dairy products have been associated with decreased risk of all-cause mortality among breast cancer patients.

Reproductive decisions influence both incidence and mortality of breast cancer. Diagnosis during pregnancy or within a short interval after delivery was associated with a threefold greater risk of dying compared with nulliparous cases. For each additional year of disease-free survival between giving birth and diagnosis, risk of death was diminished by 15%.[339] Another study of women age 45 or younger, whose last birth was within 2 years of diagnosis, indicated a similar threefold greater risk of dying than nulliparous women of similar ages and stage.[340] After controlling for stage at diagnosis, a population-based Australian study found breast cancer death increased as the interval between diagnosis and last birth decreased.[341]

Hormone use before diagnosis may have increased risk of breast cancer development, but Schairer et al. observed cases in the BCDDP screening program who had been on hormones at diagnosis were 50% less likely to develop recurrence and to die of disease.[342] The protective effect diminished 4 years after diagnosis among cases with positive axillary nodes and 12 years among node negative cases. In a more recent study by Newcomb et al. who followed a population-based series for more than 10 years, risk of death was reduced among women who were using combined estrogen-progestin therapy at time of diagnosis (HR = 0.73, 95% CI = 0.59–0.91) although not with use of estrogen alone.[222] Because the protective effect was greater after more than 5 years of use, the authors suggested less aggressive, hormonally responsive tumors develop during continued hormone use; the benefit persisted after adjusting for screening, stage of disease, and other potential confounders.[222] Aspirin use did not lower risk of breast cancer among nurses but improved survival was associated with increasing days per week of aspirin use after diagnosis.[343] Person-specific prognosis varies considerably in relation to tumor characteristics, tailored treatment, and health behaviors before cancer diagnosis.

Psychosocial Issues

Regardless of the improving statistics, women tend to fear breast cancer more than other lethal medical conditions. Numerous studies have indicated women tend to overestimate their risk of developing and dying of breast cancer. Some studies suggest the heightened fear is due to misunderstanding the one in eight statistic promoted by the ACS and widely quoted in the media. Women smokers appear to fear breast cancer more than lung cancer even though their risk of developing and dying of lung cancer far exceeds that of breast cancer.[344]

Often young women are pictured in mammography advertisements, especially during October media reports, increasing fear of the disease.[39] The Gail model calculations, genetic counseling, and *BRCA* mutation testing in the presence of a family history may be appropriate to clarify individual concerns. Quality of life has been studied by many researchers at varying times among patients after initial diagnosis. Premenopausal women noted disturbed interpersonal problems lasting up to 4 years after diagnosis including sexual functioning, body image, and partner relationships adversely affected quality of life.[345] Women who have been treated for breast cancer continually fear recurrence; however, among older women free of evidence of breast cancer, quality of life has been more adversely affected by comorbid disease.[346]

Subsequent Pregnancy

Some of the more than 23,000 women of childbearing ages diagnosed annually have experienced diminished quality of life due to temporary or permanent premature, chemotherapy-induced ovarian dysfunction, often resulting in amenorrhea with related infertility and onset of menopausal symptoms. Among young breast cancer patients, maintenance of fertility is a primary concern after diagnosis and treatment of breast cancer.[301] Petrek and colleagues surveyed 600 premenopausal patients to determine factors associated with maintenance or return

of menstrual function and identified the following: age at chemotherapy, medications prescribed, and interval since last treatment.[347] Decisions regarding future childbearing have influenced treatment options for some premenopausal patients as reported by members of the Young Survival Coalition, an international network of breast cancer survivors and supporters.[348]

Although most patients are treated with aggressive chemotherapy based on their age and stage at diagnosis, many are advised to consult gynecologists regarding fertility preservation prior to beginning treatment.[348,349] Some young patients retain or regain menstrual function and are able to achieve pregnancy;[350] prospective and retrospective studies of the prognostic influence of subsequent pregnancy indicated minimal adverse effects when compared with age and stage matched cases who did not become pregnant after diagnosis of breast cancer.[350]

Longer disease free interval before planned subsequent pregnancy may provide reassurance to young patients of the safety of their decisions for childbearing.[350] Although some women have sought ovarian stimulation and oocyte harvesting, concerns have been expressed about the risks associated with estradiol therapy. Current studies are too limited to adequately judge any adverse effects of these procedures.

Prevention Strategies

Primary prevention of breast cancer has been the goal of extensive laboratory studies and major epidemiologic research projects but limited avenues have been identified. Much research has focused on serum hormone levels that may be influenced by chemopreventive agents and lifestyle changes, including physical activity and weight control among postmenopausal women. Prophylactic mastectomy is also considered by women at increased risk or who have had unilateral breast cancer.

Prophylactic Surgery

Depending upon a woman's personal and family history, a number of options exist for primary and secondary prevention of breast cancer. In 1994, after calculating the individual risk of breast cancer associated with extensive family history, Thompson noted bilateral prophylactic mastectomy was an extreme option for women with "incapacitating" anxiety about developing the disease, although he suggested the risk may be exaggerated by women and their healthcare providers.[77] After *BRCA1* and *BRCA2* were identified, decisions regarding genetic testing became a major consideration for newly diagnosed patients and their unaffected relatives. Testing was costly until covered by health insurance and loss of privacy was a consideration until federal laws provided legal protection against discrimination based on genetic status.

Parmigiani and colleagues developed a computer-based algorithm using family history to estimate the probability of inherited risk.[103] Genetic testing necessitated guidance for women found to carry a deleterious mutation as noted in narratives from women who learned their *BRCA* status[92] and discussed among women seeking guidance through FORCE.[104] Thompson's early suggestion became a reality for a growing number of newly diagnosed women from high-risk families who were counseled to obtain genetic results through a rapid reporting program instituted by Myriad Genetics, the company owning the patent for clinical testing of the two susceptibility genes. In 1999 Hartmann et al. reported prophylactic mastectomy provided 90% protection against breast cancer[299] and bilateral oophorectomy before age 40 among *BRCA1* carriers significantly reduced breast cancer risk with OR = 0.36 (95% CI = 0.20–0.64) with protection lasting during 15 years of follow-up. Carriers of *BRCA2* may also benefit although larger samples are needed to confirm the findings.[351] Pathologic review of breast tissue from prophylactic surgery conducted at Memorial Sloan Kettering Cancer Center identified more high-risk proliferative lesions including DCIS in breast tissue of women with inherited susceptibility compared with breast tissue from women without known genetic risk.[352]

Chemoprevention

After treatment with tamoxifen was demonstrated to reduce recurrent disease and lower risk of a second breast cancer, the drug was proposed for primary prevention treatment. The first Breast Cancer Prevention Trial (BCPT) reported 49% reduction of ER-positive breast cancer among high-risk healthy women randomized to tamoxifen compared with placebo; however, potentially lethal adverse side effects occurred among some treated women, which limited acceptability.[304]

A second chemoprevention trial, Study of Tamoxifen and Raloxifene (STAR) P-2, compared the protective effect over 5 years of tamoxifen (20 mg/day) with raloxifene (60 mg/day), another selective estrogen modulator (SERM). The two drugs were equally effective at preventing breast cancer and both caused menopausal symptoms.[353] However, adverse side effects differed;[354] raloxifene caused fewer thromboembolic events and tamoxifen was associated with a threefold increased risk of endometrial cancer.[355] The FDA approved both medications as breast cancer chemopreventive agents for women at increased risk, although an estimated 95 women must be treated with either drug for 5 years to prevent diagnosis of one breast cancer.[356]

Various measures were applied to define high risk including estimates from the Gail model,[59] mammographic density,[200] circulating hormone levels,[150] benign biopsy indicating atypical hyperplasia,[16] and lobular carcinoma in situ.[304] Although both drugs reduced invasive disease by 50%, tamoxifen also lowered in situ disease by 50% compared with raloxifene.[357] Women in the STAR trial appeared to respond similarly to the two drugs in regard to their physical health, mental health, and degrees of depression.[358] However, neither tamoxifen nor raloxifene has been readily accepted by women at high risk primarily because of recognized adverse side effects.[359]

Exemestane, an aromatase inhibitor, provided a 65% breast cancer risk reduction compared with placebo in a recent RCT including 4,500 healthy postmenopausal women ages 35 or older at increased risk based on the Gail model, prior benign breast biopsy, with normal mammography before enrollment and repeated annually screening.[356] At 35 months of follow-up, invasive breast cancer was reduced 65% among treated women compared with placebo controls. In addition, exemestane was associated with reduced frequency of DCIS, proliferative breast conditions, and HER2-positive tumors.[355] Side effects included onset of hot flashes and arthritis but no cardiovascular events, bone fractures, or all-cause mortality.[356] Several other aromatase inhibitors have been developed and appear equally effective as chemopreventive agents. Davidson and Kensler noted key issues remaining include identifying appropriate women at high risk for treatment and selecting biomarkers to predict response.[357]

Lifestyle

Prevention of breast cancer is a goal of advocates and researchers alike but avenues for lowering risk are limited; however, lifestyle changes especially at young ages may contribute to lower incidence rates. Body mass index is among the first behavior factors suggested. BMI has a dual influence on risk of breast cancer with excess weight protective at younger ages often associated with hormonal aberrations; however, breast cancer increases with age and postmenopausal women may lower their risk by preventing obesity or reducing excess weight. Physical activity especially at young ages and continued across the life span has been reported to have multiple beneficial health effects by reducing fat padding and lowering levels of aromatase conversion to estrone. Aspirin may provide an avenue for reduced risk of hormone-dependent breast cancer although bleeding risks may be precipitated.[240] These combined lifestyle factors are recommended for protection against other chronic conditions and increase life expectancy in additional reduction of breast cancer risk. As genetic analyses provided by new technologies enable improved understanding of tissue specific carcinogenesis, more studies are addressing possible additional avenues to prevent breast cancer and other malignancies.

Summary

Breast cancer is a complex disease with risks and protective influences varying in association with genetic susceptibility, menopausal status, geographic distribution, and many other factors. Although most women are at average risk of developing breast cancer, fear of the disease is greater than for heart disease, diabetes, and other chronic conditions that cause considerably more morbidity and mortality. Individual women can access predictive models to obtain person-specific risk scores at differing ages but the models are based on a small number of long recognized etiologic factors without genetic assessment and without inclusion of biomarkers. Major advances in understanding the natural history and progression of breast cancer have been accomplished in recent years although additional research to identify preventive measures is needed. However, media coverage has most frequently focused on changes to screening recommendations which continue to be a source of controversy among clinicians, researchers, and the public. Fortunately, mortality rates have declined during the last 2 decades primarily associated with improved multimodality treatment and changes in personal health behaviors including avoidance of long term hormone use after menopause.

Discussion Questions

1. Screening recommendations continue to receive extensive attention in the media. Describe the earlier studies and modalities used for early detection and discuss the most recent changes that have been proposed.
2. What factors initiate malignant transformation? Who is susceptible to carcinogenesis?
3. Name factors that influence prognosis of breast cancer? Recently, mortality rates have declined. Define some factors that have been associated with improved survival.
4. How does risk differ among pre- and postmenopausal women? What role does genetics play in differentiating breast cancer diagnosed at younger versus older ages?
5. Disparities in incidence and mortality have been recognized for decades? What efforts have been undertaken limit disparities? Describe their successes and failures.
6. What role does pregnancy history play in breast cancer risk and prognosis?

References

1. American Cancer Society. *Cancer Facts and Figures 2011*. Atlanta, GA: Author; 2011.
2. Smigal C, Jemal A, Ward E, et al. Trends in breast cancer by race and ethnicity: Update 2006. *CA Cancer J Clin*. 2006;56:168–183.
3. Colditz GA, Rosner B. Cumulative risk of breast cancer to age 70 years according to risk factor status: data from the Nurses' Health Study. *Am J Epidemiol*. 2000;152:950–964.
4. Bleyer A, Welch HG. Effects of three decades of screening mammography on breast-cancer incidence. *N Engl J Med* 2012;367:1998–2005.
5. Anderson WF, Rosenberg PS, Menashe I, et al. Age-related crossover in breast cancer incidence rates between black and white ethnic groups. *J Natl Cancer Inst*. 2008;100:1804–1814.
6. Farhat GN, Cummings SR, Chlebowski RT, et al. Sex hormone levels and risks of estrogen receptor-negative and estrogen-receptor positive breast cancer. *J Natl Cancer Inst*. 2011;103:562–570.
7. Clarke CA, Glaser SL, Uratsu CS, et al. Recent declines in hormone therapy utilization and breast cancer incidence: clinical and population-based evidence. *J Clin Oncol*. 2006;24:e49–50.
8. Ganai S, Winchester DJ. Screening mammography. Bringing back into focus the value of a lifesaving intervention. *Cancer*. 2011;117:3062–3063.
9. Kerlikowske K, Miglioretti DL, Buist DS, et al. Declines in invasive breast cancer and use of menopausal hormone therapy in a screening mammography population. *J Natl Cancer Inst*. 2007;99:1335–1339. (Erratum, *J Natl Cancer Inst*. 2007;99:1493.)
10. Berry DA, Cronin KA, Plevritis SK, et al. Effect of screening and adjuvant therapy on mortality from breast cancer. *N Engl J Med*. 2005;353:1784–1792.
11. Albano JD, Ward E, Jemel A, et al. Cancer mortality in the United States by education level and race. *J Natl Cancer Inst* 2007;99:1384–1394.
12. Hershman DL, Shao T, Kushi LH, et al. Early discontinuation and nonadherence to adjuvant hormonal therapy are associated with increased mortality in women with breast cancer. *Breast Cancer Res Treat*. 2011;126:529–537.
13. Neugut AI, Murray T, Santos J, et al. Increased risk of lung cancer after breast cancer radiation therapy in cigarette smokers. *Cancer*. 1994;73:1615–1620.
14. Colditz GA, Baer HJ, Tamimi RM. Breast cancer. In: Schottenfeld D, Fraumeni JF Jr., eds. *Cancer Epidemiology and Prevention*. 3rd ed. New York: Oxford University Press; 2006:995–1012.
15. Russo IH, Russo J. Pregnancy-induced changes in breast cancer risk. *J Mammary Gland Biol Neoplasia*. 2011;16:221–233.
16. Dupont WD, Page DL. Risk factors for breast cancer in women with proliferative breast disease. *N Engl J Med*. 1985; 312:146–151.
17. Page DL, Schuyler PA, Dupont WD, et al. Atypical lobular hyperplasia as a unilateral predictor of breast cancer risk: A retrospective cohort study. *Lancet*. 2003;361:125–129.
18. Carter CL, Corle DK, Micozzi MS, et al. A prospective study of the development of breast cancer in 16,692 women with benign breast disease. *Am J Epidemiol*. 1988;128:467–477.
19. Ames BN, Gold LS, Willett WC. The causes and prevention of cancer. *Proc Nat Acad Sci*. 1995;92:5258–5265.
20. Devitt JE. Breast cancer: have we missed the forest because of the tree? *Lancet*. 1994;344:734–735.
21. Senie RT, Rosen PP, Lesser M, et al. Epidemiology of breast cancer II: factors related to the predominance of left-sided disease. *Cancer*. 1980; 46:1705–1713.
22. Russo J, Calaf G, Sohi N, et al. Critical steps in breast carcinogenesis. *Ann N Y Acad Sci*. 1993;698:1–20.
23. Virnig BA, Shamliyan T, Tuttle TM, et al. *Diagnosis and Management of Ductal Carcinoma in Situ (DCIS)*. Evidence Reports/Technology Assessments. No. 185, Rockville, MD: Agency for Healthcare Research and Quality; 2009.
24. Marshall E. Brawling over mammography. *Science*. 2010;327:938–938.
25. Reeves GK, Pirie K, Green J, et al. Reproductive factors and specific histological types of breast cancer: prospective study and meta-analysis. *Br J Cancer*. 2009;100:538–544.
26. Rosen PP, Lesser M, Senie RT, Duthie K. Epidemiology of breast carcinoma IV: age and histologic tumor type. *J Surg Oncol*. 1982;19:44–47.
27. Tamimi RM, Colditz GA, Hazra A, et al. Traditional breast cancer risk factors in relation to molecular subtypes of breast cancer. *Breast Cancer Res Treat*. 2012;131:159–167.
28. Colditz GA, Rosner BA, Chen WY, et al. Risk factors for breast cancer according to estrogen and progesterone receptor status. *J Natl Cancer Inst*. 2004;96:218–228.
29. Anders CK, Hsu DS, Broadwater G, et al. Young age at diagnosis correlates with worse prognosis and defines a subset of breast cancers with shared patterns of gene expression. *J Clin Oncol*. 2008;28:3324–3330.
30. Phipps AI, Chlebowski RT, Prentice R, et al. Reproductive history and oral contraceptive use in relation to risk of triple-negative breast cancer. *J Natl Cancer Inst*. 2011;103:470–477.
31. US Preventive Services Task Force. Screening for breast cancer: US Preventive Services Task Force Recommendation Statement. *Ann Int Med*. 2009;151: 716–726.
32. Schwartz LM, Woloshin S, Fowler FJ, Welch HG. Enthusiasm for cancer screening in the United States. *JAMA*. 2004;291:71–78.
33. Shapiro S, Venet W, Strax P, et al. Selection, follow-up, and analysis in the Health Insurance Plan Study: a randomized trial with breast cancer screening. *Natl Cancer Inst Monogr*. 1985;67:65–74.
34. Seidman H, Gelb SK, Silverberg E, et al. Survival experience in the Breast Cancer Detection Demonstration Project. *CA Cancer J Clin*. 1987;37:258–290.
35. Lerner BH. Breast cancer control after World War II. In: *The Breast Cancer Wars: Hope, Fear, and the Pursuit of a Cure in Twentieth-Century America*. New York: Oxford University Press; 2001:41–68,196–222.
36. National Breast and Cervical Cancer Early Detection Program. *Summarizing the First 12 Years of Partnerships and Progress Against Breast and Cervical Cancer*. 1991–2002 National Report. Atlanta, GA: Centers for Disease Control and Prevention; 2003.
37. Kolb TM, Lichy J, Newhouse JH. Comparison of the performance of screening mammography, physical examination, and breast US and evaluation of factors that influence them: an analysis of 27,825 patient evaluations. *Radiology*. 2002;225:165–175.
38. Ernster VL. Mammography screening for women aged 40–49—A guidelines saga and a clarion call for informed decision making. *Am J Public Health*. 1997;87:1103–1106.
39. Esserman L, Shieh Y, Thompson I. Rethinking screening for breast cancer and prostate cancer. *JAMA*. 2009;302:1685–1692.
40. Miglioretti DL, Walker R, Weaver DL, et al. Accuracy of screening mammography varies by week of menstrual cycle. *Radiology*. 2010;258:372–379.
41. White E, Velentgas P, Mendelson MT, et al. Variation in mammographic breast density by time in the menstrual cycle among women aged 40–49 years. *J Natl Cancer Inst*. 1998;17:906–910.
42. Ursin G, Parisky YR, Pike MC, Spicer DV. Mammographic density changes during the menstrual cycle. *Cancer Epidemiol Biomarkers Prev*. 2001;10: 141–142.
43. Baines C, Vidmar M, McKeown-Eyssen G, Tibshirani R. Impact of menstrual phase on false-negative mammograms in the Canadian National Breast Screening Study. *Cancer*. 1997;80:720–724.
44. Graham SJ, Stanchev PL, Lloyd-Smith JO, et al. Changes in fibroglandular volume and water content of breast tissue during menstrual cycle observed by MR imaging. *J Magn Reson Imaging*. 1995;5:695–701.
45. Mulligan D, Drife JO, Short RV. Changes in breast volume during normal menstrual cycle and oral contraceptives. *BMJ*. 1975;11:494–496.
46. DeFrank JT, Rimer BK, Gierisch JM, et al. Impact of mailed and automated telephone reminders on receipt of repeated mammograms. A randomized controlled trial. *Am J Prev Med*. 2009;36:459–467.
47. Welch HG, Black WC. Using autopsy series to estimate the disease "reservoir" for ductal carcinoma in situ of the breast: how much more breast cancer can we find? *Ann Intern Med*. 1997;127:1023–1028.

48. Rosai J. Borderline epithelial lesions of the breast. *Am J Surg Pathol.* 1991;15:209–221.

49. Wells WA, Carney PA, Eliassen MS, et al. Statewide study of diagnostic agreement in breast pathology. *J Natl Cancer Inst.* 1998;90:142–145.

50. Elmore JG, Wells CK, Lee CH, et al. Variability in radiologists' interpretation of mammograms. *N Engl J Med.* 1994;331:1493–1499.

51. Welch HG, Frankel BA. Likelihood that a women with screen-detected breast cancer has had her "life saved" by that screening. *Arch Intern Med.* 2011;Oct 24.

52. Quanstrum KH, Harward RA. Lessons from the mammography wars. *N Engl J Med.* 2010;363:1076–1079.

53. Mandelblatt JS, Cronin KA, Bailey S et al. Effects of mammography screening under different screening schedules: model estimates of potential benefits and harms. *Ann Intern Med.* 2009;151:738–747.

54. Gilbert FJ, Astley SM, Gillan MGC, et al. Single reading with computer-aided detection for screening mammography. *N Engl J Med.* 2008;359:1675–1684.

55. Fenton JJ, Abraham L, Taplin SH, et al. Effectiveness of computer-aided detection in community mammography practice. *J Natl Cancer Inst.* 2011; 103:1152–1161.

56. Berry DA. Computer-assisted detection and screening mammography: where's the beef? *J Natl Cancer Inst.* 2011;103:1139–1141.

57. Goldfrank D, Chuai S, Bernstein J, et al. Effect of mammography on breast cancer risk in women with mutations in *BRCA1* or *BRCA2*. *Cancer Epidemiol Biomarkers Prev.* 2006;15:2311–2313.

58. Saslow D, Hannan J, Osuch J, et al. Clinical breast examination: practical recommendations for optimizing performance and reporting. *CA Cancer J Clin.* 2004;54:327–344.

59. Gail MH, Brinton LA, Byer DP, et al. Projecting individualized probabilities of developing breast cancer for white females who are examined annually. *J Natl Cancer Inst.* 1989;81:1879–1886.

60. Adair FE. Clinical manifestations of early cancer of the breast. *New Engl J Med.* 1933;208:1250–1255.

61. Foster RS, Lang SP, Costanza MC, et al. Breast self-examination practices and breast cancer stage. *N Engl J Med.* 1978;299:265–270.

62. Senie RT, Rosen PP, Lesser ML, Kinne DW. Breast self-examination and medical examination related to breast cancer stage. *Am J Public Health.* 1981; 71:583–590.

63. Greenwald P, Nasca PC, Lawrence CE, et al. Estimated effect of breast self-examination and routine physician examination on breast cancer mortality. *N Engl J Med.* 1978;299:271–273.

64. Harvey BJ, Miller AB, Baines CJ, Corey PN. Effect of breast self-examination techniques on the risk of death from breast cancer. *Can Med Assoc J.* 1997; 157:1205–1212.

65. Barton MB, Harris R, Fletcher SW. Does this patient have breast cancer? The screening clinical breast examination: Should it be done? How? *JAMA.* 1999;282:1270–1280.

66. Thomas DB, Gao DL, Self SG, et al. Randomized trial of breast self-examination in Shanghai: methodology and preliminary results. *J Natl Cancer Inst.* 1997; 89:355–365.

67. Hillman M. Breast screening: making sense of the new advice. *New York Times*, November 17, 2009.

68. Borgen PI, Senie RT, McKinnon WMP, Rosen PP. Carcinoma of the male breast: analysis of prognosis compared with matched female patients. *J Surg Oncol.* 1997;4:385–388.

69. Giordano SH, Buzdar AU, Hortobagyi GN. Breast cancer in men. *Ann Int Med.* 2002;137:678–687.

70. Rosenblatt KA, Thomas DB, McTiernan A, et al. Breast cancer in men: Aspects of familial aggregation. *J Natl Cancer Inst.* 1991;83:849–854.

71. Brinton LA. Breast cancer among patients with Klinefelder syndrome. *Acta Paediatrica.* 2011;100:814–818.

72. Guinee VF, Olsson H, Moller T, et al. The prognosis of breast cancer in males. *Cancer.* 1993;71:154–161.

73. Hall IJ, Moorman PG, Millikan RC, Newman B. Comparative analysis of breast cancer risk factors among African-American women and white women. *Am J Epidemiol.* 2005;161:40–51.

74. Ziegler RG, Hoover RN, Pike MC, et al. Migration patterns ad breast cancer risk in Asian-American women. *J Natl Cancer Inst.* 1993;85:1819–1827.

75. John EM, Phipps AI, Davis A, Koo J. Migration history, acculturation, and breast cancer risk in Hispanic women. *Cancer Epidemiol Biomarkers Prev.* 2005;14:2905–2913.

76. Lynch HT, Silva E, Snyder C, Lynch JF. Hereditary breast cancer: part I. Diagnosing hereditary breast cancer syndromes. *The Breast J.* 2008;14:3–13.

77. Thompson WD. Genetic epidemiology of breast cancer. *Cancer.* 1994;74: 279–287.

78. Familial breast cancer: collaborative reanalysis of individual data from 52 epidemiological studies including 58,209 women with breast cancer and 101,986 without the disease. *Lancet.* 2001;358:1389–1399.

79. Risch N. The genetic epidemiology of cancer: interpreting family and twin studies and their implications for molecular genetic approaches. *Cancer Epidemiol Biomarkers Prev.* 2001;10:733–741.

80. Yasui Y, Newcomb PA, Trentham-Dietz A, Egan KM. Familial relative risk estimates for use in epidemiologic analyses. *Am J Epidemiol.* 2006;164:697–705.

81. Miki Y, Swensen J, Shattuck-Eiders D, et al. A strong candidate for the breast and ovarian susceptibility gene *BRCA1*. *Science.* 1994;266:66–71.

82. Wooster P, Biguell G, Lancaster J, et al. Identification of the breast cancer susceptibility gene *BRCA2*. *Nature.* 1995;378:789–792.

83. Struewing JP, Hartge P, Wacholder S, et al. The risk of cancer associated with specific mutations of *BRCA1* and *BRCA2* among Ashkenazi Jews. *N Engl J Med.* 1997;336:1401–1408.

84. Andrieu N, Easton DF, Chang-Claude J, et al. Effect of chest x-rays on the risk of breast cancer among *BRCA1/2* mutation carriers in the International BRCA1/2 Carrier Cohort Study: a report from the EMBRACE, GENEPSO, GEO-HEBON, and IBCCS Collaborators' Group. *J Clin Oncol.* 2006;24:3361–3366.

85. Antoniou A, Pharoah PDP, Narod S, et al. Average risks of breast and ovarian cancer associated with *BRCA1* or *BRCA2* mutations detected in case series unselected for family history: a combined analysis of 22 studies. *Am J Hum Genet.* 2003;72:1117–1130.

86. Berry DA, Parmigiani G, Sanchez J, et al. Probability of carrying a mutation of breast-ovarian cancer gene *BRCA1* based on family history. *J Natl Cancer Inst.* 1997;89:227–237.

87. Berry DA, Iversen ES, Gudbjartsson DF, et al. BRCAPRO validation, sensitivity of genetic testing of *BRCA1/BRCA2*, and prevalence of other breast cancer susceptibility genes. *J Clin Oncol.* 2002;20:2701–2712.

88. Huo D, Senie RT, Daly M, et al. Prediction of *BRCA* mutations using BRCAPRO model in clinic-based African American, Hispanic and other minority families in the United States. *J Clin Oncol.* 2009;27:1184–1190.

89. Claus EB, Schildkraut J, Iversen ES, et al. Effect of *BRCA1* and *BRCA2* on the association between breast cancer risk and family history. *J Natl Cancer Inst.* 1998;90:1824–1829.

90. Korde LA, Mueller CM, Loud JT, et al. No evidence of excess breast cancer risk among mutation-negative women from *BRCA* mutation-positive families. *Breast Cancer Res Treat.* 2011;125:169–173.

91. Kauff ND, Mitra N, Robson ME, et al. Risk of ovarian cancer in *BRCA1* and *BRCA2* mutation-negative hereditary breast cancer families. *J Natl Cancer Inst.* 2005;97:1382–1384.

92. Friedman E, Kotsopoulos J, Lubinski J, et al. Spontaneous and therapeutic abortions and the risk of breast cancer among *BRCA* mutation carriers. *Breast Cancer Res* 2006;8:R15 (doi:10.1186/bcr1387).

93. Klitzman RL. *Am I My Genes? Confronting Fate and Family Secrets in the Age of Genetic Testing.* New York: Oxford University Press; 2012.

94. John EM, Hopper JL, Beck JC, et al. The Breast Cancer Family Registry: an infrastructure for cooperative multinational, interdisciplinary and translational studies of the genetic epidemiology of breast cancer. *Breast Cancer Res.* 2004;6:R375–389.

95. Oddoux C, Stuewing JP, Clayton CM, et al. The carrier frequency of the *BRCA2* 6174delT mutation among Ashkenazi Jewish individuals is approximately 1%. *Nat Genet.* 1996;14:188–190.

96. Offit K, Gilewski T, McGuire P, et al. Germline *BRCA1* 185delAG mutations in Jewish women with breast cancer. *Lancet.* 1996;347:1643–1645.

97. Neuhausen S, Gilewski T, Norton L, et al. Recurrent *BRCA2* 6174delT mutations in Ashkenazi Jewish women affected by breast cancer. *Nat Genet.* 1996; 13:126–128.

98. Whittemore AS, Gong G, John EM, et al. Prevalence of *BRCA1* mutation carriers among U.S. non-Hispanic whites. *Cancer Epidemiol Biomarkers Prev.* 2004;13:2078–2083.

99. Melhem-Bertrandt A, Bojadzieva J, Ready KJ, et al. Early onset *HER-2* positive breast cancer is associated with Germline *TP53* mutations. *Cancer.* 2011 Jul 14 (Epub ahead of print).

100. Renwick A, Thompson D, Seal S, et al. *ATM* mutations that cause ataxia-telangiectasia are breast cancer susceptibility alleles. *Nat Genet.* 2006;38: 873–875.

101. Thompson D, Seal S, Schuttle M, et al. A multicenter study of cancer incidence in *Chek2* 1100delC mutation carriers. *Cancer Epidemiol Biomarkers Prev.* 2006;15:2542–2545.

102. Frank TS, Manley SA, Olopade OI, et al. Sequence analysis of *BRCA1* and *BRCA2*: Correlation of mutations with family history and ovarian cancer risk. *J Clin Oncol.* 1998;16:2417–2425.

103. Parmigiani G, Berry DA, Aguilar O. Determining carrier probabilities for breast cancer-susceptibility genes *BRCA1* and *BRCA2*. *Am J Hum Genet.* 1998;62:145–158.

104. FORCE: Facing Our Risk of Cancer Empowered. www.facingourrisk.org

105. Offit K, Kohut K, Chagett B, et al. Cancer genetic testing and assisted reproduction. *J Clin Oncol.* 2006;24:4775–4782.

106. Chen F, Chen GK, Milliken RC, et al. Fine-mapping of breast cancer susceptibility loci characterizes genetic risk in African Americans. *Human Mol Genet.* 2011;20:4491–4503.

107. Travis RC, Reeves GK, Green J, et al. Gene-environment in 7610 women with breast cancer: prospective evidence from the Million Women Study. *Lancet.* 2010;375:2143–2151.

108. Trichopoulos D. Hypothesis: does breast cancer originate in utero? *Lancet.* 1990;335: 939–940.

109. Herbst AL, Ulfelder H, Poskanzer DC. Adenocarcinoma of the vagina. Association of maternal stilbestrol therapy with tumor appearance in young women. *N Engl J Med.* 1971;284:878–881.

110. Hoover RN, Hyer M, Pfeiffer RM, et al. Adverse health outcomes in women exposed in utero to diethylstilbestrol. *N Engl J Med.* 2011;365:1304–1314.

111. Lynch HT, Reich JW. Diethylstilbestrol, genetics, teratogenesis, and tumor spectrum in humans. *Med Hypotheses.* 1985;16:315–332.

112. Colton T, Greenberg R, Noller K, et al. Breast cancer in mothers prescribed diethylstilbestrol in pregnancy. *JAMA*. 1993;269:2096–2100.

113. Palmer JR, Wise LA, Hatch EE, et al. Prenatal diethylstilbestrol exposure and risk of breast cancer. *Cancer Epidemiol Biomarkers Prev*. 2006;15:1509–1514.

114. Xue F, Michels KB. Intrauterine factors and risk of breast cancer: a systematic review and meta-analysis of current evidence. *Lancet Oncol*. 2007;8: 1088–1100.

115. Ahlgren M, Melbye M, Wohlfahrt J, Sorensen TA. Growth patterns and the risk of breast cancer in women. *N Engl J Med*. 2004;351:1619–1626.

116. Okasha M, McCarron P, Gunnell D, Smith GD. Exposures in childhood, adolescence and early adulthood and breast cancer risk: a systematic review of the literature. *Breast Cancer Res Treat*. 2003;78:223–276.

117. Wu AH, McKean-Cowdin R, Tseng CC. Birth weight and other prenatal factors and risk of breast cancer in Asian-Americans. *Breast Cancer Res Treat*. 2011;130:917–925.

118. Hankinson SE, Colditz GA, Willett WC. The lifelong interplay of genes, lifestyle, and hormones. *Breast Cancer Res*. 2004;8:213–218.

119. Michels KB, Ekbom A. Caloric restriction. Caloric restriction and incidence of breast cancer. *JAMA*. 2004;291:1226–1230.

120. Adams MJ, Dozier A, Shore RE, et al. Breast cancer risk 55+ years after irradiation for a enlarged thymus and its implioactions for early childhood medical irradiation today. *Cancer Epidemiol Biomarkers Prev*. 2010;19:48–58.

121. King MC, Marks JH, Mandell JB for the New York Breast Cancer Study Group. Breast and ovarian cancer risks due to inherited mutations in *BRCA1* and *BRCA2*. *Science*. 2003;302:643–646.

122. Brinton LA, Schairer C, Hoover RN, et al. Menstrual factors and risk of breast cancer. *Cancer Invest*. 1988;6:245–254.

123. Bernstein L, Ross RK, Lobo R, et al. The effects of moderate physical activity on menstrual cycle patterns in adolescence: Implications for breast cancer prevention. *Br J Cancer*. 1987;55:681–685.

124. Sturgeon SR, Schairer C, Grauman D, et al. Trends in cancer mortality rates by region of the United States. *Cancer Causes Control*. 2004;15:987–995.

125. Bruzzi P, Negri E, La Vecchia C, et al. Short term increase in risk of breast cancer after full term pregnancy. *BMJ*. 1988;297:1096–1098.

126. Pathak DR. Dual effect of first term pregnancy on breast cancer risk: empirical evidence and postulated underlying biology. *Cancer Causes Control*. 2002;13:295–298.

127. Lambe M, Hsieh CC, Trichopoulos D, et al. Transient increase in the risk of breast cancer after giving birth. *N Engl J Med*. 1994;331:5–9.

128. Li CI, Malone KE, Daling JR, et al. Timing of menarche and first full-term birth in relation to breast cancer risk. *Am J Epidemiol*. 2008;167:230–239.

129. Palmer JR, Wise LA, Horton NJ, et al. Dual effect of parity on breast cancer in African-American women. *J Natl Cancer Inst*. 2003;95:478–483.

130. Balogh GA, Russo J, Mailo DA, et al. Genomic signature induced by pregnancy in the human breast. *Int J Oncol*. 2006;28:399–410.

131. Terry MB, Perrin M, Salafia CM, et al. Preeclampsia, pregnancy-related hypertension, and breast cancer risk. *Am J Epidemiol*. 2007;165:1007–1014.

132. Andrieu N, Goldgar DE, Easton DF, et al. Pregnancies, breast-feeding, and breast cancer risk in the International BRCA1/2 Carrier Cohort Study (IBCCS). *J Natl Cancer Inst*. 2006;98:535–544.

133. Cullinane CA, Lubinski J, Neuhausen SL, et al. Effect of pregnancy as a risk factor for breast cancer in BRCA1/BRCA2 mutation carriers. *Int J Cancer*. 2005;117:988–991.

134. Jernstrom H, Lubinski J, Lynch HT, et al. Breast-feeding and the risk of breast cancer in BRCA1 and BRCA2 mutation carriers. *J Natl Cancer Inst*. 2004;96:1094–1098.

135. Newcomb PA, Storer BE, Longnecker MP, et al. Lactation and a reduced risk of premenopausal breast cancer. *N Engl J Med*. 1994;330:81–87.

136. Collaborative Group on Hormonal Factors in Breast Cancer. Breast cancer and breastfeeding: collaborative reanalysis of individual data from 47 epidemiological studies in 30 countries, including 50,302 women with breast cancer and 96,973 women without the disease. *Lancet*. 2002;360:187–195.

137. Titus-Ernstoff L, Egan KM, Newcomb PA, et al. Exposure to breast milk in infancy and adult breast cancer risk. *J Natl Cancer Inst*. 1998; 90:921–924.

138. Daling JR, Malone KE, Voigt LF, et al. Risk of breast cancer among young women: relationship to induced abortion. *J Natl Cancer Inst*. 1994;86: 1569–1570.

139. Newcomb PA, Storer BE, Longnecker MP, et al. Pregnancy termination in relation to risk of breast cancer. *JAMA*. 1996;275:321–322.

140. Howe HL, Senie RT, Bzduch H, Herzfeld O. Early abortion and breast cancer risk among women under age 40. *Int J Epidemiol*. 1989;18:300–304.

141. Pike MC, Henderson BE, Casagrande JT, et al. Oral contraceptive use and early abortion as risk factors for breast cancer in young women. *Br J Cancer*. 1981;43:72–76.

142. Beral V, Bull D, Doll R, et al. Breast cancer and abortion: collaborative reanalysis of data from 53 epidemiological studies, including 83,000 women with breast cancer from 16 countries. *Lancet*. 2004;363:1007–1016.

143. Henderson KD, Sullivan-Halley J, Reynolds P, et al. Incomplete pregnancy is not associated with breast cancer risk: the California Teachers Study. *Contraception*. 2008;77:391–396.

144. Huang Z, Hankinson SE, Colditz GA, et al. Dual effects of weight and weight gain on breast cancer risk. *JAMA*. 1997;278:1407–1411.

145. Kelsey JL, Bernstein L. Epidemiology and prevention of breast cancer. *Annu Rev Public Health*. 1996;17:47–67.

146. Morris PG, Hudis CA, Giri D, et al. Inflammation and increased aromatase expression occur in the breast tissue of obese women with breast cancer. *Cancer Prev Res*. 2011;4:1021–1029.

147. John EM, Sangaramoorthy M, Phipps AI, et al. Adult body size, hormone receptor status, and premenopausal breast cancer risk in a multiethnic population. The San Francisco Bay Area Breast Cancer Study. *Am J Epidemiol*. 2010;173:201–216.

148. Baer HJ, Colditz GA, Rosner B, et al. Body fattness during childhood and adolescence and incidence of breast cancer in premenopausal women: a prospective cohort study. *Breast Cancer Res*. 2005;7:R314–R325.

149. The Endogenous Hormones and Breast Cancer Collaborative Group. Endogenous sex hormones and breast cancer in postmenopausal women: reanalysis of nine prospective studies. *J Natl Cancer Inst*. 2002;94:606–616.

150. Key T, Appleby P, Barnes I, Reeves G. Endogenous sex hormones and breast cancer in postmenopausal women: reanalysis of nine prospective studies. *J Natl Cancer Inst*. 2002;94:606–616.

151. Missmer SA, Eliassen AH, Barbieri RL, Hankinson SE. Endogenous estrogen, androgen, and progesterone concentrations and breast cancer risk among postmenopausal women. *J Natl Cancer Inst*. 2004;96:1856–1865.

152. Gammon MD. John EM, Britton JA. Recreational and occupational physical activities and risk of breast cancer. *J Natl Cancer Inst*. 1998;90:100–117.

153. Anderson TJ. Mitotic activity in the breast. *J Obstet Gynecol*. 1984;4: S114–118.

154. Cancer and Steroid Hormone Study of the Centers for Disease Control and the National Institute of Child Health and Human Development. Oral contraceptive use and the risk of breast cancer. *N Engl J Med*. 1986;315: 405–411.

155. Reeves GK, Banks E, Key TJA. The impact of exogenous hormone use on breast cancer risk. In: Henderson BE, Ponder B, Ross RK, eds. *Hormones, Genes, and Cancer*. New York: Oxford University Press; 2003:130–156.

156. Marchbanks PA, Curtis KM, Mandel MG, et al. Oral contraceptive formulation and risk of breast cancer. *Contraception*. 2011 Sept 28 (Epub ahead of print)

157. Collaborative Group on Hormonal Factors in Breast Cancer. Breast cancer and hormonal contraceptives: collaborative re-analysis of individual data on 53,297 women with breast cancer and 100,239 women without breast cancer from 54 epidemiological studies. *Lancet*. 1996;347:1713–1724.

158. Marchbanks PA, McDonald JA, Wilson HG, et al. Oral contraceptives and the risk of breast cancer. *N Engl J Med*. 2002;346:2025–2032.

159. Davidson NE, Helzlsouer KJ. Good news about oral contraceptives. Editorial. *N Engl J Med*. 2002;346:2078–2079.

160. Haile RW, Thomas DC, McGuire V, et al. BRCA1 and BRCA2 mutation carriers, oral contraceptive use, and breast cancer before age 50. *Cancer Epidemiol Biomarkers Prev*. 2006;15:1863–1870.

161. Terry KL, Willett WC, Rich-Edwards JW, et al. A prospective study of infertility due to ovulatory disorders, ovulation induction, and incidence of breast cancer. *Arch Intern Med*. 2006;166:2484–2489.

162. Rossing MA, Daling JR, Weiss NS, et al. Risk of breast cancer in a cohort of infertile women. *Gynecol Oncol*. 1996;60:3–7.

163. Brinton LA, Scoccia B, Moghissi KS, et al. Breast cancer risk associated with ovulation-stimulating drugs. *Human Reprod*. 2004;19:2005–2013.

164. Venn A, Watson L, Bruinsma F, et al. Risk of cancer after use of fertility drugs with in-vitro fertilization. *Lancet*. 1999;354:1586–1590.

165. Kallen B, Finnstrom O, Lindam A, et al. Malignancies among women who gave birth after in vitro fertilization. *Human Reprod*. 2011;26:253–258.

166. Pike MC. The role of mammographic density in evaluating changes in breast cancer risk. *Gynecol Endocrinol*. 2005;21(suppl 1):1–5.

167. Trichopoulos D, Mac Mahon B, Cole P. The menopause and breast cancer risk. *J Natl Cancer Inst*. 1972;48:605–613.

168. Eisen A, Lubinski J, Klijn J, et al. Breast cancer risk following bilateral oophorectomy in BRCA1 and BRCA2 mutation carriers: an international case-control study. *J Clin Oncol* 2005;23:7491–7496.

169. Senie RT, Lobenthal SW, Rosen PP. Association of vaginal smear cytology with menstrual status in breast cancer. *Breast Cancer Res Treat*. 1985;5: 301–310.

170. Parker WH, Broder MS, Chang E, et al. Ovarian conservation at the time of hysterectomy and long-term health outcomes in the Nurses' Health Study. *Obstet Gynecol*. 2009;113:1027–1037.

171. Henderson KD. Bernstein L, Henderson B, et al. Predictors of the timing of natural menopause in the Multiethnic Cohort Study. *Am J Epidemiol*. 2008;167:1287–1294.

172. Jacoby VL, Fujimoto VY, Giudice LC, et al. Racial and ethnic disparities in benign gynecologic conditions and associated surgeries. *Am J Obstet Gynecol*. 2010; 202:514–521.

173. Grady D, Rubin SM, Petitti DB, et al. Hormone therapy to prevent disease and prolong life in postmenopausal women. *Ann Int Med*. 1992;117:1016.

174. Gorsky RD, Koplan JP, Peterson HB, Thacker SB. Relative risks and benefits of long-term estrogen replacement therapy: a decision analysis. *Obstet Gynecol*. 1994;83:161–166.

175. Barrett-Connor E, Stuenkel CA. Hormone replacement therapy (HRT)-risks and benefits. *Int J Epidemiol*. 2001;423–426.

176. Matthews KA, Kuller LH, Wing RR, et al. Prior to use of estrogen replacement therapy, are users healthier than nonusers? *Am J Epidemiol*. 1996;143: 971–978.

177. Collaborative Group on Hormonal Factors in Breast Cancer. Breast cancer and hormone replacement therapy: collaborative reanalysis of data from 51 epidemiological studies of 52,705 women with breast cancer and 108,411 women without breast cancer. *Lancet*. 1997;350:1047–1059.
178. Schairer C, Lubin J, Troisi R, et al. Menopausal estrogen and estrogen-progestin replacement therapy and breast cancer risk. *JAMA*. 2000;283:485–491.
179. Ross RK, Paganini-Hill A, Wan PC, Pike MC. Effect of hormone replacement therapy on breast cancer risk: estrogen versus estrogen plus progestin. *J Natl Cancer Inst*. 2000;92:328–332.
180. Pike MC, Spicer DV, Dahmoush L, Press MF. Estrogens, progestagen, normal breast cell proliferation, and breast cancer risk. *Epidemiol Rev*. 1993;15:17–35.
181. Newcomb PA, Titus-Ernstoff L, Egan KM, et al. Postmenopausal estrogen and progestin use in relation to breast cancer risk. *Cancer Epidemiol Biomarkers Prev*. 2002;11:593–600.
182. Shantakumar S, Terry MB, Paykin A, et al. Age and menopausal effects of hormonal birth control and hormone replacement therapy in relation to breast cancer risk. *Am J Epidemiol*. 2007;165:1187–1198.
183. Kerlikowske K, Miglioretti DL, Ballard-Barbash R, et al. Prognostic characteristics of breast cancer among postmenopausal hormone users in a screened population. *J Clin Oncol*. 2003;21:4314–4321.
184. Chlebowski RT, Kuller LH, Prentice RL, et al. Breast cancer after use of estrogen plus progestin in postmenopausal women. *N Engl J Med*. 2009;360:573–587.
185. Love SM. *Dr. Susan Love's Hormone Book*. New York: Random House; 1997.
186. Love SM. *Dr. Susan Love's Menopause and Hormone Book, Making Informed Choices*. New York: Three Rivers Press; 2003.
187. Crandall CJ, Aragaki AK, Chlebowski RT, et al. New-onset breast tenderness after initiation of estrogen plus progestin therapy and breast cancer risk. *Arch Intern Med*. 2009;169:1684–1691.
188. Crandall CJ, Aragaki AK, Cauley JA, et al. Breast tenderness after initiation of conjugated equine estrogens and mammographic density change. *Breast Cancer Res Treat*. 2012;131:969–979.
189. Chlebowski RT, Anderson G, Manson JE, et al. Estrogen alone in postmenopausal women and breast cancer detection by means of mammography and breast biopsy. *J Clin Oncol*. 2010;28:2690–2697.
190. Farhat GN, Walker R, Buist DS, et al. Changes in invasive breast cancer and ductal carcinoma in situ rates in relation to the decline in hormone therapy use. *J Clin Oncol*. 2010;28:5140–5146.
191. Robbins AS, Clarke CA. Regional changes in hormone therapy use and breast cancer incidence in California from 2001 to 2004. *J Clin Oncol*. 2007;25:3437–3439.
192. Marshall SF, Clarke CA, Deapen D, et al. Recent breast cancer incidence trends according to hormone therapy use: the California Teachers Study cohort. *Breast Cancer Res* 2010;12:R4.
193. Wolfe JN, Saftlas AF, Salane M. Mammographic parenchymal patterns and quantitative evaluation of mammographic densities: a case-control study. *Am J Radiol*. 1987;148:1087–1092.
194. Gram IT, Funkhouser E, Tabar L. The Tabar classification of mammographic parenchymal patterns. *Eur J Radiol*. 1997;24:131–136.
195. Byrne C, Schairer C, Wolfe J, et al. Mammographic features and breast cancer risk: effects of time, age, and menopausal status. *J Natl Cancer Inst* 1995;87:1622–1629.
196. Byng JW, Boyd NF, Fishell E, et al. The quantitative analysis of mammographic densities. *Phys Med Biol*. 1994;39:1629–1638.
197. Boyd NF, Martin LJ, Bronskill M, et al. Breast tissue composition and susceptibility to breast cancer. *J Natl Cancer Inst*. 2010;102:1224–1237.
198. Boyd NF, Dite GS, Stone J, et al. Heritability of mammographic density. A risk factor for breast cancer. *N Engl J Med*. 2002;347:886–894.
199. Vachon CM, Sellers TA, Carlson EE, et al. Strong Evidence of a genetic determinant for mammographic density, a major risk factor for breast cancer. *Cancer Res*. 2007;67:8412–8418.
200. Boyd NF, Lockwood GA, Martin LJ, et al. Mammographic density and risk of breast cancer among subjects with a family history of this disease. *J Natl Cancer Inst*. 1999;91:1404–1408.
201. Greendale GA, Reboussin BA, Slone S, et al. Postmenopausal hormone therapy and change in mammographic density. *J Natl Cancer Inst*. 2003;95:30–37.
202. McTiernan A, Chlebowski RT, Martin C, et al. Conjugated equine estrogen influence on mammographic density in postmenopausal women in a substudy of the Women's Health Initiative Randomized trial. *J Clin Oncol*. 2009;27:6135–6143.
203. Cuzick J, Warwick J, Pinney E, et al. Tamoxifen and breast density in women at increased risk of breast cancer. *J Natl Cancer Inst*. 2004;96:621–628.
204. Tehranifar P, Reynolds D, Flom J, et al. Reproductive and menstrual factors and mammographic density in African American, Caribbean, and white women. *Cancer Causes Control*. 2011;22:599–610.
205. Flom JD, Ferris JS, Tehranifar P, Terry MB. Alcohol intake over the life course and mammographic density. *Breast Cancer Res Treat*. 2009;117:643–651.
206. Land CE. Studies of cancer and radiation dose among atomic bomb survivors: the example of breast cancer. *JAMA*. 1995;274:402–407.
207. Hoffman DA, Lonstein JE, Morin MM, et al. Breast cancer in women with scoliosis exposed to multiple diagnostic x-rays. *J Natl Cancer Inst*. 1989;81:1307–1312.
208. Boice JD Jr, Preston D, Davis FG, et al. Frequent chest x-ray fluoroscopy and breast cancer incidence among tuberculosis patients in Massachusetts. *Radiat Res*. 1991;125:214–222.
209. Shore RE, Hildreth N, Woodard E, et al. Breast cancer among women given X-ray therapy for acute postpartum mastitis. *J Natl Cancer Inst*. 1986;77:689–696.
210. De Bruin ML, Sparidans J, van't Veer MB, et al. Breast cancer risk in female survivors of Hodgkin's lymphoma: Lower risk asfter smaller radiation volume. *J Clin Oncol*. 2009;27:4239–4246.
211. McGregor DH, Land CE, Choi K, et al. Breast cancer incidence among atomic bomb survivors, Hiroshima and Nagasaki, 1950–1969. *J Natl Cancer Inst*. 1977;59:799–811.
212. John EM, Kelsey JL. Radiation and other environmental exposures and breast cancer. *Epidemiol Rev*. 1993;15:157–162.
213. Hildreth NG, Shore RE, Dvoretsky PM. The risk of breast cancer after irradiation of the thymus in infancy. *N Engl J Med*. 1989;321:1281–1284.
214. Shore RE, Woodard E, Hempelmann LH, Pasternack BS. Synergism between radiation and other risk factor for breast cancer. *Prev Med*. 1980;9:815–822.
215. Bhatia S, Robison LL, Oberlin O, et al. Breast cancer and other second neoplasms after childhood Hodgkin's disease. *N Engl J Med*. 1996;334:745–751.
216. John EM, Phipps AI, Knight JA, et al. Medical radiation exposure and breast cancer risk: findings from the Breast Cancer Family Registry. *Int J Cancer*. 2007;121:386–394.
217. Brenner DJ. Medical imaging in the 21st century—Getting the best bang for the rad. *N Engl J Med*. 2010;362:943–945.
218. Schatzkin A, Jones DY, Hoover RN, et al. Alcohol consumption and breast cancer in the epidemiologic follow-up study of the first National Health and Nutrition Examination Survey. *N Engl J Med*. 1987;316:1169–1173.
219. Longnecker MP, Newcomb PA, Mittendorf R, et al. Risk of breast cancer in relation to lifetime alcohol consumption. *J Natl Cancer Inst*. 1995;87:923–929.
220. Horn-Ross PL, Canchola AJ, West DW, et al. Patterns of alcohol consumption and breast cancer risk in California Teachers Study cohort. *Cancer Epidemiol Biomarkers Prev*. 2004;13:405–455.
221. McDonald JA, Mandel MG, Marchbanks PA, et al. Alcohol exposure and breast cancer: results of the women's Contraceptive and Reproductive Experience Study. *Cancer Epidemiol Biomarkers Prev*. 2004;2106–2116.
222. Newcomb PA, Egan KM, Trentham-Dietz A, et al. Prediagnostic use of hormone therapy and mortality after breast cancer. *Cancer Epidemiol Biomarkers Prev*. 2008;17:864–871.
223. Li Y, Baer D, Friedman GD, et al. Wine, liquor, beer and risk of breast cancer in a large population. *Eur J Cancer*. 2009;45:843–850.
224. Li CI, Malone KE, Porter PL, et al. The relationship between alcohol use and risk of breast cancer by histology and hormone receptor status among women ages 65–79 years of age. *Cancer Epidemiol Biomarkers Prev*. 2003;12:1061–1066.
225. Kabat GC, Kim M, Shikany JM, et al. Alcohol consumption and risk of duct carcinoma in situ of the breast in a cohort of postmenopausal women. *Cancer Biomarkers Epidemiol Prev*. 2010;19:2066–2072.
226. Willett WC. Diet and breast cancer. *J Intern Med*. 2001;249:395–411.
227. Sun Q, Townsend MK, Okereka OI, et al. Alcohol consumption at midlife and successful ageing in women: a prospective cohort analysis in the Nurses' Health Study. *PloS Med*. 2011;8:Issue 9.
228. Cui Y, Miller AB, Rohan TE. Cigarette smoking and breast cancer risk: update of a prospective cohort study. *Breast Cancer Res Treat*. 2006;100:293–299.
229. MacMahon B, Trichopoulos D, Cole P, Brown J. Cigarette smoking and urinary estrogens. *N Engl J Med*. 1982; 307:1062–1065.
230. Baron JA, La Vecchia C, Levi F. The antiestrogenic effect of cigarette smoking in women. *Am J Obstet Gynecol*. 1990;162:502–514.
231. Ambrosone CB, Freudenheim JL, Graham S, et al. Cigarette smoking, N-Acetyltransferase 2 genetic polymorphisms, and breast cancer risk. *JAMA*. 1996;276:1494–1501.
232. Reynolds P, Hurley S, Goldberg DE, et al. Active smoking, household passive smoking, and breast cancer: evidence from the California Teachers Study. *J Natl Cancer Inst*. 2004;96:29–37.
233. Gammon MD, Eng SM, Teitelbaum SL, et al. Environmental tobacco smoke and breast cancer incidence. *Environ Res*. 2004;96:176–185.
234. Egan KM, Stampfer MJ, Hunter D, et al. Active and passive smoking in breast cancer: prospective results from the Nurses Health Study. *Epidemiology* 2002;13:138–145.
235. Breast Cancer Family Registry. Smoking and risk of breast cancer in carriers of mutations in *BRCA1* and *BRCA2* aged less than 50 years. *Breast Cancer Res Treat*. 2008;109:67–75.
236. Ginsburg O, Ghadirian P, Lubinski J, et al. Smoking and the risk of breast cancer in *BRCA1* and *BRCA2* carriers: an update. *Breast Cancer Res Treat*. 2009;114:127–135.
237. Schreinemachers DM, Everson RB. Aspirin use and lung, colon, and breast cancer incidence in a prospective study. *Epidemiology*. 1994;5:138–146.
238. Egan KM, Stampfer MJ, Giovannucci E, et al. Prospective study of regular aspirin use and risk of breast cancer. *J Natl Cancer Inst*. 1996;88:988–993.
239. Harris RE, Chlebowski RT, Jackson RD, et al. Breast cancer and nonsteroidal anti-inflammatory drugs: Prospective results from the Women's Health Initiative. *Cancer Res*. 2003;63:6096–6101.
240. Terry MB, Gammon MD, Zhang FF, et al. Association of frequency and duration of aspirin use and hormone receptor status with breast cancer risk. *JAMA*. 2004;291:2433–2440.
241. Marshall SF, Bernstein L, Anton-Culver H, et al. Nonsteroidal anti-inflammatory drug use and breast cancer risk by stage and hormone receptor status. *J Natl Cancer Inst*. 2005;97:805–812.

242. Jacobs EJ, Thun MJ, Connell CJ, et al. Aspirin and other nonsteroidal anti-inflammatory drugs and breast cancer incidence in a large U.S. cohort. *Cancer Epidemiol Biomarkers Prev.* 2005;14:261–264.

243. Gierach GL, Lacey JV, Schatzkin A, et al. Nonsteroidal anti-inflammatory drugs and breast cancer risk in the National Institutes of Health-AARP Diet and Health Study. *Breast Cancer Res.* 2008;10:R38. (doi:10.1186/bcr2089).

244. Takkouche B, Regueira-Mendez C, Etminan M. Breast cancer and use of nonsteroidal anti-inflammatory drugs: a meta-analysis. *J Natl Cancer Inst.* 2008;100:1439–1447.

245. Bardia A, Olson JE, Vachon CM, et al. Effect of aspirin and other NSAIDS on postmenopausal breast cancer incidence by hormone receptor status: results from a prospective study. *Breast Cancer Res Treat.* 2011;126:149–155.

246. Gates MA, Tworoger SS, Eliassen AH, et al. Analgesic use and sex steroid hormone concentrations in postmenopausal women. *Cancer Epidemiol Biomarkers Prev.* 2010;19:1033–1041.

247. Frisch RE, Wyshak G, Vincent L. Delayed menarche and amenorrhea in ballet dancers. *N Engl J Med.* 1980;303:17–19.

248. Cummings DC, Wheeler GD, Harber VJ. Physical activity, nutrition, and reproduction. *Ann NY Acad Sci.* 1994;709:55–76.

249. Frisch RE, Wyshak G, Albright NL, et al. Lower prevalence of breast cancer and cancers of the reproductive system among former college athletes compared to non-athletes. *Br J Cancer.* 1985;52:885–889.

250. Wyshak G, Frisch RE. Breast cancer among former college athletes compared to non-athletes: a 15-year follow-up. *Br J Cancer.* 2000;82:726–730.

251. Bernstein L, Henderson BE, Hanisch R, et al. Physical exercise and reduced risk of breast cancer in young women. *J Natl Cancer Inst.* 1994;86:1403–1408.

252. Maruti SS, Willett WC, Feskanich D, et al. A prospective study of age-specific physical activity and premenopausal breast cancer. *J Natl Cancer Inst.* 2008;100:728–737.

253. Tworoger SS, Sorenson B, Chubak J, et al. Effect of a 12-month randomized clinical trial of exercise on serum prolactin concentrations in postmenopausal women. *Cancer Epidemiol Biomarkers Prev.* 2007;16:895–899.

254. Friedenreich CM, Woolcott CG, McTiernan A, et al. Alberta Physical Activity and Breast Cancer Prevention Trial: sex hormone changes in a year-long exercise intervention among postmenopausal women. *J Clin Oncol.* 2010;28:1458–1466.

255. Rundle A. molecular epidemiology of physical activity and cancer. *Cancer Epidemiol Biomarkers Prev.* 2005;14:227–236.

256. Harashima E, Nakagawa Y, Urata G, et al. Time-lag estimate between dietary intake and breast cancer mortality in Japan. *Asia Pac J Clin Nutr.* 2007;16:193–198.

257. Prentice RL, Chlebowski RT, Patterson R, et al. Low-fat dietary pattern and risk of invasive breast cancer: the Women's Health Initiative Randomized Controlled Dietary Intewrvention Trial. *JAMA.* 2006;295:629–642.

258. Goldin BR, Aldercreutz H, Gorbach SL, et al. Estrogen excretion patterns ad plasma levels in vegetarian and omnivorous women. *N Engl J Med.* 1982;307:1542–1547.

259. Garland FC, Garland CF, Gorham ED, Young JF. Geographic variation in breast cancer mortality in the United States: a hypothesis involving exposure to solar radiation. *Prev Med.* 1990;19:614–622.

260. Grant WB. An ecologic study of dietary and solar ultraviolet-B links to breast carcinoma mortality rates. *Cancer.* 2002;94:272–281.

261. John EM, Schwartz GG, Dreon DM, et al. Vitamin D and breast cancer risk: The NHANES I Epidemiologic Follow-up Study, 1971–1975 to 1992 *Cancer Epidemiol Biomarkers Prev.* 1999;8:399–406.

262. Crew KD, Gammon MD, Steck SE, et al. Association between plasma 25-hydroxyvitamin D and breast cancer risk. *Cancer Prev Res.* 2009;2:598–604.

263. Bertone-Johnson ER, Chen WY, Holick MF, et al. Plasma 25-Hydroxyvitamin D and 1,25-dihydroxyvitamin D and risk of breast cancer. *Cancer Biomarkers Epidemiol Prev.* 2005;14:1991–1997.

264. Garland CF, Gorham ED, Mohr SB, et al. Vitamin D and prevention of breast cancer. Pooled analysis. *J Steroid Biochem Mol Bio.* 2007;103:708–711.

265. Chlebowski RT, Johnson KC, Kooperberg C, et al. Calcium plus vitamin D supplementation and the risk of breast cancer. *J Natl Cancer Inst.* 2007:100:1581–1591.

266. Lappe JM, Travers-Gustafson D, Davies KM, et al. Vitamin D and calcium supplementation reduces cancer risk: results of a randomized trial. *Am J Clin Nutr.* 2007;85:1586–1591.

267. Autier P, Gandini S. Vitamin D supplementation and total mortality. A meta-analysis of randomized controlled trials. *Arch Int Med.* 2007;167:1730–1737.

268. Gandini S, Boniol M, Haukka J, et al. Meta-analysis of observational studies of serum 25-hydroxyvitamin D levels and colorectal, breast, and prostate cancer and colorectal adenoma. *Int J Cancer.* 2011;128:1414–1424.

269. Fenton SE, Reed C, Newbold RR. Perinatal environmental exposures affect mammary development, function, and cancer risk in adulthood. *Annu Rev Pharmacol Toxicol.* 2012;52:455–479.

270. Russo J, Tay LK, Russo IH. Differentiation of the mammary gland and susceptibility to carcinogenesis. *Breast Cancer Res Treat.* 1982;2:5–73.

271. Teitelbaum SL, Gammon MD, Britton JA, et al. Reported residential pesticide use and breast cancer risk on Long Island, New York. *Am J Epidemiol.* 2006;165:643–651.

272. Gammon MD, Wolff MS, Neugut AI, et al. Environmental toxins and breast cancer on Long Island. II. Organochlorine compound levels in blood. *Cancer Epidemiol Biomarkers Prev.* 2002;11:686–697.

273. Wolff MS, Britton JA, Wilson VP. Environmental risk factors for breast cancer among African-American women. *Cancer.* 2003;97(suppl 1):289–310.

274. Bittner JJ. Possible relationship of the estrogenic hormones, genetic susceptibility and milk influence in the production of mammary cancer in mice. *Cancer Res.* 1942;2:710–721.

275. Holland JP, Pogo BGT. Mouse mammary tumor virus-like viral infection and human breast cancer. *Clin Cancer Res.* 2004;10:5647–5649.

276. Melana SM, Nepomnaschy I, Sakalian M, et al. Characterization of viral particles isolated from primary cultures of human breast cancer cells. *Cancer Res.* 2007;67:8960–8965.

277. Etkin PR, Stewart AFR, Wiernik PH. Mouse mammary tumor virus (MMTV)-like DNA sequences in the breast tumors of father, mother, and daughter. *Infect Agent Cancer.* 2008;3:2.

278. Johal H, Ford C, Glenn W, et al. Mouse mammary tumor like virus sequences in breast milk from healthy lactating women. *Breast Cancer Res Treat.* 2011;129:149–155.

279. Antonsson A, Spurr TP, Chen AC, et al. High prevalence of human papillomaviruses in fresh frozen breast cancer samples. *J Med Virol.* 2011;83:2157–2163.

280. Baltzell K, Buehring GC, Krishnamurthy S, et al. Limited evidence of human papillomavirus on breast tissue using molecular in situ methods. *Cancer.* 2011 Aug 5 (Epub ahead of print).

281. Costantino J, Gail MH, Pee D, et al. Validation studies for models projecting the risk of invasive and total breast cancer incidence. *J Natl Cancer Inst.* 1999;91:1541–1548.

282. Gail MH, Costantino JP, Pee D, et al. Projecting individualized absolute invasive breast cancer in African American women. *J Natl Cancer Inst.* 2007;99:1782–1792.

283. Matsuno RK, Costantino JP, Ziegler RG, et al. Projecting individualized absolute invasive breast cancer risk in Asian and Pacific Islander American women. *J Natl Cancer Inst.* 2011;103:951–961.

284. Rockhill B, Spiegelman D, Byrne C, et al. Validation of the Gail et al. Model of breast cancer risk prediction and implications for chemoprevention. *J Natl Cancer Inst.* 2001;93:358–366.

285. Bondy ML, Lustbader ED, Halabi S, et al. Validation of a breast cancer risk assessment model in women with a positive family history. *J Natl Cancer Inst.* 1994;86:620–625.

286. Tice JA, Cummings SR, Ziv E, Kerlikowske K. Mammographic breast density and the Gail model for breast cancer risk prediction in a screening population. *Breast Cancer Res Treat.* 2005;94:115–122.

287. Stovall M, Smith SA, Langholz BM, et al. Does to the contralateral breast from radiotherapy and risk of second primary breast cancer in the WECARE Study. *Int J Radiation Oncology Biol Phys.* 2008;72:1021–1030.

288. Kurian AW, Gong GD, John EM, et al. Breast cancer risk for noncarriers of family-specific *BRCA1* and *BRCA2* mutations: findings from the Breast Cancer Family Registry. *J Clin Oncol.* 2011;29:4505–4509.

289. Nsouli HH, Henson DE, Younes N, et al. Second primary breast, endometrial, and ovarian cancers in black and white breast cancer survivors over a 35-year time span: effect of age. *Breast Cancer Res Treat.* 2011;129:963–969.

290. Lehman CD, Gatsonis C, Kuhl CK, et al. MRI evaluation of the contralateral breast in women with recently diagnosed breast cancer. *N Engl J Med.* 2007;356:1295–1303.

291. Bernstein JL, Haile RW, Stovall M, et al. Radiation exposure, the ATM gene, and contralateral breast cancer in the Women's Environmental Cancer and Radiation Epidemiology Study. *J Natl Cancer Inst.* 2010;102:475–483.

292. Bertelsen L, Bernstein L, Olsen JH, et al. Effect of systemic adjuvant treatment on risk for contralateral breast cancer in the Women's Environment, Cancer and Radiation Epidemiology Study. *J Natl Cancer Inst.* 2008; 100:32–40.

293. Elkin EB, Klem ML, Gonzales AM, et al. Characteristics and outcomes of breast cancer in women with and without a history of radiation for Hodgkin's lymphoma: a multi-institutional, matched cohort study. *J Clin Oncol.* 2011;29:2466–2473.

294. Malone KE, Begg CB, Haile RW, et al. Population-based study of the risk of second primary contralateral breast cancer associated with carrying a mutation in *BRCA1* or *BRCA2*. *J Clin Oncol.* 2010;28:2404–2410.

295. Metcalfe K, Lynch HP, et al. Contralateral breast cancer in *BRCA1* and *BRCA2* mutation carriers. *J Clin Oncol.* 2004;22:2328–2335.

296. Fisher B. Role of science in the treatment of breast cancer when tumor multicentricity is present. *J Natl Cancer Inst.* 2011;103:1292–1298.

297. Tuttle TM, Jarosek S, Habermann EB, et al. Increasing rates of contralateral prophylactic mastectomy among patients with ductal carcinoma in situ. *J Clin Oncol.* 2009;27:1362–1367.

298. Dick AW, Sorbero MS, Ahrendt GM, et al. Comparative effectiveness of ductal carcinoma in situ management and the roles of margins and surgeons. *J Natl Cancer Inst.* 2011;103:92–104.

299. Hartmann LC, Sellers TA, Schaid DJ, et al. Efficacy of bilateral prophylactic mastectomy in *BRCA1* and *BRCA2* gene mutation carriers. *J Natl Cancer Inst.* 2001;93:1633–1637.

300. Beatson GT. On the treatment of inoperable cases of carcinoma of the mamma: suggestions for a new method of treatment with illustrative cases. *Lancet.* 1896;2:104–107.

301. Petrak JA, Naughton MJ, Case LD, et al. Incidence, time course, and determinants of menstrual bleeding after breast cancer treatment: a prospective study. *J Clin Oncol.* 2006;24:1045–1051.

302. Walshe JM, Denduluri N, Swain SM. Amenorrhea in premenopausal women after adjuvant chemotherapy for breast cancer. *J Clin Oncol.* 2006;24: 5769–5779.

303. Griggs JJ, Somerfield MR, Anderson H, et al. American Society of Clinical Oncology endorsement of the Cancer Care Ontario Proactice Guideline on adjuvant ovarian ablation in the treatment of premenopausal women with early-stage invasive breast cancer. *J Clin Oncol.* 2011;29:3939–3942.

304. Fisher B, Costantino JP, Wickerham JP, et al. Tamoxifen for prevention of breast cancer: report of the National Surgical Adjuvant Breast and Bowel Project P-1 Study. *J Natl Cancer Inst.* 1998;90:1371–1388.

305. Visvanathan K, Chlebowski RT, Hurley P, et al. American Society of Clinical Oncology clinical practice guideline update on the use of pharmacologic interventions including tamoxifen, raloxifene, and aromatase inhibition for breast cancer risk reduction. *J Clin Oncol.* 2009;27:3235–3258.

306. Early Breast Cancer Trialists' Collaborative Group (EBCTCG). Systemic treatment of early breast cancer by hormonal, cytoxic, or immune therapy: 133 randomized trials involving 31,000 recurrences and 24,000 deaths among 72,000 women. *Lancet.* 1992;339:1–15,71–85.

307. Early Breast Cancer Trialists' Collaborative Group (EBCTCG). Effects of chemotherapy and hormonal therapy for early breast cancer on recurrence and 15-yearsurvival:an overview of the randomized trials. *Lancet.* 2005;365:1687–1717.

308. Davidson NE. Tamoxifen—panacea or Pandora's box? *N Engl J Med.* 1992;326:885–886.

309. Bernstein L, Deapen D, Cerhan JR, et al. Tamoxifen therapy for breast cancer and endometrial cancer risk. *J Natl Cancer Inst.* 1999;91:1654–1662.

310. Early Breast Cancer Trialists' Collaborative Group (EBCTCG). Relevance of breast cancer hormone receptors and other factors to the efficacy of adjuvant tamoxifen: patient-level meta-analysis of randomised trials. *Lancet.* 2011;378:771–784.

311. Fisher B, Anderson S, Bryant J, et al. Twenty-year follow-up of a randomized trial comparing total mastectomy, lumpectomy, and lumpectomy plus irradiation for the treatment of invasive breast cancer. *N Engl J Med.* 2002;347:1233–1241.

312. Clarke M, Collins R, Darby S, et al. Effects of radiotherapy and of differences in extent of surgery for early breast cancer on local recurrence and 15-year survival: an overview of randomized trials. *Lancet.* 2005;366:2087–2106.

313. Hughes KS, Schnaper LA, Berry D, et al. Lumpectomy plus tamoxifen with or without irradiation in women 70 years of age or older with early breast cancer. *N Engl J Med.* 2004;351:971–977.

314. Petrak JA, Senie RT, Peters M, Rosen JA. Lymphedema in a cohort of breast carcinoma survivors 20 years after diagnosis. *Cancer.* 2001;92:1368–1377.

315. Mandelblatt JS, Edge SB, Meropol NJ, et al. Sequelae of axillary lymph node dissection in older women with stage 1 and 2 breast carcinoma. *Cancer.* 2002;95:2445–2454.

316. Ahmed RL, Scmitz KH, Prizment AE, Folsom AR. Risk factors for lymphedema in breast cancer survivors, the Iowa Women's Health Study. *Breast Cancer Res Treat.* 2011 Jul 15 (Epub ahead of print)

317. Helyer LK, Varnic M, Le LW, et al. Obesity is a risk factor for developing postoperative lymphedema in breast cancer patients. *Breast J.* 2010;16:48–54.

318. Szuba A, Achalu R, Rockson SG. Decongestive lymphatic therapy for patients with breast carcinoma-associated lymphedema. *Cancer.* 2002;95:2260–2267.

319. Cassileth BR, Van Zee KJ, Chan Y, et al. A safety and efficacy pilot study of acupuncture for treatment of chronic lymphedema. *Acupunct Med.* 2011;doi:10.1136.

320. McLaughlin SA, Wright MJ, Morris KT, et al. Prevalence of lymphedema in women with breast cancer 5 years after sentinel lymph node biopsy or axillary dissection: patient perceptions and precautionary behaviors. *J Clin Oncol.* 2008;26:5220–5226.

321. Le GM, O'Malley CD, Glaser SL, et al. Breast implants following mastectomy in women with early-stage breast cancer: prevalence and impact on survival. *Breast Cancer Res.* 2005;7:R184–R193.

322. Kruper L, Holt A, Xu XX, et al. Disparities in reconstruction rates after mastectomy: Patterns of care and factors associated with use of breast reconstruction in Southern California. *Ann Surg Oncol.* 2011;18:2158–2165.

323. Alderman AK, Wei Y, Birkmeyer JD. Use of breast reconstruction after mastectomy following the women's health and cancer rights act. *JAMA.* 2006;387–388.

324. Shapiro S, Venet W, Strax P, et al. Prospects for eliminating racial differences in breast cancer survival rates. *Am J Public Health.* 1982;1142–1145.

325. Henson RM, Wyatt SW, Lee NC. The National Breast and Cervical Cancer Early Detection Program: a comprehensive public health response to two major health issues for women. *J Public Health Manag Pract.* 1996;2:36–47.

326. Jones BA, Reams K, Calvocoressi L, et al. Adequacy of communicating results from screening mammograms to African American and white women. *Am J Public Health.* 2007;97:531–538.

327. Polite BN, Cirrincione C, Fleming GF, et al. Racial differences in clinical outcomes from metastatic breast cancer: a pooled analysis of CALGB 9342 abd 9840-Cancer and Leukemia Group B. *J Clin Oncol.* 2008;26:2659–2665.

328. Karliner LS, Ma L, Hofmann M, Kerlikowske K. Language barriers, location of care, and delays in follow-up of abnormal mammograms. *Med Care.* 2011;Oct. (EPub ahead of print).

329. Budman DR, Berry DA, Cirrincione CT, et al. Dose and dose intensity as determinants of outcome in the adjuvant treatment of breast cancer. The Cancer and Leukemia Group B. *J Natl Cancer Inst.* 1998;90:1205–1211.

330. Neugut AI, Subar M, Wilde ET, et al. Association between prescription co-payment amount and compliance with adjuvant hormonal therapy in women with early-stage breast cancer. *J Clin Oncol.* 2011;29:2534–2542.

331. Menasche I, Anderson WF, Jatoi I, Rosenberg PS. Underlying causes of the black-white racial disparity in breast cancer mortality: a population-based analysis. *J Natl Cancer Inst.* 2009;101:993–1000.

332. Calle EE, Miracle-McMahill HL, Thun MJ, Heath CW Jr. Cigarette smoking and risk of fatal breast cancer. *Am J Epidemiol.* 1994;139:1001–1007.

333. Scanlon EF, Suh O, Murphy SM, et al. Influence of smoking on the development of lung metastases from breast cancer. *Cancer.* 1995;75:2693–2699.

334. Senie RT, Rosen PP, Rhodes P, et al. Obesity at diagnosis of breast carcinoma influences duration of disease free survival. *Ann Int Med.* 1992;116:26–32.

335. Rock CL, Demark-Wahnefried W. Nutrition and survival after the diagnosis of breast cancer: a review of the evidence. *J Clin Oncol.* 2002;20:3302–3316.

336. Caan BJ, Emond JA, Natarajan L, et al. Post-diagnosis weight gain and breast cancer recurrence in women with early stage breast cancer. *Breast Cancer Res Treat.* 2006;99:47–57.

337. Whiteman MK, Hillis SD, Curtis KM, et al. Body mass and mortality after breast cancer diagnosis. *Cancer Epidemiol Biomarkers Prev.* 2005;14:2009–2014.

338. Lu Y, Ma H, Malone KE, et al. Obesity and survival among black women and white women 35 to 64 years of age at diagnosis with invasive breast cancer. *J Clin Oncol.* 2011;29:3358–3365.

339. Guinee VF, Olsson H, Moller T, et al. Effect of pregnancy on prognosis for young women with breast cancer. *Lancet.* 1994;343:1587–1589.

340. Olson SH, Zauber AG, Tang J, Harlap S. Relation of time since last birth and parity to survival of young women with breast cancer. *Epidemiol.* 1998;9:669–671.

341. Phillips KA, Milne RL, Friedlander ML, et al. Prognosis of premenopausal breast cancer and childbirth prior to diagnosis. *J Clin Oncol.* 2004;22:699–705.

342. Schairer C, Gail M, Byrne C, et al. Estrogen replacement therapy and breast cancer survival in a large screening study. *J Natl Cancer Inst.* 1999;91:264–270.

343. Holmes MD, Chen WY, Hertzmark E, et al. Aspirin intake and survival after breast cancer. *J Clin Oncol.* 2010;28:1467–1472.

344. Phillips KA, Glendon G, Knight JA. Putting the risk of breast cancer in perspective. *N Engl J Med.* 1999;340:141–144.

345. Avis NE, Crawford S, Manuel J. Quality of life among younger women with breast cancer. *J Clin Oncol.* 2005;23:3322–3330.

346. Ganz PA, Desmond KA, Leedham B, et al. Quality of life in long-term disease-free survivors of breast cancer: a follow-up study. *J Natl Cancer Inst.* 2002;94:39–49.

347. Petrek JA, Naughton MJ, Case LD, et al. Incidence, time course, and determinants of menstrual bleeding after breast cancer treatment: a prospective study. *J Clin Oncol.* 2006;24:1045–1051. Epub 2006 Feb 13.

348. Partridge AH, Gelber S, Peppercorn J, et al. Fertility and menopausal outcomes in young breast cancer survivors. *Clin Breast Cancer.* 2008;8:65–69.

349. Azim AA, Costantini-Ferrando M, Okay K. Safety of fertility preservation by ovarian stimulation with letrozole and gonadotropins in patients with breast cancer: a prospective controlled study. *J Clin Oncol.* 2008;26:2630–2635.

350. Kranick JA, Schaefer C, Rowell S, et al. Is pregnancy after breast cancer safe? *The Breast J.* 2010;16:404–411.

351. Eisen A, Lubinski J, Gronwald J, et al. Hormone therapy and the risk of breast cancer in *BRCA1* mutation carriers. *J Natl Cancer Inst.* 2008;100:1361–1367.

352. Kauff ND, Brogi E, Scheuer L, et al. Epithelial lesions in prophylactic mastectomy specimens from women with *BRCA* mutations. *Cancer.* 2003;97:1601–1608.

353. Vogel VG, Costantino JP, Wickerham DL, et al. Effects of tamoxifen vs raloxifene on the risk of developing invasive breast cancer and other disease outcomes. The NSABP study of tamoxifen and Raloxifene (STAR) P-2 Trial. *JAMA.* 2006;2727–2741.

354. Kinsinger LS, Harris R, Woolf SH, et al. Chemoprevention of breast cancer: a summary of the evidence for U.S. Preventive Services Task Force. *Ann Intern Med.* 2002;137:59–67.

355. DeMichele A, Toxel AB, Berlin JA, et al. Impact of raloxifene or tamoxifen use on endometrial cancer risk: a population-based case-control study. *J Clin Oncol.* 2008;26:4151–4159.

356. Goss PE, Ingle JN, Ales-Martinez JE, et al. Exemestane for breast cancer prevention in postmenopausal women. *N Engl J Med.* 2011;364:2381–2391.

357. Davidson NE, Kensler TW. "MAPping" the course of chemoprevention in breast cancer. *N Engl J Med.* 2011;364:2463–2464.

358. Land SR, Wickerham DL, Costantino JP, et al. Patient-reported symptoms and quality of life during treatment with tamoxifen or raloxifene for breast cancer prevention. The NSABP Study of Tamoxifen and Raloxifene (STAR) P-2 Trial. *JAMA.* 2006;295:2742–2751.

359. Ropka ME, Keim J, Philbrick JT. Patient decisions about breast cancer chemoprevention: a systematic review and meta-analysis. *J Clin Oncol.* 2010;28:3090–3095.

Ovarian Cancer

Ruby T. Senie, PhD

Introduction

Ovarian cancer is among the most lethal malignancies, affecting approximately 22,000 American women annually. Lower incidence rates are reported from developing nations associated with shorter life expectancy for women combined with higher parity. Having a relative diagnosed with ovarian and/or breast cancer increases ovarian cancer risk. Risk is highest among families with a genetic mutation of *BRCA1* or *BRCA2*, two susceptibility genes. High parity and oral contraceptive use provide long-term protection, including among women at high risk due to inherited susceptibility. Since current screening modalities are of limited benefit, most women are diagnosed after cancer has spread beyond the ovaries. Therefore, mortality rates have diminished only slightly in the past 30 years despite new treatment options. Research continues to focus on identifying effective and efficient early detection modalities including tumor markers and advanced imaging techniques while seeking additional avenues for disease prevention and improved treatment. This chapter provides a review of current information regarding ovarian cancer incidence and mortality, epidemiologic studies addressing risk and protective factors, clinical diagnostic procedures, and ongoing research.

U.S. Incidence and Mortality

The American Cancer Society (ACS) estimated that 21,880 women would be diagnosed with invasive ovarian cancer in 2010 and 13,850 deaths due to the disease.[1] Incidence rates increase with age from approximately 20 per 100,000 between ages 30 and 50 years to more than 40 per 100,000 among older women. Data from the Surveillance Epidemiology and End Results (SEER) program of the National Cancer Institute (NCI) indicate the mean age at diagnosis in the general population is 59 years; two-thirds of cases are older than 55 and 17% are age 40 or younger.[1,2]

Although accounting for only 3% of all malignancies among American women, the disease is the fifth highest cause of cancer-related death. Fewer than 35% survive 5 years.[1] Due to the lack of effective early detection modalities, more than 75% of women are diagnosed at stages III or IV when metastases have spread to other organs in the peritoneal cavity.[3,4] When the disease is confined to the ovaries (stage I), new therapies have enabled more than 80% to be alive at 5 years.[1] Survival is influenced by tumor aggressiveness, success of treatment, and patient's health status at time of diagnosis. Younger patients experience superior survival at each stage.[5]

Race/Ethnicity Differences in Incidence and Mortality

Ovarian cancer incidence rates have remained stable for several decades among younger white and black women and those 65 and older, although white women have experienced higher rates than black women as noted in Figure 27-1. More recent SEER data estimated that incidence between 2003 and 2007 among non-Hispanic white women, 13.9 per 100,000, was greater than among Hispanics (11.0), Asian/Pacific Islanders (9.8), and blacks and Native Americans (10.2).[2,6] Kim et al. found no stage differences at diagnosis by racial groups although survival was significantly longer for white patients.[7] Mortality is also highest among non-Hispanic white women at 9.2 per 100,000 compared with 7.2 per 100,000 among blacks and similarly lower rates for other race/ethnic groups.[2]

Biology of Ovarian Tissue at Risk

Ovarian surface epithelium, composed of a single layer of cells, invaginates with each ovulatory menstrual cycle to form clefts and inclusion cysts in the ovarian surface (Figure 27-2).[8]

The finding of inclusion cysts in healthy ovaries led some researchers to suggest cysts may precede cancer development.[9] Because of the close proximity of the fallopian tubes and fimbriae to the ovaries, Crum and colleagues carefully conducted pathologic review of tissues removed prophylactically from women at inherited risk and identified cancer in approximately 10% of ovarian and fimbrial sections of fallopian tube tissue.[10] Dubeau suggested close contact of fimbriae with ovarian epithelium during ovulation could enhance dissemination of malignant cells to adjacent ovarian and peritoneal tissue.[11]

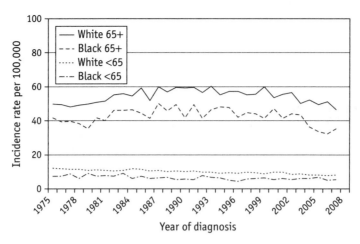

Figure 27-1 Incidence rate of ovarian cancer per 100,000 white and black women by year of diagnosis and age.

Data from National Cancer Institute, SEER Cancer Statistics Review 1975–2007.

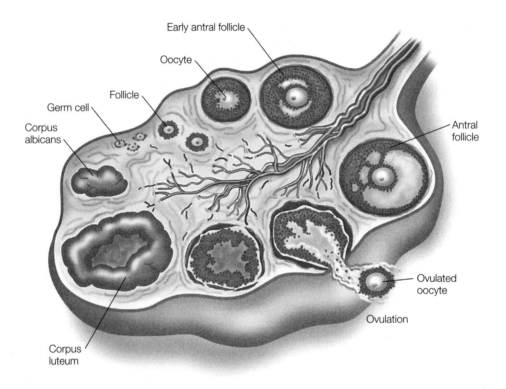

Figure 27-2 Structure of the ovary.

Characteristics differentiating the four histologic types of epithelial invasive ovarian cancer[12] include the aggressiveness of the lesion and usual symptoms. Approximately 50% classified as serous are highly lethal and often metastasize beyond the reproductive organs.[10] About 25% of ovarian tumors are endometrioid, more frequently among younger women, who may be diagnosed concurrently with endometriosis or endometrial cancer. The 10% classified as mucinous tumors are more resistant to current chemotherapeutic agents. Clear cell ovarian tumors (<10%) are most resistant to treatment. Borderline tumors of low malignant potential are diagnosed in approximately 10% of patients and are often detected during screening.[13]

Screening and Early Detection Procedures

The National Cancer Institute in 2011 advised against screening for ovarian cancer because currently available modalities do not reduce mortality[14] and have unacceptably high false positive results requiring surgery to rule out cancer.[15] In addition, the low incidence, an average of 40 cases diagnosed annually per 100,000 women older than age 50, results in screening not being feasible or cost effective. Palpation during pelvic examination has rarely been informative given the internal position of the ovaries.[16] However, for women at high risk due to genetic susceptibility or family history, ACS continues to advise annual monitoring for changes by ultrasound imaging, testing of tumor markers, and palpation.[1]

Ultrasound

In 1982, using transabdominal ultrasound, researchers identified nine ovarian cancers, including five in stage I, among more than 5,000 self-referred asymptomatic women who reported an affected relative. More than 300 false positives were identified in women who required surgery to rule out cancer.[17] The more sensitive transvaginal ultrasonography, capable of detecting small changes in ovarian volume and architecture,[16] was studied prospectively among 25,000 women who were younger than age 50 with a family history or age 50 and older considered at average risk.[18] Of the 364 who required surgery for suspicious screenings, 29 invasive cancers were identified (8%) including 14 with stage I disease.[16] Superior 5-year survival rates were noted for cases detected through screening (77%) compared with 49% following clinical diagnosis[16] although the study results were questionable because selection bias was evident and study findings were compared with historical controls.[15] Detection of changes by transvaginal ultrasound among premenopausal women is complicated by normal menstrual cycle changes of healthy ovaries,[4] requiring experienced clinicians to adequately evaluate ultrasound images.[15]

Symptom Index

In an effort to reduce mortality, ovarian cancer survivors urged clinicians to consider symptoms when referring women for screening.[19] In response, Goff and colleagues questioned patients about the frequency and severity of symptoms during the year before diagnostic surgery.[20] Their 2004 publication indentified many common symptoms including back pain, fatigue, indigestion, abdominal pain, constipation, and urinary problems. More than 90% of women had experienced at least one symptom, but 43% of cases and only 8% with benign tumors reported a combination of three specific symptoms: bloating from abdominal pressure, rapid increase in abdominal size, and urinary frequency combined with urinary urgency. These three symptoms were associated with significantly increased likelihood of ovarian cancer diagnosis (OR = 5.3; 95% CI = 2.2–12.6). Risk increased in the presence of a fourth symptom (OR = 6.2; 95% CI =2.0–18.8) suggesting a dose-response effect.[20] Daly and Ozols acknowledged that frequent symptoms should alert clinicians although they also noted similar physical complaints are frequently reported by women experiencing age-related changes or comorbid conditions.[4]

Subsequently, a symptom index created and evaluated by Goff et al. was found to have sensitivity ranging from 57% for early-stage to 80% for later-stage disease and specificity close to 90%.[21] Symptoms differed by histology; rapid abdominal enlargement associated with mucinous tumors led to diagnosis at an earlier stage. Abnormal bleeding was associated with endometrioid tumors more than other histologies. Bowel symptoms often preceded diagnosis of serous tumors due to metastases to the intestines.[22] Clinical assessment following a positive index score identified one cancer per 100 women;[23] more useful was the fact that the absence of symptoms frequently indicated an abnormal ultrasound image was benign.[24]

Biomarkers

Tumor markers, biochemical substances in blood and tissue of ovarian cancer patients, have been studied in healthy women to detect early stage disease. Since markers can be reliably and consistently measured in serum, they have been considered valuable as early detection indicators. Cancer antigen (CA-125), a frequently studied biomarker, is used to monitor response to ovarian cancer treatment.[10] However, when CA-125 was found elevated in stored serum (>35 U/mL) 18 months[25] to 3 years[26] before ovarian cancer diagnosis, the marker was not a reliable predictor of cancer due to frequent false-positive and false-negative screening results.[27] Elevated CA-125 has been associated with 80% of advanced stage disease except in patients with mucinous tumors. In addition, levels have been elevated during pregnancy, endometriosis, and pelvic inflammatory disease.[15] CA-125 may be normal among some women with early stage ovarian cancer and may rise as the malignancy progresses. Therefore, some clinicians have repeated CA-125 testing in the presence of a pelvic mass to assist clinical decision making.[28]

The combination of CA-125 with epididymis protein 4 (HE4), overexpressed by serous and endometrioid ovarian tumors, provided higher specificity among women with a palpable mass than either biomarker alone.[29] CA-125 combined with mesothelin, a tumor antigen, was more informative together than individually. Anderson et al. reported the combined high levels of three markers, CA-125, HE4 and mesothelin, were recorded 12 months before of tumor detection.[30] Among women with a detectable mass, a commercially available ovarian screening test, OVA1 (approved by the Food and Drug Administration in 2010), which includes CA-125 as one of five biomarkers, may be used. However, Muller advised the test has never been studied in a screening population although OVA1 may assist decision making before diagnostic surgery on a palpated mass.[31] The protein components of OVA1 are noted in Table 27-1 indicating the function and noting the change in serum levels associated with malignancy.

Combined Screening Modalities

Reliable screening methods would improve prognosis among older women with a positive family history[25] who might benefit from repeated CA-125 combined with transvaginal ultrasound to differentiate small pelvic masses from cysts.[32] However, a U.S. study of annual screening of women age 50 and older with CA 125 or ultrasound identified 30 false-positives for every cancer detected, judged by the authors to be unacceptably high.[33] Findings from a multimodality randomized screening trial of more than 20,000 women by Jacobs et al. included sequential steps. If CA-125 was above 30 u/mL, pelvic ultrasound was performed. If an enlarged ovary (volume > 8.8 mL) was detected, referral to a gynecologist

Table 27-1

Five serum markers of proteins associated with ovarian cancer [OVA1 test]

Protein	Apolipoprotein A1	Beta–2 microglobulin	CA–125	Prealbumin	Transferrin
Function	Cholesterol transport	Immune response	Released by tumor cells	Hormone and vitamin transport	Iron transport
Change due to ovarian cancer	Levels decline	Levels increase	Levels increase	Levels decline	Levels decline

followed. Although screen detected cases lived longer for a median of 73 months compared to 42 months among controls, the number of deaths in each group did not differ.[34]

A study combining Goff symptoms index with CA-125 followed by ultrasound had 80% sensitivity but detected cancers were too advanced.[35] Similarly, the 2009 report from the U.S. Prostate, Lung, Colorectal, and Ovarian (PLCO) Cancer Screening Trial noted 72% of ovarian cancers found were stage III or IV after four rounds of annual screening with CA 125 and transvaginal ultrasound. One invasive cancer was diagnosed for each 19 benign surgeries leading to the U.S. Preventive Services Task Force (USPSTF) not recommending routine screening with CA-125 and transvaginal ultrasound.[36] Hartge, among others, urged researchers to use new technology to improve imaging and utility of biomarkers and to reduce invasiveness of diagnostic surgery for women at high risk.[28]

Known and Suspected Risk Factors

Epidemiologic studies have been conducted to explore several hypotheses for ovarian cancer development. Highest risk has been associated with familial history and inherited susceptibility. Among nonfamilial or sporadic cases risk is increased among infertile women or women who have few children. Protective factors include oral contraceptive use, higher parity, breastfeeding, tubal ligation, and hysterectomy. Other factors with more limited and less consistent impact include history of: endometriosis, polycystic ovary syndrome, infertility treatment, postmenopausal hormone use, talc use, cigarette smoking, and central obesity (increased waist-to-hip ratio).

Hypotheses

Fathalla, in a 1971 letter in *Lancet*, suggested ovarian cancer might develop after repeated "minor trauma" caused by ovulation in the absence of pregnancy-induced "rest periods." His animal studies indicated rapid cell proliferation occurred within hours of ovulation enabling some cells to undergo malignant transformation.[37] Casagrande et al. extended this "incessant ovulation" concept noting the vulnerability of ovarian tissue to genetic mutations during DNA repair.[38] They also identified the protective effect of pregnancy and oral contraceptive (OC) use in their calculation of "ovulatory age," the interval between

menarche and menopause minus months of suppressed menstruation during pregnancy and OC use. Longer intervals of protected time were associated with slower aging of ovarian tissue and reduced ovarian cancer risk after menopause.[38]

The "gonadotropin" hypothesis, proposed by Cramer and Welch, linked cancer risk to persistent exposure of the ovaries after menopause to high levels of pituitary gonadotropins including follicle-stimulating hormone (FSH) and luteinizing hormone (LH) potentially inducing malignant transformation.[8] Among premenopausal women pituitary gonadotropins are lowered by use of oral contraceptives (OCs) and during pregnancy.[39] Risch provided an "androgen hypothesis" that unified the increased risk associated with postmenopausal elevated androgens and higher levels of androstenedione.[40] Another etiologic theory suggested deleterious mutations of several genes in the DNA repair pathways might affect risk.[41]

Family History

Before genetic susceptibility was recognized, having one or more affected relatives was the strongest recognized risk factor as noted in a case-control study of women ages 45 to 74 published in 1981.[42] The Gilda Radner Familial Ovarian Cancer Registry was organized that same year to enable researchers to study high-risk families in which a 10-year decline in ages at diagnosis occurred when daughters (49.8 yrs) and their mothers (58.5 yrs, $P<.001$) were both affected.[43] Members of families enrolled in the Radner Registry were affected with ovarian, endometrial, and colorectal cancer.

Although valuable for research, familial studies can be complicated by few blood relatives, premature death of young females, frequency of male births, and limited knowledge of cancer history of deceased relatives.[43] Accuracy of family history relies on family cohesiveness and sharing of health information; therefore, knowledge of health status may be limited to first-degree (mother, sister, or daughter) and younger second-degree relatives (aunts and female cousins). Among older generations ovarian cancer may have been misclassified as stomach or colon cancer.

The large population-based case-control Cancer and Steroid Hormone Study (CASH) confirmed the strong risk associated with having an affected mother, (RR = 3.9, 95% CI = 2.0–7.7). When multiple relatives were affected, almost 20% of cases were diagnosed before age 40.[44] Therefore, the authors noted that prophylactic oophorectomy was a reasonable option for women at such high risk,[44] although risk for primary peritoneal cancer would remain.[45]

A large meta-analysis of 15 international studies (> 6,000 cases and > 12,000 controls) enabled assessment of risk in relation to ages at diagnosis, degree of relationships, and number of affected women in the family.[46] Among women with an affected mother and sister the risk of ovarian cancer was three times greater than among women without a family history.[46] Kurian et al., using pooled data from 10 U.S. case-control studies, noted risk was similar with a first-degree relative affected by either ovarian or breast cancer (OR = 2.9, 95% CI: = 2.2–3.7);[47] family history also increased the risk of primary peritoneal cancer (OR = 3.48, 95% CI = 1.36–8.91).[48]

Genetic Predisposition

In 1991 Lynch et al. defined a hereditary syndrome involving several relatives of two or more generations diagnosed with either ovarian and/or breast cancer. The researchers determined that an autosomal dominantly inherited cancer susceptibility syndrome was operating in families with multiple cases of ovarian cancer.[49] Three separate risk groups were identified based on ages at diagnosis and other cancers among the relatives: ovarian only, breast-ovarian syndrome, and "Lynch syndrome" involving ovarian, breast, endometrial, and colon cancer.[49] Current estimates note that one in seven ovarian cancers are due to genetic susceptibility.

Although epidemiologists prefer population-based data for research, identifying specific susceptibility genes and their associated cancer risk among preselected high-risk families with multiple affected members of several generations diagnosed at young ages is most efficient. Several affected relatives may suggest inherited risk although the family may test negative for the known susceptibility genes providing resources for further gene discoveries.[45] Genetic counselors and clinicians must consider the differing family relationships and include the possibility of paternal transmission.[50] An estimated 10% of ovarian cancer cases with affected relatives carry a mutation of BRCA1 or BRCA2; risk is strongly increased among mutation carriers of either susceptibility gene although a Canadian study noted BRCA1 conferred a higher relative risk (RR = 21 (95% CI = 12.0–36.0)) than BRCA2 (RR = 7.0, 05% CI = 3.1–16.0).[51] Data from Myriad Genetics noted in Figure 27-3, the laboratory with exclusive rights to clinical BRCA genetic testing, indicates 27% to 44% of women with a BRCA mutation will develop ovarian cancer by age 70 in contrast to less than 2% of noncarriers.[52] Mutations of BRCA1 and BRCA2, tumor suppressor genes, impede DNA repair and cause chromosome instability increasing risk of malignant transformation.

BRCA mutations account for 85% of the inherited risk of breast and/or ovarian cancer; no gene has been identified with risk exclusively of ovarian cancer. However, ovarian cancer also occurs in families with hereditary nonpolyposis colorectal cancer (HNPCC) with an estimated lifetime risk of ovarian cancer among women from HNPCC families of 13%.[53]

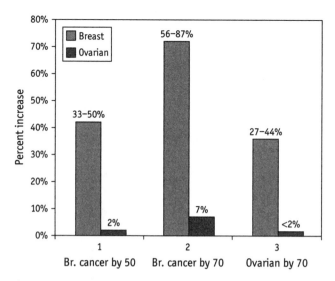

Figure 27-3 BRCA mutations increase risk of breast & ovarian cancer.

Reproduced from StatBite BRCA mutations increase risk of breast/ovarian cancer. *J Natl Cancer Inst* 2010; Courtesy of Myriad Genetics Laboratories, Inc. https://www.myriadpro.com/bracanalysis-prevalence-tables

The frequency of BRCA mutations and probability of disease differs by racial/ethnic populations although the stronger the family history of breast and ovarian cancer, the greater the likelihood of identifying a family-specific BRCA mutation.[54] One study reported 51% of families with two cases of ovarian cancer plus a relative with breast cancer had a family-specific BRCA mutation; with more affected family members the percentage of families positive for BRCA was higher (83%).[54] In Ashkenazi Jewish populations approximately 1 of 40 individuals have one of three recognized founder mutations of BRCA1 (185delAG and 5382insC) or BRCA2 (6174delT) and a small percentage have both a BRCA1 and BRCA2 mutation. Risk of developing ovarian cancer varies from 35–50% with BRCA1 and 10–30% for BRCA2.[55,56] Figure 27-4 notes the differential increased risk of having a BRCA mutation among women of Ashkenazi heritage with a relative diagnosed with ovarian cancer. The darkest bar notes the 33% increased probability of having a BRCA mutation among breast cancer patients with a family history of ovarian cancer.[52] The guidelines from USPSTF on genetic testing noted that BRCA penetrance ranged from 10% to 50% for ovarian cancer.[57] In a New York Ashkenazi family study, risk of ovarian cancer among mutation carriers reached 54% for BRCA1 and 23% for BRCA2 by age 80.[50] Higher risks were noted among women with BRCA1 born after 1940. Some clinicians encourage BRCA testing of women diagnosed with ovarian cancer in order to inform relatives of a potential increased risk of ovarian and breast cancers; in addition, if the ovarian cancer patient carriers a BRCA mutation, she may also be at risk for breast cancer although prognosis of ovarian cancer would guide further clinical treatment decisions.

Pooled data from 280 BRCA1 and 218 BRCA2 families indicated ovarian cancer was rarely diagnosed before age 30 but increased by approximately 2% yearly reaching

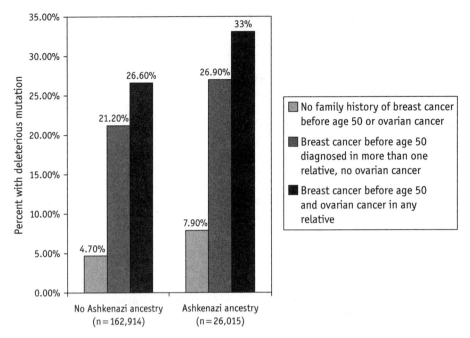

Figure 27-4 Percent of breast cancer patients <50 yrs carrying a BRCA mutations in relation to family history of breast or ovarian cancer and Ashkenazi heritage

Reproduced from StatBite BRCA mutations in breast cancer patients under age 50 tested for mutations. *J Natl Cancer Inst* 2010; DOI:10,1093. Courtesy of Myriad Genetics Laboratories, Inc. Mutation Prevalence Tables. Source : http://www.myriadpro.com/bracanalysis-prevalence-tables. Last updated Feb. 2010.

a cumulative risk of 39% (95% CI = 22%–51%) by age 80 among *BRCA1* families in contrast to 11% (95% CI = 4.1%–18%) in *BRCA2* families.[55] Overestimation of cumulative risk may result from studies exclusively among mutation carriers; however, these families provide research opportunities to understand ovarian tumor development in relation to gene–environment interactions and modifier genes that may also increase risk in broader populations.[58]

In addition to *BRCA1* and *BRCA2*, Lynch syndrome and mutations of DNA mismatch repair genes have been associated with increased risk. The most frequently acquired somatic mutations occur in the tumor protein p53 (*TP53*) gene whose functions are to maintain genomic integrity by arresting dividing cells when DNA damage has occurred, accelerating DNA repair, and regulating apoptosis, programmed cell death.[41]

Some women testing positive for either *BRCA1* or *BRCA2* have significantly lowered their risk by having prophylactic surgery to remove ovaries and fallopian tubes. Multicenter collaborations organized by the international Ovarian Cancer Association Consortium provided resources for genomewide association studies (GWAS) searching for polymorphisms in which a single nucleotide (SNP) may increase ovarian cancer risk.[59] Biologically plausible genes such as those that regulate the cell cycle but are defective in cancer cases have been explored. Although these polymorphisms may have a smaller impact on disease risk, their high prevalence in broader populations suggests they may contribute to a large percentage of the disease. Many researchers expect these large studies to significantly contribute to greater understanding of ovarian cancer development.

In the absence of a *BRCA* mutation, ovarian cancer risk is very low among women whose relatives were diagnosed with breast cancer, suggesting prophylactic bilateral oophorectomy can be avoided.[60] Others also noted the specificity of family risk suggested additional genetic markers remain to be identified among families negative for the known *BRCA* genes.[61] Clinical guidance is recommended for families with genetic susceptibility of breast, ovarian, colon and other inherited clinical conditions.

Reproductive Factors

Number of Menstrual Cycles

Reproductive decisions regarding contraception and timing of pregnancies influence ovarian cancer risk years later as more than 50% of cases are diagnosed after age 60. Ages of menarche and menopause had limited influence on risk although later onset of menses was slightly protective among premenopausal women.[62,63] Hildreth et al. reported risk was increased threefold among women with 35 or more years of menstrual cycles uninterrupted by pregnancy or OC use.[42] Similarly, John and colleagues noted increased risk (OR = 1.6) among black women who had uninterrupted menstrual cycles for 35 years or more compared with women experiencing 25 years or fewer.[64] Schildkraut et al. suggested each cycle provides an opportunity for a spontaneous, potentially carcinogenic mutation occurring during DNA repair,[65] Cramer and Welch provided an alternative biologic explanation: a greater number of ovulatory cycles provided prolonged unopposed estrogen stimulation and diminished progesterone levels, limiting the ability for apoptosis to control proliferation of transformed cells.[8]

Parity

A 1955 report noted ovarian cancer deaths were 50% higher among never-married compared to married women; however, in 1978 nulliparity rather than marital status was linked to risk of disease in a British cohort.[66] Among Connecticut women increasing parity was protective according to a 1981 publication; after four or more births, ovarian cancer risk was diminished 50%.[42] In addition, a population-based case-control study suggested risk was associated with infertility among nulliparous women.[67] The protective role of childbearing was evident (OR = 0.47; 95% CI = 0.4–0.56) when parous and nulliparous women were compared in data pooled from 12 case-control studies. Each additional term pregnancy reduced risk by 14%, although interrupted pregnancies provided less protection due to fewer missed menstrual cycles.[68] Risch also found each pregnancy, after the first, provided 14% to 16% additional risk reduction and each term pregnancy suppressed ovulation for approximately 1 year.[40]

Among black women, lower ovarian cancer risk was associated with higher parity and earlier first birth compared to white women.[65] In contrast, Adami et al. in Sweden found a 39% reduction in ovarian cancer risk when first birth occurred at age 35 or older compared to age 20.[69] These authors suggested the hormonal milieu of pregnancy among older women eliminated more transformed cells that had accumulated in the ovaries.[69] This concept was supported by another population-based study that reported increasing parity and later age at first birth provided a strong protective effect especially after OC use.[63]

Twin births are associated with increased ovulation and higher gonadotropin levels, two ovarian cancer risk factors; however, several studies have indicated multiple births lower risk. Swedish twin data indicated babies of unlike sex provided a 29% reduction[70] although similar protective results of twins without any differences by gender were found in a subsequent international study.[71] Whiteman et al. suggested higher progesterone levels associated with multiple births may contribute to lowered risk. Elevated levels of progesterone, also more frequent among older mothers, control the rate of apoptosis after childbirth.[72] These reproductive issues provide interest without firm conclusions.

Breastfeeding

Exclusive breastfeeding, known to suppress ovulation, reduced ovarian cancer risk by 1% per month; the strongest protective effect occurred during the first 6 months after childbirth.[68] Classification by ever breastfeeding was marginally protective in a case-control study although significant decreased risk (RR = 0.66, 95% CI = 0.46–0.96) was associated with 18 months or longer in analyses of pooled data from the two Nurses' Health Study cohorts.[73] Changing patterns of exclusive breastfeeding may have influenced maternal behaviors in these cohorts. Data published in 2006 indicate increased interest in breastfeeding although duration is often affected by mothers' return to employment.[74]

Infertility

Infertility, defined as 12 months of unprotected sexual intercourse without pregnancy, has been associated with increased risk. In 1992, using data from 12 case-control studies, Whittemore et al. reported a twofold increased risk associated with lack of pregnancy after 15 years of unprotected intercourse.[68] A record linkage study indicated infertile women had a threefold increased risk of borderline tumors.[75] To further assess the relationship of infertility to ovarian cancer risk, a retrospective cohort of more than 8,000 women treated for infertility was studied. Brinton et al. reported the highest ovarian cancer risk associated with infertility in this cohort was associated with a history of endometriosis (RR = 4.19, 95% CI = 2.0–7.7).[76]

Fertility Treatment

Treatment for infertility includes hormonal stimulation to enhance release of eggs. Some research has suggested these procedures may increase ovarian cancer risk, as a single stimulated cycle may produce eggs equivalent to 24 natural ovulatory cycles. In addition, many women required several treatment cycles to achieve conception.[77] Clomiphene citrate and gonadotropins are frequently prescribed medications that stimulate ovulation by raising endogenous levels of estrogen and progesterone. Therefore, some investigators have advised caution after diagnosing ovarian cancer among several women treated for infertility.[77]

An early case-control study by Whittemore et al. described previously revealed significantly increased ovarian cancer risk associated with fertility medications (OR = 2.8, 95% CI = 1.3–6.1).[68] Risk was increased after clomiphene use for 12 or more menstrual cycles;[75] others found the limited increased risk reassuring although long-term follow-up was advised.[78] After years of OC use to delay childbearing, the reduction in ovarian cancer risk may be partially reversed by the potential adverse effects of fertility treatment or stimulation for egg donation. Clinics providing infertility treatment should maintain active follow-up to detect any long-term adverse effects although conflicts of interest exist.

Tubal Ligation and Hysterectomy

The collaborative analysis by Whittemore et al. noted the protective role of hysterectomy (OR = 0.66) and tubal ligation (OR = 0.59) during the reproductive years although surgery following natural menopause had no protective effect.[68] The Nurses' Health Study also reported tubal ligation (RR = 0.33, 95% CI = 0.16–0.64) and hysterectomy (RR = 0.67, 95% CI = 0.45–1.00) lowered risk.[79] John et al. suggested the higher frequency of hysterectomy among black women may reduce ovarian cancer risk suggesting that surgery disrupted ovulatory cycles and may prevent environmental contaminants from reaching ovarian tissue.[65] Alternatively, either surgical procedure may interrupt a developing malignancy in the Fallopian tubes where some malignancies have their origin.[10] The protective effect of tubal ligation among BRCA1 mutation carriers (OR = 0.37) was even greater among women who had used OCs (OR = 0.28, 95% CI = 0.15–0.52) although *BRCA2* mutations carriers at lower risk of ovarian cancer did not receive protection from the surgery.[80]

Endogenous Hormones

Research has noted that gonadotropins, including luteinizing hormone (LH) and follicle-stimulating hormone (FSH), androgens, estrogens, and progesterone influence ovarian cancer development. However, assessment of circulating hormones is complicated among premenopausal and perimenopausal women given person-specific varying levels of endogenous hormones during each menstrual cycle.[81]

Helzlsouer et al. conducted a small study to assess cancer risk associated with prediagnostic hormone levels using serum stored more than 5 years before diagnosis of 31 ovarian cancer cases and 62 matched controls.[82] Gonadotropins, especially FSH, were lower among cases and cancer risk declined among postmenopausal women with increasing gonadotropin levels; therefore, the dose-response associations before diagnosis did not support the "gonadotropins" hypothesis.[82] However, several recognized protective factors, including multiple pregnancies and oral contraceptive use, suppress gonadotropins. Therefore, the hypothesis was supported by some epidemiologic studies but not all.[81] Pregnancy and OC use also reduce androgen levels, supporting the "androgen hypothesis" proposed by Risch. In summary, Lukanova and Kaaks noted that increased risk from the combined effect of elevated androgens and estrogen and lower levels of progesterone during more than 30 premenopausal years were more informative than measurable hormone levels at any one time point.[81]

Exogenous Hormones

Oral Contraceptives

Thirty years ago, researchers recognized that OCs reduced ovarian cancer risk[42] although studies of OCs over decades have been complicated by changing formulas, geographic differences in prescribing, and reliance on patient recall for brand and doage information. OCs prescribed before 1970, now considered high dose, usually contained 100 μg or more of estrogen. Medium-level dosages of 50 μg of estrogen became standard between 1970 and 1980, only to be replaced by low-dose preparations containing 30 μg or less of estrogen. Studies also address differing effects of specific OC formulas on ovarian tissue combined with person-specific risk factors such as age at first OC use and duration of use before a first pregnancy. Because recall of OC use varied when self-reported data and medical records were compared, Hildreth et al. instructed study interviewers to enhance memory of years of specific OCs used by constructing personal calendars on which critical life events during the reproductive years from menarche to study entry were recorded and photographs of OC containers were provided to aid recall of brands and dosages.[42] This procedure enabled more accurate and complete data collection and was used in the CASH study among others.[83] Some researchers claim

that accuracy for specific brands and dosages requires obtaining clinical records, a time-consuming and costly process in the absence of centralized datafiles.

A preliminary report in 1983 from CASH[84] followed by the 1987 publication indicated a 40% to 50% reduction in ovarian cancer risk associated with OCs containing both estrogen and progestin that were available between 1980 and 1982. Risk decreased with longer use and protection persisted for years after OCs were discontinued.[85] Although high parity reduced risk, prior use of OCs enhanced the protective effect of pregnancies. Given that OCs suppress pituitary gonadotropin levels in addition to preventing ovulation, the CASH researchers estimated that OC use may have prevented more than 1,700 ovarian cancer by 1987.[85] The diversity of OC preparations used by the large CASH study population enabled risk to be assessed by dosage. After controlling for estrogen level and other risk factors, higher potency progestin provided greater protection than lower levels.[85]

A pooled analysis from 45 international cohort and case-control studies (> 40,000 women) indicated a highly significant dose-response protective effect from longer use of OCs. For every 5 years of use, risk was reduced by 20%, preventing 200,000 new cases and 100,000 ovarian cancer deaths.[87] OC use has been credited with a recent small decline in ovarian cancer incidence among American women younger than age 60 who have had access to OCs throughout their reproductive years.[6]

Some unplanned pregnancies among OC users have questioned a potential adverse effect of obesity on OC ovarian suppression, potentially also reducing protection against ovarian cancer. However, Trussel et al. found no "convincing evidence" of obesity limiting the protective effect of OCs for either pregnancy or ovarian cancer.[88] A clinical trial conducted by Westhoff et al. reported "substantial and comparable ovarian suppression" among "consistent" OC users regardless of weight.[89] Therefore, OCs are expected to provide equal chemoprevention for consistent OC users regardless of their body mass index (BMI).

Oral Contraceptive Use by BRCA Mutation Carriers
Among women at genetic risk, OC use was protective among paired sisters who were discordant for ovarian cancer. Use of OCs significantly reduced cancer risk with OR = 0.5 (95% CI = 0.3–0.8) and protection increased with more years of use among women with a known mutation of either *BRCA1* or *BRCA2*.[90] A larger case-control study of *BRCA* mutation carriers by Narod and colleagues noted OCs use was strongly protective, especially among women who subsequently elected contraception by tubal ligation.[80] An international case-control study of *BRCA* mutation carriers found more limited protection among ever users and long-term users of OCs when compared with reductions observed in the general population.[91] Whittemore and colleagues advised women with *BRCA* mutations to consider a necessary balance between the protective effect for ovarian cancer against the potential increased breast cancer risk associated with OC use.[91]

Hormonal Therapy

Postmenopausal use of hormones, estrogen with or without progestin, prescribed for relief of symptoms and clinical conditions has been studied in relation to development of ovarian cancer. Comparisons are complicated by changing formulas over time, differing clinical prescribing patterns, varying ages at initiation and duration of use, history of natural or surgical menopause, body mass index, and international differences in preparations. Rates of hysterectomy with and without oophorectomy also influence ovarian cancer risk and must be controlled in analyses. When research revealed increased endometrial cancer following use of estrogen for menopausal symptoms, hormone therapy was modified to include both estrogen and progestin decreasing endometrial cancer risk. To assess cancer risk associated with hormone therapy, the NCI has followed women enrolled in the Breast Cancer Detection Demonstration Project (BCDDP), a breast screening program. After more than 20 years of unopposed estrogen, a threefold increased ovarian cancer risk was noted regardless of hysterectomy status.[92] Similarly a case-control study assessing current and recent unopposed estrogen use noted elevated risk in contrast to no effect of estrogen combined with progestogen.[93] However, data from the randomized Women's Health Initiative (WHI) of estrogen with progestin indicated 20 ovarian cancer cases were diagnosed in the treatment arm and 12 among those receiving placebos resulting in a nonsignificant level of risk (OR = 1.58, 95% CI = 0.77–3.24).[94] In addition, the American Cancer Society Prevention Study noted mortality following diagnosis of ovarian cancer was approximately twofold higher among women who had used estrogens for 10 or more years before diagnosis compared with nonusers.[95]

Health Behaviors and Exposures

Personal behaviors including physical activity, weight control, sun exposure, use of talc, alcohol intake, cigarette smoking, and others have been studied in relation to ovarian cancer risk. Accurate and honest self-reporting are thought to bias some epidemiologic studies that are also hampered by differing definitions and classifications. However, studies assessing risk associated with personal behaviors are important given their potential public health impact.

Physical Activity

Mixed results have been reported from studies of exercise and ovarian cancer. Physical activity assessed in a population-based case-control study indicated risk decreased as hours of leisure physical activity increased.[96] The authors noted strenuous activity often delayed menarche and produced more anovulatory cycles among young women, potentially reducing ovarian cancer risk at later ages.[96] Data on frequency and duration of exercise collected from more than 130,000 women participating in the American Association of Retired Persons (AARP) cohort ages 50–71 found no association with ovarian cancer risk. However, physical disabilities are prevalent in this cohort restricting exercise at their older ages and reported lifetime exercise patterns may have been affected by recall bias.[97]

Body Mass Index

Risk of ovarian cancer in relation to height and weight at age 18 and adulthood has been assessed in cohort and case-control studies with mixed findings, potentially reflecting differences by menopausal status. Obesity has been associated with several risk factors including low progesterone levels, high incidence of infertility, polycystic ovarian syndrome, endometriosis, high androgen levels, and inflammation. The Nurses' Health cohort reported a twofold increased risk of ovarian cancer only among premenopausal women who were obese at age 18 (BMI ≥ 30 kg/m^2).[99] Data from 12 cohort studies (> 2000 cases and > 500,000 controls) reported height greater than 5 feet 7 inches or obesity increased risk among premenopausal women suggesting a biologic effect of lowered sex hormone-binding globulin.[100] Ovarian cancer risk was increased among obese compared to normal weight women ages 50 to 70 in the AARP cohort especially those who were overweight or obese at age 18.[101] Ovarian cancer mortality was associated with obesity in the ACS Prevention Study only among women who never used postmenopausal hormones (RR = 1.36; 95% CI = 1.12–1.66).[102] The effect of BMI on ovarian cancer risk appears to be strongest at young ages many years before diagnosis.

Diet

The European Prospective Investigation into Cancer and Nutrition cohort study included 580 ovarian cancer cases diagnosed during 6 years of follow-up. Risk was not modified by total intake of fruit and vegetables nor by subgroups of vegetables (fruit, root and leafy vegetables, cabbages).[103] Pooled data from 12 U.S. and European cohort studies found no association between ovarian cancer risk and consumption of dairy foods.[104] Results of other nutritional studies have produced inconsistent findings; therefore, international incidence differences appear unrelated to diet.

Use of Perineal Powder

Studies suggest perineal powder may enter the reproductive tract and act as a chemical carcinogen; talc particles found in ovarian tissue provide evidence of such exposures. A Canadian case-control study observed increased risk after talc use on sanitary napkins or directly on genital tissue.[105] An association was also reported after powder was applied to perineal tissue and by use of genital deodorant sprays.[106] An American case-control study matched by age and geographic residence found a 60% increased risk of ovarian cancer with extensive talc use in the genital and rectal areas.[107] These consistent findings encourage research to identify specific ingredients that enable powder to reach internal organs and stimulate malignant transformation.

Radiation

Among the Japanese atom bomb survivors who were less than 20 at exposure, risk of radiation-induced ovarian cancer was significantly elevated in relation to radiation dose.[108] Another study revealing effect of radiation with a latency of 30 to 40 years is provided by follow-up after treatment for cervical cancer among women younger than age 50; risk of ovarian cancer was increased two to three fold among 100,000 cases with long term survival identified in American and European cancer registries.[109]

Analgesic Use; Nonsteroidal Anti-inflammatory Drugs (NSAIDs)

Since chronic inflammation from repeated ovulation or from endometriosis has been associated with ovarian cancer risk, researchers have studied the potential protective effect of anti-inflammatory agents. Results have not been consistent. Risk was slightly lower following use of analgesics including NSAIDS, aspirin, and acetaminophen in a 2006 review.[110] After 5 years of 4 or more doses per week of aspirin or NSAIDS, risk was reduced approximately 50% in a case-control study.[111] In contrast, data from both components of the two nurses' cohort studies reported no protective effect of analgesic agents.[112] However, two population-based case-control studies found NSAIDS protective (OR = 0.74, 95% CI = 0.59–0.92); the benefits were stronger among nulliparous women (OR = 0.47, 95% CI = 0.27–0.82) and those who never used oral contraceptives (OR = 0.58, 95% CI = 0.42–0.80).[113] Analyses of biosamples from the Nurses' Health Study indicated an inverse relationship between dose of analgesic used and hormonal levels among postmenopausal women providing modest support for a protective role of analgesics.[114]

Smoking

Jordan et al. conducted a meta-analysis of 33 international studies (910 cases and ≥ 5,500 controls) and reported smokers had a twofold greater risk of mucinous tumors but lower risk for clear cell ovarian cancer.[115] A similar positive association was noted between mucinous epithelial tumors and current (RR = 2.2, 95% CI = 1.2–4.2) and past smoking (RR = 2.0, 95% CI = 1.2–3.6) in data from the Nurses' Health Study.[116] Investigators have suggested that histologically, mucinous ovarian tumors have similar etiology to cervical cancer; both are increased among smokers.[115]

Alcohol Consumption

Alcohol, known to affect endogenous hormone levels, has not been consistently associated with ovarian cancer. No increased risk in relation to total alcohol intake or individual types of alcoholic drinks was found nor was risk modified by hormonal, environmental, or other factors in multivariate analyses of pooled data by Genkinger et al.[117] and similarly by others.[116]

Vitamin D and Sun Exposure

Ecologic studies noted higher incidence of ovarian cancer in northern U.S. states with lower levels of sun exposure, suggesting a north-south gradient that was supported by a similar international study.[118] Vitamin D has been hypothesized to control cell growth and apoptosis. However, a recent pooled analysis from seven prospective studies did not find an association between serum levels of 25-hydroxyvitamin D (25(OH)D), a reliable measure of circulating vitamin D, and development of ovarian cancer.[119]

Risk Associated with Clinical Conditions and Other Cancers

When endometrial tissue is misplaced into the peritoneal cavity during menstruation, an inflammatory response is produced stimulating increased cell proliferation and enhancing risk of endometriosis as well as malignant transformation.[120] A record linkage study by Brinton and colleagues reported a doubling of ovarian cancer among more than 20,000 Swedish women previously hospitalized for treatment of endometriosis; standardized incidence ratio for ovarian cancer increased over the 10 years of follow-up to 3.08 (95% CI = 1.8–4.9).[121] Subsequent research noted ovarian cancer was four times greater among women who became infertile due to endometriosis.[76] Contrary to these findings, the Iowa Women's Health Study did not detect an association of postmenopausal ovarian cancer among more than 1,400 women who self-reported a history of endometriosis.[122] Endometriosis and associated infertility are estimated to affect 3% to 8% of reproductive-age women although incidence is assumed to be underestimated as many women are asymptomatic.[122]

Polycystic ovarian syndrome (PCOS), a relatively common endocrine condition occurring in 5% to 10% of reproductive-age women, shares etiologic risk factors with ovarian cancer including obesity, infertility, menstrual abnormalities, and family history of PCOS. Ovarian cancer risk was increased (OR = 2.5, 95% CI = 1.0–5.9) in the CASH study among women with a history of PCOS with resulting elevated levels of androgens.[123]

Pelvic inflammatory disease (PID), a sexually transmitted condition, affects an estimated one woman in seven during reproductive years, often compromising childbearing. Inflammation associated with PID may stimulate repair mechanisms including rapid cell proliferation of ovarian tissue increasing malignant transformation. A history of recurrent episodes of PID increased ovarian cancer risk in a Canadian case-control study (OR = 1.88, 95% CI = 1.13–3.12) especially among those with PID-related infertility (OR = 3.74, 95% CI = 1.28–10.9).[124]

Women diagnosed with breast, endometrial, or cervical cancer are at increased risk for subsequent ovarian cancer associated with common genetic susceptibility, gene–environment interactions, or treatment effects such as radiation therapy for cervical cancer.[109] Using the Swedish cancer registry Bergfeldt et al. estimated ovarian cancer was increased threefold among breast cancer cases diagnosed before age 40 but when these young breast cancer patients had a family history of either breast or ovarian cancer at the time of their diagnosis, risk of subsequent ovarian cancer was significantly greater, RR = 13.9 (95% CI = 5.1– 30.1).[125] *BRCA* status was unknown but potentially contributory as an American collaborative study of 491 early stage breast cancer cases reported 10-year actuarial risk of ovarian cancer was 12.7% for *BRCA1* and 6.8% for *BRCA2*.[126]

Racial/Ethnic Risk Factor Differences

Risk factors have been studied to account for incidence differences by racial/ethnic groups. Reproductive factors are equally protective regardless of race although higher parity and greater frequency of hysterectomy among black women have contributed to their lowered risk.[65] Bilateral oophorectomy often accompanies hysterectomy although removal of the uterus may also protect retained ovaries from contaminants that might be transmitted from the vagina.[65] Ness and colleagues noted ovarian cancer incidence was 20% lower in African-American women compared with white women after controlling for parity and hysterectomy. The data from this study presented the known difference in hysterectomy by race: 9.6% of white cases, 17.9% of black cases, 11% of white controls, and 22% black controls.[127]

A population-based case-control study in North Carolina indicated risk among black women was strongly associated with greater height and weight at diagnosis. Severe obesity (BMI greater than 35) was three times as prevalent among blacks compared with whites, suggesting to Moorman and colleagues an explanation for younger mean age at ovarian cancer diagnosis among black women.[128]

Risk Factors Related to Histology

Invasive epithelial ovarian cancers are commonly classified as serous, mucinous, endometrioid, or clear cell. OC use provided protection against all four types[85] although tubal ligation reduced the risk of serous and clear cell cancers but not mucinous lesions.[47] Fewer mucinous cancers were linked to family history or genetic risk compared to serous tumors.[115] Some nonreproductive factors also differed by tumor type. First-degree family history with either breast or ovarian cancer was more strongly associated with serous and endometrioid cancer then mucinous lesions.[129] Kurian et al. reported body mass index was negatively associated with serous tumors but weakly positive for endometrioid cancer; and current smokers were at increased risk only of mucinous tumors, RR = 2.4 (95% CI = 1.5–3.8).[47]

Ness et al. noted chronic inflammation of endometriosis was associated with endometrioid and clear cell ovarian cancer.[86] A Canadian case-control study found 5 years or more of postmenopausal estrogen use increased risk of serous and endometrioid but not mucinous tumors with an OR = 2.78 (95% CI = 1.13–6.83).[130] A similar, though smaller, adverse effect of hormone use was reported from the British Million Women Study for serous compared with mucinous cancers.[131] The Nurses' Health Study also identified serous and endometrioid tumors associated with 5 years of estrogen use suggesting susceptibility to hormonal exposure differed by histologies.[132]

Pathology, Treatment, and Prognosis

Pathologic confirmation of the malignancy is essential prior to treatment or inclusion in research. Pathologic classification of cases enrolled in the CASH Study[84] conducted from 1980 to 1982 established a research standard by assembling gynecologic pathologists who independently reviewed histologic slides from cases identified by six SEER registries.[113] These experts agreed with initial diagnostic pathology reports for 98%; disagreements were noted only for the less common histologic types.

Prognosis is considered excellent following diagnosis at stage I with approximately 90% of patients alive at 5 years. Less successful outcomes have been noted among some racial/ethnic groups[7] for whom access to medical care and other social conditions may affect survival. This differential was not observed among more advanced cases where currently available treatments are minimally effective.[7]

Younger women are treated by hysterectomy with bilateral oophorectomy preventing future childbearing.[5] SEER data provided survival information of stage I cases age 50 or younger treated by bilateral oophorectomy and hysterectomy for comparison with cases who retained an unaffected ovary and the uterus; no survival differences were found.[5] Conservative surgery enabled consideration of subsequent pregnancy although adjuvant chemotherapy may impede fertility. However, some young ovarian cancer patients have become pregnant and produced healthy babies.[5] After completion of childbearing some clinicians recommend removal of the remaining ovary, fallopian tubes, and uterus to reduce the risk of recurrent cancer in these organs.[5] Ovarian conservation also avoids the long-term adverse effects of sudden estrogen depletion including rapid onset of menopausal symptoms, osteoporosis, heart disease, and psychological changes.

Familial ovarian cancer appears to have superior prognosis with 67% 5 year survival compared with 17% among nonfamilial cases.[134] Similar results were reported in 1996 when hereditary ovarian cancer cases were found to have superior survival compared to sporadic cases.[135] Longer survival has been associated with *BRCA* positive cases determined retrospectively when relatives of the deceased patients requested genetic testing to guide future clinical care of family members.[135] Building on these findings, the U.S. Preventive Services Task Force has endorsed genetic testing of women with family history of ovarian cancer in order to have the essential information available before making treatment decisions.[58]

Since a majority of newly diagnosed women with ovarian cancer have metastases to other organs, aggressive therapy achieves only 30% to 45% 5 year survival. Standard treatment protocols include extensive surgery to removal all detectable disease followed by intravenous or intraperitoneal multiagent chemotherapy.[15] A recently reported multi-institutional clinical trial compared survival among women diagnosed with stages IIIC and IV who were randomized to receive either surgery followed by multiagent chemotherapy or neoadjuvant chemotherapy prior to surgical removal of cancerous tissue; no survival differences were detected.[136] Regardless of the timing of chemotherapy, the strongest prognostic factor was the success of surgical removal of tumor tissue in the pelvic cavity.[136]

Several new options for treatment have recently prolonged survival, including inhibitors of angiogenesis (formation of new blood vessels that feed the growing tumor). Although recent results from these new modalities have been encouraging, new agents based on genetic components of specific tumor types are being developed to hopefully achieve long-term remission rather than stable disease. Recurrence and dissemination of disease remain major concerns of patients diagnosed with advanced ovarian cancer after aggressive surgery and chemotherapy. Rising CA-125 levels may be prognostic of recurrence even in the absence of symptoms or palpable abnormalities.[12]

Avenues for Prevention among Women at High Risk

Approximately 10% of ovarian cancers are believed to result from inherited susceptibility, encouraging genetic counseling referrals for newly diagnosed patients depending on ages at diagnoses and number of affected relatives. Prevention due to OC use extends to women with inherited susceptibility (OR = 0.5 (95% CI = 0.3–0.8)). Since the chemopreventive effect of OCs does not eliminate risk among mutation carriers, prophylactic removal of both ovaries and fallopian tubes was proposed several decades ago and became acceptable in the 1990s even before BRCA mutations were recognized and the degree of benefit was known.[53] Although the surgery greatly reduces risk, mutation carriers remain at risk for peritoneal cancer,[10] which is histologically identical to primary ovarian adenocarcinoma.[127] Risk-reducing surgery lowered ovarian cancer risk among BRCA mutation carriers (HR = 0.21; 95% CI = 0.12–0.39) in a meta-analysis.[138] This finding was supported by Domchek who noted benefits of risk-reducing surgery from the Prevention and Observation of Surgical Endpoints (PROSE) consortium of 18 centers in Europe and North America that followed 2,482 women with a BRCA1 or BRCA2 mutation including some women with a prior history of breast cancer who elected to undergo either prophylactic surgery or close surveillance.[139] In their 2010 publication, the authors stated that removal of ovaries and tubes reduced the risk of primary peritoneal/ovarian cancer by 85% among BRCA1 mutation carriers who were previously treated for breast cancer and lowered risk 70% for women free of breast cancer. In contrast, no cases of ovarian cancer were diagnosed among BRCA2 carriers regardless of their prior breast cancer status. All-cause mortality as well as death due to ovarian cancer was significantly reduced following risk-reducing surgery (HR = 0.40).[139] Extensive pathology review of 385 surgical specimens retrieved from prophylactic surgery revealed occult cancer in ovarian tissue or Fallopian tubes of 16 (2.4%) women of whom 12 were at genetic risk having a BRCA1 mutation.[140] Detection of malignancy was greater among women older than 40 years at time of prophylactic surgery. Having a mutation or strong family history of

ovarian cancer affecting surgery decisions must be balanced against the potential adverse effects of early, abrupt menopause, although some women have safely used hormone replacement therapy for a brief interval to diminish the symptoms associated with sudden loss of estrogen.[139]

The USPSTF noted that women who were tested and found negative for BRCA but whose family history suggested an inherited susceptibility, may also benefit from risk reducing surgery.[58] Accurate family history information is essential to guide genetic counseling before BRCA testing and to enable informed clinical decision making. Multiple marriages with children from more than one parental pair complicate genetic analyses, especially with mixed ethnicities. Although genetic guidance may be of value to women considering prophylactic surgery, not all women may have access to trained genetic testing and counseling due to lack of health insurance or coverage for these procedures.[53] Potentially, components of the new health insurance law may clarify the availability of genetic counseling and testing for women whose family history is compatible with the USPSTF guidelines.

Summary

Epidemiologic studies of ovarian cancer are challenging due to low incidence and lethal nature of the malignancy which requires rapid case identification for research. In the current era of oral contraceptive formulas, use of low-dose estrogen combined with progestin reduces ovarian cancer risk. The importance of OC use for prevention of unwanted pregnancy is obvious but young women at risk for ovarian cancer should also consider the protective role provided by these preparations. Use of OCs by the general population for cancer prevention may be less compelling. Delaying childbearing to older ages may result in women seeking treatment for infertility and potential hazards associated with hyperstimulation of the ovaries for assisted reproductive procedures. Risk associated with stimulation for egg donation should also be studied as some women have experienced these procedures several times.

Although efforts to improve early detection have been the focus of many research projects and government-sponsored trials, the results have not been encouraging. In 2010 clinicians and researchers agreed no changes are warranted to the U.S. Preventive Task Force guidelines: no current screening methods are recommended for women with familial risk or genetic susceptibility or of average risk without a family history. However, some clinicians disagree and offer a combination of screening tests for women at genetic risk.

Prophylactic surgery removing fallopian tubes and ovaries provides protection for BRCA mutation carriers although a few women will subsequently develop peritoneal carcinoma. The combined use of oral contraceptives over the past 50 years and recent decisions to undergo prophylactic surgery have been credited with a small decline in ovarian cancer incidence among women younger than age 60.

Discussion Questions

1. What avenues exist for prevention of ovarian cancer? What risks may be associated with these activities and exposures?
2. What percentage of ovarian cancer is believed to be due to inherited susceptibility? Is family history an indicator? Describe some of the familial patterns that implicate genetic risk.
3. What symptoms might be associated with ovarian cancer? Why are they inadequate for early detection?
4. Describe some screening modalities that have been studied. Why does the USPSTF not recommend any of these on a routine basis?
5. What types of studies are most useful for identifying risk factors? Why are these most valuable?

References

1. Jemal A, Siegel R, Ward EM. American Cancer Society. *Cancer Facts & Figures 2010*. Atlanta, GA: 2010.
2. SEER Cancer Statistics Review 1975–2007. Surveillance Epidemiology and End Results. Table 21.11. http://seer.cancer.gov/statfacts/html/ovary.html. (Accessed August 2010.)
3. Brescia RJ, Dubin N, Demopoulos RI. Endometrioid and clear cell carcinoma of the ovary. Factors affecting survival. *Int J. Gynecol Pathol* 1989;8:132–138.
4. Daly MB, Ozols RF. Symptoms of ovarian cancer—Where to set the bar? *JAMA*. 2004;291:2755–2756.
5. Wright JD, Shah M, Mathew L, et al. Fertility preservation in young women with epithelial ovarian cancer. *Cancer*. 2009;115:4118–4126.
6. Mink PJ, Sherman ME, Devesa SS. Incidence patterns of invasive and borderline ovarian tumors among white women and black women in the United States. *Cancer*. 2002;95:2380–2389.
7. Kim S, Dolecak TA, Davis FG. Racial differences in stage at diagnosis and survival from epithelial ovarian cancer: a fundamental cause of disease approach. *Soc Sci Med*. 2010;71:274–281.
8. Cramer DW, Welch WR. Determinants of ovarian cancer risk. II. Inferences regarding pathogenesis. *J Natl Cancer Inst*. 1983;71:717–721.
9. Mittal KR, Zeleniuch-Jacquotte A, Cooper JL, Demopoulos RI. Contralateral ovary in unilateral ovarian carcinoma: a search for preneoplastic lesions. *Int J Gynecol Pathol*. 1993;12:59–63.
10. Crum CP, Drapkin R, Kindelberger D, et al. Lessons from BRCA: the tubal fimbria emerges as an origin for pelvic serous cancer. *Clin Med Res*. 2007;5:35–44.
11. Dubeau L. The cell of origin of ovarian epithelial tumours. *Lancet Oncology*. 2008;9:1191–1197.
12. Cannistra SA. Cancer of the ovary. *N Engl J Med*. 2004;351:2519–2529.
13. Glud E, Kjaer SK, Troisi R, Brinton LA. Fertility drugs and ovarian cancer. *Epidemiol Reviews*. 1998;20:237–257.
14. National Cancer Institute. Ovarian cancer screening (PDQ®). CA 125 levels, Transvaginal ultrasound, and pelvic examinations. Statement of benefit. http://www.cancer.gov/cancertopics/pdq/screening/ovarian/healthprofessional. Accessed January 20, 2011.
15. Clarke-Pearson D. Screening for ovarian cancer. *N Engl J Med*. 2009;361:170–177.
16. van Nagell JR Jr, DePriest PD, Ueland FR, et al. Ovarian cancer screening with annual transvaginal sonography: findings of 25,000 women screened. *Cancer*. 2007;109:1887–1896.
17. Campbell S, Bhan V, Royston P, et al. Transabdominal ultrasound screening for early ovarian cancer. *BMJ*. 1989;299:1363–1367.
18. Pavik EJ, DePriest PD, Gallion HH, et al. Ovarian volume related to age. *Gynecol Oncol*. 2000;77:410–412.
19. Black SS, Butler SL, Goldman PA, Scoggins MJ. Ovarian cancer symptom index. Possibilities for earlier detection. *Cancer*. 2007;109:167–169.
20. Goff BA, Mandel LS, Melancon CH, Muntz HG. Frequency of symptoms of ovarian cancer in women presenting to primary care clinics. *JAMA*. 2004;291:2705–2712.
21. Goff BA, Mandel LS, Drescher CW, et al. Development of an ovarian cancer symptoms index. Possibilities for earlier detection. *Cancer*. 2007;109:221–227.
22. Lurie G, Wilkens LR, Thompson PJ, et al. Symptom presentation in invasive ovarian carcinoma by tumor histology type and grade in a multiethnic population: a case analysis. *Gynecol Oncol*. 2010;119:278–284.
23. Rossing MA, Wicklund KG, Cushing-Haugen KL, Weiss NS. Predictive value of symptoms for early detection of ovarian cancer. *J Natl Cancer Inst*. 2010;102:222–229.
24. Pavlik EJ, Saunders BA, Doran S, et al. The search for meaning-symptoms and transvaginal sonography screening for ovarian cancer. *Cancer*. 2009;115:3689–3698.
25. Zurawski VR Jr, Orjaseter H, Andersen A, et al. Elevated serum CA 125 levels prior to diagnosis of ovarian cancer neoplasia: relevance for early detection of ovarian cancer. *Int J Cancer*. 1988;42:677–680.
26. Helzlsouer KJ, Bush TL, Alberg AJ, Bass KM, Zacer H, Comstock GW. Prospective study of serum CA-125 levels as markers of ovarian cancer. *JAMA*. 1993;269:1123–1126.
27. Daly MB, Ozols RF. The search for predictive patterns in ovarian cancer: Proteomics meets bioinformatics. *Cancer Cell*. 2002;1:111–112.
28. Hartge P. Designing early detection programs for ovarian cancer. *J Natl Cancer Inst*. 2009;102:3–4.
29. Moore RG, McMeekin DS, Brown AK, et al. A novel multiple marker bioassay utilizing HE4 and CA125 for the prediction of ovarian cancer in patients with a pelvic mass. *Gynecol Oncol*. 2009;112:40–46.
30. Anderson GL, McIntosh M, Wu L, et al. Assessing lead time of selected ovarian biomarkers: a nested case-control study. *J Natl Cancer Inst*. 2010;102: 26–38.
31. Muller CY. Doctor, should I get this new ovarian cancer test—OVA1? *Obstet Gynecol*. 2010;116:246–247.
32. Bourne TH, Cambell S, Reynolds K, et al. The potential role of serum CA 125 in an ultrasound-based screening program for familial ovarian cancer. *Gynecol Oncol*. 1994;52:379–385.
33. Carlson KJ, Skates SJ, Singer DE. Screening for ovarian cancer. *Ann Intern Med*. 1994;121:124–132.
34. Jacobs IJ, Skates SJ, MacDonald N, et al. Screening for ovarian cancer: a pilot randomized controlled trial. *Lancet*. 1999;353:1207–1210.
35. Anderson MR, Goff BA, Lowe KA, et al. Combining a symptoms index with CA 125 to improve detection of ovarian cancer. *Cancer*. 2008;113:484–489.
36. Partridge E, Kreimer AR, Greenlee RT, et al. Results from four rounds of ovarian cancer screening in a randomized trial. *Obstet Gynecol*. 2009;113:775–782.
37. Fathalla MF. Incessant ovulation—A factor in ovarian neoplasia? *Lancet*. 1971;2:163.
38. Casagrande JT, Louie EW, Pike MC, et al. "Incessant ovulation" and ovarian cancer. *Lancet*. 1979;2:170–173.
39. Jeppsson S, Rannevik G, Thorell JL, et al. Influence of LH/FSH releasing hormones (LRH) on the basal secretion of gonadotropins in relation to plasma levels of oestradiol, progesterone and prolactin during post-partum period in lactating and non-lactating women. *Acta Endorinol*. 1977;84:713–728.
40. Risch HA. Hormonal etiology of epithelial ovarian cancer, with a hypothesis concerning the role of androgens and progesterone. *J Natl Cancer Inst*. 1998;90:1774–1786.
41. Schildkraut JM, Iversen ES. Wilson MA, et al. Association between DNA damage response and repair genes and risk of invasive serous ovarian cancer. *PloS One*. 2010;5:e10061.
42. Hildreth NG, Kelsey JL, LiVolsi VA, et al. An epidemiologic study of epithelial carcinoma of the ovary. *Am J Epidemiol*. 1981;114:398–405.
43. Piver MS, Baker TR, Jishi MF, et al. Familial ovarian cancer. A report of 658 families from the Gilda Radner Familial Ovarian Cancer Registry 1981–1991. *Cancer*. 1993;71:582–588.
44. Amos CI, Shaw GL, Tucker MA, Hartge P. Age at onset for familial epithelial ovarian cancer. *JAMA*. 1992;268:1896–1899.
45. Rubin SC. Chemoprevention of hereditary ovarian cancer. Editorial. *N Engl J Med*. 1998;339:469–471.
46. Stratton JF, Paroah P, Smith SK, Easton D, Ponder BA. A systematic review and meta-analysis of family history and risk of ovarian cancer. *Br J Obstet Gynaecol*. 1998; 105:493–499.
47. Kurian AW, Balise RR, McGuire V, Whittemore AS. Histologic types of epithelial ovarian cancer: have they different risk factors? *Gynecol Oncol*. 2005: 520–530.
48. Grant DJ, Moorman PG, Akushevich L, et al. Primary peritoneal and ovarian cancers: an epidemiological comparative analysis. *Cancer Causes Control*. 2010;21:991–998.
49. Lynch HT, Watson P, Bewira C, et al. Hereditary ovarian cancer. Heterogeneity in age at diagnosis. *Cancer*. 1991;67:1460–1466.
50. King MC, Marks JH, Mandell JB for the New York Breast Cancer Study Group. Breast and ovarian cancer risks due to inherited mutations in BRCA1 and BRCA2. *Science*. 2003;302:643–646.
51. Risch HA, McLaughlin JR, Cole DEC, et al. Population BRCA1 and BRCA2 mutation frequencies and cancer penetrance: a kin-cohort study in Ontario, Canada. *J Natl Cancer Inst*. 2006;98:1694–1706.
52. StatBite: BRCA mutations increase risk of breast/ovarian cancer. *J Natl Cancer Inst*. 2010:102:755.
53. South SA, Vance H, Farrell C, et al. Consideration of hereditary nonpolyposis colorectal cancer in BRCA mutation-negative familial ovarian cancers. *Cancer*. 2008;115:324–333.
54. Ramus SJ, Harrington PA, Pye C, et al. Contribution of BRCA1 and BRCA2 mutations to inherited ovarian cancer. *Hum Mutat*. 2007;28:1207–1215.
55. Antoniou A, Pharoah PDP, Narod S, et al. Average risks of breast and ovarian cancer associated with BRCA1 or BRCA2 mutations detected in case series unselected for family history: a combined analysis of 22 studies. *Am J Hum Genet*. 2003;72:1117–1130.

56. Boyd J. Specific keynote: hereditary ovarian cancer. What we know. *Gynecol Oncol.* 2003;88:S8–S10. Discussion S11–S13.

57. U.S. Preventive Services Task Force. Genetic risk assessment and *BRCA* mutation testing for breast and ovarian cancer susceptibility: recommendation statement. *Ann Intern Med.* 2005;143:355–361.

58. Olopade OI. Genetics in clinical care– The future is now. *N Engl J Med.* 1996;335:1455–1456.

59. Fasching PA, Gayther S, Pearce L, et al. Role of genetic polymorphisms and ovarian cancer susceptibility. *Molecular Oncol.* 2009;3:171–181.

60. Kauff ND, Mitra N, Robson ME. et al. Risk of ovarian cancer in BRCA1 and BRCA2 mutation-negative hereditary breast cancer families. *J Natl Cancer Inst.* 2005;97:1382–1384.

61. Lee JS, John EM, McGuire V, et al. Breast and ovarian cancer in relatives of cancer patients, with and without BRCA mutations. *Cancer Epidemiol Biomarkers Prev.* 2006;15:359–363.

62. Schildkraut JM, Cooper GS, Halabi S, et al. Age at natural menopause and risk of epithelial ovarian cancer. *Obstet Gynecol.* 2001;98:85–90.

63. Titus-Ernstoff L, Perez K, Cramer DW, et al. Menstrual and reproductive factors in relation to ovarian cancer risk. *British J Cancer.* 2001;84:714–721.

64. John EM, Whittemore AS, Harris R, et al. Characteristics relating to ovarian cancer risk: Collaborative analysis of seven US case-control studies. Epithelial ovarian cancer in black women. *J Natl Cancer Inst.* 1993;85:142–147.

65. Schildkraut JM, Bastos E, Berchuck A. Relationship between lifetime ovulatory cycles and over-expression of mutant p53 in epithelial ovarian cancer. *J Natl Cancer Inst.* 1997;89:932–938.

66. Beral V, Fraser P, Chilvers C. Does pregnancy protect against ovarian cancer? *Lancet.* 1978;1:1083–1087.

67. Nasca PC, Greenwald P, Chorost S, et al. An epidemiologic case-control study of ovarian cancer and reproductive factors. *Am J Epidemiol.* 1984;119:705–713.

68. Whittemore AS, Harris R, Intyre J, Collaborative Ovarian Cancer Group. Characteristics relating to ovarian cancer risk: collaborative analysis of twelve US case-control studies. II. Invasive epithelial ovarian cancer in white women. *Am J Epidemiol.* 1992; 136:1184–1203.

69. Adami HO, Hsieh CC, Lambe M, et al. Parity, age at first childbirth, and risk of ovarian cancer. *Lancet.* 1994;344:1250–1254.

70. Lambe M, Wuu J, Rossing MA, Hsieh CC. Twinning and maternal risk of ovarian cancer. *Lancet.* 1999;353:1941.

71. Whiteman DC, Murphy MFG, Cook LS, et al. Multiple births and risk of epithelial ovarian cancer. *J Natl Cancer Inst.* 2000;92:1172–1177.

72. Whiteman DC, Siskind V, Purdie DM, Green AC. Timing of pregnancy and risk of epithelial ovarian cancer. *Cancer Epidemiol Biomarkers Prev.* 2003;12:42–46.

73. Danforth KN, Hecht JL, Colditz GA. Breastfeeding and risk of ovarian cancer in two prospective cohorts. *Cancer Causes Control.* 2007;18:517–523.

74. Ryan AS, Zhou W, Arensberg MB. The effect of employment status on breastfeeding in the United States. *Womens Health Issues.* 2006;16:243–251.

75. Rossing MA, Daling JR, Weiss NS, et al. Ovarian tumors in a cohort of infertile women. *N Engl J Med.* 1994;331:771–776.

76. Brinton LA, Lamb EJ, Moghissi KS, et al. Ovarian cancer risk associated with varying causes of infertility. *Fertil Steril.* 2004;82:405–414.

77. Fishel S, Jackson P. Follicular stimulation for high tech pregnancies: are we playing it safe? *BMJ.* 1989;299:309–311.

78. Brinton LA, Lamb EJ, Moghissi KS, et al. Ovarian cancer risk after the use of ovulation-stimulating drugs. *Obstet Gynecol.* 2004;103:1194–1203.

79. Hankinson SE, Hunter DJ, Colditz GA, et al. Tubal ligation, hysterectomy, and risk of ovarian cancer. A prospective study. *JAMA.* 1993;270:2813–2818.

80. Narod SA, Sun p, Ghadirian P, et al. Tubal ligation and risk of ovarian cancer in carriers of BRCA1 and BRCA2 mutations: a case-control study. *Lancet.* 2001;357:1467–1470.

81. Lukanova A, Kaaks R. Endogenous hormones and ovarian cancer: epidemiology and current hypotheses. *Cancer Epidemiol Biomarkers Prev.* 2005;14:98–107.

82. Helzlsouer KJ, Alberg AJ, Gordon GB, et al. Serum gonadotropins and steroid hormones and the development of ovarian cancer. *JAMA.* 1995;274:1926–1930.

83. Wingo PA, Tong T, Bolden S. Cancer statistics, 1995. *CA Cancer J Clin.* 1995;45:8–30.

84. Oral contraceptive use and the risk of ovarian cancer: the Centers for Disease Control Cancer and Steroid Hormone Study. *JAMA.* 1983;249:1596–1599.

85. The Cancer and Steroid Hormone Study of the Centers for Disease Control and the National Institute of Child Health and Human Development. The reduction in risk of ovarian cancer associated with oral contraceptive use. *N Engl J Med.* 1987;316:650–655.

86. Ness RB, Grisso JA, Klapper J, et al. Risk of ovarian cancer in relation to estrogen and progestin dose and use characteristics of oral contraceptives. *Am J Epidemiol.* 2000;152:233–241.

87. Collaborative Group on Epidemiological Studies of Ovarian Cancer; Beral V, Doll R, et al. Ovarian cancer and oral contraceptives: collaborative reanalysis of data from 45 epidemiological studies including 23,257 women with ovarian cancer and 87,303 controls. *Lancet.* 2008;371:303–314.

88. Trussell J, Schwarz EB, Guthrie K. Obesity and oral contraceptive failure. *Contraception.* 2009;79:334–338.

89. Westhoff CL, Torgal AH, Mayeda ER, et al. Ovarian suppression in normal-weight and obese women during oral contraceptive use. *Obstet Gynecol.* 2010;116:275–283.

90. Narod SA, Risch H, Moslehi R, et al. Oral contraceptives and the risk of hereditary ovarian cancer. *N Engl J Med.* 1998;339:424–428.

91. Whittemore AS, Balise RR, Pharoah PDP, et al. Oral contraceptive use and ovarian cancer risk among carriers of BRCA1 and BRCA2 mutations. *Br J Cancer.* 2004;91:1911–1915.

92. Lacey JV, Mink PJ, Lubin JH, et al. Menopausal hormone replacement and risk of ovarian cancer. *JAMA.* 2002;288:334–341.

93. Rossing MA, Cushing-Haugen KL, Wicklund KG, et al. Menopausal hormone therapy and risk of epithelial ovarian cancer. *Cancer Epidemiol Biomarkers Prev.* 2007;16:2548–2556.

94. Anderson GL, Judd HL, Kaunitz AM, et al. Effects of estrogen plus progestin on gynecologic cancers and associated diagnostic procedures. The Women's Health Initiative Randomized Trial. *JAMA.* 2003;290:1739–1748.

95. Rodriguez C, Patel AV, Calle EE, et al. Estrogen replacement therapy and ovarian cancer mortality in a large prospective study of US women. *JAMA.* 2001;285:1460–1465.

96. Cottreau CM, Ness RB, Kriska AM. Physical activity and reduced risk of ovarian cancer. *Obstet Gynecol.* 2000;96:609–614.

97. Leitzmann LF, Koebnick C, Moore SC, et al. Prospective study of physical activity and risk of ovarian cancer. *Cancer Causes Control.* 2009;20:765–773.

98. Olsen CM, Green AC, Whiteman DC, et al. Obesity and the risk of epithelial ovarian cancer: a systematic review and meta-analysis. *European J Cancer.* 2007;43:690–709.

99. Fairfield KM, Willett WC, Rosner BA, et al. Obesity, weight gain, and ovarian cancer. *Obstet Gynecol.* 2002;288:296.

100. Schouten LJ, Rivera C, Hunter DJ, et al. Height, body mass index, and ovarian cancer: a pooled analysis of 12 cohort studies. *Cancer Epidemiol Biomarkers Prev.* 2008;17:902–912.

101. Leitzmann LF, Koebnick C, Danforth KN, et al. Body mass index and risk of ovarian cancer. *Cancer.* 2009;115:812–822.

102. Rodriguez C, Calle EE, Fakhrabadi-Shokoohi D, et al. Body mass index, height, and risk of ovarian cancer mortality in a prospective cohort of post-menopausal women. *Cancer Epidemiol Biomarkers Prev.* 2002;11:822–828.

103. Schulz M, Lahmann PH, Boeing H, et al. Fruit and vegetable consumption and risk of epithelial ovarian cancer: the European Prospective Investigation into Cancer and Nutrition. *Cancer Epidemiol Biomarkers Prev.* 2005;14:2531–2535.

104. Genkinger JM, Hunter DJ, Spiegelman D et al. Dairy products and ovarian cancer: a pooled analysis of 12 cohort studies. *Cancer Epidemiol Biomarkers Prev.* 2006;15:364–372.

105. Chang S, Risch HA. Perineal talc exposure and risk of ovarian carcinoma. *Cancer.* 1997;79:2396–2401.

106. Cook LS, Kamb ML, Weiss NS. Perineal powder exposure and the risk of ovarian cancer. *Am J Epidemiol.* 1997;145:459–465.

107. Cramer DW, Liberman RF, Titus-Ernstoff L, et al. Genital talc exposure and risk of ovarian cancer. *Int J Cancer.* 1999;81:351–356.

108. Tokuoka S, Kawai K, Shimizu Y, et al. Malignant and benign ovarian neoplasms among atomic bomb survivors, Hiroshima and Nagasaki, 1950–80. *J Natl Cancer Inst.* 1987;79:47–51.

109. Chaturvedi AK, Engels EA, Gilbert ES, et al. Second cancers among 104,760 survivors of cervical cancer: evaluation of long-term risk. *J Natl Cancer Inst.* 2007;99:1634–1343.

110. Hankinson SE, Danforth KN. Ovarian cancer. In: Schottenfeld D, Fraumeni JF, Jr., eds. *Cancer Epidemiology and Prevention.* 3rd ed. New York: Oxford University Press; 2006:1013–1026.

111. Rosenberg L, Palmer JR, Rao S, et al. A case-control study of analgesic use and ovarian cancer. *Cancer Epidemiol Biomarkers Prev.* 2000;9:933–937.

112. Pinheiro SP, Tworoger SS, Cramer DW, et al. Use of nonsteroidal anti-inflammatory agents and incidence of ovarian cancer in 2 large prospective cohorts. *Am J Epidemiol.* 2009;169:1378–1387.

113. Wernli KJ, Newcomb PA, Hapton JM, et al. Inverse association of NSAID use and ovarian cancer in relation to oral contraceptive use and parity. *Br J Cancer.* 2008;98:1781–1783.

114. Gates MA, Tworoger SS, Eliassen H, et al. Analgesic use and sex steroid hormone concentrations in postmenopausal women. *Cancer Epidemiol Biomarkers Prev.* 210;19:1033–1041.

115. Jordan SJ, Whiteman DC, Purdie DM, et al. Does smoking increase risk of ovarian cancer? A systematic review. *Gynecol Oncol.* 2006;103:1122–1129.

116. Tworoger SS, Gertig DM, Gates MA, et al. Caffeine, alcohol, smoking and the risk of incident epithelial ovarian cancer. *Cancer.* 2008;112:1169–1177.

117. Genkinger JM, Hunter DJ, Spiegelman D, et al. Alcohol intake and ovarian cancer risk: a pooled analysis of 10 cohort studies. *Br J Cancer.* 2006;94:757–762.

118. Garland CF, Mohr SB, Gorham ED, et al. Role of ultraviolet B irradiance and vitamin D in prevention of ovarian cancer. *Am J Prev Med.* 2006;31:512–514.

119. Zheng W, Danforth KN, Tworoger SS, et al. Circulating 25-hydroxyvitamin D and risk of epithelial ovarian cancer. Cohort consortium vitamin D pooling project of rarer cancers. *Am J Epidemiol.* 2010;172:70–80.

120. Ness RB, Modugno F. Endometriosis as a model for inflammation-hormone interactions in ovarian and breast cancers. *Eur J Cancer.* 2006;42:691–703.

121. Brinton LA, Gridley G, Persson I, et al. Cancer risk after a hospital discharge diagnosis of endometriosis. *Am J Obstet Gynecol.* 1997;176:572–579.

122. Olson JE, Cerhan JR, Janney CA, et al. Postmenopausal cancer risk after self-reported endometriosis diagnosis in the Iowa Women's Health Study. *Cancer.* 2002;94:1612–1618.

123. Schildkraut J, Schwingl PJ, Bastos E, et al. Epithelial ovarian cancer risk among women with polycystic ovarian syndrome. *Obstet Gynecol.* 1996;88:549–554.

124. Risch HA, Howe GR. Pelvic inflammatory disease and risk of epithelial ovarian cancer. *Cancer Epidemiol Biomarkers Prev.* 1995;4:447–451.

125. Bergfeldt K, Rydh B, Granath F et al. Risk of ovarian cancer in breast cancer patients with a family history of breast or ovarian cancer. A population-based cohort study. *Lancet.* 2002;360:891–894.

126. Metcalfe KA, Lynch HT, Ghadirian P, et al. The risk of ovarian cancer after breast cancer in BRCA1 and BRCA2 carriers. *Gynecol Oncol.* 2005;96:222–226.

127. Ness RB, Grisso JA, Klapper J, Vergona R. Racial differences in ovarian cancer risk. *J Natl Med Assoc.* 2000;92:176–182.

128. Moorman PG, Palmieri RT, Akushevich L, et al. Ovarian cancer risk factors in African-American and white women. *Am J Epidemiol.* 2009;170:598–606.

129. Schildkraut JM, Thompson WD. Relationship of epithelial ovarian cancer to other malignancies within families. *Genetic Epidemiol.* 1988;5:355–367.

130. Risch HA, Marrett LD, Jain M, Howe GR. Differences in risk factors for epithelial ovarian cancer by histologic type. results of a case-control study. *Am J Epidemiol.* 1996;144:363–372.

131. Beral V, Bull D, Green J, Reeves G. Ovarian cancer and hormone replacement therapy in the Million Women Study. *Lancet.* 2007;369:1703–1710.

132. Gates MA, Rosner BA, Hecht JL, Tworoger SS. Risk factors for epithelial ovarian cancer by histologic subtype. *Am J Epidemiol.* 2010;171:45–53.

133. Tyler CW, Lee NC, Robboy SJ, et al. The diagnosis of ovarian cancer by pathologists: how often do diagnoses by contributing pathologists agree with a panel of gynecologic pathologists? *Am J Obstet Gynecol.* 1991;164:65–70.

134. Buller RE, Anderson B, Connor JP, Robinson R. Familial ovarian cancer. *Gynecol Oncol.* 1993;51:160–166.

135. Rubin SC, Benjamin I, Behbakht K, et al. Clinical and pathological features of ovarian cancer in women with germ-line mutations of BRCA1. *N Engl J Med.* 1996;335:1413–1416.

136. Vergote I, Trope CG, Armant F, et al. Neoadjuvant chemotherapy or primary surgery in stage IIIC or IV ovarian cancer. *N Engl J Med.* 2010;363:943–953.

137. Piver MS, Jishi MF, Tsukada Y, Nava G. Primary peritoneal carcinoma after prophylactic oophorectomy in women with a family history of ovarian cancer. *Cancer.* 1993;71:2751–2755.

138. Rebbeck TR, Kauff ND, Domcheck SM. Meta-analysis of risk reduction estimates associated with risk-reducing salpingo-oophorectomy in *BRCA1* or *BRCA2* mutation carriers. *J Natl Cancer Inst.* 2009;101:80–87.

139. Domchek SM, Friebel TM, Singer CF, et al. Association of risk-reducing surgery in *BRCA1* or *BRCA2* mutation carriers with cancer risk and mortality. *JAMA.* 2010;304:967–975.

140. Domchek SM, Friebel TM, Garber JE, et al. Occult ovarian cancers identified at risk-reducing salpingo-oophorectomy in a prospective cohort of *BRCA1/2* mutation carriers. *Breast Cancer Res Treat.* 2010;124:195–203.

Endometrial Cancer

Susan R. Sturgeon, DrPH, MPH and Aimee Kroll-Desrosiers, MS

Introduction

Endometrial and cervical cancers both arise in the uterus; however, they differ dramatically in pathophysiology and etiology. The major cause of cervical cancer is the sexually transmitted human papilloma virus (HPV); endometrial cancer results from hormonal carcinogenesis. This chapter focuses on the epidemiology of endometrial cancer.

Endometrial cancer develops in the body, or corpus, of the uterus as indicated in Figure 28-1. The most common histologic type of endometrial cancer is endometrioid adenocarcinoma, which develops from the glandular cells of the endometrium (the inner lining of the uterus). Less common but more aggressive histologic types of endometrial cancer include clear cell carcinoma, papillary serous carcinoma, poorly differentiated carcinoma, mucinous carcinoma, and squamous cell carcinoma. Another histologic type, uterine sarcoma, forms in the muscle layer of the body of the uterus.[1]

Endometrial hyperplasia, a precursor to endometrioid adenocarcinoma, is a thickening of the endometrium that occurs in response to estrogenic stimulation unopposed by progesterone. The likelihood that endometrial hyperplasia will progress to cancer depends on the extent of cellular atypia (abnormal cells), ranging from 1% for women with simple hyperplasia to nearly 30% for women with complex atypical hyperplasia. Conversely, nonendometrioid carcinomas, which consist primarily of papillary serous and clear cell carcinomas, probably develop by a pathway that does not involve stimulation by estrogen or the hyperplasia precursor.[2]

Descriptive Epidemiology

Endometrial cancer is primarily a disease of industrialized countries. Incidence rates in North America are nearly double those in Europe and almost 10 times higher than in parts of Africa. Worldwide, the age-standardized incidence

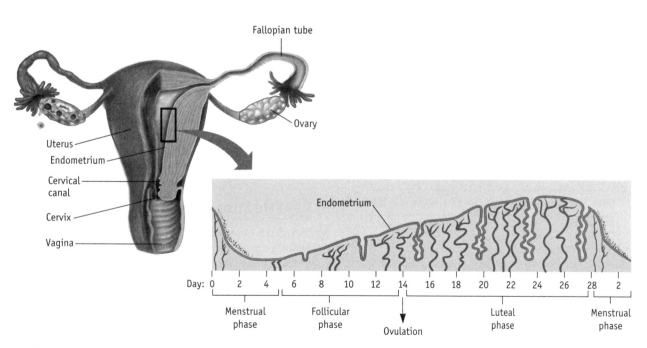

Figure 28-1 Uterus, endometrial lining, ovaries and fallopian tubes.

rate in 2002 was the highest at 22.8 per 100,000 in the United States compared to a low of 2.2 per 100,000 in Western Africa. Mortality rates are substantially lower than incidence rates, due to generally favorable prognoses. Age-standardized mortality rates in 2002 were highest in parts of the Caribbean (4.3 per 100,000) and in Central and Eastern European countries (3.6 per 100,000) compared to 2.6 per 100,000 in the United States.[3]

Endometrial cancer is the fourth most common cancer diagnosed in American women after cancers of the lung, colorectum, and breast.[4] Over 49,000 women are estimated to be diagnosed with endometrial cancer in 2013.[5] Non-Hispanic white women have consistently higher incidence rates than women of other racial/ethnic groups in the United States (Figure 28-2). From 1997 to 2006, the most recent time period for which data are available, the incidence decreased slightly in non-Hispanic white women but not in other racial/ethnic groups.[5]

Each year in the United States about 8,000 women die from endometrial cancer. That number has remained relatively unchanged for the past 2 decades (Figure 28-2). Although blacks experience a lower incidence of endometrial cancer, they are more than twice as likely to die from the disease as non-Hispanic whites. Some possible reasons for this striking disparity in mortality rates include

barriers to access to care, inequalities in treatment, greater number of comorbid conditions complicating cancer treatment, and a higher prevalence of more aggressive histologic types of endometrial cancer.[6]

One must exercise some caution in interpreting incidence and mortality rates for endometrial cancer because population estimates typically do not account for the proportion of women who have had surgical menopause. According to one study, if the prevalence of hysterectomy in the United States were taken into account, the incidence rate for endometrial cancer would rise by approximately two-thirds.[7] Rates also may be affected by the fact that uterine cancer can be classified as uterine cervix or uterine corpus, and a small proportion of cases may even be classified ambiguously as "uterine-part not specified."[8]

About 75% of endometrioid adenocarcinomas are diagnosed at a localized stage when over 90% of cases are highly curable with life expectancy exceeding 10 years or longer. Prognosis is less favorable for women with other histologic types of endometrial cancer and for women with more extensive disease at diagnosis. For example, the 5-year survival rates for clear cell and papillary serous cancers range from 60% to 70%, and the 5-year survival rates for women diagnosed with regional or metastatic disease range from 29% to 80%.[9]

Age at Diagnosis

Endometrial cancer occurs most commonly in postmenopausal women with an estimated median age at diagnosis of 62 years. Approximately 80% of cases are diagnosed between 45 and 74 years and fewer than 10% develop endometrial cancer before age 45.[10]

Detection Methods and Screening Patterns

When a woman presents with unexplained uterine spotting, bleeding, or discharge, endometrial cancer may be the cause. To make a formal diagnosis, an endometrial biopsy or dilation and curettage procedure is performed in order to obtain tissue essential for pathologic review. Currently, no routine screening test exists for endometrial cancer that is comparable to the Papanicolaou test for cervical cancer. The American Cancer Society recommends that only high-risk women who have inherited nonpolyposis colorectal cancer (HNPCC) syndrome should undergo annual screening beginning at age 35 with endometrial biopsy and/or transvaginal ultrasound.[5]

Genetic Susceptibility

Hereditary nonpolyposis colorectal cancer syndrome, or HNPCC, is a rare genetic defect that impedes repair of DNA damage. Women with this rare syndrome have a 50% increased lifetime risk of developing endometrial cancer, accounting for only about 5% of endometrial cancer cases.[11] A first-degree family history of endometrial cancer correlates with a modest elevation in endometrial cancer risk (RR = 1.5 to 2.0), likely due to shared environmental factors rather than genetics.[12] Many small association studies have

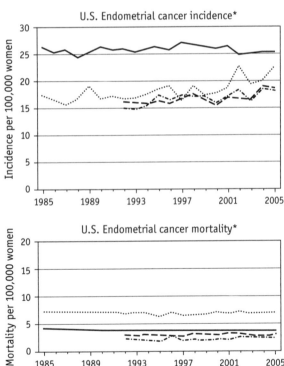

Figure 28-2 Incidence and mortality of endometrial cancer by race/ethnicity, United States, 1985–2005.

Source: Reproduced from National Cancer Institute. A Snapshot for Endometrial Cancer. www.cancer.gov/aboutnci/servingpeople/endometrial-snapshot.pdf Accessed June 25, 2012.

examined allelic variants in hormone receptors and in enzymes that are involved in the biosynthesis and metabolism of steroid hormones or other candidate pathways.[13] However, a true understanding of genetic susceptibility to endometrial cancer will require large, collaborative genome-wide studies with greater attention to statistical methods that address multiple comparisons, as well as the independent verification of the findings of such studies.[14–15]

Risk Factors

Hormones

The "unopposed estrogen hypothesis" provides a compelling explanation for the etiology of most endometrial cancer.[16] Estrogen exposure, without the moderating presence of progesterone or progestin, stimulates uncontrolled cell division increasing the likelihood of deleterious DNA mutations that may initiate endometrial cancer. Increased estrogen exposure or deficits in progesterone exposure is associated with many common risk factors for endometrial cancer, including body fatness and infertility.

Endogenous Estrogens

There is strong support in the literature for the "unopposed estrogen hypothesis." For example, women who have medical conditions associated with elevated levels of endogenous estrogens, including granulosa cell tumors of the ovary and polycystic ovary syndrome, are at higher risk of endometrial cancer.[17,18] In addition, several cohort studies report that postmenopausal women with serum estrogen levels in the highest quartile are twice as likely to develop endometrial cancer than women in the lowest quartile.[19–21] Conversely, data on premenopausal women indicate that concentrations of serum sex hormones do not have a measurable effect on endometrial cancer risk.[19]

Exogenous Estrogens

Oral Contraceptives

Early sequential oral contraceptives consisted of potent synthetic estrogens with low-dose progestin for only a few days of each cycle. These medications were removed from the market in the 1970s when users were found to have a substantially elevated risk of endometrial cancer.[22] By contrast, the oral contraceptives now used widely combine estrogen and progestin and have consistently been associated with a *reduction* in endometrial cancer risk. These preparations combine lower doses of synthetic estrogen and progestin taken continuously during the monthly treatment cycle. Aggregated data from 11 epidemiologic studies demonstrate a greater reduction in risk with increasing years of use, with relative risks of 0.44, 0.33, and 0.28 for use of combined oral contraceptives for 4, 8, and 12 years, respectively.[23] Studies also indicated that women benefit from reduced risk for 2 decades after last use of combined oral contraceptives compared to women who never used these preparations.[23] The observed associations are biologically plausible because women who take oral contraceptives are exposed to progesterone on more days of the monthly cycle compared to nonusers, and women who have taken oral contraceptives have lower serum estrogen levels after menopause.[24,25] Additional studies are needed to evaluate the effect of newer, very low-dose estrogen-progestin oral contraceptives on endometrial cancer risk.

Estrogen Therapy Alone

Many studies have confirmed that menopausal estrogen use increases the risk of endometrial cancer.[26] In the United States estrogen prescribed for menopausal symptoms is most often taken as 0.625 mg of nonconjugated equine estrogen tablets. Among users of menopausal estrogens, the overall risk of developing endometrial cancer is more than twice that of nonusers, based on a meta-analysis of nearly 40 studies conducted by Grady and colleagues.[27] Risk of endometrial cancer increased with duration of use, so that use for less than 1 year confers a small increase in risk; however, among women reporting 10 or more years of estrogen use, risk was increased almost tenfold. Furthermore, a twofold increased risk persists for at least 5 years after use is discontinued. Risk elevations have been observed at all doses of estrogen examined, including doses as low as 0.3 mg per day. As a result of such research findings, a causal link was acknowledged between menopausal estrogen use and endometrial cancer, leading to a rapid decline in number of prescriptions, and a striking decrease in the number of newly diagnosed endometrial cancer cases, further strengthening the case for a causal link (Figure 28-3).[28]

Of historical interest, early epidemiologic studies that implicated estrogens in the development of endometrial cancer were controversial. Critics contended that being under the care of a physician while taking estrogens may lead to the detection of endometrial cancer that otherwise might have remained occult, given that uterine bleeding is a side effect of menopausal estrogen use. Horwitz and Feinstein[29] reported that endometrial cancer risks associated with estrogen use were greatly attenuated in case-control studies by the use of alternative control groups to compensate for the alleged detection bias, such as women with benign uterine conditions. However, the relative risk estimates based on studies with alternative controls were subsequently determined to be biased downward because women diagnosed with benign uterine conditions and who have uterine bleeding were more likely to be estrogen users and thus were inappropriate as control subjects.[29–31]

Combined Estrogen-Progestin Therapy

Because estrogen use alone was shown to increase the risk of endometrial cancer, combined estrogen-progestin regimens were introduced in the 1980s for women with intact uteri. Both estrogen use and estrogen-progestin use declined precipitously in 2002–2003 after the Women's Health Initiative randomized trial reported unexpected adverse effects on cardiovascular disease, breast cancer, and dementia for the combined regimen (conjugated estrogens 0.625 mg/d plus medroxyprogesterone acetate 2.5 mg/d in one tablet), and an increased risk of stroke for estrogens alone (conjugated estrogens, 0.625 mg/d).[32,33]

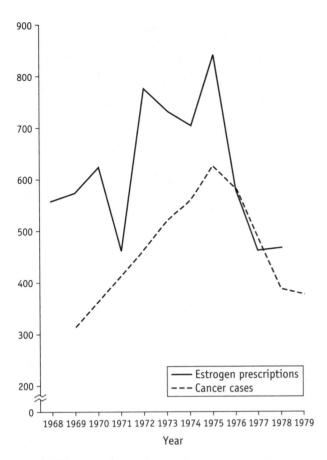

Figure 28-3 Annual number of estrogen prescriptions to women ages 50–74 in western region sample, 1968–78, and annual number of new cases of endometrial cancer among white women ages 50–74 in San Francisco–Oakland, CA 1969–1979.

Source: Reproduced from Austin DF, Roe KM. The decreasing incidence of endometrial cancer: Public health implications. Am J Public Health 1982;72:65–68 with kind permission. © American Public Health Association.

Current guidelines recommend hormone therapy at the lowest possible dose for the shortest period of time to achieve relief of menopausal symptoms.[34]

Two of the most widespread types of combined therapy involve estrogen with cyclical or continuous progestin treatment. In cyclical regimens, 0.625 mg of conjugated estrogen is taken daily, with 5–10 mg of progestin added on 10 to 14 days each month. In continuous regimens, both estrogen and progestin (typically 2.5 mg/day) are taken daily. According to the National Cancer Institute, the risk of endometrial cancer with estrogen-progesterone treatment is much less than with estrogen alone, although still increased relative to nonusers.[35] The ability to quantify the effects of combined estrogen-progestin therapy on endometrial cancer risk in epidemiologic studies has proved complicated. Challenges include small sample sizes, different formulations of progesterone in terms of dose and days taken per month, and limited information concerning long-term use. In addition, women who take progesterone frequently experience bleeding, which can lead to testing and treatments such as endometrial biopsies and hysterectomy.[36]

In the first treatment approach, cyclical regimens, risk appears to be inversely associated with the number of days progesterone is taken and is positively associated with increasing years of use.[37] Some studies report that taking progestin for at least 10 days a month does not confer an increased risk.[38–41] However, other reports indicate some elevation of risk among women taking progestin for 10 days or more per month, especially with increasing years of use.[42] A large case-control study from Sweden reported a significant elevation of the summary relative risk among women taking 10 or more days of cyclic progesterone per month compared to nonusers (RR = 2.0; 95% CI = 1.4−2.7);[43] with risk rising to threefold after 5 or more years of use (RR = 2.9; 95% CI = 1.8−4.6).[44] The association between continuous regimens and endometrial cancer risk is less clear. Studies to date have yielded conflicting results, with some studies indicating possible increases,[37,40,45] some showing decreases[39,41–44] and still others reporting null effects.[36,38] The Women's Health Initiative randomized trial reported no increase in endometrial cancer risk among women receiving 5 years of treatment with a combined continuous regimen (RR = 0.81; 95% CI = 0.4−1.2). However, this finding may have been influenced by the extensive surveillance and treatment of endometrial hyperplasia during the study. [32,36]

Low-Potency Menopausal Estrogens and Other Routes of Administration

Although much less studied than oral medium-potency estrogens, use of unopposed low-potency estrogens (e.g., oral estriol and vaginal estriol and estradiol) and higher potency estrogen use in patch or gel form also appear to increase the risk of endometrial cancer.[46]

Diethylstilbesterol (DES)

A potent oral synthetic estrogen, DES, was promoted from 1938 to 1971 to reduce the risk of spontaneous abortion and premature delivery. This medication did not prevent miscarriage but did adversely affect both mother and developing fetus. Although no excess risk of endometrial cancer has been reported, breast cancer risk is increased based on long-term follow-up studies of mothers and their daughters exposed to DES during pregnancy.[47,48]

Tamoxifen and Raloxifene

Use of tamoxifen, a selective estrogen receptor modulator (SERM) prescribed for the treatment and prevention of breast cancer, has consistently been shown to double the risk of endometrial cancer within 2 to 5 years of use.[49] This risk increased with prior postmenopausal estrogen use and, to a lesser extent, if a woman is obese.[50] In most cases, endometrial cancer in tamoxifen users tends to be diagnosed at an early readily treatable stage. Raloxifene, another SERM, has antiestrogen effects on the breast similar to tamoxifen and has not been linked with increased risk of endometrial cancer.[49]

Obesity

Obesity is one of the strongest and most well-established risk factors for endometrial cancer, with nearly half of all endometrial cancer cases attributed to excess weight for height.[51] In the Million Women Cohort Study, a 10 kg/m² increase in body weight was associated with a threefold increased risk, with a greater increase in postmenopausal compared to premenopausal women.[52] According to a recent review, abdominal obesity likely contributes to endometrial cancer risk independent of its association with overall body fatness.[53] The importance of obesity in the etiology of endometrial cancer is consistent with the "unopposed estrogen" hypothesis. The main source of endogenous estrogens in postmenopausal women is from the conversion of adrenal androgens to estrogens in fat tissue. In premenopausal women with functioning ovaries, obesity is associated with chronic anovulatory menstrual cycles and progesterone deficiency. A recent study also has implicated other biologic mechanisms to explain the correlation between obesity and endometrial cancer in postmenopausal women, including hyperinsulinemia and inflammation.[19]

Physical Activity

The relationship between physical activity and the risk of endometrial cancer has been examined in many studies. Overall, the data suggest a modest inverse association. For example, 10 cohort studies compared women in the highest category of physical activity to those in the lowest category and found relative risks ranging from 0.74 to 0.85, with two exceptions.[12,54] These cohort studies have assessed different aspects of activity, including total,[55] occupational,[56–58] recreational,[54,59,60] vigorous,[61,62] and unspecified physical activity.[12] These cohort studies indicate that different types of physical activity can reduce endometrial cancer risk. A consistent but modest inverse association has been observed even among studies that account for body mass index.[12,54,55,59–63] A number of case-control studies have suggested a stronger decreased risk with recent years of activity compared to activity in adolescence or childhood.[58,64–66]

Moderate-to-vigorous physical exercise correlates with lower levels of endogenous estrogens due to menstrual cycle irregularities and reduced excess adipose tissue. Physical activity may reduce the risk of hyperinsulinemia as well as lower the risk of endometrial cancer.[67] Other biologic mechanisms under study include increased circulating levels of anti-inflammatory cytokines, enhanced estrogen metabolism, and improved activation of cell-signaling pathways.[68]

Reproductive Factors

Parity and Timing of Birth

Numerous studies show that parous women are at lower risk than nulliparous women of developing endometrial cancer, and risk further decreases with each additional birth.[66,69–83] Reduced risk was also reported following a recent birth and among women with an older age at last birth. A recent analysis of data from the Nurses' Health Study cohort indicated women who had their last child at 40 years or older had a 50% lower risk compared with women who had their last child when they were between the ages of 25 and 29 years. In addition, an inverse association between risk and increasing number of births was substantially attenuated after adjustment for age at last birth.[37] Several biological mechanisms have been proposed for the decreased risk in parous women, including the shedding of malignant epithelial cells present in the endometrium during delivery,[84] decreases in mitotic activity during pregnancy, and increased production of progesterone during pregnancy.[75]

Age at Menarche and Menopause

Most studies indicate that women who have an earlier age at menarche or a later age at menopause have a modestly increased risk of endometrial cancer. Participants in the Nurses' Health cohort who began menstruating at age 15 or older had a 34% lower risk of endometrial cancer compared with women who began menstruating at age 11 or younger. Consistent with the hypothesis of risk associated with longer duration of exposure to endogenous estrogen, nurses who reached menopause after age 55 years or older had a 53% higher risk compared with women whose menopause occurred between ages 45 and 49.[37]

Infertility

In a large cohort study, women with impaired fertility related to an imbalance of endogenous estrogens and progesterone who had not used infertility treatments were found to have more than a threefold increase in endometrial cancer risk.[85] Several other studies have also found an increased risk of endometrial cancer associated with impaired fertility.[86] The relation between fertility treatments and risk also has been of interest. Recently, a large cohort study with extensive follow-up time suggested that infertile women treated with gonadotropins, clomiphene, or human chorionic gonadotropin also have an increased risk of endometrial cancer.[87]

Other Reproductive Factors

Results from two recent cohort studies indicate no association between lactation and endometrial cancer risk, although inverse associations have been observed in several case-control studies conducted in developing countries where the duration of breastfeeding tends to be longer.[25,80] There is no consistent evidence that spontaneous or induced abortions are associated with risk of endometrial cancer.[66,71,75,77]

Alcohol

Several cohort studies have evaluated the risk of endometrial cancer associated with alcohol intake. In a multiethnic cohort in the United States, women who consumed more than two drinks per day experienced a twofold increase in risk compared to nondrinkers.[88] In a Netherlands cohort, women who consumed three or more drinks per day had an approximate doubling of risk compared to nondrinkers.[89] Risk was not elevated in women consuming fewer drinks per day in either of these studies. Three other cohort studies reported no relationship between alcohol intake and endometrial cancer risk.[12,90–91] However, these studies had a very narrow range of alcohol intake among drinkers. A biological mechanism has not been established, although alcohol intake has been linked to higher estrogen levels.[92,93]

Cigarette Smoking

Surprisingly, a meta-analysis by Zhou and colleagues[94] including 10 prospective and 24 case-control studies reported a *decreased* risk of endometrial cancer among women who ever smoked. The association was observed in both prospective (RR = 0.81; 95% CI = 0.74−0.88) and case-control studies (RR = 0.72; 95% CI = 0.66−0.79). In the Nurses' Health Study cohort, women with the highest intensity and duration of smoking had the lowest risk, although the trend was not significant.[95] Conversely, some data indicate that smoking is associated with adverse effects on endometrial cancer in premenopausal women.[94] For example, the European Prospective Investigation into Cancer and Nutrition cohort study found that among premenopausal women, current smokers with long duration (30–39 years) and high intensity (more than 15 cigarettes per day) had more than a twofold increase in risk.[96] The biologic explanation for the effects of cigarette smoking on endometrial cancer risk is not clear. Cigarette smoking has not been shown to alter circulating levels of estrogens in premenopausal or postmenopausal women.[95] Cigarette smoking has been associated with anovulatory menstrual cycles typified by low progesterone levels, providing a possible explanation for the increased risk observed among premenopausal women.[96]

Other Medical Conditions and Medications

Inflammation

Inflammation has been proposed to play a role in the development of endometrial cancer, suggesting that anti-inflammatory medications might decrease endometrial cancer risk.[97] However, overall null associations have been observed between the use of aspirin and other nonsteroidal anti-inflammatory drug use and risk of endometrial cancer in two recent cohort studies.[98,99]

Diabetes and Hyperinsulinemia

Because insulin resistance is common in heavier women, insulin has been hypothesized to play a role in endometrial carcinogenesis. Insulin could promote development of endometrial cancer either directly as a mitogen or indirectly through its effects on estrogen production and availability. Friberg and colleagues[67] reported a summary risk estimate of 2.10 (95% CI = 1.8−2.7) for diabetes mellitus (primarily type 2) and risk of endometrial cancer based on 3 cohort studies and 13 case-control studies. Whether the association with diabetes implicates insulin

in the development of endometrial cancer has been more difficult to establish. Three cohort studies have observed only modestly elevated risks for diabetes ranging from 1.4 to 1.9, after adjustment for weight or body mass index.[12,67,100] Two cohort studies observed positive associations with fasting blood levels of insulin and C-peptide, but only one suggested an independent effect of insulin after controlling for obesity and serum estrogen levels.[101,102] Conversely, the observation that a history of type 1 diabetes, a condition that is not typically associated with obesity or hyperinsulinemia, is associated with substantially elevated risk of endometrial cancer deserves further investigation.[67]

Hypertension

Although women with hypertensive disease are more likely to develop endometrial cancer, hypertension is not generally found to be an independent risk factor after accounting for obesity. A recent large cohort study confirmed the absence of correlation between hypertension and endometrial cancer risk, although it did suggest a possible link between risk and thiazide diuretics used to treat hypertension, plausibly due to an estrogenic mechanism.[103]

Intrauterine Devices

The use of an intrauterine device (IUD) has been shown consistently to protect against endometrial cancer. In a meta-analysis of 10 case-control studies, all but one reported an inverse association between IUD use and endometrial cancer, and risk decreased with increasing years of use. The overall relative risk was 0.54 (95% CI = 0.47−0.63), regardless of type of IUD. Because 8 out of the 10 studies examined women who were diagnosed with endometrial cancer prior to 1993, their exposure was most likely due to nonhormonal IUDs, as IUDs containing progesterone were not available until 1990.[104] Nonhormonal IUDs may alter the endometrial response to hormones by changing the endometrial environment.[104] Copper IUDs have been shown to reduce endometrial mitotic activity and estrogen receptor concentration, mechanisms that possibly may protect against endometrial cancer.[104]

Endometriosis and Uterine Fibroids

Endometriosis is a condition of endometrial tissue growth outside the uterus as a result of retrograde menstruation. For certain types of ovarian cancer, endometriosis is considered to be a precursor lesion.[105] Although some studies report an association between endometriosis and risk of endometrial cancer, this finding may result from shared estrogenic influence on both conditions.[83] Uterine fibroids, benign tumors that form in the muscle layer of the uterus, are not considered precursors of endometrial cancer.

Diet

Beyond the convincing link with body fatness, few conclusions can be made on the relationship between diet and endometrial cancer. Studies are relatively sparse and most have employed only case-control study designs.

A comprehensive review of the literature, undertaken as part of the American Institute for Cancer Research Expert Report, concluded that red meat consumption may increase risk, and that risk may be lower in women who consume more nonstarchy vegetables.[53] Potential inverse associations between risk and higher intake of coffee, black or green tea, soy, grains, and cruciferous vegetables warrant further investigation.[53,106–107] A greater attained body height, a marker of early life exposures including diet, also has been inversely associated with endometrial cancer.[53]

Occupation and Environment

Few occupational or environmental risk factors have been explored.[108,109] No clear associations have emerged from the few studies that have examined risk and exposure to chemicals with possible estrogenic effects, such as cadmium[110] or organochlorines.[111] Work in the textile industry is linked with increased risk in one study.[112] The hypothesis that night shift workers may have a higher risk of developing endometrial cancer has been gaining some traction.[113] Such an association is plausible as melatonin levels are lower in nightshift workers, and melatonin is reported to have antiestrogenic and antiaromatase activities.[113]

Treatment and Prevention

Treatment is dependent on the extent of disease. Women with localized disease are generally curable with surgery alone. Other treatment options include radiation and chemotherapy.[114] Avenues for endometrial cancer prevention include maintaining a healthy body weight, increasing physical activity, and using postmenopausal hormone therapy for as short a time as possible, if at all. Seeking prompt medical attention for unexplained uterine bleeding is important for reducing morbidity and mortality.

Summary

Endometrial cancer occurs most commonly after menopause. The history of this cancer presents an interesting epidemiologic sequence. The development of synthetic estrogen provided medical relief of menopausal symptoms and led to increased incidence of the disease. Once the relationship between hormone use and cancer was recognized, women ceased use of the medication and the incidence of endometrial cancer declined rapidly as noted in Figure 28-3. Estrogen was then recognized as a cancer promoter. The subsequent change in postmenopausal therapy to include both estrogen and progestin enabled women to again use hormones for prevention of menopausal symptoms although for a limited time to avoid other chronic conditions hormones may stimulate. Incidence and mortality of the disease differ by race/ethnicity primarily due to limited access to health care, more aggressive disease at diagnosis, and higher rates of obesity. When diagnosed at early stages, endometrial cancer can be readily treated by surgery.

Discussion Questions

1. Describe the incidence and mortality patterns of endometrial cancer in the United States.
2. Discuss how hysterectomy practices may impact comparisons of endometrial cancer incidence by person, place, and time.
3. What is the unopposed estrogen hypothesis? Explain how established risk factors for endometrial cancer support or refute the unopposed estrogen hypothesis.
4. Compare and contrast the association between endometrial cancer risk and use of menopausal estrogen use alone, cyclic estrogen-progestin use, and continuous estrogen-progestin use.
5. Explain how the strong association between obesity and endometrial cancer complicates the investigation of other hypothesized risk factors, such as hyperinsulinemia and physical activity.

References

1. Mendivil A, Schuler KM, Gehrig PA. Non-endometrioid adenocarcinoma of the uterine corpus: A review of selected histological subtypes. *Cancer Control.* 2009;16:46–52.
2. Furness S, Roberts H, Marjoribanks J, et al. Hormone therapy in postmenopausal women and risk of endometrial hyperplasia. *Cochrane Database Syst Rev.* 2009;CD000402.
3. International Agency for Research on Cancer. GLOBOCAN 2002 I. Crude and age-standardised (world) rates, per 100,000 corpus uteri.
4. U.S. Cancer Statistics Working Group. United States cancer statistics: 1999–2005 incidence and mortality web-based report. http://apps.nccd.cdc.gov/uscs/. Accessed August 26, 2012.
5. American Cancer Society. *Cancer Facts & Figures 2013.* Atlanta: American Cancer Society; 2013.
6. Allard JE, Maxwell GL. Race disparities between black and white women in the incidence, treatment, and prognosis of endometrial cancer. *Cancer Control.* 2009;16:53–56.
7. Sherman ME, Carreon JD, Lacey JV, Jr, Devesa SS. Impact of hysterectomy on endometrial carcinoma rates in the united states. *J Natl Cancer Inst.* 2005;97:1700–1702.
8. Percy CL, Horm JW, Young JL, Jr, Asire AJ. Uterine cancers of unspecified origin—a reassessment. *Public Health Rep.* 1983;98:176–180.
9. Kosary CL. Cancer of the corpus uteri. Ries LAG, Young JL, Keel GE, et al., eds. *SEER Survival Monograph: Cancer Survival Among Adults: U.S. SEER Program, 1988–2001, Patient and Tumor Characteristics.* Bethesda, MD: National Cancer Institute, SEER Program; 2007:123–132. NIH publication 07–6215.
10. Horner MJ, Ries LAG, Krapcho M, et al. SEER cancer statistics review, 1975–2006. http://seer.cancer.gov/csr/1975_2006/.
11. Meyer LA, Broaddus RR, Lu KH. Endometrial cancer and lynch syndrome: Clinical and pathologic considerations. *Cancer Control.* 2009;16:14–22.
12. Terry P, Baron JA, Weiderpass E, et al. Lifestyle and endometrial cancer risk: a cohort study from the Swedish Twin Registry. *Int J Cancer.* 1999;82:38–42.
13. Meyer LA, Westin SN, Lu KH, Milam MR. Genetic polymorphisms and endometrial cancer risk. *Expert Rev Anticancer Ther.* 2008;8:1159–1167.
14. Setiawan VW, Doherty JA, Shu XO, et al. Two estrogen-related variants in CYP19A1 and endometrial cancer risk: a pooled analysis in the epidemiology of endometrial cancer consortium. *Cancer Epidemiol Biomarkers Prev.* 2009;18:242–247.
15. Olson SH, Chen C, De Vivo I, et al. Maximizing resources to study an uncommon cancer: E2C2—epidemiology of endometrial cancer consortium. *Cancer Causes Control.* 2009;20:491–496.
16. Key TJ, Pike MC. The dose-effect relationship between 'unopposed' oestrogens and endometrial mitotic rate: its central role in explaining and predicting endometrial cancer risk. *Br J Cancer.* 1988;57:205–212.
17. Bjorkholm E, Silfversward C. Granulosa- and theca-cell tumors. incidence and occurrence of second primary tumors. *Acta Radiol Oncol.* 1980;19:161–167.
18. Chittenden BG, Fullerton G, Maheshwari A, Bhattacharya S. Polycystic ovary syndrome and the risk of gynaecological cancer: a systematic review. *Reprod Biomed Online.* 2009;19:398–405.
19. Allen NE, Key TJ, Dossus L, et al. Endogenous sex hormones and endometrial cancer risk in women in the European Prospective Investigation into Cancer and Nutrition (EPIC). *Endocr Relat Cancer.* 2008;15:485–497.
20. Lukanova A, Lundin E, Micheli A, et al. Circulating levels of sex steroid hormones and risk of endometrial cancer in postmenopausal women. *Int J Cancer.* 2004;108:425–432.

21. Zeleniuch-Jacquotte A, Akhmedkhanov A, Kato I, et al. Postmenopausal endogenous oestrogens and risk of endometrial cancer: Results of a prospective study. *Br J Cancer.* 2001;84:975–981.

22. Henderson BE, Casagrande JT, Pike MC, et al. The epidemiology of endometrial cancer in young women. *Br J Cancer.* 1983;47:749–756.

23. Collins JA, Schlesselman JJ. Perimenopausal use of reproductive hormones effects on breast and endometrial cancer. *Obstet Gynecol Clin North Am.* 2002;29:511–525.

24. Chan MF, Dowsett M, Folkerd E, et al. Past oral contraceptive and hormone therapy use and endogenous hormone concentrations in postmenopausal women. *Menopause.* 2008;15:332–339.

25. Dossus L, Allen N, Kaaks R, et al. Reproductive risk factors and endometrial cancer: The European Prospective Investigation into Cancer and Nutrition. *Int J Cancer.* 2009.

26. International Agency for Research on Cancer, ed. *Hormonal Contraception and Postmenopausal Hormone Therapy.* Lyon, France: International Agency for Research on Cancer; 1999. IARC Monographs on the Evaluation of Carcinogenic Risks to Humans; No. 72.

27. Grady D, Gebretsadik T, Kerlikowske K, Ernster V, Petitti D. Hormone replacement therapy and endometrial cancer risk: a meta-analysis. *Obstet Gynecol.* 1995;85:304–313.

28. Austin DF, Roe KM. The decreasing incidence of endometrial cancer: public health implications. *Am J Public Health.* 1982;72:65–68.

29. Horwitz RI, Feinstein AR, Stremlau JR. Alternative data sources and discrepant results in case-control studies of estrogens and endometrial cancer. *Am J Epidemiol.* 1980;111:389–394.

30. Antunes CM, Strolley PD, Rosenshein NB, et al. Endometrial cancer and estrogen use. report of a large case-control study. *N Engl J Med.* 1979;300: 9–13.

31. Spengler RF, Clarke EA, Woolever CA, Newman AM, Osborn RW. Exogenous estrogens and endometrial cancer: a case-control study and assessment of potential biases. *Am J Epidemiol.* 1981;114:497–506.

32. Rossouw JE, Anderson GL, Prentice RL, et al. Risks and benefits of estrogen plus progestin in healthy postmenopausal women: principal results from the Women's Health Initiative Randomized Controlled Trial. *JAMA.* 2002;288:321–333.

33. Hendrix SL, Wassertheil-Smoller S, Johnson KC, et al. Effects of conjugated equine estrogen on stroke in the Women's Health Initiative. *Circulation.* 2006;113:2425–2434.

34. Rossouw JE. Postmenopausal hormone therapy for disease prevention: have we learned any lessons from the past? *Clin Pharmacol Ther.* 2008;83:14–16.

35. National Cancer Institute Fact sheet. Menopausal hormone replacement therapy and cancer. http://www.cancer.gov/cancertopics/factsheet/Risk/menopausal-hormones.

36. Anderson GL, Judd HL, Kaunitz AM, et al. Effects of estrogen plus progestin on gynecologic cancers and associated diagnostic procedures: The Women's Health Initiative Randomized Trial. *JAMA.* 2003;290:1739–1748.

37. Karageorgi S, Hankinson SE, Kraft P, De Vivo I. Reproductive factors and postmenopausal hormone use in relation to endometrial cancer risk in the nurses' health study cohort 1976–2004. *Int J Cancer.* 2009;126:208–216.

38. Pike MC, Peters RK, Cozen W, et al. Estrogen-progestin replacement therapy and endometrial cancer. *J Natl Cancer Inst.* 1997;89:1110–1116.

39. Beral V, Bull D, Reeves G. Million Women Study Collaborators. Endometrial cancer and hormone-replacement therapy in the million women study. *Lancet.* 2005;365:1543–1551.

40. Newcomb PA, Trentham-Dietz A. Patterns of postmenopausal progestin use with estrogen in relation to endometrial cancer (United States). *Cancer Causes Control.* 2003;14:195–201.

41. Strom BL, Schinnar R, Weber AL, et al. Case-control study of postmenopausal hormone replacement therapy and endometrial cancer. *Am J Epidemiol.* 2006;164:775–786.

42. Doherty JA, Cushing-Haugen KL, Saltzman BS, et al. Long-term use of postmenopausal estrogen and progestin hormone therapies and the risk of endometrial cancer. *Am J Obstet Gynecol.* 2007;197:139.e1–139.e7.

43. Beresford SA, Weiss NS, Voigt LF, McKnight B. Risk of endometrial cancer in relation to use of oestrogen combined with cyclic progestagen therapy in postmenopausal women. *Lancet.* 1997;349:458–461.

44. Weiderpass E, Adami HO, Baron JA, et al. Risk of endometrial cancer following estrogen replacement with and without progestins. *J Natl Cancer Inst.* 1999;91:1131–1137.

45. Lacey JV, Jr, Leitzmann MF, Chang SC, et al. Endometrial cancer and menopausal hormone therapy in the National Institutes of Health-AARP Diet and Health Study Cohort. *Cancer.* 2007;109:1303–1311.

46. Epstein E, Lindqvist PG, Olsson H. A population-based cohort study on the use of hormone treatment and endometrial cancer in southern Sweden. *Int J Cancer.* 2009;125:421–425.

47. Troisi R, Hatch EE, Titus-Ernstoff L, et al. Cancer risk in women prenatally exposed to diethylstilbestrol. *Int J Cancer.* 2007;121:356–360.

48. Hoover RN, Hyer M, Pfeiffer RM, et al. Adverse health outcomes in women exposed in utero to diethylstilbestrol. *N Engl J Med.* 2011;365:1304–1314.

49. Nelson HD, Fu R, Griffin JC, et al. Systematic review: comparative effectiveness of medications to reduce risk for primary breast cancer. *Ann Intern Med.* 2009;151:703–15, W-226–35.

50. Bernstein L, Deapen D, Cerhan JR, et al. Tamoxifen therapy for breast cancer and endometrial cancer risk. *J Natl Cancer Inst.* 1999;91:1654–1662.

51. Key TJ, Spencer EA, Reeves GK. Symposium 1: Overnutrition: consequences and solutions obesity and cancer risk. *Proc Nutr Soc.* 2009;69:86–90.

52. Reeves GK, Pirie K, Beral V, et al. Cancer incidence and mortality in relation to body mass index in the million women study: Cohort study. *BMJ.* 2007;335:1134–1145.

53. World Cancer Research Fund/American Institute for Cancer Research. *Food, Nutrition, Physical Activity and Prevention of Cancer: A World Perspective.* Washington, DC: American Institute of Cancer Research; 2007.

54. Schouten LJ, Goldbohm RA, van den Brandt PA. Anthropometry, physical activity, and endometrial cancer risk: results from the Netherlands Cohort Study. *J Natl Cancer Inst.* 2004;96:1635–1638.

55. Colbert LH, Lacey JV, Jr, Schairer C, et al. Physical activity and risk of endometrial cancer in a prospective cohort study (United States). *Cancer Causes Control.* 2003;14:559–567.

56. Zheng W, Shu XO, McLaughlin JK, et al. Occupational physical activity and the incidence of cancer of the breast, corpus uteri, and ovary in shanghai. *Cancer.* 1993;71:3620–3624.

57. Pukkala E, Kyyronen P, Sankila R, Holli K. Tamoxifen and toremifene treatment of breast cancer and risk of subsequent endometrial cancer: a population-based case-control study. *Int J Cancer.* 2002;100:337–341.

58. Moradi T, Weiderpass E, Signorello LB, et al. Physical activity and postmenopausal endometrial cancer risk (Sweden). *Cancer Causes Control.* 2000;11:829–837.

59. Patel AV, Feigelson HS, Talbot JT, et al. The role of body weight in the relationship between physical activity and endometrial cancer: Results from a large cohort of US women. *Int J Cancer.* 2008;123:1877–1882.

60. Furberg AS, Thune I. Metabolic abnormalities (hypertension, hyperglycemia and overweight), lifestyle (high energy intake and physical inactivity) and endometrial cancer risk in a Norwegian cohort. *Int J Cancer.* 2003;104: 669–676.

61. Conroy MB, Sattelmair JR, Cook NR, et al. Physical activity, adiposity, and risk of endometrial cancer. *Cancer Causes Control.* 2009;20:1107–1115.

62. Gierach GL, Chang SC, Brinton LA, et al. Physical activity, sedentary behavior, and endometrial cancer risk in the NIH-AARP Diet and Health Study. *Int J Cancer.* 2009;124:2139–2147.

63. Voskuil DW, Monninkhof EM, Elias SG, et al Task Force Physical Activity and Cancer. Physical activity and endometrial cancer risk, a systematic review of current evidence. *Cancer Epidemiol Biomarkers Prev.* 2007;16:639–648.

64. Olson SH, Vena JE, Dorn JP, et al. Exercise, occupational activity, and risk of endometrial cancer. *Ann Epidemiol.* 1997;7:46–53.

65. Levi F, La Vecchia C, Negri E, Franceschi S. Selected physical activities and the risk of endometrial cancer. *Br J Cancer.* 1993;67:846–851.

66. Shu XO, Brinton LA, Zheng W, et al. A population-based case-control study of endometrial cancer in Shanghai, China. *Int J Cancer.* 1991;49:38–43.

67. Friberg E, Mantzoros CS, Wolk A. Diabetes and risk of endometrial cancer: a population-based prospective cohort study. *Cancer Epidemiol Biomarkers Prev.* 2007;16:276–280.

68. Cust AE, Armstrong BK, Friedenreich CM, et al. Physical activity and endometrial cancer risk: a review of the current evidence, biologic mechanisms and the quality of physical activity assessment methods. *Cancer Causes Control.* 2007;18:243–258.

69. Albrektsen G, Heuch I, Wik E, Salvesen HB. Parity and time interval since childbirth influence survival in endometrial cancer patients. *Int J Gynecol Cancer.* 2009;19:665–669.

70. Albrektsen G, Heuch I, Tretli S, Kvale G. Is the risk of cancer of the corpus uteri reduced by a recent pregnancy? A prospective study of 765,756 Norwegian women. *Int J Cancer.* 1995;61:485–490.

71. Brinton LA, Berman ML, Mortel R, et al. Reproductive, menstrual, and medical risk factors for endometrial cancer: results from a case-control study. *Am J Obstet Gynecol.* 1992;167:1317–1325.

72. Hemminki K, Bermejo JL, Granstrom C. Endometrial cancer: population attributable risks from reproductive, familial and socioeconomic factors. *Eur J Cancer.* 2005;41:2155–2159.

73. Kalandidi A, Tzonou A, Lipworth L, et al. A case-control study of endometrial cancer in relation to reproductive, somatometric, and life-style variables. *Oncology.* 1996;53:354–359.

74. Mogren I, Stenlund H, Hogberg U. Long-term impact of reproductive factors on the risk of cervical, endometrial, ovarian and breast cancer. *Acta Oncol.* 2001;40:849–854.

75. McPherson CP, Sellers TA, Potter JD, et al. Reproductive factors and risk of endometrial cancer. the Iowa women's health study. *Am J Epidemiol.* 1996;143:1195–1202.

76. Neale RE, Darlington S, Murphy MF, et al. The effects of twins, parity and age at first birth on cancer risk in Swedish women. *Twin Res Hum Genet.* 2005;8:156–162.

77. Parazzini F, Negri E, La Vecchia C, et al. Role of reproductive factors on the risk of endometrial cancer. *Int J Cancer.* 1998;76:784–786.

78. Pfeiffer RM, Mitani A, Landgren O, et al. Timing of births and endometrial cancer risk in Swedish women. *Cancer Causes Control.* 2009;20(8):1441–1449.

79. Salazar-Martinez E, Lazcano-Ponce EC, Gonzalez Lira-Lira G, et al. Reproductive factors of ovarian and endometrial cancer risk in a high fertility population in Mexico. *Cancer Res.* 1999;59:3658–3662.

80. Wernli KJ, Ray RM, Gao DL, et al. Menstrual and reproductive factors in relation to risk of endometrial cancer in Chinese women. *Cancer Causes Control.* 2006;17:949–955.

81. Xu WH, Xiang YB, Ruan ZX, et al. Menstrual and reproductive factors and endometrial cancer risk: Results from a population-based case-control study in urban Shanghai. *Int J Cancer.* 2004;108:613–619.

82. Epplein M, Reed SD, Voigt LF, et al. Risk of complex and atypical endometrial hyperplasia in relation to anthropometric measures and reproductive history. *Am J Epidemiol.* 2008;168:563–570; discussion 571–576.

83. Zucchetto A, Serraino D, Polesel J, et al. Hormone-related factors and gynecological conditions in relation to endometrial cancer risk. *Eur J Cancer Prev.* 2009;18:316–321.

84. Kvale G, Heuch I, Nilssen S. Reproductive factors and cancers of the breast and genital organs—are the different cancer sites similarly affected? *Cancer Detect Prev.* 1991;15:369–377.

85. Modan B, Ron E, Lerner-Geva L, et al. Cancer incidence in a cohort of infertile women. *Am J Epidemiol.* 1998;147:1038–1042.

86. Klip H, Burger CW, Kenemans P, van Leeuwen FE. Cancer risk associated with subfertility and ovulation induction: a review. *Cancer Causes Control.* 2000;11:319–344.

87. Jensen A, Sharif H, Kjaer SK. Use of fertility drugs and risk of uterine cancer: results from a large Danish population-based cohort study. *Am J Epidemiol.* 2009;170:1408–1414.

88. Setiawan VW, Monroe KR, Goodman MT, et al. Alcohol consumption and endometrial cancer risk: The Multiethnic Cohort. *Int J Cancer.* 2008;122:634–638.

89. Loerbroks A, Schouten LJ, Goldbohm RA, van den Brandt PA. Alcohol consumption, cigarette smoking, and endometrial cancer risk: results from the Netherlands Cohort Study. *Cancer Causes Control.* 2007;18:551–560.

90. Friberg E, Wolk A. Long-term alcohol consumption and risk of endometrial cancer incidence: a prospective cohort study. *Cancer Epidemiol Biomarkers Prev.* 2009;18:355–358.

91. Gapstur SM, Potter JD, Sellers TA, et al. Alcohol consumption and postmenopausal endometrial cancer: results from the Iowa Women's Health Study. *Cancer Causes Control.* 1993;4:323–329.

92. Purohit V. Moderate alcohol consumption and estrogen levels in postmenopausal women: a review. *Alcohol Clin Exp Res.* 1998;22:994–997.

93. Mahabir S, Baer DJ, Johnson LL, et al. The effects of moderate alcohol supplementation on estrone sulfate and DHEAS in postmenopausal women in a controlled feeding study. *Nutr J.* 2004;3:11.

94. Zhou B, Yang L, Sun Q, et al. Cigarette smoking and the risk of endometrial cancer: a meta-analysis. *Am J Med.* 2008;121:501–508.e3.

95. Viswanathan AN, Feskanich D, De Vivo I, et al. Smoking and the risk of endometrial cancer: results from the Nurses' Health Study. *Int J Cancer.* 2005;114:996–1001.

96. Al-Zoughool M, Dossus L, Kaaks R, et al. Risk of endometrial cancer in relationship to cigarette smoking: results from the EPIC study. *Int J Cancer.* 2007;121:2741–2747.

97. Modugno F, Ness RB, Chen C, Weiss NS. Inflammation and endometrial cancer: a hypothesis. *Cancer Epidemiol Biomarkers Prev.* 2005;14:2840–2847.

98. Danforth KN, Gierach GL, Brinton LA, et al. Nonsteroidal anti-inflammatory drug use and endometrial cancer risk in the NIH-AARP Diet and Health study. *Cancer Prev Res (Phila Pa).* 2009;2:466–472.

99. Viswanathan AN, Feskanich D, Schernhammer ES, Hankinson SE. Aspirin, NSAID, and acetaminophen use and the risk of endometrial cancer. *Cancer Res.* 2008;68:2507–2513.

100. Anderson KE, Anderson E, Mink PJ, et al. Diabetes and endometrial cancer in the Iowa Women's Health Study. *Cancer Epidemiol Biomarkers Prev.* 2001;10:611–616.

101. Cust AE, Allen NE, Rinaldi S, et al. Serum levels of C-peptide, IGFBP-1 and IGFBP-2 and endometrial cancer risk; results from the European Prospective Investigation into Cancer and Nutrition. *Int J Cancer.* 2007;120:2656–2664.

102. Gunter MJ, Hoover DR, Yu H, et al. A prospective evaluation of insulin and insulin-like growth factor-I as risk factors for endometrial cancer. *Cancer Epidemiol Biomarkers Prev.* 2008;17:921–929.

103. Fortuny J, Sima C, Bayuga S, et al. Risk of endometrial cancer in relation to medical conditions and medication use. *Cancer Epidemiol Biomarkers Prev.* 2009;18:1448–1456.

104. Beining RM, Dennis LK, Smith EM, Dokras A. Meta-analysis of intrauterine device use and risk of endometrial cancer. *Ann Epidemiol.* 2008;18:492–499.

105. Kurman RJ, McConnell TG. Precursors of endometrial and ovarian carcinoma. *Virchows Arch.* 2010;456:1–12.

106. Tang NP, Li H, Qiu YL, Zhou GM, Ma J. Tea consumption and risk of endometrial cancer: A metaanalysis. *Am J Obstet Gynecol.* 2009;201:605.e1–605.e8.

107. Friberg E, Orsini N, Mantzoros CS, Wolk A. Coffee drinking and risk of endometrial cancer—A population-based cohort study. *Int J Cancer.* 2009;125(10):2413–2417.

108. MacArthur AC, Le ND, Abanto ZU, Gallagher RP. Occupational female breast and reproductive cancer mortality in British Columbia, Canada, 1950–94. *Occup Med (Lond).* 2007;57:246–253.

109. Weiderpass E, Pukkala E, Vasama-Neuvonen K, et al. Occupational exposures and cancers of the endometrium and cervix uteri in Finland. *Am J Ind Med.* 2001;39:572–580.

110. Akesson A, Julin B, Wolk A. Long-term dietary cadmium intake and postmenopausal endometrial cancer incidence: a population-based prospective cohort study. *Cancer Res.* 2008;68:6435–6441.

111. Sturgeon SR, Brock JW, Potischman N, et al. Serum concentrations of organochlorine compounds and endometrial cancer risk (United States). *Cancer Causes Control.* 1998;9:417–424.

112. Wernli KJ, Ray RM, Gao DL, et al. Occupational risk factors for endometrial cancer among textile workers in Shanghai, China. *Am J Ind Med.* 2008;51:673–679.

113. Viswanathan AN, Hankinson SE, Schernhammer ES. Night shift work and the risk of endometrial cancer. *Cancer Res.* 2007;67:10618–10622.

114. National Cancer Institute. Endometrial cancer treatment. http://www .cancer.gov/cancertopics/pdq/treatment/endometrial/HealthProfessional/ page5. Accessed January 31, 2009.

Cervical Cancer

Ruby T. Senie, PhD

Introduction

Early in the 20th century, cervical cancer was the leading cause of cancer death of America women; however, in the past 40 years, incidence and mortality rates have decreased 67% after screening with Pap tests, which has led to early diagnosis and treatment of precancerous lesions and lower rates of *in situ* and invasive disease.[1] Although incidence and mortality rates of cervical cancer differ by race/ethnicity with a greater burden among minority and low-income women, in 2010 this disease is surpassed by lung, breast, and other malignancies among all American women.

Recent epidemiologic and molecular studies have detected human papillomaviruses (HPV) in cervical tissue, which is now recognized as the etiologic agent transmitted from males to females.[2] Research now recognizes HPV is *necessary* for development of cervical abnormalities but not *sufficient* to cause disease, because HPV infection rates are high, especially among young women, but invasive cancer rarely develops. Current epidemiologic studies now focus on potential cofactors that enable persistent and progressive HPV infections.

Two HPV vaccines were approved by the Food and Drug Administration (FDA) in 2006, providing an avenue for primary prevention of cervical cancer. The combination of the HPV vaccine with Pap smear testing has lowered cervical cancer incidence and mortality. This chapter reviews cervical cancer statistics, research that identified HPV, epidemiologic studies of cofactors, vaccine development and administration, the history of screening, and current screening guidelines.

Incidence and Mortality Rates

The American Cancer Society (ACS) estimated 12,200 new invasive cervical cancer cases and 4,210 deaths from cervical cancer would occur in 2010. In contrast to the lifelong risk of breast cancer estimated to affect 1 in 8 American women, the risk of cervical cancer is 1 in 147.[3] Surveillance Epidemiology End Results (SEER) data indicate decreasing age-adjusted incidence and mortality rates over the past 30 years from an average of 14.8 per 100,000

in 1975 to an average of 8.1 cases per 100,000 in 2007. However, the averages hide the disparity in incidence among black and Hispanic women compared with white and Asian, which was significant in 1993 but remains to a lesser extent in 2009 (Figure 29-1), although mortality differences by race have diminished (Figure 29-2).[4] Since 1999, SEER has included American Indian/Alaskan native data, and the most recent rates for the five primary racial/ethnic groups are noted in Table 29-1.[4]

The median age of cervical cancer diagnosis between 2004 and 2008 reported by SEER was 48 years. Cervical cancer is rarely diagnosed before age 20 or after age 65. Incidence declines as women approach menopause. The peak incidence of invasive disease, 20 cases per 100,000 women, occurs between ages 35 to 39; *in situ* lesions are more prevalent between ages 25 to 35 at a rate of 130 per 100,000.[4]

In the absence of public health education and screening, estimated incidence rates of invasive disease would be two to three times higher. The rates could be lower if cytology screening were more sensitive because approximately 30% of cervical cancers are associated with lack of reliable cytopathology assessments and 10% due to inadequate follow-up after abnormal findings.[5] Currently, cervical cancer is the 14th most common cause of cancer death for U.S. women; in contrast, cervical cancer is the second most common cause of cancer death for women in developing nations.[4]

The estimated age-adjusted mortality rate for cervical cancer is 2.5 per 100,000, which differs geographically with clusters of higher than average death rates in rural southern regions and some cities including Washington, DC (Figure 29-3). These are the same regions noted on maps associated with high rates of sexually transmitted infections and human immunodeficiency virus/acquired immune deficiency syndrome (HIV/AIDS). To assess factors distinguishing these clusters, Du and colleagues conducted an ecologic study with data from SEER, Behavioral Risk Factor Surveillance System, chlamydia rates reported from the Centers for Disease Control and Prevention (CDC), and county-specific descriptors of socioeconomic and education levels.[6] Mortality rates were threefold higher (OR = 3.39, 95% CI = 1.9–5.9) in counties characterized by greater than 10% non-Hispanic

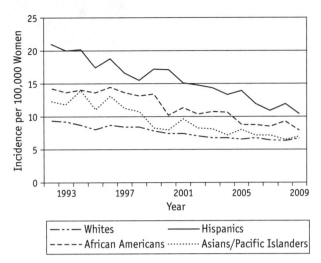

Note: Insufficient data available for time trend analysis for American Indians/Alaska Natives.

Figure 29-1 Cervical cancer incidence rates by race/ethnicity, United States, 1993–2009.

Modified from National Cancer Institute, October 2012. A Snapshot of Cervical Cancer. http://www.cancer.gov/aboutnci/servingpeople/snapshots/Cervical-Snapshot.pdf

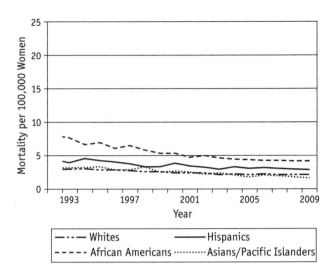

Note: Insufficient data available for time trend analysis for American Indians/Alaska Natives.

Figure 29-2 Cervical cancer mortality rates by race/ethnicity, United States, 1993–2009.

Modified from National Cancer Institute, October 2012. A Snapshot of Cervical Cancer. http://www.cancer.gov/aboutnci/servingpeople/snapshots/Cervical-Snapshot.pdf

Table 29-1

SEER Cervical Cancer Incidence and Mortality Rates, per 100,000 by race/ethnicity, 2004–2007[4]

Race/Ethnicity	Incidence	Mortality
White	8.0	2.2
Black	10.0	4.4
Asian/Pacific Islander	7.3	2.1
American Indian/Alaskan	7.8	3.4
Hispanic	11.1	3.1

Source: Reproduced from SEER Cancer Statistics Review, 1975-2007, National Cancer Institute. http://seer.cancer.gov/csr/1975_2007/. US Mortality Files, National Center for Health Statistics, Centers for Disease Control and Prevention.

blacks, higher rates of poverty, lower educational levels, less frequent Pap testing, greater percentage of smokers, and higher prevalence of chlamydia (substituting for the lack of HPV surveillance data). Of these, the strongest factor was the percentage of non-Hispanic black women.[6]

Cervical Anatomy: Tissue at Risk

Cervical tissue, the lower portion of the uterus extending into the vagina, is composed of two distinct types of cells: squamous epithelium, similar to the vagina, and mucus-secreting columnar epithelium derived from the endometrium (Figure 29-4). Hormonal stimulation of puberty and early adulthood causes maturation of cervical tissue creating the transformation zone, where the tissue is composed of two kinds of epithelium that are uniquely susceptible to HPV infection and histologic changes.[1] Approximately 80% of invasive disease is squamous cell

carcinomas, reflecting the epithelial origin; the remaining 20% are classified as adenocarcinomas.

Cervical tissue at risk for HPV infection vacillates between normal histology and dysplasia with an alternating pattern of progression and regression over many years. In the past, clinicians assumed once tissue indicated a change from normal, a *unidirectional* progression would follow, with premalignant stages including the development of intraepithelial lesions before invasive disease.[8] Research has clarified the natural history of cervical changes with an estimated 95% of cervical cancers having a long preinvasive phase rarely progressing to invasive cancer during 10 to 20 years of follow-up. The natural history depicted in Figure 29-5 indicates transient infection is normally cleared by immune response unless a woman's immune system is compromised. Therefore, most clinicians recognize that treatment of preinvasive lesions will

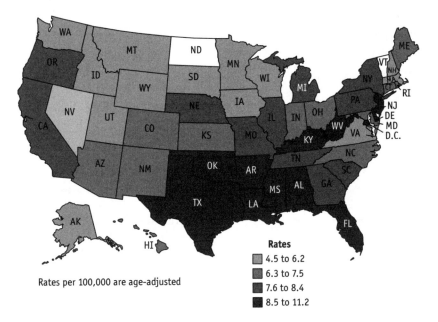

Rates
- ⬜ 4.5 to 6.2
- 🟪 6.3 to 7.5
- ⬛ 7.6 to 8.4
- ⬛ 8.5 to 11.2

Rates per 100,000 are age-adjusted

Figure 29-3 Cervical cancer incidence rates by state 2007.

Source: Reproduced from U.S. Cancer Statistics Working Group, Centers for Disease Control and Prevention, Cervical Cancer Rates by State.

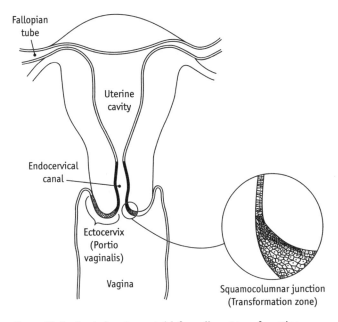

Figure 29-4 Cervical anatomy at risk for malignant transformation.

Source: Reproduced from Schottenfeld D, Fraumeni JF. Cancer Epidemiology and Prevention, Third Edition, Oxford University Press, 2006, with kind permission.

interrupt progression of disease and reduce risks of invasive cancer although many cervical changes regress with minimal intervention.[8]

Identification and Prevalence of Human Papillomavirus

Studies conducted in the 1980s in which cervical cancer samples and premalignant lesions were tested led to the identification of more than 150 types of HPV that grow in skin or surface epithelium. A majority of HPV types are classified as low risk, associated with benign warts and other nonmalignant conditions. However, 2 of 15 high-risk or carcinogenic types, HPV16 and HPV18, were more frequently identified in both *in situ* and invasive cervical cancers diagnosed in New Mexico and reported to SEER between 1985 and 1999. HPV16 was detected in 53.2% of invasive lesions and 56.3% of *in situ* cases; in contrast, HPV18 was detected in 13.1% of invasive tumors and few *in situ* cases. Other HPV types were far less common.[9]

Between 1985 and 1997 Munoz and colleagues collected vaginal smears from 11 international cervical cancer case-control studies to assess prevalence of HPV DNA; 13.4% of control samples were positive in contrast to 90.7% of smears from cases for an extremely high odds ratio (OR = 75.7, 95% CI = 32.9−174.2) linking HPV with cervical cancer risk.[10] In their accompanying editorial, Wright and Schiffman noted that persistent HPV infection was present in almost all squamous cell carcinomas tested. Therefore, in the absence of persistent infection, cancer risk was very low suggesting to clinicians that longer intervals between routine cytologic testing would be safe if combined with HPV analyses.[8]

To estimate the national burden of HPV infection, CDC collected samples from family planning and sexually transmitted diseases (STD) clinics; high-risk HPV types were detected among 20% of women with sexually transmitted infections and 15% of patients attending family planning clinics.[11] Additional HPV DNA seroprevalence data were obtained from biologic samples collected from National Health and Nutrition Examination Survey (NHANES) participants between 2003 and 2004. Figure 29-6 notes infection with any of four HPV types 6, 11, 16, and 18 (now included in the quadrivalent vaccine) was significantly higher at all ages among women than men.[11]

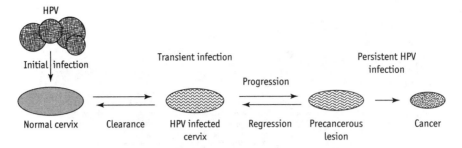

Figure 29-5 Natural history of cervical cancer.

Source: Adapted from Wright TC, Schiffman M. Adding a test for human papillomavirus DNA to cervical cancer screening. N Engl J Med. 2003;348:489-490.

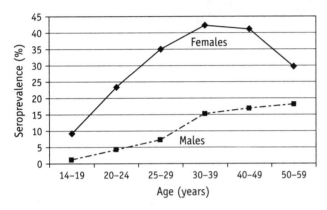

Figure 29-6 Seroprevalence of any human papillomavirus vaccine type (type 6, 11, 16, or 18) among males and females, by age group, in the National Health and Nutrition Examination Survey 2003–2004.

Source: Reproduced from Markowitz LE, Sternberg M, Dunne EF, et al. Seroprevalence of human papillomavirus Types 6,11,16, and 18 in the United States : National Health and Nutrition Examination Survey 2003-2004. J Inf Dis. 2009;200:1059-1067.

Both high-risk (carcinogenic) and low-risk (associated with benign lesions) types of HPV were found in the samples from female NHANES participants; detection differed by age group (Figure 29-7). HPV infection with any type

of virus was highest, 44.8%, among women ages 20–24.[12] Prevalence of HPV DNA among women was also associated with race/ethnicity, poverty level, marital status, and sexual behavior. Multivariate analyses indicated infection risk was fourfold greater among women with three or more sexual partners in the year of specimen donation, OR = 4.12 (95% CI = 1.72−9.85).[12]

Epidemiologic Risk Factors for Cervical Cancer and HPV Infection

Detection of highly prevalent HPV infection and low incidence of cervical cancer encouraged investigators to search for potential cofactors associated with persistent infection and subsequent cancer. Some cofactors studied included age, sexual habits, other sexually transmitted diseases, race/ethnicity noted previously, smoking behaviors, male circumcision, hormone use, high parity, and genetic susceptibility. Preinvasive cervical cancer rarely produces symptoms; however, when disease invades cervical and adjacent tissue, pain and bleeding may be experienced during or after sexual intercourse, and heavier than usual bleeding may occur during menstruation, between cycles, or after menopause.

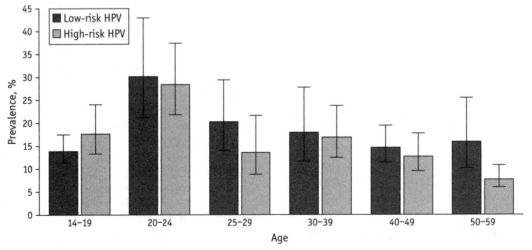

NOTE: Error bars indicate 95% confidence intervals. Both high-risk and low-risk HPV types were detected in some females.

Figure 29-7 Human papillomavirus (HPV)—Prevalence of high-risk and low-risk types among females 14 to 59 years of age from a national survey, 2003–2004.

Source: Reproduced from Centers for Disease Control and Prevention. Sexually Transmitted Disease Surveillance, 2008. Atlanta, GA: U.S. Department of Health and Human Services; November 2009.

Age

Soon after becoming sexually active, young women usually experience concurrent and sequential infections with different oncogenic and benign types of HPV.[13] Although adolescents have the highest rates of high-risk HPV cervical abnormalities, their cervical cancer rates are low.[13] Focus is primarily on young sexually active women at childbearing ages. However, a British study was conducted to assess potential progression over a 3-year follow-up interval among older compared to younger women. Archived cervical smears free of cytologic abnormalities were tested for HPV DNA for comparison with smears collected 3 years later. Positivity rate was highest, 23%, among 20-year-olds and declined with age to 10.5% among women in their 50s. However, after 3 years of follow-up, some older women had higher HPV infection rates and more older women had persistent infections.[14] The authors suggested older women may have acquired HPV from new sexual partners, through partner infidelity, or persistent infection due to reduced immune function.[14]

Sexual Behavior

Since the 19th century, when cervical cancer was a frequent disease of prostitutes but not nuns, sexual transmission was a recognized risk factor. New technology enabled identification of HPV as the agent transmitted during sexual activity between couples, including during oral sex, vaginal intercourse, and touching of genitals.[15] Barrier methods of contraception lower the risk of cervical cancer, but HPV infection may still occur as condoms and diaphragms do not cover external genital tissue. Women who identify as lesbians are at equal risk of HPV infection in relation to their partners' exposures to the virus. HPV infection was identified in 90% of cervical swabs and 75% of urine samples from sexually active teenage patients at an STD clinic; the presence of an intraepithelial lesion was associated with the number of HPV types detected.[16]

Having 10 or more lifetime sexual partners was associated with a threefold excess risk of invasive squamous cell cervical cancer in a case-control study published in 1987.[17] Shields and colleagues analyzed archived data and sera for HPV and also noted among controls 10 or more sexual partners significantly increased risk of HPV positivity compared to women reporting only one partner (OR of 7.7 (95% CI = 3.4–17.0); once infected, however, the number of partners was not a risk factor for cervical cancer.[18] Therefore, the earlier studies noting risk associated with number of sexual partners was a surrogate for multiple opportunities for HPV acquisition.

Among students in a Seattle study persistent HPV infection was associated with having more than one new sexual partner compared to monogamous peers (adjusted hazard ratio of 6.9 [95% CI = 2.9–16.0]), especially monogamous couples using condoms at each sexual encounter.[19] Some students with HPV infections reported only nonpenetrative sexual contact.[19] Other nonsexual HPV infections with high- and low-risk types were found in vaginal swabs from young girls obtained during gynecologic examinations prior to initiation of sex. After ruling out sexual abuse, investigators suggested HPV may be acquired during birth.[20]

Given the transient nature of HPV infections, prospective studies are required to understand the varying infection patterns, as in a Canadian study with repeated cervical smears during 2 years of follow-up when changes in sexual behavior may influence prevalence of infection. HPV was detected at least once among 52.7%, and among 48%, a prior infection was cleared. Interestingly, several factors were associated with clearance of HPV including routine condom use, becoming a nonsmoker, and increased vegetable consumption.[21]

Coinfection with Other Sexually Transmitted Conditions

Human Immunodeficiency Virus

In 2010, CDC estimated women account for 27% of AIDS cases in the United States. Since sexual transmission of HPV and HIV was recognized to significantly increase invasive cervical cancer risk, CDC expanded the AIDS surveillance case definition.[22] A 1992 review noted that *in situ* or invasive cervical lesions were five times more frequently identified among HIV-infected than noninfected women (OR = 4.9 [95% CI = 3.0–8.2]).[23] HPV infections among women in the HIV Epidemiology Research Study (HERS) persisted rather than being cleared and recurrent infections were more frequent than among controls, varying by type of HPV infection and immunosuppression as measured by CD4+ level.[24] Among sexually inactive HIV-positive women reactivation of HPV was noted as CD4+ counts decreased.[25] Data linking cancer and HIV/AIDS registries noted greater risk of cervical cancer after AIDS diagnosis (RR = 5.3, 95% CI = 2.0–12) than before (RR = 2.6, 95% CI = 1.6–3.9).[26] Immunosuppresssion similarly increased risk of cervical cancer among HIV positive and transplant patients.[27] Treatment with highly active antiretroviral therapy (HAART) has improved clinical status and survival of HIV-infected women; however, risk of HPV infections and cervical cancer remain elevated and may increase as the population ages.[23,28] Cytologic screening followed by treatment of cervical abnormalities among high-risk women may also reduce the risk of acquiring HIV, which is two to three times greater among women with a history of persistent HPV infection.[29]

Chlamydia, Herpes Simplex Virus Type 2

An increased risk of squamous but not adenocarcinoma of the cervix was associated with evidence of *Chlamydia trachomatis* infection;[30] however, other researchers suggested chlamydia may be associated with chronic cervical inflammation rather than an independent risk factor.[6] Both HPV and chlamydia are frequently detected in young sexually active women. However, Daling and colleagues noted herpes simplex type 2 (HSV-2) was associated with cervical cancer in the absence of HPV infection.[31] Both HSV-2 and HPV are sexually transmitted resulting in potential coinfection at different stages of disease development.

Male Circumcision

A study by the International Agency for Research on Cancer (IARC) noted that circumcision reduced HIV infection of men and penile HPV infection, a preventive intervention recommended for high-risk populations.[32] Prevalence of HPV infection was significantly greater among uncircumcised men (19.6%) compared to circumcised men (5.5%). Both HPV infection and cervical cancer risk were significantly reduced when partners were circumcised and less likely to transmit HPV.[33] Castellsagué and colleagues suggested circumcision enables better personal hygiene and causes penile tissue to become thicker, resistant to abrasion and less susceptible to HPV infection.[33]

Hormonal Exposure: Contraception and Postmenopausal

Prior to HPV identification a twofold increased risk of both adenocarcinoma and squamous cell cervical cancer was noted after oral contraceptive (OC) use for 5 or more years, especially pills of high estrogen content.[34] Increased risks were reported from a similarly designed study of women who began using OCs before age 18 (RR = 2.3 [95% CI = 1.4−3.8]).[31] Analyses by Beral and colleagues indicated cervical cancer was increased after 5 years or more of OC use (RR = 1.9) and risk declined 10 years after OCs were discontinued.[35] In contrast to these findings, two reviews reported conflicting findings: Green and colleagues reported no evidence of a strong positive or negative impact OCs[36] whereas Smith et al. noted a twofold increased risk of cervical cancer among HPV-positive women after 10 years of OC use compared to nonusers (RR = 2.5, 95% CI = 1.6−3.9).[37] Studies of OC use are complicated by changing hormonal composition as well as environmental and personal risk factors. One of the few studies addressing risk associated with menopausal hormone use noted unopposed estrogen increased the risk of estrogen-sensitive adenocarcinoma but not squamous carcinoma; in contrast, estrogen combined with progestin had no adverse effect on cervical cancer risk.[38]

Parity

High parity after controlling for number of sexual partners was associated with elevated cervical cancer risk prior to assessment for HPV.[17] Increased risk specifically of squamous cell cervical cancer was greater among women with high parity by Munoz et al. who analyzed data from nine international case-control studies.[39] Another international investigation restricted to HPV-positive women, found parity of seven or more increased risk compared with nulliparous women with an adjusted OR = 3.8 (95% CI = 2.7−5.5) or women with one or two term pregnancies (OR = 2.3 [95% CI = 1.6−3.2]). Among parous women, cesarian deliveries were associated with lower risk than vaginal births, indicating that effects late in pregnancy or method of birth may affect HPV progression.[39] The authors speculated that the decline in parity among American women may partially explain lower squamous-cell cervical cancer incidence during recent decades.[39]

Obesity

Among HPV-positive women obesity increased risk of cervical cancer differently by histology. Body mass index (BMI) greater than 30 elevated adenocarcinoma risk (OR = 2.1 [95% CI = 1.1−3.8]) but not squamous cell cervical cancer.[40] Adenocarcinomas were stimulated by elevated endogenous estrogen levels associated with obesity and with estrogen use for menopausal symptoms noted previously.

Genetic and Familial Susceptibility

Familial clustering of cervical abnormalities may be associated with genetic susceptibility, shared environment, or similar personal behavior patterns. Inherited susceptibility has been suggested although specific genes have not been identified. Environmental factors rather than genetics were noted in a Scandinavian twin registry study that reported a twofold increased risk associated with an affected first-degree relative.[41] Similar findings were reported from the Swedish Family-Cancer Database and the Netherlands: a twofold increased risk was noted for daughters and sisters of affected women.[42,43] A cohort study in Costa Rica and an American case-control study reported cervical cancer history in a first-degree relative increased risk of in situ or invasive squamous cell carcinoma by similar magnitudes: RR = 3.2 for Costa Rica and OR = 2.6 in the U.S. study.[44]

Cigarette Smoking

Increased cervical cancer risk due to chemical carcinogens from smoking was hypothesized in 1977 by Winkelstein and supported by numerous studies.[45] After controlling for sexual behavior, many subsequent studies supported the association revealing a dose-response relationship with odds ratios ranging from 2.5 to 4.5.[46] Extensive exposure to passive cigarette smoke at home also increased risk twofold among nonsmokers.[47] Chemical analysis of cervical mucus provided convincing evidence; mucus from smokers contained higher levels of nicotine, cotinine, and tobacco-related carcinogens than did mucus of nonsmokers.[48]

Studies linking smoking, HPV infection, and cervical lesions found higher HPV DNA viral levels among current smokers compared with never smokers. However, viral levels were comparable when former and never smokers were compared, suggesting smoking cessation may reduce HPV susceptibility, thus lowering risk of cervical disease.[49] Among HPV-infected women cancer risk was increased among current smokers varying by years of smoking and number of cigarettes smoked per day (RR = 2.0–4.0). Cessation of smoking for 6 years or longer reduced the risk.[18] Ho and colleagues found that risk of high-grade cervical lesions was two- to three-fold greater among smokers than nonsmokers suggesting smoking may enable HPV-infected cells to undergo malignant transformation.[50] Others noted risk due to smoking differed by histology; an inverse association was found for adenocarcinoma in contrast to significantly increased risk of invasive squamous cell carcinoma (OR = 3.0 [95% CI = 1.7–5.3]).[51]

The antiestrogenic effect of smoking may have influenced the carcinogenic impact of HPV on cervical tissue resulting in decreased risk of estrogen-associated adenocarcinoma lesions of the cervix.

Prenatal in Utero Exposure to Diethylstilbestrol

From the 1940s to the 1970s, the synthetic estrogen diethylstilbestrol (DES) was prescribed to more than 4 million pregnant American women under the misguided belief that estrogen would reduce risks of miscarriage and other pregnancy complications. Although a carefully designed clinical trial revealed *increased* rather than decreased risk of miscarriage among exposed women,[52] use continued until 1971 when Herbst and colleagues reported a highly significant case-control study indicating an association between in utero DES exposure with vaginal and cervical cancer among 7 young women ages 13 to 22.[53] Through long-term follow-up, approximately 4,000 women prenatally exposed to DES were found to have gynecologic abnormalities, including enlargement of the transformation zone of the cervix (identified in Figure 29-4), increasing their risk of malignant transformation of cervical cells. DES daughters were found to be at two- to fourfold increased risk of cervical dysplasia and cancer.[54] Although some researchers have suggested incidence may be increased due to greater use of early detection modalities among known DES-exposed women, a biologically plausible association was confirmed from a 20-year follow-up study that reported risk was highest among women exposed during the first 7 weeks of fetal development (RR = 2.8 [95% CI = 1.4–5.5]).[55]

Tubal Sterilization

Reduced cervical cancer following tubal ligation has been reported by some but not all researchers, who have suggested the association may be due to detection bias. However, linked files enabled a Danish study to detect a slight decline in cervical cancer, although risk of severe dysplasia was slightly higher among more than 65,000 women following tubal sterilization compared with national incidence rates.[56] Similar results, a slight decline for 5 years after tubal ligation, were reported by Li and Thomas from an international hospital-based case-control study. The authors noted cervical tissue responds to ovarian estrogens, which are reduced following tubal ligation.[57]

Cervical Cancer Screening

In 1943, Dr. George Papanicolaou reported premalignant cervical changes preceding cervical cancer could be detected by exfoliated vaginal cells. He proposed screening for cervical abnormalities, enabling intervention before the condition advanced. Although his concept was initially rejected by clinicians who questioned the ability to microscopically detect individual cancer cells from vaginal smears, doctors were eventually convinced and patients accepted Pap testing.[1] However, a new healthcare

professional was required to meet the expanding number of Pap tests performed; cytotechnologists were trained to identify Pap smears with abnormal cells for subsequent pathology review.

In 1974, endorsement by the ACS and the National Cancer Act Amendments reflected a change in public health policy from programs benefitting all members of a community, such as mass vaccine administration, to personalized procedures. Foltz and Kelsey in 1978 critiqued the 30-year history of annual Pap smears for all women age 20 and older, noting the statistical odds of high false-positive screening of women at minimal risk when prevalence rates are low. False-positive tests, especially among young women, were often treated aggressively by hysterectomy, preventing future childbearing.[58] The screening program created a public health paradox: incidence of cervical cancer increased, but mortality decreased, as most patients were cured by aggressive surgery for early stage disease.[59] A randomized trial was not conducted to evaluate the efficacy of the procedure, but case-control studies conducted internationally reported Pap testing reduced invasive cervical cancer by 60% to 90% with the benefit varying by the interval between screenings. Protection seemed to diminish as the interval exceeded 3 years.[5]

To address the continuing debate over the value of routine cervical cancer screening, Eddy developed statistical models using published cohort data to estimate incidence rates by age of first screen and frequency of subsequent testing based on two assumptions:[5] 1) cervical cancer developed after a lengthy preinvasive phase and 2) few cases of dysplasia or *in situ* disease become invasive cancer. His complex models predicted screening initiated at ages 20 or 23 with rescreening every 3 years after three negative tests would be safe.[5] In an earlier publication Eddy noted 250/100,000 women of average risk would develop invasive cervical cancer in their lifetime and 118/100,000 might die of the disease in the absence of Pap screening.[5] In contrast, current SEER data estimated 8.1/100,000 American women would be diagnosed in 2010 and 2.5/100,000 would die of cervical cancer.[4]

Controversy also surrounds age at ending routine Pap testing because risk varies considerably by age, sexual history, smoking behaviors, comorbid conditions, and prior screening history. Therefore, person-specific characteristics were needed to guide recommendations,[60] especially for older immigrant women who may have never been screened before migrating to the United States.[61] The National Health Interview Survey of the CDC questioned women on recency of Pap testing, providing the data presented in Figure 29-8. Reported screening varied by age group and education level. The oldest and least educated women had lowest rates of Pap testing although they may have been at highest risk. Public health messages have been appropriately directed to communities with low screening rates in which advanced stage cervical cancer has been diagnosed; however, continued efforts are required to overcome education-related disparities noted in Figure 29-8.[60]

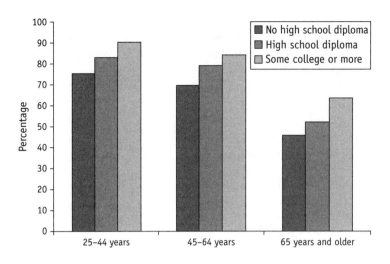

Figure 29-8 Percentage of women ages 25 and older who had a Pap test in the 3 years before interview by education level, 2005.

Source: Reproduced from National Center for Health Statistics. Health, United States, 2007 With Chartbook on Trends in the Health of Americans. Hyattsville, MD: 2007.

Reliability of Pap Tests

Although screening of presumably healthy women is intended to differentiate suspicious from normal cytology, considerable variability has been reported among clinicians evaluating Pap smears. The false-negative rate has varied from 5% to 50% regardless of the stage of disease: dysplasia, *in situ* cancer, or invasive cervical cancer with detection failures possibly due to inadequate cervical sampling and mishandling of specimens.[62] Falsely negative screens may be hazardous for women who may ignore signs and symptoms that develop between routine Pap tests. To reduce false-negative readings some researchers have proposed reevaluation of 10% of normal vaginal smears whereas others have applied computer-assisted scanning to identify grossly abnormal smears for clinical review.[62] Automated liquid-based cytology has replaced traditional Pap smears in many institutions although similar deficits have been identified with the newer technique.[63]

False-positive diagnoses of dysplasia or *in situ* disease are often followed by unnecessary and costly reexaminations and potentially harmful treatment. Large investigations have documented spontaneous regression of lesions in 6% to 60% of cases over 10 to 20 years. Therefore, periodic screening should provide numerous opportunities for diagnosis without overtreating early-stage disease.[5] To compare false-positive and false-negative screenings 20,000 slides were reviewed by two independent laboratories. Failure to identify *in situ* or invasive cancer ranged from 34% to 57%, varying by individual laboratory standards.[63] Diagnoses of cytology smears by expert referral pathologists compared with community-based pathologists revealed more aggressive readings by community clinicians, with kappa agreement (the proportion of agreement beyond chance) of 0.46 (95% CI = 0.43−0.49).[64] Although methods to reduce false-negative and false-positive Pap tests are being developed, conventional Pap smears continue to be performed with little concern for

low rates of sensitivity (58%) and specificity (69%). Given these estimates of efficacy, clinicians rely on repeat screens to detect any previously missed abnormalities and must be cautious to avoid overtreatment.[62]

Current Screening Recommendations for Cervical Cancer

Although clinicians and researchers have greater understanding of HPV and cervical disease, debates continue over screening guidelines. Balancing benefits of early detection with risks of overtreatment receives little attention. Sawaya noted evidence-based decisions guided the 2009 published recommendations of the American Congress of Obstetricians and Gynecologists (ACOG)[65] including limited but important reductions compared with those of ACS, which were initially published in 2002 (Table 29-2). Differences exist in relation to age at initiating screening, intervals between follow-up screenings, and age at discontinuation.[66] Screening recommendations noted in Table 29-2 are for women with prior history of normal screening; any clinically suspicious findings would necessitate more frequent examinations.[7]

The 2002 ACS updated guidelines included optional HPV DNA testing[7] but other details differed when compared with ACOG recommendations regarding age at first screening and frequency of repeat screening. More frequent screening was recommended for women at higher risk due to in utero exposure to DES (noted previously) or among women who are immune compromised following organ transplant or diagnosis of HIV/AIDS. Specialized guidelines for some at higher than average risk were recommended.[7] Revisions to the guidelines are anticipated as more research compares detection by HPV DNA analyses with cytology screening.

A randomized trial of 10,000 Canadian women who received both procedures compared the sensitivity of HPV DNA analyses with cytology screening for detection of

Table 29-2

Pap smear screening recommendations of the American Cancer Society and the American College of Obstetricians & Gynecologists

Screening Protocols	American Cancer Society 2002[7] & 2010[66]	American College Obstetricians & Gynecologists 2009[65]
Age at first test	3 years after first sexual intercourse	Not before age 21
Screening interval women age < 30 years	Annual with standard Pap; every 2 years with liquid Pap	Every 2 years
Screening interval women age ≥ 30 years	Every 2–3 years	Every 3 years
Age to discontinue screening	Age 70 after 3 negative tests in last 10 years	Age 65–70 after 3 negative tests in last 10 years
After hysterectomy	Discontinue screening if hysterectomy for benign condition	Discontinue screening if hysterectomy for benign condition
Additional screening options	Standard Pap test or liquid cytology; HPV DNA testing at age 30; repeat every 3 years	Standard Pap test or liquid cytology; HPV DNA testing at age 30; repeat every 3 years

cervical abnormalities; HPV testing was more sensitive than cytology (39.2% differences) and only 2.7% less specific in detecting cervical intraepithelial neoplasia (CIN) or more advanced lesions. However, data combined from both provided sensitivity of 100% and specificity of 92% reducing false positives and referrals for colposcopy.[67] Additional data from several European studies assessed the efficacy of screening by HPV DNA with and without liquid-based cytology or Pap smear screening, HPV DNA analyses detected persistent high-grade lesions earlier, providing a longer interval for intervention but younger women were overdiagnosed with lesions known to regress.[68]

The American Society for Colposcopy and Cervical Pathology recommends women with a positive HPV and negative cytology to receive colposcopy only if the infection persists. A proposed triage system would use cytology screening and HPV to identify women at highest risk for referral for colposcopy. Castle and colleagues, who noted clinicians inappropriately screen adolescents before they have initiated sexual activity, called for adherence to evidence-based guidelines for the benefit of patients to avoid adverse events among mostly healthy women.[64]

Molecular testing has recently been included in screening programs especially when cytology evaluation was indeterminate.[8] However, Wright and Schiffman cautioned against overuse of HPV analyses in clinical care because most infections are transient.[8] HPV DNA may needlessly classify young women as high risk causing them anxiety, unnecessary repeat assessments, potentially harmful overtreatment, and extra expense.[8] The challenge remains to balance the benefits of new technology while avoiding adverse effects of scheduling reexaminations following any minimally suspicious findings.[8]

Patients rely on physician guidance for screening, which increases the responsibility for doctors to keep current with professional recommendations.[69] Although some

clinicians and researchers have proposed discontinuing screening of older women, based on their research findings, Grainge and colleagues suggest Pap tests for older women should be determined by patient-specific risk factors and past screening history.[14] Mandelblatt and colleagues noted that 10% of invasive cervical cancers occur in older women, many of whom had never been screened.[60]

Clinical Adherence to Guidelines

A national survey of primary care physicians who provide Pap smears was conducted by Yabroff and colleagues in 2006–2007 to assess adherence to 2002–2003 revised screening guidelines. The survey included attitudinal questions, practice-specific data, participant demographics, and patient vignettes describing age and sexual behaviors.[70] Responses differed by practice specialty with an average of fewer than 30% following published guidelines pertaining to age at beginning, ending, and frequency of screening. Most responders were screening more frequently and beginning screening earlier than guidelines advised.[70] Women, infected with HIV and considered at high risk of cervical cancer may be one population not receiving adequate Pap testing.[71] Physician and patient education as well as reimbursement policy changes may be required to improve adherence to science-based clinical guidelines. Screening guidelines will again need modifications as more young women are protected by the HPV vaccine.[67]

Cost Estimates Associated with Pap Testing and Prevention Modalities

Although early detection modalities are assumed to be cost effective, potential savings must be balanced with added treatment expenses for lesions that have the potential to spontaneously regress. Over the past decades Pap smear screening has been a costly public health program. Eddy used his modeling methodology to note that initiating screening at age 18 versus 20 with annual rather than less frequent repeat screenings increased expenses but provided limited benefit.[5] Cost savings could occur through follow-up assessments performed on self-collected vaginal specimens, which have been shown to be acceptable to patients, their healthcare providers, and laboratory technicians.[72]

Cervical Cancer Screening in Relation to Sexual Orientation

Sexual orientation may influence frequency and acceptability of cervical cancer screening among women. Tracy and colleagues assessed the relationship between screening practices and barriers among self-identified lesbians recruited through national lesbian-oriented newspapers and websites using an online multidisciplinary survey for data collection.[73] Mean age of the 225 respondents was 41 years, and a majority were well-educated white women. Less than optimal screening frequency was associated with poor understanding of recommendations, low perception of benefits, and more barriers than noted by other women who reported more frequent Pap tests. Regardless of sexual orientation, knowledge and attitudes about cancer screening rely on education and receptivity of clinical care providers. However, lesbian women have considered themselves at lower risk than heterosexual or bisexual women because sex with men has been a recognized risk factor for cervical cancer.[73]

Assumptions about sexual practices among lesbians may have contributed to lower frequency of screening, although HPV analyses have indicated transmission may occur between women who reported no heterosexual contacts themselves and their partners, some of whom previously experienced sex with men.[74] In addition to HPV spread by skin contact, transmission may occur by shared sex toys and digital-vaginal contact, although the observed presence of HPV infection was lower among women who never had sex with men or whose last contact was greater than 10 years before study samples were obtained.[74] Marrazzo et al. also noted that increasing numbers of sexual partners, regardless of gender, was associated with greater positivity for HPV infection.[74] Lesbians may be at increased cervical cancer risk because of high prevalence of smoking and rates of obesity.[73]

Treatment Options for Preinvasive and Invasive Disease

When cervical cancer was the leading cause of cancer death, treatment options were limited to aggressive surgery and radiation therapy. Pap smear screening has enabled early detection followed by treatment using colposcopy to administer cryosurgery and laser treatment.[60] However, Trimble et al. used SEER data to assess cervical cancer treatment and noted a lack of consensus among institutions.[75] Clinicians now recognize that early detection of mild HPV infections are often cleared without any treatment and rarely progress to invasive disease.[75] Among adolescents, over 90% of infections of CIN1 and 60% of CIN2 lesions will regress within 3 years.[8] Despite

efforts by International Federation of Gynecology and Obstetrics (FIGO) to develop standardized algorithms, physician- and institution-specific significant differences in treatment approaches remain.[75]

Adverse Effects of Treatment of Dysplasia and Cervical Intraepithelial Neoplasia

Screening among women younger than 21 years has received special attention as infection rates are high but progression infrequently occurs. Overtreatment may complicate subsequent pregnancies when small dysplastic lesions are treated by conization or loop electrosurgical excision procedure (LEEP), which uses low-voltage electrical current. This treatment of mild to moderate dysplasia may adversely affect cervical tissue resulting in a two- to threefold increased risk of adverse pregnancy outcomes. The amount of tissue destroyed and depth of the surgical incision may adversely affect maintenance of a future pregnancy.[76]

A retrospective cohort of colposcopy patients treated in Auckland, New Zealand, between 1988 and 2000 were followed to determine pregnancy outcomes after treatment of CIN by conization, laser ablation, or LEEP procedures.[77] Comparisons of treated and untreated women noted rates of preterm delivery differed marginally; however, a significantly higher incidence of premature rupture of membranes occurred among 8% of treated and 3.5% of untreated women ($P < .004$).[77] In addition, preterm delivery was increased by smoking during pregnancy, prior preterm birth, and more aggressive histology of cervical lesions.[77] Similar results were reported from a Norwegian study of more than 15,000 women whose birth and treatment records were linked. Increased preterm deliveries occurred after conization procedures compared to deliveries of women whose pregnancies preceded conization and women not requiring treatment. The risk of preterm births decreased as treatment procedures changed, reducing the amount of cervical tissue removed.[78] Continuing concern regarding pregnancy outcomes led to a meta-analysis of data from studies published between 1960 to 2007. Significantly increased perinatal mortality was observed among women treated by conization (RR = 2.87, 95% CI = 1.42−5.81), the most damaging of excisional procedures.[76] Decisions on treatment modalities for women diagnosed with CIN are based on the size and location of the lesion, the aggressiveness of the abnormality and any evidence of microinvasion. These combined factors influence the amount of cervical tissue excised.

HPV Vaccine for Prevention of Cervical Cancer

A major public health event of 2006 was approval by the FDA of two HPV prophylactic vaccines, quadrivalent (including types 6, 11, 16, and 18) and bivalent (types 16 and 18), for administration to females ages 9–26 to ultimately provide primary prevention against 90% of genital warts and 70% of cervical cancers. Current guidelines indicate full protection requires three doses of the vaccine administered several months apart. A new genital HPV infection is estimated to occur among 6 million Americans annually; the newly licensed vaccines are expected to protect women against 70% of cervical cancers that might have developed years after the initial infection.[79]

Among more than 50,000 young women who participated in one of several international controlled trials testing the efficacy of either the quadrivalent or bivalent vaccine, 97% seroconverted with prevention of 90% of cervical lesions caused by HPV16 or HPV18 compared with controls.[80] Although the primary goal of preventing cervical cancer will not be detectable for several decades, reduced cervical infections and precancerous lesions are serving as intermediate markers of the vaccine's efficacy.[81,82] In trials required for FDA approval, the vaccine was shown to be effective for more than 3 years after the initial dose protecting against the specific HPV types included in the specific vaccine administered.[65] Additional data from two large international placebo-controlled clinical trials documented the statistically significant reduction in cervical changes detected by cytology including benign lesions and genital warts. Fewer referrals for diagnostic colposcopy and other therapeutic interventions were required reducing morbidity.[83]

To assess the cost effectiveness of the expensive vaccine, Kim and Goldie developed a model to predict long-term cost savings following widespread distribution, if the vaccine provides lifelong protection and if the rate of cytologic screening is reduced.[81] However, ACS has advised routine Pap testing regardless of having received the vaccine because some high-risk HPV types were not included. Also, education was recommended to inform people that the vaccine does not protect against other STDs.[7,66] Additional research is required to determine the length of protection and the potential benefit of the vaccine among individuals previously infected with HPV. Clinical studies are also needed to assess the effectiveness and safety of the vaccine for immunocompromised women.[84]

HPV Vaccine among Males

Giuliano et al. argued that males should also receive the vaccine because HPV infection has been found in 50% to 70% of some male populations although the most common HPV types differed by gender (Figure 29-6).[85] A large international placebo-controlled, double-blind clinical trial was conducted using the quadrivalent vaccine among more than 4,000 males ages 16 to 26 from 18 countries. External genital lesions were significantly reduced among vaccinated males compared to controls.[85] Risk from use of the quadrivalent vaccine among males associated with infection due to HPV16, HPV18, and other HPV types include anal cancer, malignancies of other sites, and benign anogenital warts.[85] Giuliano et al. noted the difficulty of assessing the efficacy of HPV vaccine among males, complicating assessment of cost effectiveness of gender-neutral administration.[85]

A review of the literature noted male college students were more accepting of the vaccine (74–78%) than a con-venience sample of community members in Georgia; the vaccine was more acceptable to men with multiple sex partners. Parents of sons and physicians indicated high acceptance of HPV vaccine for males although the lack of recognizable benefit for males was cited by those opposed.[86] A survey of clinicians indicated support for a gender-neutral HPV vaccine program providing opportunities for discussing sexual health. Greater education about vaccine benefits for both women and men might counter some opposition from physicians and male patients.

Potential Vaccine Side Effects

Adverse side effects of vaccination reported to CDC among the more than 23 million doses of the quadrivalent vaccine administered in the United States by the end of 2008 totaled 12,000. Most were common to any vaccine administrations and were not considered serious; 700 events were investigated by the FDA and CDC but none were related to the HPV vaccine. Current guidelines define who should be excluded from receiving the vaccine; as additional data accumulate from vaccine recipients, the guidelines will be revised.[80] Although rates of miscarriage did not differ by vaccine status among the 3,500 women unaware of their pregnancy at time of receiving the vaccine,[87] pregnant women will remain excluded until more research has been reported. Cancers with viral causes provide the opportunity for vaccine development and primary prevention as shown with hepatitis B vaccine and lowered liver cancer; however, some questions remain to be addressed: Will the vaccine clear persistent infections or interrupt progression to cancer among women with dysplasia or CIN? Among immune-compromised women, will the vaccine cause harm or be protective?[80,88]

Age at Vaccine Administration

The Advisory Committee on Immunization Practices encourages initial vaccination among girls 11 and 12 as well as catch-up for those ages 13 to 26.[89] Kahn also encourages continued cytology screening as HPV infection may have preceded vaccination and infections may have been caused by an HPV type not included in either vaccine.[80] A 2010 *Morbidity and Mortality Weekly Report* from CDC noted that approximately 44.3% of American girls between the ages of 13 and 17 have received at least the first dose of the HPV vaccine and 26.7% had received all three doses.[90] Although these data indicate a considerable number of American girls have received the HPV vaccine, limited research has been conducted to assess parental acceptance of this cancer prevention modality. Within the year after the vaccines were licensed, many states were considering mandates to increase vaccine administration providing educational programs, allocation of public funds to cover vaccine costs, and encouragement of insurance coverage.[91] However, a survey of political and scientific controversies that arose indicated that questions remain regarding adequate testing for safety, fears of government coercion, parental fears associated with adolescent sexual behaviors, and other issues.[91]

Increased educational programs are considered essential to promote acceptance of this cancer prevention modality.

Advertising of the "anticancer" vaccine has avoided the sexual transmission component of the disease given the low risk of young adolescents who are the current target population for vaccination.[92] Rather than promoting the vaccine to high-risk young Hispanic and black women, the health message implies all were at equal risk, which is not supported by data. An additional concern regarding marketing is the acceptance of financial support by several professional organizations from vaccine manufacturers to develop educational programs for colleagues to encourage vaccine administration and to promote state and federal agencies to cover the cost of the series.[92] Garner, a researcher affiliated with Merck, reviewed the history of vaccine development and acknowledged the manufacturer emphasized cancer prevention to counter parental fears of changed sexual behavior after their daughters received HPV vaccine.[93]

Parental acceptance of the vaccine is essential for successful widespread administration, requiring public health, personal physicians, and the media to address anticipated benefits and parental fears of side effects.[94] To assess parental attitudes toward vaccine administration, educational material and a questionnaire were mailed to randomly selected members of an American group health cooperative.[95] Acceptance of the vaccine program was associated with personal health beliefs and older ages at proposed administration rather than the specific protection provided by the vaccine. A survey of high school girls conducted in California found 48.4% participated in making the decision about the HPV vaccine, indicating that education for students and parents was essential for successful dissemination.[96]

Given the long legacy from initial HPV infection to malignant transformation, the efficacy of the vaccine as measured by reduced incidence will not be evident for decades; however, reduced incidence of cervical abnormalities may be an earlier indicator of protection provided by the vaccine. With implementation of medical record databases, linkage of vaccine histories with cytology screening information will provide early evidence of protection against early-stage cervical changes not reported to cancer registries. Long-term assessment of women receiving the vaccine will require cytologic confirmation of continued protection.

Summary

With the release in July 2011 of the consensus report from the Institute of Medicine (IOM) titled *Clinical Preventive Services for Women: Closing the Gap*, cervical cancer has received more attention as screening for early detection was the first preventive service identified in need of improvement.[97] Screening for this malignancy can now benefit from detection of HPV seroprevalence, persistence of infections, and greater appreciation of the natural history of cervical disease. Major revisions to screening guidelines have been published by ACS, ACOG, and others in past 5 to 10 years and renewed interest stimulated by the IOM report will enhance opportunities for future modifications,

especially after more young women and men received the HPV vaccine and benefits of vaccination are reported. Clinicians should augment protection against cervical cancer by stressing the importance of personal health behaviors including avoiding smoking, using condoms during sexual encounters, and eating nutritious foods including fruit and vegetables. These health behaviors developed at young ages may contribute to lower risks of sexually transmitted infections and other chronic conditions. Among young women caution is required in treating early stages of cervical abnormalities as damage to the cervix may increase risk of premature births. Screening protocols addressing the specific needs of women by age, family history, health behaviors, and future childbearing decisions are needed for appropriate patient-specific care. The future role of genetic risk to early detection and treatment decisions await further research to identify disease-specific susceptibility genes.

Discussion Questions

1. Describe the controversies associated with cervical cancer screening. How do recommendations vary regarding age at first screening and frequency of rescreening?

2. How do men influence the risk of cervical cancer among women? Why do rates of disease vary by age, education, and race/ethnicity?

3. Describe the research needed to identify the virus that is associated with cervical cancer. Does the viral infection always lead to cancer?

4. How has the identification of HPV influenced clinical understanding of cervical cancer development? Is the presence of the virus essential for cervical cancer development?

5. How does the incidence and mortality associated with cervical cancer compare with these rates for lung cancer, breast cancer, colon cancer, and endometrial cancer?

References

1. Schiffman MH, Hildesheim A. Cervical cancer. In: Schottenfeld D, Fraumeni JF. *Cancer Epidemiology and Prevention*. 3rd ed. New York: Oxford University Press; 2006.
2. Adami HO, Trichopoulos D. Cervical cancer and the elusive male factor. *N Engl J Med*. 2002;346:1160–1161.
3. American Cancer Society. *Cancer Facts & Figures 2010*. Atlanta, GA: Author; 2010. http://www.cancer.org/acs/groups/content/@nho/documents/document/acspc-024113.pdf
4. Surveillance, Epidemiology and End Results (SEER). Cancer of the cervix uteri (invasive). http://seer.cancer.gov/csr/1975_2007/results_merged/sect_05_cervix_uteri.pdf. (Accessed) May 5, 2011.
5. Eddy DM. Screening for cervical cancer. *Ann Int Med*. 1990;113:214–236.
6. Du P, Lemkin A, Kluhsman B, et al. The roles of social domains, behavioral risk, health care resources, and chlamydia in spatial clusters of US cervical cancer mortality: not all the clusters are the same. *Cancer Causes Control*. 2010;21:1669-83. Epub 2010 Jun 8.
7. Saslow D, Castle PE, Cox JT, et al. American Cancer Society guideline for Human Papillomavirus (HPV) vaccine use to prevent cervical cancer and its precursors. *CA Cancer J Clin*. 2007;57:7–28.
8. Wright TC Jr, Schiffman M. Adding a test for human papillomavirus DNA to cervical-cancer screening. *N Engl J Med*. 2003;348:489–490.
9. Wheeler CM, Hunt WC, Joste NE, et al. Human papillomavirus genotype distributions: implications for vaccination and cancer screening in the United States. *J Natl Cancer Inst*. 2009;101:475–487.
10. Munoz N, Bosch FX, de Sanjose S, et al. Epidemiologic classification of human papillomavirus types associated with cervical cancer. *N Engl J Med*. 2003;348:518–27.
11. Markowitz LE, Sternberg M, Dunne EF, et al. Seroprevalence of human papillomavirus types 6,11,16, and 18 in the United States: National Health and Nutrition Examination Survey 2003–2004. *J Infect Dis*. 2009;200:1059–1067.

12. Dunne EF, Unger ER, Sternberg M, et al. Prevalence of HPV infection among females in the United States. *JAMA*. 2007;297:813–819.

13. Wright TC, Massad S, Dunton CJ, et al. 2006 consensus guidelines for the management of women with cervical intraepithelial neoplasia or adenocarcinoma in situ. *Am J Obstet Gynecol*. 2007; 197:340–345.

14. Grainge MJ, Seth R, Coupland C, et al. Human papillomavirus infection in women who develop high-grade cervical intraepithelial neoplasia or cervical cancer: a case-control study in the UK. *Br J Cancer*. 2005;92:1794–1799.

15. Widdice LE, Breland DJ, Jonte J, et al. Human papillomavirus concordance in heterosexual couples. *J Adolesc Health*. 2010;47:151–159.

16. Jacobson DL, Womack SD, Peralta L, et al. Concordance of human papillomavirus in the cervix and urine among inner city adolescents. *Pediatr Infect Dis J*. 2000;19:722–728.

17. Brinton LA, Hamman RF, Huggins GR, et al. Sexual and reproductive risk factors for invasive squamous cell cervical cancer. *J Natl Cancer Inst*. 1987;79:23–30.

18. Shields TS, Brinton LA, Burk RD, et al. A case-control study of risk factors for invasive cervical cancer among US women exposed to oncogenic type of human papillomavirus. *Cancer Epidemiol Biomarkers Prev*. 2004;13: 1574–1582.

19. Winer RL, Hughes JP, Feng Q, et al. Condom use and the risk of genital human papillomavirus infection in young women. *N Engl J Med*. 2006;354:2645–2654.

20. Doerfler D, Bernhaus A, Kottmel A, et al. Human papilloma virus infection prior to coitarche. *Am J Obstet Gynecol*. 2009;200:487.e1–5

21. Richardson H, Abrahamowicz M, Tellier PP, et al. Modifiable risk factors associated with clearance of type-specific cervical human papillomavirus infections in a cohort of university students. *Cancer Epidemiol Biomarkers Prev*. 2005;14:1149–1156.

22. Centers for Disease Control and Prevention. 1993 revised classification system for HIV infection and expanded surveillance case definition for AIDS among adolescents and adults. *MMWR Morb Mortal Wkly Rep*.1992;41:1–17.

23. Mandelblatt JS, Fahs M, Garibaldi K, et al. Association between HIV infection and cervical neoplasia: implications for clinical care of women at risk for both conditions. *AIDS*. 1992;6:173–178.

24. Theiler RN, Farr SL, Karon JM, et al. High-risk human papillomavirus reactivation in human immunodeficiency virus-infected women. Risk factors for cervical viral shedding. *Obstet Gynecol*. 2010;115:1150–1158.

25. Strickler HD, Burk RD, Fazzari M, et al. Natural history and possible reactivation of human papillomavirus in human immunodeficiency virus-positive women. *J Natl Cancer Inst*. 2005;97:577–586.

26. Engels EA, Biggar RJ, Hall HI, et al. Cancer risk in people infected with human immunodeficiency virus in the United States. *Int J Cancer*. 2008;123:187–194.

27. Gurlich AE, van Leeuwen MT, Falster MO, Vajdic CM. Incidence of cancers in people with HIV/AIDS compared with immunosuppressed transplant recipients: a meta-analysis. *Lancet*. 2007;370:59–67.

28. Bratcher LF, Sahasrabuddhe VV. The impact of antiretroviral therapy on HPV and cervical intraepithelial neoplasia: current evidence and directions for future research. *Infect Agents Cancer*. 2010;5:8

29. Smith-McCune KK, Shiboski S, Chirenje MZ, et al. Type-specific cervico-vaginal human papillomavirus infection increases risk of HIV acquisition independent of other sexually transmitted infections. *PLoS One*. 2010;5:e10094.

30. Madeleine MM, Anttila T, Schwartz SM, et al. Risk of cervical cancer associated with *Chlamydia trachomatis* antibodies by histology, HPV type and HPV cofactors. *Int J Cancer*. 2006;120:650–655.

31. Daling JR, Madeleine MM, McKnight B, et al. The relationship of human papillomavirus-related cervical tumors to cigarette smoking, oral contraceptive use, and prior herpes simplex virus type 2 infection. *Cancer Epidemiol Biomarkers Prev*. 1996;5:541–548.

32. Weiss HA, Hankins CA, Dickson K. Male circumcision and risk of HIV infection in women: a systematic review and meta-analysis. *Lancet Infect Dis*. 2009;9:669–677.

33. Castellsagué X, Bosch FX, Muñoz N, et al. Male circumcision, penile human papillomavirus infection, and cervical cancer in female partners. *N Engl J Med*. 2002;346:1105–1112.

34. Brinton LA, Huggins GR, Lehman HF, et al. Long-term use of oral contraceptives and risk of cervical cancer. *Int J Cancer*. 1986;38:339–344.

35. Beral V, Franceschi S, and the International Collaboration of Epidemiological Studies of Cervical Cancer. Cervical cancer and hormonal contraceptives: collaborative reanalysis of individual data from 16,573 women with cervical cancer and 35,509 women without cervical cancer from 24 epidemiological studies. *Lancet*. 2007;370:1609–1621.

36. Green J, Berrington de Gonzalez A, Smith JS, et al. Human papillomavirus infection and use of oral contraceptives. *Br J Cancer*. 2003;88:1713–1720.

37. Smith JS, Green J, Berrington de Gonzalez A, et al. Cervical cancer and use of hormonal contraceptives: a systematic review. *Lancet*. 2003;361:1159–1167.

38. Lacey JV, Brinton LA, Barnes WA, et al. Use of hormone replacement therapy and adenocarcinomas and squamous cell carcinomas of the uterine cervix. *Gynecol Oncol*. 2000;77:149–154.

39. Muñoz N, Franceschi S, Bosetti C, et al. Role of parity and human papillomasvirus in cervical cancer: the IARC multicentric case-control study. *Lancet*. 2002;359:1093–1101.

40. Lacey JV, Swanson CA, Brinton LA, et al. Obesity as a potential risk factor for adenocarcinomas and squamous cell carcinomas of the uterine cervix. *Cancer*. 2003;98:814– 821.

41. Lichtenstein P, Holm NV, Verkasalo PK, et al. Environmental and hereditable factors in the causation of cancer. Analyses of cohorts of twins from Sweden, Denmark and Finland. *N Engl J Med*. 2000;343:78–85.

42. Hemminki K, Li X, Mutanen P. Familial risks in invasive and in situ cervical cancer by histological type. *Eur J Cancer Prev*. 2001;10:83–89.

43. Zoodsma M, Sijmons RH, de Vries EGE, van der Zee AGJ. Familial cervical cancer: case reports, review and clinical implications. *Hered Cancer Clin Pract*. 2004;2:99–105.

44. Zelmanowicz A, Schiffman M, Herrero R, et al. Family history as a co-factor for adenocarcinoma and squamous cell carcinoma of the uterine cervix: results from two studies conducted in Costa Rica and the United States. *Int J Cancer*. 2005;116:599–605.

45. Winkelstein W Jr. Smoking and cervical cancer—current status: a review. *Am J Epidemiol*. 1990;131:945–957.

46. Brinton LA, Schairer C, Haenszel W, et al. Cigarette smoking and invasive cervical cancer. *JAMA*. 1986;255:3265–3269.

47. Slattery ML, Robison LM, Schuman KL, et al. Cigarette smoking and exposure to passive smoke are risk factors for cervical cancer. *JAMA*. 1989;261:1593–1598.

48. Prokopczyk B, Cox JE, Hoffmann D, Waggoner SE. Identification of tobacco-specific carcinogen in the cervical mucus of smokers and non-smokers. *J Natl Cancer Inst*. 1997;89:868–873.

49. Xi LF, Koutsky L, Castle PE, et al. Relationship between cigarette smoking and human papilloma virus types 16 and 18 DNA load. *Cancer Epidemiol Biomarkers Prev*. 2009;18:3490–3496.

50. Ho GYF, Kadish AS, Burk RD, et al. HPV16 and cigarette smoking as risk factors for high-grade cervical intra-epithelial neoplasia. *Int J Cancer*. 1998;78:281–285.

51. Lacey JV, Frisch M, Brinton LA, et al. Associations between smoking and adenocarcinomas and squamous cell carcinomas of the uterine cervix (United States). *Cancer Causes Cont*. 2001;12:153–161.

52. Dieckmann WJ, Davis ME, Rynkiewicz LM, Pottinger RE. Does the administration of diethylstilbestrol during pregnancy have therapeutic value? *Am J Obstet Gynecol*. 1953;66:1062–1075.

53. Herbst AL, Ulfeder H, Poskanzer DC. Adenocarcinoma of the vagina: association of maternal stilbestrol therapy with tumor appearance in young women. *N Engl J Med*. 1971;284:878–881.

54. Robboy SJ, Noller KL, O'Brien P, et al. Increased incidence of cervical and vaginal dysplasia in 3980 diethylstilbestrol-exposed young women. Experience of the National Collaborative Diethylstilbestrol Adenosis Project. *JAMA*. 1984;252:2979–2983.

55. Hatch EE, Herbst AL, Hoover RN, et al. Incidence of squamous neoplasia of the cervix and vagina in women exposed prenatally to diethylstilbestrol (United States). *Cancer Causes Control*. 2001;12:837–845.

56. Kjaer SK, Mellemkjaer L, Brinton LA, et al. Tubal sterilization and risk of ovarian, endometrial and cervical cancer. A Danish population-based follow-up study of more than 65,000 sterilized women. *Int J Epidemiol*. 2004;33:596–602.

57. Li H, Thomas DB. Tubal ligation and risk of cervical cancer. *Contraception*. 2000;61:323–328.

58. Foltz AM, Kelsey JL. The annual Pap test: a dubious policy success. *Milbank Mem Fund Q Health Soc*. 1978;56:426–62.

59. Morabia A, Zhang FF. History of medical screening: from concept to action. *Postgrad Med J*. 2004;80:463–469.

60. Mandelblatt J, Lawrence W, Yi B, King J. The balance of harms, benefits and costs of screening for cervical cancer in older women. *Arch Intern Med*. 2004;164:245–247.

61. Taylor VM, Yasui Y, Burke N, et al. Pap testing adherence among Vietnamese American women. *Cancer Epidemiol Biomarkers Prev*. 2004;13:613–619.

62. Nanda K, McCrory DC, Myers ER, et al. Accuracy of the Papanicolaou test in screening for and follow-up of cervical cytologic abnormalities: a systematic review. *Ann Intern Med*. 2000;132:810–819.

63. Yobs AR, Plott AE, Hicklin MD, et al. Retrospective evaluation of gynecologic cytodiagnosis: II. Interlaboratory reproducibility as shown in rescreening large consecutive samples of reported cases. *Acta Cytol*. 1987;31:900–910.

64. Castle PE, Stoler MH, Solomon D, Schiffman M. The relationship of community biopsy-diagnosed cervical intraepithelial neoplasia grade 2 to the quality control pathology-reviewed diagnoses. *Am J Clin Pathol*. 2007;127:805–815.

65. Sawaya GF. Cervical-cancer screening—New guidelines and the balance between benefits and harms. *N Engl J Med*. 2009;361:2503–2505.

66. Smith RA, Cokkinides V, Brooks D, et al. Cancer screening in the United States, 2010: A review of current American Cancer Society guidelines and issues in cancer screening. *CA Cancer J Clin*. 2010;60:99–119.

67. Mayrand MH, Duarte-Franco E, Rodrigues I, et al. Human papillomavirus DNA versus Papanicolaou screening tests for cervical cancer. *N Engl J Med*. 2007;357:1579–1588.

68. Ronco G, Giorgi-Rossi P, Carozzi F, et al. Efficacy of human papillomavirus testing for the detection of invasive cervical cancers and cervical intraepithelial neoplasia: a randomized controlled trial. *Lancet Oncol*. 2010;11:249–257.

69. Caughlin SS, Beslau ES, Thompson T, Benard VB. Physician recommendation for Papanicolaou testing among US women, 2000. *Cancer Epidemiol Biomarkers Prev.* 2005;14:1143–1148.

70. Yabroff KR, Saralya M, Meissner HI, et al. Specialty differences in primary care physician reports of Papanicolaou test screening practices: a national survey, 2006-2007. *Ann Intern Med.* 2009;151:602–611.

71. Logan JL, Khambaty MQ, D'Souza KM, Menezes LJ. Cervical cancer screening among HIV-infected women in a health department setting. *AIDS Patient Care STDS.* 2010;24:471–475.

72. Anhang R, Nelson JA, Telerant R, et al. Acceptability of self-collection of specimens for HPV DNA testing in an urban population. *J Womens Health (Larchmt).* 2005;14:721–728.

73. Tracy JK, Lydecker AD, Ireland L. Barriers to cervical cancer screening among lesbians. *J Womens Health (Larchmt).* 2010;19:229–237.

74. Marrazzo JM, Koutsky LA, Kiviat NB, et al. Papanicolaou test screening and prevalence of genital human papillomavirus among women who have sex with women. *Am J Public Health.* 2001;91:947–952.

75. Trimble EL, Harlan LC, Gius D, et al. Patterns of care for women with cervical cancer in the United States. *Cancer.* 2008;113:743–749.

76. Arbyn M, Kyrgiou M, Simoens C, et al. Perinatal mortality and other severe adverse pregnancy outcomes associated with treatment of cervical intraepithelial neoplasia: meta-analysis. *BMJ.* 2008;337:a1284.

77. Sadler L, Saftlas A, Wang W, et al. Treatment for cervical intraepithelial neoplasia and risk of preterm delivery. *JAMA.* 2004;291:2100–2106.

78. Albrechtsen S, Rasmussen S, Thoresen S, et al. Pregnancy outcome in women before and after cervical conization: population based cohort study. *BMJ.* 2008;337:a1343.

79. Steinbrook R. The potential of human papillomavirus vaccines. *N Engl J Med.* 2006;354:1109–1112.

80. Kahn JA. HPV Vaccination for the prevention of cervical intraepithelial neoplasia. *N Engl J Med.* 2009;361:271–278.

81. Kim JJ, Goldie SJ. Health and economic implications of HPV vaccination in the United States. *N Engl J Med.* 2008;359:821–832.

82. Haug CJ. Human papillomavirus vaccination—Reasons for caution. *N Engl J Med.* 2008;359:861–862.

83. Muñoz N, Kjaer SK, Sigurdsson K, et al. Impact of human papillomavirus (HPV)-6/11/16/18 vaccine on all HPV-associated genital disease in young women. *J Natl Cancer Inst.* 2010;102:325–339.

84. Palefsky JM, Gillison ML, Strickler HD. Chapter 16: HPV vaccines in immunocompromised women and men. *Vaccine.* 2006;24S3:S3/140–146.

85. Giuliano AR, Palefsky JM, Goldstone S, et al. Efficacy of quadrivalent HPV vaccine against HPV infection and disease in males. *N Engl J Med.* 2011;364:401–411.

86. Liddon N, Hood J, Wynn BA, Markowitz LE. Acceptability of human papillomavirus vaccine for males: a review of the literature. *J Adolesc Health.* 2010;46:113–123.

87. Wacholder S, Chen BE, Wilcox A, et al. Risk of miscarriage with bivalent vaccine against human papilloma virus (HPV) types 16 and 18: pooled analysis of two randomized controlled trials. *BMJ.* 2010;340:c712

88. Finn OJ, Edwards RP. Human papillomavirus vaccine for cancer prevention. *N Engl J Med.* 2009;361:1899–1901.

89. Markowitz LE, Dunne EF, Saraiya M, et al. Quadrivalent human papillomavirus vaccine: recommendations of the Advisory Committee on Immunization Practices (ACIP). *MMWR Morb Mortal Wkly Rep Recomm Rep.* 2007;56 (RR-2):1–24.

90. CDC. National, state and local vaccination coverage among adolescents aged 13-17 years—United States, 2009. *MMWR Morb Mortal Wkly Rep.* 2010;59:1018–1023.

91. Cosgrove J, Abiola S, Mello MM. HPV vaccination mandates—lawmaking amid political and scientific controversy. *N Engl J Med.* 2010;363:785–791.

92. Rothman SM, Rothman DJ. Marketing HPV vaccine. Implications for adolescent health and medical professionalism. *JAMA.* 2009;302:781–786.

93. Garner EIO. A case study: Lessons learned from human papillomavirus vaccine development: approval of a vaccine for use in children and young adolescents for prevention of an adult disease. *J Acquir Immune Defic Syndr.* 2010;54,(suppl 1):S50–S52.

94. Goldstein MA. Human papillomavirus vaccine in males. *N Engl J Med.* 2008;359:862–863.

95. Dempsey AF, Zimet GD, David RL, Koutsky L. Factors that are associated with parental acceptance of human papillomavirus vaccines: a randomized intervention study of written information about HPV. *Pediatrics.* 2006;117:1486–1493.

96. Mathur MB, Mathur VS, Reichling DB. Participation in the decision to be vaccinated against human papillomavirus by California high school girls and the predictors of vaccine status. *J Pediatr Health Care.* 2010;24:14.

97. Institute of Medicine. *Clinical Preventive Services for Women: Closing the Gaps.* Washington, DC: National Academies Press; 2011.

Colorectal Cancer

Julie Ruckel Kumar, MPH; Sidney J. Winawer, MD; and Ann G. Zauber, PhD

Introduction

Colorectal cancer (CRC) accounts for almost 9% of all cancer deaths nationwide and is the third most common cause of cancer death in women; approximately 25,220 women will have died from this cancer in 2012.[1] However, colorectal cancer is one of the few cancers that can be prevented in women through regular screening and removal of adenomatous polyps.

Provider recommendations are the most effective way to ensure that average-risk individuals undergo screening.[2] Because most women receive primary care through gynecologists,[3] these providers play a critical role in recommending colorectal cancer screening for women. In addition, cancer screening is often a routine and familiar medical task for women beginning with Papanicolaou tests for cervical cancer and mammographies for breast cancer detection.[4] Screening rates for breast (76% every 2 years) and cervical (83% every 3 years) cancer are also notably higher than for CRC (49% for either yearly fecal occult blood test or colonoscopy every 10 years).[5] Advocating colorectal cancer screening as part of a comprehensive cancer prevention and detection plan by providers may increase the CRC screening rate to the levels currently seen in breast and cervical cancer.

Unique and important differences exist for women compared with men in colorectal cancer etiology, screening, and diagnosis. For example, studies have shown that estrogen protects women against CRC development.[6] In terms of risk, the long-term adverse effects of smoking in women are only now being appreciated. Finally, as women age, adenoma incidence increases, making screening increasingly important.[7]

Biology Overview

Three known biological pathways lead to colorectal cancer development. The main pathway through which most neoplasia originates is the adenoma-carcinoma pathway based on evidence from clinical, epidemiologic, autopsy, and genetic studies.[8,9] In this pathway colorectal cancer usually arises as a small adenomatous polyp. Left-sided or distal polyps are located in the rectum, sigmoid and descending colon up to and including the splenic flexure whereas right-sided or proximal polyps are found in the transverse colon, hepatic flexure, and ascending colon up to the cecum.[10,11] As noted in Figure 30-1 during colonoscopy, regardless of polyp classification, all visualized polyps are removed and histologically classified.[12] Adenomas are commonly found in adults over age 50 and are estimated to take an average of 10 or more years to transform into a cancer.[13,14] Less than 2% of women develop colon cancer between the ages of 50 and 69 years.[15] Risk factors associated with adenomas include increasing age, male gender, and family history.[16] The prevalence of adenomatous polyps among asymptomatic women and men has been estimated to be between 15% and 33% based on screening trials.[7,17–19] Several gene mutations have been associated with this pathway of polyp formation including adenomatous polyposis coli (APC).[13,20]

A second pathway to colon cancer is the serrated polyp pathway not associated with APC mutations.[12–14] The third biological pathway occurs in hereditary nonpolyposis colorectal cancer (HNPCC), in which microsatellite instability results in DNA repair gene mutations and facilitation of adenoma growth.[14,20]

Removal of adenomas interrupts the carcinoma sequence reducing colorectal cancer incidence and mortality. The National Polyp Study prospectively followed 1,418 patients for 10 years after adenoma polypectomy. A 76–90% reduction in colorectal cancer incidence was found when incidence in the screened cohort was compared with three referent groups.[21] Other studies found similar observations.[22,23] Although adenomatous polyps (and hyperplastic polyps in the serrated pathway) can be precursors to colorectal cancer, identification and removal of these polyps through screening tests prevents cancerous growth.

Incidence and Survival Rates

Incidence and mortality rates for colorectal cancer are falling and survival rates are increasing.[24] In the average-risk population, a rise in CRC incidence usually begins after age 50.[13] The median age at colorectal cancer diagnosis for 2002–2006 was 71 years. Incidence rates among women are higher in African Americans and lowest in

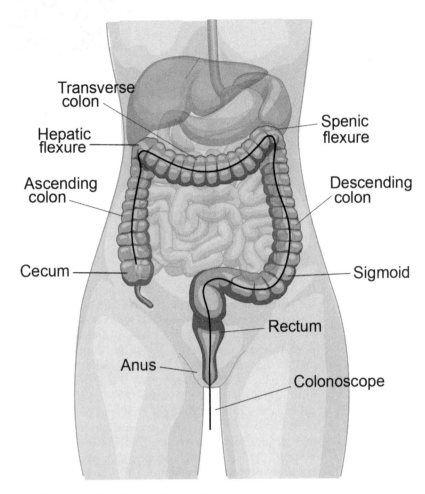

Figure 30-1 Large intestine indicating position of colonoscopy

Transverse colon
Spenic flexure
Hepatic flexure
Ascending colon
Descending colon
Cecum
Sigmoid
Rectum
Anus
Colonoscope

Figure 30-2 Colon polyp detectable during colonoscopy

Reproduced from Colon cancer screening. Basic Fact Sheet. Centers for Disease Control and Prevention's Screen for Life: National Colorectal Cancer Action Campaign. http://www.cdc.gov/cancer/colorectal/pdf/Basic_FS_Eng_Color.pdf

Hispanics (Table 30-1). Both women and men have a 5.2% lifetime chance of being diagnosed with CRC based on 2004–2006 rates.[15]

In the United States, more CRC cases are being diagnosed at a localized stage[24] according to Surveillance, Epidemiology and End Results (SEER) data, which has a 5-year relative survival of 91%.[15] However, African Americans are often diagnosed at later stages with lower survival rates than white patients.[25] In addition, men have been shown to have higher rates of advanced cancers of the colon than women.[7,19]

The annual age-adjusted death rate for CRC is 18.2 per 100,000 Americans based on 2002–2006 SEER data with a median age at death of 75 years. Overall, the CRC 5-year relative survival rate for all stages combined exceeds 60%.[20] As of January 1, 2006, over 1.1 million Americans—specifically over 567,000 women—had active CRC or were cured after effective treatment.[15]

Screening Methods

A screening test is performed on "asymptomatic individuals" without signs or symptoms of a disease or illness.[26] CRC symptoms may include diarrhea or constipation lasting more than a few days, blood in the stool, or cramping and abdominal pain.[27] Screening is the key component in preventing colorectal cancer and finding cancer at an early stage. Currently, a number of noninvasive and invasive screening methods are recommended. Stool-based tests primarily enable cancer detection and structural tests detect adenomas as well as cancers. Standard screening guidelines and timelines for persons of average risk and high risk have been developed by the American Cancer Society(ACS), the U.S. Multi-Society Task Force on Colorectal Cancer (USMSTF), the U.S. Preventive Services Task Force (USPSTF),[28] and the American Congress of Obstetricians and Gynecologists (ACOG).[29,30]

Colonoscopy

Colonoscopy is a one-step method that can prevent cancer by removal of adenomatous polyps. Furthermore, colonoscopy is the diagnostic test for a positive fecal occult blood test (FOBT), a positive finding on computed tomographic colonography (CTC), or flexible sigmoidoscopy. During colonoscopy, the endoscopist meticulously inspects the entire colon, from rectum to cecum, through use of a colonoscope and performs biopsies and polyp removal as needed. An effective colonoscopy is also dependent on a patient's ability to adequately perform the bowel preparation.

Table 30-1

Age-Adjusted Colorectal Cancer Incidence & Mortality Rates per 100,000 by Race/Ethnicity & Gender (SEER 2002-2006)

Incidence Rates per 100,000		Race/Ethnicity	Mortality Rates per 100,000	
Female	Male		Female	Male
42.8	57.3	All Races	15.4	21.9
53.5	69.3	African American	21.6	31.4
41.2	43.1	American Indian/Alaska Native[†]	13.7	20.0
34.6	46.9	Asian/Pacific Islander	10.0	13.8
32.2	46.3	Hispanic[‡]	10.7	16.1
42.1	56.9	White	14.9	21.4

(SEER data)[†]=Incidence and mortality data from American Indian/Alaska Native are based on the CHSDA (Contract Health Service Delivery Area) counties;
[‡]=Hispanic death rates exclude deaths from the District of Columbia, Minnesota, New Hampshire, and North Dakota.[15]
Reproduced from SEER Stat Fact Sheets Cancer: Colon and Rectum. 2009; http://seer.cancer.gov/statfacts/html/colorect.html. Accessed March 2, 2010.

Often considered the most difficult aspect of the procedure for the patient, a day prior to the colonoscopy the patient adopts a liquid diet and ingests oral laxative solutions to ensure a clean bowel. During the procedure, patients are often given a sedative to prevent discomfort. Currently, colonoscopy is recommended once every 10 years starting at age 50 for those at average risk (no personal history of polyps or colorectal cancer and no family history of CRC).[29]

The evidence for colonoscopy and polypectomy effectiveness has come from a variety of studies including randomized controlled trials (RCT) of other screening modalities with positive findings.[31–33] The National Polyp Study showed that colonoscopy reduced the incidence of CRC by 76–90%, suggesting primary prevention through polypectomy.[21] Furthermore, a case-control study of endoscopic procedures found veterans who had a colonoscopy had more than a 50% reduction in colorectal cancer incidence.[34] The magnitude of protection is uncertain as no long-term RCTs of screening colonoscopy in the general population have been completed.[29]

Quality issues include adequacy of the bowel preparation and time taken to examine the colon during withdrawal of the colonoscope.[35] Barclay et al. found that clinicians whose withdrawal time was over 6 minutes, the minimum amount of time for adequate mucosal inspection, had greater rates of adenoma detection compared with more rapid withdrawal of less than 6 minutes.[17] The USMSTF guidelines stress that key components of an effective colon examination by appropriately trained clinicians include careful assessment during withdrawal to provide adequate time by appropriately trained clinicians to perform a complete examination.[29]

Complications are rare as noted in a large screening study.[7] The greatest procedural risk is colon perforation, which was noted as 0.2%, or 2 per 1,000 patients, among a random sample of Medicare patients. This rate has declined recently, which suggests improvement in technology and technique.[36] Other rare but serious conditions (as well as additional limitations of colonoscopy) are listed in Table 30-2.

Studies consistently indicate that approximately 67–82% of patients who undergo colonoscopy will not have neoplastic findings (nonadvanced adenoma, advanced adenoma, or cancer).[7,17–19] A study of 1,463 asymptomatic, average-risk women referred for colonoscopy from four military medical centers revealed a 4.9% rate of advanced neoplasia (adenomas $\geq$ 1 cm, villous adenoma, advanced adenoma, and cancer), which increased significantly with age; women aged 70–79 had a higher risk, RR = 3.56, (95% CI = 1.70–7.58) than women aged 50–59.[19] Regula et al. observed that more women in various age groups (40–66 years of age) needed to be screened to detect an advanced neoplasia compared with similarly aged men.[7]

Flexible Sigmoidoscopy

Flexible sigmoidoscopy examines the distal or lower third of the colon and rectum, requires less extensive bowel preparation, and can be performed by a nonspecialist physician or nurse practitioner. Current recommendations suggest rescreening every 5 years.[29]

Research indicates sigmoidoscopy is effective for screening the distal colon. A case-control screening study at Kaiser Permanente found a 60% mortality reduction associated with sigmoidoscopy screening.[37] Similar results were reported by other sigmoidoscopy case-control studies.[34,38] The efficacy of flexible sigmoidoscopy is currently being evaluated through the U.S. multicenter, Prostate, Lung, Colorectal, Ovary (PLCO) trial supported by the National Cancer Institute; the United Kingdom Flexi-Scope trial; and the Italian multicenter randomized controlled trial, Screening for Colon Rectum (SCORE). Efficacy is reported for the Flexi-Scope study (May 2010) with 23% reduction of incidence and 31% reduction of mortality in intention-to-treat analyses.[39–43]

If distal adenomas are found by sigmoidoscopy, a follow-up colonoscopy is recommended to examine the entire colon. Two studies that used colonoscopy to model flexible sigmoidoscopy results reported distal adenomas

Table 30-2

Advantages and disadvantage of colorectal screening modalities

Test & Frequency	Benefits	Limitations
Colonoscopy *Every 10 years*	• Entire colon/rectum examined • Proximal and distal polyp(s) removed as necessary	• Potential perforation of the colon (very low risk) • Possible bleeding from polypectomy • Potential cardiopulmonary complications (very low risk) • Extensive bowel preparation procedures • A half or entire day for procedure and recovery • Chaperone for transportation • Dependent on endoscopist's skill
Sigmoidoscopy *Every 5 years*	• Distal colon examined with polyp removal • No sedation • Easier bowel preparation • Nurse practioners and other clinicians can perform • Can be done in office-based settings • Mortality benefit in RCT	• Proximal colon unexamined • Patient discomfort • Perforation of the colon (very low risk) • Follow-up colonoscopy recommended with positive findings
CT Colonography *Unknown; Possibly every 5 years*	• 2-D and 3-D visual of the entire colon/rectum • Less invasive than colonoscopy • No sedation • Extracolonic findings	• Missed flat and small polyps • Exposure to low-dose radiation • Bowel preparation procedures • Perforation (very low risk) • Not cost effective and often not reimbursed • Uncertain screening intervals • Follow-up colonoscopy recommended with positive findings
gFOBT Hemoccult II Hemoccult Sensa *Yearly*	• Tests with increased sensitivity available • Mortality benefit in RCT • Convenient, performed at home • Noninvasive	• Sensitivity and specificity test variations • Low sensitivity for detecting advanced adenomas • Dietary and drug restrictions • Prone to inadequate sample collection • Variations in lab interpretation • Follow-up colonoscopy recommended with positive findings
iFOBT/FIT *Yearly*	• Increased sensitivity and specificity compared to gFOBT • No dietary or medication restrictions • Noninvasive • Higher sensitivity for advanced adenomas than for gFOBT	• Test characteristics differ by FIT versions • Follow-up colonoscopy recommended with positive findings
Fecal DNA *Unknown*	• Identification of DNA mutations associated with CRC • One-time collection • Convenient, performed at home	• Test does not contain all CRC markers • Collection of entire stool; frozen 8 hours before shipment • High cost compared to other tests • Efficacy of test unknown • Not FDA approved • Further management with positive fecal DNA findings but negative colonoscopy

increased the risk for proximal advanced adenomas. In a Veterans Administration study, more than 3,000 patients who had distal adenomas were more likely to have advanced proximal neoplasia, OR = 3.4 (95% CI = 1.8–6.5) compared to those without distal adenomas.[18] Imperiale et al. also found distal polyps and adenomas increased risk for proximal advanced adenomas in an employer-based population.[44] Furthermore, Schoenfeld et al. studied polyp detection by colonoscopy to estimate detection by sigmoidoscopy in average-risk women and noted sigmoidoscopy alone would have missed 65% of the advanced neoplasms. This finding suggested a potential right-sided adenoma prevalence, making colonoscopy a preferable screening modality for women.[19] In the United States, flexible sigmoidoscopy has not been very popular because of the exclusive focus on the distal colon and the lack of identification of proximal neoplasia.[18,29]

CT Colonography ("Virtual" Colonoscopy)

As a minimally invasive form of screening, computed tomographic (CT) colonography (sometimes referred to as "virtual colonoscopy"), provides the radiologist a visual 2-D and 3-D computer image of the entire colorectum. For appropriate visualization, patients undergo the same colon preparation as colonoscopy and often receive an oral contrast fluid. Air or carbon dioxide is instilled by rectum during the procedure. CTC screening is recommended beginning at age 50 but subsequent time intervals have yet to be determined.[29] Efficacy of CTC is being studied although some performance data have been reported including sensitivity and specificity percentages (see Table 30-3.)

Extracolonic clinically significant findings have been reported in numerous studies and require an additional diagnostic workup.[29,45] Additional CTC concerns are that small and flat adenomas are often missed and the procedure includes exposure to low-dose radiation and extracolonic findings are uncovered that require diagnostic work-up.[29] Compared with all other modalities, CT colonography is not a cost-effective alternative to colonoscopy.[46] CTC is a new, evolving technology for CRC screening that requires further study.

Stool Blood Tests

Stool blood tests, able to detect occult blood or microscopic amounts of blood in stool, detect cancers and large adenomas (>1 cm) that have a tendency to bleed. The two main types of tests are the Guaiac Fecal Occult Blood Test and the Fecal Immunohistochemical Test.

Guaiac FOBT (gFOBT)

Recommended annually, the gFOBT detects the presence of blood in stool through a chemical reaction involving guaiac and the heme of hemoglobin. The test is performed at home usually using two samples of three consecutive bowel movements smeared on test cards. These six stool samples are needed to increase sensitivity because bleeding of cancer and polyps tend to be intermittent. Prior to gFOBT testing, individuals interrupt use of aspirin and other nonsteroidal anti-inflammatory drugs as well as avoid eating red meat, all of which may increase false-positive results. To avoid increasing false-negative results, patients should avoid vitamin C. Test cards are returned to a laboratory or the patient's physician for evaluation. A positive gFOBT test should always be followed up with a colonoscopy.[29]

RCTs of FOBT indicate that CRC mortality is reduced by 33% and incidence by 20% following gFOBT testing with a high sensitive slide and done every year for many years compared with individuals who did not undergo

Table 30-3

Sensitivity and specificity of screening tests

Screening Test	Sensitivity	Specificity
Colonoscopy[16]	≈95% for cancer and large adenomas (≥ 10 mm)	≈90% for cancer and large adenomas
Flexible Sigmoidoscopy[16]	≈95% for cancer and large adenomas only within reach	≈92% for colon and rectal area within reach
CT Colonography[45,55–56]	85–90% for large adenomas (≥ 9–10 mm) 35–90% for adenomas (≥ 6mm)	86% for large adenomas (≥ 10 mm)
gFOBT[49,57]	*Hemoccult Sensa:* 64% for cancer 20–40% for detecting advanced adenomas *Hemoccult II:* 37% for cancer detection	*Hemoccult Sensa:* 90% for cancer 91% for adenomas *Hemoccult II:* 98% for cancer detection
FIT[49–51]	82–88% for cancer 36–44% for advanced adenomas	86–97% for cancer 86–97% for advanced adenomas
Genetic Stool Tests[52,58]	52–88% for cancer 18–46% for advanced adenomas	82–94% for cancer

screening.[33,47] However, sensitivity and specificity of the test (see Table 30-3) varies greatly based on a number of factors such as test type, sample number, collection method, and analytic procedures including rehydration.[29]

Although posing little risk, and considered by some to be easier and more convenient for patients compared to colonoscopy, the gFOBT is encouraged for annual screening, which provides programmatic sensitivity for cancer detection greater than 90% if done yearly for more than ten years.[48]

Fecal Immunohistochemical Test (FIT)

More sensitive than the gFOBT test Hemoccult II, FIT detects the protein globin in human hemoglobin. The FIT, recommended for annual screening, requires smears of fecal samples on a testing card, in a tube, or on long-handled brush to swish in the toilet to collect consecutive samples that are then sent to a designated testing laboratory. The FIT test does not require dietary or medication changes prior to the procedure.[29]

The effectiveness of FIT was compared with the sensitivity of gFOBT with FIT in a screening cohort (and in one study a small symptomatic diagnostic group), which demonstrated that sensitivity for detecting cancers and advanced adenomas was substantially higher for FIT.[29,49,50] Greenberg et al. reviewed a variety of fecal blood tests and found FIT had significantly greater sensitivity rates for cancer and large adenomas than various gFOBT tests (see Table 30-3).[51] The greater sensitivity and specificity and the lack of dietary restrictions with FIT make this an attractive alternative to the gFOBT.

Genetic Stool Tests

Recently developed stool tests focus on analyzing specific DNA mutations and epigenetic alterations in the adenoma-carcinoma sequence from stool. A noninvasive test, stool DNA involves a one-time collection and is administered at home. For testing, the entire stool is collected in an ice pack and kept frozen at least 8 hours before shipment to a laboratory. Efficacy of DNA screening tests is preliminary but the ACS and USMSTF have deemed this test an acceptable screening method,[29] although the USPSTF analyses of available data found insufficient evidence to recommend this test at this time.[42] Imperiale et al. showed greater sensitivity for cancer and advanced adenomas (defined as a tubular adenoma at least 1 cm in diameter, a polyp with villous histological appearance or with high-grade dysplasia) and comparable specificity for the DNA test than the older, less sensitive Hemoccult II gFOBT.[52] These results were lower than expected due to breakdown of the DNA integrity assay in this study; improved DNA testing material has increased sensitivity and specificity.[35]

Cost is a barrier to increased use of these new genetic tests compared with established screening methods.[53] Furthermore, a majority but not all genetic markers of CRC are included in this test. If an individual is found with a positive genetic finding but a colonoscopy does not show abnormalities, it is unclear how to guide future screening of the patient. The recommended 5-year

screening interval promoted by the manufacturer has not been evaluated sufficiently,[29] and the genetic stool test has not received Food and Drug Administration (FDA) approval, but preliminary results show promise and will require further study.

Other Tests

The double contrast barium enema (DCBE) and the digital rectal exam, older colon examination tests, are used less frequently than in the past. Although USMSTF continues to suggest DCBE as a screening option if other tests are not available every 5 years for average-risk women, it is not recommended by USPSTF. The digital rectal exam is no longer recommended as a screening exam by either the USMSTF or the USPSTF.[28,29,54]

Screening Rates and Adherence Patterns

Screening rates vary by gender, race/ethnicity, income, insurance coverage, and geographic region.[59,60] According to the National Health Interview Survey (NHIS), self-reported screening rates (either FOBT or endoscopy) for men and women have increased since 2000. However, 50.4% of women and 49.2% of men reported screening for CRC in 2005.[61] Another self-reported nationwide survey, the statewide Behavioral Risk Factor Surveillance System (BRFSS) survey of 2008 found that 21% of respondents indicated having an FOBT in the past 2 years and 62% reported either a sigmoidoscopy or colonoscopy at least once in their lifetime.[5] Data from both BRFSS and Medicare indicate whites and individuals with insurance, higher education, and higher income had higher screening rates.[59,62] The Medicare data also note African Americans and Hispanics had lower rates of endoscopy screening than whites.[60]

Analyses of Medicare coverage for CRC screening between 1998 and 2005 showed that less than half (47.2%) had complied with recommendations despite authorized screening coverage for FOBT, sigmoidoscopy, and barium enema for average-risk individuals since 1998 and colonoscopy since 2001 (Federal Registry Bill No. 66 FR 55329). However, the frequency of colonoscopy has increased yearly since 2003,[60] whereas FOBT and sigmoidoscopy have declined in the Medicare population.[62]

Among women one estimate noted more than 23 million eligible women have not been screened (of the 42 million unscreened in total).[63] The BRFSS showed that 61.8% of women reported having had a colonoscopy or sigmoidoscopy in their lifetime whereas nearly 40% had never had one.[5] Trivers et al. also found the greatest screening disparities among women who were Hispanic or uninsured and rates for both these groups have not increased over the last 5 years. Compared to whites, African American women had lower screening rates, although Asians have the lowest of any racial/ethnic group.[64,65] Although CRC screening rates, especially use of colonoscopy have increased over the last decade, screening disparities by race, gender, insurance, and socioeconomic status still exist.

Table 30-4

List of risk and protective factors for colorectal cancer

Potential Risk Factors	Evidence*
Smoking	Increased risk of adenomas and potentially also associated with colon cancer among current and long-term smokers
Alcohol	Suggestive positive association for total alcohol intake
High BMI/Abdominal Fatness	Consistent positive association with high BMI especially among premenopausal women
	Greater positive association with abdominal fatness compared to high BMI

Potential Protective Factors	Evidence
Diet	Inconclusive; some suggestive protective association of diet rich in vegetables and fruit and suggestive lowered risk associated with high fiber
Increased Physical Activity	Convincing evidence of negative association
Aspirin and NSAIDS	*Aspirin:* Protective against adenomas but increased risk of gastrointestinal bleeding and renal impairment
	COX-2 NSAIDS: Protective association with COX-2 inhibitors but increased risk of cardiovascular events
Folate	Negative association for those with low folate levels; however high doses of folates may increase risk of carcinoma formation
Calcium and Vitamin D	Suggestive protective effect for calcium and Vitamin D
Hormone Replacement Therapy	Evidence suggests hormones are protective for colon cancer but increase risk of breast cancer and cardiovascular events
Statins	Overall little evidence of a negative association

*See text for references

Risk and Protective Factors

Significant, known, and/or well-studied potential risks and protective factors are discussed in Table 30-4.

Risk Factors

Familial/Genetic

Approximately 75% of CRC cases are in average-risk individuals who do not have a hereditary syndrome or family history. More aggressive screening and surveillance are advised for the 25% of Americans who are at increased risk due to a family history of CRC, a hereditary cancer syndrome, inflammatory bowel disease and/or a prior history of colon neoplasia.[20] A patient's family history is an important identifier of risk status: having one first- and/or two second-degree relatives with CRC increases CRC risk. An estimated 5–10% of additional colorectal cancer cases arise from a hereditary syndrome. Two syndromes have been identified: hereditary nonpolyposis colorectal cancer and familial adenomatous polyposis (FAP). HNPCC is a rare disease due to germline mutations in mismatch-repair genes. Adenomatous polyps begin to develop in an individual by the age of 20, usually leading to cancer by age 45. FAP is extremely rare, due to a mutation in the tumor suppressor gene APC, which causes hundreds of

adenomas to grow in an individual beginning as early as the teen years. A person with FAP will usually develop colon cancer by age 40 and treatment consists of resecting or removal of the colon. Because both diseases are autosomally dominant, children have a 50% chance of inheriting FAP or HNPCC from an affected parent.[14,20,54] A family history is critical for the identification of high-risk patients so they can be appropriately referred for genetic counseling and testing to further assess their risk and provide appropriate screening and management.

Race/Ethnicity

As shown previously, African Americans have higher CRC incidence rates than any other racial or ethnic group. Comparing African Americans and whites for the years 2002 to 2006, incidence rates were higher and survival rates were lower in African Americans than whites. Incidence rates for African American women were shown to stabilize whereas for African American men the rate increased during the time period 1975–2000.[64] This survival discrepancy is partially attributed to later stage of disease at diagnosis and increased comorbidities reflecting greater underlying upstream risk factors such as poverty, lack of access to diagnosis, treatment, and follow-up care.[66,67] A study at Harlem Hospital, a New York City municipal hospital serving a predominately poor African American neighborhood, showed that 70% of CRC patients presented with an incurable form or late stage of CRC resulting in higher mortality rates than national averages.[25] Census data show the poverty rate is three times higher among African Americans than whites; lower socioeconomic status is also associated with higher prevalence of CRC risk factors including smoking and sedentary lifestyle.[64,68]

Studies suggest that African Americans may have a higher prevalence of proximal adenomas and cancers compared to historical controls.[64,69] This anatomic distribution pattern may result from lack of screening, especially by colonoscopy, as the National Colonoscopy Study showed no statistically significant differences in the prevalence of adenomas, advanced adenomas, or right-sided-adenomas between African Americans and whites.[70] The American College of Gastroenterology recommends beginning screening at age 45 among African Americans[68] although this recommendation is not shared by others. A study using microsimulation modeling or computerized statistical projections of risk suggested that shortened screening intervals would be beneficial for African Americans.[71]

Hispanics and Asians have been found to have more distal disease compared to whites.[29] In addition, about 6% of Ashkenazi Jews (whose ancestors migrated from Eastern Europe) have twofold increased risk of CRC associated with a mutation in the tumor suppressor gene APC.[54] Racial and ethnic differences for screening and anatomic distribution require future studies as findings may affect screening guidelines.

Smoking

Although smoking is a risk factor for adenomas, the effect on cancer risk is unclear. The most recent Surgeon General's report stated smoking is not a causal factor in CRC although some evidence suggests a link; in contrast, the International Agency for Research on Cancer (IARC) has reported sufficient evidence exists to conclude smoking is a causal factor in colon cancer.[72–74] Genetic damage from smoking occurs slowly in the colorectal mucosa; often a lag time of 35–40 years is needed before detection of adverse effects. Many American women started smoking in the 1940s and 1950s, possibly explaining the lower incidence of colon cancer among women earlier in the 20th century.[75,76] The Nurses' Health Study (NHS) reported RR = 2.0 (95% CI = 1.14–3.49) and RR = 1.63 (95% CI = 1.14–2.33) for cancer for women who smoked at least 45 years and for those who smoked 40 to 44 years respectively.[77] The Women's Health Initiative (WHI) found that current smokers had an increased risk of rectal cancer, HR = 1.95, (95% CI = 1.10–3.47) but not for colon cancer, a finding supported in other studies.[78,79] Risk increases with greater number of years and number of cigarettes smoked, indicating a dose-response relationship. Lieberman et al. showed current smoking status had a similar risk for CRC and large adenomas as having a first-degree relative with CRC.[80]

Furthermore, cigarette smoking may increase the growth of adenomas especially high-risk adenomas in the early formation phase.[81,82] A review of 22 studies assessing long-term, heavy cigarette smoking found a two- to three-fold increase of adenomas in almost every study.[75] Therefore, the evidence quite clearly suggests that smoking has a deleterious effect on adenoma formation and possibly promotes progression to cancer, thus adding to the long list of smoking's negative effects.

Alcohol Intake

Research suggests an association of alcohol intake with increased CRC risk. A meta-analysis of alcohol in 16 case-control and 6 cohort studies found generally inconsistent results for an association with CRC although a modest dose-response increase for CRC risk was noted; RR = 1.08 (95% CI = 1.06–1.10) for 25 g/day, RR = 1.18 (95% CI = 1.14–22) for 50 g/day and RR = 1.38 (95% CI = 1.29–1.49) for 100 g/day. (Two drinks equal about 30 grams.)[83,84] Of note, the estimates across the studies were heterogenous. Looking exclusively at women, an NHS dietary intake study found women who drank 30 g/day had increased adenoma risk, RR 1.84 (95% CI = 1.19–2.86).[84] Furthermore, intake of 30 g/day or more was associated with elevated CRC risk in a pooled cohort study that included the NHS and Iowa Women's Health Study.[85]

High BMI/Abdominal Fatness

Higher body mass index (BMI) is associated with CRC risk more strongly among men than women although an international meta-analysis of 56 publications identified an increase in risk of higher BMI levels among both genders; BMI increase of 5 kg/m^2 increased risk by 18% with the highest level, ≥30 kg/m^2 showing a 41% increased risk.[86] Furthermore, Terry et al. documented elevated BMI was associated with a twofold higher risk only among premenopausal women and not among postmenopausal women.[87] Among postmenopausal women estrogen, a known CRC protective factor, is produced by adipose tissue after menopause; higher BMI could then result in a higher estrogen concentration, thus conferring some added protection against CRC.[87,88] Rectal cancer, of note, does not seem to be affected by BMI. Furthermore, greater visceral adipose distribution or greater waist circumference (waist-to-hip ratio) also affects CRC and adenoma risk.[89]

Type 2 diabetes, associated with high BMI and hyperglycemia, an excess of insulin in the bloodstream, has been shown to increase adenoma and CRC risk.[89] A meta-analysis revealed a 43% increased risk of CRC for both men and women and a 33% risk of rectal cancer.[90] One NHS study and other research reported higher elevated CRC risk associated with insulin-like growth factor (IGF) levels, a known tumor promoter.[89,91] Although risk for CRC has been shown to decrease as women with high BMI grow older, encouraging dietary and behavioral adjustments still remains critical in preventing colon cancer and other chronic diseases for women with high BMI.

Potential Protective Factors

Diet and Physical Activity

Although some studies suggest that a diet rich in fruits, vegetables (nonstarchy), and fiber may protect against colorectal cancer, results are still inconclusive. The World Cancer Research Fund, investigating a large body of cohort studies, concluded that diets high in vegetables and fruit contribute to lower colorectal cancer although supporting evidence is limited.[92] A pooled multivariate analysis of 14 prospective studies demonstrated that total fruit and vegetable intake lowered colon cancer risk when high intake ≥800 g/day was compared with lower consumption (<200 g/day), RR = 0.74 (95% CI = 0.57–0.95).[93] However, CRC risk was not significantly influenced by quantity of either fruit or vegetable consumption among NHS or the Health Professionals' Follow-up Study (HPFS) participants of either gender.[95] The American Institute for Cancer Research identified convincing evidence that fiber is a protective mechanism against colorectal cancer. High fiber intake is known to reduce stool transit time, dilute fecal contents, and increase stool weight. Review of 16 cohort studies suggested a dose-response relationship between increasing fiber intake and modestly reduced CRC risk.[92]

In contrast to assessment of dietary intake in relation to risk of CRC, consumption of five or more daily servings of fruit (specifically citrus fruit) significantly lowered adenoma prevalence (OR = 0.60, 95% CI = 0.44–0.81) among more than 34,000 NHS participants with a history of either colonoscopy or sigmoidoscopy. Vegetable consumption was not similarly protective.[94]

The World Cancer Research Fund found convincing evidence for the protective role of physical activity though the effect is stronger for colon than rectal cancer. Increased intensity and frequency (or dose-response) of exercise greatly reduces CRC risk.[92] Women who exercised more than 21.5 metabolic equivalent hours (MET) per week (1.0 MET is given for sitting) had the greatest effect, RR = 0.77 (95% CI = 0.58–1.01), especially on distal adenomas. Women who walk at least 1 hour per week had reduced risk.[96] Moreover, an NHS report indicated women who engaged in over 21 MET/per week of physical activity showed a 46% reduction. However, women who report more physical activity are also less likely to smoke, less likely to be obese, and more likely to eat a healthier diet.[97] Furthermore, Slattery et al. noted that women who were physically inactive, had high energy intake levels, and higher BMI had the greatest risk for CRC, OR = 3.35 (95% CI = 2.09–5.35). In older women, this risk appears lower.[98]

Aspirin and Nonaspirin Nonsteroidal Anti-inflammatory Drugs (NSAIDS)

When taken for pain relief and inflammation control, aspirin and NSAIDS may play a role in preventing adenoma and colorectal cancer development by inhibiting cyclooxygenase-1 (COX-1) or cyclooxygenase-2 (COX-2) that may be overexpressed in adenomas and CRC.[99,100] In an NHS study, risk of colorectal cancer was reduced by 23%

after 20 years or more of routine aspirin use (≥ 2 standard 325-mg tablets per week) compared to nonregular users; the protective effect was observed only after 10 years of use.[101] A systematic review of 33 studies supported these findings but also noted gastrointestinal complications such as bleeding with higher aspirin intake.[102] A WHI Observational Study however found no reduction in CRC incidence with any aspirin use although the dose (100 mg every other day) and duration (10 years) may have been too limited to produce any benefit.[103]

Studies demonstrate a reduction in adenoma formation with use of selective COX-2 inhibitors; however, this class of NSAIDS drugs significantly increases cardiovascular events. The Adenoma Prevention with Celecoxib RCT trial, showed a 33% reduction in recurrent adenomas among individuals receiving 200 mg twice daily of celecoxib and a 45% reduction with a higher dose, 400 mg celecoxib twice daily. However, cardiovascular events including myocardial infarction, stroke and congestive heart failure were increased among participants receiving either low RR = 2.6 (95% CI = 1.1–6.1) or high-dose RR = 3.4 (95% CI = 1.5–7.9).[99] Aspirin may benefit average-risk patients but the adverse cardiovascular effect of NSAIDS led the USPSTF to not recommend these chemopreventive agents for the general public.[104] High-risk patients are exempt from this recommendation.

Folates

A diet low in folic acid could result in increased adenoma growth and cancer development due to lack of protection from DNA mutations and low DNA methylation (which allows for normal control of proto-oncogenes).[84] Vegetables, fruits, and supplemental folate are all sources of the vitamin; in 1998 folate fortification of the U.S. food supply became mandatory.[84,105] The NHS showed a reduced risk of adenoma formation with an increase in folate intake, RR = 0.66 (95% CI = 0.46–0.95) even after control of other vitamins thought to lower risk.[84] In addition, a 3-year RCT involving daily intake of 5 mg of folic acid for patients with a history of adenomas demonstrated a 64% decrease in recurrence compared to the placebo.[106] Furthermore, a low-folate diet in addition to alcohol intake may compound the risk of cancer development as alcohol has a deleterious effect on folate metabolism.[84] In contrast, the large Aspirin/Folate Polyp Prevention RCT indicated folic acid, compared to placebo, did not prevent but instead slightly elevated rates of adenomas. Participants who took 1 mg per day had increased risk of three or more adenomas, RR = 2.32 (95% CI = 1.23–4.35). The authors suggest the mandatory fortification of foods with folate could have affected their results, suggesting that supplemental folic acid may increase risk of colorectal cancer.[107] Moreover, very high supplemental folate levels have been shown to promote cancer growth when folate is increased *after* microscopic preclinical carcinoma in the mucosa is present.[108] Folate may therefore play a role in primary prevention before adenoma genesis but not in secondary prevention.[109] However, Wolpin et al. tested prediagnostic plasma folate samples from participants with CRC in the NHS and HPFS and observed no association between prediagnostic higher folate levels and increased CRC mortality rates.[105] Folate therefore is not innocuous nor as beneficial as initially thought; supplementation may have deleterious effects.

Calcium and Vitamin D

Although results are not yet definitive, growing evidence suggests that calcium and dairy foods may have a protective effect. Calcium may reduce colon epithelial cell growth and risk of recurrent adenomas through binding to secondary bile acids and ionized fatty acids. Vitamin D assists with calcium absorption and may play a role in colon cancer prevention. The Calcium Polyp Prevention RCT found a statistically significant 17% decrease in adenomas formation for those who took 1200 mg per day of elemental calcium for 4 years; the protective effect extended for 5 years after the trial was completed.[110] An inverse association with increased calcium intake and colorectal cancer risk among women and men was also observed in a pooled analysis of 10 cohort studies[111] and a combined NHS and HPFS cohort study showed a negative association with calcium intake only for distal colon cancer. A threshold effect was noted for calcium intake with dosage beyond 700 mg per day having minimal protective effect.[112]

The combined effects of calcium and vitamin D reduced risk of adenoma reoccurrence with OR = 0.56 (95% CI = 0.39–0.80) whereas supplemental and dietary vitamin D did not have a significant effect.[113] An RCT from the WHI also showed no effect for vitamin D and calcium separately and combined although critiques of the study state the design and short duration could have contributed to the null findings.[35,114,115] Vitamin D alone was assessed in a review of both oral intake and solar ultraviolet B (UVB) exposure; higher serum levels (≥38 ng/ml) of vitamin D in the body were linked to 55% reduction of CRC risk compared to lower levels.[116] Calcium and vitamin D intake are of special interest to women (especially in terms of osteoporosis) and these supplements may have additional benefit against adenoma formation.

Postmenopausal Hormone Therapy

Female hormones used after menopause may reduce colorectal cancer by acting on the colon mucosa or reducing the amount of harmful liver proteins.[117,118] In one component of the WHI, CRC was measured as a secondary outcome among women aged 50 and older who were randomized to receive estrogen plus progestin or a placebo. During the 5.2 years of follow-up CRC rates were reduced by 37% with results showing benefits beginning in the third year (HR = 0.63, 95% CI = 0.74–0.86). Due to adverse health risks identified among women randomized to combined hormone therapy including increased incidence of breast cancer, coronary heart disease, stroke and pulmonary embolism, the clinical trial was stopped.[6] Observational studies continue and other studies of postmenopausal hormone use have supported the WHI lowered CRC risk. A meta-analysis of 18-studies reported a 20% reduction in colon cancer risk and a 19% reduction in rectal cancer risk among current users of hormones.[119] Of note, a WHI estrogen-alone RCT of women post surgical menopause found no protective effect of hormone use, which was further supported by findings from a population-based case-control study in which estrogen only use had no effect on risk.[120,121]

Additional follow–up of WHI observation studies showed that hormone use was associated with more advanced stage at diagnosis of CRC compared with cases among women in the placebo group.[122] A nested-case control study within the NYU Women's Health study cohort also demonstrated higher levels of endogenous estrone increased colorectal cancer risk.[118] Furthermore, an additional analysis of the WHI observed no CRC mortality benefit compared to the placebo after an average 8-year treatment and follow-up period.[120] Observational studies continue to monitor the effects of hormone therapy on colorectal cancer. Women who have taken hormones should consider discussing risk of CRC with their provider regarding frequency and types of screening. Despite promising chemopreventive results, hormone therapy is not recommended as a protective agent against CRC.

Statins

Statins are prescribed to lower low-density lipoprotein (LDL) cholesterol for those with or at risk of cardiovascular disease. Although a few studies have demonstrated statin use may lower CRC risk, the growing body of literature suggests statins are not protective. A case-control study conducted in 2004 noted statin usage for 5 years or more was associated with a significant reduction in colorectal cancer incidence, OR = 0.50 (95% CI = 0.40–0.63), after adjusting for as aspirin use, physical activity, and family history.[123] Despite these findings additional research has been inconsistent and inconclusive. A case-control study of women observed no effect on CRC risk, in contrast to a meta-analysis of case-control studies which reported a small decreased risk (RR = 0.91, 95% CI = 0.87–0.96).[124–126] Overall, findings do not support statin usage as a chemopreventive agent for colorectal cancer.

Treatment

Most colorectal cancers are detected at an early stage when neoplasia is localized or with regional lymph node involvement. Treatment options vary by stage at diagnosis. Stage I has a 91% cure rate; underscoring the impact of regular and timely screening.[127] Differences exist between treatment for colon and rectal cancer. Surgical resection is the primary treatment for patients diagnosed at an early stage; partial colectomy removes cancerous tissue, the margins (or surrounding area of normal tissue), and regional lymph nodes. The remaining sections of the colon are anatomically reconnected. A colostomy, or opening in the skin to allow fecal discharge, is usually not permanent.[54]

An estimated 20% of patients will have liver metastasis at diagnosis,[11] which may be resectable. Five-year survival rate is 25–40%.[127] Other common sites of CRC metastasis are lung and intra-abdominal organs, including the pelvic organs (ovaries) in women (Sidney J. Winawer, MD, personal communication, 2010). Follow-up after resection is important to detect and treat recurrence.[35]

For rectal cancer, a combination of surgery, chemotherapy, and radiation therapy is commonly prescribed. Postoperative chemotherapy and radiation have been beneficial as adjuvant therapies.[11,128] Cancers of the midrectum and upper rectum allow sphincter preservation.[11] For cancers close to the anal opening involving the sphincter muscles, a permanent colostomy may be required, although medical and surgical advances have recently eliminated this for many patients (Sidney J. Winawer, MD, personal communication, 2010).

Postoperative chemotherapy is usually given for stage III colon cancer (with positive lymph nodes). Chemotherapy for stage II is controversial as overall survival benefit is only 2–4% with benefit reserved for patients at high risk for recurrence. Advanced cancers at stage IV require chemotherapy. The drug 5-fluorouracil (5-FU) and variants are the primary agents, which may be combined with leucovorin and oxaliplatin. Capecitabine, an oral drug, is converted to 5-FU in the body at the tumor site and shows equivalent effectiveness to intravenous 5-FU; it generally has fewer side effects including vomiting, nausea, and diarrhea. In addition to 5-FU, capecitabine, and oxaliplatin, irinotecan, bevacizumab, cetuximab, and panitumumab comprise the seven FDA approved CRC drugs.[127] Although treatment for CRC has improved over the past decades, routine screening is essential to prevent cancer and discover it at a curable stage.

Summary

Colorectal cancer is diagnosed in 1 of 20 women reaching age 85; however, the number of women receiving colorectal cancer screening remains lower than screening for breast or cervical cancer. One national estimate shows only 49% of women have been screened despite the high survival rate for early detected CRC and the known fact that this cancer is preventable by removing adenomatous polyps. Looking specifically at colorectal cancer effects on women, a few key observations emerge. Evidence has shown that women develop more advanced neoplasia more often as they get older. Furthermore, postmenopausal women, especially those who have used hormone therapy, may have reduced risk of CRC although the need for screening remains.

Screening rates for women have risen in recent years as educational programs and public health measures have increased awareness. Rates have increased in New York City from 42% reporting having had a colonoscopy in 2003 to 68% in 2010. In addition, screening disparity rates by race/ethnicity have almost been eliminated. A portion of this increase is attributable to the efforts of the Citywide Colon Cancer Control Coalition and the New York City Department of Health and Hygiene including the introduction of Patient Navigators, individuals who guide patients through screening procedures and the healthcare system of city hospitals.[129] Furthermore, in 2008, the American College of Obstetricians and Gynecologists (ACOG) partnered with the Jay Monahan Center for Gastrointestinal Health to educate patients about colorectal screening. The aim is to make women as aware of CRC as they are of breast and cervical cancer and bring screening test rates up to the levels of the mammogram and Pap test.[130] In addition, ACOG also recommended colonoscopy as the preferred screening method for women although all screening options need to be discussed with individual patients.[30] Through such partnerships and education programs, women's increased awareness of colorectal cancer and screening methods should improve screening rates and reduce the incidence and mortality of this highly preventable cancer.

Discussion Questions

1. Why are colorectal cancer screening rates so low in women, especially African American women, compared to breast and cervical cancer screening rates? How can this be increased?
2. Should the current screening guidelines for average-risk patients be changed for women? How should they be changed?
3. Is there enough evidence to suggest women should undergo screening with colonoscopy? What are the limitations and the benefits with other screening tests? What additional research is needed to motivate women to begin screening?
4. What pros and cons should a woman of average risk for CRC consider when deciding whether to begin hormone replacement therapy?
5. Which, if any, of the chemoprevention measures should average-risk women adopt? What additional research is needed to clarify risks and benefits of these measures?
6. How can women be made aware of the impact of knowing their family medical history on CRC risk?

References

1. American Cancer Society. *Cancer Facts and Figures 2012*. Atlanta, GA: Author; 2009. http://www.cancer.org/acs/groups/content/@epidemiologysurveilance/documents/document/acspc-031941.pdf. Accessed January 13, 2013.
2. Klabunde CN, Lanier D, Nadel MR, et al. Colorectal cancer screening by primary care physicians: recommendations and practices, 2006-2007. *Am J Prev Med.* 2009;37:8–16.
3. Menees SB, Patel DA, Dalton V. Colorectal cancer screening practices among obstetrician/gynecologists and nurse practitioners. *J Womens Health (Larchmt).* 2009;18:1233–1238.
4. Killackey M. Partnering with the OB-GYN Community: ACOG's District II/NY Cancer Prevention and Detection Initiative. Paper presented at the 6th Annual Citywide Colon Cancer Control Coalition (C5) Summit: Increasing High Quality CRC Screening in NYC; June 11, 2009, 2009; New York, NY.
5. Behavioral Risk Factor Surveillance System. [Web Page]. 2008. http://www.cdc.gov/brfss/index.htm. Accessed February 26, 2010.
6. Rossouw JE, Anderson GL, Prentice RL, et al. Risks and benefits of estrogen plus progestin in healthy postmenopausal women: principal results from the Women's Health Initiative randomized controlled trial. *JAMA* 2002;288:321–333.
7. Regula J, Rupinski M, Kraszewska E, et al. Colonoscopy in colorectal-cancer screening for detection of advanced neoplasia. *N Engl J Med.* 2006;355:1863–1872.
8. Morson BC. The evolution of colorectal carcinoma. *Clin Radiol.* 1984;35:425–431.
9. Vogelstein B, Fearon ER, Hamilton SR, et al. Genetic alterations during colorectal-tumor development. *N Engl J Med.* 1988;319:525–532.

10. Bleeker WA, Hayes VM, Karrenbeld A, et al. Impact of KRAS and TP53 mutations on survival in patients with left- and right-sided Dukes' C colon cancer. *Am J Gastroenterol.* 2000;95:2953–2957.

11. Winawer SJ, ed. *Management of Gastrointestinal Diseases.* New York: Gower; 1992.

12. Huang CS, O'Brien M J, Yang S, Farraye FA. Hyperplastic polyps, serrated adenomas, and the serrated polyp neoplasia pathway. *Am J Gastroenterol.* 2004;99:2242–2255.

13. Hawk ET, Limburg PJ, Viner JL. Epidemiology and prevention of colorectal cancer. *Surg Clin North Am.* 2002;82:905–941.

14. Lynch HT, de la Chapelle A. Hereditary colorectal cancer. *N Engl J Med.* 2003;348:919–932.

15. Surveillance, Epidemiology and End Results. SEER stat fact sheets: Colon and rectum. 2012. http://seer.cancer.gov/statfacts/html/colorect.html. Accessed January 13, 2013.

16. Zauber AG, Lansdorp-Vogelaar I, Knudsen AB, et al. Evaluating test strategies for colorectal cancer screening: a decision analysis for the US Preventive Services Task Force. *Ann Intern Med.* 2008;149:659–669.

17. Barclay RL, Vicari JJ, Doughty AS, Johanson JF, Greenlaw RL. Colonoscopic withdrawal times and adenoma detection during screening colonoscopy. *N Engl J Med.* 2006;355:2533–2541.

18. Lieberman DA, Weiss DG, Bond JH, et al. Use of colonoscopy to screen asymptomatic adults for colorectal cancer. Veterans Affairs Cooperative Study Group 380. *N Engl J Med.* 2000;343:162–168.

19. Schoenfeld P, Cash B, Flood A, et al. Colonoscopic screening of average-risk women for colorectal neoplasia. *N Engl J Med.* 2005;352:2061–2068.

20. Weitz J, Koch M, Debus J, et al. Colorectal cancer. *Lancet.* 2005;365:153–165.

21. Winawer SJ, Zauber AG, Ho MN, et al. Prevention of colorectal cancer by colonoscopic polypectomy. The National Polyp Study Workgroup. *N Engl J Med.* 1993;329:1977–1981.

22. Citarda F, Tomaselli G, Capocaccia R, et al. Efficacy in standard clinical practice of colonoscopic polypectomy in reducing colorectal cancer incidence. *Gut.* 2001;48:812–815.

23. Thiis-Evensen E, Hoff GS, Sauar J, et al. Population-based surveillance by colonoscopy: effect on the incidence of colorectal cancer. Telemark Polyp Study I. *Scand J Gastroenterol.* 1999;34:414–420.

24. National Cancer Institute. Cancer trends progress report—2007 Update. 2007. http://progressreport.cancer.gov/trends-glance.asp. Accessed March 3, 2010.

25. Freeman HP, Alshafie TA. Colorectal carcinoma in poor blacks. *Cancer.* 2002;94:2327–2332.

26. Achengrau A, Seage GR. *Essentials of Epidemiology for Public Health.* Sudbury, MA: Jones and Bartlett; 2003.

27. American Cancer Society. All About Colon and Rectum Cancer. 2010. http://www.cancer.org/docroot/CRI/CRI_2x.asp?sitearea=&dt=10. Accessed March 4, 2010.

28. Screening for colorectal cancer: US Preventive Services Task Force recommendation statement. *Ann Intern Med.* 2008;149:627–637.

29. Levin B, Lieberman DA, McFarland B, et al. Screening and surveillance for the early detection of colorectal cancer and adenomatous polyps, 2008: a joint guideline from the American Cancer Society, the US Multi-Society Task Force on Colorectal Cancer, and the American College of Radiology. *Gastroenterology.* 2008;134:1570–1595.

30. American College of Obstetricians and Gynecologists Committee on Gynecologic Practice Committee Opinion Number 482. Colonoscopy and Colorectal Cancer Screening Strategies. *Obstet Gynecol* 2011;117:766–771.

31. Hardcastle JD, Chamberlain JO, Robinso MH, et al. Randomised, controlled trial of faecal occult blood screening for colorectal cancer. *Lancet.* 1989;1:1160–1164.

32. Kronborg O, Fenger C, Olsen J, et al. Randomised study of screening for colorectal cancer with faecal-occult-blood test. *Lancet.* 1996;348:1467–1471.

33. Mandel JS, Bond JH, Church TR, et al. Reducing mortality from colorectal cancer by screening for fecal occult blood. Minnesota Colon Cancer Control Study. *N Engl J Med.* 1993;328:1365–1371.

34. Muller AD, Sonnenberg A. Protection by endoscopy against death from colorectal cancer. A case-control study among veterans. *Arch Intern Med.* 1995;155:1741–1748.

35. Kahi CJ, Rex DK, Imperiale TF. Screening, surveillance, and primary prevention for colorectal cancer: a review of the recent literature. *Gastroenterology.* 2008;135:380–399.

36. Gatto NM, Frucht H, Sundararajan V, et al. Risk of perforation after colonoscopy and sigmoidoscopy: a population-based study. *J Natl Cancer Inst.* 2003;95:230–236.

37. Selby JV, Friedman GD, Quesenberry CP, Jr., Weiss NS. A case-control study of screening sigmoidoscopy and mortality from colorectal cancer. *N Engl J Med.* 1992;326:653–657.

38. Newcomb PA, Norfleet RG, Storer BE, et al. Screening sigmoidoscopy and colorectal cancer mortality. *J Natl Cancer Inst.* 1992;84:1572–1575.

39. Ransohoff DF. Lessons from the UK sigmoidoscopy screening trial. *Lancet.* 2002;359:1266–1267.

40. Schoen RE, Pinksy PF, Weissfeld JL, et al. Colorectal-cancer incidence and mortality with screening flexible sigmoidoscopy. *N Engl J Med.* 2012 Jun 21;366:2345–2357.

41. O'Brien B, Nichaman L, Browne JE, et al. Coordination and management of a large multicenter screening trial: the Prostate, Lung, Colorectal and Ovarian (PLCO) Cancer Screening Trial. *Control Clin Trials.* 2000;21(6 suppl):310S–328S.

42. Segnan N, Armaroli P, Bonelli L, et al. Once-only sigmoidoscopy in colorectal cancer screening: follow-up findings of the Italian Randomized Controlled Trial—SCORE. *J Natl Cancer Inst.* 2011 Sep 7;103:1310–1322.

43. Atkin WS, Edwards R, Kralj-Hans I, et al. Once-only flexible sigmoidoscopy screening in prevention of colorectal cancer: a multicentre randomised controlled trial. *Lancet.* 2010;375:1624–1633.

44. Imperiale TF, Wagner DR, Lin CY, et al. Risk of advanced proximal neoplasms in asymptomatic adults according to the distal colorectal findings. *N Engl J Med.* 2000;343:169–174.

45. Johnson CD, Chen MH, Toledano AY, et al. Accuracy of CT colonography for detection of large adenomas and cancers. *N Engl J Med.* 2008;359:1207–1217.

46. Lansdorp-Vogelaar I, van Ballegooijen M, Zauber AG, et al. At what costs will screening with CT colonography be competitive? A cost-effectiveness approach. *Int J Cancer.* 2009;124:1161–1168.

47. Mandel JS, Church TR, Bond JH, et al. The effect of fecal occult-blood screening on the incidence of colorectal cancer. *N Engl J Med.* 2000;343:1603–1607.

48. Church TR, Ederer F, Mandel JS. Fecal occult blood screening in the Minnesota study: sensitivity of the screening test. *J Natl Cancer Inst.* 1997;89:1440–1448.

49. Allison JE, Sakoda LC, Levin TR, et al. Screening for colorectal neoplasms with new fecal occult blood tests: update on performance characteristics. *J Natl Cancer Inst.* 2007;99:1462–1470.

50. Smith A, Young GP, Cole SR, Bampton P. Comparison of a brush-sampling fecal immunochemical test for hemoglobin with a sensitive guaiac-based fecal occult blood test in detection of colorectal neoplasia. *Cancer.* 2006;107:2152–2159.

51. Greenberg PD, Bertario L, Gnauck R, et al. A prospective multicenter evaluation of new fecal occult blood tests in patients undergoing colonoscopy. *Am J Gastroenterol.* 2000;95:1331–1338.

52. Imperiale TF, Ransohoff DF, Itzkowitz SH, Turnbull BA, Ross ME. Fecal DNA versus fecal occult blood for colorectal-cancer screening in an average-risk population. *N Engl J Med.* 2004;351:2704–2714.

53. Song K, Fendrick AM, Ladabaum U. Fecal DNA testing compared with conventional colorectal cancer screening methods: a decision analysis. *Gastroenterology.* 2004;126:1270–1279.

54. Pochapin MB. *What Your Doctor May Not Tell You About Colorectal Cancer.* New York: Warner; 2004.

55. Cotton PB, Durkalski VL, Pineau BC, et al. Computed tomographic colonography (virtual colonoscopy): a multicenter comparison with standard colonoscopy for detection of colorectal neoplasia. *JAMA.* 2004;291:1713–1719.

56. Fenlon HM, Nunes DP, Schroy PC 3rd, et al. A comparison of virtual and conventional colonoscopy for the detection of colorectal polyps. *N Engl J Med.* 1999;341:1496–1503.

57. Allison JE, Tekawa IS, Ransom LJ, Adrain AL. A comparison of fecal occult-blood tests for colorectal-cancer screening. *N Engl J Med.* 1996;334:155–159.

58. Itzkowitz S, Brand R, Jandorf L, et al. A simplified, noninvasive stool DNA test for colorectal cancer detection. *Am J Gastroenterol.* 2008;103:2862–2870.

59. Centers for Disease Control and Prevention. Use of colorectal cancer tests—United States, 2002, 2004, and 2006. *Morb Mortal Wkly Rep.* 2008;57:253–258. http://www.cdc.gov/mmwr/preview/mmwrhtml/mm5710a2.htm. Accessed March 1 2010.

60. Schenck AP, Peacock SC, Klabunde CN, et al. Trends in colorectal cancer test use in the Medicare population, 1998–2005. *Am J Prev Med.* 2009;37:1–7.

61. Shapiro JA, Seeff LC, Thompson TD, et al. Colorectal cancer test use from the 2005 National Health Interview Survey. *Cancer Epidemiol Biomarkers Prev.* 2008;17:1623–1630.

62. Doubeni CA, Laiyemo AO, Reed G, et al. Socioeconomic and racial patterns of colorectal cancer screening among Medicare enrollees in 2000 to 2005. *Cancer Epidemiol Biomarkers Prev.* 2009;18:2170–2175.

63. Seeff LC, Manninen DL, Dong FB, et al. Is there endoscopic capacity to provide colorectal cancer screening to the unscreened population in the United States? *Gastroenterology.* 2004;127:1661–1669.

64. Agrawal S, Bhupinderjit A, Bhutani MS, et al. Colorectal cancer in African Americans. *Am J Gastroenterol.* 2005;100:515–523; discussion 514.

65. Trivers KF, Shaw KM, Sabatino SA, et al. Trends in colorectal cancer screening disparities in people aged 50–64 years, 2000–2005. *Am J Prev Med.* 2008;35:185–193.

66. American Cancer Society. *Cancer Facts and Figures for African Americans 2007–2008.* Atlanta, GA: American Cancer Society; 2008.

67. Bach PB, Schrag D, Brawley OW, et al. Survival of blacks and whites after a cancer diagnosis. *JAMA.* 2002;287:2106–2113.

68. Early colorectal cancer screening for African Americans. *Lancet.* 2009;373:980.

69. Rex DK, Khan AM, Shah P, Newton J, Cummings OW. Screening colonoscopy in asymptomatic average-risk African Americans. *Gastrointest Endosc.* 2000;51:524–527.

70. Close G, Zauber AG, Mills G, Jordan PA, et al. African-Americans have the same prevalence and proximal distribution of adenomas as whites in the National Colonoscopy Study. *Gastroenterology.* 2010; 138(5 Suppl 1):S–190.

71. Lansdorp-Vogelaar I, van Ballegooijen M, Zauber AG, et al. Individualizing colonoscopy screening by sex and race. *Gastrointest Endosc*. 2009;70:96–108, 108 e101–124.

72. International Agency for Research on Cancer. *Tobacco Smoke and Involuntary Smoking*. Lyon, France: International Agency for Research on Cancer; 2004. IARC Monographs on the Evaluation of Carcinogenic Risks to Humans; vol. 83.

73. *The Health Consequences of Smoking: A Report from the Surgeon General*. Atlanta, GA: National Center for Chronic Disease and Prevention and Health Promotion, Centers for Disease Control and Prevention; 2004.

74. Secretan B, Straif K, Baan R, et al. A review of human carcinogens—part E: tobacco, areca nut, alcohol, coal smoke, and salted fish. *Lancet Oncol*. 2009;10:1033–1034.

75. Giovannucci E. An updated review of the epidemiological evidence that cigarette smoking increases risk of colorectal cancer. *Cancer Epidemiol Biomarkers Prev*. 2001;10:725–731.

76. Limburg PJ, Vierkant RA, Cerhan JR, et al. Cigarette smoking and colorectal cancer: long-term, subsite-specific risks in a cohort study of postmenopausal women. *Clin Gastroenterol Hepatol*. 2003;1:202–210.

77. Giovannucci E, Rimm EB, Stampfer MJ, et al. A prospective study of cigarette smoking and risk of colorectal adenoma and colorectal cancer in US men. *J Natl Cancer Inst*. 1994;86:183–191.

78. Paskett ED, Reeves KW, Rohan TE, et al. Association between cigarette smoking and colorectal cancer in the Women's Health Initiative. *J Natl Cancer Inst*. 2007;99:1729–1735.

79. Tsoi KK, Pau CY, Wu WK, et al. Cigarette smoking and the risk of colorectal cancer: a meta-analysis of prospective cohort studies. *Clin Gastroenterol Hepatol*. 2009;7:682–688 e681–685.

80. Lieberman DA, Prindiville S, Weiss DG, Willett W. Risk factors for advanced colonic neoplasia and hyperplastic polyps in asymptomatic individuals. *JAMA*. 2003;290:2959–2967.

81. Botteri E, Iodice S, Raimondi S, et al. Cigarette smoking and adenomatous polyps: a meta-analysis. *Gastroenterology*. 2008;134:388–395.

82. Terry MB, Neugut AI. Cigarette smoking and the colorectal adenoma-carcinoma sequence: a hypothesis to explain the paradox. *Am J Epidemiol*. 1998;147:903–910.

83. Bagnardi V, Blangiardo M, La Vecchia C, Corrao G. A meta-analysis of alcohol drinking and cancer risk. *Br J Cancer*. 2001;85:1700–1705.

84. Giovannucci E, Stampfer MJ, Colditz GA, et al. Folate, methionine, and alcohol intake and risk of colorectal adenoma. *J Natl Cancer Inst*. 1993;85:875–884.

85. Cho E, Smith-Warner SA, Ritz J, et al. Alcohol intake and colorectal cancer: a pooled analysis of 8 cohort studies. *Ann Intern Med*. 2004;140:603–613.

86. Ning Y, Wang L, Giovannucci EL. A quantitative analysis of body mass index and colorectal cancer: findings from 56 observational studies. *Obes Rev*. 2010;11:19–30.

87. Terry PD, Miller AB, Rohan TE. Obesity and colorectal cancer risk in women. *Gut*. 2002;51:191–194.

88. Giovannucci E. Obesity, gender, and colon cancer. *Gut*. 2002;51:147.

89. Giovannucci E, Michaud D. The role of obesity and related metabolic disturbances in cancers of the colon, prostate, and pancreas. *Gastroenterology*. 2007;132:2208–2225.

90. Larsson SC, Orsini N, Wolk A. Diabetes mellitus and risk of colorectal cancer: a meta-analysis. *J Natl Cancer Inst*. 2005;97:1679–1687.

91. Wei EK, Ma J, Pollak MN, et al. A prospective study of C-peptide, insulin-like growth factor-I, insulin-like growth factor binding protein-1, and the risk of colorectal cancer in women. *Cancer Epidemiol Biomarkers Prev*. 2005;14:850–855.

92. World Cancer Research Fund/American Institute for Cancer Research. *Food, Nutrition, Physical Activity, and the Prevention of Cancer: A Global Perspective*. Washington, DC: AICR; 2007.

93. Koushik A, Hunter DJ, Spiegelman D, et al. Fruits, vegetables, and colon cancer risk in a pooled analysis of 14 cohort studies. *J Natl Cancer Inst*. 2007;99:1471–1483.

94. Michels KB, Giovannucci E, Chan AT, et al. Fruit and vegetable consumption and colorectal adenomas in the Nurses' Health Study. *Cancer Res*. 2006;66:3942–3953.

95. Michels KB, Giovannucci EL, Joshipura KJ, et al. Prospective study of fruit and vegetable consumption and incidence of colon and rectal cancers. *J Natl Cancer Inst*. 2000;92:1740–1752.

96. Wolin KY, Lee IM, Colditz GA, et al. Leisure-time physical activity patterns and risk of colon cancer in women. *Int J Cancer*. 2007;121:2776–2781.

97. Martinez ME, Giovannucci E, Spiegelman D, et al. Leisure-time physical activity, body size, and colon cancer in women. Nurses' Health Study Research Group. *J Natl Cancer Inst*. 1997;89:948–955.

98. Slattery ML, Potter J, Caan B, et al. Energy balance and colon cancer—beyond physical activity. *Cancer Res*. 1997;57:75–80.

99. Bertagnolli MM, Eagle CJ, Zauber AG, et al. Celecoxib for the prevention of sporadic colorectal adenomas. *N Engl J Med*. 2006;355:873–884.

100. Imperiale TF. Aspirin and the prevention of colorectal cancer. *N Engl J Med*. 2003;348:879–880.

101. Chan AT, Giovannucci EL, Meyerhardt JA, et al. Long-term use of aspirin and nonsteroidal anti-inflammatory drugs and risk of colorectal cancer. *JAMA*. 2005;294:914–923.

102. Dube C, Rostom A, Lewin G, et al. The use of aspirin for primary prevention of colorectal cancer: a systematic review prepared for the US Preventive Services Task Force. *Ann Intern Med*. 2007;146:365–375.

103. Cook NR, Lee IM, Gaziano JM, et al. Low-dose aspirin in the primary prevention of cancer: the Women's Health Study: a randomized controlled trial. *JAMA*. 2005;294:47–55.

104. Psaty BM, Potter JD. Risks and benefits of celecoxib to prevent recurrent adenomas. *N Engl J Med*. 2006;355:950–952.

105. Wolpin BM, Wei EK, Ng K, et al. Prediagnostic plasma folate and the risk of death in patients with colorectal cancer. *J Clin Oncol*. 2008;26:3222–3228.

106. Jaszewski R, Misra S, Tobi M, et al. Folic acid supplementation inhibits recurrence of colorectal adenomas: a randomized chemoprevention trial. *World J Gastroenterol*. 2008;14:4492–4498.

107. Cole BF, Baron JA, Sandler RS, et al. Folic acid for the prevention of colorectal adenomas: a randomized clinical trial. *JAMA*. 2007;297:2351–2359.

108. Kim YI. Folate, colorectal carcinogenesis, and DNA methylation: lessons from animal studies. *Environ Mol Mutagen*. 2004;44:10–25.

109. Ulrich CM, Potter JD. Folate and cancer—timing is everything. *JAMA*. 2007;297:2408–2409.

110. Grau MV, Baron JA, Sandler RS, et al. Prolonged effect of calcium supplementation on risk of colorectal adenomas in a randomized trial. *J Natl Cancer Inst*. 2007;99:129–136.

111. Cho E, Smith-Warner SA, Spiegelman D, et al. Dairy foods, calcium, and colorectal cancer: a pooled analysis of 10 cohort studies. *J Natl Cancer Inst*. 2004;96:1015–1022.

112. Wu K, Willett WC, Fuchs CS, Colditz GA, Giovannucci EL. Calcium intake and risk of colon cancer in women and men. *J Natl Cancer Inst*. 2002;94:437–446.

113. Martinez ME, Marshall JR, Sampliner R, et al. Calcium, vitamin D, and risk of adenoma recurrence (United States). *Cancer Causes Control*. 2002;13:213–220.

114. Forman MR, Levin B. Calcium plus vitamin D3 supplementation and colorectal cancer in women. *N Engl J Med*. 16 2006;354:752–754.

115. Wactawski-Wende J, Kotchen JM, Anderson GL, et al. Calcium plus vitamin D supplementation and the risk of colorectal cancer. *N Engl J Med*. 2006;354:684–696.

116. Garland CF, Gorham ED, Mohr SB, Garland FC. Vitamin D for cancer prevention: global perspective. *Ann Epidemiol*. 2009;19:468–483.

117. Calle EE, Miracle-McMahill HL, Thun MJ, Heath CW, Jr. Estrogen replacement therapy and risk of fatal colon cancer in a prospective cohort of postmenopausal women. *J Natl Cancer Inst*. 1995;87:517–523.

118. Clendenen TV, Koenig KL, Shore RE, et al. Postmenopausal levels of endogenous sex hormones and risk of colorectal cancer. *Cancer Epidemiol Biomarkers Prev*. 2009;18:275–281.

119. Grodstein F, Newcomb PA, Stampfer MJ. Postmenopausal hormone therapy and the risk of colorectal cancer: a review and meta-analysis. *Am J Med*. 1999;106:574–582.

120. Prentice RL, Pettinger M, Beresford SA, et al. Colorectal cancer in relation to postmenopausal estrogen and estrogen plus progestin in the Women's Health Initiative clinical trial and observational study. *Cancer Epidemiol Biomarkers Prev*. 2009;18:1531–1537.

121. Newcomb PA, Zheng Y, Chia VM, et al. Estrogen plus progestin use, microsatellite instability, and the risk of colorectal cancer in women. *Cancer Res*. 2007;67:7534–7539.

122. Chlebowski RT, Wactawski-Wende J, Ritenbaugh C, et al. Estrogen plus progestin and colorectal cancer in postmenopausal women. *N Engl J Med*. 2004;350:991–1004.

123. Poynter JN, Gruber SB, Higgins PD, et al. Statins and the risk of colorectal cancer. *N Engl J Med*. 2005;352:2184–2192.

124. Bonovas S, Filioussi K, Flordellis CS, Sitaras NM. Statins and the risk of colorectal cancer: a meta-analysis of 18 studies involving more than 1.5 million patients. *J Clin Oncol*. 2007;25:3462–3468.

125. Coogan PF, Smith J, Rosenberg L. Statin use and risk of colorectal cancer. *J Natl Cancer Inst*. 2007;99:32–40.

126. Shadman M, Newcomb PA, Hampton JM, et al. Non-steroidal anti-inflammatory drugs and statins in relation to colorectal cancer risk. *World J Gastroenterol*. 2009;15:2336–2339.

127. National Cancer Institute. Colon cancer treatment (PDQ®). 2008. http://www.cancer.gov/cancertopics/pdq/treatment/colon/healthprofessional. Accessed March 4, 2010.

128. National Cancer Institute. Rectal cancer treatment (PDQ®). 2009. http://www.cancer.gov/cancertopics/pdq/treatment/rectal/HealthProfessional. Accessed March 4, 2010.

129. Pochapin Mark B. MD., CRC Screening in Women: C5 and ACOG. Presentation: 6th Annual Citywide Colon Cancer Control Coalition (C5) Summit June 11, 2009; New York, NY. http://www.nyc.gov/html/doh/downloads/pdf/cancer/cancer-2009-pochapin.pdf Accessed December 27, 2012.

130. ACOG District II. Focus on Female Cancers: Colorectal Cancer. 2010; http://mail.ny.acog.org/ Accessed Dec 27, 2012.

Chronic Conditions

Women and Cardiovascular Disease

Mary Kilty, MBA, MPH, MPhil; Heidi Mochari Greenberger, PhD, MPH, RD; and Moise Desvarieux, MD, PhD

Introduction

Cardiovascular disease (CVD) caused 68% of American deaths in 2007, and more than a million Americans are diagnosed annually. Recent awareness of CVD among women has increased attention to gender-specific differences in clinical presentation, disease processes, and outcomes. Improved treatment and reduction of some risk factors have enabled significant declines in CVD death for women and men; however disparities among Americans exist when rates are compared by race/ethnicity and geographic region. The purpose of this chapter is to review the epidemiology of CVD among women, including factors associated with risk and prevention such as the use of postmenopausal hormones, highlighting gender-specific differences and commonalities.

Cardiovascular Disease

CVD includes diseases of the heart and circulatory system.[1] CVD includes coronary heart disease (CHD), acute myocardial infarction (MI), angina pectoris, atherosclerotic CVD, and other cardiac conditions.[2,3] Between 1997 and 2007 the mortality rate for this complex of conditions declined 28%. However, CVD affects one in four American adults, caused 34% of all deaths in 2007, approximately 2,200 deaths daily, of which one-third occurred prematurely before age 75.[2]

Although the overall mortality rate in 2007 from CVD was 251.2 per 100,000, significant differences were noted by gender and race: mortality risk per 100,000 was highest in black men (405.9) followed by white men (294); white women had the lowest mortality from CVD (205.7) compared with black women (286.1). Among women age 65 and older, diseases of the heart were the leading causes of death, followed by cancer and stroke.[2] Among the 813,804 U.S. CVD deaths in 2007, almost 50% were caused by CHD and 16.9% by stroke.[2]

Characteristics of Cardiovascular Disease

CHD develops as the coronary arteries supplying the heart are blocked by plaque.[4] A stroke occurs when a blood vessel in the brain either ruptures (hemorrhagic stroke) or is blocked by a mass and/or blood clot (ischemic stroke) depriving the brain of oxygen.[4] Although clinical manifestations of CVD occur primarily in middle-aged and elderly adults, many people with atherosclerosis lack traditional risk factors. CVD is now understood to be a progressive disease that increases with age: modifiable risk factors for CVD may be present in utero,[5] and classic risk factors for CVD, including early stages of subclinical disease, are found in children and teens.[6,7] The primary underlying disease processes in CVD are atherosclerosis and hypertension.[1]

Atherosclerosis

Atherosclerosis is a systemic disease in which fatty deposits composed of cholesterol, fat, and other blood components form plaque in the arteries.[4] Over the life span plaque builds, causing narrowing and hardening of the arteries obstructing blood flow from the heart to other parts of the body.[8] Figure 31-1 presents the developmental stages of atherosclerosis that include the following:

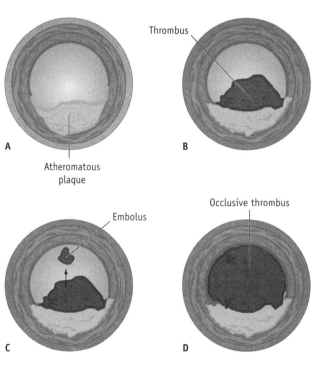

Figure 31-1 Stages in the development of atherosclerosis.

- Lesions in arterial walls attract macrophages and other blood components.[9,10]
- Fatty material is deposited in the lining of the artery wall, narrowing the lumen.
- Narrowed arteries become blocked, forming atheromas.
- Arteries may be occluded by a blood clot or plaque, becoming vulnerable to rupture.[1,2,4]

Atherosclerosis, an inflammatory process[9], is most damaging when plaques become fragile and rupture enabling clot formation that obstructs blood flow.[11–13] Blood clots in coronary arteries cause myocardial infarction (heart attack); a stroke is the result of obstructed blood flow to the brain.[14,15]

Hypertension (High Blood Pressure)

Hypertension is harmful when elevated arterial blood pressure is sustained.[16] Data from the National Health and Nutrition Examination Survey (NHANES) of 2005–2008 indicated 52% of women were receiving medication for hypertension and 28.7% had uncontrolled hypertension; fewer men used antihypertensive medication (38.6%) but 30.6% were hypertensive when examined for NHANES.[17] Untreated hypertension may cause arterial narrowing and damage to target organs including brain, kidneys, and heart and may also lead to heart failure or stroke.[18]

U.S. and Global CVD Burden in Women

Cardiovascular Disease in the United States

Across all ages approximately one in three American adults has some form of CVD; approximately 50% are age 60 or older.[2] Data for 2008 estimated 16.3 million Americans were diagnosed with either angina or myocardial infarc-

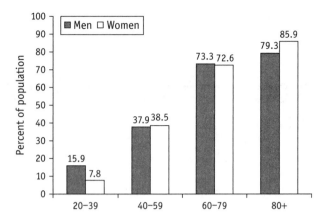

Figure 31-2 Prevalence of cardiovascular disease by age and gender, United States, 2005–2008.

Source: Data from National Health and Nutrition Examination Survey: 2005–2008, National Center for Health Statistics (NCHS). Hyattsville, MD: U.S. Department of Health and Human Services, Centers for Disease Control and Prevention.

tion and 7 million with stroke. Among men and women CVD prevalence rises with age (Figure 31–2).[14] Heart disease prevalence is estimated to be 6.1% for women and 8.3% for men.[2] Black women have proportionally more CHD (7.6%) compared to non-Hispanic white (5.8%) and Mexican-American (5.6%) women.[2]

The average annual incidence rate of first CVD events among women ages 45–54 years is estimated to be 3/1000; rates are similar for men ages 35–44.[2] Before age 75 a higher proportion of CVD events due to CHD occurs in males, although more women experience strokes.[2] In recent decades the CVD death rates have declined for women and men.[2] Almost half of this decrease has been attributed to improved medical therapies and half related to reduction in risk factors resulting from changes in lifestyle and environmental exposures.[20] CVD mortality rates are higher for black females compared to white females.

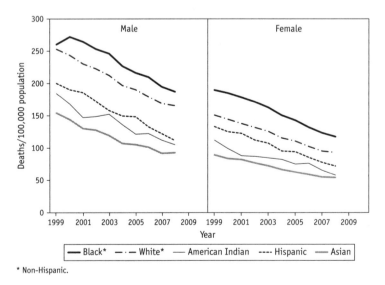

Figure 31-3 Age-adjusted death rates for coronary heart disease by race/ethnicity and sex, U.S., 1999–2008.

Reproduced from Morbidity & Mortality: 2012 Chart book on cardiovascular, lung, and blood diseases. National Institutes of Health, National Heart, Lung, and Blood Institute, 2012.

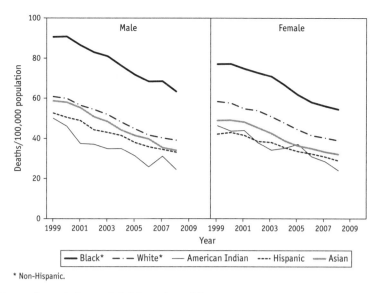

Figure 31-4 Age-adjusted death rates for stroke by race/ethnicity and sex, U.S., 1999–2008.

Reproduced from Morbidity & Mortality: 2012 Chart book on cardiovascular, lung, and blood diseases. National Institutes of Health, National Heart, Lung, and Blood Institute, 2012.

Declining mortality rates between 1999 and 2009 for CHD (Figure 31-3) and stroke (Figure 31-4) indicate women and men of all race/ethnicities have benefited from improved survival.[2]

International Burden of Cardiovascular Disease in Women

Half of the deaths among adult women globally are caused by noncommunicable diseases, particularly CVD.[21] Although CVD was once characterized as a "western" disease of affluence, high levels of CVD mortality are found across the globe at all stages of economic development.[22,23] The World Health Organization's Global Burden of Disease estimated CVD is the leading cause of death in the world, specifically among women;[24] globally, CVD caused approximately 32% of deaths in women and 27% in men in 2004.[24] The total burden of CVD adversely affects productivity as measured by disease-adjusted life years (DALYs).[21,23] In 2004, ischemic heart disease and cerebrovascular disease were the second and third leading causes of DALYs in middle- and high-income countries globally; in contrast, ischemic heart disease is the ninth leading cause of DALYs in low-income countries.[24]

The growing prevalence of CVD in developing countries reflects the epidemiologic transition in which morbidity and mortality from chronic diseases increase as childhood mortality from infectious disease declines.[21,25] In recent decades deaths from cardiovascular conditions have been rising in developing countries, with 50% occurring before age 70, in contrast to declining mortality rates in developed nations.[25] CVD prevalence in developing countries has been attributed to urbanization accompanied by changing lifestyles such as increased food supply, less nutritious diet, lowered physical activity levels, and greater affluence among young and middle-aged adults.[26]

Between 1990 and 2020, ischemic heart disease mortality is expected to increase by 120% in women and 137% in men in developing countries, a greater increase than projected for developed nations (29% in women and 48% in men).[26] CVD mortality rates vary globally from low rates in Africa with 9% of total deaths in 2002 to 50% of mortality in Eastern and Western Europe.[23]

Risk Factors for Coronary Heart Disease and Stroke in Women

Although heart disease is a major public health burden, some personal behaviors may reduce the risk of disease.[27] The INTERHEART, a global case-control study of CVD risk factors, identified nine risk factors associated with 90% of CVD in women, including hypertension, dyslipidemia, diabetes, obesity, physical inactivity, poor diet, smoking, stress, and excess alcohol consumption.[28] The probability of disease was positively associated with the total number of number of risk factors reported. Table 31-1 notes factors that may be modifiable and risks remaining that cannot be readily controlled including inherited susceptibility, increasing age, race/ethnicity, etc.[28]

Inherited Susceptibility

CVD clusters in families due to shared genes, environment, lifestyle, and customs. Having a family history including a parent with premature CVD (father before age 45, mother before age 55) was an independent risk factor for offspring with an age-adjusted OR = 2.3 (95% CI = 1.3–4.3).[32] Recognition of familial risk led to a family-based prevention program to lower risk by lifestyle modifications among relatives of CVD patients. Recent work has documented effectiveness of the interventions to modify personal behaviors including improved diet and increased exercise.[33,34]

Table 31-1

Heart disease risk factors

Modifiable	Nonmodifiable
Hypertension	Aging
Elevated blood cholesterol	Genetic susceptibility
Smoking	Family history
Diabetes	Race/ethnicity
Obesity	Personal history of CVD
Lack of physical activity	
Stress	
Diet high in saturated fats	
Excess alcohol consumption	

Risk differs by race/ethnicity; U.S. black women have higher CHD and stroke rates than white women.[30] This relationship may be partially attributable to higher prevalence of specific risk factors among black women compared to white women, including hypertension, diabetes, and obesity.[35,36] NHANES data indicate obesity is higher among non-Hispanic black women compared with Mexican American or non-Hispanic white women.[36] Comparing CVD risk among ethnic groups is complicated by geographic location, with highest rates among Asian women in India compared with those in the United Kingdom, Japan, and Korea.[37]

History of CVD

Women with a personal history of a CVD event such as a heart attack, stroke, or transient ischemic attack (TIA) are at risk for recurrent disease. Carotid artery disease and atrial fibrillation are two vascular disorders specifically linked to increased stroke risk;[38] during 5 years of follow-up after a first CVD episode, 20% of women aged 40–69 years are at risk for a second heart attack or stroke.[30]

Increasing Age

As women age, atherosclerosis advances and cholesterol accumulates in lining of the arteries forming plaques with their potential for rupture resulting in elevated risk of CHD and stroke.[31] Figure 31-5 notes age related risk of death among females by race/ethnicity. Mortality within the first weeks after a heart attack appears greater for older women than older men.[31] With each decade after age 55, stroke risk doubles, potentially associated with reduced physical activity, increasing blood pressure, and weight gain.[38]

Elevated Blood Lipid Levels

Elevated blood cholesterol is a major risk factor for both CHD and stroke. Among participants in a prospective study in Finland, for each mmol/L increase in total blood cholesterol risk of developing and dying from CHD was increased 20% among women.[39] High levels of low-density lipoprotein cholesterol (LDL-C) were predictive of atherosclerosis across different populations.[31] Research has found LDL-C levels are higher among women aged 55 years and older than among similarly aged men;[30] LDL-C levels below 100 mg/dL are considered optimal.[40]

High-density lipoprotein cholesterol (HDL-C), the "good" cholesterol, has been associated with lower CVD

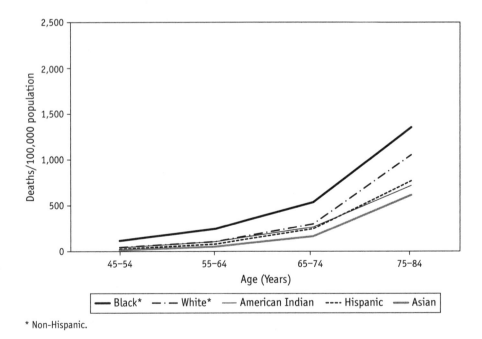

Figure 31-5 Death rates for heart disease in females by age and race/ethnicity, U.S., 2008.

Reproduced from Morbidity & Mortality: 2012 Chart book on cardiovascular, lung, and blood diseases. National Institutes of Health, National Heart, Lung, and Blood Institute, 2012.

risk, which may be more predictive among women than men.[30] Among women, low HDL cholesterol was shown to be more closely related to CVD than LDL-C.[41] High HDL-C is particularly important for women as 1 mg/dL increase was associated with a 3% reduction compared to only a 2% risk reduction in men.[42] Triglycerides are the chemical forms of fat circulating in the body. High triglyceride levels equal to 150 mg/dL accompany low HDL-C, higher LDL-C, and increased risk of diabetes, but triglyceride levels are not included as major independent CHD risk factors.[30,31,40]

Diabetes

Both type 1 and 2 diabetes independently increase risk of CHD and stroke causing three of four deaths among diabetics.[35,38,43] Regardless of age or menopausal status, women with diabetes are at greater risk of CVD.[42] The impact of diabetes on CHD among Framingham participants was greater among women than men regardless of age, and women were more likely to experience angina, myocardial infarction, and sudden death.[42] After 20 years follow-up, female Framingham participants who developed diabetes were at greater risk of CVD (RR = 2.8) than women without diabetes.[44] Diabetes also increased risk of myocardial infarction more strongly among women than men in the INTERHEART study; risk was elevated among women with a history of gestational diabetes who subsequently developed type 2 diabetes.[45,46]

Hypertension

Elevated blood pressure is associated with risk of stroke and CHD among women and men at younger and older ages.[31,38] Blood-pressure control has been linked to decline in rate of death from stroke.[38] Hypertension is more likely diagnosed among women with a family history of elevated blood pressure, those who developed elevated blood pressure during pregnancy, while taking certain types of birth control pills, after menopause, or among obese women with very high body mass index (BMI).[30]

Hypertension has been defined as systolic blood pressure equal to or greater than 140 mm Hg and a diastolic pressure equal or greater than or to 90 mm Hg. In the United States current treatment with antihypertensive medication is also considered evidence of hypertension.[31,47] However, systolic blood pressure values between 120 to 140 have also been associated with increased risk.[31,47] Hypertension raises the risk of heart attack more strongly among women than men.[45] Data from a large Finnish cohort of WHO-MONICA participants show a risk ratio of 1.11 (95% CI = 1.04–1.18) for CHD incidence in women for each 10 mm Hg increase in systolic blood pressure.[39]

Overweight and Obesity

Excess body fat independently and combined with high blood pressure, abnormal blood lipid levels, and diabetes increases CHD and stroke risk.[30] Excess central obesity, fat located in the abdomen, has specifically been linked to increased CVD risk among women.[30,31,35,48] Inactivity coupled with large waist circumference significantly increases risk of developing CHD compared to active women with a low waist circumference.[49] Waist–hip ratio has also been associated with increased CVD mortality, even among women of normal weight.[50] In the Framingham population, the age-adjusted risk ratio for CVD was increased in overweight women (RR = 1.20; 95% CI = 1.03–1.41), and obese women (RR = 1.64; 95% CI = 1.37–1.98) compared to normal weight women.[51] CVD prevention guidelines recommend women maintain or achieve a BMI of less than 25 and a waist circumference less than 35 inches.[40]

Cigarette Smoking

Smoking is the single most preventable cause of death in the United States and a major cause of CVD in women.[30] Among participants in the Nurses' Health Study (NHS) initiated in 1976 smoking 25 cigarettes or more per day was associated with fatal CHD or nonfatal myocardial infarction at a rate of 125 cases/100,000 women and an age-adjusted RR = 6.0 (95% CI = 4.6–8.1) compared with nonsmokers.[52] Risk of stroke was twofold greater among smokers compared to nonsmokers[53] especially among smokers who use birth control pills.[30] Regular exposure to secondhand tobacco smoke has been implicated in increasing CVD risk among female nonsmokers as well.[30]

Physical Inactivity

Low levels of physical activity increase the risk of CHD and stroke more strongly among women than men.[30,45,54] A statistically significant inverse association between amount and intensity of physical activity and coronary events was documented in the NHS; the decline ranged from RR = 0.77 to RR = 0.46 with a highly significant trend ($P < 0.001$).[54] Protection is provided by exercise-induced decline in blood pressure, elevated LDL cholesterol, and lowered HDL cholesterol.[31] CVD prevention guidelines encourage a minimum of 150 minutes/week of moderate exercise, 75 minutes/week of vigorous exercise, or an equivalent combination of moderate- and vigorous-intensity aerobic physical activity.[40]

Diet and Alcohol Consumption

Ecologic and prospective studies have linked dietary patterns with CVD risk. The Seven Countries Study was among the first to note a consistent correlation between average intake of saturated fat and long-term CVD incidence rates.[55–58] An ecologic association was demonstrated by a parallel decline in CVD mortality and average saturated fat intake in the United States between 1970 and 2000.[59–61] Cohort studies including the Nurses' Health Study also linked diet with CVD risk. Increased CVD mortality was noted among women consuming a "western diet" including high consumption of red and processed meat, refined grains, french fries, and sweet desserts.[62] Several randomized controlled trials supported a protective role of low dietary saturated fat and reduced CVD.[63–66] However, the recently reported Women's Health Initiative (WHI) Randomized Controlled Dietary Modification Trial testing reduction of dietary fat to 20%

of total calories accompanied by increased intake of vegetables, fruit, and grains did not significantly lower risk of CHD, stroke, or CVD in older postmenopausal women[67] compared with the usual diet of controls. The intensive behavior modification program included group instruction and individual counseling in contrast to limited educational guidance from a federal diet publication provided to the comparison group. During the trial, repeated food frequency questionnaire data measured changes in dietary patterns. Women receiving the intervention reported lower intake of fat and increased consumption of fruit, vegetables, and grains; however, no significant changes were detected in levels of triglycerides, HDL-C levels or other serum markers. After 8 years of follow-up, the number of CHD events did not differ by diet assignment.[67] Suggested explanations for the unanticipated findings that differed from other randomized trials and observational studies included:

- possible counterbalancing of positive dietary changes with potentially adverse effects of others (e.g., replacing saturated fats with carbohydrates from refined grains)[68]
- possible insufficient duration of diet change to affect CVD risk[67,68]
- low adherence to prescribed diet in the intervention arm (i.e., insufficient reduction in saturated fat or inaccurate reporting on food questionnaire).[68]

The comparison group was found to have a lower than estimated risk of CVD, limiting the ability to detect diet-related differences. In addition, dietary patterns affecting CVD risk may be most protective when initiated at younger ages before progression of atherosclerosis associated with aging. Dietary recommendations include five to six servings daily of fruit and vegetables, whole grain, high-fiber foods, and fish (especially oily fish) at least twice a week in addition to low sodium and sugar consumption and no trans fats.[40]

Moderate alcohol consumption was associated with reduced risk of CVD primarily by raising HDL cholesterol levels; however, excessive alcohol intake raised blood pressure and risk of heart failure and stroke.[35,38,69] The association between alcohol consumption and CVD risk is similar for men and women. CVD risk is slightly higher among nondrinkers, risk declines among light to moderate drinkers, and rises with heavy intake forming a J-shaped risk curve with the nadir at a lower dose for women than for men.[69] Current guidelines recommend women consume no more than one alcoholic beverage per day (12 ounces of beer, 4 ounces of wine, or 1.5 ounces of spirits).[40,70]

Recently Identified CVD Risk Factors

Inflammation

Atherosclerosis, once thought to be a disease of blood lipid storage, is now recognized as an inflammation process with measurable biomarkers as potential correlates of CVD in women and men.[71,72] Markers of inflammation, studied among participants in the Nurses' Health Study, indicated elevated relative risks of CHD ranging from 1.92 to 2.57 were associated with highest marker levels compared with lowest levels.[72] These estimates were attenuated following adjustment for parental history of CHD, alcohol intake, level of physical activity, ratio of total to HDL cholesterol, body mass index, and use of postmenopausal hormone therapy.[72] Obesity has been consistently associated with higher levels of inflammatory markers as well as increased risk of CVD; however, the biologic mechanisms linking obesity with inflammation and CVD risk are not fully understood.[74] The recent discovery that some fat cells release inflammatory markers contributing to their measured levels makes assessment of these relationships of special interest.[75]

Psychosocial Factors

In recent decades research has documented CVD risk in both men and women associated with several psychosocial factors classified into three psychosocial domains including (1) negative emotional states (e.g., depression), (2) psychosocial stressors (e.g., caregiving and job-related strain), and (3) problematic social factors (e.g., lack of social ties and social support).[76] Examples from each domain are discussed next:

Depression

Several studies documented an association between depression or depressive symptoms and CVD risk more strongly among women than men in diverse populations. The increased risk of CHD associated with depression was identified in two meta-analyses[77,78] with the stronger impact for clinical depression, RR = 2.69, than depressed moods, RR = 1.49.[57] The INTERHEART study reported odds ratios for acute myocardial infarction among depressed women (OR = 1.60) and men (OR = 1.53).[79] Comparisons of myocardial infarction cases with controls from 54 countries revealed an elevated odds ratio for depression (OR = 1.5).[79] The 10-year NHANES I Follow-Up Study reported depression among women and men raised the risk of nonfatal CHD (RR = 1.73).[83] However, the WHI Observational Study noted depressive symptoms predicted cardiovascular mortality (RR = 1.5) but not CHD incidence patterns.[84]

Psychosocial Stress

The INTERHEART study assessed four domains of stress and major life events during the year before study entry; higher prevalence of all stress factors was significantly associated with acute myocardial infarction ($P < 0.0001$).[79] "Job strain" has been defined as "jobs characterized by high psychological workload demands' combined with 'low decision latitude; decision latitude', a measure of control that includes both job decision-making and use of skills.[86,87] Many studies conducted over 30 years have reported an association between job strain and CVD risk.[87] Among women intermediaries between work-related stress and risk of heart disease was proposed due to increases in BMI, smoking intensity, and elevated blood pressure.[88] Conflicting results in the scientific literature have questioned potential confounding factors linking job strain and CVD risk. Among females enrolled in the Framingham Offspring cohort, job strain was not significantly associated with incident CHD over a 10-year period; low versus high job strain was assessed before and after adjusting for blood pressure, body mass index, cigarette smoking, diabetes, and blood cholesterol (RR = 1.63, 95% CI = 0.57–4.67).[89] However, among apparently healthy participants in the WHI, job strain increased risk of heart disease independent of age, race, education, and income (RR = 1.40, 95% CI = 1.06–1.86).[90] Potential explanations for conflicting results include older employees who may experience less job strain, thus diluting the effect on CVD,[91] and data from cross-sectional studies provide only single-time assessment rather than long-term follow-up necessary for assessment of long-term (chronic) job strain.[92] Chronic job strain has been linked to recurrent CHD events in middle-aged women and men independent of recognized CVD risk factors, suggesting a direct effect of chronic job strain on the cardiovascular system.[93]

An estimated one in three American households have an unpaid family member providing care to one or more relatives (e.g., child, spouse, parent) and the majority of caregivers (66%) are women.[94] Not surprisingly, the strain and burdens associated with caregiving increased risk of CVD among women.[94–96] Among participants in the NHS during a 4-year follow-up period, caring for small healthy children 20 hours or more per week or for grandchildren 9 or more hours per week was associated with an increased risk of CHD (RR = 1.59 and 1.55 respectively).[97] Data from the NHS also indicated providing care to an ill spouse increased CHD in women after adjustment for age, smoking, exercise, alcohol, body mass index, hypertension, diabetes, and other covariates (RR = 1.82; 95% CI = 1.08–3.05).[95] Similarly, high in-home caregiving to a disabled spouse increased stroke risk 23%.[96] Current research is evaluating CVD risk among caregivers of spouses or blood relatives.[98]

Social Network
Measures of social ties and social networks were established as correlates of CVD morbidity and mortality in the Women's Ischemia Syndrome Evaluation study (WISE); among the 503 participants with suspected coronary artery disease (CAD), subsequent disease was greater among women with lower frequency of social contacts.[99] Larger social network scores were associated with reduced CVD risk factors and less severe CAD measured by angiogram.[99] Social support is defined as support from other people arising through interpersonal relationships.[100] Emotional support (i.e., providing empathy, caring, love, trust, esteem, concern, and listening), a component of social support, has been linked to lower levels of CVD and is important for people who are ill. Among hospitalized myocardial infarction patients risk of death was threefold greater for patients with low levels of emotional support.[101] Elderly hospitalized patients with heart failure who received no emotional support had an OR = 2.4 of recurrent disease during the year after hospital discharge, especially among women.[102] The Stockholm Female Coronary Risk Study reported higher levels of social support were associated with less progression of atherosclerosis as measured by artery luminal diameter.[103]

Life Course
Life-course studies investigate influences on health outcomes across the life span based on two concepts: (1) exposures at critical or sensitive stages of growth during gestation, childhood, adolescence and young adulthood combine with health behaviors at later ages and interact with (2) accumulated adverse environmental conditions, socioeconomic factors, and health damaging behaviors to have a significant impact on health status among adults.[104]

Higher traditional CVD risk factors during childhood increase atherosclerosis progression at later ages, independent of adult risks.[6] The Cardiovascular Risk in Young Finns study showed significant associations between childhood levels of systolic blood pressure, LDL cholesterol, cigarette smoking, and body mass index at ages 12 to 18 and adult carotid intima-media thickness (a measure of atherosclerosis progression).[6,103]

Similarly, the Bogalusa Heart Study of 486 adults aged 25–37 from a semirural community in Louisiana detected increased carotid intima-media thickness, which related to measures during childhood of LDL cholesterol (OR = 1.42; 95% CI = 1.14–1.78) and BMI (OR = 1.25, 95% CI = 1.01–1.54) compared to participants with lower levels and independent of risk factors measured in adulthood.[105] The Muscatine Study, a cohort of children followed through adulthood in Iowa, found cholesterol levels of girls and childhood body mass index at ages 8 to 11 independently and positively associated with carotid intima-media thickness when measured as young adults.[106]

A developmental model postulates that nutrition from the fetal stage through early childhood establishes functional capacity of organs and establishes metabolic processes and future responses to environmental exposures; the example presented by Barker et al. notes the consequences of undernutrition in utero and low birth weight followed by rapid weight gain in childhood predisposed members of the Helsinki cohort to heart disease in adulthood.[5,107] Although the exact physiological mechanisms are not known, two CVD risk factors develop from this growth pattern: insulin resistance and hypertension.[108–111] In the NHS, a one kilogram increase in birth weight was associated with significantly reduced risk of heart disease but not risk of stroke.[112] Hazard rate for stroke among Finnish adults was found to be inversely associated with weight gain between birth and age 2, which was not influenced by weight at older ages.[113] In contrast, adult risk of CHD was increased in relation to low weight gain from birth to age 2 followed by rapid weight gain after age 2.

Socioeconomic and Neighborhood Factors
Socioeconomic status (SES) during childhood and adulthood contributes to adult heart disease mortality.[114] For example, a direct association between birth weight and hypertension was found in a large cohort, but was limited

to those persons whose fathers were laborers or lower middle class.[115] A subset of Finnish men born at a low ponderal index (birth weight/length³), had higher rates of CHD if they were in a low income tax bracket.[116] A review of the epidemiologic studies suggested low socioeconomic circumstances during childhood increased risk of CVD morbidity and mortality, independent of their circumstances as adults.[117] Among studies addressing disease risk associated with socioeconomic status in childhood, several focused on women including the mothers of the 1958 Birth Cohort whose mortality due to CHD, stroke, and respiratory diseases was influenced by both adult and childhood social class, although risk was attenuated after adjustment for adult BMI and smoking.[118] This finding was consistent with female participants of lower economic status in the Alameda County, California, cohort who experienced 30% excess CVD mortality.[119] Another prospective study confirmed these findings; nurses of the NHS whose fathers were manual laborers had 50% excess risk of CHD and nonfatal myocardial infarction compared to women whose fathers were professionals.[120]

The link between socioeconomic status and health was established in many studies. SES has many definitions but the primary classification includes income, education level, and/or occupation.[121] Marmot and others studied the risk of heart disease in five job classifications in England noting higher rates of CHD among women and men in the lower social classes.[122] Between 1980 and 1989 among men ages 45–59 at death in 11 western European countries, risks of dying differed by country, social class, and specific causes; however, men of higher income had an advantage independent of the specific disease or associated risk factors.[123]

Income and education were each independently inversely associated with risk of death over 10 years of follow-up among more than 530,500 women and men age 25 or older selected for the American National Longitudinal Mortality Study.[124] In addition, blacks between ages 25 and 44 had twice the mortality rate of whites; other factors associated with greater mortality in this large cohort were being unemployed, having lower level occupations, being less educated, and being single rather than married.[124]

U.S. census data from 1990 linked with mortality files from the Centers for Disease Control and Prevention (CDC) indicated the size of the inequality gap between wealthy and less fortunate individuals was associated with age-adjusted death from CHD that varied by state within the United States; therefore, federal policies regarding income distribution may contribute to the state-based measures of health.[125] The strongest direct health effects of income inequality were observed among the American states with aggregate-level data noting higher proportions of blacks in the population, lower investments in education, and more limited healthcare availability. Figure 31-6 indicates the southern states that have been classified as the "stroke belt" by CDC and other agencies.[1] These factors associated with low income collectively influence state-specific health

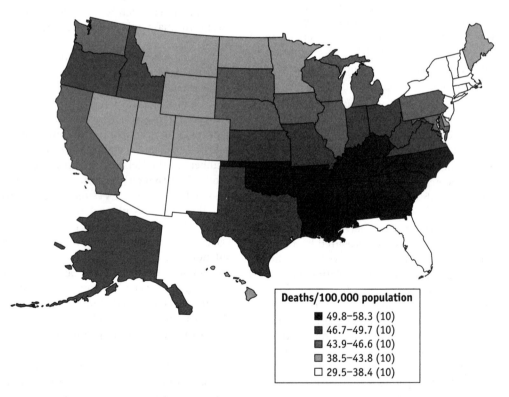

Figure 31-6 Age-adjusted death rate for stroke, by state, U.S., 2005–2007.

Reproduced from Morbidity & Mortality: 2012 Chart book on cardiovascular, lung, and blood diseases. National Institutes of Health, National Heart, Lung, and Blood Institute, 2012.

risks including CVD mortality although some limitations of the association followed adjustment for individual risk factor data.[126]

Studies have documented associations between CVD risk and neighborhood socioeconomic characteristics such as opportunities for safe physical activity, local food availability, and community resources for social support in addition to individual circumstance.[127] Another study relying on census data, the Atherosclerosis Risk in Communities Study, indicated higher CVD incidence occurred after 9 years of follow-up among residents of disadvantaged neighborhoods even after controlling for personal income, education level, and occupation.[128] The British Women's Heart and Health study showed that CHD prevalence in women was related to area deprivation defined by male unemployment, household overcrowding, car ownership, and the proportion of household members in semiskilled or unskilled manual occupations.[129] In the WISEWOMAN project conducted by the CDC, residential environment and socioecologic characteristics were associated with BMI and CHD risk among low-income women; BMI and CHD risk were lower in relation to environments of "mixed land use" (i.e., parks, bike paths) compared to more racially segregated areas that lacked public amenities.[130] Other neighborhood characteristics shown to affect biological risk factors for CVD include air pollution, noise, density, walkability, and access to physical activity venues.[127]

Hormone Replacement Therapy

Perhaps the most controversial women's cardiovascular health topic in the past half century is whether hormone replacement therapy (HRT) confers protection against CVD. Several epidemiological observations indicated cyclical female hormones were protective against CVD including:

- lower CVD rates in premenopausal women compared to men,
- increased CVD incidence in women after menopause, and
- decreased CVD risk among women with early menopause receiving hormone replacement therapy.

Historically, a perception existed that women were excluded from research in part due to risks associated with hormone cycles; guidelines issued by the Food and Drug Administration in 1977 discouraged inclusion of women of childbearing age in drug trials following the recognition of in utero exposures adversely affecting the future health of the developing fetus. In addition, major studies of heart disease focused on middle-aged men whose risk of premature death was steadily increasing.[131] However, from its initiation the Framingham heart study included women, and several cohorts formed in the 1970s focused on women's health including the first Nurses' Health Study.

Other investigations of women's health included the Lipid Research Clinics study, which provided evidence of a protective effect of hormone use by postmenopausal women with and without established risks[132] and the Postmenopausal Estrogen/Progestin Interventions (PEPI) clinical trial testing the comparative effect of unopposed estrogen, estrogen with progestin, or placebo on four markers of risk of heart disease among women ages 46–64.[133] Estrogen alone or combined with progestin improved lipoprotein and fibrinogen levels but did not influence blood pressure. An adverse outcome of the trial was estrogen alone was associated with endometrial hyperplasia, frequently requiring hysterectomy.[133] The question remained: Would the differences in markers produced by estrogen use translate to lower cardiovascular disease? A review of the systemic impact of HRT noted protective effects on the blood vessels as progression of atherosclerosis was slower; however, some nonvascular adverse effects were thought to reduce the benefits.[134]

The Heart and Estrogen/progestin Replacement Study (HERS), another randomized controlled trial (RCT), tested the effect of combined therapy versus placebo on risk of death from myocardial infarction or CHD among 2,763 postmenopausal women with established CHD during more than 4 years of follow-up.[135] No significant reduction in deaths was observed among treatment or placebo groups although a significant time trend noted more CHD events in year 1 among treated than control women; this greater incidence associated with hormone exposure was reversed in years 4 and 5 when risk increased among controls.[135] Based on their findings, the authors advised against initiating hormone treatment for women with heart disease.[135] The HERS study also noted the intervention compared to placebo did not reduce the risk of transient ischemic attack or stroke, either fatal or nonfatal.[136]

One suggested explanation for the lack of benefit from hormone exposure in the HERS trial was inadequate duration of follow-up; however, CHD deaths did not differ after longer follow-up when the living members of HERS from both treated and control groups were recruited to HERS II and followed for an average of 6.8 years.[137] The lack of secondary prevention in the HERS trial and the limited benefit for heart disease markers among women in the PEPI trial led to reexamination of observational study data with careful assessment of potential sources of confounding or selection bias. Several research teams noted women prescribed HRT tended to be of higher socioeconomic status, had greater access to health care, and were healthier and more physically active than nonusers.[138,139]

In 2001 Grodstein et al. published a study based on data from the Nurses' Health Study to identify women with coronary heart disease, some of whom were taking hormones, in order to compare the risk of recurrent disease with HERS study findings.[140] Results paralleled the HERS trial; short-term use increased risk of recurrent disease but longer use reduced risk of death.[140]

The timing of initiating hormone use after menopause was questioned by some researchers who suggested use concurrently with menopause might protect against development of heart disease. This question and others were addressed among 16,608 postmenopausal women aged 50–79 in the clinical trial component of the Women's Health Initiative who were randomized to receive estrogen plus progestin or placebo. After a mean duration of 5.2 years, the study was terminated (planned duration 8.5 years) due to increased incidence of CHD events among women assigned to the estrogen plus progestin arm compared to placebo (HR = 1.24; 95% CI = 1.00–2.54). The adverse effect of hormone exposure was most apparent during the first year of the trial.[141] Study authors concluded that the combination of estrogen and progestin did not protect generally healthy postmenopausal women from developing heart disease.[141] WHI also tested the association between HRT and CHD risk in unopposed estrogen versus placebo trial in women who had undergone hysterectomy; hormone exposure increased risk of stroke and venous thromboembolism after a median of 5.9 years; risk diminished with discontinued hormone use.[142]

Although short-term hormone use was known to provide relief of menopausal symptoms among women electing to take the medication, the RCT was essential to assess the impact of treatment on randomly assigned healthy women. Results of long-term cohort studies are also needed to provide measures of the interaction of hormone use and personal behavior changes associated with aging.[143] Some scientists have continued to question the potential cardioprotective role of HRT reported from observational research with initiation of treatment during the menopausal transition.[144] The majority of WHI participants were more than a decade post menopause (mean age at randomization was 63 years) and likely had underlying atherosclerotic disease at time of randomization.[145] Clinical research is ongoing to determine whether initiation of HRT specifically at the onset of menopause is cardioprotective in women without CVD [146]

Antioxidant Supplements

Antioxidant vitamin supplements (e.g., vitamins E, C, and beta-carotene) are not currently recommended for the primary or secondary prevention of CVD in women based on evidence from randomized trials showing no association between antioxidant vitamin supplementation and risk of CVD.[147,148] The Women's Antioxidant Cardiovascular Study was one of the first to examine interactions among antioxidant vitamins and vitamin C (ascorbic acid) on CVD risk in women. The study used a 2 × 2 × 2 factorial design to test the effects of ascorbic acid, vitamin E, and beta-carotene on the combined outcome of myocardial infarction, stroke, coronary revascularization or CVD death among 8,171 female health professionals aged 40 years or older with CVD or three or more CVD risk factors.[148] Participants were followed 1995–2005; no overall effect of ascorbic acid, vitamin E, or beta-carotene was noted on combined or individual outcomes.[148] Therefore, dietary supplements are not recommended; antioxidant vitamins should be consumed from fruits and vegetables.[31,40]

Folic Acid and B Vitamins

Some researchers hypothesized that folic acid, vitamin B6, vitamin B12, or a combination might provide benefit by reducing CVD risk. Prospective cohort data from the NHS indicate women with higher intake of folate and B6 from food and supplements have lower CHD risk;[149] and folic acid and B vitamin supplementation have also been shown to reduce levels of homocysteine, an amino acid directly linked to CVD risk.[150] However, this finding has not been supported by RCT data including a recent large-scale randomized trial conducted solely in women at high risk for CVD, the Women's Antioxidant and Folic Acid Cardiovascular Study (WAFACS).[151] The WAFACS trial initiated in 1998 enrolled more than 5,400 women with history of CVD aged 42 and older who were randomized to the combination of folic acid, vitamin B6, and vitamin B12 or placebo. The trial was a component to the Women's Antioxidant Cardiovascular Study. After 7.3 years of treatment and follow-up, no beneficial effect on CVD risk was observed among women who received the combination pill compared with controls.[151] Based on this and other current research suggesting lack of CVD benefit, folic acid supplementation (with or without vitamin B6 and B12) is not recommended for women;[152,153] although folic acid supplementation is recommended during childbearing years to prevent neural tube defects.[40]

Vitamin D

Animal studies, prospective human studies, and small randomized controlled trials suggest vitamin D insufficiency is associated with increased risk of CVD. Vitamin D deficiency has been directly linked to CVD risk in the Framingham Heart Study cohort[154] and to CVD risk factors in the Multi-Ethnic Study of Atherosclerosis (MESA) cohort.[155] More recently, a RCT component to the WHI randomized controlled trial investigated the effect of vitamin D supplementation versus placebo on CVD risk among 36,282 postmenopausal women aged 50–79; after 7 years of follow-up, calcium plus vitamin D supplementation had no detectable effect CVD risk.[156] The null findings could indeed indicate vitamin D does not affect pathways leading to CVD outcomes; alternatively, some researchers have speculated that:[157,158]

- the vitamin D dose provided in WHI (400 IU/day) was not sufficient.
- WHI cohort was not vitamin D deficient at study entry.
- Vitamin D intake among controls was high, diluting any effects.

Given the uncertainty until additional research is available, vitamin D supplementation is not recommended for CVD prevention.[40]

Barriers to CVD Prevention in Women
Sex Bias in Medical Management

Gender differences in management of patients with CVD could contribute to disparities in CVD prevention and treatment among men compared with women. Survey and clinical studies suggest physicians may be more likely to categorize women at lower CVD risk compared to men with similar risk profiles. Recent research conducted among medical students, residents, internists, and family physicians found that identical CHD symptoms presented in the context of a stressful life event were more likely to be identified as psychogenic in origin in female versus male patients resulting in lower CHD diagnosis and referrals to cardiologist for female patients.[159,160]

Although differential risk assessment may predict medical management by gender, multiple factors other than gender alone may contribute. For example, women are older at the onset of CVD and have been shown to have less severe obstructive coronary artery disease compared to men.[161,162] Although research conducted in the United States and abroad suggests women with clinical signs of CVD, such as angina, may be less likely to be referred to coronary intervention or to receive preventive treatment compared to men even after accounting for differences in risk factors.[163–170] Much of the research highlighting gender differences in CVD evaluation, referral and treatment was conducted 10 or more years ago; there is a need for follow-up evaluation to determine whether these gender differences persist today.[161]

Women's Knowledge and Awareness about CVD

Since 1997, the American Heart Association has conducted national surveys with representative sample of women aged 25 years and older to assess knowledge and awareness of CVD.[171] Increasing awareness about CHD being the leading cause of death has been noted since 1997; however, awareness remains at only 54% and is significantly lower among black and Hispanic women compared to white women.[171] Since knowledge is a known antecedent to preventive action, lack of awareness contributes to overall CHD risk and disparities in risk by race/ethnicity.[171,172]

Barriers to CVD prevention most commonly reported by American women include family obligations, confusion in the media, and a belief that God or a higher power determines health.[172] In addition, when asked whose health is most important to them, women often note their child or a spouse/partner.[172] In a recent American Heart Association national survey (2009), women under age 50 years were more likely than older women to report barriers to living a "heart-healthy lifestyle" including their perception of being at low risk for heart disease, being too stressed, and/or lacking time to take care of themselves.[171]

Low Enrollment in Clinical Trials

In the past women of childbearing age were excluded from clinical drug trials and several major CVD studies were conducted exclusively among men; however, this policy was changed by the National Institutes of Health as federal studies are required to include a balance of participants by gender unless the condition occurs only in men or only in women.[173] The past practices created a shortage and delay of evidence-based practices for clinical guidance of CVD care of women. Recent guidelines for cardiovascular disease prevention in women are based on many studies in which women represented only one-third of the study sample.[174,175] Although participation of women in clinical trials has increased during the past several decades, the proportion of women in clinical trials remains much lower than the proportion of women in the diseased population,[175] with the exception of trials sponsored by the National Heart Lung Blood Institute in which rates of enrollment of women have been proportional to sex-specific prevalence of CHD since the mid 1980s.[176]

Symptoms of CVD in Women

Clinical presentation of CHD differs between men and women; CHD in women commonly includes symptoms such as back pain, fatigue, indigestion, nausea, shortness of breath, and weakness, which are not frequently reported by men who generally present with severe chest pain.[178] Differing symptom presentation has been documented as a reason for gender differences resulting in treatment delay potentially associated with gender disparities in hospitalization and treatment outcomes.[179]

Summary

This chapter provides a brief overview of CVD morbidity and mortality, risk factors, current issues, and some barriers to prevention of risk and death among women. Onset of heart disease occurs at older ages among women compared to men although CVD is the leading cause of death of women and men. American and international data consistently identified personal behaviors, inherited risks, and neighborhood and personal socioeconomic factors associated with adult heart disease that may relate to development in utero and during early childhood. Although men and women share the same major CVD risk factors, gender differences in symptom presentation have delayed recognition of disease severity and onset of treatment among women. Changes associated with menopause, questionable effect on heart disease associated with use of hormones for relief of menopausal symptoms, and emotional burdens of caregiving responsibilities added to the uncertainty of knowledge among women about heart disease risk have contributed to disparities by gender, race/ethnicity, and economic status.

Discussion Questions

1. How do the major causes of death compare among women and men in the United States? Describe geographic differences and potential explanations for these data.
2. Describe disparities is disease outcomes by race/ethnicity, economic status, residential setting, and personal behaviors.
3. Name several modifiable and nonmodifiable risk factors for cardiovascular disease.
4. How might job-related stress affect heart disease risk differently among women and men?
5. Does diet influence risk? What are possible explanations for conflicting results?
6. Why are randomized trials valuable in comparison to case-control and cohort studies for studying heart disease?

References

1. *Morbidity & Mortality: 2009 Chart Book on Cardiovascular, Lung, and Blood Diseases*. Rockville, MD: National Institutes of Health. National Heart, Lung, and Blood Institute; 2009.
2. Roger VL, Go AS, Lloyd-Jones DM, et al. Heart disease and stroke statistics 2011 update: A report from the American Heart Association. *Circulation*. 2011;123;e18–e209.
3. Vaccarino V, Badimon L, Corti R, et al. Ischaemic heart disease in women: are there sex differences in pathophysiology and risk factors? *Cardiovasc Res.* 2011;90:9–17.
4. Centers for Disease Control and Prevention. About heart disease. Coronary artery disease. www.cdc.gov/heartdisease/coronary_ad.htm. (Accessed)June 10, 2011.
5. Barker DJP, Osmond C, Forsen TJ, et al. Trajectories of growth among children who have coronary events as adults. *N Engl J Med.* 2005;353:1802–1809.
6. Raitakari OT, Juonala M, Kähönen M et al. Cardiovascular risk factors in childhood and carotid artery intima-media thickness in adulthood: the Cardiovascular Risk in Young Finns Study. *JAMA.* 2003;290:2277–2283.
7. Olsen RE. Atherogenesis in children: implications for the prevention of atherosclerosis. *Adv Pediatr.* 2000;47:55–78.
8. Seshadri S, Beiser A, Kelly-Hayes M, et al. The lifetime risk of stroke. Estimates from the Framingham study. *Stroke.* 2006;37:345–350.
9. Ross R. Atherosclerosis—an inflammatory disease. *N Eng J Med.* 1999;340:115–126.
10. Linton MF, Fazio S. Macrophages, inflammation, and atherosclerosis. *Int J Obes Relat Metab Disord,* 2003;27(suppl 3):S35–S40.
11. Stary HC. Natural history and histological classification of atherosclerotic lesions: an update. *Arterioscler Thromb Vasc Biol.* 2000;20:1177–1178.
12. Richardson PD. Biomechanics of plaque: progress, problems, and new frontiers. *Ann Biomed Eng.* 2002;30:524–536.
13. Stary HC, Chandler AB, Dinsmore RE, et al. A definition of advanced types of atherosclerotic lesions and a histological classification of atherosclerosis. A report from the Committee on Vascular Lesions of the Council on Arteriosclerosis, American Heart Association. *Circulation.* 1995;92:1355–1374.
14. American Heart Association. Atherosclerosis. http://www.heart.org/HEARTORG/Conditions/Cholesterol/WhyCholesterolMatters/Atherosclerosis_UCM_305564_Article.jsp. Accessed August 26, 2012.
15. Kumar V, et al. *Basic Pathology.* 5th ed. Philadelphia, W.B. Saunders Co.; 1992.
16. American Heart Association. What is high blood pressure? www.heart.org/HEARTORG/Conditions/HighBloodPressure/AboutHighBloodPressure/What-is-High-Blood-Pressure_UCM_301759_Article.jsp. Accessed February 15, 2011.
17. Keenan NL, Rosenforf KA. Prevalence of hypertension and controlled hypertension—United States, 2005–2008. *MMWR Surveill Summ.* 2011;60(01 suppl)94–97.
18. National Heart Lung and Blood Institute. What is high blood pressure? Diseases and conditions index. www.nhlbi.nih.gov/health/dci/Diseases/Hbp/HBP_WhatIs.html. Accessed February 7, 2011.
19. Lloyd-Jones D, Adams RJ, Brown TM, et al. Executive summary: heart disease and stroke statistics 2010 update: a report from the American Heart Association. *Circulation.* 2010;121:948-954;121:e259.
20. Ford ES, Ajani UA, Croft JB, et al. Explaining the decrease in U.S. deaths from coronary disease, 1980–2000. *N Engl J Med.* 2007;356:2388–2398.
21. World Health Organization. *Women and Health. Today's Evidence, Tomorrow's Agenda.* Geneva, Switzerland: Author; 2009. http//whqlibdoc.who.int/publications/2009/9789241563857_eng.pdf. Accessed February 8, 2011.
22. Ezzati M, Vander Hoorn S, Lawes CM, et al. Rethinking the "diseases of affluence" paradigm: global patterns of nutritional risks in relation to economic development. *PLoS Med.* 2005;2:e133.
23. World Health Organization. The World Health Report: 2003: shaping the future. 2003. http://www.who.int/whr/2003/en/. Accessed February 14, 2011.
24. Yusuf S, Reddy KS, Ôunpuu S, Anand S. Global burden of cardiovascular diseases. Part I: general considerations, the epidemiologic transition, risk factors, and impact of urbanization. *Circulation.* 2001;104;2746–2753.
25. Reddy KS, Yusuf S. Emerging epidemic of cardiovascular disease in developing countries. *Circulation.* 1998;97:596–601.
26. Yusuf S, Reddy S, Ôunpuu S, Anand S. Global burden of cardiovascular diseases. Part II. Variations in cardiovascular disease by specific ethnic groups and geographic regions and prevention strategies. *Circulation.* 2001;104:2855–2864.
27. Wong ND, Black HR, Gardin JM. *Preventive Cardiology: A Practical Approach.* 2nd ed. New York: McGraw-Hill; 2005.
28. Yusuf S, Hawken S, Ounpuu S, et al. Effect of potentially modifiable risk factors associated with myocardial infarction in 52 countries (the INTERHEART study): case control study. *Lancet.* 2004;364:937–952.
29. Stampfer MJ, Hu FB, Manson JE, et al. Primary prevention of coronary heart disease in women through diet and lifestyle. *N Engl J Med.* 2000;343:16–22.
30. Mendis S. The contribution of the Framingham Heart Study to the prevention of cardiovascular disease: a global perspective. *Prog Cardiovasc Dis.* 2010;53:10–14.
31. National Cholesterol Education Program (NCEP) Expert Panel on Detection, Evaluation, and Treatment of High Blood Cholesterol in Adults (Adult Treatment Panel III). Third Report of the National Cholesterol Education Program (NCEP) Expert Panel on Detection, Evaluation, and Treatment of High Blood Cholesterol in Adults (Adult Treatment Panel III) final report. Circulation. 2002;106:3143–3421. *JAMA.* 2003;289:2560–2572.
32. Lloyd-Jones DM, Nam BH, D'Agostino RB Sr, Levy D, Murabito JM, et al. Parental cardiovascular disease as a risk factor for cardiovascular disease in middle-aged adults: a prospective study of parents and offspring. *JAMA.* 2004;291:2204–2211.
33. Mosca L, Mochari H, Liao M, et al. A novel family-based intervention trial to improve heart health (FIT Heart): results of a randomized controlled trial. *Circ Cardiovasc Qual Outcomes.* 2008;1:98–106.
34. Wood DA, Kotseva K, Connolly S, et al. EUROACTION Study Group. Nurse-coordinated multidisciplinary, family-based cardiovascular disease prevention programme (EUROACTION) for patients with coronary heart disease and asymptomatic individuals at high risk of cardiovascular disease: a paired, cluster-randomized controlled trial. *Lancet.* 2008;371:1999–2012.
35. American Heart Association. Risk factors and coronary heart disease. http://www.heart.org/HEARTORG/Conditions/More/MyHeartandStrokeNews/Coronary-Artery-Disease—The-ABCs-of-CAD_UCM_436416_Article.jsp. Accessed August 26, 2012.
36. Taylor AL, Bellumkonda L. Minority women and cardiovascular disease. In: Ferdinand KC, Armani A, eds. *Contemporary Cardiology: Cardiovascular Disease in Racial and Ethnic Minorities.* New York: Humana Press; 2009.
37. Hu D, Yu D. Epidemiology of cardiovascular disease in Asian women. *Nutr Metab Cardiovasc Dis.* 2010;20:394–404.
38. The Emerging Risk Factors Collaboration. Lipoprotein (a) concentration and the risk of coronary heart disease, stroke, and nonvascular mortality. *JAMA.* 2009;302:412–423.
39. Jousilahti P, Vartiainen E, Tuomilehto J, Puska P. Sex, age, cardiovascular risk factors, and coronary heart disease. A prospective follow-up study of 14,786 middle-aged men and women in Finland. *Circulation.* 1999;99:1165–1172.
40. Mosca L, Benjamin EJ, Berra K, et al. Effectiveness-based guidelines for the prevention of cardiovascular disease in women 2011 update: a guideline from the American Heart Association. *J Am Coll Cardiol.* 2011;57:1404–1423.
41. Jacobs DR, Melbane IL, Bangdiwaia SI, et al. High density lipoprotein cholesterol as a predictor of cardiovascular disease mortality in men and women: the follow-up study of the lipid research clinics prevalence study. *Am J Epidemiol.* 1990;131:32–47.
42. Legato MJ. Dyslipidemia, gender, and the role of high-density lipoprotein cholesterol: implications for therapy. *Am J Cardiol.* 2000;86:(suppl 1):15–18.
43. Gajula S, Reddy A, Kurukulasuriya LR, Manrique C, Lastra G, Sowers JR. Cardiovascular disease in women with diabetes. In: Tsatsoulis A, Wyckoff J, Brown, FM, eds. *Diabetes in Women: Pathophysiology and Therapy.* New York: Humana Press; 2009.
44. Kannel WB, McGee DL. Diabetes and cardiovascular disease. The Framingham Study. *JAMA,* 1979;241:2035–2038.
45. Anand SS, Islam S, Rosengren A, et al. Risk factors for myocardial infarction in women and men: insights from the INTERHEART study. *Eur Heart J.* 2008;29:932–940.
46. Shah BR, Retnakaran R, Booth GL. Increased risk of cardiovascular disease in young women following gestational diabetes mellitus. *Diabetes Care.* 2008;31:1668–1669.
47. Chobanian AV, Bakris GL, Black HR, Cushman WC, Green LA, et al; National Heart, Lung, and Blood Institute Joint National Committee on Prevention, Detection, Evaluation, and Treatment of High Blood Pressure; National High Blood Pressure Education Program Coordinating Committee. The Seventh Report of the Joint National Committee on Prevention, Detection, Evaluation, and Treatment of High Blood Pressure: the JNC 7 report. *Hypertension.* 2003;42:1206.
48. Lee LV, Foody JM. Cardiovascular disease in women. *Curr Atheroscler Rep.* 2008;10:295–302.
49. Arsenault BJ, Rana JS, Lemieux I, et al. Physical inactivity, abdominal obesity and risk of coronary heart disease in apparently healthy men and women. *Int J Obes.* 2010; 34:340–347.
50. Zhang C, Rexrode KM, van Dam RM, et al. Abdominal obesity and risk of all-cause cardiovascular and cancer mortality. Sixteen years of follow up in US women. *Circulation.* 2008;117;1658–1667.
51. Wilson PWF, D'Agostino RB, Sullivan L, Parise H, Kannel WB. Overweight and obesity and determinants of cardiovascular risk. The Framingham experience. *Arch Intern Med.* 2002;162:1867–1872.
52. Willett WC. Green A, Stampfer MJ. Relative and absolute excess risks of coronary heart disease among women who smoke cigarettes. *N Engl J Med.* 1987;317:1303–1309.
53. Kenfield SA, Wei EK, Rosner BA, et al. Burden of smoking on cause-specific mortality: application to the Nurses' Health Study. *Tob Control.* 2010;19: 248–254.
54. Manson JE, Hu FB, Rich-Edwards JW, et al. A prospective study of walking as compared with vigorous exercise in the prevention of coronary heart disease in women. *N Engl J Med.* 1999;341:650–658.
55. Keys A, Aravanis C, Van Buchem F, et al. The diet and all causes death rate in the Seven Countries Study. *Lancet.* 1982;2:58–61.
56. Keys A, Menotti A, Karvonen MJ, et al. The diet and 15-year death rate in the Seven Countries Study. *Am J Epidemiol.* 1986;124:903–915.

57. Kromhout D, Menotti A, Bloemberg B, et al. Dietary saturated and trans fatty acids and cholesterol and 25-year mortality from coronary heart disease: The Seven Countries Study. *Prev Med.* 1995;24:308–315.

58. Menotti A, Kromhout D, Blackburn H, et al. Food intake patterns and 25-year mortality from coronary heart disease: cross cultural correlations in the Seven Countries Study. *Eur J Epidemiol.* 1999;15:507–515.

59. Ernst ND, Sempos CT, Briefel RR, Clark MB. Consistency between US dietary fat intake and serum cholesterol concentrations: the National Health and Nutrition Examination Surveys. *Am J Clin Nutr.* 1997;66:965S–972S.

60. Achievements in public health, 1990–1999: decline in deaths from heart disease and stroke—United States, 1990–1999. *MMWR Morb Mortal Wkly Rep.* August 6, 1999;48:649–656.

61. Wright JD, Wang CY, Kennedy-Stephenson J, Ervin RB. Dietary intake of ten key nutrients for public health, United States: 1999–2000. Advance data from vital and health statistics; no. 334. Hyattsville, MD: National Center for Health Statistics; 2003.

62. Heidemann C, Schulze MB, Franco OH, et al. Dietary patterns and risk of mortality from cardiovascular disease, cancer, and all causes in a prospective cohort of women. *Circulation.* 2008;118:230–237.

63. Turpeinen O, Karvonen MJ, Pekkarinen M, et al. Dietary prevention of coronary heart disease: the Finnish Mental Hospital Study. *Int J Epidemiol.* 1979;8:99–118.

64. Leren P. The Oslo diet-heart study. Eleven-year report. *Circulation.* 1970;42:935–942.

65. De Lorgeril M, Selan P, Martin J, et al. Mediterranean Diet, traditional risk factors, and the rate of cardiovascular complications after myocardial infarction. Final report of the Lyon Diet Heart Study. *Circulation.* 1999;99:779–785.

66. Kris-Etherton P, Eckel RH, Howard BV, et al. Lyon Diet Heart Study. Benefits of a Mediterranean-style, national cholesterol education program/American Heart Association Step I dietary pattern on cardiovascular disease. *Circulation.* 2001;103:1823–1825.

67. Howard BV, Van Horn L, Hsia J, et al. Low-fat dietary pattern and risk of cardiovascular disease: the Women's Health Initiative Randomized Controlled Dietary Modification Trial. *JAMA.* 2006;295:655–666.

68. Mozaffarian D. Low-fat diet and cardiovascular disease. *JAMA.* 2006;296:279–280.

69. Hoekstra T, Beulens JW, van der Schouw YT. Cardiovascular disease prevention in women: impact of dietary interventions. *Maturitas.* 2009;63:20–27.

70. Lichtenstein AH, Appel LJ, Brands M, et al. Diet and lifestyle recommendations revision 2006: a scientific statement from the American Heart Association Nutrition Committee. *Circulation.* 2006;114;82–96.

71. Libby P. Inflammation and cardiovascular disease mechanisms. *Am J Clin Nutr.* 2006;83:456S–4560S.

72. Ridker PM, Hennekens CH, Buring JE, et al. C-reactive protein and other markers of inflammation in the prediction of cardiovascular disease in women. *N Eng J Med.* 2000;342:836–843.

73. Danesh J, Whincup P, Walker M, et al. Low grade inflammation and coronary heart disease: prospective study and updated meta-analyses. *BMJ.* 2000;321:199–204.

74. Franks PW. Obesity, inflammatory markers and cardiovascular disease: distinguishing causality from confounding. *J Hum Hyperten.* 2006;20:837–840.

75. Hansson GK. Inflammation, atherosclerosis and coronary artery disease. *N Engl J Med.* 2005;352:1685–1695.

76. Everson-Rose SA, Lewis TT. Psychosocial factors and cardiovascular diseases. *Ann Rev Public Health.* 2005;26:469–500.

77. Wulsin LR, Singal BM. Do depressive symptoms increase the risk for the onset of coronary disease? A systematic quantitative review. *Psychosom Med.* 2003;65:201–210.

78. Rugulies R. Depression as a predictor for coronary heart disease: a review and meta-analysis. *Am J Prev Med.* 2002;23:51–61.

79. Rosengren A, Hawken S, Ounpuu S, et al. Association of psychosocial risk factors with risk of acute myocardial infarction in 11119 cases and 13648 controls from 52 countries (the INTERHEART study): case-control study. *Lancet.* 2004;364:953–962.

80. Everson SA, Roberts RE. Depressive symptoms and increased risk of stroke mortality over a 29-year period. *Arch Intern Med.* 1998;158:1133–1138.

81. Jonas BS, Mussolino ME. Symptoms of depression as a prospective risk factor for stroke. *Psychosom Med.* 2000;62:463–471.

82. Ohira T, Iso H Satoh S, et al. Prospective study of depressive symptoms and risk of stroke among Japanese. *Stroke.* 2001;32:903–908.

83. Ferketich AK, Schwartzbaum JA, Frid DJ, Moeschberger ML. Depression as an antecedent to heart disease among women and men in the NHANES I Study. *Arch Intern Med.* 2000;160:1261–1268.

84. Wassertheil-Smoller S, Shumaker S, Ockene J, et al. Depression and cardiovascular sequelae in postmenopausal women. The Women's Health Initiative (WHI) *Arch Intern Med.* 2004;164:289–298.

85. Karasek RA. Job demands, job decision latitude, and mental strain: implications for job redesign. *Adm Sci Q.* 1979;24:285–308.

86. Karasek R, Theorell T. *Healthy Work: Stress, Productivity and the Reconstruction of Working Life.* New York: Basic Books, Inc.; 1990.

87. Schnall PL, Landsbergis PA, Baker D. Job strain and cardiovascular disease. *Annu Rev Public Health.* 1994;15:381–411.

88. Hellersted WL, Jeffery RW. The associations of job strain and health behaviors in men and women. *Int J Epidemiol.*1997;26:575–583.

89. Eaker ED, Sullivan LM, Kelly-Hayes M, et al. Does job strain increase the risk of coronary heart disease or death in men and women? The Framingham Offspring Study. *Am J Epidemiol.* 2004;159:950–958.

90. Conen D, Chae CU, Glynn RJ, et al. Risk of death and cardiovascular events in initially healthy women with new-onset atrial fibrillation. *JAMA.* 2011:305:2080–2087.

91. Kivimaki M, Theorell T, Westerlund H, et al. Job strain and ischemic disease: does the inclusion of older employees in the cohort dilute the association? The WOLF Stockholm Study. *J Epidemiol Community Health.* 2008;62:372–374.

92. Kivimaki M, Head J, Ferie JE, et al. Why is evidence of job strain and coronary heart disease mixed? An illustration of measurement challenges in the Whitehall II Study. *Psychosom Med.* 2006;68:398–401.

93. Aboa-Eboule C, Brisson C, Maunsell E, et al. Job strain and risk of acute recurrent coronary heart disease events. *JAMA.* 2007;298:1652–1660.

94. National Alliance for Caregiving and AARP. Caregiving in the U.S., 2009. http://www.caregiving.org/data/Caregiving_in_the_US_2009_full_report.pdf. Accessed February 17, 2011.

95. Lee S, Colditz GA, Berkman LF, Kawachi I. Caregiving and risk of coronary heart disease in US women. *Am J Prev Med.* 2003;24:113–119.

96. Haley WE, Roth DL, Howard G, Safford MM. Caregiving strain and estimated risk for stroke and coronary heart disease among spouse caregivers. Differential effects by race and sex. *Stroke.* 2010;41:331–336.

97. Lee S, Colditz FA, Berkman LF, et al. Caregiving to children and grandchildren and risk of coronary heart disease in women. *Am J Public Health.* 2003;93:1939–1944.

98. Mosca L, Mochari-Greenberger H, Aggarwal B, et al. Patterns of caregiving among patients hospitalized with cardiovascular disease. *J Cardiovasc Nurs.* 2011;26(4):305–311.

99. Rutledge T, Reis SE, Olson M et al. Social networks are associated with lower mortality rates among women with suspected coronary disease: The National Heart, Lung, and Blood Institute-Sponsored Women's Ischemia Syndrome Evaluation Study. *Psychosom Med.* 2004;66:882–888.

100. Cooke BD, Rossman MM, McCubbin HI, Patterson JM. Examining the definition and assessment of social support: a resource for individuals and families. *Family Relations.* 1988;37:211–216.

101. Berkman LF, Leo-Summers L, Horwitz RI. Emotional support and survival after myocardial infarction. A prospective, population-based study of the elderly. *Ann Intern Med.* 1992;117:1003–1009.

102. Krumholz HM, Butler J, Miller J et al. Prognostic importance of emotional support for elderly patients hospitalized with heart failure. *Circulation.* 1998;97:958–964.

103. Wang HW, Mittleman MA, Orth-Gomer K. Influence of social support on progression of coronary artery disease in women. *Soc Sci Med.* 2005;60:599–607.

104. Kuh D, Ben-Shlomo Y, Lynch J, et al. Life course epidemiology. *J Epidemiol Community Health.* 2003;57:778–783.

105. Li S, Chen W, Srinivasan SR, et al. Childhood cardiovascular risk factors and carotid vascular changes in adulthood. *JAMA.* 2003;290:2271–2276.

106. Davis PH, Dawson JD, Riley WA, et al. Carotid intimal-medial thickness is related to cardiovascular risk factors measured from childhood through middle age: The Muscatine Study. *Circulation.* 2001;104:2815–2819.

107. Barker DJ, Osmond C, Forsén TJ, et al. Trajectories of growth among children who have coronary events as adults. *N Engl J Med.* 2005;353:1802–1809.

108. Hales CN, Barker DJP, Winter PD, et al. Early growth and death from cardiovascular disease in women. *BMJ.* 1991;303:1019–1022.

109. Huxley RR, Schiell AW, Law CM. The role of size at birth and postnatal catch-up growth in determining systolic blood pressure: a systematic review of the literature. *J Hypertens.* 2000;18:815–831.

110. Lithell HO, McKeigue PM, Berglund L, et al. Relation of size at birth to non-insulin dependent diabetes and insulin concentration in men aged 50–60 years. *BMJ.* 1996;312:406–410.

111. Newsome CA, Shiell AW, Fall CH, et al. Is birthweight related to later glucose and insulin metabolism? A systematic review. *Diabetes Med.* 2003;20: 339–348.

112. Rich-Edwards JW, Kleinman K, Michels KB, et al. Longitudinal study of birth weight and adult body mass index in predicting risk of coronary heart disease and stroke in women. *BMJ.* 2005; doi:10.1136/bmj.38434.629630.E0

113. Osmond C, Kajantie E, Forsén TJ, et al. Infant growth and stroke in adult life: the Helsinki birth cohort study. *Stroke.* 2007;38:264–270.

114. Galobardes B, Lynch JW, Smith DG. Childhood socioeconomic circumstances and cause-specific mortality in adulthood: systematic review and interpretation. *Epidemiol Reviews.* 2004;26:7–21.

115. Barker DJ, Forsén TJ, Eriksson JG, et al. Growth and living conditions in childhood and hypertension in adult life: a longitudinal study. *J Hypertension.* 2002;20:1951–1956.

116. Barker DJ, Forsén TJ, Uutela A, et al. Size at birth and resilience to the effects of poor living conditions in adult life: longitudinal study. *BMJ.* 2001;323:1273–1276.

117. Galobardes B, Smith DG, Lynch JW. Systematic review of the influence of childhood socioeconomic circumstances on risk for cardiovascular disease in adulthood. *Ann Epidemiol.* 2006;16:91–104.

118. Power C, Hyppönen E, Smith GD. Socioeconomic position in childhood and early adult life and risk of mortality: a prospective study of the mothers of the 1958 British birth cohort. *Am J Public Health.* 2005;95:1396–1402.

119. Beebe-Dimmer J, Lynch JW, Turrell G, et al. Childhood and adult socioeconomic conditions and 31-year mortality risk in women. *Am J Epidemiol.* 2004;159:481–490.

120. Gliksman MD, Kawachi I, Hunter D, et al. Childhood socioeconomic status and risk of cardiovascular disease in middle aged US women: a prospective study. *J Epidemiol Community Health.* 1995;49:10–15.

121. Adler NE, Boyce T, Chesney MA, et al. Socioeconomic status and health. The challenge of the gradient. *Am Psychol.* 1994;49:15–24.

122. Marmot MG, Shipley MJ, Rose G. Inequalities in death—specific explanations of a general pattern? *Lancet.* 1984;i:1003–6.

123. Kunst AE, Groenhof F, Mackenbach JP, Health EW. Occupational class and cause specific mortality in middle aged men in 11 European countries: comparison of population based studies. EU Working Group on Socioeconomic Inequalities in Health. *BMJ.* 1998;316:1636–1642.

124. Sorlie PD, Backlund E, Keller JB. US mortality by economic, demographic, and social characteristics: the National Longitudinal Mortality Study. *Am J Public Health.* 1995;85:949–956.

125. Kennedy BP, Kawachi I, Prothrow-Stith D. Income distribution and mortality: cross sectional ecological study of the Robin Hood index in the United States. *BMJ.* 1996;312:1004–1007.

126. Lynch J, Smith GD, Harper S, et al. Is income inequality a determinant of population health? Part 2. U.S. National and regional trends in income inequality and age- and cause-specific mortality. *Milbank Q.* 2004;82:355–400.

127. Diez Roux AV. Residential environments and cardiovascular risk. *J Urban Health.* 2003;80:569–589.

128. Diez Roux AV, Merkin SS, Arnett D, et al. Neighborhood of residence and incidence of coronary heart disease. *N Engl J Med.* 2001;345:99–106.

129. Lawlor DA, Smith DG, Patel R, et al. Life-course socioeconomic position, area deprivation, and coronary heart disease: findings from the British Women's Heart and Health Study. *Am J Public Health.* 2005;95:91–97.

130. Mobley LR, Root ED, Finkelstein EA, et al. Environment, obesity, and cardiovascular disease risk in low-income women. *Am J Prev Med.* 2006;30:327–332.

131. Meinert CL. The inclusion of women in clinical trials. *Science.* 1995;269:795–796.

132. Bush TL, Barrett-Connor E, Cowan LD, et al. Cardiovascular mortality and noncontraceptive use of estrogen in women: results for the Lipid Research Clinics Program Follow-up Study. *Circulation.* 1987;75:1102–1109.

133. The Writing Group for the PEPI Trial. Effects of estrogen on heart disease risk factors in post menopausal women. *JAMA.* 1995;273:199–208.

134. Mendelsohn ME, Karas RH. The protective effects of estrogen on the cardiovascular system. *N Engl J Med.* 1999;340:1801–1811.

135. Hulley S, Grady D, Bush T, et al. Randomized trial of estrogen plus progestin for secondary prevention of coronary heart disease in postmenopausal women. Heart and Estrogen/progestin Replacement Study (HERS) Research Group. *JAMA.* 1998;280:605–613.

136. Simon JA, Hsia J, Cauley JA, et al. Postmenopausal hormone therapy and risk of stroke: the Heart and Estrogen/progestin Replacement Study (HERS). *Circulation.* 2001;103:638–642.

137. Grady D, Herrington D, Bittner V, et al. Cardiovascular disease outcomes during 6.8 years of hormone therapy. Heart and estrogen/progestin replacement study follow-up (HERS II). *JAMA.* 2002;288:49–57.

138. Nelson HD, Humphrey LL, Nygren P, et al. Postmenopausal hormone replacement therapy. *JAMA.* 2002;288:872–881.

139. Stampfer MJ, Colditz GA. Estrogen replacement therapy and coronary heart disease: a quantitative assessment of the epidemiologic evidence. *Prev Med.* 1991;20:41–63.

140. Grodstein F, Manson JE, Stampher MJ. Postmenopausal hormone use and secondary prevention of coronary events in the Nurses' Health Study a prospective observational study. *Ann Intern Med.* 2001;135:1–8.

141. Manson JE, Hsia J, Johnson KC, et al. Estrogen plus progestin and risk of coronary heart disease. *N Engl J Med.* 2003;349:523–534.

142. LaCroix AZ, Chlebowski RT, Manson JE, et al. Health outcomes after stopping conjugated equine estrogens among postmenopausal women with prior hysterectomy. A randomized controlled trial. *JAMA.* 2011;305:1305–1314.

143. Whittemore AS, McGuire V. Observational studies and randomized trials of hormone replacement therapy: what can we learn from them? *Epidemiol.* 2003;14:8–10.

144. Miller VM, Black DM, Brinton EA, et al. Using basic science to design a clinical trial: baseline characteristics of women enrolled in the Kronos Early Estrogen Prevention Study (KEEPS). *J Cardiovasc Transl Res.* 2009;2:228–239.

145. Grodstein F, Manson JE, Stampfl MJ. Hormone therapy and coronary heart disease: the role of time since menopause and age at hormone initiation. *J Womens Health.* 2006;15:35–44.

146. Harman SM, Brinton EA, Cedars M, et al. KEEPS: The Kronos Early Estrogen Prevention Study. *Climacteric.* 2005;8:3–12.

147. Kris-Etherton PM, Lichtenstein AH, Howard BV, et al. Antioxidant vitamin supplements and cardiovascular disease. *Circulation.* 2004;110:637–641.

148. Cook NR, Albert CM, Gaziano JM, et al. A randomized factorial design trial of vitamins C and E and beta carotene on the secondary prevention of cardiovascular events in women: results from the Women's Antioxidant Cardiovascular Study. *Arch Intern Med.* 2007;167:1610–1618.

149. Rimm EB, Willett WC, Hu FB, et al. Folate and vitamin B6 from diet and supplements in relation to risk of coronary heart disease among women. *JAMA.* 1998;279:359–364.

150. Boushey CJ, Beresford SA, Omenn GS, Motulsky AG. A quantitative assessment of plasma homocysteine as a risk factor for vascular disease. Probable benefits of increasing folic acid intakes. *JAMA.* 1995;274:1049–1057.

151. Albert CM, Cook NR, Gaziano JM, et al. Effect of folic acid and B vitamins on risk of cardiovascular events and total mortality among women at high risk for cardiovascular disease. A randomized trial. *JAMA.* 2008;299:2027–2036.

152. Miller ER 3rd, Juraschek S, Pastor-Barriuso R, et al. Meta-analysis of folic acid supplementation trials on risk of cardiovascular disease and risk interaction with baseline homocysteine levels. *Am J Cardiol.* 2010;106:517–527.

153. Armitage JM, Bowman L, Clarke RJ, et al. Effects of homocysteine-lowering with folic acid plus vitamin B12 vs placebo on mortality and major morbidity in myocardial infarction survivors: a randomized trial. *JAMA.* 2010;303;2486–2494.

154. Wang PJ, Pencina MJ, Booth SL, et al. Vitamin D deficiency and risk of cardiovascular disease. *Circulation.* 2008;117:503–511.

155. de Boer IH, Kestenbaum B, Shoben AB, et al. 25-hydroxyvitamin D levels inversely associate with risk for developing coronary artery calcification. *J Am Soc Nephrol.* 2009;20:1805–1812.

156. Hsia J, Heiss G, Ren H, et al. Calcium/vitamin D supplementation and cardiovascular events. *Circulation.* 2007;115:846–854.

157. Michos ED, Blumenthal RS. Vitamin D supplementation and cardiovascular disease risk. *Circulation.* 2007;115:827–828.

158. Thadhani R, Manson JE. Vitamin D for cardiovascular disease prevention in women: state of the evidence. *Curr Cardio Risk Rep.* 2010;4:216–221.

159. Chiaramonte GR, Friend R. Medical students' and residents' gender bias in the diagnosis, treatment, and interpretation of coronary heart disease symptoms. *Health Psych.* 2006;25:255–266.

160. Chiaramonte GR, Friend R, Jaffe AS, et al. Gender bias in the diagnosis, treatment, and interpretation of CHD symptoms: two experimental studies with internists and family physicians. *Abstract: Transcatheter Cardiovascular Therapeutics* (TCT) *Scientific Symposium.* New York: Cardiovascular Research Foundation; 2008.

161. Vaccarino V. Ischemic heart disease in women. Many questions, few facts. *Circ Cardiovasc Qual Outcomes.* 2010;3:111–115.

162. Lerner DJ, Kannel WB. Patterns of coronary heart disease morbidity and mortality in the sexes: a 26-year follow-up of the Framingham population. *Am Heart J.* 1986;111:383–390.

163. Daly C, Clemens F, Lopez Sendon JL, et al. Gender differences in the management and clinical outcome of stable angina. *Circulation.* 2006;113:490–498.

164. Murphy NF, Simpson CR, MacIntyre K, et al. Prevalence, incidence, primary care burden, and medical treatment of angina in Scotland: age, sex, and socioeconomic disparities: a population-based study. *Heart.* 2006;92:1047–1054.

165. Tobin JN, Wassertheil-Smoller S, Wexler JP, et al. Sex bias in considering coronary bypass surgery. *Ann Intern Med.* 1987;107:19–25.

166. Ayanian JZ, Epstein AM. Differences in the use of procedures between women and men hospitalized for coronary heart disease. *N Engl J Med.* 1991;325:221–225.

167. Steingart RM, Packer M, Hamm P, et al. Sex differences in the management of coronary artery disease. Survival and Ventricular Enlargement Investigators. *N Engl J Med.* 1991;325:226–230.

168. Shaw LJ, Miller DD, Romeis JC, et al. Gender differences in the noninvasive evaluation and management of patients with suspected coronary artery disease. *Ann Intern Med.* 1994. 120:559–566.

169. Chang AM, Mumma B, Sease KL, et al. Gender bias in cardiovascular testing persists after adjustment for presenting characteristics and cardiac risk. *Acad Emerg Med.* 2007;14:599–606.

170. Schulman KA, Berlin JA, Harless W, et al. The effect of race and sex on physician's recommendations for cardiac catheterization. *N Engl J Med.* 1999;340:618–626.

171. Mosca L, Mochari-Greenberger H, Dolor RJ, et al. Twelve year follow-up of American women's awareness of cardiovascular disease risk and barriers to heart health. *Circ Cardiovasc Qual Outcomes.* 2010;3:120–127.

172. Mosca L, Mochari H, Christian A, et al. National study of women's awareness, preventive action, and barriers to cardiovascular health. *Circulation.* 2006;113:525–534.

173. Schenck-Gustafsson K. Risk factors for cardiovascular disease in women. *Maturitas.* 2009;63:186–190.

174. Mosca L, Banka CL, Benjamin EJ, et al. Evidence-based guidelines for cardiovascular disease prevention in women: 2007 update. *Circulation.* 2007;115:1481–1501.

175. Melloni C, Berger JS, Wang TY, Gunes F, Stebbins A, et al. Representation of women in randomized clinical trials of cardiovascular disease prevention. *Circ Cardiovasc Qual Outcomes.* 2010;3:135–142.

176. Harris DJ, Douglas PS. Enrollment of women in cardiovascular clinical trials funded by the National Heart, Lung, and Blood Institute. *N Engl J Med.* 2000;343:475–480.

177. Leuzzi C, Modena MG. Coronary artery disease: clinical presentation, diagnosis, and prognosis in women. *Nutr Metab Cardiovasc Dis.* 2010:20: 426–435.

178. Shaw LJ, Bairy Merz CN, Pepine CJ, Reis SE, Bittner V, et al., for the WISE investigators. Insights from the NHLBI-sponsored Women's Ischemia Syndrome Evaluation (WISE) Study. *J Am Coll Cardiol.* 2006;47:4S–20S.

179. Lefler LL, Bondy KN. Women's delay in seeking treatment with myocardial infarction. A meta-synthesis. *J Cardiovasc Nurs.* 2004;19:251–268.

Migraine in Women

Mark W. Green, MD

Introduction

There are many forms of migraine recognized by the International Headache Society, but the most prevalent and best studied are migraine without aura and migraine with aura. Migraine is a phenotypic expression of a familial condition. Only three clear genetic profiles have yet been identified, and they are associated with familial hemiplegic migraine, a rare form of the condition.

Hormonal changes influence the attack frequency, quality, and severity of migraines. Since these span the lifetime of women, these influences will alter treatment recommendations. Several other pain conditions including irritable bowel syndrome, fibromyalgia, back pain, temporomandibular dysfunction and arthritis are disproportionately more frequent among women.

Epidemiology of Migraine

Two American migraine studies reveal a 1-year prevalence of migraine as 18% in women and 6% in men. Prior to puberty, the rate among boys outnumbers that of girls; however, after the late teens the ratio changes to reflect the 3:1 female: male ratio. The incidence rate among girls rises rapidly between menarche and reproductive years; after reaching highest incidence around age 40, the rate then declines.[1] In women ages 20–40, the incidence of migraine may reach 20% with only 6–9% of similarly aged men affected.

Despite the frequency of migraine headaches, the diagnosis rate in the United States is poor. Only half of those fulfilling all of the criteria of the International Headache Society for the diagnosis of migraine are correctly diagnosed. Of the undiagnosed migraine sufferers, 32% were diagnosed as having "tension headaches" and 42% were diagnosed as having "sinus headaches."[2] Women remaining undiagnosed experience frequent disabling attacks.[3]

Migraines have a significant impact, both personally and economically, because the condition affects people during their most productive years.[2] The World Health Organization has listed migraine as the 19th highest cause of disability, and the 12th highest in women.[4] Migraine has significant direct and indirect costs. More than two-thirds

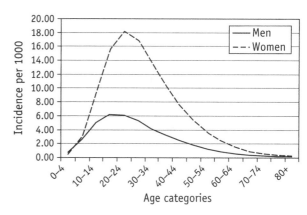

Figure 32-1 Prevalence of migraine by age and gender.

Source: Data from Stewart WF, Wood C, Reed ML, et al. Cumulative lifetime migraine incidence in women and men. Cephalalgia 2008;28:1170–1178.

of children with migraine interrupt their activities, and almost a million migraineurs between the ages of 6–18 in the United States missed 329,000 school days/month.[5] A downward socioeconomic drift is noted in migraine sufferers as their work attendance and work performance suffer.

Genetic and Environmental Risk Factors

Although most cases are likely to be genetically driven, what appears to be inherited is a low threshold for the development of attacks. The brains of migraineurs appear to be intolerant to changes, such that variations in sleep cycles, hormones, stress, meals, and other factors can trigger attacks in this population. Migrainous triggers often involve change (oversleeping and undersleeping, stress and relaxation following stress, missing meals). The tendency to avoid new and unknown situations might offer an evolutionary advantage to migraineurs (curiosity killed the cat). There are comorbidities of migraine with several psychiatric conditions; notably depression, bipolar disease, and social phobias. Depression, drug dependence, and antisocial behavior are highly associated with migraine in adolescent girls.[6]

Pathophysiology of Migraine

Assuming there could be multiple genetic determinants of migraine, the final common pathway to an attack remains to be determined. There is evidence that migraineurs possess a cerebral cortex that is hyperexcitable and more easily activated.[7] For example, when a transcranial magnetic stimulator is applied over the visual cortex of the occiput, phosphenes (sensations of light produced by mechanical or electrical stimulation) are generated at a much lower threshold in migraineurs.[8] However, after the cortex is activated, there is evidence that a wave of cortical spreading depression (CSD) is triggered. This is an electrical event, which may be initiated in various parts of the cortex and spreads anteriorly at a speed of 3–4 mm/minute. Cortical spreading depression triggers nociceptors (nerves sensing and transmitting pain) in the meninges, which are innervated by the first division of trigeminal nerve (V1).[9] The pulsatile pain of migraine is likely caused by the normal pulsations of the dura, usually painless, becoming painful in the setting of activated nociception. There is good evidence that this event underlies the auras of migraine, but may also be present without auras. Neurons are initially activated, probably accounting for the positive phenomena often noted in migraine auras, such as scintillations and tingling. As these neurons enter a refractory period after this initial stimulation, negative phenomena reflecting the absence of cortical neuronal activity such as blind spots and numbness are experienced.

Some evidence suggests that migraine may be harmful to the brain. Deep white matter lesions, suggesting infarcts, correlate with the number of attacks independent of age and comorbidities. Women who experience migraine with or without aura have an increased load of such lesions.[10] Iron deposition in the periaqueductal gray, an area that is activated during migraine, correlates with the burden of migraine. The suggestion is that iron, per se, is not the cause, but reflects free radical cellular damage occurring in this region.[11] Similar accumulations have been identified in other deep brain nuclei that are involved in pain processing as well.[12]

Clinical Presentations of Migraine

As there are many forms of migraine, there may be many presentations. In migraine with aura, visual, sensory, or motor phenomena may be noted and generally precede pain. Visual phenomena include scintillations, blind spots, and teichopsia (transient visual sensation of bright shimmering colors). The blind spots often begin as a small region of the visual field, expanding over time, often lasting 20–30 minutes or as long as an hour. Sensory complaints of tingling followed by numbness in the extremities and lips are common. In most cases there will not be an aura, although prodromal symptoms commonly occur up to a day before the attack begins and are often unrecognized as a part of the attack. Subtle indicators include yawning, mood changes such as euphoria or depression, cold extremities, food cravings, frequent urination, and many others.

Headaches in migraine attacks are not invariable, but when they occur they most commonly follow the resolution of the aura or prodrome. The pain of migraine can be pulsatile or pressure-like; it can be unilateral or bilateral. Neck pain commonly occurs, often confusing a migraine attack with a tension-type headache. The pain of migraine is accompanied by autonomic phenomena, most commonly photophobia (abnormal sensitivity to light) and phonophobia (morbid fear of loud sounds), but osmophobia (abnormal response to odor) can also occur. Nausea and occasionally vomiting may accompany the attack. Routine exertion enhances the pain. Attacks typically last 4–72 hours and may be followed by a postdromal period of fatigue and anorexia.

In the pediatric population with migraine, girls have greater frequency and longer lasting headaches than those experienced by boys. Girls also are more likely to report the pain as sharp and being posterior in the head.[13]

Treatment of Migraine

The successful management of migraine often involves both trigger management and acute treatment. Many triggers such as weather changes can be identified by the sufferer, but have no treatment implications. Hormonal triggers, if reliable, can be useful in some cases where miniprophylaxis can be offered. Since migrainous brains do poorly with change, an environmental milieu of constancy is preferable. Both undersleeping and oversleeping can trigger attacks, so the sleep schedule should not vary during the course of the week, if possible. Multiple food triggers might be identified. The most common is alcohol, but foods containing tyramine, monosodium glutamate, and many others may precede attacks. Missing meals is one of the most common food triggers, and migraineurs are encouraged to eat multiple small meals daily. Dehydration is a common trigger and adequate hydration is therefore important, particularly during warm weather. Although stress may be a trigger, relaxation following prolonged periods of stress may also stimulate a migraine.

Most migraine attacks require the use of acute medications. Although over-the-counter preparations are sometimes effective, it is essential to question whether they are blunting the attack and whether they relieve all of the symptoms of the migraine including head pain, photophobia, phonophobia, nausea, and vomiting.

High doses of nonsteroidal anti-inflammatory drugs might be sufficient to terminate an attack. As with all acute antimigraine agents, if they are administered very early in the attack, they will have greater efficacy. The most commonly recommended prescription agents for migraine are triptans. Several are currently marketed in the United States, all having similar, but not identical receptor targets, side effect profiles, and efficacies. All are contraindicated in those with cerebrovascular and cardiovascular disease and uncontrolled hypertension. Fortunately, the highest prevalence of migraine occurs in women of childbearing years, a group with a low cardiovascular risk profile. Ergots, in particular, dihydroergotamine, may be alternatives. Opioids are occasionally used in the acute management of migraine. However, these rarely terminate an attack entirely, as these medications often increase nausea and are sedating, limiting the chance for the patient to return to normal function. Furthermore, opioids can be proinflammatory, enhancing neurogenic inflammation, which can potentiate the attack. There is also evidence that opioids block the clearance of glutamine, the most powerful excitatory amino acid in the brain, preventing the resolution of cortical spreading depression.

Butalbital-containing medications are commonly employed for the acute treatment of migraine. These agents are not approved by the Food and Drug Administration (FDA) for migraine and have very little supportive data for migraine treatment. Their short duration of action coupled with a long half-life might be responsible for the high incidence of medication overuse headache caused by these drugs.

In addition, all barbiturates have a risk of enhancing depression, a common comorbidity with migraine and individuals might self-treat anxiety and panic attacks with these medications, increasing their chance of abuse. Migraineurs often recognize that early intervention with their acute agents is desirable. However, in the face of a high frequency of attacks, early treatment may not be feasible. The "migraine-specific" agents tend to be costly and medical insurance plans generally limit the amounts that can be dispensed.

The overuse of acute antimigraine agents can also precipitate a condition where the attacks become more frequent with a baseline of headache rather than freedom from pain. With "medication overuse headache," frequent use of these acute agents will worsen the condition, increasing the frequency of disabling attacks, a higher headache baseline, and decreased responsiveness to the acute treatments. The number of days these agents are administered per week is more important than the actual total numbers used as the frequency of use resulted in sustained elevated blood levels. The incidence of chronic headache in the general population is 4%;[14] and in a headache clinic population can represent 80% of patients. There is evidence that this disorder is largely limited to migraineurs. When patients who do not experience migraines take similar analgesics for pain sources other than headache, they do not appear to develop headaches de novo and do not develop chronic daily headaches.[15]

Preventive Treatments

Preventive agents may be underused.[16] If headache frequency is high, these are always appropriate. There is limited agreement about what constitutes high frequency, but a reasonable number might be around six attacks monthly. The degree of disability and the responsiveness of attacks to acute drugs should also be considered. Those successfully treated with preventive agents often show an increased responsiveness to acute medications. The most effective acute medications are vasoconstrictors, which are contraindicated in the presence of vascular disease; therefore, patients with vascular disease may require

prophylaxis even with a modest frequency of attacks. There is some suggestion that the use of such medications can modify the disease, reducing the progression of migraine, but this has not yet been proven. Long-term studies are needed to document whether the deep white matter lesions or the iron deposition in the periaqueductal gray matter are markers of migraine progression and are modified by the use of the preventive agents.

The mechanism of prophylactic antimigraine agents is uncertain. They do not show more than a 50% reduction of headaches in clinical trials. Recent research suggests that agents shown to prevent migraine also reduce cortical spreading depression in animals.[17] If this mechanism of action proves to be valuable, it will be a useful laboratory marker assisting in the future development of better preventive agents.

A limited number of preventive drugs are available with grade A clinical evidence for efficacy: propranolol, timolol, amitriptyline, divalproex, and topiramate. All take several weeks of daily administration before they begin to effectively prevent attacks; therefore, patients need to be informed of this fact or compliance suffers. Amitriptyline is a tricyclic antidepressant but its efficacy in migraine is not predicted by the presence or absence of depression because the usual doses are far lower than those used to treat depression. Divalproex and topiramate, the most recent agents to be approved by the Food and Drug Administration for migraines, have the most robust data. Divalproex is commonly associated with weight gain, which is also seen with the beta-blockers and tricyclic antidepressants. This medication is contraindicated during pregnancy as it has been shown to cause neural tube defects in the developing fetus. Topiramate is associated with weight loss, rather than weight gain, a nearly unique aspect of this agent. It can, however, cause cognitive complaints and nephrolithiasis (kidney stone formation), which may limit its utility.

Conditions that are often comorbid with migraine initially determine the choice of preventive agents. Some beta-blockers have antimigraine effects; in particular propranolol, nadolol, timolol, atenolol, metoprolol, and perhaps nebivolol. The beta-blockers might be useful in an individual with hypertension but poor choices with comorbid asthma, depression, or in athletes. Amitriptyline might be of benefit to an individual with a coexisting insomnia, but the sleep pattern in such patients is abnormal. The doses used for migraine are rarely adequate to treat depression. Furthermore, migraine is commonly comorbid with bipolar disease and antidepressants can "flip" a bipolar individual into acute mania. Divalproex is an effective mood stabilizer, which might be a better choice in such an individual. Topiramate might have some antianxiety properties. An interaction may occur with contraceptives containing estrogen, although only with doses exceeding 200 mg daily; most women with migraine are managed on 100 mg or less.[18]

Emerging data suggests that some antiepileptic agents used long term by women with a history of migraine may negatively affect bone health, in particular, affecting bone mineral density. Medications that induce cytochrome p450 are most frequently implicated. An exception is valproate, an inhibitor of that enzyme, which might also be problematic and is also one of the two antiepileptic drugs (AEDs) FDA approved for migraine prophylaxis.[19] It does not appear that topiramate, the other AED used for migraine, leads to bone disease.[20]

Some migraineurs with aura have been shown to have decreased levels of magnesium in the cerebral cortex, increasing the likelihood of cortical spreading depression. Blood magnesium levels are not reflective of brain levels. However, some migraineurs benefit from magnesium supplementation.[21]

Nonmedication Migraine Treatments

Although many nonmedication methods are employed in the prevention of migraines, only cognitive behavioral therapy, relaxation techniques, and electromyographic (EMG) biofeedback have shown evidence of efficacy.[22] It is wise to teach women these skills in advance of pregnancy if possible, as pregnant women treated with physical therapy, biofeedback, and relaxation showed 80% efficacy in reducing attacks, and improvement was maintained in 68% up to a year after delivery.[23]

Hormones in Migraine

Each menstrual cycle has a single progesterone peak and two peaks of estrogen. The second estrogen peak is somewhat coincident with the progesterone peak. Somerville showed that declining estrogen levels triggered a migraine. When the hormone decline was postponed by supplementary estradiol, the migraine was also prevented.[24] The progesterone drop coincides with the beginning of menstruation; progesterone supplements at this time postponed menstruation but not headache in this early study.[25] Therefore, with the decrease in both estrogen and progesterone late in the luteal phase of the menstrual cycle triggering migraines, the condition is linked to menstruation.

Martin charted the prevalence of migraines over the course of a menstrual cycle and showed the lowest prevalence during the midluteal interval coinciding with the highest progesterone peak.[26] Estrogen elevations decrease the number of 5-HT1 receptors, the site of action of triptans, and increase trigeminal mechanoreceptor fields. However, elevated estrogen levels also increase pain tolerance.[27] In animals, estrogen withdrawal decreases central opioid concentrations and increases the reactivity of cerebral vessels to serotonin. Low estrogen levels lead to a bradykinin-induced release of calcitonin gene-related peptide from sensory neurons and enhances neurogenic inflammation in meningeal vessels. Tryptophan hydroxylase, the rate-limiting enzyme for serotonin synthesis, is highest with the highest estrogen levels. Therefore serotonin levels cycle with the estrous cycle and serotonin drops are correlated with migraines.

Estrogen levels appear to play a role specifically in migraine with aura as elevated levels increase the likelihood of aura. Women having migraine with aura show significantly higher mean estradiol levels during a typical menstrual cycle compared to women without a history of migraine and those with migraine without aura.[28] This effect has also been noted in male to female transsexuals who are treated with high doses of estrogens: 26% had migraine and 54% had aura whereas normally only 6% of males have migraine and 20% of migraineurs have aura.[29] The effects of progestins on migraine are unpredictable. Oral progestins can prevent menstrual migraines, but injectable medroxyprogesterone and levonorgestrol implants trigger attacks of headaches, suggesting that the effect of progesterone on migraine is more complex than initially reported.[26]

Menstrual Migraine: Definitions and Management

Menarche in the United States typically begins at age 12.[30] An association of migraine and menses begins with menarche in one-third of migrainous women, and two-thirds of women with migraine report that migraines occur in association with their menses.[31] The International Headache Society defines menstrual migraine without aura occurring between 2 days before and 3 days after menses begins in two-thirds of menstrual cycles.[32] The major mechanism is presumed to be the cyclical, rapid decline of endogenous estrogen levels among susceptible women rather than sex hormone level abnormalities. Most menstrual migraines occur without aura.[33]

Many migrainous women report an increase in migraines during menstruation, but headaches may also occur at other times of the month. Although this observation is generally accurate, it is clouded by recall bias as medical illnesses may be more readily associated and recalled during menstruation. Menstrual migraine, when attacks occur only perimenstrually, is relatively uncommon, occurring in 7–14% of migraine cases.[31]

Although it is often stated that menstrual migraine is more difficult to treat, little evidence supports this in the triptan era. However, menstrual migraine attacks often appear to be longer in duration and are more likely to be severe.[34] The treatment of menstrual migraine is often the same as with other triggers, usually with triptans or nonsteroidal anti-inflammatory agents. The predictable nature of such attacks can present some therapeutic opportunities aside from the usual acute therapies of such attacks. The preemptive treatment with nonsteroidal anti-inflammatory agents (Sanses) or with triptans (off label for prevention) might be successful.[35–38] Alternatively, a brief course of corticosteroids might also prevent such attacks. Blunting the withdrawal of estrogen with estrogen supplementation during the late luteal phase is sometimes of value although small studies have not supported this therapy.

Use of Birth Control in Migraineurs

Combination oral contraceptives (OCs) block the midcycle surge of luteinizing hormone. When the prescribed pills include a placebo week characterized by declining levels of estrogen and progesterone, migraines often occur. However, high levels of estrogen have also been implicated in triggering migraines.[39] The effect of estrogen-containing contraceptives on migraine attacks is variable and unpredictable in relation to the dose of progestin in the contraceptive prescribed. OCs may induce, alter, or alleviate headaches. Among 30–35% of cases migraine frequency and severity may be improved by OC use although 18–50% of cases may experience a worsening of migraines. Since migraines can be triggered by estrogen withdrawal, in order to reduce the chance of these agents adversely affecting migraines, oral contraceptives containing low-dose estrogen are recommended. Eliminating the placebo week can also reduce the number and severity of attacks.[39] Increased estrogen levels are accompanied by migraine with aura, in particular. Estrogen-containing OCs can enhance migraine with aura as well as being associated with auras occurring without headaches (acephalic migraines).

There are several circumstances where OCs should be discontinued in migraineurs: the de novo development of daily headaches (new daily persistent headache), new onset of migraine with aura, a worsening of the frequency, severity of attacks or their refractoriness to treatment, and prolonged aura symptoms.

Migraine, Cardiovascular Disease, and Stroke

Several studies have varied conclusions, but a recent report suggested an association of migraine and cardiovascular disease only in women with aura.[40] The relationship between migraines and increased risk of ischemic stroke was recently reported among women who experienced migraine attacks weekly.[40] The risk is most pronounced in women under the age of 45, where the average risk for stroke is very low among healthy women. A meta-analysis of several studies evaluating the association of migraine and ischemic stroke, myocardial infarction, and cardiovascular death has revealed that migraine with aura conferred a greater than twofold increased risk of ischemic stroke (RR = 2.16, 95% CI = 1.31–2.39).[41]

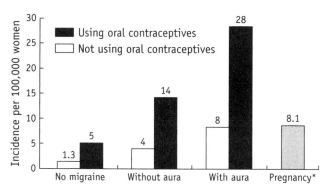

Figure 32-2 Expected incidence of ischemic stroke per 100,000 women per year aged 25–34 by oral contraceptive use.

Source: Reproduced from MacGregor EA, de Lignieres B. The place of combined oral contraceptives in contraception. Cephalalgia 2000;20: 157–163. With permission.

A more serious consideration in the use of estrogen-containing oral contraceptives by migraineurs is the increased incidence of ischemic stroke as noted in Figure 32-2. Among women who have aura with migraines and smoke cigarettes, the OR for stroke may rise above 30.[42] Progestin-only oral contraceptives do not carry this high risk of stroke but are not preferred for other reasons, such as their association with excessive bleeding and the necessity of taking the pill at the same time daily. Reported odds ratios for risk of stroke are derived from extensive meta-analyses of studies conducted over many years including old formulations of OCs with estrogen doses often substantially higher than in most currently available products; therefore, risks may be lower with newer low-dose oral contraceptives.

Pregnancy and Postpartum
In Vitro Fertilization and Migraine

The treatment with hormonal stimulation required for in vitro fertilization (IVF) may be associated with an exacerbation of migraines and may even induce attacks in nonmigrainous women. One study revealed that 27% of migraineurs and 18% of nonmigraineurs developed headaches, 81% of which were disabling during IVF treatment procedures.[43]

Impact of Migraine on Pregnancy

Significant changes in migraine frequency often accompany pregnancy and lactation; however, migraine history does not affect outcomes of pregnancy.[44] In the general population, the risk of birth defects is 3–5%, the rate is the same for migraineurs. However, women with hyperemesis gravidarum may have severe migraines with vomiting and develop hypotension and metabolic abnormalities as a consequence of prolonged emesis. There is also a comorbidity of migraine and preeclampsia; both conditions increase the risk of stroke.[45] Migraine does appear to increase the risk of preeclampsia and gestational hypertension, although the biologic link remains to be identified.[46]

Impact of Pregnancy on Migraine

Commonly, migraines improve during pregnancy; in particular during the third trimester; 58% of women with migraine had complete resolution of their attacks during pregnancy.[47] The sustained elevated estrogen levels during gestation are generally protective against migraine triggers. The Head-HUNT study suggested that this relationship occurred only in nulliparous women. Even in nonpregnant women, nulliparous pregnant women had a lower attack frequency compared to those with previous pregnancies.[48] Pain thresholds are, in general, increased with pregnancy levels of estrogens and progesterone. Beta-endorphin levels also increase with pregnancy; research suggests that opiate-active beta-endorphin may increase the ability of women to tolerate acute pain during labor.[49]

Treatment of Migraine in Pregnancy

Since 50% of pregnancies are unplanned, fetal exposure to medications is very common.[50] A World Health Organization International Survey on Drug Utilization in Pregnancy revealed that 86% of women reported medication use during pregnancy with an averaged of 2.9 prescriptions per woman without including over-the-counter and herbal preparations.[51] Clearly, it is preferable to avoid the use of all medications during pregnancy given their unknown effect on the developing fetus. Nonpharmacological approaches to treatment of migraines with ice, bed rest, fluid replacement, and biofeedback often provide relief. Milder attacks that may be self-managed might respond to various nonsteroidal anti-inflammatory agents (Category B by the Food and Drug Administration), although these are Category D in the third trimester.

However, there are circumstances where migraines are severe and disabling and treatment with medication is necessary. The Food and Drug Administration's drug labeling rules address known risks of medications during pregnancy.[52] Also, some migraine attacks are associated with vomiting and subsequent hypotension, which may have adverse effects on a developing fetus. Comorbidity has been noted of migraine with hyperemesis gravidarum (HG), with a 20-fold increase in HG in migraineurs and a twofold increase in the incidence of hyperemesis with routine migraines.[53] Intravenous chlorpromazine or prochlorperazine are generally effective in treating both the pain and vomiting and should be administered with ample fluid replacement. These agents are Category C in pregnancy as opposed to metoclopramide (Category B), so metoclopramide might be tried first, although it is a less effective antimigraine agent. Occasionally, intravenous magnesium may be of value.[54] Corticosteroids may help reduce headache recurrence following an acute therapy. Prednisone is preferred in this setting being Category B in pregnancy, as opposed to dexamethasone (Category C). Dihydroergotamine, often used in the emergency room to treat migraine, is contraindicated during pregnancy. Opioids are not clearly teratogenic, but there is always a risk of dependency in the mother and the developing fetus.

As previously mentioned, opioids are frequently not effective in migraine but may play a particular role during pregnancy when fewer options are available. Meperidine and morphine are Category B, as opposed to butorphanol, codeine, and propoxyphene, which are Category C. All become Category D during the third trimester. Combination agents with butalbital are commonly recommended during pregnancy. These are not FDA approved for migraine headache. Acetaminophen is category B and butalbital is C, but becomes category D during the third trimester.

Postpartum Management of Migraine

During pregnancy, particularly during the second and third trimesters, migraine frequency is often reduced. Following delivery when estrogen levels fall rapidly, migraines may return to the original pattern or even be more severe and debilitating. In addition, stress, sleep deprivation, and dietary changes may contribute to worsen migraine frequency and severity. In the absence of breastfeeding, the usual preventive and acute medications can be used.

Acute and Preventive Treatment with Lactation

Most nonsteroidal anti-inflammatory agents and some opioids appear to be safe during lactation, if their use is limited. Sumatriptan, the least lipophilic triptan, is compatible with lactation if the breast is pumped 2 hours following the use of this drug. Ergotamine suppresses lactation and is contraindicated with breastfeeding. Due to the complexity of this subject and the multiple agents that are used in migraine, it is important to understand the manufacturer's recommendation and FDA labeling before lactating women are treated with antimigraine drugs.

Menopause and Migraine

The menopausal transition associated with cessation of ovulation generally occurs over a 4-year period during which extreme fluctuations of sex hormones occur.[55] The natural history of migraine shows an increase in prevalence among women around age 42 declining with aging. Surgical menopause characterized by the sudden drop in circulating hormones, as opposed to natural menopause, is more commonly associated with a worsening of migraines. Two-thirds of migraineurs improve following natural menopause, but two-thirds worsen following hysterectomy when bilateral oophorectomy is also performed resulting in sudden loss of endogenous hormones. Some years after menopause low estrogen levels (<50 pg/ml) and high follicle stimulating hormone levels (>30 mIU/ml) are associated with low prevalence of migraine.[56]

Estrogen replacement therapy following menopause is not used as often as in the past since publication of the Women's Health Initiative in 2002. Alternative applications of estrogen may be used for treatment of menopausal symptoms relief including vaginal rings and percutaneous administration of estradiol.

Obesity

Although obesity is not a problem peculiar to women, excess body mass may have profoundly increase the frequency of migraine attacks.[57] Those with episodic headaches and obesity are five times more likely to develop chronic daily headaches.[58] Morbidly obese women have been shown to have a high incidence of migraine with aura, as is seen with other hyperestrogenic states. Extraovarian estrogen synthesis in adipose tissue was hypothesized to be the mechanism for this finding.[59] Hyperemesis gravidarum, which can be comorbid with migraine, is also more prevalent in women with higher body mass indices.[60]

Summary

Migraine is highly prevalent in women. This condition reflects an underlying sensitivity to headaches. The attacks in women are often influenced by fluctuating estrogen levels as migraines often coincide with premenstrual falls in estrogen, by placebo tablets taken in oral contraceptive regimens, and immediately after giving birth. During pregnancy and lactation women at risk for migraines require specialized management. Greater understanding of exposures that trigger migraines have encourage preventive modalities and have led to improvement in treatment options.

Discussion Questions

1. What is the relationship of estrogen and progesterone to migraine attacks?
2. What are the safety issues of estrogen containing oral contraceptives in migraine?
3. Under what circumstances are migraines treated with medications during pregnancy?
4. How can menstrual migraines be managed?

References

1. Stewart WF, Wood C, Reed ML, et al. Cumulative lifetime migraine incidence in women and men. *Cephalalgia.* 2008;28:1170–1178.
2. Lipton RB, Stewart WF, Diamond S, et al. Prevalence and burden of migraine in the United States: data from the American Migraine Study II. *Headache.* 2001;41:646–657.
3. Lipton RB, Diamond S, Reed M, et al. Migraine diagnosis and treatment: results from the American Migraine Study II. *Headache.* 2001;41:638–645.
4. World Health Organization. World health report 2001. http://www.who.int/whr/2001/en/index.html.
5. Robertson WC. Migraine headache: pediatric perspective. WebMD. http://www.emedicine.com/neuro/topic529.htm.
6. Marmorstein NR, Iacono WG, Markey CN. Parental psychopathology and migraine headaches among adolescent girls. *Cephalalgia.* 2009;29:38–47.
7. Welch KMA, D'Andrea G, Tepley N, et al. The concept of migraine as a state of central neuronal hyper excitability. *Headache.* 1990;8:817–828.
8. Aurora SK, Ahmad BK, Welch KMA, et al. Transcranial magnetic stimulation confirms hyper excitability of occipital cortex in migraine. *Neurology.* 1998;50:1111–1114.
9. Moskowitz M. The neurobiology of vascular head pain. *Ann Neurol.* 1984;16:157–168.
10. Kruit MC, van Buchem MA, Hofman PAM, et al. Migraine as a risk factor for subclinical brain lesions. *JAMA.* 2004;291:427–434.
11. Welch KM, Nagesh V, Aurora SK, Gelman N. Periaqueductal gray matter dysfunction in migraine: cause or the burden of illness? *Headache.* 2001;41:629–637.
12. Kruit MC, Launer LJ, Overbosch J, et al. Iron accumulation in deep brain nuclei in migraine: a population-based magnetic resonance imaging study. *Cephalalgia.* 2009:29:351–359.
13. Slater S, Crawford MJ, Kabbouche MA, et al. Effects of gender and age of paediatric headache. *Cephalalgia.* 2009;29:969–973.
14. Castillo J, Munoz P, Guitera V, Pasqual J. Epidemiology of chronic daily headache in the general population. *Headache.* 1999;39:190–196.
15. Lance J, Parkes C, Wilkinson M. Does analgesic abuse cause headaches de novo? *Headache.* 1988;38:61–62.
16. Diamond S, Bigal M, Silberstein S, et al. Patterns of diagnosis and acute and preventive treatment for migraine in the United States: results from the American Migraine Prevalence and Prevention Study. *Headache.* 2006;47:355–363.
17. Ayata C, Jin H, Kudo C, Dalkara, Moskowitz M. Suppression of cortical spreading depression in migraine prophylaxis. *Ann Neurol.* 2006;59:652–661.
18. Silberstein SD, Goadsby PJ. Migraine: Preventive treatment. *Cephalalgia.* 2002;22:491–512.
19. Sato Y, Dondo I, Ishida S et al. Decreased bone mass and increased bone turnover with valproate therapy in adults with epilepsy. *Neurology.* 2001;57: 445–449.
20. Stephen LJ, McLellan AR, Harrison JH, et al. Bone density and epileptic drugs: a case-controlled study. *Seizure.* 1999;8:339–342.
21. Piekert A, Wilimzig C, Kihne-Volland R. Prophylaxis of migraine with oral magnesium: results from a prospective, multicenter, placebo-controlled and double blind randomized study. *Cephalalgia.* 1996;16:257–263.
22. American Headache Society. US Headache Consortium Guidelines. http://www.americanheadachesociety.org/professional_resources/us_headache_consortium_guidelines/.
23. Scharff L, Marcus DA, Turk, DC. Maintenance of effects in the non-medical treatment of headaches during pregnancy. *Headache.* 1996;36: 285–290.
24. Somerville BW. The role of estradiol withdrawal in the etiology of menstrual migraine. *Neurology.* 1972;22:355–365.
25. Somerville BW. The role of progesterone in menstrual migraine. *Neurology.* 1971;21:853–859.
26. Martin V. Ovarian hormones and migraine headache: understanding mechanisms and pathogenesis—Part 2. *Headache.* 2006;46:365–386.
27. Bawson-Basoa MB, Gintzler AR. 17-beta estradiol and progesterone modulate an intrinsic opioid analgesic system. *Brain Res.*1993;601:241–245.
28. Nagel-Leiby S, Welch KMA, Grunfeld S, D'Andrea G. Ovarian steroid levels in migraine with and without aura. *Cephalalgia.* 1990;10:147–152.
29. Pringsheim T, Gooren L. Migraine prevalence in male to female transsexuals on hormone therapy. *Neurology.* 2004;63:593–594.
30. Anderson SE, Must A. Interpreting the continued decline in the average age at menarche: results from two nationally representative surveys of U.S. girls studied 10 years apart. *J Pediatr.* 2005;147:753–760.
31. Kornstein SG, Parker AJ. Menstrual migraines: Etiology, treatment, and relationship to premenstrual syndrome. *Curr Opin Obstet Gynecol.* 1997;9:154–159.
32. International Headache Society. The International Classification of Headache Disorders 2nd Ed. *Cephalalgia.* 2004;24(suppl 1):1–151.
33. Stewart WF, Lipton RB, Chee E, et al. Menstrual cycle and headache in a population sample of migraineurs. *Neurology.* 2000;55:1517–1523.
34. Granella F, Sances G, Allais E, et al. Characteristics of menstrual and non-menstrual attacks in women with menstrually related migraine referred to headache centers. *Cephalalgia.* 2004;24:707–716.
35. Newman LC, Lipton RB, Lay CL, Solomon S. A pilot study of oral sumatriptan as intermittent prophylaxis of menstruation-related migraine. *Neurology.* 1998;51:307–309.
36. Newman L, Mannix LK, Landy S, Neto W. Naratriptan as short-term prophylaxis of menstrually associated migraine: a randomized, double-blind, placebo-controlled study. *Headache.* 2001;41:248–256.
37. Silberstein SD, Elkind AH, Schreiber C, Keywood C. A randomized trial of frovatriptan for the intermittent prevention of menstrual migraine. *Neurology.* 2004;63:261–269.
38. Tuchman M. Oral zolmitriptan 2.5 mg demonstrates high efficacy and good tolerability in the prophylactic treatment of menstrual migraine headaches [abstract OR713] *Headache.* 2005;45:771–772.
39. Sulak P, Willis S, Kuehl T, et al. Headaches and oral contraceptives: Impact of eliminating the standard 7-day placebo interval. *Headache.* 2007;47:27–37.
40. Kurth T, Schürks M, Logroscino G, Buring J. Migraine frequency and risk of cardiovascular disease in women. *Neurology.* 2009;73:581–588.
41. Schürks M, Rist P, Bigal M, et al. Migraine and cardiovascular disease: a systemic review and meta-analysis. *BMJ.* 2009 Oct 27;339:b3914.
42. MacGregor EA, de Lignieres B. The place of combined oral contraceptives in contraception. *Cephalalgia.* 2000;20:157–163.
43. Amir B, Yaacov B, Guy B, et al. Headaches in women undergoing in vitro fertilization and embryo-transfer treatment. *Headache.* 2005;45:215–219.
44. Sances G, Granella F, Nappi RE, et al. Course of migraine during pregnancy and postpartum: A prospective study. *Cephalalgia.* 2003;23:197–205.
45. Adeney KL, Williams MA, Miller RS, et al. Risk of preeclampsia in relation to maternal history of migraine headaches. *J Matern Fetal Neonatal Med.* 2005;18:167–172.
46. Facchinetti F, Allais G, Nappi RE, et al. Migraine is a risk factor for hypertensive disorders in pregnancy: a prospective cohort study. *Cephalalgia.* 2009;29:286–292.
47. Estresvag JM, Zwart JA, Helde G, et al. Headache and transient focal neurological symptoms during pregnancy, a prospective cohort. *Acta Neurol Scand.* 2005;111:233–237.
48. Aegidius K, Zwart JA, Hagen K, Stovner L. The effect of pregnancy and parity on headache prevalence: The Head-HUNT study. *Headache.* 2009;49: 851–859.
49. Cahill CA. Beta-endorphin levels during pregnancy and labor: a role in pain modulation? *Nurs Res.* 1989;38:200–203.
50. Aubé M. Migraine in pregnancy. *Neurology.* 1999;53(4 suppl 1):S26–S28.
51. Yaffe SJ, ed. *Drugs in Pregnancy and Lactation.* 6th ed. Philadelphia: Lippincott, Williams & Wilkins; 2002.
52. Physicians Desk Reference 2010.
53. Heinrichs L. Linking olfaction with nausea and vomiting of pregnancy, recurrent abortion, hyperemesis gravidarum, and migraine headache. *Am J Obstet Gynecol.* 2002;186:S215–219.
54. Bigal ME, Bordini CA, Tepper SJ, Speciali JG. Intravenous magnesium sulfate in the acute treatment of migraine without aura and migraine with

aura. A randomized, double-blind, placebo-controlled study. *Cephalalgia.* 2002;22:345–353.

55. McKinlay SM. The normal menopause transition: an overview. *Maturitas.* 1996;23:137–145.

56. Wang SJ, Fuh JL, Lu SR, Huang KD, Wang PH. Migraine prevalence during menopausal transition. *Headache.* 2003;43:470–478.

57. Bigal ME, Lieberman JN, Lipton RB. Obesity and migraine: a population study. *Neurology.* 2006;66:545–550.

58. Scher AI, Stewart WF, Ricci JA, Lipton RB. Factors associated with the onset and remission of chronic daily headache in a population-based study. *Pain.* 2003;106:81–89.

59. Horev A, Wirguin I, Lantsberg L, Ifergane G. A high incidence of migraine with aura among morbidly obese women. *Headache.* 2005;45:936–938.

60. Depue RH, Bernstein L, Ross RK, et al. Hyperemesis gravidarum in relation to estradiol levels, pregnancy outcome, and other maternal factors: a seroepidemiologic study. *Am J Obstet Gynecol.* 1987;156:1137–1141.

CHAPTER 33

Epidemiology of Chronic Pain and Chronic Pain-Related Conditions

Thelma J. Mielenz, PT, PhD, OCS and Kimberly J. Alvarez, MPH

Introduction

Demographic trends and an increase in the prevalence of chronic diseases in recent years have led to a greater susceptibility for nonmalignant musculoskeletal pain.[1] Literature rarely discusses pain as a condition in and of itself; rather, it is viewed as a symptom of another condition.[2] Nonetheless, pain affects both physical and mental functioning, which greatly influences a person's quality of life. Women are disproportionally affected by pain not only because the prevalence of pain-related musculoskeletal conditions is higher among women, but also because women are more likely to suffer comorbidities that have been shown to exacerbate the pain, both in duration and severity.[3] All persons experience pain at some time during their lives. This pain can last for days or even weeks, suddenly offering brief relief, only to return again. One in four U.S. adults reports pain in at least one region of the body in any given month.[3] Furthermore, 1 in 10 state that the pain lasts a year or longer.

The direct and indirect costs of chronic pain are numerous and include physician visits for diagnosis and treatment, therapies, drugs, overall loss of productivity, and increased periods of sick leave from work. The total economic burden of chronic pain is approximately more than $215 billion U.S. dollars each year.[4] The associated costs of pain not only highlight the great financial burden on both the individual and the healthcare system, but also magnify the inadequate methods of preventing and treating chronic pain and chronic pain-related conditions. Furthermore, the great variety of interventions, from physical activity promotion to addressing psychosocial factors, suggests the enormous difficulty in treating pain effectively. A mainstay of treatment to decrease pain is oral nonsteroidal anti-inflammatory drugs (NSAIDs). There is mounting evidence that many selective NSAIDs can expose adults to adverse events such as cardiac risk, gastrointestinal bleeding, and ulcerations.[5,6]

Pain-related research has demonstrated that gender differences exist between men and women. For example, Figure 33-1 shows how women were more likely to be diagnosed with low back pain (30.2% versus 26.0%) or to report chronic joint symptoms (30.5% virus 26.5%) compared to men.[7,8] To address this issue, this chapter reviews the rapidly growing body of literature on chronic pain and chronic pain-related conditions (i.e., fibromyalgia and

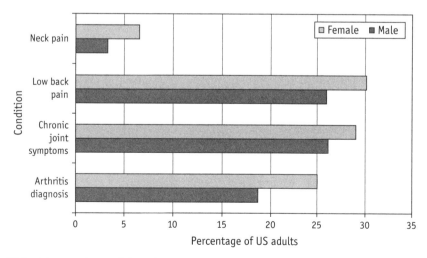

Figure 33-1   Percentage of U.S. adults reporting conditions related to pain, 2009.

Data from Pleis JR, Ward BW, Lucas JW. Summary health statistics for U.S. adults: National Health Interview Survey, 2009. National Center for Health Statistics. Vital Health Stat 10(249). 2010. http://www.cdc.gov/nchs/data/series/sr_10/sr10_249.pdf

spine pain) on women's health. The role of nonmalignant musculoskeletal pain on health are considered over the life course, focusing on the role of gender and how women are differentially affected by pain. This chapter topic is broad and far reaching. Although several topics of interest have been selected, it is inevitable that many interesting subtopics will remain unexplored (e.g., chronic headache and chronic fatigue syndrome).[9]

Background

Pain is defined as a sensory and emotional experience, continuously unpleasant, and associated with actual or potential damage to the systems of the body.[10] The duration and characteristics of pain depend on the severity of the illness or injury. Pain may be continuous or periodic, last for several minutes or several years, be sharp or dull, throbbing or piercing, limited to a small area or widespread, and eventually, tolerable or intolerable. Overall, 25.8% of adults over the age of 20 report pain lasting for 24 hours or more in a given month; 27.1% are women and 24.4% are men.[11]

Although the literature states that pain is secondary to primary insults to the body, there are several conditions that are characterized by the specific types of pain they produce. Researchers are beginning to recognize that pain is not merely a symptom but in some cases a disease in itself. Fibromyalgia and spine pain are good examples of conditions that researchers have identified and are seeking to improve understanding of risk factors and opportunities for prevention. This chapter focuses on these conditions. It has been well documented that the pain experienced with these chronic pain-related conditions is severe and persistent adversely affecting overall quality of life across all domains (Figure 33-2).[3] In addition to physical disability, pain can have important psychological consequences. For example, fibromyalgia has been documented to have a significant impact on quality of life, including increased rates of sleep disorders, anxiety,

and depression.[12] These relationships are discussed in the following sections.

Fibromyalgia

Fibromyalgia is a nonarticular rheumatic syndrome characterized by chronic and diffuse musculoskeletal pain[13] that is associated with generalized muscular pain and fatigue, loss of sleep, and stiffness.[7,13] The causes of fibromyalgia are unknown, yet researchers hypothesize that genetics and certain stressors (specifically, physical and emotional stressors) contribute to the development of this condition.[8] As a result of its unknown etiology, fibromyalgia is difficult to diagnose because several of the clinical symptoms overlap with other diseases.[8]

Diagnostic criteria for fibromyalgia include a combination of physical symptoms and features of the pain.[14] These symptoms include fatigue, difficulty thinking clearly, headaches, gastrointestinal discomfort, and numbness or tingling. Overall body pain is the defining characteristic of fibromyalgia and, therefore, the most important diagnostic criterion for medical professionals. Unfortunately, there are no specific diagnostic tests for this condition. Diagnostic procedures for fibromyalgia are distinct from other rheumatic disorders because of the use of a severity scale of symptoms including a physical examination to assess tenderness points on the body (Figure 33-3).[14] In addition, fibromyalgia may be differentiated from other conditions based on blood tests that indicate specific pain-producing conditions such as thyroid stimulating hormone.[15]

Epidemiology of Fibromyalgia

In 2009, an estimated 5 million adults reported suffering from fibromyalgia.[13] This figure is debated and has been considered a gross underestimation of the true prevalence rate because several of its symptoms may be associated with other conditions, such as chronic fatigue syndrome

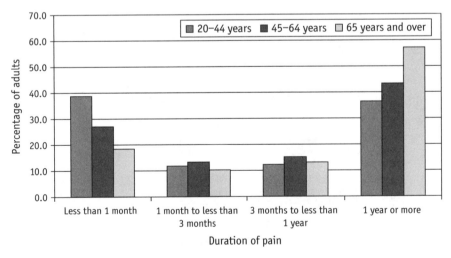

Figure 33-2 Duration of overall reported pain among adults, 2002.

Source: Data from National Center for Health Statistics Health, United States, 2006 With Chartbook on Trends in the Health of Americans Hyattsville, MD: 2006. http://www.cdc.gov/nchs/data/hus/hus06.pdf

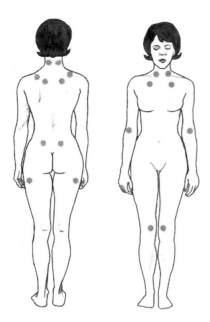

Figure 33-3 An anterior and posterior view of the "tender points" used to aid in the diagnosis of fibromyalgia.

Source: Courtesy of National Institute of Arthritis and Musculoskeletal and Skin Diseases.

and migraines.[16] Therefore, it is difficult to disentangle primary and secondary disease diagnoses and to assign symptoms to fibromyalgia especially among those who suffer from multiple comorbidities.

Prevalence studies in the United States indicate that fibromyalgia affects about 3% to 5% of adult women and about 0.5% of adult men.[13] Most individuals diagnosed with fibromyalgia are middle aged although prevalence increases with age.[8] Women are also differentially affected by fibromyalgia compared to men, in both severity and duration.[12,13]

Risk Factors of Fibromyalgia

Fibromyalgia risk factors among women include established autoimmune disorders and individuals with systemic inflammatory conditions such as lupus, rheumatoid arthritis, and ankylosing spondylitis.[13] In addition, fibromyalgia is significantly more common in women with endometriosis in the U.S. population.[17]

Interventions for Fibromyalgia

Hospitalizations, medications, and therapies for women with fibromyalgia have been increasing over the years. A woman with fibromyalgia will have approximately one hospitalization every 3 years to control pain symptoms with an average annual cost (both direct and indirect) of $5,945 per person.[8] Direct medical costs include medications, complementary and alternative therapies, and diagnostic tests. As a result of the physical consequences of the illness, women with fibromyalgia are three times more likely to develop major depression than those without the disease.[18] Therefore, medical and psychiatric comorbidities have been strong determinants of high physician use compared to functional comorbidities.[8]

Moreover, a diagnosis of fibromyalgia has been associated with low levels of physical activity although increased

activity has been shown to reduce pain and improve quality of life.[12,17,19] Specifically, recommendations include increasing physical activity and exercise for individuals with fibromyalgia to improve general fitness, physical function, and emotional well-being rather than affecting actual pain.[19] Unfortunately, published studies consistently indicate that the debilitating pain experienced by women with fibromyalgia prevent them from fulfilling the daily-recommended levels of physical activity, and as a consequence, these patients often have the highest rates of physical inactivity.[12,17,19]

Spine Pain

Spine pain, including low back and neck pain, is one of the most common medical problems today, with more than 80% of the population experiencing an episode of low back pain at some point during their lives.[10,20] Low back and neck pain are the second most common causes of disability among U.S. adults after arthritis.[7,20] As a result, women are frequently unable to work resulting in an estimated loss of 149 million days of work per year.[2,21]

Consistent with the literature, low back and neck pain are symptoms of diverse medical conditions including mechanical problems, injuries, acquired conditions, and diseases.[10] Research has identified many medical problems associated with back pain that affect women disproportionally compared to men, including various forms of arthritis, pregnancy, endometriosis, and fibromyalgia.[10]

Epidemiology of Spine Pain

Low Back Pain

Low back pain has a 1-year prevalence in approximately 15% of adults and a lifetime prevalence among more than 70% in developed countries.[22–27] The natural history of low back pain tends to be self-limiting with 70% to 80% of patients recovering by 1 month and approximately 90% returning to work after 2–3 months.[24,28,29] The small percentage (5–9%) of low back pain cases that persist for a year or longer accounts for approximately three-fourths of the overall cost.[24,30] Recurrences of low back pain are common, with a 1-year prevalence of 20% to 44% and lifetime prevalence of recurrence of approximately 85%.[24,31] Patients with low back pain seek relief not just from primary care physicians but also from specialists (e.g., orthopedists, neurologists, and rheumatologists) and other health practitioners (e.g., physical therapists and chiropractors) and account for a significant proportion of these specialists' caseloads.[29] Low back pain is a large burden to society from both direct treatment costs (~$24 billion) and indirect work loss costs (~$266 billion).[24]

Women consistently report higher percentages of low back pain, compared to men, across all age groups (Figure 33-4), as well as consequences due to low back pain, such as longer periods of sick leave from work.[4] Women of all income levels reported low back pain more often compared to men at the same income levels.[10] In addition, women of lower socioeconomic status (SES) were more likely to report low back pain compared to

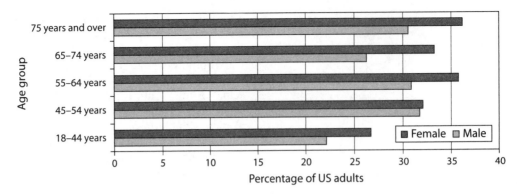

Figure 33-4 Percentage of U.S. adults reporting low back pain, 2009.

Source: Data from Pleis JR, Ward BW, Lucas JW. Summary health statistics for U.S. adults: National Health Interview Survey, 2009. National Center for Health Statistics. Vital Health Stat 10(249). 2010. http://www.cdc.gov/nchs/data/series/sr_10/sr10_249.pdf

women of higher SES.[10] Gender differences persist with age, race, and ethnicity.[3] Among adults aged 65 and older, 33% of women reported low back pain. Non-Hispanic African American women document low back pain about 30% more often than their male counterparts and Hispanic women 40% more often. Interestingly, non-Hispanic white women and men had a higher prevalence of low back pain compared to any other race/ethnic group with women having a higher prevalence than men.[3]

Neck Pain

The prevalence of neck pain in adults ranges from 30% to 50% and the lifetime prevalence is similar to low back pain at 70%.[32,33] For the majority of people, neck pain will not be disabling and will subside over time. For those who experience disabling neck pain, the 1-year prevalence in adults ranges from 2% to 11%.[32] Recurrences of neck pain are also common, with a 1- to 5-year prevalence of recurrence of 50–85%.[32] Neck pain has a point prevalence of 19%, paralleling low back pain as a large burden to society.[32–34]

Risk Factors for Spine Pain

Low Back Pain

Risk factors for low back pain are multidimensional and include several domains, such as age (a first attack of low back pain typically occurs between the ages of 30 and 40), fitness level (low back pain is more common among those who are not physically fit), race (African American women are two to three times more likely than white women to develop spondylolisthesis, which leads to low back pain), presence of other diseases (many diseases can cause or contribute to low back pain and neck pain, such as osteoarthritis, spinal stenosis, and osteoporosis), psychological state, and occupational environmental factors.[10,29]

Neck Pain

Nonmodifiable risk factors for neck pain include female gender and age (peaks in middle-aged adults and then declines).[32] Modifiable risk factors include behaviors such as not smoking and routine physical activity as well as positive mental health.[32]

Interventions for Spine Pain

Low Back Pain

Interventions for low back pain include surgery, drug therapy, and noninvasive treatments, which are summarized extensively in systematic reviews in the literature.[35] Subgrouping of low back pain patients into effective therapeutic approaches is gaining momentum and this approach may improve treatment effectiveness in the coming years.[36] Broadly speaking, effective noninvasive interventions have focused on nonspecific low back pain as a symptom and have included exercise (encompassing physical activity, cardiovascular fitness, strengthening, and stretching), multidisciplinary treatment and behavioral therapy.[37,38]

Treatment interventions for low back pain are often focused on three types of defined pain: (1) acute: <6 weeks, (2) subacute (6–12 weeks), and (3) chronic (>12 weeks).[35] For example, exercise as an intervention is somewhat effective in decreasing chronic low back pain. In subacute low back pain, graded exercise is effective and in "acute low back pain, exercise therapy is as effective as either no treatment or other conservative modalities."[35]

Neck Pain

For nonspecific neck pain, best-evidence noninvasive treatments include therapeutic exercise, manual therapies, and a focus on self-management.[32] For neck pain from a nerve root impingement, there is evidence that corticosteroid injections and decompression surgery help with short-term relief but the long-term benefit is unclear.[32] Further evidence is needed in the form of large well-executed randomized controlled trials for the treatment of chronic neck pain with and without radicular symptoms including interventions such as mechanical traction, massage, and electrotherapies.[39–41]

Chronic Pain

Chronic pain management is a multidisciplinary field affecting people of all ages, with interactions between medical, psychological, and socioeconomic factors. Close to 56 million adults (28% of the adult population) in the

United States experience chronic pain; this includes low back pain, arthritis, migraine pain, neuropathic pain, and jaw and lower-facial pain.[11] What encompasses chronic pain complaints and definitions are broad ranging and may occur in the absence of an injury[42] although chronic pain is often a symptom of a more serious condition, such as arthritis or fibromyalgia.[12] Research studies consistently document that chronic pain experienced in association with other health conditions is often more severe, longer in duration, and difficult to identify and treat, especially in women.[12,43,44]

Pain is generally divided into two distinct categories: acute and chronic. Acute pain, more commonly referred to as short-term pain, usually lasts for several days to several weeks and gradually subsides.[45] In contrast, pain is classified as chronic when duration exceeds 3 months[45] and is distinguished from acute pain by its progressive nature and difficulty in determining its cause.

Epidemiology of Chronic Pain

Chronic pain is a common phenomenon, advancing with age and differentially affecting women compared to men (10% versus 7%).[11] Chronic pain is associated with more severe mobility difficulty especially among older women. As a result, use of healthcare services among women has substantially increased over the years, especially with a rise in the use of spinal injections, surgery, and medications to treat pain symptoms.[3] For example, in 2002, 4.2% of adults reported taking a narcotic drug to alleviate pain, compared to 3.2% recorded in 1994.[10]

Gender Differences in Chronic Pain

According to 2009 data collected by the Centers for Disease Control and Prevention, the four most widely reported types of chronic pain for both men and women include migraine or severe headache, pain in the neck, pain in the lower back, and pain in the face or jaw.[11] Women are more likely than men to have experienced a higher rate of pain in all four categories. Specifically, women experience a greater rate of pain in the neck (17.5% versus 12.6%) and pain in the lower back (30.2% versus 26.0%) compared to men of the same age categories.[3] The pain experienced by women not only differs in degree of severity and duration, but direct costs of treating low back and neck pain are often greater, as women are more likely to seek treatment.[46]

Women are eight times more likely to be diagnosed with fibromyalgia and to experience a greater number of tender points on the body that correspond to pain locations compared to men.[12] An important difference by gender is that overall pain is more frequently reported in women than in men and the threshold of pain differs significantly by gender.[7]

A cross-sectional study nested in a prospective cohort completed in the Netherlands evaluated lumbar radiographs in 1,204 men and 1,615 women.[46] In women, disc space narrowing was more prevalent especially located in the lower lumbar levels whereas in men, osteophytes were more common. Disc space narrowing rather than osteophytes was reported to be more strongly associated with low back pain although this association was stronger in men (OR = 1.9; 95% CI = 1.4–2.8). Further exploration of this hypothesis may explain the differential seen in low back pain among women.

Several explanations for the disproportionate rates of chronic pain among men and women have been explored. First, several chronic pain conditions are unique to reproductive organs and also are associated with endogenous or exogenous sex hormone changes. Among women, this includes labor pains, migraines, and dysmenorrheal.[47] Second, sex differences have been reported in pain perception and responses. For example, women often report lower pain thresholds and tolerances compared to men.[48] This could be a function of the sex differences in immune responses to pain sensitivity. Finally, women are more likely to seek pain-related care compared to men.[49] Furthermore, among those who seek care for pain-related symptoms, there are a variety of diagnostic tests and treatments available, although evidence suggests men and women may be offered different tests and treatments, which could thereby influence the reporting of pain duration, severity, and recovery.[50]

Although keeping oneself healthy and preventing chronic diseases begin early in life by simple behaviors such as maintaining a healthy weight, regular physical activity, and seeking prompt medical care when ill or injured, the real challenge is creating an effective intervention post pain onset to increase quality of life among pain sufferers. Unfortunately, most pain interventions are not gender specific. This is an important issue because women suffer from different chronic pain-related conditions than men and they also experience unique symptoms and respond to treatments differently. Some studies suggest that women respond to pain interventions better than men and experience better clinical outcomes,[51] although others report no gender differences.[52] The conflicting literature warrants future research on the effectiveness of pain management and reduction among women.

Interventions for Chronic Pain

Traditionally, prevention programs to reduce pain have focused on targeting specific conditions related to causes of pain; however, with the increase in the number of individuals who experience pain over the life course and the attendant increase in medical expenditures associated with the onset of several major chronic pain causing conditions, researchers are beginning to focus on primary prevention, wellness, and promotion of healthy behavior. Researchers consistently document the health benefits of physical activity, especially among those suffering from pain. Regular exercise may prevent certain chronic conditions, reducing both pain and risk of mortality.[19] Exciting new findings are pointing to a potential strong link between chronic pain and abdominal fat in older adults, again supporting the importance of weight management in chronic pain patients.[53] Ray and colleagues found in a cross-sectional study that central obesity had a strong association with chronic pain (OR = 1.70, 95% CI = 1.05–2.75).[54]

The methods for treatment interventions for chronic pain range from therapeutic to medicinal, with recent literature suggesting a focus on reducing or eliminating psychosocial factors that predispose individuals to chronic pain.[55] Several of these interventions suggest focusing less on the actual pain than increasing the amount of meaningful activity to increase satisfaction in one's life. For example, being surrounded by a high level of social support encourages positive behaviors and provides a means for coping, which results in better quality of life.[55] Overall, interventions that focus on eliminating psychosocial risk factors for pain do so because studies consistently document a positive association between strong social support, coping behaviors, overall satisfaction, and meaning in life.[43,55–57]

More recently, the use of cognitive-behavioral therapy including relaxation, pleasurable activity scheduling, and activity pacing, has been incorporated into physical therapy.[58] The effectiveness of this treatment, coupled with an exercise program, is especially apparent among older adults.

Summary

The underlying goal of research in chronic pain and chronic pain-related conditions is to assess how pain affects quality of life and to create interventions that will alleviate and/or improve these symptoms. Pain-related research has demonstrated that differences do exist between men and women. Increasingly, studies are being refined to show that chronic pain and chronic pain-related conditions differentially affect women. To achieve this, studies of chronic pain and chronic pain-related conditions must include not only healthy women but also those who are affected by pain and chronic pain-related conditions.

There is no doubt that chronic pain affects health. Collectively, the research completed for chronic pain and chronic pain-related conditions is quite promising and shows the potential for improvements in behaviors to mitigate changes associated with chronic pain. The chronic pain field is growing rapidly, and new advances and applications for pain interventions are emerging with increasing regularity. Regular physical activity, for example, is low cost, produces positive side effects, is available to all age groups, and can have a tremendous influence on those who choose to partake in it.

Discussion Questions

1. What are the most prevalent nonmalignant musculoskeletal pain conditions affecting women?
2. Why are women more susceptible to chronic pain and chronic pain-related conditions compared to men?
3. What interventions may relieve pain?
4. What does social support provide to women with chronic pain?

References

1. Karjalainen K, Malmivaara A, van Tulder M, et al. Multidisciplinary rehabilitation for fibromyalgia and musculoskeletal pain in working age adults. *Cochrane Database Syst Rev.* 2000;(2):CD001984.
2. Stewart W, Ricci J, Chee E, Morganstein D, Lipton R. Lost productive time and cost due to common pain conditions in the US workforce. *JAMA.* 2003;290:2443–2454.
3. Centers for Disease Control and Prevention. *Health, United States, 2006 with Chartbook on Trends in the Health of Americans.* Hyattsville, MD: National Center for Health Statistics; 2006. www.cdc.gov/nchs/data/hus/hus06.pdf. Accessed March 1, 2011.
4. Leboeuf-Yde C, Fejer R, Nielsen J, et al. Consequences of spinal pain: do age and gender matter? A Danish cross-sectional population-based study of 34,902 individuals 20–71 years of age. *BMC Musculoskelet Disord.* 2011;12:39.
5. Lopez-Pintor E, Lumbreras B. Use of gastrointestinal prophylaxis in NSAID patients: a cross sectional study in community pharmacies. *Int J Clin Pharm.* 2011;33(2):155–164.
6. Matsui H, Shimokawa O, Kaneko T, et al. The pathophysiology of nonsteroidal anti-inflammatory drug (NSAID)-induced mucosal injuries in stomach and small intestine. *J Clin Biochem Nutr.* 2011;48:107–111.
7. Arthritis Foundation. Arthritis in women. 2011. http://www.arthritis.org/women.php. Accessed March 1, 2011.
8. Centers for Disease Control and Prevention. Arthritis: Fibromyalgia. 2010. http://www.cdc.gov/arthritis/basics/fibromyalgia.htm. Accessed March 1, 2011.
9. Veehof MM, Oskam MJ, Schreurs KM, Bohlmeijer ET. Acceptance-based interventions for the treatment of chronic pain: a systematic review and meta-analysis. *Pain.* 2011;152:533–542.
10. National Institute of Arthritis and Musculoskeletal and Skin Diseases. Back pain. 2010. http://www.niams.nih.gov/Health_Info/Back_Pain/default.asp. Accessed March 1, 2011.
11. Centers for Disease Control and Prevention. Key statistics from NHANES: Chronic pain. 2009. http://wwwn.cdc.gov/nchs/nhanes/bibliography/key_statistics.aspx. Accessed March 1, 2011.
12. Barsante Santos A, Schulze Burti J, Lopes JB, et al. Prevalence of fibromyalgia and chronic widespread pain in community-dwelling elderly subjects living in São Paulo, Brazil. *Maturitas.* 2010;67:251–255.
13. Arthritis Foundation. Fibromyalgia: what is it? 2011. http://www.arthritis.org/disease-center.php?disease_id=10. Accessed March 1, 2011.
14. Wolfe F, Clauw DJ, Fitzcharles M-A, et al. The American College of Rheumatology preliminary diagnositic criteria for fibromyalgia and measurement of symptom severity. *Arthritis Care Res.* 2010;62:600–610.
15. American College of Rheumatology. Fibromyalgia. 2010. http://www.rheumatology.org/practice/clinical/patients/diseases_and_conditions/fibromyalgia.asp. Accessed March 14, 2011.
16. Evans RW, Johnston JC. Migraine and medical malpractice. *Headache.* 2011;51:434–440.
17. Sinaii N, Cleary S, Ballweg et al. High rates of autoimmune and endocrine disorders, fibromyalgia, chronic fatigue syndrome and atopic diseases among women with endometriosis: a survey analysis. *Human Reprod.* 2002;17:2715–2724.
18. Adams H, Thibault P, Davidson N, et al. Depression augments activity-related pain in women but not in men with chronic musculoskeletal conditions. *Pain Res Manag.* 2008;13:236–242.
19. McBeth J, Nicholl BI, Cordingley L, et al. Chronic widespread pain predicts physical inactivity: results from the prospective EPIFUND study. *Eur J Pain.* 2010;14:972–979.
20. Freburger JK, Holmes GM, Agans RP, et al. The rising prevalence of chronic low back pain. *Arch Intern Med.* 2009;169:251–258.
21. Ricci J, Stewart W, Chee E, et al. Back pain exacerbations and lost productive time in United States workers. *Spine.* 2006;31:3052–3060.
22. van Tulder M, Koes B. Chronic low back pain. *Am Fam Physician.* 2006;74:1577–1579.
23. Andersson G. The epidemiology of spinal disorders. In: JW Frymoyer et al., eds. *The Adult Spine: Principles and Practice.* 2nd ed. New York: Raven Press; 1997:93–141.
24. Krismer M, van Tulder M. Strategies for prevention and management of musculoskeletal conditions: low back pain (non-specific). *Best Pract Res Clin Rheumatol.* 2007;21:77–91.
25. Andersson G. Low back pain. *J Rehabil Res Dev.* 1997;34:ix–x.
26. Loney P, Stratford P. The prevalence of low back pain in adults: a methodological review of the literature. *Phys Ther.* 1999;79:384–396.
27. Walker B. The prevalence of low back pain: a systematic review of the literature from 1966 to 1998. *J Spinal Disord.* 2000;13:205–217.
28. Carey T, Garrett J, Jackman A, et al. The outcomes and costs of care for acute low back pain among patients seen by primary care practitioners, chiropractors, and orthopedic surgeons. The North Carolina Back Pain Project. *N Engl J Med.* 1995;333:913–917.
29. Rubin D. Epidemiology and risk factors for spine pain. *Neurol Clin.* 2007;25:353–371.

30. Hashemi L, Webster B, Clancy E, Courtney T. Length of disability and cost of work-related musculoskeletal disorders of the upper extremity. *J Occup Environ Med*. 1998;40:261–269.

31. Anderson R. A case study in integrative medicine: alternative theories and the language of biomedicine. *J Altern Complement Med*. 1999;5:165–173.

32. Haldeman S, Carroll L, Cassidy JD. Findings from the bone and joint decade 2000 to 2010 task force on neck pain and its associated disorders. *J Occup Environ Med*. 2010;52:424–427.

33. Carlesso LC, Macdermid JC, Santaguida LP. Standardization of adverse event terminology and reporting in orthopaedic physical therapy: application to the cervical spine. *J Orthop Sports Phys Ther*. 2010;40:455–463.

34. Bovim G, Schrader H, Sand T. Neck pain in the general population. *Spine*. 1994;19:1307–1309.

35. Hayden JA, van Tulder MW, Malmivaara A, Koes BW. Exercise therapy for treatment of non-specific low back pain. *Cochrane Database Syst Rev*. 2005:CD000335.

36. Browder DA, Childs JD, Cleland JA, Fritz JM. Effectiveness of an extension-oriented treatment approach in a subgroup of subjects with low back pain: a randomized clinical trial. *Phys Ther*. 2007;87:1608–1618; discussion 1577–1609.

37. Walker BF, French SD, Grant W, Green S. A Cochrane review of combined chiropractic interventions for low-back pain. *Spine*. 2011;36:230–242.

38. van Middelkoop M, Rubinstein SM, Kuijpers T, et al. A systematic review on the effectiveness of physical and rehabilitation interventions for chronic non-specific low back pain. *Eur Spine J*. 2011;20:19–39.

39. Graham N, Gross A, Goldsmith CH, et al. Mechanical traction for neck pain with or without radiculopathy. *Cochrane Database Syst Rev*. 2008:CD006408.

40. Ezzo J, Haraldsson BG, Gross AR, et al. Massage for mechanical neck disorders: a systematic review. *Spine*. 2007;32:353–362.

41. Kroeling P, Gross A, Goldsmith CH, et al. Electrotherapy for neck pain. *Cochrane Database Syst Rev*. 2009:CD004251.

42. National Institute of Neurological Disorders and Stroke. NINDS chronic pain information page. 2011. http://www.ninds.nih.gov/disorders/chronic_pain/chronic_pain.htm. Accessed March 14, 2011.

43. Scascighini L, Toma V, Dober-Spielmann S, Sprott H. Multidisciplinary treatment for chronic pain: a systemic review of interventions and outcomes. *Rheumatology*. 2008;47:670–678.

44. Eggermont LH, Shmerling RH, Leveille SG. Tender point count, pain, and mobility in the older population: the mobilize Boston study. *J Pain*. 2010;11:62–70.

45. National Institutes of Health. Low back pain fact sheet. 2011. http://www.ninds.nih.gov/disorders/backpain/detail_backpain.htm. Accessed March 1, 2011.

46. de Schepper EI, Damen J, van Meurs JB, et al. The association between lumbar disc degeneration and low back pain: the influence of age, gender, and individual radiographic features. *Spine*. 2010;35:531–536.

47. Silberstein SD. Headache and female hormones: what you need to know. *Curr Opin Neurol*. 2001;14:323–333.

48. Riley JL, 3rd, Robinson ME, Wise EA, Myers CD, Fillingim RB. Sex differences in the perception of noxious experimental stimuli: a meta-analysis. *Pain*. 1998;74:181–187.

49. Barsky AJ, Peekna HM, Borus JF. Somatic symptom reporting in women and men. *J Gen Intern Med*. 2001;16:266–275.

50. Weisse CS, Sorum PC, Sanders KN, Syat BL. Do gender and race affect decisions about pain management? *J Gen Intern Med*. 2001;16:211–217.

51. Jensen IB, Bergstrom G, Ljungquist T, Bodin L, Nygren AL. A randomized controlled component analysis of a behavioral medicine rehabilitation program for chronic spinal pain: are the effects dependent on gender? *Pain*. 2001;91:65–78.

52. Mannion AF, Junge A, Taimela S, et al. Active therapy for chronic low back pain: part 3. Factors influencing self-rated disability and its change following therapy. *Spine*. 2001;26:920–929.

53. Somers TJ, Wren AA, Keefe FJ. Understanding chronic pain in older adults: abdominal fat is where it is at. *Pain*. 2011;152:8–9.

54. Ray L, Lipton RB, Zimmerman ME, et al. Mechanisms of association between obesity and chronic pain in the elderly. *Pain*. 2011;152:53–59.

55. Jensen MP, Moore MR, Bockow TB, et al. Pyschosocial factors and adjustment to chronic pain in persons with physical disabilities: a systemic review. *Arch Phys Med Rehabil*. 2011;92:146–160.

56. Molton IR, Graham C, Stoelb BL, Jensen MP. Current psychological approaches to the management of chronic pain. *Curr Opin Anaesthesiol*. 2007;20:485–489.

57. Dworkin RH, Turk DC, Wyrwich KW, et al. Interpreting the clinical importance of treatment outcomes in chronic pain clinical trials: IMMPACT recommendations. *J Pain*. 2008;9:105–121.

58. Beissner K, Henderson CR, Jr., Papaleontiou M, Olkhovskaya Y, Wigglesworth J, Reid MC. Physical therapists' use of cognitive-behavioral therapy for older adults with chronic pain: a nationwide survey. *Phys Ther*. 2009;89:456–469.

Osteoarthritis and Rheumatoid Arthritis

Laura Robbins, DSW

Introduction

Arthritis and rheumatic conditions are major public health concerns because of their high prevalence, costs, lifetime risk, serious complications, and risks of disabilities, all of which have a huge impact on quality of life for millions of people. More than 100 different conditions and diseases have been grouped under the term "arthritis"; all involve systemic inflammation of the joints and surrounding tissues with varying degrees of pain ranging from mild to severe. Osteoarthritis is the most common; other important forms include rheumatoid arthritis (also discussed in this chapter), fibromyalgia, and lupus.

The National Health Interview Survey (NHIS) conducted from 2007 to 2009 and reported in 2010 indicated approximately 50 million Americans aged 18 and older, about one in five adults, reported doctor-diagnosed arthritis. Arthritis is now one of the most prevalent, and costly, health conditions in the United States; 1 million additional adults were diagnosed annually during the years of the survey.[1] Age-adjusted prevalence indicates more women (25.9%) than men (18.3%) are affected.[1] Comorbid conditions including cardiovascular disease contribute to the burden of morbidity and mortality associated with these conditions.

Arthritis is more prevalent among Caucasians (25.4%) than African Americans (20.2%).[1] Previous estimates had noted Hispanics had rates far lower that whites or African Americans, although among Hispanic subgroups prevalence varied from 11.7% among Cuban Americans to 21.8% among Puerto Ricans.[2]

Prevalence of age-adjusted arthritis is almost double among obese compared to normal-weight individuals as noted in Figure 34-1; risk associated with obesity is more prevalent among women than men, and increasing weight was associated with greater likelihood of arthritis related disabilities.[1]

Although 25 million Americans were projected to be diagnosed with arthritis by 2030, considerably more cases may develop as life expectancy increases and rates of obesity continue to rise. More than 50% of cases are diagnosed after age 65, and about one-third among working-age adults.[1,3] Arthritis is the leading cause of disability and activity limitations (42.3% of women and 38.8% of men).[4] Weight loss and increased physical activity significantly reduce morbidity, lower the risk of disability, and reduce costs for comprehensive care. Work limitations due to arthritis were reported by 5.3% (6.9 million) of American adults ages 18 to 64 participating in the NHIS of 2002.[1] Among persons with arthritis, work limitations were reported by approximately 30%, or one in three affected working adults. Prevalence was highest among individuals in the lowest income bracket and lower education level.[5]

This chapter describes the two main types of arthritis: osteoarthritis and rheumatoid arthritis. These conditions manifest unique symptoms, diagnostic procedures, and treatment. Clinicians specializing in rheumatology have advanced medical knowledge of treatment options but now focus on reducing morbidity though lifestyle changes and appropriate intervention soon after diagnosis to limit development of disabilities. Such measures are crucial to avoid the crippling consequences of these devastating diseases and their impact on quality of life.

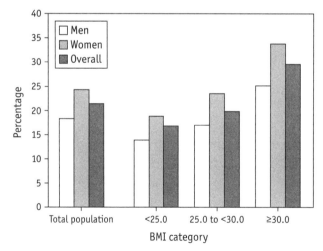

Figure 34-1 Age-adjusted* prevalence of doctor-diagnosed arthritis among adults, by gender and body mass index [BMI]** category–National Health Interview Survey, United States, 2007–2009.
Source: Reproduced from Centers for Disease Control and Prevention. *MMWR* 2010;59:1261–1264.
*Age-adjusted to the 2000 U.S. adult population, using age groups: 18–44 yrs, 45–64 yrs, and >65 yrs.
**BMI = weight [kg]/height (m2). Categorized as follows: underweight/normal [<25.0], overweight [25–29.9], obese [>30].

Osteoarthritis Prevalence

Osteoarthritis (OA) affected approximately 26.9 million adults in 2005: 14% of Americans aged 25 and older and 34% over 65.[6] The National Arthritis Data Workgroup recognized that prevalence of specific rheumatic conditions are estimates because reporting of new diagnoses is not mandated by national health agencies; therefore, the workgroup applied the frequencies from three studies conducted in defined populations to U.S. 2005 census data to calculate estimates of national prevalence rates.[6] The three studies included the Framingham Osteoarthritis Study;[7] the Johnston County Osteoarthritis Project, which included African American and white adults age 60 and older living in rural North Carolina;[8] and the National Health and Nutrition Examination Study (NHANES) III conducted from 1991 to 1994.[9] Presence of disease was assessed by radiography among 70% of the total participants. However, some adults with radiographic evidence of OA remain asymptomatic. Prevalence data are presented in Table 34-1 with differences noted by age, gender, and joint affected. Hands and knees were more frequently affected among women than men. African Americans in the NHANES and Johnson County studies were more likely than whites to have radiographic knee[6] and hip OA.[10] Data presented in Table 34-1 were assembled from several publications to provide estimated prevalence for comparisons by gender and affected joint.

The workgroup noted that osteoarthritis cases had increased to 27 million in the 10 years reflected in National Hospital Discharge Survey data for 2006 presented in Table 34-2, which indicated 773,000 hospitalizations due to OA or related disorders had occurred, including 231,000 hip replacements and 542,000 knee replacements with women affected more than men. The rate of knee replacement for those aged 65 years and older increased 46% between 2000 and 2006; the rate doubled among those aged 45–64 during the same time period.[11] The 2004 costs for knee replacements were $6.3 billion and for hip replacements $5.3 billion.[12]

Table 34-1

Prevalence of osteoarthritis diagnosed radiographically in hands, knees, and hips, by age and gender estimated from population-based studies*

Site	Age [yrs]	Source	Ref	Male	Female	Total
				Prevalence		
Hands	≥26	Framingham 2002	48	25.9	28.2	27.2
Knees	≥26	Framingham 1987	49	14.1	13.7	13.8
	≥45	Framingham 1987	49	18.6	19.3	19.2
	≥45	Johnston County OA 2007	6	24.3	30.1	27.8
	≥60	NHANES III 2007	7	31.2	42.1	37.4
Hips	≥45	Johnson County OA project 2003	50	25.7	26.9	27.0

Source: Reproduced from Lawrence RC, et al., and National Arthritis Data Workgroup. Estimates of the prevalence of arthritis and other rheumatic conditions in the United States: Part II. *Arthritis Rheum*. 2008;58:26–35.

*Estimates represent prevalence per 100 individuals age-standardized to projected 2000 census except, NHANES III which are adjusted for 1980 census.

Table 34-2

Numbers of hip and knee replacements by age and sex, 2006

Type	15–44 yrs	45–64 yrs	≥65 yrs	All Ages
Hip	13,000	92,000	126,000	231,000
Knee	11,000	204,000	328,000	542,000
	Male	**Female**	**Both**	
Hip	102,000	129,000	231,000	
Knee	199,000	344,000	542,000	

Source: Data from Buie VC, Owings MF, DeFrances CJ, Golosinskiy A. National Hospital Discharge Survey: 2006 summary. *Natl Center Health Statistics. Vital Health Stat*. 2010;13.[11]

Osteoarthritis Risk Factors

Although the etiology of OA is not completely understood, mechanical, cellular, and biomechanical factors have been associated with the condition. Risk factors differ among racial/ethnic populations in which physical activity, body habitus, and diet affect OA development as populations age. Risk is elevated following developmental abnormalities of infancy and childhood that leave joints misshapen, increasing stress on cartilage as children grow taller and heavier. These adverse growth problems of youth increase risk of OA at older ages many years later.

Genetics

Genetic predisposition is known to influence OA risk and appears to differ by joint affected; 50% of OA involving hip and hand joints appears to reflect family patterns, in contrast to OA of the knee, which is less heritable.[13] Although inherited risk for OA has been suspected with greater frequency among women than men, new large studies have confirmed a marker of genetic predisposition (GDF5 rs143383 polymorphism) specifically for knee OA with a smaller effect than previously considered.[14] Racial and ethnic diversity among study populations may be influencing the weaker associations observed, which suggests that other genetic factors remain to be identified.

Gender

Men are more often affected before age 50 in contrast to women who experience increased risk after age 50, suggesting an influence of hormonal changes associated with menopause. Although numerous studies have provided inconsistent results.[15] Women experience more hand, foot, and knee OA in contrast to men who are more frequently affected in the hip.[13] Reasons for this gender difference have not been clarified.

Hormonal Therapy

Some researchers using radiographic evidence of OA have noted lower prevalence among women who used menopausal estrogen therapy; however, a recent review of 19 studies noted inconsistent associations between postmenopausal hormone therapy and OA, with some studies indicating an adverse effect and others a protective role.[16] Some investigators have considered studies of hormone replacement potentially biased as women prescribed hormones tend to be healthier. Unfortunately, data from the randomized controlled trials (RCTs) of the Women's Health Initiative (WHI) was not presented independently but instead was merged with the observational components of the WHI; the combined data indicated a 30% increased risk of OA among hormone-exposed women, which may include biased prescribing patterns.[17]

A large cohort study from a retirement community noted 64% of the more than 1,000 women studied had used postmenopausal hormones for at least 1 year (average 14 years).[18] Age-adjusted prevalence of OA was 34.5% among women who had used hormones compared with 30.9% among those who never used the medications or used them for less than 1 year ($P = 0.02$). After adjusting for potential confounding variables including age, body mass index (BMI), smoking, and routine exercise, women who used estrogen for 1 year or longer had a slightly higher odds ratio (OR) for OA of any site (OR = 1.5, 95% CI = 1.1–2.0) and risk was increased with longer duration of estrogen use.[18] Factors associated with diverse research findings in hormone use studies may relate to prescribing patterns of estrogen with or without progestins of differing types at differing dosages and for varying durations.

Aging

Women age 70 and older in the WHI were at considerably increased risk of OA compared to younger postmenopausal women, OR = 2.79, 95% CI = 2.60–2.78.[17] Felson in his review of the extensive literature pertaining to OA risk factors noted the primary factor affecting joint vulnerability was increasing age. Vulnerability was due to loss of muscle strength and slowed response time to daily physical activity.[13] Chondrocytes, the cells in cartilage, lose their responsiveness, limiting their ability to repair normal damage to cartilage. Since people 75 and older report less pain associated with their diminished physical activity, weight-bearing activity is assumed to be necessary for OA to develop.

Bone Density and Osteoporosis

An inverse relationship between OA and osteoporosis has been reported, as high bone density has been associated with increased prevalence of hip, hand, and knee OA. Higher bone density may increase bone stiffness and facilitate cartilage damage. A longitudinal study of pre- and perimenopausal women with newly diagnosed OA indicated greater radiographic evidence of bone loss during 3 years of follow-up compared to women without OA.[19]

Women with high exposure to endogenous and exogenous estrogen have high bone mass associated with OA of the knee and hip. Estrogen exposure may slow bone changes and bone turnover reducing the risk of progression of OA. Therefore, studies indicate estrogen has a potentially conflicting role in OA as it does in other clinical conditions such as heart disease and cancer. Biomarkers of bone turnover are being studied in hopes that indicators of high risk of occurrence and progression can be identified to improve disease management.

Obesity

National survey data indicated obesity significantly increases OA of the knees especially among older women (OR = 2.80, 95% CI = 2.63–2.99).[1] Every pound of excess weight increases OA risk three- to sixfold; weight loss has been shown to lower risk and reduce symptoms among those affected. Interestingly, weight is not associated with OA of hip joints.[13] Among obese postmenopausal women OA may be aggravated by higher endogenous estrogen levels associated with aromatization of androstenedione to estrogen in adipose tissues. Researchers have questioned whether being overweight preceded or was a consequence of immobility often caused by OA. Prospective studies have now confirmed that obesity precedes and increases the likelihood of OA development.[20]

Framingham Study data indicated that OA would decrease by more than 50% if weight loss programs enabled modest declines in BMI.[20] Cartilage breakdown due to mechanical overloading of the knee and hip joints results in OA with each pound of increased weight raising the force on knees by two to three pounds.[21] Given obesity affects joints differently, Felson suggested metabolic and inflammatory factors may accompany risk associated with obesity.[13]

Race/Ethnicity

Significant differences in prevalence of OA by race/ethnicity were noted among WHI participants with African American, Hispanic, and American Indian women having higher rates than white women. Two characteristics separated the 44% of WHI participants with OA from those without the disease: being in the oldest age group (70–79) and having the highest BMI (≥ 40).[17] The combination of highest BMI and African American heritage increased risk of OA with an OR = 3.31, 95% CI = 2.79–3.91.[17] Since African American women are known to have higher bone density than women of other ethnic groups, their risk of OA is significantly increased by obesity, and they experience more disabling effects of the disease.[17]

Trauma

Regular physical activity at moderate levels protects against OA development in contrast to participation in competitive sports that may increase risk. Participation by young women in sports requiring physical contact with other players may cause trauma to joints leading to an increase in OA many years later.[21] Protective sports equipment reduces risk but cannot eliminate the damage that may occur during intense competition.

Major injuries from sports or other accidents, including fractures, may cause permanent damage to the biomechanics of joints, increasing local stresses and susceptibility to OA development. Lower limb misalignment increases stress on joints; similarly, trauma may cause misshaped joints increasing local stress and vulnerability to cartilage damage. Occupational settings that overwork the joints and fatigue muscles also increase risk of OA. Repetitive movements related to employment over many hours each workday strain joints, leaving them vulnerable to damage. Work that requires knee bending and heavy lifting predisposes men and women to OA of the knee and hip.

Nutrition

Bone formation and bone resorption (replacement of old bone tissue) occur across the life span influenced by nutrition and exercise. At younger ages bone formation exceeds bone resorption; the process is reversed after peak bone mass is reach around age 35. As people age, resorption occurs at an increasingly faster rate and among women acceleration of bone loss occurs after menopause when ovarian estrogen production declines.[22]

Researchers have suggested that continuous exposure to oxidants contributes to age-related conditions including osteoarthritis. Antioxidants provide protection against tissue injury; therefore, high dietary intake of these micronutrients may provide protection against OA. Vitamins necessary for bone health and protection against OA or disease progression include ascorbic acid or vitamin C, vitamin E, vitamin D, beta-carotene, and vitamin K.[22] Since vitamin D is essential for normal bone metabolism and differentiation of cytokine-producing lymphocytes,[19] low tissue levels of vitamin D may impede essential joint repair of day-to-day damage. This concept was supported in the Framingham study; lower vitamin D levels were associated with significantly increased risk of knee OA progression with an OR = 4.0, 95% CI = 1.4–11.6.[23] Lane et al. found high levels of vitamin D protected against incident and progressive hip OA.[24] McAlindon and colleagues noted a threefold reduction in risk of progressive radiographic evidence of OA among individuals taking large doses of vitamin C; knee pain was also reduced.[23]

Pathophysiology of OA

OA causes irreversible damage to soft tissue of joints, cartilage deterioration, and bony changes resulting in pain, stiffness, loss of motion in the affected joints, and disability. Protection of the joints from injury during daily activities is provided by muscles and tendons and other structural components. However, OA develops when injury causes the rate of cartilage degeneration to overwhelm repair mechanisms.

Mechanical environmental factors influence OA development, which are noted when anatomic differences of the knee are studied in relation to gender. Since approximately 70% of adults with knee OA are female, women's knees have been found to experience greater ligament laxity, displacement, or rotation of the tibia with respect to the femur. Therefore, women are predisposed to OA as their structural alignment between the hip and ankle is less straight and neuromuscular strength is weaker.[25]

Osteoarthritis of the hands was more frequently detected among women (26.2%) compared with men (13.4%) among the more than 1,080 participants (64% female) in the Framingham osteoarthritis study of subjects aged 71 to 100 years.[26] Hand radiographs and assessment of grip strength were performed during a biennial examination in 1992–1993. OA of the hands was more frequent among women than men; limitations were noted in grip strength, difficulty writing, and handling small objects.

Obesity aggravates the condition by affecting mobility, especially walking, and mechanical overloading. Pain leads to decreased use of the joint and lowered stimulation of cartilage cells (chondrocytes), leading to greater impaired function. Inflammation of the synovium (joint lining) caused by cartilage breakdown leads to production of cytokines and enzymes that further damage the cartilage. The knees, hips, hands, and spine are the joints most commonly affected.

Diagnosis

Diagnosis relies on a combination of clinical history, physical examination, x-rays, magnetic resonance imaging (if x-ray findings are not conclusive), blood tests to rule out other disorders, and possibly joint aspiration (Table 34-3). Regardless of specific joints with evidence of OA on x-ray, some people will have no symptoms whereas others will have severe pain, although radiologically the disease may appear mild.[13] Therefore, the correlation between structural disease and severity is limited. Pain stems from joint swelling and edema of bone marrow, presumably resulting from repeated bone trauma.[13]

Treatment

Treatment for OA is limited and usually involves pain relief (using drugs that unfortunately have severe side effects), followed by joint replacement surgery, if necessary. There is a growing feeling among rheumatologists that modification of the joint structure by physical therapy and other means is vastly underused and that obesity needs to be addressed more intensively.[27]

Nonpharmacologic Therapy

The American College of Rheumatology guidelines for the medical management of OA of the hip and knee state that nonpharmacologic measures should be the first and most important elements of treatment for OA.[28] Patient education encouraging self-management is essential with a focus on the following: weight control, good nutrition, low-impact aerobic fitness exercises for strength and flexibility training, regularly scheduled rest from joint stress, and appropriate footwear when physically active to ensure alignment of joints. Some patients may require assistive devices for ambulation and activities of daily living. Non-drug pain relief techniques using heat or cold have provided relief; other patients find massage helpful as well as transcutaneous electrical nerve stimulation (TENS). A recent report on more than 2,500 knee OA patients who are part of the ongoing Osteoarthritis Initiative trial found that those with the highest levels of physical activity also had the highest levels of function.[29]

Drug Therapy

Drug therapy for pain relief is most effective when combined with nonpharmacologic measures. Oral medications include acetaminophen (first-line therapy; no more than 4 g/day), cyclo-oxygenase 2 (COX-2)-specific inhibitors, nonacetylated salicylate, nonsteroidal anti-inflammatory drugs (NSAIDs) plus misoprostol or a proton pump inhibitor for those at risk for the upper gastrointestinal adverse side effects of NSAIDs, which include bleeding and ulcers.

Preparations applied topically may provide relief; capsaicin (hot pepper) cream and methylsalicylate applied to knees have helped some patients. Intra-articular treatment with glucocorticoids or hyaluronic acid may improve knee symptoms.

Surgical Therapy

Patients with severe pain and limitation in activities of daily living not relieved by self-management and therapy-assisted techniques may need referral to an orthopedic surgeon. Osteotomy, surgical sectioning of bone, or total joint replacement may be necessary to obtain marked pain relief and functional improvement. Knee replacement is three times more frequently performed on women although they are less likely than men to be referred for the procedure, possibly through physician bias.[30] In addition, by the time knee replacement is performed, women have worse symptoms and physical function than men and may never "catch up."[31,32]

Complementary/Alternative Therapy

Serious side effects associated with conventional OA pain control treatment may result in OA patients seeking relief through alternative medications and techniques. Framingham Study researchers noted antioxidants significantly reduced knee OA progression compared to the lowest intake, middle (OR = 0.3, 95% CI = 0.1–0.8) and highest tertiles (OR = 0.3, 95% CI = 0.1–0.6) of vitamin C intake.[33]

Table 34-3

Diagnostic methods and findings for osteoarthritis

Method	Finding
History	Pain or tenderness increased by activity and relieved by rest
	Morning stiffness and functional limitation
	Asymmetric involvement of the knee, hip, spine, or fingers
	Weather changes may affect symptoms
Physical	Crepitus, sound produced by rubbing bone against irregular cartilage surfaces
	Joint swelling with pain, stiffness, and limitation of movement
	Deformity and bony enlargement
X-rays	Osteophytes, cartilage space narrowing, and sclerosis below rib cartilage

Source: Data from Hart D, Spector T, Brown P, et al. Clinical signs of early osteoarthritis: reproducibility and relation to x-ray changes in 541 women in the general population. *Ann Rheum Dis*. 1991;50:467–470.

The role of glucosamine and/or chondroitin sulfate was assessed in a meta-analysis of current studies that reported one brand was effective in reducing the pain of moderate to severe knee OA, improving function, and slowing progression of joint space narrowing.[34] Medications from reputable manufacturers are more active compared with less costly brands, which may lack quality control. Ginger extract provided moderate benefit in pain reduction,[35] and a meta-analysis found conclusive evidence that avocado/soybean unsaponifiables (ASU), that have been widely doctor prescribed and monitored in France but not the United States, can reduce knee OA pain.[36] Oxygen radicals play a role in the destruction of connective tissue and cartilage.[19] A randomized trial in Italy found the antioxidant pcynogenol (from pine bark) reduced OA joint pain by 55%, medication use by 58%, stiffness by 53%, physical function scores by 57%, gastrointestinal complications by 63%, and pain medication use by 58% in OA patients compared with controls.[37]

The National Center for Complementary and Alternative Medicine (NCCAM) and the National Institute of Arthritis and Musculoskeletal and Skin Diseases (NIAMS) funded a randomized clinical trial of acupuncture for knee OA.[38] Among patients who received 26 weeks of true acupuncture, pain decreased 40% and function increased by almost 40% compared with patients randomized to 'sham' control procedures.[38] A form of tai chi specifically developed for OA patients was also effective in lessening pain, improving balance, and physical functioning.[39] A larger, recent study using the tai chi program of the Arthritis Foundation found that after 8 weeks, OA patients had improvements in pain, fatigue, stiffness, reach, balance, and sense of well-being.[40] A meta-analysis of studies on balneotherapy (mineral baths) noted pain may be lessened with certain minerals added such as Dead Sea salts. [41]

Prevention of OA

Exercise

Routine exercise across the life span may reduce risk of muscle weakness with aging that often results in falls among older adults, increasing risk of OA. Joint movement maintains healthy cartilage; aerobic fitness exercise including swimming, running, and race-walking are recommended. To protect against developing disabilities, patients are advised to maintain agility through range of motion exercises, stretching such as yoga, and strength training. A 14-year controlled study of the impact of aerobic exercise on musculoskeletal pain in older men and women concluded that consistent long-term exercise balanced with muscle relaxation is associated with about 25% less musculoskeletal pain than in more sedentary controls.[42]

Nutrition

A diet rich in fruits, vegetables, whole grains, beans, and essential fatty acids (particularly flaxseed and fish oils, which contain omega-3) and low in animal products to lessen acidity and potentially inflammation (i.e., the Mediterranean diet) is advised for OA patients.

Avoidance of Repetitive Movement

Repeated stressful motions at work or during sports may contribute to cartilage deterioration. Employment requiring squatting or kneeling for many hours may increase risk of OA; employers should be informed of the adverse effect of such physically demanding activities, which may subsequently cause a need for medical care for employees. The *OA Agenda* recommends that policies for prevention of joint injuries be promoted for worksites, and programs for self-management education and physical activity at the workplace should be encouraged.

Prevention has been the most recent focus for decreasing the enormous public health burden of OA. Reducing obesity is an important target, with recognition of ethnic differences.

In 2010 the Centers for Disease Control and Prevention (CDC) and the Arthritis Foundation launched *A National Public Health Agenda for Osteoarthritis* to focus public policy on disease management and preventive measures.[43] This *OA Agenda* is a "blueprint for action" that sets forth three main goals to be achieved by 2013: (1) provide all Americans who have OA with information on intervention strategies (self-management, exercise, weight management, and healthy nutrition); (2) establish supportive government and community alliances and initiatives including state programs; and (3) initiate the research needed to better understand the public health burden of OA, its risk factors, and more effective intervention strategies.

Rheumatoid Arthritis

Rheumatoid arthritis (RA) is a multisystemic disorder of unknown etiology characterized by chronic proliferative inflammation of joints accompanied by bone destruction. This autoimmune disease has a variable course and outcome affecting an estimated 1.3 million American adults in 2005 (0.6% of the adult population), a decrease from an estimated 2.1 million noted in 1995.[44] The decrease may reflect more stringent diagnostic criteria.[45,46] Incidence data are available from limited targeted studies; one of the most reliable sources for incidence of RA is available from ongoing monitoring in Olmstead County, Minnesota. A cohort of RA patients was followed from initial diagnosis through 2000 for the analysis reported by Doran and colleagues. The age at diagnosis differed by gender; incidence among 164 men was low until age 35, when a steady increase through age 85 was noted. In contrast, incidence among the 445 women rose until ages 55–64 and then declined.[45]

After having steadily declined for more than 40 years, recent data indicated rates of RA rose only among women between 1995 to 2007.[47] The prevalence of RA in each decade in Olmstead County indicated women were affected twice as frequently as men.[44] Approximately 44% of RA patients are unable to work 15 years after onset of disease.[48] Significantly increased levels of fibrinogen are detected among RA increasing their risk of death due to cardiovascular disease.[49] RA causes 22% of all deaths from arthritis and related disorders.[50]

Rheumatoid Arthritis Risk Factors

Rheumatoid arthritis is believed to develop through an interaction of multiple factors, including hormonal, dietary, microbial, environmental, and genetic–environment interaction. Progression of RA can be slowed by early diagnosis and adequate treatment to limit joint destruction; assessment of risk factors may assist in early diagnosis.

Genetic Susceptibility

Familial aggregation of RA has been recognized for many years and has been confirmed in repeated studies of multi-case families [51] including known autosomal dominant inheritance among monozygotic twins. Genetic susceptibility accounted for approximately 60% of disease among identical twin pairs with nongenetic health behaviors and environmental factors accounting for the balance; risk among twins did not vary by gender, age at diagnosis, or disease severity.[52] The major histocompatibility or human leukocyte antigens (HLA), encoded by genes located on the chromosome 6, is directly related to immune response.[51] HLA antigens have been associated with a number of immune-mediated conditions including RA. More than 30 genetic regions have been identified although only HLA genes and PTPN22 have been reported from several studies.[53] Although certain genes have been associated with the disease, not everyone who has these genes will develop RA because personal health behaviors and environmental factors contribute to risk.[54]

Fetal Origin

Life-course epidemiologic studies have identified in utero and early life exposures related to adult onset diseases. Birth weight, reflecting the fetal environment, has been studied among cases of RA reported by women enrolled in both components of the Nurses' Health Study. High birth weight, ≥ 4.54 kg vs. 3.2–3.85 kg, was associated with a twofold increased risk of RA in an adjusted multivariate model: RR = 2.0 (95% CI = 1.3–3.0) and after restriction to cases with positive rheumatoid factor.[55]

Age

Prevalence rises with age and is highest among women older than age 65 although the reported average age of patients has been increasing steadily, from 63.3 years in 1965 to 66.8 years in 1995.[29] Incidence rates range from 5 to 50 cases per 100,000 adults.[53] RA is truly a devastating disease, and early diagnosis and treatment are crucial in an attempt to slow progression and joint destruction.

Gender

Differences by gender in prevalence, age of onset, and autoantibody production have been reported;[56] hormonal and behavioral factors of women compared to men also influence susceptibility. Most RA patients are middle-aged women, usually more than 70% in any RA cohort studied.[57] Compared with men, the immune systems of women are more enhanced, increasing their susceptibility to autoimmune disease.[58] After 4 decades of declining

RA, 2005 age-adjusted incidence rates increased among women from 53.1 cases to 104 cases per 100,000, highest among women between ages 65 and 74.[45]

Oral Contraceptives

Many epidemiologic studies have noted reduced risk of RA among women who used oral contraceptives (OCs); a meta-analysis of nine studies including six case-control and three cohort studies indicated a pooled OR = 0.73 (95% CI = 0.61–0.85).[59] Incidence rates of RA among women declined following introduction of OCs and remained stable for years until recently. Some have suggested reduced doses of estrogen in current OCs may be related to the previously noted diminished risk. The suggested protective effect of OCs was questioned by other researchers reviewing the meta-analyses, although the authors agreed that OCs use prior to diagnosis reduced the severity of RA.[60]

Parity

The immune suppression of pregnancy is known to induce remission of RA and may also reduce risk of RA, as nulliparous women are at increased risk. Pregnancy-related factors were compared among newly diagnosed RA cases and controls in an American study. Among the more than 1,300 parous women, 213 developed RA (16%) compared with 23% of the 296 nulliparous women (68 cases and 228 controls). Parity was associated with significantly reduced risk (RR = 0.61, 95% CI = 0.43–0.86).[61] Risk reduction associated with pregnancy diminished with increasing years since last childbirth, although lowered risk continued for more than 10 years. Interrupted pregnancies provided no protection against RA.

Since the elevated hormones of pregnancy diminish rapidly after parturition, RA relapse is known to occur within months of childbirth among more than 60% of parous patients. A French study of RA cases was conducted to assess the effects of pregnancy and breastfeeding on the course of RA. Higher parity and breastfeeding prior to diagnosis were both associated with more severe RA although use of OCs before childbirth and RA diagnosis was associated with less severe disease.[62] Increasing rates of RA among women in a study from the Mayo Clinic included lower rates of breastfeeding associated with lower parity, combined with increased smoking in past decades, lower serum levels of vitamin D as women hesitate to be exposed to sunlight fearing skin cancer, and increased obesity.[63]

Smoking

Smoking is the dominant environmental risk factor, doubling the likelihood of disease compared with nonsmokers, primarily among women with rheumatoid factor.[53] Smoking has been associated with increased risk of several autoimmune conditions due to its effect on the immune system by reducing natural killer cells, depressing circulating hormones, and dysfunction of T lymphocytes.[64] Although smoking increases risk of RA more among men than women, current and former female smokers are at 20% to 30% increased risk of disease. In a meta-analysis of 16 studies on the role of smoking, the summary odds ratio for 20 or more pack-years of smoking was 2.31 (95% CI = 1.55–3.41) for men and 1.75 (95% CI = 1.52–2.02) for women.[64] Smoking is the only risk factor that has shown a consistent association with RA.

Geographic Residence

Prevalence of RA varies geographically being more common in northern Europe and North America compared with other regions.[53] Within the United States 122,000 women in the Nurses' Health Study 800 participants were diagnosed with RA during 28 years. In 1992 a follow-up question asked their residences at critical ages from birth, at age 15 and 30. Compared with women residing in western states, the relative risk of diagnosis with RA was 37% to 45% higher among women who had ever lived in the New England region,[65] and mean age at RA diagnosis was at a significantly younger age among women residing in eastern (57.3 yrs) compared with western (60.1 yr) states.[65] Suggested explanations for geographic patterns of RA include potential locally based infectious agents, ultraviolet light exposure, environmental exposures, and socioeconomic factors. Climate differences across the nation may influence lifestyle, especially exercise and diet. In addition, availability of rheumatology specialists may be associated with diagnosis.

Infectious Agents

Many organisms have been considered potentially involved with the development of RA. Doran and colleagues noted temporal and cyclical patterns in RA incidence in Olmstead County, which suggested an infectious etiology although subsequent studies have not confirmed any specific agent.[45] However, the incidence differences between men and women argue against a common infectious agent.

Clinical Manifestation

Laboratory analyses detecting rheumatoid factor (RF), an autoantibody marker of RA, combined with traditional radiographic abnormalities confirm the diagnosis. This antibody found in about 80% of RA patients was more significantly associated with diagnosis among men (OR = 3.02, 95% CI = 2.35–3.88) than among women, (OR = 1.34, 95% CI = 0.99–1.80). The authors speculated hormonal influences increase risk among women, although the antiestrogenic effect of smoking may lower the likelihood of RF detection among women.[64]

Pathophysiology of RA

Symptoms of RA, ranging from mild to severe, are due to inflammation of joints causing stiffness, swelling, pain, and loss of function often causing anemia and producing feelings of fatigue and malaise. The natural history of RA is known to be quite variable. About 10% of newly diagnosed patients experience spontaneous remission within the first 6 months, some affected individuals experience recurrence of serious attacks followed by quiescent periods; however, most patients develop persistent progressive disease that waxes and wanes in intensity. Systemic manifestations involving cardiopulmonary, neurologic, and ocular systems occur in some patients. RA can be aggressive and debilitating and may increase risk of myocardial infarction, stroke, and lymphoma. Mortality in RA patients is twice that of the general population (http://www.cdc.gov/arthritis/basics/rheumatoid.htm#8).

A 25-country analysis of gender differences in RA disease activity, characteristics, and treatment found that women had lower scores than men in all RA measures.[57] A report from the Netherlands noted that women were referred later than men for assessment of symptoms that lead to delay in diagnosis and initiation of appropriate treatment.[66] Remission rates were higher for men (30%) than women (17%).

Recent research has shown that naturally occurring anti-inflammatory factors are overwhelmed by proinflammatory agents. The inflamed synovium progressively erodes bone and cartilage within the joint, often significantly within a year of onset.[53] One aspect of the inflammatory sequence includes overproduction and overexpression of tumor necrosis factor, which causes the joint destruction. Researchers have debated whether the disease begins with bone and moves to the joint or the reverse although evidence for initiation in joints is probable as the disease moves between joints leading to polyarthritis.

Diagnosis of Rheumatoid Arthritis

Diagnosis of RA depends upon the variability in type and severity of symptoms often resembling other rheumatic conditions. In the early stages, only a few symptoms may be present. The American College of Rheumatology diagnostic criteria guidelines are included in Table 34-4.

Treatment
Drugs

No cure exists for RA; however, to avoid irreversible joint damage that may occur early in the disease process, antirheumatic drugs are often recommended.[66] The goals of treatment are to relieve pain, decrease joint inflammation, slow or stop bone erosion, improve functioning, and enhance quality of life. Early versus later initiation of antirheumatic therapy was studied in the Netherlands by Lard and colleagues between 1993 and 1995 among 109 patients. Less radiologic joint damage was observed 2 years after early treatment started within 15 days of diagnosis than among patients with delayed treatment of more than 100 days.[66] With early detection, new drugs early in the course of treatment may slow or even stop disease progression. The immunologic benefit increases women's resistance to many infectious agents that may occur during biologic treatment for RA.[67]

Symptoms diagnostic for rheumatoid arthritis

1. Symmetric polyarthritis of the small joints of the hands and feet

2. Involvement of the wrists and metacarpophalangeal (MCP) joints

3. Persistent inflammation for more than a few months, ruling out postviral inflammation

4. Fatigue that limits function

5. Morning stiffness

6. X-ray changes with periarticular osteopenia, joint space narrowing, or marginal erosions (or synovitis or erosion on ultrasound or magnetic resonance study) in conjunction with clinical and laboratory findings indicated RA

7. Laboratory findings:

   - Complete blood count: thrombocytosis, normochromic, normocytic anemia

   - Erythrocyte sedimentation rate > 30 mm/h

   - Elevated C-reactive protein

   - Positive rheumatoid factor (but can be negative in 30% of early stage disease)

   - Positive anticyclic citrullinated peptides (anti-CCPs; found in more than 60% of cases, but less very early in disease)

   - Negative antinuclear antibodies (ANAs)

   - Joint fluid with 5,000 to more than 50,000 WBC/mm^3, with at least 50% neutrophils; no crystals and negative culture.

Source: Adapted from the ACR *Guidelines for the Management of Rheumatoid Arthritis* by Hospital for Special Surgery/Weill Medical College of Cornell University and used with permission.[28]

Treatment often starts aggressively with NSAIDs (including COX-2 inhibitors), a short-course of prednisone, and disease-modifying antirheumatic drugs (DMARDs) such as methotrexate. Newer drugs termed biologic DMARDs have produced rapid improvements. Since all drugs have serious side effects, patients receiving pharmacologic treatment must be monitored for onset of gastrointestinal bleeding, cardiovascular events, liver toxicity, and susceptibility to infection.[66]

Nonpharmacologic Therapy

Lifestyle changes may enable patients with RA to function better, maintain mobility, and enhance their quality of life. Routine exercise and rest in a good balance are essential and may be supplemented with physical therapy including range of motion and strengthening exercises. Protection of joints from damage with self-help devices may avoid trauma. Stress reduction is recommended to reduce fear, anger, and depression especially among women who may benefit from psychosocial support through group involvement.

Surgical Therapy

Drug therapy is the mainstay of RA treatment, but several kinds of surgery are used routinely for advanced disease. These include replacement of deteriorated hips and knees as well as shoulders, feet, ankles, and hand joints. Fusion and tendon reconstruction are additional surgical therapies.

Complementary/Alternative Therapy

Certain complementary modalities seem to show promise for RA patients, among them the anti-inflammatory agents. Omega-3 fatty acids (found in flax and fish oils) were found by NCCAM to have promising pain relief properties.[68] Other anti-inflammatory agents such as turmeric, boswellia serrata, ginger, and green tea have been studied in small trials with good results.[69] An NCCAM-funded study using a mouse model found that pomegranate extract (an antioxidant) was effective in reducing inflammation and destruction of bone and cartilage.[70]

RA patients require nutrient-dense foods while limiting refined and processed foods to reduce risk of heart disease and diabetes. Food intolerance (such as to gluten) may play a role, and special diets have provided relief for some RA patients, possibly a susceptible subset.[71,72] The decrease in symptoms found by fasting (under medical supervision) may be due to elimination of allergens.[71] Several European trials have shown that vegetarian/vegan diets (low/no animal products) can decrease pain, inflammation, and disease activity.[71] A randomized, controlled trial of the Mediterranean diet showed a 56% decrease in disease activity (joint swelling, tenderness, and pain) in RA patients compared with controls, and more studies are planned.[73]

Mind–body therapies like tai chi, relaxation, meditation, biofeedback, and guided imagery may provide special benefit to RA patients coping with stress and depression. Mind–body studies have shown promising results in terms of function, pain, emotional state, and ability to cope.[74] The recent University of North Carolina tai chi study previously discussed found improvements in OA as well as RA patients with decreased pain, fatigue, and stiffness as well as improved reach, balance, and sense of well-being.[75]

Research assessing the role of mineral baths for RA has reported positive findings although a meta-analysis indicated methodological flaws prevented accurate assessment.[76] The role of acupuncture is still unclear.

Prevention of RA

Smoking cessation is important, but other aspects of prevention are not as clear. In the first trial to evaluate a preventive role for aspirin in RA, a component of the Women's Health Study, low-dose aspirin (100 mg every other day) did not reduce women's risk of developing RA.[77] However, high consumption of oily fish modestly reduced the risk of RA development in a large Swedish epidemiologic study.[78] Health behaviors play an important preventive role; risk of RA is reduced among women and men who exercise routinely, avoid psychosocial stress, and consume a balanced diet rich in fruits and vegetables, omega-3 fatty acids, anti-inflammatory agents, and antioxidants.[79]

Summary

Osteoarthritis and rheumatoid arthritis are major disabling diseases that increase with age and often compromise the quality of life of women during their senior years. Given the major societal burden these conditions are anticipated to create for health care in the next few decades, emphasis should be placed on health behaviors during youth and young adulthood to protect against or delay onset of these debilitating conditions. Community-based interventions to promote routine exercise across the life span coupled with nutritional education, smoking cessation, and weight loss activities may prevent onset of rheumatic conditions. These activities may reduce morbidity and control progression of disease among OA and RA patients.

Employment limitations due to arthritis affect more than 5% of Americans ages 18 to 64. Onsite exercise facilities and health-related programs provided by employers may reduce morbidity associated with physically demanding activity, which may decrease use of sick leave. Important advances have been made in the early diagnosis and treatment of both OA and RA, and much more knowledge is available today while researchers continue searching for additional genetic markers, risk factors, and environmental causes of these two conditions.

Discussion Questions

1. What factors distinguish osteoarthritis from rheumatoid arthritis?
2. How are these conditions and their symptoms similar?
3. What are the primary risk factors of each disease?
4. What characteristics may affect incidence and prevalence rates of different types of rheumatoid conditions?

Additional information is available from the following websites:

American College of Rheumatology (http://www .rheumatology.org)
Arthritis Foundation (http://www.arthritis.org),
NIAMS (http://www.niams.nih.gov), and the CDC (http://www.cdc.gov).

The Arthritis Foundation has listed many of the supplements available in a useful *Supplement Guide* describing the properties, doses, and safety profiles of many nutrients and herbs with anti-inflammatory action.

Acknowledgments

Dr. Robbins thanks her assistant, Phyllis Tower, for help in preparing this chapter.

References

1. Chang YJ, Hootman JM, Murphy LB, et al. Prevalence of doctor-diagnosed arthritis and arthritis-attributable activity limitation—United States, 2007–2009. *MMWR Morb Mortal Wkly Rep*. 2010;59:1261–1264.
2. Murphy LB, Hootman JM, Langmaid GA, et al. Prevalence of doctor-diagnosed arthritis and arthritis-attributable effects among Hispanic adults, by Hispanic subgroup—United States, 2002, 2003, 2006, and 2009. *MMWR Morb Mortal Wkly Rep*. 2011;60:167–171.
3. Hootman JM, Helmick CG. Projections of US prevalence of arthritis and associated activity limitations. *Arthritis Rheum*. 2006;54:226–229.
4. Centers for Disease Control and Prevention. Prevalence of disabilities and associated health conditions among adults—United States, 1999. *MMWR Morb Mortal Wkly Rep*. 2001;50:120–125.
5. Theis KA, Murphy L, Hootman JM, et al. Prevalence and correlates of arthritis-attributable work limitation in the US population among persons ages 18–64: 2002 National Health Interview Survey Data. *Arthritis Rheum*. 2007;57:355–363.
6. Lawrence RC, Felson DT, Helmick CG, et al.; for the National Arthritis Data Workgroup. Estimates of the prevalence of arthritis and other rheumatic conditions in the United States. Part II. *Arthritis Rheum*. 2008;58:26–35.
7. Zhang Y, Niu J, Kelly-Hayes M, et al. Prevalence of symptomatic hand osteoarthritis and its impact on functional status among elderly: the Framingham Study. *Am J Epidemiol*. 2002;156:1021–1027.
8. Jordan JM, Helmick CG, Renner JB, et al. Prevalence of knee symptoms and radiographic and symptomatic knee osteoarthritis in African-Americans and Caucasians: the Johnston County Osteoarthritis Project. *J Rheumatol*. 2007;34:172–180.
9. Dillon CF, Rasch EK, Gu Q, Hirsch R. Prevalence of knee osteoarthritis in the United States: arthritis data from the third National Health and Nutrition Examination Survey 1991–1994. *J Rheumatol*. 2006;33:2271–2279.
10. Jordan JM, Helmick CG, Renner JB, et al. Prevalence of hip symptoms and radiographic and symptomatic hip osteoarthritis in African Americans and Caucasians: The Johnston County Osteoarthritis Project. *J Rheumatol*. 2009;36:809–815.
11. Buie VC, Owings MF, DeFrances CJ, Golosinskiy A. National Hospital Discharge Survey: 2006 summary. *Natl Center Health Statistics. Vital Health Stat*. 2010;13.
12. Merrill C, Elixhauser A. *Hospital Stays Involving Musculoskeletal Procedures, 1997–2005*. Rockville, MD: Agency for Healthcare Research and Quality; July 2007. HCUP Statistical Brief #34. http://www.hcup-us.ahrq.gov/reports/statbriefs/sb34.pdf. Accessed September 6, 2010.
13. Felson DT. Risk factors for osteoarthritis: understanding joint vulnerability. *Clin Orthop Rel Res*. 2004;427S:S16–S21.
14. Evangelou E, Chapman K, Meulenbelt I, et al. Large-scale analysis of association between GDF5 and FRZB variants and osteoarthritis of the hip, knee, and hand. *Arthritis Rheum*. 2009;60:1710–1721.
15. Stevens-Lapsley JE, Kohrt WM. Review: osteoarthritis in women: effects of estrogen, obesity and physical activity. *Future Med*. 2010;6:601–615.
16. de Klerk BM, Schiphofl D, Groeneveld FPMJ, et al. Limited evidence for a protective effect of unopposed estrogen therapy for osteoarthritis of the hip: a systematic review. *Rheumatology*. 2009;48:104–112.
17. Wright NC, Riggs GK, Liss JR, Chen Z; Women's Health Initiative. Self-reported osteoarthritis, ethnicity, body mass index, and other associated risk factors in postmenopausal women—results from the Women's Health Initiative. *J Am Geriatr Soc*. 2008;56:1736–1743.

18. von Muhlen D, Morton D, von Muhlen CA, Barrett-Connor E. Postmenopausal estrogen and increased risk of clinical osteoarthritis at the hip, hand and knee in older women. *J Womens Health Gend Based Med.* 2002;11:511–518.

19. Sowers MF. Epidemiology of risk factors for osteoarthritis: system factors. *Curr Opin Rheum.* 2001;13:447–451.

20. Felson DT, Zhang Y, Hannan MT, et al. Risk factors for incident radiographic knee osteoarthritis in the elderly: the Framingham Study. *Arthritis Rheum.* 1997;40:718–733.

21. Felson DT, Lawrence RC, Dieppe PA, et al. Osteoarthritis: new insights. *Ann Internal Med.* 2000;133:635–646.

22. Sanghi DS, Avasthi S, Srivastava RN, Singh A. Nutritional factors and osteoarthritis: a review article. *Internet J Med Update.* 2009;4:42–53. www.akspublication.com/Paper08_Jan2009_.pdf. Accessed September 6, 2010.

23. McAlindon TE, Felson DT, Zhang Y, et al. Relation of dietary intake and serum levels of vitamin D to progression of osteoarthritis of the knee among participants in the Framingham Study. *Ann Intern Med.* 1996;125:353–359.

24. Lane NE, Gore LR, Cummings SR, et al. Serum vitamin D levels and incident changes of radiographic hip osteoarthritis: a longitudinal study. Study of Osteoporotic Fractures Research Group. *Arthritis Rheum.* 1999;42:854–860.

25. Huston LJ, Greenfield ML, Wojtys EM. Anterior cruciate ligament injuries in the female athlete. Potential risk factors. *Clin Orthop Relat Res.* 2000;372:50–63.

26. Zhang Y, Niu J, Kelly-Hayes M, et al. Prevalence of symptomatic hand osteoarthritis and its impact on functional status among elderly: the Framingham Study. *Am J Epidemiol.* 2002;156:1021–1027.

27. Hunter DJ. Focusing osteoarthritis management on modifiable risk factors and future therapeutic prospects. *Ther Adv Musculoskel Dis.* 2009;1:35–47.

28. American College of Rheumatology Subcommittee on Osteoarthritis Guidelines. Recommendations for the medical management of osteoarthritis of the hip and knee. 2000. http://www.rheumatology.org/practice/clinical/guidelines/oa-mgmt.asp. Accessed September 26, 2010.

29. Dunlop DD, Song J, Semank PA, Sharma L, Chang RW. Physical activity levels and functional performance in the Osteoarthritis Initiative: a graded relationship. *Arthritis Rheum.* 2001;63:127–136.

30. Hawker GA, Wright JG, Coyte PC, et al. Differences between men and women in the rate of use of hip and knee arthroplasty. *N Engl J Med.* 2000;342:1016–1022.

31. Petterson SC, Raisis L, Bodenstab A, Snyder-Mackler L. Disease-specific gender differences among total knee arthroplasty candidates. *J Bone Joint Surg Am.* 2007;89:2327–2333.

32. Singh JA, Gabriel S, Lewallen D. The impact of gender, age, and preoperative pain severity on pain after TKA. *Clin Orthop Relat Res.* 2008;466:2717–2723.

33. McAlindon TE, Jacques P, Zhang Y, et al. Do antioxidant micronutrients protect against the development and progression of knee osteoarthritis? *Arthritis Rheum.* 1996;39:648–656.

34. Towheed TE, Maxwell L, Anastassiades TP, et al. Glucosamine therapy for treating osteoarthritis (Cochrane Review). In: *The Cochrane Library*, Issue 4. Chichester, UK: John Wiley & Sons, Ltd.; 2007.

35. Altman RD, Marcussen KC. Effects of a ginger extract on knee pain in patients with osteoarthritis. *Arthritis Rheum.* 2001;44:2531–2538.

36. Little CV, Parsons T, Logan S. Herbal therapy for treating osteoarthritis (Cochrane Review). In: *The Cochrane Library*, Issue 1. Chichester, UK: John Wiley & Sons, Ltd.; 2001.

37. Belcaro G, Cesarone MR, Errichi C, et al. Treatment of osteoarthritis with pycnogenol. The SVOS (San Valentino Osteo-Arthrosis) Study. Evaluation of signs, symptoms, physical performance and vascular aspects. *Phytother Res.* 2008;22:518–523.

38. Berman BM, Lao L, Langenberg P, et al. Effectiveness of acupuncture as adjunctive therapy in osteoarthritis of the knee: a randomized, controlled trial. *Ann Intern Med.* 2004;10:36–43.

39. Song R, Lee EO, Lam P, Bae SC. Effects of tai chi exercise on pain, balance, muscle strength, and perceived difficulties in physical functioning in older women with osteoarthritis: a randomized clinical trial. *J Rheumatol.* 2003;30:2039–2044.

40. University of North Carolina School of Medicine. Tai chi relieves arthritis pain, improves reach, balance, well-being, study suggests. *Science Daily.* November 8, 2010. http://www.sciencedaily.com/releases/2010/11/101107202140.htm. Accessed December 6, 2010.

41. Verhagen AP, Bierma-Zeinstra SMA, Boers M, et al. Balneotherapy for osteoarthritis (Cochrane Review). In: *The Cochrane Library*, Issue 1. Chichester, UK: John Wiley & Sons, Ltd.; 2007.

42. Bruce B, Fries JF, Lubeck DP. Aerobic exercise and its impact on musculoskeletal pain in older adults: a 14 year prospective longitudinal study. *Arthritis Res Ther.* 2005;7:R1263–1270.

43. Centers for Disease Control and Prevention. *A National Public Health Agenda for Osteoarthritis.* Atlanta, GA: Author; 2010. http://www.cdc.gov/arthritis/docs/OAagenda.pdf. Accessed September 13, 2010.

44. Helmick CG, Felson DT, Lawrence RC, et al.; for the National Arthritis Data Workgroup. Estimates of the prevalence of arthritis and other rheumatic conditions in the United States. Part I. *Arthritis Rheum.* 2008;58:15–25.

45. Doran MF, Pond GR, Crowson CS, et al. Trends in incidence and mortality in rheumatoid arthritis in Rochester, Minnesota, over a forty-year period. *Arthritis Rheum.* 2002;46:625–631.

46. Hochberg MC. Changes in the incidence and prevalence of rheumatoid arthritis in England and Wales, 1970–1982. *Semin Arthritis Rheum.* 1990;19:294–302.

47. Myasoedova E, Crowson CS, Kremers HM, et al. Is the incidence of rheumatoid arthritis rising? Results from Olmsted County, Minnesota, 1955–2007 *Arthritis Rheum.* 2010;62:1576–1582.

48. Eberhardt K, Larsson B-M, Nived K, Lindqvist E. Work disability in rheumatoid arthritis—development over 15 years and evaluation of predictive factors over time. *J Rheumatol.* 2007;34:481–487.

49. Rooney T, Scherzer R, Shigenage JK, et al. Levels of plasma fibrinogen are elevated in well-controlled rheumatoid arthritis. *Rheumatology (Oxford).* 2011;50:1458–1465.

50. Sacks JJ, Helmick CG, Langmaid G. Deaths from arthritis and other rheumatic conditions, United States, 1979–1998. *J Rheumatol.* 2004;31:1823–1828.

51. Kelsey JL, Hochberg MC. Epidemiology of chronic musculoskeletal disorders. *Ann Rev Public Health.* 1988;9:379–401.

52. MacGregor AJ, Snieder H, Rigby AS, et al. Characterizing the quantitative genetic contribution to rheumatoid arthritis using data from twins. *Arthritis Rheum.* 2000;43:30–37.

53. Scott DL, Wolfe F, Huizinga TWJ. Rheumatoid arthritis. *Lancet.* 2010;376:1094–1108.

54. Hochberg MC, Spector TD. Epidemiology of rheumatoid arthritis: update. *Epidemiol Rev.* 1990;12:247–252.

55. Mandl LA, Costenbader KH, Simard JF, Karlson EW. Is birthweight associated with risk of rheumatoid arthritis? Data from a large cohort study. *Ann Rheum Dis.* 2009;68:514–518.

56. Jawaheer D, Lum RF, Gregersen PK, Criswell LA. Influence of male sex on disease phenotype in familial rheumatoid arthritis. *Arthritis Rheum.* 2006;54:3087–3094.

57. Sokka T, Toloza S, Cutolo M, et al; for the QUEST-RA Group. Women, men, and rheumatoid arthritis: analyses of disease activity, disease characteristics, and treatment in the QUEST-RA Study. *Arthritis Res Ther.* 2009;11:R7.

58. Cannon JG, St Pierre BA. Gender differences in host defense mechanisms. *J Psychiatr Res.* 1997;31:99–113.

59. Spector TD, Hochberg MC. The protective effect of the oral contraceptive pill on rheumatoid arthritis: an overview of the analytic epidemiological studies using meta-analysis. *J Clin Epidemiol.* 1990;43:1221–1230.

60. Pladevail-Vila M, Delclos GL, Varas C, et al. Controversy of oral contraceptives and risk of rheumatoid arthritis: meta-analysis of conflicting studies and review of conflicting meta-analyses with special emphasis on analysis of heterogeneity. *Am J Epidemiol.* 1996;144:1–14.

61. Guthrie KA, Dugowson CE, Voigt LF, et al. Does pregnancy provide vaccine-line protection against rheumatoid arthritis? *Arthritis Rheum.* 2010;62:1842–1848.

62. Jorgensen C, Picot MC, Bologna C, Sany J. Oral contraception, parity, breast feeding, and severity of rheumatoid arthritis. *Ann Rheum Dis.* 1996;55:94–98.

63. Myasoedova E, Crowson CS, Kremers HM, et al. Is the incidence of rheumatoid arthritis rising? Results from Olmsted County, Minnesota, 1955–2007 *Arthritis Rheum.* 2010;62:1576–1582.

64. Sugiyama D, Nishimura K, Tamaki K, et al. Impact of smoking as a risk factor for developing rheumatoid arthritis: a meta-analysis of observational studies. *Ann Rheum Dis.* 2010;69:70–81.

65. Costenbader KH, Chang S-C, Laden F, et al. Geographic variation in rheumatoid arthritis incidence among women in the United States. *Arch Intern Med.* 2008;168:1664–1670.

66. Lard LR, Visser H, Speyer I, et al. Early versus delayed treatment in patients with recent-onset rheumatoid arthritis: comparison of two cohorts who received different treatment strategies. *Am J Med.* 2001;111:446–451.

67. Burmester GR, Mariette S, Montecucco C, et al. Adalimumab along and in combination with disease-modifying antirheumatic drugs for the treatment of rheumatoid arthritis in clinical practice: the Research in Active Rheumatoid Arthritis (ReAct) trial. *Ann Rheum Dis.* 2007;66:732–739.

68. National Center for Complementary and Alternative Medicine. *Research Report: Rheumatoid Arthritis and Complementary and Alternative Medicine.* http://nccam.nih.gov/health/RA/RA.pdf. Accessed September 20, 2010.

69. University of Maryland Medical Center. Rheumatoid arthritis. http://www.umm.edu/altmed/rheumatoid-arthritis-000142.htm. Accessed September 24, 2010.

70. Shukla M, Gupta K, Rasheed Z, et al. Consumption of hydrolyzable tannin-rich pomegranate extract suppresses inflammation and joint damage in rheumatoid arthritis. *Nutrition.* 2008;24:733–743.

71. Haaz S. Complementary and alternative medicine for patients with rheumatoid arthritis. http://www.hopkinsarthritis.org/patient-corner/disease-management/ra-complementary-alternative-medicine/. Accessed September 20, 2010.

72. Hvatum M, Kanerud L, Hallgren R, Brandtzaeg P. The gut-joint axis: cross reactive food antibodies in rheumatoid arthritis. *Gut.* 2006;55:1240–1247.

73. Skoldstam L Hagfors L, Johansson G. An experimental study of a Mediterranean diet intervention for patients with rheumatoid arthritis. *Ann Rheum Dis.* 2003;62:208–214.

74. National Center for Complementary and Alternative Medicine. *Research Report: Rheumatoid Arthritis and Complementary and Alternative Medicine.* http://nccam.nih.gov/health/RA/RA.pdf. Accessed September 20, 2010.

75. University of North Carolina School of Medicine. Tai chi relieves arthritis pain, improves reach, balance, well-being, study suggests. *Science Daily*. November 8, 2010. http://www.sciencedaily.com/releases/2010/11/101107202140.htm. Accessed December 6, 2010.

76. Verhagen AP, Bierma-Zeinstra SM, Boeers M, et al. Balneotherapy for rheumatoid arthritis. *Cochrane Database of Systematic Reviews*. 2009;(1)CD000518.

77. Shadick NA, Karlson EW, Cook NR, et al. Low-dose aspirin in the primary prevention of rheumatoid arthritis: the Women's Health Study. *Arthritis Care Res*. 2010;62:545–550.

78. Wesley RM, Klareskog L, Alfredsson L. and the EIRA study group. Dietary fish and fish oil and the risk of rheumatoid arthritis. *Epidemiology*. 2009;20:896–901.

79. Cerhan JR, Saag KG, Merlino LA, et al. Iowa Women's Health Study. Antioxidant micronutrients and risk of rheumatoid arthritis in a cohort of older women. *Am J Epidemiol*. 2003;157:345–354.

Osteoporosis: Epidemiology and Consequences

Jeri W. Nieves, PhD

Introduction

Osteoporosis is a skeletal disorder characterized by decreased bone mass and deterioration in the microarchitecture of bone, resulting in an increased risk of fracture.[1] These fractures can cause debilitating pain, reduced mobility, a diminished quality of life, and increased mortality. The microarchitectural changes include thin and porous cortices and fewer, thinner trabeculae that are less connected than they are in normal bone (Figure 35-1). The World Health Organization (WHO) operationally defines osteoporosis as a bone density that falls 2.5 standard deviations (SD) below the mean for young, healthy adults of the same gender—also referred to as a *T-score* of –2.5.[1] Postmenopausal women who fall at the lower end of the young normal range (a T-score of > 1 SD below the mean) are defined as having low bone density.

Osteoporosis, a major public health problem, has significant adverse effects on women's health affecting

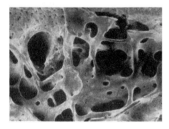

Figure 35-1A   Normal bone.

Source: Photo Insolite Realite/Photo Researchers, Inc.

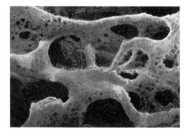

Figure 35-1B   Osteoporotic bone.

Source: Professor Pietro M. Motta/Photo Researchers, Inc.

mobility and the quality of life at older ages. Options for prevention and treatment to avoid fractures are discussed in this chapter.

Pathophysiology

Bone is a living and growing tissue that, throughout the life span, is constantly being renewed in a process called remodeling.[2] The remodeling process is complex but includes two main types of cells, osteoclasts and osteoblasts. Osteoclasts break down or remove bone and prepare the bone for remodeling (Figure 35-2). Osteoclasts release enzymes and acids that break down bones for resorption, releasing calcium, phosphorus, and other components of bone into the blood for use by the body. After the osteoclasts remove a small amount of bone, the bone surface is prepared for the osteoblasts. The osteoblasts are the cells responsible for bone formation.[3] Bone building occurs when more bone is laid down than is removed. During growth, the skeleton increases in size by linear growth and by apposition of new bone tissue on the outer surfaces of the cortex. This is called *modeling*, a process that also allows the long bones to adapt in shape to the stresses placed upon them. Increased sex hormone production at puberty is required for skeletal maturation, which reaches maximum mass in early adulthood. Heritability estimates of 50–80% for bone mass and size have been derived based on twin studies.[4] Heaney diagrammed the changes in bone mass by age noting peak bone mass maximized during growth and perhaps also in the early adult years through factors such as normal endocrine function, adequate dietary intake (particularly calcium), and adequate exercise, which can modify this genetic potential that an individual may achieve.

In young adults, resorbed bone is replaced by an equal amount of new bone tissue. Thus, the mass of the skeleton remains constant after peak bone mass is achieved in the late teens or early 20s. After age 30–45, however, the resorption and formation processes become imbalanced, and resorption exceeds formation.[5–7] This imbalance may begin at different ages and varies at different skeletal sites; it becomes exaggerated in women approaching menopause. In adults, bone remodeling is the principal metabolic

Modeling

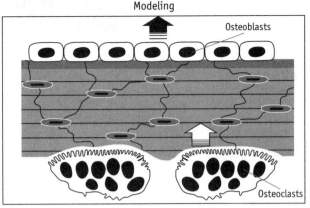

In bone modeling, osteoblast and osteoclast actions are not linked and rapid changes can occur in the amount, shape, and position of bone.

Remodeling

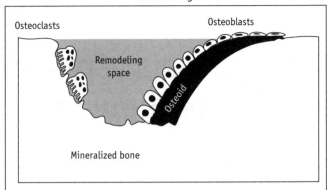

In remodeling, osteoblast action is coupled to prior osteoclast action. Net changes in shape of bone are minimal unless there is a remodeling imbalance.

Figure 35-2 Bone modeling and remodeling.

Source: Reproduced from Bone Health and Osteoporosis: A Report of the Surgeon General. http://www.surgeongeneral.gov/library/reports/bonehealth/chapter_2.html. Adapted from Rauch F, Glorieux FH. Osteogenesis imperfecta. The Lancet 2004;1377–1385, with permission from Elsevier.

skeletal process. Bone remodeling has two primary functions: (1) to repair microdamage within the skeleton to maintain skeletal strength, and (2) to supply calcium from the skeleton to maintain serum calcium. Remodeling may be activated by microdamage to bone as a result of excessive or accumulated stress or by lowered serum calcium. Bone mass is maintained when bone building equals bone removal. Bone loss occurs when more bone is removed than replaced.[4] As this happens, the bones lose minerals (such as calcium). This makes bones thinner, weaker, and more likely to break or fracture, even after a minor injury. Osteoporosis results from bone loss due to age-related

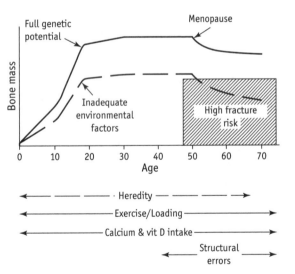

Note: This diagrammatic representation of bone mass life-line indicates individuals who achieve full genetic potential for skeletal mass and those who do not. [The magnitude of the difference between the curves is not to scale. Factors noted below are known to impact bone density].

Figure 35-3 Bone mass in relation to age.

Source: Courtesy of Robert P Heaney, used with permission. In: Heaney RP, Abrams S, Dawson-Hughes B, et al. Peak bone mass. *Osteoporosis Int* 2000;11:985–1009.

changes in the process of bone remodeling as well as other factors that can exaggerate this process.

The factors that modify the rate of bone loss include endocrine, environmental, genetic, and a variety of local factors. Women experience a rapid period of bone loss at the time of menopause that is related to a declining estrogen levels and an increase in the number of remodeling units activated per unit time. Decreased estrogen leads to an increase in bone resorption throughout the skeleton and subsequent bone loss. In fact, women can lose up to 20% of their bone mass in the first 5–7 years after the onset of menopause.[5-7] Slower bone loss continues as women grow older.[8] The imbalance between osteoclasts and osteoblasts may occur when more aggressive osteoclasts cause an increase in resorption depth, less efficient osteoblasts, or a combination of these processes. Another possibility is that the osteoclasts actually penetrate the trabeculae so that there is no template for the osteoblasts to build bone upon.

Epidemiology

In the United States, approximately 8 million women and 2 million men have osteoporosis, defined as having a bone mass T-score < –2.5. An additional 18 million individuals have bone mass levels that put them at increased risk of developing osteoporosis (defined as bone mass T-score < –1.0).[9,10] Although osteoporosis affects more than 10 million individuals in the United States, only a small proportion with fractures are diagnosed and treated. Osteoporosis occurs and progresses with increasing age, as bone tissue is steadily lost. In women, the loss of ovarian function at menopause (average age 51) precipitates rapid bone loss such that most women meet the diagnostic criterion for osteoporosis by age 70–80. These measures of decreased bone density (low bone mass and osteoporosis) are clearly related to fracture risk both in postmenopausal women,[11] and older men.[12] Numerous studies have reported a strong relationship between bone density and risk of fracture that increases as the bone density goes down.[13–19] Bone density is a measure of skeletal fragility and low bone density is believed to be responsible for 80–95% of hip and spine fractures in white women, depending on age.[20] An analysis of peripheral bone mineral density (BMD) and fractures in over 200,000 women (The National Osteoporosis Risk Assessment, or NORA, study) suggested that at least half of all fragility fractures occurs in the low bone mass group without recognized osteoporosis.[21–26]

The most serious consequence of osteoporosis is fracture, which may be the first visible sign of osteoporosis in patients. The most common sites of fractures related to osteoporosis are the hip, wrist, and vertebrae.[5] Osteoporosis was a contributing factor in more than 2 million fractures in 2005, including approximately 297,000 hip fractures, 547,000 vertebral fractures, 397,000 wrist fractures, 135,000 pelvic fractures, and 675,000 fractures at other sites.[27–29] Overall osteoporosis-related fracture frequency increases with age, is greater in females than in males, and typically occurs with moderate trauma. Fracture rates vary by gender and at each fracture site there is at least a twofold increase in incidence among women even after adjusting for age.[30]

The epidemiology of fractures follows the trend for bone density loss. Fractures of the distal radius increase in frequency before age 50 and plateau by age 60, with only a modest age-related increase thereafter.[15,31] In contrast, incidence rates for hip fractures double every 5 years after age 70. This distinct epidemiology may be related to the pattern of falls as age advances, with fewer falls on an outstretched hand and more falls directly on the hip (Figure 35-4) more hip fractures occurring to women after menopause require hospitalization and surgical intervention, increasing the risk of deep vein thrombosis and pulmonary embolism (20–50%).[32]

There are about 600,000 vertebral crush fractures per year in the United States; however, most are relatively asymptomatic. Only a fraction of these are recognized clinically after being incidentally detected during radiography for other purposes. Vertebral fractures rarely require

hospitalization but are associated with long-term morbidity and a slight increase in mortality, primarily related to pulmonary disease. Multiple vertebral fractures lead to height loss (often of several inches), kyphosis, and secondary pain and discomfort related to altered biomechanics of the back. Thoracic fractures can be associated with restrictive lung disease, whereas lumbar fractures are associated with abdominal symptoms including distention, early satiety, and constipation. Approximately 400,000 wrist fractures and 135,000 pelvic fractures occur in the United States each year. Fractures of other bones (with an estimated annual rate of 675,000) also occur with osteoporosis, which is not surprising given that bone loss is a systemic phenomenon. Fractures of the pelvis and proximal humerus are clearly associated with osteoporosis. Although some fractures are the result of major trauma, the threshold for fracture is reduced for an individual with osteoporosis.

The prevalence of osteoporosis is going to increase significantly as the population ages. In the United States, the number of people age 65 and older is expected to rise from 35 to 86 million between 2000 and 2050, and the number age 85 and older will increase from 4 to 20 million.[33,34] Much of this increase will occur in the next 25 years as the "baby boomers" reach their 70s and 80s. By 2020, one in two Americans over age 50 is expected to have or be at risk of developing osteoporosis of the hip although even more elderly will be at risk of developing osteoporosis at any site in the skeleton.[35]

Risk and Impact of Osteoporosis-Related Fractures

A substantial portion of the population faces a serious risk of experiencing a fragility fracture in their lifetime. In fact, 4 in 10 white American women age 50 or older will experience a hip, spine, or wrist fragility fracture sometime during the remainder of their lives.[32] The latest estimates are that 50% of women and 25% of men will suffer an osteoporosis-related fracture within their lifetime. In fact the lifetime risk for hip, spine, and wrist fracture is similar to the risk of coronary heart disease in women. Men and women of other ethnic groups have a slightly lower but still substantial risk for fracture; 5% of African-American women aged 50 years or older are estimated to have osteoporosis and an additional 35% are estimated to have low bone mass.[28,29,36]

Hip fractures are the most serious threat, as 17% white women and 6% of white men age 50 and older will suffer a hip fracture sometime during the remainder of their life.[32] Although the rates of hip fracture are lower in African Americans, the consequences following a hip fracture are greater than in Caucasians. Approximately 10% to 20% of hip fracture patients die within a year of the fracture.[37,38] Mortality is high for individuals who were ambulatory and not living in nursing homes at the time of their hip fracture; these patients have a 2.8-fold increased risk of dying within 3 months of the fracture. Those with poor prefracture health have higher mortality rates.[39] Hip fractures are

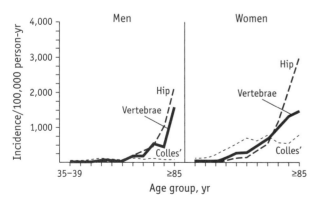

Figure 35-4 Age-specific incidence rates for hip, vertebral, and wrist fractures in Rochester, MN for men and women.

Source: Reproduced from Cooper C, Melton L. Epidemiology of osteoporosis. *Trends Endocrinol Metab.* 1992;3:224–229 with permission from Elsevier.

by far the most devastating type of fracture and frequently lead to disability; after experiencing a hip fracture[32] an estimated 50% of individuals will be unable to walk without assistance and one out of five will require long-term nursing home care.[40,41]

An estimated 25% of women older than 65 years may have sustained an asymptomatic vertebral fracture. The female-to-male ratio of vertebral fracture is estimated to be between 2 and 8 to 1.[42–44] Spine fractures are less devastating than hip fractures, with only 1 in 10 patients requiring hospitalization and less than 2% requiring nursing home care.[45] However, recent studies have shown up to 20% increased mortality after spine fractures as well as hip fractures.[46–50]

One of the most important consequences of a fracture is the dramatically increased risk of subsequent fractures (fracture begets fracture). Following the first spine fracture, there is an increased risk of a second spine fracture. In fact, one in five women will have a second fracture within a year of a first spine fracture.[51] In a review of the literature, a history of wrist fracture increased the risk of another wrist fracture by 40%, a spine fracture by 4.4-fold and a hip fracture by 2.3-fold; a prior hip fracture increased the risk of a spine fracture by 2.5-fold and of a second hip fracture by 2.3-fold.[50,52,53]

Osteoporosis-related fractures create a heavy economic burden that has led to 500,000 hospitalizations, more than 800,000 emergency room encounters, greater than 2.5 million physician office visits, and nursing home placement of nearly 180,000 individuals, according to the Surgeon General.[10] Based on a statistical model, American women age 45 and older could experience 5.2 million fractures of the hip, spine, or forearm, resulting in 2 million person-years of disability over a 10-year period.[54] Studies show that annual direct care expenditures for osteoporosis-related fractures range from $12.2–$17.9 billion per year in 2002 dollars.[41,55,56]

Risk Factors for Osteoporosis

Many of the risk factors for osteoporosis and fractures are modifiable, enabling women and men to reduce their risk through healthful behaviors (Table 35-1).[57,58]

Nutrition

Adequate nutrition plays a major role in the prevention and treatment of osteoporosis; the nutrients of greatest importance are calcium and vitamin D. The other micronutrient needs for optimizing bone health can be easily met by a healthy diet that is high in fruits and vegetables to ensure adequate intakes for magnesium, potassium, vitamin C, vitamin K, and other potentially important nutrients. Peak bone mass may be impaired by inadequate nutrition, primarily calcium intake but also inadequate calories, protein, and other vitamins and minerals during growth.

During the adult phase of life, insufficient calcium intake causes an increase in the rate of bone remodeling removing calcium from bones in order to maintain normal serum calcium levels. Although homeostatic responses are important to maintain serum calcium, the long-term effects on bone remodeling are detrimental to the skeleton and accelerate bone loss. All individuals should obtain an adequate intake of dietary calcium (at least 1,200 mg per day, including supplements if necessary) throughout life to attain maximal peak bone mass and prevent bone loss at older ages. Food is the preferred source to maintain calcium balance because there are other essential nutrients that are found in foods with high calcium content. For those individuals whose calcium intake from diet is inadequate, supplemental calcium can be used. Supplemental or dietary calcium should be spread out throughout the day with 500 mg or less being consumed at each meal in order to optimize absorption. Intakes in excess of 1,200 to 1,500 mg per day have limited potential for benefit and may possibly increase the risk of developing kidney stones or cardiovascular disease.

Vitamin D plays a major role in calcium absorption, bone health, muscle performance, and balance lowering the risk of falling. Severe vitamin D deficiency causes rickets in children or osteomalacia in adults. There is accumulating evidence that vitamin D insufficiency is more prevalent than previously thought, particularly among the elderly in addition to those living in northern latitudes and individuals with poor nutritional habits, conditions causing malabsorption, or chronic liver or renal disease. Dark-skinned individuals are also at high risk of vitamin D deficiency. Reduced fracture rates have

Table 35-1

Risk factors for fracture

• Low BMD	• **Estrogen deficiency at an early age (< 45 yrs) or hypogonadism**
• **Age**	• Discontinuation of estrogen therapy
• **History of fracture as an adult**	• Dementia
• **Family history of fracture**	• Poor health status/frailty/low physical activity
• Body weight /BMI	• Recent falls
• **Smoker**	• Poor mobility
• **Use of glucocorticoids**	• Lifelong low calcium/vitamin D intakes
• Impaired vision	• **Alcohol**
• Weakness	• **Rheumatoid arthritis and other secondary causes**
• Medications (narcotics, sedatives, diuretics)	

*Bold-faced risk factors are those taken into account by the FRAX risk assessment tool.

been documented among individuals who have greater vitamin D intake and have higher 25-hydroxyvitamin D [25(OH)D] serum levels. Vitamin D adequacy may also affect risk and/or severity of other diseases including cancers (colorectal, prostate, and breast), heart disease, autoimmune diseases, and diabetes. Vitamin D intakes of 800 IU to 1000 IU each day for people over 50 are recommended by the National Osteoporosis Foundation. Vitamin D from foods, supplements, and/or multivitamins can be used to meet the vitamin D requirement. Food sources of vitamin D are limited and include milk (100 IU per glass), salt-water fish, and liver. Some calcium supplements and most multivitamin tablets also contain vitamin D.

Tobacco and Excessive Alcohol Consumption

The risk of falling among elderly people is higher in smokers than in nonsmokers significantly increasing the lifetime risk from about 12% to 19% in women up to age 85[59,60] and from 22% to 37% to the age of 90.[61] The effect of smoking on hip fracture is most evident among thin, elderly female smokers older than 50 years; the excess risk of hip fracture was 50% among women with body mass index < 20 kg/m² (less than optimum). Among women and men the risk of hip fracture among smokers was increased threefold relative to nonsmokers.[62] In a recent analysis including 51 studies with 512,000 people, current smoking was associated with higher risk of any fracture, hip and spine fractures but not wrist fractures.[63] Previous smoking was associated only with increased risk of hip fracture.[63] The authors of a recent report studied risk of fractures associated with smoking internationally among 59,232 men and women (74% female) from 10 prospective cohorts followed for a total of 250,000 person-years. Current smoking was associated with a significantly increased risk of any fracture compared to nonsmokers (RR = 1.25; 95% CI = 1.15–1.36), with only a moderate reduction in the RR after controlling for bone mineral density. Low BMD accounted for only 23% of the smoking-related risk of hip fracture. Past smoking significantly increased risk of fracture compared with individuals who never smoked but the risk ratios were lower than for current smokers.[64]

Alcohol

The negative effects of alcohol consumption on bone have long been recognized. Chronic heavy drinking has been identified as a significant risk factor for various diseases, including osteoporosis. Chronic and heavy alcohol consumption is known to contribute to low bone mass, decreased bone formation, an increased incidence of fractures, and delays in fracture healing. Moderate alcohol consumption may actually have a modest favorable effect on bone density, particularly in postmenopausal women, although not all studies agree. However, alcohol intake of three or more drinks per day is detrimental to bone health and increases the risk of falling.

Physical Activity

In adulthood, physical activity can modestly increase bone mass, reduce bone loss, improve posture, promote balance to prevent falls, and increase muscle mass to cushion bones in the event of a fall. Beneficial exercise includes weight-bearing, muscle-strengthening, postural, and balance exercises to improve agility, strength, posture, and balance. Weight-bearing exercise, physical activity in which feet and legs are supporting or carrying weight, will build bone mass in youth and maintain bone mass in adulthood. Some examples of weight-bearing exercises include walking, racquet sports, team sports, dancing, and climbing stairs but not swimming and bicycling. Muscle strengthening exercises include lifting weights, using resistance bands, and exercising on resistance machines to strengthen muscle. Postural training exercises promote correct posture and proper body alignment, potentially minimizing stooped posture resulting from osteoporosis. Balance exercises, such as tai chi, may reduce the risk of falling. Inactivity, such as prolonged bed rest or paralysis, results in significant bone loss. Skeletal growth is most marked when the stimulus begins before puberty. Adults are less capable than children of increasing bone mass following restoration of physical activity. Epidemiologic data support the beneficial effects on the skeleton of chronic high levels of physical activity. Fracture risk is lower in rural communities and in countries where physical activity is maintained into old age. However, when exercise is initiated during adult life, the effects of moderate exercise on the skeleton are modest, with a bone mass increase of 1–2% in short-term studies of less than 2 years' duration.

Fall Prevention

Everyone is at risk of falling although falls are especially concerning in the older adult population. Among community-dwelling men and women aged 65 and older between 30% and 40% fall each year with about one-third resulting in serious injury. Approximately 90% to 95% of hip fractures result from falls. Strategies to reduce falls include, but are not limited to, checking and correcting vision and hearing, evaluating any neurological problems, reviewing prescription medications for side effects that may affect balance, and improving safety at home. It is important to do a home safety check on a regular basis to identify and modify falling hazards. Using a checklist can assist individuals in safe-proofing their homes.[65,66]

Body Mass Index

Although no ideal weight-to-height ratio has been set for reducing osteoporosis and fracture risk, higher range of body mass index (BMI) > 26–28 kg/m² offers protection, whereas a slender body habitus of < 22–24 kg/m² increases risk.[67] A BMI of about 30 kg/m² is associated with a 4–8% greater spine bone mineral density, 8–9% greater hip density, and 25% greater radial density compared to thinner women with BMI of 20 kg/m². Furthermore, a BMI of 30 kg/m² compared with BMI of 20 kg/m² is associated with one-half the loss in spine density during early postmenopausal years.[68–71] Two prospective cohort studies, the Framingham[72] and the Rancho Bernardo population,[73] noted both body weight and BMI explained a substantial proportion of the variance in BMD at various skeletal sites, and this relationship was stronger at weight-bearing sites.[73,74]

Low body mass index is a consistent risk factor for future fracture although the strength of this association is unclear. A recent meta-analysis of almost 60,000 women and men from 12 cohorts was used to quantify this relationship and it was found that the contribution of BMI to fracture risk was more marked at low values of BMI such that BMI of 25 kg/m^2 versus 20 kg/m^2 was associated with a nearly twofold increase in risk (RR = 1.95, 95% CI = 1.71, 2.22) compared with a 17% reduction in risk when BMI of 30 was compared to BMI = 25.[75] The BMI fracture risk relationship was independent of age and gender; however, the relationship is, at least in part, dependent on BMD.[75]

Estrogen Status

Estrogen deficiency can lead to bone loss by (1) activation of new bone remodeling sites, and (2) imbalance between bone formation and resorption. The increase in remodeling sites in the skeleton increases the probability that trabeculae will be penetrated, eliminating the template upon which new bone can be formed. The most frequent estrogen-deficient state is the cessation of ovarian function at the time of menopause, which occurs on average at the age of 51. Thus, with current life expectancy, an average woman will spend about 30 years without ovarian estrogens in addition to periods of amenorrhea experienced by some younger women.

Chronic Disease and Medications

Numerous causes of secondary osteoporosis include diseases of endocrine, gastrointestinal, renal, rheumatologic, and hematologic systems. Some medications, especially those required after organ transplantation, as well as treatments required for other diseases may lead to bone loss.[76–80] Medications that are implicated in bone loss include glucocorticoids, aromatase inhibitors, depo-medroxyprogesterone, gonadotropin-releasing hormone agonists, long-term heparin, anticonvulsants, lithium, cancer chemotherapeutic drugs, and immunosuppressants. Medications that may have a possible association with bone loss and fractures include proton pump inhibitors and selective serotonin reuptake inhibitors/serotonin-norepinephrine reuptake inhibitors (SSRIs/SNRIs) and thiazolidinediones (TZDs). Mechanisms that contribute to bone loss are unique for each disease and typically result from multiple factors including nutrition, reduced physical activity levels, and hormonal and cytokine factors that affect bone-remodeling rates.

Bone Density Testing

Fracture risk at any age is predicted primarily by skeletal mass, which is determined by the maximum mass achieved at maturity (peak bone mass) and the subsequent rate and duration of bone loss. Before the first fracture, bone density measurements are considered the gold standard for diagnosing osteoporosis; however, increasing awareness of osteoporosis and improved treatment has led to more frequent bone density assessments and increased demand for preventive treatment. In addition, more reliable testing for osteoporosis may identify fractures that might not have been clinically recognized. The World Health Organization defined osteoporosis as a bone mineral density value more than 2.5 standard deviations below the mean reference value for young women.[81] A reduction of one standard deviation in femoral BMD is comparable to a 14-year increase in age on the risk for hip fracture.[82] Roughly 10 million individuals over age 50 in the United States have osteoporosis of the hip based on a bone mineral density test and 33.6 million Americans over age 50 have low bone mass at the hip, increasing their risk of fracture and progression to osteoporosis.[29,39,83]

Many organizations advocate the use of a BMD test to diagnose osteoporosis in order to avoid the clinical sequelae associated with a fracture. In general, BMD testing should be performed on all women aged 65 and older regardless of risk factors, younger postmenopausal women with one or more risk factors (other than being white, postmenopausal, and female), postmenopausal women who present with fractures and men over the age of 70. According to the American College of Rheumatology, central measurement of BMD using dual energy x-ray absorptiometry (DXA) remains the gold standard for the diagnosis of osteoporosis and low bone mass.

The Fracture Risk Assessment Tool (FRAX®)[84] has recently been developed by the World Health Organization to evaluate fracture risk in patients. It combines femoral neck BMD with clinical risk factors to evaluate fracture risk in individuals, particularly those with low bone mass (T from –1 to –2.5) in an attempt to identify those who might be at greatest risk of fracture. The selection of these risk factors was based on the review of data from cohorts in Europe, North America, Asia, and Australia and the result of using the FRAX® tool,[57,85] is a 10 year probability of hip fracture and a 10-year probability of a major osteoporosis related fracture (clinical spine, forearm, hip or shoulder). The risk factors that come into play in the FRAX® tool are highlighted in bold print in Table 35-1. The projected FRAX® fracture probability is for individuals who have not received any treatment and is dependent on the accurate determination of the risk factors listed in the FRAX® calculator.

In order to monitor osteoporosis therapy, BMD is usually repeated after the first test 2 years after initiating treatment and then every 2 years thereafter. The determination of any change in bone density requires an understanding of the minimal difference that can be clinically detected; this value is between 3 and 6% depending on the technologist, dual energy x-ray absorptiometry equipment and skeletal site.

Treatment for Osteoporosis

Clearly, the personal and economic consequences of osteoporosis dictate that measures be taken to prevent and treat it. The latest *Clinician's Guide to Prevention and Treatment of Osteoporosis* states that treatment should be considered for persons with a prior fracture at the spine or hip, individuals with osteoporosis of the hip by bone density, or persons with low bone mass with additional risk factors leading to a sufficiently high risk of a hip or major osteoporosis-related fracture.[86]

Although there is no cure for osteoporosis, several medications have been approved that have been demonstrated to improve bone density and to reduce the risk of fracture. It is important that all people at risk or requiring treatment for osteoporosis follow certain strategies for prevention and treatment. All patients should be counseled to consume a healthy diet with adequate intake of protein, fruit, and vegetables.[87] In addition, each person should consume 1,200 mg of calcium from the combination of diet and supplemental calcium intake. Vitamin D intake should be at least 800 to 1,000 IU per day and if serum vitamin D levels are sufficiently low, higher supplements of vitamin D may be recommended. Serum vitamin D levels should be above 30 ng/ml; serum levels lower than 20 ng/ml may require 50,000 IU once or twice weekly for at least 8 weeks.[88] Drugs with sedative effects can be eliminated or a lower dose can be prescribed.

In the 2008 publication of National Osteoporosis Foundation *Clinician's Guide to Prevention and Treatment of Osteoporosis*,[86,89] treatment guidelines were based on the following:

The Food and Drug Administration (FDA)-approved medical therapies in postmenopausal women and men aged 50 years and older, are based on the following:

- A hip or vertebral (clinical or morphometric) fracture
- T-score ≤ –2.5 at the femoral neck or spine after appropriate evaluation to exclude secondary causes
- Low bone mass (T-score between –1.0 and –2.5 at the femoral neck or spine) and a 10-year probability of a hip fracture ≥ 3% or a 10-year probability of a major osteoporosis-related fracture ≥ 20% based on the U.S.-adapted WHO algorithm
- Clinician's judgment and/or patient preferences may indicate treatment for people with 10-year fracture probabilities above or below these levels

There are numerous treatments available for the prevention and treatment of osteoporosis in postmenopausal women and men as well as for glucocorticoid-induced osteoporosis. The indications for these medications are shown in Table 35-2. The goals of osteoporosis therapy are to maintain bone mineral density and to prevent fractures. However, no treatment has been shown to reduce fractures by much more that 50%; therefore, a fracture in a treated individual should not be considered a treatment failure. The efficacy of treatment for osteoporosis must be balanced with the effects on other organ systems for drugs such as raloxifene and estrogen therapy.

Table 35-2

FDA-approved medications for osteoporosis

	Dose
Estrogen	Variable
Raloxifene	60 mg daily
Calcitonin	200 U daily
Alendronate	5/10 mg daily, 35/70 mg weekly
Risedronate	5 mg daily 35 mg weekly 75 mg 2CDM 150 mg monthly
Ibandronate	150 mg monthly 3 mg IV q3 months
Zoledronic Acid	5 mg IV yearly
Parathyroid Hormone	20 mcg SC daily
Denosumab	60 mg SC every 6 months

Estrogens

Clinical trial data indicate that various types of estrogens (conjugated equine estrogens, estradiol, estrone, esterified estrogens, ethinyl estradiol, and mestranol) reduce bone turnover; produce increases in bone mass of the spine, hip, and total body; and reduce the risk of vertebral, hip, and all clinical fractures. The effects of estrogen are seen in women with natural or surgical menopause and in late postmenopausal women with or without established osteoporosis. When estrogens are discontinued, bone remodeling increases, to levels that might exceed those before treatment, and bone loss ensues rapidly. Epidemiologic data indicate that women who take estrogen replacement have a 50% reduction on average of fractures, including hip fractures. The beneficial effect of estrogen against fractures is lost after discontinuation. The Women's Health Initiative was a large clinical trial in generally healthy postmenopausal women, with a low prevalence of osteoporosis. The estrogen-progestin (EP) arm of the WHI involving more than 16,000 postmenopausal healthy women indicated that hormone therapy reduces the risk of hip and clinical spine fracture by 34% and all clinical fractures by 24%.[90] The estrogen-only arm (involving more than 10,000 women with a history of hysterectomy) showed fairly similar protective results against fractures. The risks of EP therapy include venous thrombosis, stroke, coronary heart disease events, breast cancer, and gallbladder disease.

Estrogen Agonist Antagonists

Raloxifene (60 mg/d) is approved for prevention and treatment of osteoporosis and prevention of breast cancer and has effects on bone turnover and bone mass that are estrogenic. The effect of raloxifene on bone density (+1.4–2.8% versus placebo in the spine, hip, and total body) is somewhat less than that seen with standard doses of estrogens.[91,92] Raloxifene reduces the occurrence of vertebral fracture by 30–50%, depending on the population; however, there are no data confirming that raloxifene can reduce the risk of non-vertebral fractures over 8 years of observation.[91,92]

Bisphosphonates

Alendronate, risedronate, ibandronate, and zoledronic acid are approved for the prevention and treatment of postmenopausal osteoporosis. Alendronate, risedronate, and zoledronic acid are approved for treatment of osteoporosis in men. Alendronate has been shown to decrease bone turnover and increase bone mass in the spine by up to 8% versus placebo and by 6% versus placebo in the hip over 3 years of study.[93] Vertebral fracture risk is reduced by about 50%, multiple vertebral fractures by up to 90%, and hip fractures by up to 50%.[93–96] Risedronate also reduces bone turnover and increases bone mass. Clinical trials have demonstrated 40–50% reduction in vertebral fracture risk over 3 years, accompanied by a 40% reduction in clinical nonspine fractures. Risedronate reduced hip fracture risk in women in their 70s with confirmed osteoporosis by 40%, but was not effective at reducing hip fracture occurrence in older women (80+ years) without proven osteoporosis. Ibandronate reduces vertebral fracture risk by ~40% but with no overall effect on nonvertebral fractures, except in a subgroup of women with a femoral neck T-score of –3 or below where this risk was reduced by ~60%. Zoledronic acid is a potent bisphosphonate with unique administration, once yearly intravenous (IV) therapy. In a study of >7,700 women followed for 3 years, zoledronic acid (5 mg as a single IV infusion annually) reduced the risk of vertebral fractures by 70%, nonvertebral fractures by 25%, and hip fractures by 40%.[97] These results were associated with less height loss and disability. There was also a reduction in mortality in this study (29%) that is not completely explained by the reduction in hip fracture incidence

Calcitonin

Calcitonin is a polypeptide hormone produced by the thyroid gland. Calcitonin preparations are approved by the FDA for osteoporosis in women more than 5 years past menopause. A nasal spray containing calcitonin (200 IU/d) is available for treatment of osteoporosis in postmenopausal women. One study suggests that nasal calcitonin produces small increments in bone mass and a small reduction in new vertebral fractures in calcitonin-treated patients versus those on calcium alone. There has been no proven effectiveness of any calcitonin preparation against nonvertebral fractures.

Parathyroid Hormone

Endogenous parathyroid hormone (PTH) is an 84-amino-acid peptide that is largely responsible for calcium homeostasis. Although chronic elevation of PTH, which occurs in hyperparathyroidism, is associated with bone loss (particularly cortical bone), PTH elevation can also exert anabolic effects on trabecular bone. An exogenous PTH analogue (1-34hPTH; teriparatide) is approved for the treatment of established osteoporosis in both men and women. In the pivotal study (median, 19 months' duration), 20 μg PTH(1-34) daily by subcutaneous injection reduced vertebral fractures by 65% and nonvertebral fractures by 45%.[98] Treatment is administered as a single daily injection given for a maximum of 2 years. Teriparatide produces increases in bone mass and mediates architectural improvements in skeletal structure.

Denosumab

A novel agent, given twice yearly by subcutaneous administration in a randomized controlled trial in postmenopausal women with osteoporosis, denosumab has been shown to increase BMD in the spine, hip, and forearm and reduce vertebral, hip, and nonvertebral fractures over a 3-year period by 70%, 40%, and 20% respectively.[99] Denosumab was approved in 2010.

Treatment Duration

In some cases the treatment duration has been established such as the 2 years for teriparatide. However, the continued use of bisphosphonates beyond a treatment period of 3 to 5 years should be reevaluated annually based on pertinent medical history including bone density and fracture history. It has been suggested that consideration should be given to stopping—at least temporarily—bisphosphonate therapy in patients without incident fractures and with a T-score of greater than –2 and no other major risk factors.[89]

Summary

Osteoporosis is clearly a public health problem with many personal consequences to the individual. It is important to know the risk factors for osteoporosis to identify those at risk for future fracture. The use of a bone density test to diagnose osteoporosis before a fracture is an important step in prevention. In addition many organizations have developed treatment guidelines for women with osteoporosis or at sufficient risk for fracture. Treatment of an individual with a prior fracture or sufficiently low bone mass can reduce fracture risk by 50% for the spine and hip skeletal sites and by about 20% in the combined category of nonspine fractures. In conclusion, there are many studies that demonstrate that osteoporosis is a serious disease with potential impact on an individual's mobility, morbidity, and mortality. There are also personal and economic consequences of osteoporosis. It is important to prevent and treat osteoporosis in those at risk of fracture.

Discussion Questions

1. Bone is living tissue. Describe the process of modeling and remodeling of bone.
2. How do the bones of women compare with men? Describe how changes occur over time by gender.

3. Many risk factors increase the likelihood of fractures over the life span. Which are modifiable?

4. What treatments have been proposed to prevent osteoporosis and to reduce progression of the condition?

5. What is implied by "peak bone mass"? How is this measured? Is it a stable measure or does bone mass change over time?

References

1. NIH Consensus Development Panel on Osteoporosis Prevention, Diagnosis, and Therapy. Osteoporosis prevention, diagnosis, and therapy. *JAMA* 2001;286:785–795.

2. Dempster DW, Shane E, Horbert W, Lindsay R. A simple method for correlative light and scanning electron microscopy of human iliac crest bone biopsies: qualitative observations in normal and osteoporotic subjects. *J Bone Miner Res.* 1986;1;15–21.

3. Rauch F, Glorieux FH. Osteogenesis imperfecta. *Lancet* 2004;363(9418); 1377–1385.

4. Dempster DW. Bone remodeling. In: Coe FL, Favus M, eds. *Disorders of Bone and Mineral Metabolism.* Philadelphia: Lippincott, Williams and Wilkins; 2002.

5. Nieves J, Cosman F, Lindsay R. Primary osteoporosis. In: Coe FL, Favus M, eds. *Disorders of Bone and Mineral Metabolism.* Philadelphia: Lippincott Williams and Wilkins; 2002;805–830.

6. Nilas L, Christiansen C. Rates of bone loss in normal women: evidence of accelerated trabecular bone loss after the menopause. *Eur J Clin Invest.* 1988;18;529–534.

7. Heaney RP, Abrams S, Dawson-Hughes B, et al. Peak bone mass. *Osteoporosis Int.* 2000;11;985–1009.

8. Greenspan SL, Maitland LA, Myers ER, Krasnow MB, Kido TH. Femoral bone loss progresses with age: a longitudinal study in women over age 65. *J Bone Miner Res.* 1994;9;1959–1965.

9. National Osteoporosis Foundation. *America's Bone Health: The State of Osteoporosis and Low Bone Mass in Our Nation.* Washington, DC: National Osteoporosis Foundation; 2002.

10. *Bone Health and Osteoporosis; A Report of the Surgeon General.* Washington, DC: US Department of Health and Human Services, Office of the Surgeon General; 2004.

11. Stone KL, Seeley DG, Lui LY, et al. BMD at multiple sites and risk of fracture of multiple types: long-term results from the Study of Osteoporotic Fractures. *J Bone Miner Res.* 2003;18;1947–1954.

12. Nguyen TV, Eisman JA, Kelly PJ, Sambrook PN. Risk factors for osteoporotic fractures in elderly men. *Am J Epidemiol.* 1996;144;255–263.

13. Nelson HD, Rizzo J, Harris E, et al. Osteoporosis and fractures in postmenopausal women using estrogen. *Arch Intern Med.* 2002;162;2278–2284.

14. Cummings SR, Nevitt MC, Browner WS, et al. Risk factors for hip fracture in white women. Study of Osteoporotic Fractures Research Group. *N Engl J Med.* 1995;332(12);767–773.

15. De Laet CE, Van Hout BA, Burger H, Weel AE, Hofman A, Pols HA. Hip fracture prediction in elderly men and women: validation in the Rotterdam study. *J Bone Miner Res.* 1998;13;1587–1593.

16. Black DM, Cummings SR, Genant HK, Nevitt MC, Palermo L, Browner W. Axial and appendicular bone density predict fractures in older women. *J Bone Miner Res.* 1992;7;633–638.

17. Nevitt MC, Johnell O, Black DM, Ensrud K, Genant HK, Cummings SR. Bone mineral density predicts non-spine fractures in very elderly women. Study of Osteoporotic Fractures Research Group. *Osteoporos Int.* 1994;4;325–331.

18. Duboeuf F, Hans D, Schott AM, et al. Different morphometric and densitometric parameters predict cervical and trochanteric hip fracture: the EPIDOS Study. *J Bone Miner Res.* 1997;12;1895–1902.

19. Schott AM, Cormier C, Hans D, et al. How hip and whole-body bone mineral density predict hip fracture in elderly women: the EPIDOS Prospective Study. *Osteoporos Int.* 1998;8(3);247–254.

20. Melton LJ, 3rd, Thamer M, Ray NF, et al. Fractures attributable to osteoporosis; report from the National Osteoporosis Foundation. *J Bone Miner Res.* 1997;12;16–23.

21. Siris ES, Miller PD, Barrett-Connor E, et al. Identification and fracture outcomes of undiagnosed low bone mineral density in postmenopausal women;results from the National Osteoporosis Risk Assessment. *JAMA.* 2001;286;2815–2822.

22. Schuit SC, van der Klift M, Weel AE, et al. Fracture incidence and association with bone mineral density in elderly men and women: the Rotterdam Study. *Bone.* 2004;34;195–202.

23. Siris ES, Simon JA, Barton IP, McClung MR, Grauer A. Effects of risedronate on fracture risk in postmenopausal women with osteopenia. *Osteoporos Int.* 2008;19;681–686.

24. Sornay-Rendu E, Garnero P, Munoz F, Duboeuf F, Delmas PD. Effect of withdrawal of hormone replacement therapy on bone mass and bone turnover: the OFELY study. *Bone.* 2003;33;159–166.

25. Wainwright SA, Marshall LM, Ensrud KE, et al. Hip fracture in women without osteoporosis. *J Clin Endocrinol Metab.* 2005;90;2787–2793.

26. Sanders KM, Nicholson GC, Watts JJ, et al. Half the burden of fragility fractures in the community occur in women without osteoporosis. When is fracture prevention cost-effective? *Bone.* 2006;38;694–700.

27. Burge R, Dawson-Hughes B, Solomon DH, Wong JB, King A, Tosteson A. Incidence and economic burden of osteoporosis-related fractures in the United States, 2005–2025. *J Bone Miner Res.* 2007;22;465–475.

28. Aloia JF, Talwar SA, Pollack S, Yeh J. A randomized controlled trial of vitamin D3 supplementation in African American women. *Arch Intern Med.* 2005;165;1618–1623.

29. National Osteoporosis Foundation. Fast Facts on Osteoporosis. http://medschool.creighton.edu/fileadmin/user/medicine/images/Creighton_FIRST/Osteo_Spotlight/Fast_Facts.pdf

30. Cooper C, Melton L. Epidemiology of osteoporosis. *Trends Endocrinol Metab.* 1992;3;224–229.

31. Black DM, Cooper C. Epidemiology of fractures and assessment of fracture risk. *Clin Lab Med.* 2000;20;439–453.

32. Cummings SR, Melton LJ. Epidemiology and outcomes of osteoporotic fractures. *Lancet.* 2002;359(9319);1761–1767.

33. Anderson SL, Zager K, Hetzler RK, Nahikian-Nelms M, Syler G. Comparison of Eating Disorder Inventory (EDI-2) scores of male bodybuilders to the male college student subgroup. *Int J Sport Nutr.* 1996;6;255–262.

34. U.S. Census Bureau.U.S. Interim Projections by Age, Sex, Race, and Hispanic Origin. Washington, DC: U.S. Census Bureau, Population Division, Populations Projection Branch; 2009.

35. National Osteoporosis Foundation. *America's Bone Health: The State of Osteoporosis and Low Bone Mass in Our Nation.* Washington, DC National Osteoporosis Foundation; 2002.

36. Looker AC, Orwoll ES, Johnston CC, Jr., et al. Prevalence of low femoral bone density in older U.S. adults from NHANES III. *J Bone Miner Res.* 1997;12(11);1761–1768.

37. Cauley JA, Thompson DE, Ensrud KC, et al. Risk of mortality following clinical fractures. *Osteoporos Int* 2000;11;556–561.

38. Leibson CL, Tosteson AN, Gabriel SE, et al. Mortality, disability, and nursing home use for persons with and without hip fracture: a population-based study. *J Am Geriatr Soc.* 2002;50;1644–1650.

39. Richmond J, Aharonoff GB, Zuckerman JD, Koval KJ. Mortality risk after hip fracture. 2003. *J Orthop Trauma.* 2003;17(8 suppl);S2–S5.

40. Magaziner J, Fredman L, Hawkes W, et al. Changes in functional status attributable to hip fracture: a comparison of hip fracture patients to community-dwelling aged. *Am J Epidemiol.* 2003;157;1023–1031.

41. Ray NF, Chan JK, Thamer M, Melton LJ, 3rd. Medical expenditures for the treatment of osteoporotic fractures in the United States in 1995: report from the National Osteoporosis Foundation. *J Bone Miner Res.* 1997;12;24–35.

42. Melton LJ, 3rd. Epidemiology of fractures. In: Riggs BL, Melton LJ, eds. *Osteoporosis Etiology, Diagnosis and Management.* 2nd ed. Philadelphia: Lippincott-Raven; 1995;225–248.

43. Melton LJ, 3rd. Epidemiology of spinal osteoporosis. *Spine.* 1997;22(24 suppl);2S–11S.

44. Ross PD, Davis JW, Epstein RS, Wasnich RD. Pre-existing fractures and bone mass predict vertebral fracture incidence in women. *Ann Intern Med.* 1991;114;919–923.

45. Chrischilles EA, Butler CD, Davis CS, Wallace RB. A model of lifetime osteoporosis impact. *Arch Intern Med.* 1991;151;2026–2032.

46. Johnell O, Kanis JA, Oden A, et al. Mortality after osteoporotic fractures. *Osteoporos Int.* 2004;15;38–42.

47. Kanis JA, Johansson H, Oden A, et al. A family history of fracture and fracture risk: a meta-analysis. *Bone.* 2004;35;1029–1037.

48. Kado DM, Duong T, Stone KL, et al. Incident vertebral fractures and mortality in older women; a prospective study. *Osteoporos Int.* 2003;14;589–594.

49. Kado DM, Browner WS, Palermo L, Nevitt MC, Genant HK, Cummings SR. Vertebral fractures and mortality in older women: a prospective study. Study of Osteoporotic Fractures Research Group. *Arch Intern Med.* 1999;159; 1215–1220.

50. Black DM, Arden NK, Palermo L, et al. Prevalent vertebral deformities predict hip fractures and new vertebral deformities but not wrist fractures. Study of Osteoporotic Fractures Research Group. *J Bone Miner Res.* 1999;14;821–828.

51. Lindsay R, Burge RT, Strauss DM One year outcomes and costs following a vertebral fracture. *Osteoporos Int* 2005;16;78–85.

52. Klotzbuecher CM, Ross PD, Landsman PB, Abbott TA, 3rd, Berger M. Patients with prior fractures have an increased risk of future fractures: a summary of the literature and statistical synthesis. *J Bone Miner Res.* 2000;15;721–739.

53. Johnell O, Kanis JA, Oden A, et al. Fracture risk following an osteoporotic fracture. *Osteoporos Int.* 2004;15;175–179.

54. Chrischilles E, Shireman T, Wallace R. Costs and health effects of osteoporotic fractures. *Bone.* 1994;15;377–386.

55. Tosteson A. Economic impact of fractures. In: Orwoll ES, ed. *Osteoporosis in Men: The Effects of Gender on Skeletal Health.* San Diego: Academic Press, 1999;15–27.

56. Gabriel SE, Tosteson AN, Leibson CL, et al. Direct medical costs attributable to osteoporotic fractures. *Osteoporos Int.* 2002;13;323–330.

57. Kanis JA, Borgstrom F, De Laet C, et al. Assessment of fracture risk. *Osteoporos Int.* 2005;16;581–589.

58. National Osteoporosis Foundation. *The State of Osteoporosis and Low Bone Mass in the US.* Washington, DC: National Osteoporosis Foundation; 2005.

59. Ensrud KE, Nevitt MC, Yunis C, et al. Correlates of impaired function in older women. *J Am Geriatr Soc.* 1994;42;481–489.

60. Nelson HD, Nevitt MC, Scott JC, Stone KL, Cummings SR. Smoking, alcohol, and neuromuscular and physical function of older women. Study of Osteoporotic Fractures Research Group. *JAMA.*1994;272;1825–1831.

61. Law MR, Hackshaw AK. A meta-analysis of cigarette smoking, bone mineral density and risk of hip fracture: recognition of a major effect. *BMJ.* 1997;315(7112);841–846.

62. Forsen L, Bjorndal A, Bjartveit K, et al. Interaction between current smoking, leanness, and physical inactivity in the prediction of hip fracture. *J Bone Miner Res.* 1994;9;1671–1678.

63. Vestergaard P, Mosekilde L. Fracture risk associated with smoking: a meta-analysis. *J Intern Med.* 2003;254;572–583.

64. Kanis JA, Johnell O, Oden A, et al. Smoking and fracture risk: a meta-analysis. *Osteoporosis Int* 2005;16;155–162.

65. Centers for Disease Control and Prevention. What You Can D to Prevent Falls. http://www.cdc.gov/HomeandRecreationalSafety/pubs/English/brochure_Eng_desktop-a.pdf. Accessed December 2012

66. National Osteoporosis Foundation. Preventing Falls. http://nof.org/articles/17. Accessed December 2012

67. Wardlaw GM. Putting body weight and osteoporosis into perspective. *Am J Clin Nutr.* 1996;63(3 suppl);433S–436S.

68. Haffner SM, Bauer RL. The association of obesity and glucose and insulin concentrations with bone density in premenopausal and postmenopausal women. *Metabolism.* 1993;42;735–738.

69. Ribot C, Tremollieres F, Pouilles JM, et al. Obesity and postmenopausal bone loss: the influence of obesity on vertebral density and bone turnover in postmenopausal women. *Bone.* 1987;8;327–331.

70. Shiraki M, Ito H, Fujimaki H, Higuchi T. Relation between body size and bone mineral density with special reference to sex hormones and calcium regulating hormones in elderly females. *Endocrinol Jpn.* 1991;38;343–349.

71. Tremollieres FA, Pouilles JM, Ribot C. Vertebral postmenopausal bone loss is reduced in overweight women: a longitudinal study in 155 early postmenopausal women. *J Clin Endocrinol Metab.* 1993;77;683–686.

72. Felson DT, Zhang Y, Hannan MT, Anderson JJ. Effects of weight and body mass index on bone mineral density in men and women: the Framingham study. *J Bone Miner Res.* 1993;8;567–573.

73. Edelstein SL, Barrett-Connor E. Relation between body size and bone mineral density in elderly men and women. *Am J Epidemiol.* 1993;138;160–169.

74. Yano K, Wasnich RD, Vogel JM, Heilbrun LK. Bone mineral measurements among middle-aged and elderly Japanese residents in Hawaii. *Am J Epidemiol.* 1984;119;751–764.

75. De Laet C, Kanis JA, Oden A, et al. Body mass index as a predictor of fracture risk: a meta-analysis. *Osteoporos Int.* 2005;16;1330–1338.

76. Osteoporosis prevention, diagnosis, and therapy. *NIH Consensus Statement.* 2000;17;1–45.

77. Prevention and management of osteoporosis. *World Health Organ Tech Rep Ser.* 2003;921;1–164, back cover.

78. *Bone Health and Osteoporosis: A Report of the Surgeon General.* Washington, DC: US Department of Health and Human Services, Office of the Surgeon General; 2004.

79. Cummings S, Cosman F, Jamal S, eds. *Osteoporosis: An Evidence-Based Guide to Prevention and Management.* Philadelphia: American College of Physicians; 2002.

80. Adachi JD, Olszynski WP, Hanley DA, et al. Management of corticosteroid-induced osteoporosis. *Semin Arthritis Rheum.* 2000;29;228–251.

81. World Health Organization. *Prevention and Management of Osteoporosis.* Technical Report Series 921. Geneva, Switzerland: World Health Organization; 2003.

82. Melton LJ, 3rd, Atkinson EJ, O'Fallon WM, Wahner HW, Riggs BL. Long-term fracture prediction by bone mineral assessed at different skeletal sites. *J Bone Miner Res.* 1993;8;1227–1233.

83. Looker AC, Wahner HW, Dunn WL, et al. Updated data on proximal femur bone mineral levels of US adults. *Osteoporos Int.* 1998;8;468–489.

84. FRAX®. WHO Fracture Risk Assessment Tool. Sheffield, UK: WHO Collaborating Centre for Metabolic Bone Diseases; 2010.

85. Kanis JA, McCloskey EV, Johansson H, Strom O, Borgstrom F, Oden A. Case finding for the management of osteoporosis with FRAX—assessment and intervention thresholds for the UK. *Osteoporos Int.* 2008;19;1395–1408.

86. National Osteoporosis Foundation. *Clinician's Guide for Prevention and Treatment of Osteoporosis.* Washington, DC;National Osteoporosis Foundation; 2008.

87. Nieves JW. Nutritional therapies (including fosteum). *Curr Osteoporos Rep.* 2009;7;5–11.

88. Holick MF. Sunlight and vitamin D for bone health and prevention of autoimmune diseases, cancers, and cardiovascular disease. *Am J Clin Nutr.* 2004;80(6 suppl);1678S–188S.

89. Nieves JW, Cosman F. Atypical subtrochanteric and femoral shaft fractures and possible association with bisphosphonates. *Curr Osteoporos Rep.* 2010;8;34–39.

90. Effects of hormone therapy on bone mineral density;results from the postmenopausal estrogen/progestin interventions (PEPI) trial. The Writing Group for the PEPI. *JAMA.* 1996;276;1389–1396.

91. Delmas PD, Ensrud KE, Adachi JD, et al. Efficacy of raloxifene on vertebral fracture risk reduction in postmenopausal women with osteoporosis: four-year results from a randomized clinical trial. *J Clin Endocrinol Metab.* 2002;87;3609–3617.

92. Ettinger B, Black DM, Mitlak BH, et al. Reduction of vertebral fracture risk in postmenopausal women with osteoporosis treated with raloxifene: results from a 3-year randomized clinical trial. Multiple Outcomes of Raloxifene Evaluation (MORE) Investigators. *JAMA.* 1999;282;637–645.

93. McClung M, Clemmesen B, Daifotis A, et al. Alendronate prevents postmenopausal bone loss in women without osteoporosis. A double-blind, randomized, controlled trial. Alendronate Osteoporosis Prevention Study Group. *Ann Intern Med.* 1998;128;253–261.

94. Black DM, Thompson DE, Bauer DC, et al. Fracture risk reduction with alendronate in women with osteoporosis: the Fracture Intervention Trial. FIT Research Group. *J Clin Endocrinol Metab.* 2000;85;4118–4124.

95. Black DM, Thompson DE. The effect of alendronate therapy on osteoporotic fracture in the vertebral fracture arm of the Fracture Intervention Trial. *Int J Clin Pract Suppl.* 1999;101;46–50.

96. Cummings SR, Black D, Barrett-Connor E, Scott J, Wallace RB. Alendronate and fracture prevention. *JAMA* 1999;282;324–325.

97. Black DM, Delmas PD, Eastell R, et al.;Once-yearly zoledronic acid for treatment of postmenopausal osteoporosis. *N Engl J Med.* 2007;356;1809–1822.

98. Neer RM, Arnaud CD, Zanchetta JR, et al. Effect of parathyroid hormone (1–34) on fractures and bone mineral density in postmenopausal women with osteoporosis. *N Engl J Med.* 2001;344;1434–1441.

99. McClung MR, Lewiecki EM, Cohen SB, et al. Denosumab in postmenopausal women with low bone mineral density. *N Engl J Med.* 2006;354;821–831.

Aging

Clinical Changes Experienced by Older Women

Ruby T. Senie, PhD

Introduction

As life expectancy continues to increase in the United States, the number of women and men aged 65 and older has grown substantially, creating complex medical and social challenges for individuals, their relatives, communities, and healthcare providers. Census data for 2008 indicated older women accounted for 58% of the population aged 65 and older, increasing to 67% by age 85.[1] Between 2010 and 2030, the population between ages 25 and 64 is predicted to increase 9.4% in contrast to growth of 79.2% among people aged 65 and older. Public health workers and policy analysts have used these projections to estimate increased healthcare costs for the aging baby boom generation born between 1946 and 1964. These Americans are considered unique due to their large numbers (78 million), significant spending power, and independent spirit.

More than 50 years ago, recognition of this large postwar birth cohort stimulated studies of biologic changes associated with aging. The federal government funded several cohorts that led to the creation of the National Institute of Aging (NIA). Some researchers focused on predictors of health preservation, avoidance of debilitating chronic diseases, maintenance of energy levels, and ability of older adults to continue living independently. The concepts of life-course epidemiology emphasized the influence of lifelong behaviors on age-related changes at the molecular, cellular, and tissue levels. Protective and deleterious factors were identified through comparisons of healthy and disabled older women and men. This chapter reviews some age-related health changes that may be delayed or avoided by protective routine health behaviors established at younger ages that influence the quality of life as older women approach their last decades.

Changing Demographics and Associated Health Needs

In 2006, 13% of the U.S. population was age 65 or older, having grown to 39 million from 3 million in 1900. Figure 36-1 notes the additional years of life estimated for Americans at ages 65 and 85 from decennial census data collected between 1900 and 2006.[1] Compared

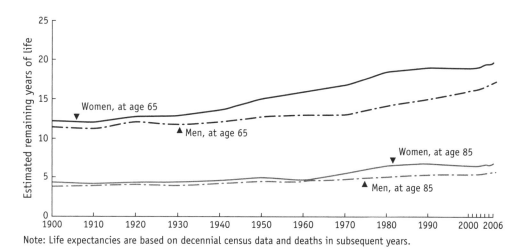

Note: Life expectancies are based on decennial census data and deaths in subsequent years.

Figure 36-1 Life expectancy between 1900 and 2006 at age 65 and age 85 by gender for selected years, United States.

Source: Reproduced from Federal Interagency Forum on Aging-Related Statistics. Older Americans 2010: Key Indicators of Well-Being. Federal Interagency Forum on Aging-Related Statistics. Washington, DC: U.S. Government Printing Office. July 2010. Page 24. http://www.agingstats.gov/agingstatsdotnet/Main_Site/Data/2010_Documents/docs/OA_2010.pdf.

with an estimated 100,000 elderly age 85 alive in 1900, 5.7 million Americans reached age 85 in 2010. The U.S. Census Bureau has projected further growth to 19 million by 2050. The estimated number of remaining years of life for seniors of these ages has continued to increase, although slight dips are noted for women in the earliest years of the 21st century.

Over the past 110 years, life expectancy from birth has increased by more than 30 years. Earlier in the 20th century more than 80% of increased life expectancy occurred before age 65, when most American males and many American females were employed.[2] Improved medical care and preventive modalities have lowered risks of death before age 65, resulting in more Americans living longer after retirement when they are financially dependent on pensions, savings, and Social Security.[2] As of 2009 life expectancy for the total U.S. population reached 78.2 years; however, white females lived longer (80.9 years) than black women (77.4 years).[3] Tabulations for 2002 indicated that 37% of women who survived to age 80 reached age 90, compared with 15% in 1950,[4] suggesting to Christensen et al. that babies born in the 21st century are likely to celebrate their 100th birthdays.[5] Their prediction is supported by the significant decline in mortality over the course of the 20th century, reflecting the Epidemiologic Transitions Theory Omran described in 1971; greater longevity, he stated, was due to replacement of infectious conditions with chronic diseases diagnosed at older ages.[6] This progress was attributed to improvements in public health programs, including sanitation and housing, in addition to greater attention to personal hygiene, food handling, better nutrition, immunizations, and enhanced health education, especially for women, leading to reduced maternal and infant mortality.[7]

Figure 36-2 notes the significant increases in life expectancy during the past 35 years among white and black women and men.[8] Among Hispanics, life expectancy varies by country of origin: Americans from Puerto Rico had shorter life expectancy than immigrants from Central and South America.[9] Limited data are currently available for the more diverse racial and ethnic immigrant populations now residing in the United States.

In 1985 Rowe considered America unprepared for the "explosion of elderly" who have benefitted from advances in medical care, enabling longer life expectancy after retirement.[10] He predicted that by 2015, women and men aged 60 and older would outnumber children aged 15 and younger.[10] The population in the United States is expected to be 50% larger in 2050 than in 1990, with 70 million Americans aged 65 or older, compared with 35 million in 2000.[11] These estimates were based on fertility rates, life expectancy, mortality rates, and immigration patterns, each of which could remain constant, increase, or decrease over the next 2 decades altering the age distribution of the actual population in 2050.

Age-adjusted mortality rates declined 45% for all demographic subgroups between 1960 (1339.2 per 100,000) and 2009 (741.0 per 100,000) significantly reducing long-standing disparities in mortality (Figure 36-3).[3] In 1975 women lived almost 8 years longer than men, but the gender gap declined to 5 years by 2007, the same year in which the smallest disparity in life expectancy by race was recorded.[9] The black–white differential fell to 4.8 years from the high point of almost 8 years in 1989. Mortality reductions in the past 2 decades have been attributed to lower incidence rates and improved treatment of heart disease, cancer, stroke, and respiratory diseases.

Beginning in the 1960s, declining premature mortality of infants and adult minority populations were reflected in longer life expectancy, which Kreiger et al. attributed to civil rights legislation that provided improved health benefits for populations of color coupled with the federal "War on Poverty," which provided increased economic opportunities. Figure 36-3 notes the adverse effect of the widening economic differential that occurred in the 1980s before more recent progress became evident among black populations.[12] These authors stated that 14% of white

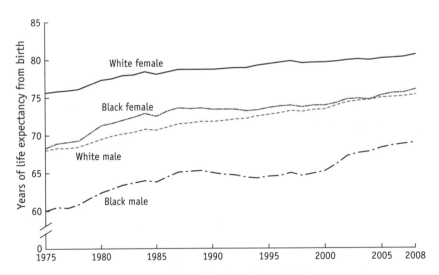

Figure 36-2 Life expectancy at birth by race and gender, United States, 1975–2007, 2008 preliminary.

Source: Reproduced from Miniño AM, Xu JQ, Kochanek KD. Deaths: Preliminary data for 2008. National Vital Statistics Reports; vol. 59 no. 2. Hyattsville, MD: National Center for Health Statistics. 2010. Page 4. http://www.cdc.gov/nchs/data/nvsr/nvsr59/nvsr59_02.pdf.

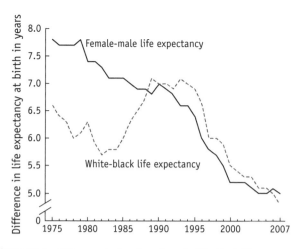

Figure 36-3 Differences in female-male and white-black life expectancies: United States, 1975–2007.

Source: Reproduced from Xu JQ, Kochanek KD, Murphy SL, Tejada-Vera B. Deaths: Final data for 2007. National vital statistics reports; vol 58 no 19. Hyattsville, MD: National Center for Health Statistics. 2010. Page 8. http://www.cdc.gov/NCHS/data/nvsr/nvsr58/nvsr58_19.pdf.

premature deaths and 30% of premature deaths among populations of color would not have occurred between 1960 and 2002 if the same age-specific mortality rates of the wealthiest whites had pertained to all Americans.[12] Continued disparities in life expectancy are less likely to be associated with race/ethnicity than one or more of the following: limited access to high-quality clinical care, low level of education, or lack of insurance to cover high costs of medical treatment, including prescription drugs. For example, mortality from cardiovascular disease was more significantly associated with low socioeconomic status than race/ethnicity among participants in the National Health and Nutrition Examination Survey (NHANES) survey of 2001–2006.[13]

Health of Aging Americans

Population projections suggest that most women age 65 in 2010 will live to age 85, retaining their high energy level and mobility, although 10% to 15% of older women will be burdened with arthritis and other pain-causing conditions. Rowe noted that the media often depict older adults as frail and disabled, not recognizing the heterogeneity of health status and cognitive functioning within the aging population.[10] Cross-sectional studies frequently reported high rates of physical and mental deficits among elderly participants; however, researchers recognized the importance of prospective studies to document normal age-related changes in health status and intellectual functioning in representative populations.[14] One of the earliest cohorts, the Baltimore Longitudinal Study of Aging (BLSA) initiated in 1958, recruited 1,400 men between ages 20 and 90 for intensive physical assessments. During their follow-up of the cohort from middle age to senior years, the scientists recorded physiologic markers that provided detailed assessments of aging.[7] Ten years later, Congress created the Gerontology Research Center in Baltimore, which became the foundation for the NIA.

Between 1989 and 1990, a two-stage sampling process was used in four regions of the United States for recruitment of women and men ages 65 and older to the Cardiovascular Health Study (CHS) to study health changes associated with aging in a multi-institutional population-based cohort. Important differences were identified when older adults meeting entry criteria and agreeing to participate in the CHS were compared with those who refused. The complexities of prospective recruitment of older adults complicates interpretation of research findings during long-term follow-up.[15] With a mean age of 73 years (ranging from 65 to 101), clinical assessments identified at baseline enabled creation of a "prognostic score" for each participant that was predictive of mortality during the following 5 years.[16] This landmark study established important standards for prospective assessment of clinical aspects of aging.

Several other cohorts also provided major sources of data including the Health and Retirement Study (HRS) conducted by the University of Michigan's Institute for Social Research under a cooperative agreement with NIA. In 1992 a representative sample of 12,600 Americans born between 1931–1941 were enrolled.[1] Phone and in-person interviews scheduled biennially continue to provide interdisciplinary data for researchers, policy analysts, and program planners. Through monitoring of age-associated changes in physical functioning and cognitive health, the HRS study has guided development of appropriate programs, allocation of funds to meet specific needs, and advised expansion of access to clinical care as the Medicare population increased.[1] HRS data has been included in several sections of this chapter.

Many aging women fear loss of physical mobility, serious illness, frailty, dependency, and mental decline. This negative view of growing older was rejected in 1980 by Fries, who predicted a shortened duration of infirmity was achievable before a "more natural death" at a relatively fixed upper age of 85 (Figure 36-4).[17] The change in life expectancy between 1900 and 1980 predicted by Fries is clearly demonstrated in his projected "rectangularization" of the survival curve.[17] Thirty years after his landmark publication, research has documented the lifelong benefits of initiating healthy behaviors during youth and maintaining these patterns throughout adult years, successfully delaying onset of adverse effects of aging while minimizing vulnerability to acute illness and trauma.[10,17,18] Concepts of life-course epidemiology suggest health status at older ages may be partially established during in utero development, when maternal exposures may interact with genetic susceptibility to influence fetal growth and the future health of newborns. Subsequent health behaviors developed during childhood, adolescence, and reproductive years influence health status along the life course especially of older women.[19]

Epidemiologic studies have further emphasized that successful aging is characterized by maintaining high levels of mental and physical functioning while preventing or delaying onset of chronic and disabling medical conditions. Rowe specified several key features of successful aging: being at low risk of major chronic diseases,

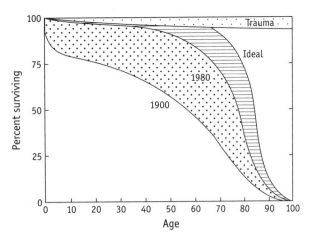

Figure 36-4 Rectangularization of the survival curve.

Source: Reproduced from Fries JF. Aging, natural death, and the compression of morbidity. *N Engl J Med* 1980;303:130–135. With permission. © 1980 Massachusetts Medical Society. All rights reserved.

avoiding disease-related disability, maintaining optimum mental and physical functioning, and remaining actively engaged in meaningful activities.[10] Technologic advances coupled with greater understanding of human biology are expected to further enhance successful aging in the 21st century.

Recognition of the burden of chronic diseases that frequently occur at older ages and often cause disability encouraged Fries to predict that morbidity could be replaced by years of ideal aging following adoption of preventive behaviors during younger ages[17] (Figure 36-4). Data from 2006–2008 indicate 75% of adults aged 65 and older report their health as good to excellent.[1] Although lifestyle interventions could not prevent some age-related clinical changes such as hardening of the arteries, cataract formation, hearing loss, decline in kidney function, and diminished skin elasticity, Fries proposed the elderly could live successfully with some unavoidable disabilities or limitations.[20,21] His "compression of morbidity" hypothesis was initially dismissed as "dangerous optimism" by some policy analysts charged with projecting future healthcare needs and their anticipated costs associated with the changing demographics of America.[7] Research has confirmed Fries' prediction in some populations who have experienced shorter intervals of health deterioration. House et al. found socioeconomically advantaged elders benefitted from compressed morbidity in contrast to the least advantaged whose health and functional status steadily declined with age.[22] Others feared declining mortality would result in higher prevalence of disease with more elderly burdened by disabilities due to multiple comorbid chronic conditions.

Crimmins and Beltran-Sanchez questioned the "fixed limit" component of Fries' theory as increasing numbers of women and men have lived beyond 100 years, often with multiple chronic conditions.[23] For example, reduced cardiovascular disease (CVD) mortality has contributed 60% to increased longevity. After a heart attack or stroke older patients are often burdened with functional limitations and prescriptions for multiple pharmaceutical agents.[23] Over the 8 years of their study, incidence rates of diseases and chronic debilitating conditions had not substantially changed, they noted, although longer survival led to elderly experiencing increased comorbid conditions with higher healthcare costs but not meeting the authors' definition of healthy life without disease. Therefore, they questioned whether health was improving with each generation or if instead therapeutic interventions had increased the number of Americans treated for chronic conditions living longer lives with increasing disabilities rather than prolonged years of "compressed morbidity."[23]

As more people approached the "maximum" biologic life span predicted by Fries, interindividual variability appeared to diminish. Women and men surviving to their 90s may have inherited protective genetic markers or shared preventive behavior patterns. Many experienced greater satisfaction with life events and had psychological characteristics enabling balanced acceptance of age-related health changes.[20] Baltes and Smith distinguished between young-old and old-old populations through cohort comparisons noting recent gains in physical and mental functioning of individuals in their 70s who exhibit comparable qualities of earlier cohorts at younger ages. Especially evident were gains in cognitive reserve, termed "self-plasticity" by the authors, enabling many to remain employed or active in community organizations.[24] As new technology has enhanced health maintenance and disease prevention, Olshansky et al. suggested interventions to slow the aging process are scientifically plausible, extending years of youthful vigor, and enabling continued employment at older ages.[25]

Older Women in the Workforce

Employment of older women has increased during the past 4 decades (Figure 36-5).[26] In 2008, 42% of women aged 62 to 64 were employed compared with 29% in 1990; at ages 65 to 69, 26% were employed in 2009, compared with 17% in 1990.[27] Some employers have offered phased retirement, inducing workers to continue either full- or part-time employment; this practice was encouraged by the Pension Protection Act of 2006 and the Senior Citizens Freedom to Work Act of 2000, permitting pension benefits and Social Security payments to employed workers regardless of earned income. Employer-sponsored health promotion programs open to workers of all ages have documented improved health status as well as reduced health care costs.[28]

Depending upon the working environment, continued employment affects women's health. In contrast to the positive aspects of social involvement and improved sense of self worth associated with employment, some recent data indicate working women may experience increased morbidity associated with asthma, chronic bronchitis, diabetes, congestive heart failure, and arthritis.[29] Many factors, in addition to health status, guide individual decision-making of older women, especially general economic conditions. Lower income older workers in service and agricultural jobs may require continued employment

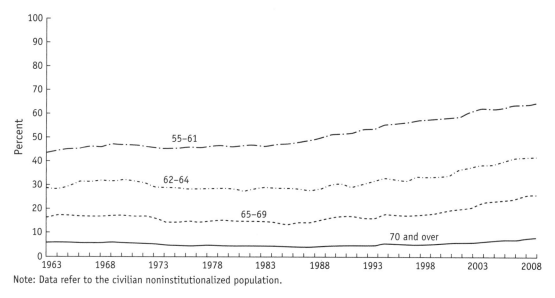

100
90
80
70
60
50   55–61
40
Percent
30   62–64
20
10   65–69
                                                        70 and over
0
1963   1968   1973   1978   1983   1988   1993   1998   2003   2008

Note: Data refer to the civilian noninstitutionalized population.

Figure 36-5   Annual averages of women age 55 and older employed by age group, United States,1963–2008.

Source: Reproduced from Federal Interagency Forum on Aging-Related Statistics. Older Americans 2010: Key Indicators of Well-Being. Federal Interagency Forum on Aging-Related Statistics. Washington, DC: U.S. Government Printing Office. July 2010. Page 19. http://www.agingstats.gov/agingstatsdotnet/Main_Site/Data/2010_Documents/docs/OA_2010.pdf.

due to lack of pensions or limited funds for basic needs, including health insurance. In addition, some pension programs are lowering their support of retirees whose former employers are unable to maintain financial commitments.[27] Older women more than men experience the death of their spouse, often resulting in loss of financial support. Of necessity, they may continue working long hours even though the physical demands of the work may jeopardize their health or cause severe pain from arthritis or other conditions.[30] Costs to employers providing health benefits may increase when older workers require more clinical care than younger employees. Some companies have achieved significantly lowered costs by providing onsite clinical care as well as exercise facilities and educational programs to improve the health of their workforce while controlling expenses.[31]

Social and Behavioral Determinants of Health of Older Women

Although disease prevention and health promotion are frequently merged as public health goals, prevention modalities avoid onset of diseases or conditions by encouraging appropriate vaccinations and avoidance of risky exposures such as smoking and obesity.[28] In contrast, health promotion includes early detection of clinical problems through screening and/or physical and social assessment followed by essential appropriate treatment to reduce morbidity and increase life expectancy.[28]

Promoting Healthy Behaviors

Epidemiologic studies have confirmed the long-term benefits of healthy behaviors across the life span, lowering the risk of morbidity and premature mortality. For example, among more than 3,000 University of Pennsylvania

alumni recruited in 1962 at a mean age of 43 and followed for 30 years by annual mailed questionnaires, smoking, high body-mass index, and/or limited routine exercise at midlife were associated with disability onset by age 75 or death prior to last follow-up.[14] Among participants with healthier lifestyles at time of enrollment, longevity was greater and onset of disability was postponed by 5 or more years before the end of life (P <.0001). Increasing evidence has documented accumulated benefits that healthier lifestyles adopted at older ages also have benefits.[28] The primary causes of preventable premature deaths identified by Danaei et al. included smoking and hypertension before age 65 followed by excess body mass and lack of routine physical activity.[32]

Social Support

Social and lifestyle factors were found to affect the health and well-being of older Americans as group pressure encourages flu vaccinations, participation in physical activity, and smoking cessation.[1] Berkman and Syme, among others, emphasized the role of social interactions and support as preventive medicine, especially for older women.[33] As noted in Figure 36-5, more women age 55 and older were employed in 2008 than in any previously reported year.[1] Continued employment provides workers not only with access to health care but benefits of social involvement and personal satisfaction, in contrast to retirement, which may lead to feelings of isolation following disruption of a woman's social network. To evaluate the role of social support among aging participants in the Alameda County, California study, Berkman and Syme created a social network index derived from baseline questionnaire data, including marital status, numbers of relatives and friends, religious involvement, and other group affiliations. Follow-up 9 years later revealed threefold greater risk of mortality among similarly aged women with the fewest social network contacts compared with the highest index level.[33] Berkman suggested social ties provided a sense of belonging, intimacy for sharing personal feelings, expression of similar goals, sense of integration, and self worth, although she noted some downsides could exist when social contacts encourage or accept poor health habits such as smoking.[33] Recent research by Christakis and Fowler based on participants in the Framingham Heart Study noted similar social network influences in the spread of smoking behavior and subsequently smoking cessation.[34]

Due to the importance of social networks to older women and men, death of loved ones and friends, or forced relocation may trigger health problems as these disruptive life events may terminate comfortable relationships and support systems.[35] Therefore, community organizations, religious groups, and voluntary agencies have created support groups for older women and men who express need for and find comfort among others with similar life experiences.

Smoking Cessation

Following the first Surgeon General's report in 1964, smoking was targeted by public health workers as a primary disease-causing behavior, although tobacco companies countered scientific evidence linking smoking to lung cancer and other adverse health outcomes with extensive and expensive advertising.[36] Although the prevalence has diminished among Americans, smoking remains the most common preventable cause of premature death.[37] In 2010, approximately 450,000 deaths were due to smoking and 8 million Americans were sickened or disabled from current or past active or passive smoking. More than 10% of recent responders to the National Health Interview Survey (NHIS) age 65 or older indicated they were active smokers. The prevalence was higher among men than women of lower education and income who lacked health insurance.[38]

Unfortunately the residual adverse effects of past smoking may continue to cause disease and shorten the life span (Figure 36-6);[39] national survey data indicate 55% of men and 31% of women age 65 or older are former smokers.[1] Rates declined sharply during the last decades of the 20th century occurring more rapidly among men than women resulting in comparable rates by gender in the youngest birth cohorts. The decline was primarily orchestrated by laws controlling cigarette advertising, increased taxes raising cigarette costs, and prohibition of smoking in public buildings.[40] Analyses by Wang and Preston revealed risk of death remains elevated for many years after quitting. In addition, older female smokers have increased risk of several major chronic conditions including arthritis, cardiovascular disease, and cancer of several organs.[41] Risk of death due to cancer of the lung, mouth, throat, pancreas, and other organs increases with age; smokers have twice the risk of nonsmokers.[42]

Although the percentage of active smokers significantly declined between 1965 and 2008 among both female and male Americans, Figure 36-6 documents the

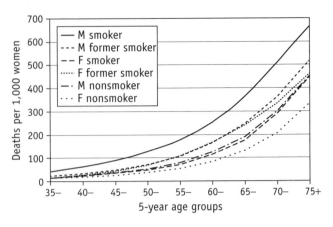

Figure 36-6   Risk of death within 10 years per 1,000 men and women by 5-year age groups.

Source: Adapted from Woloshin S, Schwartz LM, Welch HG. The risk of death by age, sex, and smoking status in the United State: Putting health risks in context. J Natl Cancer Inst 2008;100:845–853.

relationship of smoking history by gender with risk of death at all ages. Responding to some older adults who questioned health benefits from quitting smoking, Goetzel et al. presented convincing evidence of improved quality of life as well as longevity when seniors reduced modifiable risk factors including, smoking and weight control during their remaining years,[28] and Breslow advised adults that it was never too late to stop smoking, to eat nutritious meals, and to participate in routine exercise.[18] Figure 36-6 notes current male smokers at the oldest ages have the highest mortality compared with former or never smokers of both genders;[39] female nonsmokers had the lowest mortality rate. Several cohort studies have confirmed smoking cessation even at older ages reduced risk of cancer or heart disease development or disease progression.[43,44]

Goetzel et al. proposed health behavior programs for Medicare participants designed to meet physical and cognitive needs rather than based on age or birth cohort, reflecting Rowe's earlier concept of heterogeneity of functional status among the elderly.[10,28] Health promotion activities, defined by Goetzel et al., related to personal prevention behaviors, including routine exercise, fitness training, weight control, consuming a healthy diet, receiving appropriate immunizations, practicing safe sex, drinking moderately, enrolling in stress reduction activities, being active in social support programs, and being alert as pedestrians or motor vehicle drivers.[28] They noted that the Centers for Medicare and Medicaid Services (CMS) developed the Healthy Aging Initiative to identify and test promising evidence-based health promotion strategies, determine their cost, and promote acceptance by older subscribers. Medicare preventive programs were successful in convincing seniors to stop smoking, lose weight, increase physical activity, and reduce risks of falling. These efforts resulted in lowered blood pressure, improved diabetes control, and mental health benefits. These authors suggested community-based volunteers could enhance health benefits of these programs.[28] In addition, the Senior Risk Reduction Demonstration (SRRD) assessed health promotion programs including behavior change and self-help activities developed in private care settings (General Motors and Bank of America).[28,31] A random sample of older adults received tailored health messages and interactions with research staff. Results will be available in 2013. Employers are providing health maintenance facilities to working adults to encourage healthful behaviors reducing morbidity especially among older employees planning retirement.

Physical Activity

Research has repeatedly indicated that physical activity is essential for the maintenance of health among older adults, reducing the risks of several chronic conditions, relieving symptoms of depression, maintaining independent living, providing social interaction, and enhancing overall quality of life.[1] Among participants in the Cardiovascular Health Study, continuing physical activity at all ages provided a dose-response protective effect against death 5 years after enrollment.[16] Mobility and physical functioning can be improved through routine exercise such as swimming and balance training (Figure 36-7).

In 2008 the U.S. Department of Health and Human Services revised physical activity recommendations to include 75 minutes per week for muscle strengthening and increased heart and breathing rates. To assess exercise duration in a random sample of Americans, the Behavioral Risk Factor Surveillance System survey collected data from responders age 65 and older; 51% reported exercise levels meeting recommendations. Although duration of time spent active is important, Studenski et al. found walking speed an important clinical indicator of multiple organ systems functioning.[45] Among 34,500 community-based residents age 65 or older from nine cohort studies in which walking speed had been recorded, faster speed was associated with diminished risk of mortality 5 years after study entry.

The findings from the Americans Changing Lives (ACL), a cohort study of almost 4,000 adults aged 25 years and older recruited in 1986 and followed for 19 years, indicated the lowest level of physical activity among participants ages 55 and older was associated with increased risk of dying (HR = 2.65, 95% CI = 2.01−3.49) after controlling for predictive factors including body mass index (BMI).[46] Inactivity was among the most important findings of the ACL study, as sedentary lifestyle has increased in America, with more hours spent watching television or using computers and other electronic devices. Lack of routine exercise accelerates loss of skeletal muscle leading to sarcopenia, age-related changes in muscle fiber quantity and quality, reduction in flexibility, and physical decline, with the onset of frailty and ultimately loss of ability to remain living independently.[47] Improved protein intake and increasing physical activity may correct some of the loss of muscle strength.[47]

Some studies indicated health behaviors of older adults who spend more time in their local communities may be influenced by physical and social factors prevalent in their residential environment.[48] Therefore, neighborhood characteristics such as safety, available parks, and recreational facilities may affect the frequency and types of physical activity of elderly residents. To investigate the suggested perception of neighborhood problems influencing the reporting of activity levels, Beard et al. linked disability information reported by residents aged 65 and older during the 2000 U.S. Census by New York City tract data with neighborhood physical and social characteristics.[48] The findings indicated more physical disabilities and less time spent outside the home among residents living in less residential stable communities of low socioeconomic status.

Major health consequences result from low physical activity. A dose-response relationship between exercise and cognitive decline leading toward Alzheimer's disease was suggested by findings from a population-based study conducted in northern Manhattan.[49] In addition to amount of routine exercise, other lifestyle factors, including consumption of a Mediterranean style diet, contributed to mental functioning and successful aging.[49] King reviewed community-based programs and suggested physicians should recommend increased

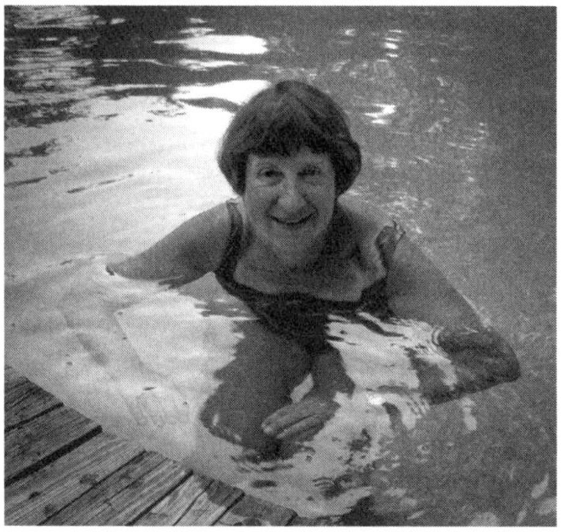

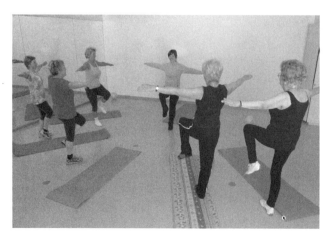

Figure 36-7a Swimming is a recommended exercise for seniors.

Figure 36-7b Balance training lowers risk of falling.

© iStockphoto/Thinkstock

exercise among the elderly while administering influenza, pneumococcal, and other preventive vaccines. She suggested carefully targeted programs should meet the physical and cultural needs of subgroups by physical abilities or race/ethnicity.[50] With increased activity level, nutritional intake improved and psychological well-being was enhanced.

Nutritional Requirements of Elderly Women

Appropriate nutritional intake is essential for health maintenance among older women to avoid frailty, loss of bone mass, and muscle weakness. A healthy diet also reduces the risk of hypertension, diabetes, and obesity. The Surgeon General's report of 2004 emphasized the need for increased intake of vitamin D by elderly women to support bone health and lower the risk of osteoporosis and hip fracture (Figure 36-8).[51] The link between lean body mass and nutritional intake was studied among more than 2,700 community-dwelling healthy women and men ages 70 to 79 in the Health, Aging and Body Composition Study (Health ABC). Baseline diet history was collected by trained interviewers using a food frequency questionnaire (FFQ).[52] Three years later, all participants had lost some lean body mass although the highest consumption of protein was most protective and lowered risk by 40%.[53]

Additional research from the Women's Health Initiative (WHI) observational study confirmed the importance of adequate dietary protein for older adults noting a strong, independent, dose-responsive protective effect against development of frailty.[54] Dietary deficiencies of protein detected in almost 4,000 WHI participants (5.5%) were associated with diagnosis of anemia. Inadequate nutrient intake was more frequent among blacks (15%) and Hispanics (16%) than white women (7%).[55]

Poor diet is a major contributor to onset of physical and mental conditions among the elderly. Malnutrition, often associated with poor health in developing countries, may occur among older Americans who experience some of the risk factors in Table 36-1.[56] Careful assessment, preferably through home visits, may identify at-risk elderly lacking adequate or appropriate nutrition toward the end of life.

Table 36-1

Risk factors for malnutrition among the elderly

Poverty	Disability
Social isolation	Bereavement
Depression	Dementia
Use of multiple drugs	Alcoholism
Surgical procedures	Malabsorption
Loss of taste or smell	Oral health problems
Acute or chronic illness	Institutionalization

Energy level can be maintained and low blood sugar levels avoided by consumption of small, more frequent meals, each including small amounts of protein.[47] Fasting for many hours may be life-threatening for the elderly, as the resulting hypoglycemia may cause dizziness, anxiety, cardiac palpitations, blurred vision, and loss of consciousness.[22] Water consumption is also essential especially following exercising to avoid feelings of fatigue that accompany dehydration. Coffee, a stimulant, may increase energy level and alertness but may also induce insomnia. Moderate alcohol consumption, defined as one drink per day for women and two for men, was protective in the ACL study.[22] In contrast, excessive alcohol drinking reduces energy level and mental alertness but may impede mobility and mental competence.

Clinical Care and Health Maintenance of Elderly Women

Health promotion through early detection by screening followed by appropriate treatment limits morbidity and increases life expectancy. Tinetti and Fried suggested that acute infections resulting in chronic disease among the elderly often led to overtreatment, undertreatment, or mistreatment.[57] Undertreatment resulted from clinicians hesitating to prescribe remedies for the elderly whose symptoms, complicated by age-related impairment, did not meet diagnostic criteria. They also noted that aging

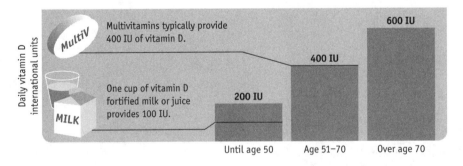

Figure 36-8 Vitamin D requirements increase with aging.

Source: Reproduced from U.S. Department of Health and Human Services. The 2004 Surgeon General's Report on Bone Health and Osteoporosis: What It Means To You. U.S. Department of Health and Human Services, Office of the Surgeon General, 2004.

patients required longer clinical time to adequately assess their physical and emotional symptoms.[57] Tinetti and Fried stated "the disease model of diagnosis and treatment" was outdated and potentially harmful to aging Americans. Instead they proposed clinical decisions needed to be personalized to meet the biologic, social, economic, and cultural needs and desires of individuals.[57]

Detecting hypertension, obesity, malnutrition, and elevated biomarkers followed by comprehensive multimodality treatment has lengthened survival of older patients.[28] The Medicare Modernization Act of 2003 provided a prescription plan with preventive physical examinations including screening for diabetes and cardiovascular disease. With increasing life expectancy, clinicians and professional organizations have debated having upper age limits for routine screening, especially for breast and cervical cancer. Detection of these diseases at very early stages in elderly women may result in overtreatment for conditions that may never become lethal during the women's remaining lifetime while potentially causing serious, life-threatening, and costly consequences that may adversely affect the quality of their remaining years of life.[58]

Genetic Predisposition

Unusually long, healthy lives are assumed to reflect a combination of lifestyle choices, inheritance of protective genes, and lower prevalence of disease-causing mutations. Shared environmental exposures and healthy behaviors, especially at young ages, within families may interact to either reduce or augment inherited genetic predisposition to longevity and/or susceptibility to clinical conditions.[19] Inheritance was evident among sibling participants in the New England Centenarian Study, whose life expectancy, even at very old ages, was far greater than the average life span of members of the same U.S. birth cohorts.[19] To identify specific protective genes, several research groups have undertaken molecular genetic analyses of available relatives from families distinguished by exceptional longevity.[59] These authors noted the members of the Ashkenazi population with exceptional longevity reported similar health behaviors to those reported by participants in the NHANES I survey from the same birth cohort. Therefore, the researchers suggested shared environment and lifestyle within families may have also contributed to longevity. However, many of the Jewish study participants were immigrants to the United States whose experiences, health behaviors, and exposures prior to migration may have influenced their exceptional longevity rather than protective genetics. This study may be based on a selected population whose cultural patterns and health status enabled immigration to the United States. Therefore, subsequent generations of these exceptional families may not enjoy equally long lives.

Advancing technology has enabled identification of specific single nucleotide polymorphisms (SNPs) through genomewide association studies (GWAS) that confer modest elevations of risk of common chronic disorders and cancers in large study populations. In the near future the genetic information should enable clinicians to provide guidance for health behaviors and/or therapeutic interventions to delay or prevent onset of disease, although many unanswered questions remain to be addressed before findings will be applicable to personalized clinical care.

Oral Health

Oral health screening coupled with personal oral hygiene and maintenance of healthy teeth are essential for consumption of adequate nutrition to support immune function and avoid diseases that occur more frequently among older women. Healthy teeth are necessary for chewing, speaking clearly, avoiding pain, and enjoying social interaction.[60] Physicians are encouraged to coordinate their clinical assessments of older adults with dentists to assure appropriate oral care for their elderly patients.

Oral pathogens associated with periodontal infections are known to increase the risk of bacterial pneumonia and/or heart disease among the elderly. A Japanese randomized trial among nursing home patients (mean age of 82) assessed the role of intensive oral hygiene on avoidance of pneumonia. Yoneyama et al. reported the control patients receiving usual clinical care were 2.5 times more likely to develop and die of pneumonia than patients receiving the intervention.[61] Subsequent implementation of preventive oral hygiene in Japanese nursing homes lowered the risk of acquiring a systemic infection related to oral bacteria.

National data indicate by age 65, 30% of the American adults have lost all their teeth. Among 826 women aged 70−79 followed by Semba et al., 63.5% used dentures, which often caused difficulty chewing, resulting in more malnutrition, frailty, and lower 5-year survival rates (HR = 1.43, 95% CI = 1.05−1.99).[62] Physical immobility and diminished sight may impede some elderly from maintaining healthy teeth and gums; assistance may be required to adequately cleanse the mouth. Changes in the quantity of saliva caused by medications may lead to greater tooth decay, increasing tooth loss, and reducing dietary options. In addition, taste and palatability of some foods may be diminished by intensive treatments such as chemotherapy.

Racial/ethnic disparities in oral health among elderly Americans were detailed in the Surgeon General's report of 2000. Wu and colleagues analyzed the magnitude of the disparities in NHANES data collected during in-home interviews and examinations between 1999 and 2004.[63] Their results noted minority elders compared with whites had significantly worse oral health with more missing and decayed teeth. More blacks (19%) and Hispanics (20%) than whites (7%) reported needing teeth to be extracted.[63]

Common Health Conditions and Impairments Affecting Older Women

Older women experience a number of acute and chronic health conditions and impairments that may adversely affect their quality of life, impede their functioning, and limit their independence. The biologic impact of loss of endogenous estrogens and other hormones following natural or surgical menopause strongly influences the subsequent health of aging women. Some classic symptoms often reported or detected clinically include sleep disturbances, ocular changes, osteoporosis, atherosclerosis, elevated blood pressure, and lowered energy levels among other discomforts.

Comorbidity has become quite prevalent among aging American women and men. The 2010 publication of the U.S. Department of Health and Human Services indicated 25% of all Americans including 66% of those age 65 or older require continuing medical care for two or more chronic conditions.[1] The presence of comorbid conditions may not be detected until a health crisis develops if clinical care is limited and assessment inadequate. Signs and symptoms of new health problems often differ among older patients compared with younger women experiencing the same pathologic conditions. Delayed detection may limit treatment options while enabling disease progression. Diagnostic procedures and treatment planning may also be complicated when a patient exhibits loss of mental clarity, an early sign of dementia. Continuity of care in addition to electronic medical record-keeping could avoid the need for repeated review of past history and potentially avoid treatment errors.

Obesity

Obesity rates in the United States had remained stable for decades until a rapid rise in prevalence occurred in the 1980s and 1990s; currently more than 60% of adults are overweight or obese. Figure 36-9 indicates changing percentages of obesity among women aged 65 to 74 and 75 or older between 1988 and 2008. With the expanding obesity epidemic, some researchers have predicted a decline in life expectancy as well as more disability from diabetes, arthritis, stroke, asthma, and other respiratory conditions.[64] Research has already reported reduced longevity averaging 5 to 10 years among the most severely obese. Danaei et al. found obesity was responsible for 1 in 10 premature deaths among women.[32] Risk of diabetes is increased 30% to 40% among obese women, shortening life expectancy by about 13 years.[64] Risk of breast, colon, and endometrial cancers are increased among women who gain weight after menopause, and recent studies have associated obesity, especially centrally distributed fat, with increased risk of dementia (HR = 2.8, 95% CI = 2.3−3.3).[65]

Future health risks associated with obesity are predicted based on current and anticipated continued increased incidence of obesity. Research has linked being overweight or obese with many chronic conditions; however, some studies have noted **reduced** mortality among overweight (HR=0.81, 95% CI=0.69–0.96) or obese (HR = 0.73, 95% CI=0.59–0.90) women aged 55 and older compared with normal weight women.[46] For some elderly women, higher BMI provides protection against trauma, frailty, and wasting syndromes. In addition, fat padding associated with excess weight provides a source of endogenous estrogen through androstenedione conversion in adipose tissue. The ACL baseline data was collected before the obesity epidemic began; therefore, the authors expressed concern that long-term obesity from childhood might affect mortality differently from weight gain only at older ages.[46] Flegal et al. used NHANES data to report increased mortality among underweight and extreme levels of obesity. However, among men and women ages 60−69 and 70 or older, being overweight or slightly obese did not significantly increase risk of mortality. The authors suggested their findings reflected improved medical care for heart disease, the primary cause of death at older ages.[66]

Hypertension and Cardiovascular Disease

As Figure 36-10 indicates, heart disease is the leading cause of death among American women age 65 and older; hypertension, defined as systolic blood pressure 140 mm Hg or higher and diastolic greater than 90, increases with

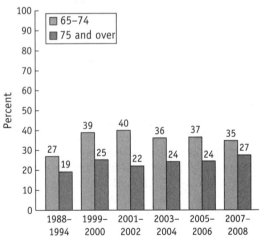

Note: Data are based on measured height and weight among participants in the National Health and Nutrition Examination Survey (NHANES)

Figure 36-9 Percentage of American women age 65 and older who were obese during selected years, 1988–2008.

Source: Reproduced from Federal Interagency Forum on Aging-Related Statistics. Older Americans 2010: Key Indicators of Well-Being. Federal Interagency Forum on Aging-Related Statistics. Washington, DC: U.S. Government Printing Office. July 2010. Page 40. http://www.agingstats.gov/agingstatsdotnet/Main_Site/Data/2010_Documents/docs/OA_2010.pdf.

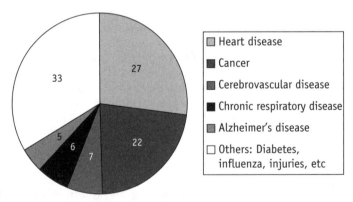

Figure 36-10 Percent of leading causes of death among American women aged 65 and over, 2010.

Source: Reproduced from Miniño AM, Murphy SL. Death in the United States, 2010. NCHS data brief, no 99. Hyattsville, MD: National Center for Health Statistics. 2012. Page 4. http://www.cdc.gov/nchs/data/databriefs/db99.pdf.

age and raises the risk of cardiovascular disease. Studies indicate many Americans have undetected or inadequately treated hypertension that, according to data from the original Framingham study, increases lifetime risk of stroke to one in six or higher among women aged 55 to 75. Risk was 50% lower for women with normal blood pressure (120/80) compared with similarly aged women with hypertension (≥140/90).[67] Elevated blood pressure was among the primary modifiable causes of preventable deaths analyzed by Danaei et al. using National Center for Health Statistics (NCHS) data.[32] They noted the number of deaths caused by each factor: smoking (1 in 5 deaths), hypertension (1 in 6 deaths) and obesity, high blood glucose level, and physical inactivity each were responsible for 1 in 10 deaths.

Gender-specific analyses indicated 19% of deaths among women were due to hypertension- related cardiovascular disease (CVD), which reflected high salt intake and limited physical activity.[32] In contrast to the adverse effects of excessive alcohol intake, moderate drinking reduced deaths from heart disease and diabetes.[32] Interventions have successfully reduced blood pressure by encouraging routine exercise, weight control, and low sodium diet reducing water retention.[68] Some studies have identified dietary patterns and moderate alcohol intake, especially red wine, as protective against death from heart disease.[69,70] Great progress has been accomplished in extensive cardiovascular disease research, enabling the significant reduction in mortality that has occurred over the past 4 decades.

Arthritis and Osteoporosis

Arthritis and musculoskeletal conditions often cause chronic pain and disabilities that limit mobility resulting in isolation. The prevalence of disabilities due to fibromyalgia, arthritis, osteoporosis, and musculoskeletal conditions is expected to increase in coming decades with more women affected (24%) than men (18%).[71] Centers

for Disease Control and Prevention (CDC) data indicated 34% of women compared with 25% of men were obese in 2010; the higher prevalence of arthritis in women could be attributable to greater weight combined with current or recent smoking history and lower rates of physical activity. Obesity is strongly linked with osteoarthritis of the knee increasing the likelihood of total knee replacement. For women with multiple comorbid conditions, surgery for joint replacement may be complicated. Community-based health interventions have addressed obesity by stimulating greater physical activity to control development of arthritis among aging adults.[71]

Women have lower bone density than men and experience greater bone loss as they age, resulting in significantly higher rates of osteoporosis. Normal bone resorption and formation become unbalanced from diminished estrogen levels associated with menopause. To lower the risk of hip fractures, which occur twice as frequently among women over the age of 75 compared with men, increased consumption of calcium and vitamin D and routine weight-bearing exercises are encouraged. The Surgeon General's report of 2004 addressed bone health and osteoporosis noting the disparity between self-reported hip fractures and osteoporosis and assessment by physical examination of Americans included in NHANES (Table 36-2).[51]

Diabetes

The epidemiology of diabetes across the life span notes the disease increases with age and is greater in women of color. An estimated 1 in 10 American women had diabetes in 2010. If not monitored and treated, diabetes increases the risk of heart disease, stroke, kidney failure, leg amputation, nerve damage, and blindness; diabetes is also the sixth leading cause of death in women 65 and older. Among the dire predictions for coming decades is increased incidence of diabetes among elderly women associated with the increasing prevalence of obesity. By

Table 36-2

Prevalence of osteoporosis and hip fracture per 100 men and women aged 65 and older

| Gender and Age | Self-Reported | | Tested |
	Hip Fracture %	Osteoporosis %	Osteoporosis %
Male	2.3	1.3	3.8
65–74 yrs	2.1	1.3	2.0
75–84 yrs	2.4	1.3	6.4
85 yrs and older	4.1	1.6	13.7
Female	6.1	11.1	26.1
65–74 yrs	4.5	10.9	19.0
75–84 yrs	7.3	12.1	32.5
85 yrs and older	11.8	9.7	50.5

Modified from Praemer A, Furner S, Rice DP. Musculoskeletal conditions in the United States. Rosemont, IL: American Academy of Orthopaedic Surgeons. 1999:182. In: *Bone Health and Osteoporosis: A Report of the Surgeon General.* U.S. Department of Health and Human Services, Office of the Surgeon General, 2004.

2050 an estimated 29 million Americans will have diabetes. Dentists often identify undiagnosed diabetes; a strong correlation was reported between the number of missing teeth and extent of periodontal disease in older adults with undiagnosed diabetes.[72] Therefore, improved access to dental care, especially for older minority women, could increase early detection of diabetes among those shown to be at highest risk; timely treatment could prevent diabetic complications that lead to disability, loss of independence, and death.[72]

Urinary Incontinence

Urinary incontinence and an overactive bladder are estimated to affect 13 million elderly women, approximately 5% to 20% of those living independently and about 40% of nursing home residents.[10] Women often report stress incontinence associated with physical exertion or when sneezing or coughing. Quality of life is often adversely affected by the social stigma and embarrassment associated with incontinence, a topic rarely discussed with healthcare providers.[73] Factors associated with incontinence among older women include obesity, recurrent urinary tract infections (UTIs), history of hysterectomy, depression, and impaired functional status. Research indicates neurologic deficits do not cause incontinence in most women, although prevalence is greater among female stroke patients and women diagnosed with multiple sclerosis.

To study the prevalence, precipitating factors, and potential interventions associated with incontinence, Brown et al. studied 8,000 women aged 65 and older enrolled in the Heart and Estrogen/Progestin Replacement Study (HERS); 41% reported occasional urine loss and 14% experienced daily incontinence.[74] Symptoms worsened among women randomized to combined hormonal therapy.[75] Prevalence increased 30% with each 5 years of advancing age, especially among women with a history of UTIs, diabetes, obesity, and/or major depression. Moore et al. reported 60% of postmenopausal women who developed a UTI during their longitudinal study experienced incontinence twice as often (4.7 times/month) as similarly aged women without a history of UTI.[76] Diabetes, especially requiring insulin, was significantly associated with both UTI and incontinence. Diabetics reported difficulty controlling urination, were unable to completely empty the bladder, and required pads to protect clothing.[77] Severe incontinence was reported by 50% of nurses older than age 50 with type 2 diabetes; Lifford et al. suggested the neurologic complications associated with diabetes may have impaired bladder control.[78]

Obesity independently increased both the risk of incontinence (OR = 1.6, 95% CI = 1.4 − 1.7) and onset of diabetes.[74] A 6-month weight loss intervention trial, the Program to Reduce Incontinence by Diet and Exercise (PRIDE), successfully helped women lose 8% of body weight accompanied by 70% reduction in incontinence compared with control subjects who received usual clinical care.[79] Some women experience incontinence after hysterectomy or hormone use, either oral or vaginal cream.[80] Nygaard has advised consistent routine exercises to strength pelvic floor muscles, use of electrical stimulation of the muscles, or medication to help control incontinence.[73]

Sleep Disorders

Advances in technology have enabled confirmation of self-reported frequencies of sleep disturbances among aging adults. Sleep difficulties were often associated with reduced physical activity, medical conditions, and/or psychosocial concerns.[81] As in other aspects of aging, daily sleep-wake patterns and age-related changes vary greatly among older adults. At all ages sleep includes two different physiological states: rapid eye movement sleep (REM), when muscles are most relaxed and dreaming occurs, and intervals of nonrapid eye movement (NREM). NREM is now divided into Stage N1 and N2, defined by light sleep with greater potential for arousal, in contrast to Stage N3 characterized by deeper sleep.[82] Sleep cycles are generally 90 minutes long with deeper Stage N3 occurring in the first half of the night and REM sleep in the second half. brief or prolong awakenings interrupt the sleep-wake patterns. Older adults experience shorter durations of REM sleep and more frequent awakenings associated with physiologic, psychological, and environmental factors.[82]

Elderly women reported increased insomnia (75%) and reduced sleep quality (71%) from frequent nocturia, which may be due to diminished sphincter control from vaginal atrophy.[83] Among commonly reported sleep disorders of older adults are insomnia (20–40%), obstructive sleep apnea (50–60%), and restless leg syndrome (10%).[82] In addition, some prescribed and over-the-counter medications may adversely affect sleep patterns. Researchers have identified sleep disruptions associated with familial patterns and obesity.[84] During lighter sleep of NREM stages, osteoarthritis pain disturbed sleep of 50% of adults surveyed. Taibi and Vitiello proposed a pilot study testing yoga for pain relief before sleep; the successful pilot is leading to a randomized trial to test the behavior in a broader population.[85]

Many clinicians are not familiar with the strong bidirectional relationship between disturbed sleep and serious medical conditions among elderly patients including hypertension, depression, and cardiovascular and cerebrovascular diseases.[82] Some conditions result in sleepiness during waking periods with desire for napping; however, older adults fear napping may increase wakefulness at night. Napping did not alter total sleep time or the quality of nighttime sleep under experimental conditions designed by Campbell et al. In addition, enhanced cognitive and psychomotor performance was observed after an afternoon nap, an effect that extended to the following day.[81]

Depression and Depressive Symptoms

Hormonal depletion during the menopausal transition and psychosocial stressors at that critical time in women's lives increase risk of depression in older women. During the past several decades, rates of clinical depression have remained stable with women reporting depression (20%)

more than men (10%). Although depressive symptoms were more prevalent among women, despression increases with aging among both men and women.[1]

Socioeconomic Status

During 15 years of follow-up of the ACL population, the strongest determinants of health maintenance or deterioration were socioeconomic status and related educational level.[22] House et al. found socioeconomically advantaged elders benefitted from compressed morbidity in contrast to the least advantaged whose health and functional status steadily declined with age.[22] Although health disparities were largely explained by economic, behavioral, and biomedical determinants, the researchers found improvements had occurred over time. Younger ACL participants were healthier than similarly aged cohort members had been 15 years earlier.[22] The impact of socioeconomic status varied across the life span; adverse effects were limited at young ages, increased during middle ages, but declined among the elderly, reflecting the protective role of federal and state social health and welfare programs.[22]

Sexual Health of Older Women

The media rarely depict sexual attraction among older members of society, suggesting enjoyment of intimacy declines with age; however, many older Americans consider sexuality a vital aspect of their lives, although comfortable patterns of sexual expression may require some adjustments. Age-related neurologic and hormonal changes may affect physiologic responses of women and men to sexual arousal;[86] however, health professionals can provide clinical options for older patients seeking optimum quality of sexual health, including medications to treat male erectile dysfunction and products to ease female discomforts.[87] Videos and mechanical devices in addition to products designed to stimulate sexual desire are promoted to enable older couples to achieve sexual pleasure.[89]

Lindau and Gavrilova analyzed data from two population-based national surveys to assess health status in relation to sexual activity and quality of sexual life. Between ages 75 and 85 more men (38.5%) were sexually active in the past year than women (16.7%) and the gender difference increased with age. Among the sexually active elderly respondents, good health was significantly associated with the frequency, quality, and interest in sexual expression by both men and women.[87] Partner availability is obviously a factor; among the elderly age 85 and older, the ratio of males to females is approximately 1:2.5.[86] Understandably, sexual activity differs by partner status; more men (78%) than women (40%) reported a regular partner.[87]

Sexual response includes a complex of emotional, cultural, and physical aspects that may necessitate differing methods of arousal and stimulation as women age. Illness reduces desire or impedes ease of familiar aspects of sexual expression as reflected in national data that indicated 50% of older men and women had at least one sexual problem.[86] Side effects of some medications interfere with or reduce sexual functioning. Chronic pain from arthritis or immobility after a stroke may require special planning

for partners to achieve comfortable and satisfying sexual experiences. Lindau and Gavrilova indicated 34% of men experienced erectile difficulties and 14% had used drugs to enhance sexual function.[87] Among older women, 43% expressed limited desire for sexual intercourse, 39% experienced vaginal discomfort, and 34% were unable to achieve climax. Vaginal changes such as decreasing elasticity, thinning of vaginal walls, and shortening of vaginal canal may cause physical discomforts which may be relieved with nonprescription lubricants. When applied by the woman's partner, lubricants may reduce discomfort while stimulating desire.[88] Some women, after surgery with significant body image changes, have reported sexual dysfunction, especially discomfort with a new partner.[88]

Comparable data regarding sexual activity among older adults were reported from another national survey of more extensive questions including sexual orientation; same sex partners were reported by 9% of men and 2% of women during the most recent sexual experience.[89] These researchers also noted that many older women and men experienced partner loss due to divorce, death, or serious illness, resulting in new sexual partnering. Although the experience may heighten arousal and enhance likelihood of orgasm, new intimacy may rekindle fears of sexually transmitted infections, although survey data indicated 20% had used condoms.[89]

Factors Associated with Morbidity and Mortality among Older Women

The biologic impact of loss of endogenous estrogens and other hormones following natural or surgical menopause strongly influences the subsequent health of aging women. Some classic symptoms often reported or detected clinically include sleep disturbances, ocular changes, osteoporosis, atherosclerosis, elevated blood pressure, and lowered energy levels among other discomforts. The following section addresses some findings from studies of aging women that may guide future interventions to reduce the risk of chronic diseases and associated disabilities that diminish the quality of life at older ages.

Socioeconomic Status and Education

The ACL longitudinal study indicated higher mortality was associated with low income and low education level linked with high-risk behaviors. However, Lantz and colleagues noted that, regardless of economic and education level, death occurred among participants aged 55 and older more frequently among ACL participants who were current or past smokers, nondrinkers, severely underweight (BMI < 18.5), and participated in very limited physical activity. These behaviors were more prevalent among those with low income and low education.[46] Light alcohol intake was more protective among the older than younger study participants. The authors encouraged policymakers to address social and behavioral determinants of health using the media to encourage smoking prevention (or cessation) and increased physical activity, the two strongest mortality predictors identified.[46]

Physical Limitations of Aging

Compared with men, women's longer life expectancy lengthens the number of years they are living with functional limitations.[7] Figure 36-11 identifies the chronic conditions causing physical limitations by age group per 1,000 recorded by the NHIS conducted by CDC, indicating the personal needs requiring care provider assistance for women and men. In 2008–2009 the NHIS noted 15% of women and 10% of men aged 80 and older needed assistance with personal care activities such as eating, bathing, and dressing; however, these self-reported data of functional impairment may be an underestimate. Despite the increasing frequency of chronic disease and use of medications by Americans of all ages, the percentage of disabled older adults ages 65 to 74 decreased from 14.2% in 1982 to 8.9% in 2004–2005, declining 1.5% per year among participants in National Long-Term Care Surveys (NLTCS). This trend extended the declining rate detected in an earlier analysis of the NLTCS data from 1982 thru 1994 by Singer and Manton.[90] Significant declines in institutionalization were also reported for Americans age 75 and older from 8.1% to 4.2% and from 27.7% to 15.6% of elders age 85 and older.[91]

Onset of poor health or functional decline is a critical negative transition in older adulthood. Independence, a positive state, is associated with the ability to perform all activities of daily living (ADL) without having to resort to help from others in contrast to dependency, a negative state, that implies helplessness and powerlessness.[92] Aging-associated losses of autonomy and control contribute to emotional distress, potentiate the impact of physiologic changes, and diminish quality of life. Accumulating adverse life events such as loss of loved ones may compound anxiety associated with increasing disability. Fillit and Butler suggested preparation for the transition to greater dependence and acceptance of physical limitations by the caregivers, family members, and aging individuals

may encourage adaptive responses rather than feelings of grief for lost independence.[93]

In 2007 approximately 66% of older adults with one or more ADL received personal assistance and/or used specialized equipment to function within their home with the need increasing slightly with aging. More than 70% of the elderly age 85 and greater received personal assistance with ADL, often from family caregivers, enabling chronically disabled elders to reside in the community rather than a long-term care facility. However, 67% of older adults with three or more ADL limitations were residents of nursing homes.[1] More diverse residential facilities have been developed recently providing housing and supportive services, although limited data are available on the number of residential settings and types of services offered. Licensing and certification requirements vary by state law. To address the deficiencies regarding knowledge of the number of facilities, the varied levels of supportive services available, the housing arrangements, and the costs of maintaining elders in such facilities will be obtained from the newly created National Survey of Residential Care Facilities.[1]

Hearing Impairment

The NHIS asked respondents about their ability to hear without listening devices. Diminished hearing was reported with increasing age by both women and men from less than 30% at age 65 to more than 60% at age 85 or older. Approximately 35% of older adults reported using hearing aids.

Visual Impairment

Blindness or low vision affects approximately 1 in 28 Americans older than age 40 according to the Eye Diseases Prevalence Research Group.[94] Figure 36-11 presents NHIS data indicating vision problems by age group among Americans 65 and older; the percentage of older women reporting vision problems increased from 17% at age 65 to 28%

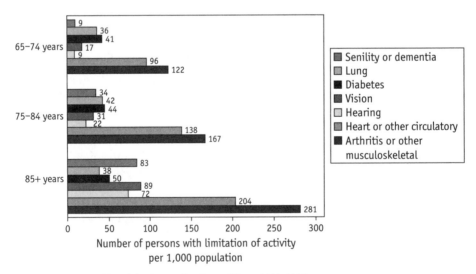

Figure 36-11 Activity limitations among older adults due to chronic conditions, 2003–2004.

Source: Reproduced from National Center for Health Statistics. Health, United States, 2009: With Special Feature on Medical Technology. Hyattsville, MD. 2010. http://www.cdc.gov/nchs/data/hus/hus09.pdf

by age 85.[1] The prevalence of unrecognized but correctable visual impairment has been estimated to range from 7% to 34% in the United States; therefore, Evans and Rowlands suggested general practitioners should assess vision during annual health exams in conjunction with blood pressure and diabetes screening of Medicare patients.[95]

Cataracts

Cataracts, the most common age-related cause of visual impairment, are correctable by surgical extraction. The surgery, performed more than a million times annually, is the most common surgical procedure covered by Medicare.[96] Age-related cataracts are associated with diabetes, excessive exposure to ultraviolet light, smoking, and passive exposure to tobacco smoke. To understand the natural history of cataract development and macular degeneration, the Age-Related Eye Disease Study (AREDS) enrolled 4,400 participants aged 55 to 80 years at 11 U.S. eye centers.[97] Postmenopausal women were at greater risk than similarly aged men unless they were using hormonal replacement therapy, which significantly lowered risk of cataracts.[97] Twin studies conducted in England indicated heritability accounted for 48% of nuclear cataract development, 38% was age related, and only 14% was associated with smoking history or other environmental factors.[96]

Age-Related Macular Degeneration

Age-related macular degeneration (AMD) causes progressive damage to the macula, the central portion of the retina that enables clear vision. Blurred sight may be the first indication of degeneration which progressed to loss of central vision while peripheral vision is retained. This irreversible condition restricts the ability of an affected individual to handle activities of daily living and to function independently. Tomany and colleagues merged international data to assess risk factors of AMD and reported cigarette smoking was associated with nearly a threefold increased risk and diagnosis occurred approximately 10 years earlier among smokers than nonsmokers.[98]

The Eye Diseases Prevalence Research Group, based on data from international population-based studies applied to age-specific U.S. census records has estimated almost 1 million Americans aged 40 or older are blind and another 2.5 million have impaired vision.[94] Although visual impairment increases with aging, routine eye examinations enable detection of impending problems before permanent deficits occur. As eye conditions progress, patients often adjust to slow deterioration reducing their ability to detect serious changes.

Cardiovascular Disease and Stroke

Incidence of CVD among the elderly has increased although mortality has declined, raising the prevalence of older Americans living longer after earlier diagnosis and improved treatment.[5] Incidence and mortality rates vary by race/ethnicity and gender. All subgroups have benefited from improved treatment of hypertension and changes in health behaviors although disparities remain including striking geographic differences within the United States.

The national Health and Retirement Study (HRS) followed more than 19,000 stroke-free adults for 8 years and identified predictors of first stroke among participants aged 50 and 64. Independent factors included lower socioeconomic status and education level.[99] The authors suggested age-related differences reflected clinical care available for Medicare recipients, The HRS also noted increased stroke incidence associated with residence at birth and during childhood in a southeastern state, the "stroke belt".[100] Geographic residence may influence access to medical care, social and cultural norms affecting behaviors, socioeconomic conditions, dietary patterns, and psychosocial pressures.[100]

Some elderly people experience dizziness and frequent falls from postural hypotension, a sudden drop in blood pressure as they quickly standup following prolonged inactivity.[101] In addition, dehydration and some medications may increase risk of postural hypotension. Falls among the elderly, especially in the bathroom, have resulted in the need for hospital emergency department assessment often associated with hip fracture. Careful studies have provided insight into the causes of falling and opportunities for prevention. Among preventive measures to avoid falls are: improving safety of home environments with grab bars in bathrooms, wearing vision correcting glasses, maintaining exercise to improve balance, using a cane or walker for security, wearing supportive shoes, and avoiding drug interactions.

Malignancies

Cancer incidence rises with age although incidence patterns vary among malignancies of different sites, which may reflect susceptibility by family history, genetics, personal health behaviors, environmental factors, and preventive modalities. The number of newly diagnosed malignancies rises with age; after age 65 cancer is the second leading cause of death of older American women following cardiovascular disease. Given the estimated growth of the aging population, oncologists are estimating a 65% increase in diagnoses in the next few decades.[102] Among women, the three most frequent cancer sites are the breast, colon, and lung. Smith et al. encouraged expansion of prevention strategies, including vaccination for hepatitis B and human papilloma virus, chemoprevention for women at risk of breast cancer, and elimination of smoking.[102]

Controversies regarding routine mammography among women ages 75 and older are frequently debated in the media as recommendations by American and international professional and voluntary organizations differ concerning age at which screening can be discontinued. Many researchers and the public have questioned the value of mammography to reduce breast cancer mortality among older women, especially those with comorbid conditions.[103] Others have noted the difficult logistics associated with accessing screening facilities especially for women with physical disabilities. In addition, treatment of very early stage disease detected by mammography carries potential risks of overtreatment.[58] After thoroughly reviewing all available literature, the U.S. Preventive Services Task Force reported the benefit-to-harm ratio for screening mammography peaks between ages 60 to 69.[104] Analysis of breast cancer survival data among Medicare recipients revealed higher mortality was associated with comorbid conditions than from metastatic cancer.

Data presented in the American Cancer Society 2012 Cancer Facts and Figures indicated mortality has declined for several cancers.[42] However, other malignancies diagnosed among older women lack early detection modalities such as pancreatic, ovarian, and lung cancers and therefore remain highly lethal. Screening options to detect lung cancer among smokers have been studied in a clinical trial conducted between 2002 and 2004. Participants were randomized to either three annual low-dose spiral scans using computed tomography (CT) or chest x-ray. Although fewer lung cancer deaths occurred among participants who received CT scans compared to chest x-ray, significant risks were associated with the large number of false-positive screens that required highly invasive lung biopsies to rule out malignancy.[105]

Medication Use and Misuse

Prescription drugs have significantly contributed to controlling chronic clinical conditions among older adults by relieving symptoms, improving quality of life, and increasing longevity of America's aging population. During the past 10 years the National Health and Nutrition Examination Survey (NHANES) data indicated an increase in drug prescribing patterns between 1999 and 2008 (Figure 36-12). Among men and women age 60 or older, 88% were prescribed at least one medication, 76% were on two medications, and more than 37% were prescribed 5 or more drugs.[106] (Figure 36-13). Older American women (53%) were more frequently prescribed medications by their clinicians than older men (43.2%).[106] An estimated 35% of all prescribed medications are used by

people age 60 and older who are also heavy consumers of over-the-counter drugs, vitamins, and minerals as well as herbal preparations and supplements. The percentage of older adults using prescribed medications was associated with having a regular source of healthcare and prescription benefits included in their health insurance.

Multiple medication use creates significant challenges for elderly patients, who often have coexisting disorders that each requires medication. Decreasing cognitive ability may augment the risk of therapeutic errors when patients take the wrong medication or at the wrong dose. However, adverse reactions may also occur when medications are taken as prescribed by the physician and pharmaceutical company.[107] Adherence to physician prescribed protocols is known to decrease as the number of medications and frequency of use per day is increased,[112] which may be accompanied by higher prevalence of dangerous drug-related side effects.[106] Elderly patients using generic medications for treatment of chronic condition may be confused by the legal requirements of drug companies to diversity the color and markings for the same bioequivalent medication, a requirement instituted to prevent the sale of counterfeit drugs.[109] Illiteracy is rarely mentioned as a hazard but some elderly patients, especially first generation immigrants, may be unable to read either English or their native language.

Calls to poison information centers often seek help with drug poisoning among elderly patients. Patients over age 65 were at twice the risk of experiencing an adverse drug event which resulted in hospitalization 7 times more frequently than for younger patients.[108] Zhang et al. analyzed national prescribing patterns from the Healthcare Effectiveness Data and Information Set (HEDIS) to determine the frequency of use of drugs considered high-risk for elderly patients with one or more of three conditions: dementia, hip or pelvic fracture, or chronic renal failure.[108] Large geographic differences were observed in the quality of prescribing patterns and subsequent frequency of adverse drug reactions with greater inappropriate medication use in southeastern states.[108]

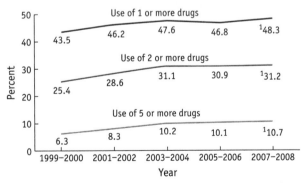

Note: Age-adjusted to 2000 U.S. population. Significant linear trend of increased use.

Figure 36-12 Trends in prescription drug use in the United States from 1999–2000 through 2007–2008.

Source: Reproduced from Gu Q, Dillon CF, Burt VL. Prescription drug use continues to increase: U.S. prescription drug data for 2007–2008. NCHS data brief, no 42. Hyattsville, MD: National Center for Health Statistics. 2010. Page 1. http://www.cdc.gov/nchs/data/databriefs/db42.pdf.

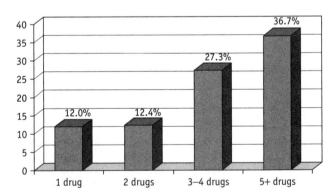

Figure 36-13 Percentage of Americans age 60 and older by number of prescription drugs used within past month, United States, 2007–2008.

Source: Modified from Gu Q, Dillon CF, Burt VL. Prescription drug use continues to increase: U.S. prescription drug data for 2007–2008. NCHS data brief, no 42. Hyattsville, MD: National Center for Health Statistics. 2010. Page 2. http://www.cdc.gov/nchs/data/databriefs/db42.pdf.

Thousands of Americans are injured or die annually from preventable adverse drug reactions presenting a significant public health burden.[111] Skarupski et al. suggested drug interactions among the elderly is a "silent epidemic."[107] Data obtained from chart review of a national representative sample of 266,000 emergency department visits by patients aged 65 or older indicated 37.5% resulted in subsequent hospitalizations due to allergic reactions, undesirable effects at recommended doses, or unintentional overdose from prescribed and over-the-counter medications, vaccines, and/or dietary supplements.[113] The risk of drug related hospitalization was 3.5 times greater among patients 85 or older compared with ages 65–69.[113] Some data suggests avoidable hospitalizations occur more readily among those who do not adhere to medical advice including consistent use of prescribed drugs; therefore, various monitoring, tracking and reminder methodologies are being developed to increase consistent use of prescribed medications with an ultimate goal of maintaining health and avoiding hospitalizations. Unintended interaction and adverse drug reactions occur with increasing frequently as women age due to changes in drug metabolism influencing dose requirements, vision problems causing patient confusion, forgetfulness and cognitive deficits associated with bereavement or illness, and increasing comorbid conditions.

New regulations were promoted by the FDA in 2006 to increase patient safety and decrease confusion for prescribing clinicians.[114] Although extensive lists of potential side effects are mandated on drug labels and package inserts, Avorn and Shrank noted a delay of several years between the reporting of newly recognized adverse drug effects and inclusion of the information on package inserts or in the Physician Desk Reference while manufacturers conduct post marketing studies.[114] Online information was also mandated by the new regulations although the use of the web-based information by physicians, before prescribing a new drug had not been assessed.[114]

Anergia

Complaints of lack of energy (anergia) by elderly patients are often dismissed as a normal age-related problem; however, Cheng et al. considered this complaint a potential indicator of an underlying treatable condition. Among more than 2,000 multiethnic community-dwelling elderly in New York, 18% met their criteria for anergia; 22% were female and 12% male.[110] Anergia was associated with presence of comorbid conditions indicating interactions of biologic, psychological, and social factors necessitating more healthcare facilities and resulting in higher mortality during follow-up.[110]

Frailty

Frailty, characterized by slowness of motion, weakness, fatigue, and unintentional weight loss, is a wasting syndrome of aging resulting from comorbid physical disorders and functional impairments. Fries noted that physiologic decline in organ function gradually increases with aging but accelerates to frailty in the presence of

comorbid conditions.[21] With accumulating physical and cognitive deficits, older adults become less able to adapt to age-related physical and social changes.[115] Frail elderly are at increased risk of falling, cognitive decline, increased dependency on others, and greater risk of mortality than similarly aged men and women who continue to thrive.[7] Twin studies have suggested genetics may contribute to risk of frailty, and men are less likely to become frail, possibly due to male hormones maintaining muscle strength.[7]

Because definitions vary, estimates of the prevalence of frailty are approximate ranging from 7.3% to 16.3% of the elderly U.S. population. Some researchers define frailty by observing elderly with difficulties in two or more areas including physical, nutritive, cognitive, or sensory.[116] Others advocate using biomarkers of nutrient levels and inflammatory responses to measure degree of frailty and enable more consistent classifications across studies.[117] Fillit and Butler coined the term "frailty identity crisis" representing the psychological effect to a dependent status for previously robust seniors.[93] The concept specified body image changes including shortened stature, less steady balancing, wrinkled skin, and declining muscle often accompanied by depression.[93]

Two population-based cross-sectional studies, the Women's Health and Aging Studies, conducted by Fried et al. assessed frailty among female residents of Baltimore, Maryland, aged 70–79 years. Five criteria used to classify participants with/without frailty were weakness (low grip strength), slow walking speed, low physical activity, unintentional weight loss, and self-reported exhaustion.[115] Frailty required three or more criteria; women with one or two factors were labeled prefrail. A cascade effect appeared to begin with unintentional weight loss (10 pounds over 12 months) resulting in physical limitations including slowed walking and reduced energy. Risk of frailty was positively associated the number of chronic comorbid conditions detected during clinical evaluation.

The onset of frailty in adults in Alameda County, California, during 30 years of follow-up was predicted by such behavioral factors as heavy drinking, cigarette smoking, physical inactivity, depression, social isolation, and prevalence of chronic disease. Frailty was self-reported by 3,298 (13.5%) of the 24,000 women aged 65 to 79 enrolled in the WHI observational study who indicated low levels of physical functioning, exhaustion, and unintended weight loss.[54]

Assistance Needed for Activities of Daily Living

Many baby boomers are also members of the "sandwich generation," who have been caretakers for aging parents while raising children and developing their careers. They observed progression of age-related dependencies and deficits while aware of the heterogeneity among older relatives and friends whose mental competency and physical functioning remained intact. However, activity limitations and deficits accumulated over passing years as readily noted in Figure 36-14. The self-reported data may underestimate the full measure of functional impairment

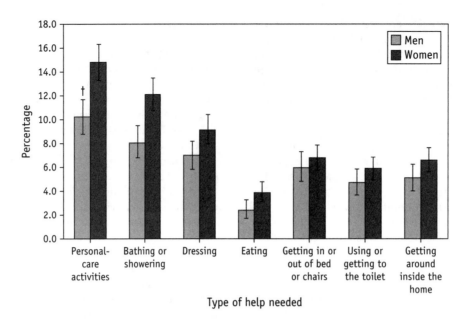

Figure 36-14 Percentage of noninstitutionalized adults age 80+ needing help with personal care by gender, United States, 2008–2009.

Source: Reproduced from QuickStats: Percentage of noninstitutionalized adults age >80 years who need help with personal care, by sex—United States, 2008–2009. Morbidity and Mortality Weekly Report 2011;60:819. http://www.cdc.gov/mmwr/preview/mmwrhtml/mm6024a5.htm

because some older adults may accept physical changes as indicative of normal aging[10] even though they may need assistance with some activities of daily living (ADLs).[1]

Other measures of physical functioning include stooping or kneeling, reaching over head, walking two or three blocks, lifting 10 pounds, and ability to write.[1] Between 1991 and 2007 the percentage of women enrolled in Medicare who needed help with one or more ADLs remained comparable with 32% of women and 19% of men unable to perform at least one of five indicators of physical disability. In 2008–2009 NHIS noted 15% of women and 10% of men aged 80 and older needed assistance with personal care activities such as eating, bathing, and dressing often provide by family members;[118] an estimated 1.3 million home health aides are providing essential services for very ill and frail elderly patients in their homes. With ever-increasing life expectancy, elderly often require physical therapy, visiting nurse services, and other personal services required to continue living independently. Home health care grew rapidly following extended coverage by Medicare in 1987. An American survey indicated 30% of households had at least one member (66% were female) who provided unpaid care to a sick or elderly relative with physical and/or emotional problems.

Gershon and colleagues assessed experiences encountered by home health aides in New York City. After signing the study consent form promising anonymity, more than 1,500 employed aides completed the questionnaire.[118] Most responders were female (95%), mean age of 43 years, 90% had received training, and averaged 8 years experience providing care in private homes or assisted living facilities. Aides reported diverse personal hazards including unsanitary conditions, abuse from patients or family members, and racial or ethnic discrimination. Abuse of the patient by relatives was also noted. Often

professional nursing expertise rather than skills of aides was needed.[118] The authors suggested greater oversight of home health aides is required to ensure protection of vulnerable patients and their caretakers.[118]

Self-Neglect Syndrome

Pavlou and Lachs in their literature review of self-neglect syndrome, a geriatric behavior pattern characterized by persistent neglect of personal hygiene and poor maintenance of their residence, creating hazardous conditions that threaten personal safety coupled with refusal to accept services to improve quality of life. Self-neglect was often associated with comorbid clinical conditions necessitating several medications accompanied by dementia, depression, or other mental disorders leading to social isolation and fear of losing independence.[119] Aging-associated loss of autonomy and control often create emotional and physiologic changes with diminishing quality of life.

Accumulating adverse life events such as loss of loved ones, diminished eyesight, hearing loss, and need for dentures may compound anxiety associated with increasing disability.[1] Community-residing adults may avoid medical care until an emergency occurs or neighbors detect a growing problem. Pavlou and Lachs presented an algorithm for intervention by a multidisciplinary team to provide the patient with essential services and treatment. Estimates from Adult Protective Services suggest 5–10% of elderly may be diagnosed with self-neglect syndrome.[119] Naik and colleagues conducted a comprehensive physical and mental assessment in the homes of 200 study participants to characterize this geriatric syndrome: 100, identified by Adult Protective Services as self-neglecting, to be compared with 100 adults of similar ages recruited through a local geriatric clinic.[120] Ability to handle activities of daily living differentiated the two populations. Vulnerable elderly in this study were more often frail and in need of basic medical care. The authors encouraged additional research to identify factors precipitating onset of the syndrome and avenues to interrupt the progression of self-neglect to avoid personal harm and danger to others.[120]

Self-neglect syndrome and onset of depression among aging women may be components of the continuum known to exist from normal aging to severely affected brain function leading to dementia and Alzheimer's disease.

Elder Abuse and Domestic Violence

As women age, their vulnerability to elder abuse and domestic violence increases. These abusive acts occur in domestic settings, such as private homes, and are hidden by family members.[122] Elder abuse may include intentional actions by a caregiver or person in a position of trust that causes harm or leaves the older person at risk of harm. Abuse may result from omission of needed life-sustaining food or medicine or may take the form of overt acts that threaten the patient's safety and well being.[121] Data reported in 2005 by the National Center on Elder Abuse (NCEA) was compiled from numerous studies and population-based surveys that included several categories: physical abuse, sexual abuse, emotional abuse, financial exploitation, neglect, and abandonment. State-reported data has shown a 150% increase between 1986 (117,000 reports) and 1996 (293,000). More than 1 million elders were victims excluding self-neglecting elders and an estimated 18,000 reports of financial exploitation were submitted by states to NCEA in 2001; 58% of the victims were female and 65% were aged 66 or older.[122] Among the recommendations included in the Institute of Medicine report titled *Clinical Preventive Services for Women* was an annual "well-woman preventive care" visit including culturally sensitive screening for evidence of domestic violence.[123] The signs of elder abuse are often not recognized resulting in underestimates of the prevalence.[123] Mouton and Carter-Nolan suggested elders who become isolated within their communities are at risk of abuse, as they lack a social network for support and protection. The social isolation, they noted, enabled family violence to remain hidden. As women age and experience cognitive impairment progressing toward dementia and other mental problems, they are more likely to be victimized.[121]

Technology-Enhanced Monitoring

Technology has provided new avenues for social contact heavily used by youth but also readily accessed by many seniors, who enjoy online communication and access to health-related information. Security has been provided to housebound older people through electronic devices that alert emergency personnel; computerized medication dispensers prevent some confusion with drugs, and household motion detectors have been developed to monitor routines of elderly living alone. The Food and Drug Administration has encouraged continued development of medical applications for smart phones and other mobile communications devices that enable healthcare professionals to improve patient care such as alerting patients to timely administration of medications and providing individuals with calorie content of specific foods. FDA monitors newly developed applications to ensure patient safety and to reject any that may present potential risks to patients if the applications do not function as intended.

A British pilot study conducted by the National Health Service called Safe Mobile Care provides healthcare professionals with electronic monitoring of home-based patients with chronic conditions.[124] The equipment enables personalized care that can readily be updated by mobile phone connections, fostering a sense of independence while ensuring a safe home environment for elderly patients. The British have a centrally based communication system that can rapidly respond to emergency occurrences.[124]

End of Life Issues

The last year or months of an older person's life are often complicated by many family and personal decisions about medical care, potential changes in living arrangements, access to caregivers, and other factors. Clinical care, especially symptom control and pain relief, has often been hampered by inadequate communication among healthcare providers of diverse backgrounds and between clinicians and their patients resulting in insufficient attention to patient preferences.[1] Americans of all ages are encouraged to prepare a living will indicating personal decisions regarding life-sustaining care should trauma or illness impair an individual's ability to communicate.

Summary

Although the aging of the baby boomer cohort has created anxiety among public health workers and politicians concerned with rising healthcare costs associated with the increasing numbers of retired Americans, some researchers have promoted the benefits of new technology providing greater longevity with delayed or diminished disease and disability resulting from healthier lifestyles during younger years. Genetics have been shown to contribute to exceptional longevity enhanced by personal health behaviors including routine exercise, nutritious diets rich in fruit and vegetables, weight control in relation to height, and social networking. Education and financial well-being were predictors of healthful longer life spans and racial/ethnic disparities have lessened but remain to be overcome. Careful clinical management of chronic conditions is encouraged to limit progression of morbidity and diminish painful symptoms enhancing the quality of senior years. Future research must be directed to understanding the biology of aging especially the onset of cognitive deficits that precede progression to Alzheimer's disease.

Discussion Questions

1. Researchers include a wide variety of physical and psychological parameters to define "successful aging." Describe the concepts presented by several leading investigators and compare their definitions of aging with yours.

2. What public health programs have had the greatest impact on life expectancy? On average women live longer than men. What factors contribute to differences by gender?

3. How do exercise, diet, weight control, and other health behaviors contribute to morbidity and mortality at older ages?

4. Community and social involvement has been found to influence the health of aging women. What benefits are gained from such activities?

5. What does "compression of morbidity" refer to? How can this be achieved?

References

1. Federal Interagency on Aging-Related Statistics. *Older Americans 2010. Key Indicators of Well-Being.* Federal Interagency Forum on Aging-Related Statistics. Washington, DC: U.S. Government Printing Office; 2010.
2. Fuchs VR. New priorities for future biomedical innovations. *N Engl J Med.* 2010;363:704–706.
3. Minino AM. Death in the United States, 2009. Atlanta, GA: Centers for Disease Control and Prevention; 2011. NCHS Data Brief No. 64.
4. Rau R, Soroko E, Jasilionis D, Vaupel JW. Continued reductions in mortality at advanced ages. *Popul Dev Rev.* 2008;34:747–68.
5. Christensen K, Doblhammer G, Rau R, Vaupel JW. Ageing populations: the challenges ahead. *Lancet.* 2009;374:1196–1208.
6. Omran AR. The epidemiologic transition. A theory of population change. *Milbank Mem Fund Q.* 1971;49:509–538.
7. Satariano WA. *Epidemiology of Aging: An Ecological Approach.* Sudbury, MA: Jones and Bartlett; 2006.
8. Kochanek KD, Xu J, Murphy SL, et al. Deaths: preliminary data for 2009. *Natl Vital Stat Rep.* 2011;59:4.
9. Xu J, Kochanek KD, Murphy SL, et al. Deaths: final data for 2007. *Natl Vital Stat Rep.* 2010;58:19.
10. Rowe JW. Health care of the elderly. *N Engl J Med.* 1985;312:827–835.
11. Day JC. National Population Projections. Population Profile of the United States. Washington, DC: U.S. Census Bureau; 1995. http://www.census.gov/prod/1/pop/profile/95/2_ps.pdf.
12. Krieger N, Rehkopf DH, Chen JT, et al. The fall and rise of US inequities in premature mortality: 1960–2002. *PloS Med.* 2008;5:e46:227–240.
13. Karlamangia AS, Merkin SS, Crimmins EM, Seeman TE. Socio-economic and ethnic disparities in cardiovascular risk in the United States, 2001–2006. *Ann Epidemiol.* 2010;20:617–628.
14. Vita AJ, Terry RB, Hubert HB, Fries JF. Aging, health risks, and cumulative disability. *N Engl J Med.* 1998;338:1035–1041.
15. Tell GS, Fried LP, Hermanson B, et al. Recruitment of adults 65 years and older as participants in The Cardiovascular Health Study. *Ann Epidemiol.* 1993;3:358–366.
16. Fried LP, Kronmal RA, Newman AB, et al. Risk factors for 5-year mortality in older adults. The Cardiovascular Health Study. *JAMA.* 1998;279:585–592.
17. Fries JF. Aging, natural death, and the compression of morbidity. *N Engl J Med.* 1980;303:130–135.
18. Breslow L. From disease prevention to health promotion. *JAMA.* 1999;281:1030–1033.
19. Perls TT, Wilmoth J, Levenson R, et al. Life-long sustained mortality advantage of siblings of centenarians. *Proc Natl Acad Sci USA.* 2002;99:8442–8447.
20. Fries JF. The compression of morbidity. *Milbank Mem Fund Q.* 1983;61:397–419.
21. Fries JF. Frailty, heart disease, and stroke. The Compression of Morbidity paradigm. *Am J Prev Med.* 2005;29:164–168.
22. House JS, Lantz PM, Herd P. Continuity and change in the social stratification of aging and health over the life course: evidence from a nationally representative longitudinal study from 1986 to 2001/2002 (Americans' Changing Lives Study). *J Gerontology.* 2005;60B(special issue II):15–26.
23. Crimmins EM, Beltran-Sanchez H. Mortality and morbidity trends: is there compression of morbidity? *J Gerontol Soc Sci.* 2011;66B:75–86.
24. Baltes PB, Smith J. New frontiers in the future of aging: from successful aging of the young old to the dilemmas of the fourth age. *Gerontology.* 2003;49:123–135.
25. Olshansky SJ, Perry D, Miller RA, Butler RN. Pursuing the longevity dividend scientific goals for an aging world. *Ann NY Acad Sci.* 2007;1114:11–13.
26. Mosisa A, Hipple S. *Trends in Labor Force Participation in the United States.* Current Population Survey. Washington, DC: US Department of Labor, Bureau of Labor Statistics; 2006.
27. Purcell P. *Older Workers: Employment and Retirement Trends.* Washington, DC: Congressional Research Service; 2009. Report for Congress 7–5700.
28. Goetzel RZ, Shechter D, Ozminkowski RJ, et al. Can health promotion programs save Medicare money? *Clin Interv Aging.* 2007;2:117–122.
29. Bhattacharya J, Choudhry K, Lakdawalla D. Chronic disease and trends in severe disability in working age populations. *Med Care.* 2008;46:92–100.
30. Caban-Martinez AJ, Lee DJ, Fleming LE, et al. Arthritis, occupational class, and the aging US workforce. *Am J Public Health.* 2011:e1-e6.doi:10.2105/; *Am J Public Health.* 2011.300173.
31. Leigh JP, Richardson N, Beck R, et al. Randomized controlled study of a retiree health promotion program. The Bank of America Study. *Arch Intern Med.* 1992;152:1201–1206.
32. Danaei G, Ding EL, Mozaffarian D, et al. The preventable causes of death in the United States: comparative risk assessment of dietary, lifestyle, and metabolic risk factors. *PLoS Med.* 2009;6:e1000058
33. Berkman LF, Syme SL. Social networks, host resistance, and mortality: a nine-year follow-up study of Alameda Count. *Am J Epidemiol* 1979;109:186–204.
34. Christakis NA, Fowler JH. The collective dynamics of smoking in a large social network. *N Engl J Med.* 2008;358:2249–2258.
35. Rowe JW, Kahn RL. Human aging: usual and successful. *Science.* 1987;237:143–149
36. Brandt AM. *The Cigarette Century. The Rise, Fall, and Deadly Persistence of the Product that Defined America.* New York: Basic Books; 2007.
37. Schroeder SA, Warner KE. Don't forget tobacco. *N Engl J Med.* 2010;363:201–204.
38. Syamlal G, Mazurek JM, Malarcher AM. Current cigarette smoking prevalence among working adults—United States, 2004–2010. *MMWR Morb Mortal Wkly Rep.* 2011;60:1305–1309.
39. Woloshin S, Schwartz LM, Welch HG. The risk of death by age, sex, and smoking status in the United States: putting health risks in context. *J Natl Cancer Inst.* 2008;100:845–853.
40. Cosgrove J, Bayer R, Bachynski KE. Nowhere left to hide? The banishment of smoking from public spaces. *N Engl J Med.* 2011;364:2375–2377.
41. Wang H, Preston SH. Forecasting United States mortality using cohort smoking histories. *Proc Natl Acad Sci USA.* 2009;106:393–98.
42. American Cancer Society. *Cancer Facts & Figures, 2012.* Atlanta, GA: American Cancer Society; 2012. http://www.cancer.org/acs/groups/content/@epidemiologysurveilance/documents/document/acspc-031941.pdf
43. Hermanson B, Omenn GS, Kronmal RA, et al. Beneficial six-year outcome of smoking cessation in older men and women with coronary artery disease. *N Engl J Med.* 1988;319:1365–1369.
44. LaCroix AZ, Lang J, Scherr P, et al. Smoking and mortality among older men and women in three communities. *N Engl J Med.* 1991;324:1619–1625.
45. Studenski S, Perera S, Patel K, et al. Gait speed and survival in older adults. *JAMA.* 2011;305:50–58.
46. Lantz PM, Golberstein E, House JS, Morenoff J. Socioeconomic and behavioral risk factors for mortality in a national 19-year prospective study of U.S. adults. *Soc Science Med.* 2010;70:1558–1566.
47. Waters DL, Baumgartner RN, Garry PJ, Vellas B. Advantages of dietary, exercise-related, and therapeutic interventions to prevent and treat sarcopenia in adult patients: an update. *Clin Intervent Aging.* 2010;5:259–270.
48. Beard JR, Blaney S, Cerda M, et al. Neighborhood characteristics and disability in older adults. *J Gerontol B Psychol Sci Soc Sci.* 2009;64B:252–257.
49. Scarmeas N, Luchsinger JA, Schupf N, et al. Physical activity, diet, and risk of Alzheimer Disease. *JAMA.* 2009;302:627–637.
50. King AC. Interventions to promote physical activity by older adults. *J Gerontol A Biol Sci Med Sci.* 2001;56A:36–46.
51. *Bone Health and Osteoporosis: A Report of the Surgeon General.* Rockville, MD: Office of the Surgeon General, US Department of Health and Human Services; 2004.
52. Willett WC, Sampson L, Stampfer MJ, et al. Reproducibility and validity of a semiquantitative food frequency questionnaire. *Am J Epidemiol.* 1985;122:51–65.
53. Houston DK, Nicklas BJ, Ding J, et al. Dietary protein intake is associated with lean mass change in older, community-dwelling adults: the Health, Aging, and Body Composition (HEALTH ABC) Study. *Am J Clin Nutr.* 2008;87:150–155.
54. Beasley JM, LaCroix AZ, Neuhouser ML, et al. Protein intake and incident frailty in the Women's Health Initiative observational study. *J Am Geriatr Soc.* 2010;58:1063–1071.
55. Thomson CA, Stanaway JD, Neuhouser ML, et al. Nutrient intake and anemia risk in the Women's Health Initiative Observational Study. *J Am Diet Assoc.* 2011;111:532–541.
56. Chernoff R. Nutrition and health promotion in older adults. *J Gerontol A Biol Sci Med Sci.* 2001;56A:47–53.
57. Tinetti ME, Fried T. The end of the disease era. *Am J Med.* 2004;116:179–185.
58. Welch HG, Schwartz LM, Woloshin S. *Overdiagnosed. Making People Sick in the Pursuit of Health.* Boston, MA: Beacon Press; 2011.
59. Rajpathak SN, Liu Y, Ben-David O, et al. Lifestyle factors of people with exceptional longevity. *J Am Geriatr Soc.* 2011;59:1509–1512.
60. Studen-Pavlovich D, Ranalli DN. Evolution of women's oral health. *Dental Clinic N Am.* 2001;45:433–442.
61. Yoneyama T, Yoshida M, Ohrui T, et al. Oral care reduces pneumonia in older patients in nursing homes. *J Am Geriat Soc.* 2003;50:430–433.
62. Semba RD, Blaum CS, Bartali B, et al. Denture use, malnutrition, frailty, and mortality among older women living in the community. *J Nutr Health Aging.* 2006;10:161–167.
63. Wu B, Plassman BL, Liang J, et al. Differences in self-reported oral health among community-dwelling black, Hispanic, and white elders. *J Aging Health.* 2011;23:267–287.

64. Olshansky SJ, Passaro DJ, Hershow RC, et al. A potential decline in life expectancy in the United States in the 21st century. *N Engl J Med.* 2005;352:1138–1145.

65. Whitmer RA, Gustafson DR, Barrett-Connor E, et al. *Neurology.* 2008;71: 1057–1064.

66. Flegal KM, Graubard BI, Williamson DF, Gail MH. Excess deaths associated with underweight, overweight, and obesity. *JAMA.* 2005;293:1861–1867.

67. Seshadri S, Beiser A, Kelly-Hayes M, et al. The lifetime risk of stroke. Estimates from the Framingham study. *Stroke.* 2006;37:345–350.

68. Morrison AC, Ness RB. Sodium intake and cardiovascular disease. *Ann Rev Public Health.* 2011;32:71–90.

69. Maselko J, Bates LM, Avendano M, Glymour MM. The intersection of sex, marital status, and cardiovascular risk factors in shaping stroke incidence: results from the Health and Retirement Study. *J Am Geriatr Soc.* 2009;57:2293–2009.

70. Mukamal KJ, Chen CM, Rao SR, Breslow RA. Alcohol consumption and cardiovascular mortality among US adults, 1987 to 2002. *J Am Coll Cardiol.* 2010;55:1328–1335.

71. Cheng YJ, Hootman JM, Murphy LB, et al. Prevalence of doctor-diagnosed arthritis and arthritis-attributable activity limitations—United States 2007-2009. *MMWR Morb Mortal Wkly Rep.* 2010;59:1261–1265.

72. Lalla E, Papapanou PN. Diabetes mellitus and periodontitis: a tale of two common interrelated diseases. *Nat Rev Endocrinol.* 2011;7:738–748.

73. Nygaard I. Idiopathic urgency urinary incontinence. *N Engl J Med.* 2010;363:1156–1162.

74. Brown JS, Grady D, Ouslander JG, et al. Prevalence of urinary incontinence and associated risk factors in postmenopausal women. Heart & Estrogen/Progestin Replacement Study (HERS) Research Group. *Obstet Gynecol.* 1999;94:66–70.

75. Grady D, Brown JS, Vittinghoff E, et al. Postmenopausal hormones and incontinence: the Heart and Estrogen/Progestin Replacement Study. *Obstet Gynecol.* 2001;97:116–120.

76. Moore EE, Jackson SL, Boyko EJ, et al. Urinary incontinence and urinary tract infection: temporal relationships in postmenopausal women. *Obstet Gynecol.* 2008;111:317–323.

77. Jackson SL, Scholes D, Boyko EJ, et al. Urinary incontinence and diabetes in postmenopausal women. *Diabetes Care.* 2005;28:1730–38.

78. Lifford KL, Curhan GC, Hu FB, et al. Type 2 diabetes mellitus and risk of developing urinary incontinence. *J Am Geriatr Soc.* 2005;53L1851–57.

79. Subak LL, Wing R, West DS, et al. Weight loss to treat urinary incontinence in overweight and obese women. *N Engl J Med.* 2009;260:481–490.

80. Brown JS, Seeley DG, Fong J, et al. Urinary incontinence in older women: who is at risk? Study of Osteoporotic Fractures Research Group. *Obstet Gynecol.* 1996;87:715–721.

81. Campbell SS, Murphy PJ, Stauble TN. Effects of a nap on nighttime sleep and waking function in older subjects. *J Am Geriatr Soc.* 2005;53:48–53.

82. Bloom HG, Ahmed I, Alessi CA, et al. Evidence-based recommendations for the assessment and management of sleep disorders in older persons. *J Am Geriatr Soc.* 2009;57:761–789.

83. Bliwise DL, Foley DJ, Vitiello MV, et al. Nocturia and disturbed sleep in the elderly. *Sleep Med.* 2009;10:540–548.

84. Watson NF, Buchwald D, Vitiello MV, et al. A twin study of sleep duration and body mass index. *J Clin Sleep Med.* 2010;6:11–17.

85. Taibi DM, Vitiello MV. A pilot study of gentle yoga for sleep disturbances in women with osteoarthritis. *Sleep Med.* 2011;12:512–517.

86. Bancroft JHJ. Sex and aging. *N Engl J Med.* 2007;357:820–822.

87. Lindau ST, Gavrilova N. Sex, health, and years of sexually active life gained due to good health: evidence from two US population based cross sectional surveys of ageing. *BMJ.* 2010;340:c810.

88. Holzapfel S. Aging and sexuality. *Can Fam Physician.* 1994;40:748–766.

89. Schick V, Herbenick D, Reece M, et al. Sexual behaviors, condom use, and sexual health of Americans over 50: implications for sexual health promotion for older adults. *J Sexual Med.* 2010;7(suppl 5):315–329.

90. Singer BH, Manton KG. The effects of health changes on projections of health service needs for the elderly population of the United States. *Proc Natl Acad Sci USA.* 1998;95:15618–15622.

91. Manton KG, Gu XL, Lamb VL. Change in chronic disability from 1982 to 2004/2005 as measured by long-term changes in function and health in the US elderly population. *Proc Natl Acad Sci USA.* 2006;103:18374–18379.

92. Baltes MM, Carstensen LL. The process of successful ageing. *Ageing Soc.* 1996;16:397–422.

93. Fillit H, Butler RN. The frailty identify crisis. *J Am Geriatr Soc.* 2009;57:348–352.

94. The Eye Diseases Prevalence Research Group. Causes and prevalence of visual impairment among adults in the United States. *Arch Ophthalmol.* 2004;108:1400–1408.

95. Evans BJW, Rowlands G. Correctable visual impairment in older people: a major unmet need. *Ophthal Physiol Opt.* 2004;24:161–180.

96. Hammond CJ, Snieder H, Spector TD, Gilbert CE. Genetic and environmental factors in age-related nuclear cataracts in monozygotic and dizygotic twins. *N Engl J Med.* 2000;342:1786–1790.

97. Age-Related Eye Disease Study Research Group (AREDS). Risk factors associated with age-related nuclear and cortical cataract. *Ophthalmol.* 2001;108:1400–1408.

98. Tomany SC, Wang JJ, van Leeuwen R, et al. Risk factors for incident age-related macular degeneration. Pooled findings from 3 continents. *Ophthalmol.* 2004;111:1280–1287.

99. Glymour MM, Avendano M. Can self-reported strokes be used to study stroke incidence and risk factors? Evidence from the Health and Retirement Study. *Stroke.* 2009;40:873–879.

100. Glymour MM, Avendano M, Berkman LF. Is the "Stroke Belt" worn from childhood? Risk of first stroke and state of residence in childhood and adulthood. *Stroke.* 2007;38:2415–2421.

101. Stevens JA, Haas EN, Haileyesus T. Nonfatal bathroom injuries among persons aged ≥15 years. *J Safety Res.* 2011;42:311–315.

102. Smith BD, Smith GL, Hurria A, et al. Future of cancer incidence in the United States: Burdens upon an aging, changing nation. *J Clin Oncol.* 2009;27:2758–2765.

103. Berry DA, Baines CJ, Baum M, et al. Flawed inferences about screening mammography's benefit based on observational data. *J Clin Oncol.* 2009;27:639–640.

104. US Preventive Services Task Force. Screening for breast cancer: US Preventive services Task Force recommendation statement. *Ann Intern Med.* 1009;151:716–726.

105. De Gonzalez AB, Curtis RE, Kry SF, et al. Proportion of second cancers attributable to radiotherapy treatment in adults: a cohort study in the US SEER cancer registries. *Lancet Oncol.* 2011;12:353–360.

106. Gu Q, Dillon CF, Burt VL. Prescription drug use continues to increase: US prescription drug data for 2007–2008. *NCHS Data Brief.* 2010;42.

107. Skarupski KA, Mrvos R, Krenzelok EP. A profile of calls to a poison information center regarding older adults. *J Aging Health.* 2004;16:228–247.

108. Zhang Y, Baicker K, Newhouse JP. Geographic variation in the quality of prescribing. *N Engl J Med.* 2010;363:1985–1988.

109. Greene JA, Kesselheim AS. Why do the same drugs look different? Pills, trade dress, and public health. *N Engl J Med.* 2011;365:83–89.

110. Cheng H, Gurland BJ, Maurer MS. Self-reported lack of energy (anergia) among elders in a multiethnic community. *J Gerontol* 2008;63:707–714.

111. Bain KT, Holmes HM, Beers MH, et al. Discontinuing medications: a novel approach for revising the prescribing stage of the medication-use process. *J Am Geriatr Soc.* 2008;56:1946–1952.

112. Boyd CM, Darer J, Boult C, et al. Clinical practice guidelines and quality of care for older patients with multiple comorbid diseases. *JAMA.* 2005;294:716–724.

113. Budnitz DS, Lovegrove MC, Shehab N, Richards CL. Emergency hospitalizations for adverse drug events in older Americans. *N Engl J Med.* 2011;365:2002–2012.

114. Avorn J, Shrank W. Highlights and a hidden hazard—The FDA's new labeling regulations. *N Engl J Med.* 2006;354:2409–2411.

115. Fried LP, Xue QL, Cappola AR, et al. Nonlinear multisystem physiological dysregulation associated with frailty in older women: implications for etiology and treatment. *J Gerontology.* 2009;64A:1049–1057.

116. Strawbridge WJ, Shema SJ, Balfour JL, et al. Antecedents of frailty over three decades in an older cohort. *J Gerontol B Psychol Sci Soc Sci.* 1998;53:S9–S16.

117. Ferrucci L, Cavazzini C, Corsi A, et al. Biomarkers of frailty in older persons. *J Endocrinol Invest.* 2002;25 (suppl 10): 10–15.

118. Gershon RRM, Pogorzelska M, Qureshi KA, et al. Home health care patients and safety hazards in the home: preliminary findings. In: Henriksen K, Battles JB, Keyes MA, Grady ML, eds. *Advances in Patient Safety: New Directions and Alternative Approaches* (Vol. 1: Assessment). Rockville, MD: Agency for Healthcare Research and Quality; 2008.

119. Pavlou MP, Lachs MS. Self-neglect in older adults: A primer for clinicians. *J Gen Intern Med.* 2008;23:1841–1816.

120. Naik AD, Lai JM, Kunik ME, Dyer CB. Assessing capacity in suspected cases of self-neglect. *Geriatrics.* 2008;63:24–31.

121. Mouton CP, Carter-Nolan PL. Elder abuse. In: Fife RS, Schrager S, eds. *Family Violence. What Health Care Providers Need to Know.* Sudbury, MA: Jones & Bartlett Learning; 2012.

122. National Center on Elder Abuse. *Elder Abuse Prevalence and Incidence Fact Sheet.* Washington, DC; National Center on Elder Abuse; 2005.

123. Institute of Medicine. *Clinical Preventive Services for Women: Closing the Gaps.* Washington, DC: National Academies Press; 2011. http://www.iom.edu/Reports/2011/Clinical-Preventive-Services-for-Women-Closing-the-Gaps.aspx.

124. British National Health Service. Safe Mobile Care. http://www.safepatientsystems.com/products/safemobilecare.ashx.

Subjective Well-Being of Midlife and Older Women

Victoria H. Raveis, PhD

Introduction

The well-being of middle-aged and older women is of significant public health concern, given advances in medical care, nutrition, and lifestyle have enabled women to live longer, healthier lives. Over the last 50 years, while the birth rate has declined, the average life expectancy for both men and women has increased by about 10 years, contributing to the graying of the population being experienced not just in the United States but on a global scale.[1]

By 2050, over one-fifth of the U.S. population will be 65 and older. The greatest rate of increase will be among the oldest-old group—those 85 and above who in 2000 represented 1.5% of the population. By 2050, estimates project this population to increase to approximately 19 million, almost 5% of the U.S. population with more than 60% women.[2] Subjective well-being is an important social indicator for informing public health policies and practices about critical health resources and supportive services needed for this steadily increasing aging population.[3]

Subjective Well-Being

Subjective well-being or positive affect is broad and multidimensional, encompassing various aspects of quality of life, the positive domains. Negative states such as poor mental and physical health and negative affect are not discussed in this chapter.

Cognitive and behavioral elements as well as evaluative or affective aspects are components of subjective well-being that may be represented as a global state such as happiness, life satisfaction, meaning in life, high morale, positive self-esteem or perceived self-worth, and satisfaction with achievement of specific life goals.[3–12]

A variety of social indicators have been used to assess subjective well-being, including the Bradburn Affect Balance Scale (NAS),[13] the Life Satisfaction Index,[14] the Philadelphia Geriatric Center Morale Scale,[15] Rosenberg Self-Esteem Scale,[7] and a number of single item measures of overall life satisfaction and happiness.[16] Indicators of domain-specific satisfaction can be found in Andrews and Withey.[4]

Extensive research has demonstrated that health states are an important determinant of subjective well-being,[12,17–21] with longitudinal studies documenting the adverse impact of illness and physical functioning on subjective well-being.[22] A growing number of investigations indicate that this relationship is likely bidirectional; subjective well-being has been shown to have a beneficial impact on health and longevity.[22–24] In a recent meta-analysis of experimental, ambulatory, and longitudinal studies that examined the association of subjective well-being and physical health, subjective well-being was found to have a positive impact on short-term and long-term health outcomes as well as a buffering effect on disease-related decline.[24] Prospective cohort investigations have also established an association between positive well-being and decreased mortality among both healthy and diseased members of study populations in a meta-analysis.[23] Based on pooled results in their meta-analysis, Howell et al.[24] estimated that a high level of subjective well-being increased the probability of living longer by 14% compared to that of persons with low subjective well-being. Among elderly with chronic illness, survival was increased by 10% when a patient's subjective well-being level was high. Two landmark studies that have informed this body of work, the Nun Study and the Twins Study, are discussed in Box 37-1.

Understanding the complex route by which subjective well-being may influence health and disease outcomes of older adults is limited, although a meta-analysis indicated the beneficial impact of well-being on health was through promotion of healthy lifestyles associated with cardiovascular and physiological reactivity.[24] Pressman and Cohen[22] proposed two models to guide further scientific inquiry on this relationship—the main effect model and the stress buffering model. In the main effect model, positive well-being directly affects disease incidence, severity, recovery, and recurrence through various mediating behaviors (i.e., health practices and social ties) and physiological responses (i.e., endogenous opioids, autonomic nervous system, and hypothalamic-pituitary-adrenal activities). In the stress buffering model, the health benefit of subjective well-being is expressed by ameliorating the adverse physiological consequences of stressful events and situations (e.g., attenuating inflammatory responses, lowering cortisol output, and regulating cardiovascular reactivity).

Gender and Subjective Well-Being

Most research investigating gender differences in subjective well-being have noted men report slightly higher levels of life satisfaction and positive affect over the life course than women. However, meta-analyses of these investigations have determined that gender, though a statistically significant predictor, accounts for very little of the variance.[31,32] After controlling for social class factors that could have affected subjective well-being (i.e., composite socioeconomic status, occupational status, and income), the mean effect size was minimal. Pinquart and Sorensen[32] examined gender differences separately for life satisfaction, happiness, and self-esteem in a meta-analysis. The mean affect size for gender noted women score slightly lower on subjective well-being including life satisfaction and self-esteem. Based on additional analyses the authors found physical health, competence, and socioeconomic status influenced gender differences in subjective well-being, leading them to conclude that gender-differences are linked to the accumulated disadvantages older women experienced across their life course related to socioeconomic status, social resources, and health. Smith and Baltes[33] acknowledge: "Gender is a carrier variable for life context factors such as marital status, education, multimorbidity, and functional capacity that contribute to individual differences."

Age and Subjective Well-Being

For both men and women, aging is associated with declines and losses in the physical, cognitive, and social domains.[1] The Berlin Aging Study, which included institutionalized adults, documented that the prevalence of chronic illness, frailty, and incapacity doubled after age 85 compared with those 70 to 84.[9] Although women's life expectancy significantly exceeds that of men, older women experience higher levels of morbidity. Compared with similarly aged men, older women have a 1.6 times higher risk for physical frailty that is likely to have an impact on psychological functioning.[33]

Coexisting with these age-linked trends in morbidity is an expanding body of literature indicating that across the life course, men and women retain high levels of positive affect and subjective well-being. Most investigations have documented negligible differences in subjective well-being across groups of young, middle-aged, and older adults.[34–36] A number of studies have even shown relatively higher levels of happiness and satisfaction for older adults compared to younger age groups.[37,38]

Although a drop in subjective well-being has been observed among the very old, the declines were not as strong as would have been predicted, given the losses and adverse physical and mental changes experienced by many older people.[39] For example, some researchers[40] reported a small but significant decline in positive affect over a 20-year period when individuals were followed longitudinally from their 60s into their 80s. Similarly, in a community-dwelling sample of older adults, life satisfaction was high for people ages 60–89, dropping slightly for those 90 and older.[41] Evidence from long-term longitudinal national samples (United States, Great Britain, Germany, and Israel) suggested precipitous deterioration in subjective well-being occurred in late life associated with terminal decline and impending death.[42,43]

Studies examining gender differences in subjective well-being across the life span have been limited by gender differences in longevity. Samples that include the oldest-old tend to be primarily female, with the oldest men representing a selected subgroup of their birth cohort. Future efforts to understand gender differences across the life course need to take into consideration sampling issues and the contribution of other factors that are gender linked.

Pinquart and Sorensen's meta-analysis of subjective well-being and gender was restricted to investigations that included adults 55 and older.[32] They observed the strongest gender differences at higher mean ages when older women's subjective well-being was significantly lower than that of similarly aged men. The Berlin Aging Study oversampled older men and persons 85 and older, permitting a comprehensive examination of gender-linked variables on subjective well-being in the oldest-old population. As has been found in other research, older women had a small, but significantly lower level of subjective well-being compared

Box 37-2 Gendered Nature of Inequalities Affecting Subjective Well-Being at Older Ages

Gender in Western culture and historical time determines constraints and opportunities, played out mainly through social status and education, which impinge on life careers. This impingement most likely does not have the same saliency and weight at all phases of the life course, and some subgroups may have more or fewer possibilities to buffer the impact. At older ages, individuals have to live with the accumulation of the constraints through their social class and education. These constraints may be enhanced by differences in marital status and health as women age. In general, men appear to have accumulated more of the advantages and resources to better cope with the demands of aging.[33]

Source: Reproduced from Smith J, Baltes MM. The role of gender in very old age: Profiles of functioning and everyday life patterns. Psychol Aging 1998;13:691.

to older men. However, when various life context factors were controlled, the unique effect for gender on the life satisfaction subscale was eliminated.[33] These findings illustrate the cumulative disadvantages linked to gender over the life course are reflected in the larger gender differences in subjective well-being at older ages (see Box 37-2).

Gender and Social Integration

Women's subjective well-being is embedded in the social context of their lives at all ages as women tend to prioritize social relationships with family and friends in contrast to men who are generally more focused on financial concerns.[44] Middle-aged and older women often have larger social networks and more extensive social resources than men,[45] and these stronger social patterns have been related to life satisfaction and happiness for women.[46]

Family responsibilities are known to be the primary focus in the social construction of women's lives.[47] The respondents in Ryff's study of middle-aged and older adults identified family and social relationships as their main sources of life satisfaction.[38] Similarly, a sample of older women indicated their feelings of general life satisfaction were more strongly influenced by social relationships than health status.[48] Heidrich and Ryff also observed in a sample of women aged 65 and older living in the community that the social domain, holding positive perspectives of age-related normative behavior, was associated with increased life satisfaction.[49]

Happiness in marriage was a stronger predictor of global happiness for women than men.[50] Among older community residents, Strawbridge and Wallhagen observed gender differences in meaningful activities among those who rated themselves as aging successfully.[51] Specifically, women scored higher on activities that denoted social integration, i.e., growing spiritually, being involved with friends and social organizations, and being helpful to others. Men scored higher on being athletic and enjoying intimacy.

Given the centrality of social integration and relationships in older women's lives, their subjective well-being may be adversely affected by life-course transitions such as reduced mobility that limit social participation. In studies of community residents by Farquhar,[52] more negative quality of life was reported by those 85 and older compared with younger seniors, reflecting the loss of social relationships and reduced social contacts. The research of Ryff[38] and others[53] has noted that the social domain retains its importance as women grow older, although the impact of diminishing health maintenance increases with each passing year.

Gender, Stress, and the Life Course

A more comprehensive understanding of what is meaningful for women and important for their subjective well-being as they grow older is provided by two intellectual traditions—life-course perspectives and the social origins of stress. These theoretical frameworks provide important insights to women's social circumstances.

Life-Course Perspectives

The life-course perspective informs the gender-related nature of the experiences that are contributing to older women's subjective well-being.[47] This framework focuses on stability and change over time in people's lives, emphasizing that experiences at one point in time shape the subsequent life course. Such transitions include movements into and out of various roles and statuses; the timing of these events impose direction on the life course and influence life conditions that affect subjective well-being.[54,55]

Analyses of life histories indicate women are at higher risk than men of experiencing numerous entry and exit transitions during middle and late adulthood, such as caregiving, widowhood, and loss of functional independence. These transitions may adversely alter personal, social, and economic resources affecting their subjective well-being. Interestingly, when men and women undergo the same transition, the experiences differ greatly by gender.[47] For example, women transition into old age with fewer tangible resources, limited savings, and lower or no retirement benefits than men as a consequence of gender-associated inequities including lower income and shorter employment histories due to family responsibilities.[56,57] This gender-linked economic vulnerability is particularly evident in older age cohorts. In 2007, more than 13% of women 75 and older in the United States were living in poverty compared with 7% of men in this age group.[1]

Social Origins of Stress

Life strains arising from persistent problems, chronic frustrations, and hardships are sources of stress embedded in social roles of day-to-day activities including the burdens of caregiving.[58] Life strains arouse distress but can also develop from the changes in social circumstances precipitated by life transitions, such as marriage or the birth of a child, and nonnormative disruptive events including divorce or being fired from a job.[54,55,59] The social origins of stress also include resource inequities that women experience, which contribute to differential exposures and responses to life stresses.[54,59]

Social Determinants of Subjective Well-Being

Compared with men of their generation, women are more likely to encounter socially challenging events and situations as they and their loved ones experience functional decline.[1] These life circumstances generate social disadvantages and stresses, factors that may have an adverse impact on women's subjective well-being.

Caregiving

Assuming caregiving responsibilities for dependent or infirm relatives is a significant life transition women encounter more frequently than men. With the aging of the population and decreasing family size, women may simultaneously be providing care to multiple family members of differing generations or experience sequential caregiving responsibilities that can continue longer than parenting duties.

Adult children caregivers have been described as the "sandwich generation" and "women in the middle"[60] because of the pressures that many experience in trying to balance the demands of elder care with employment and childcare. Assuming caregiving tasks can bring about long-term interruptions in women's social activities and life circumstances.

Although caregiving is a socially valued role, the chronic and acute strains of the responsibilities may precipitate declines in the physical health and well-being of caregivers. Older women, especially grandparent caregivers, are at increased risk for adverse health consequences. Three decades of caregiving research have noted the harmful physical and mental health effects associated with this primarily female role.[62,63]

Caregiving may limit work efficiency and threaten employment potentially affecting caregivers' economic resources. A MetLife study of informal caregivers[64] estimated that the impact of care provision on total wealth lost over a lifetime is substantial due to lost wages, Social Security, and pension benefits. In addition to loss in economic productivity, hidden costs associated with caregiving encompass out-of-pocket expenditures in care provision and lifestyle changes necessitated by providing care such as a change in residence or frequent travel for care-related visits.

The demands of caregiving compete with the day-to-day role responsibilities of the caregiver's own life, particularly when caregiving is long lasting and intense, as commonly occurs with dementia and Alzheimer's disease.[58] Role overload is commonplace, disrupting daily routines, imposing restrictions on other activities, and precipitating losses in social relationships.[65] Longitudinal studies indicate that although various domains of caregiving may diminish over time, the burden does not completely subside,[66] instead the detrimental impact on the social context of the caregiver may endure.[67]

Widowhood

Given women's greater longevity, widowhood is more common among women than men. In 2008 American women age 65 and older were three times more likely than similarly aged men to be widowed. At ages 85 and older over three-quarters of women were widowed.[1] Widowhood is a multiple jeopardy status, as the social loss often precipitates a number of significant and enduring changes in women's life circumstances.[68] Wives are commonly involved in the provision of emotional and practical assistance to their husbands. When elderly widows face challenges caring for their husbands at the end of life, they often ignore their own health. For some women their own health-limiting conditions may have impeded their ability to provide ongoing care; for others ignoring clinical symptoms may delay diagnosis and treatment of major medical conditions. Performing repetitive tasks over a protracted and intensive period could also have increased their risk of a subsequent decline in well-being.[69] Indeed, bereavement can predispose women to physical and mental illness, aggravate existing conditions, and cause death.[70]

Even though dependency, declining health, and impending death are anticipated life events in the elderly, widowhood is a particularly potent and stressful transition for older women. In bereavement they may be mourning an altered future following the loss of a life-long companion, confidant, and supporter. Widowhood increases the risk of social isolation in older women. Widowhood can also generate severe lifestyle changes and financial strains. Expenses associated with a husband's care prior to his death could have depleted the couple's financial resources.[71] Elderly women may also experience a loss of or reduction in their husband's pension and other benefits at his death.[56] In some instances, this diminution of economic resources may necessitate an undesired change in residence, either shortly following the death or at a later point in the widow's life course. The longer lifespan of women coupled with higher rates of morbidity put women at increased risk for experiencing a residential transition.

Loss of Independence

Onset of poor health or functional decline is a critical negative transition in older adulthood. Remaining independent is associated with the ability to perform all activities of daily living (ADL) without resorting to help from others; dependency, a negative state, implies helplessness and powerlessness.[72] Older women have a higher prevalence of functional impairment than older men and experience greater dependency. In 2007, almost 60% of women aged 85 and older in the United States compared with 40% of the men were unable to perform even one of five activities reflecting physical functioning including being able to walk two to three blocks, reach up over one's head, or grasp small objects.[1] The loss of functional independence often leads to a need for residence in a long-term care facility. Diminished financial and support resources of women reduce the likelihood of older women receiving needed long-term care while remaining in their own residence. Therefore, the development of physical and mental conditions that diminish women's capacity to live independently mark an additional transition point with severe implications for women's well-being and quality of life.[73]

For most, residing in a long-term care facility is an undesirable life circumstance. In comparison to older community residents remaining in their private homes, institutionalized elders report lower levels of positive affect.[9] In 2007 women 65 and older were almost twice as likely as men of the same age to be living in a long-term care facility (4.5% vs. 2.5%).[1] However, healthy seniors with adequate finances are now finding comfortable alternatives to remaining in former private homes; senior residences with private accommodation but shared dining, specialized health, and entertainment facilities provide an attractive alternative for some who wish to relinquish the burdens of private home living while maintaining their physical independence.

Paradox of Subjective Well-Being in Aging

Happy Life Expectancy vs. Active Life Expectancy

Although life events and losses occur at all ages, adverse health changes and other negative transitions accelerate in old age when the resources needed for coping and adaptation are more limited. Nonetheless, allowing for measurement differences, research has documented that both men and women maintain their subjective well-being levels into advanced age. Recent analyses to estimate age-specific prevalence rates of happiness using population life expectancy estimates and mortality rates, combined with responses to subjective well-being questions from large-scale national representative surveys, provide compelling evidence that morbidity and debility in old age are not always equated with poor life quality. Happy Life Expectancy is a population-level social indicator that estimates the number of years a member of the life table cohort would be happy given age-specific rates of mortality and happiness.[74] Using national surveys conducted with U.S. populations in 1970, 1980, 1990, and 2000, Yang[74] determined the number of years of life members of the cohort could expect to be in good health, free of disability. Her analysis indicated that white women had longer years of total life and happy expectations at most ages than black women. Racial differences diminished at older ages although disparities persisted.[74]

Optimal and Successful Aging

In light of the cumulative disadvantages that can occur as people age, the absence of significant declines in subjective well-being is a social phenomenon that has been termed a paradox.[75] The body of scientific and theoretical work on optimal or successful aging addresses this conundrum.[75–79] Rowe and Kahn[78,80] defined a multidimensional concept of successful or 'ideal' aging as consisting of three components: avoidance of disease and disease-related disability, high mental and physical functioning, and active engagement with life. This model provides a framework for healthy aging, encouraging health promotion and disease prevention behaviors to improve or maintain physical and mental capacities across the life course.[80] Although all three components are necessary for successful aging, these authors recognized that individual variability exists on each of these components and acknowledged notable exemplars, such as Mother Teresa, who was able to personify engagement with life even when experiencing disease and disability. Despite severe health issues in her later years, Mother Teresa successfully continued her ministry of service to the poor and disenfranchised until her death in 1997 at age 87. Periodic media coverage of healthy and active older women has reassured many seniors as they approach their 80s and 90s.

Although the Rowe and Kahn model emphasizes the importance of healthy behavior in maximizing ideal aging, Baltes and Baltes[75] have outlined the principles for adaption to aging, acknowledging the gains and losses that occur throughout life, recognizing the unique experiences of individuals, and the role of cultural variations. Specifically, the Selective Optimization with Compensation (SOC) model suggests successful aging can be achieved through the interplay of three related strategies—selection, compensation and optimization—in which individuals select and concentrate on high-priority activities or life goals that optimize their individual skills, capacity, and motivation while compensating for deficits and identifying alternative means to reach desired objectives (see Box 37-3).

Since its inception, the SOC model remains a leading framework with growing interest as reviewed by Ouwehand and colleagues.[79] Freund and Baltes[81,83] confirmed the utility of this model to predict global subjective well-being, indicative of successful aging, in cross-sectional data drawn from the Berlin Aging Study. The model may also offer an explanation for the decline in subjective well-being that has been observed in the oldest populations. Additional analyses of data from the Berlin Aging Study suggest that women aged 85 and older may be particularly vulnerable to a decline in subjective well-being as they experience higher rates of cognitive deterioration, limiting their ability to engage in key elements of the SOC process.[81,83]

Summary

Loss is more frequent in later life and the oldest-old are likely to experience changes in health status, deterioration in physical and cognitive functioning, loss of relatives and friends, and more limited economic resources. Such undesirable changes can adversely affect quality of life. On a number of social and health indicators current cohorts of older women are more disadvantaged than older men. Compared to men 65 and older, older women have lower per capita income, are more likely to be widowed or living alone, and have a higher probability of living in long-term care facilities due to more functional impairments and chronic health conditions. These gender differences are most apparent in the oldest age groups. Although women live longer than men, the gender-linked disadvantages across the life span are compounded by decline in health status that occurs with aging and is reflected in women's lower levels of subjective well-being.

It merits noting, however, that the lifestyles and economic and social conditions of aging women living in the 21st century in the United States are different from experiences of women in earlier birth cohorts. As a consequence of the historical changes in women's educational, marital, and employment patterns occurring over the latter half of the 20th century, present gender-linked vulnerabilities of old age may decrease as subsequent cohorts of women grow older. By 2030, the baby boomer generation born between 1946 and 1964 will be older than 65 years old. The influences on subjective well-being associated with later age at marriage, higher divorce rates and fewer children, coupled with higher education and expanded labor force participation, will continue to be topics for study in relation to gender-related differences associated with aging.

An additional resource, the World Database of Happiness (www.worlddatabaseofhappiness.eur.nl), is a repository of international scientific research on the subjective indicators of well-being including information on over 600 social indicators that tap happiness as well as an extensive data archive on responses to questions from national survey studies.

Box 37-3 Successful Aging and the Selective Optimization with Compensation Model

Selective Optimization with Compensation (SOC) Model. The selective optimization with compensation (SOC) model developed by Baltes and Baltes[75,76] outlines the principles of an adaptive process for successful aging. The model provides a general framework for understanding the changes that occur over the life span taking into consideration the gains and losses, incorporating objective and subjective criteria, and recognizing individual heterogeneity in the cultural context. Successful aging is achieved through the interplay of three component processes or strategies—selection, compensation, and optimization in which the individual selects and concentrates on high-priority domains or goals that represent the optimal convergence of individual skills, capacity, and motivation with environmental demands. It is a life management strategy to promote "the maximization and attainment of positive (desired) outcomes and the minimization and avoidance of negative (undesired) outcomes."[81]

A basic tenet of the model is that measurement of successful outcomes needs to be multidimensional and multilevel, to reflect what an individual regards as personally meaningful and important. Baltes and Baltes[75] note further that although selective optimization with compensation is a process that individuals may implement at any age in any context, this adaptation strategy attains new importance at advanced ages, when losses and restrictions in the biological, cognitive, and social domains are common.

The renowned concert pianist Arthur Rubinstein was 80 years old when he was asked how he was able to continue to perform in concerts so well. As Baltes and Smith[82] observed, his answer provided a compelling example of the SOC model: "He reduced his repertoire (i.e., selection). This gave him the opportunity to practice each piece more (i.e., optimization). And finally, he used contrasts in speed to hide his loss in mechanical finger speed, a case of compensation" (p. 132).

Discussion Questions

1. What are the limitations that characterize research studies examining gender and age variations in subjective well-being?
2. What are some of the knowledge gaps concerning the ways in which gender influences health and subjective well-being in old age?
3. What resources and environmental conditions would be instrumental in reducing the gender-linked disparities in subjective well-being?

4. What societal changes are occurring that are likely to affect the life-course experiences of today's younger women?

References

1. Federal Interagency Forum on Aging-Related Statistics. *Older Americans 2010: Key Indicators of Well-Being*. Federal Interagency Forum on Aging-Related Statistics. Washington, DC: US Government Printing Office; July, 2010.
2. Siegel J. Aging into the 21st century. National Aging Information Center. 1996. http://www.aoa.gov/AoARoot/Aging_Statistics/future_growth/aging21/preface.aspx. Accessed August 16, 2010.
3. Andrews FM. Population issues and social indicators of well-being. *Popul Environ.* 1983;6:210–230.
4. Andrews FM, Withey SB. *Social Indicators of Well-being: Americans' Perceptions of Life Quality.* New York: Plenum; 1976.
5. Campbell A, Converse PE, Rodgers WL. *The Quality of American Life: Perceptions, Evaluations, and Satisfactions.* New York: Russell Sage Foundation; 1976.
6. Diener E, Emmons RA. The independence of positive and negative affect. *J Pers Soc Psychol.* 1985;47:1105–1117.
7. Rosenberg M. *Society and the Adolescent Self-Image.* Princeton, NJ: Princeton University Press; 1965.
8. Sheldon KM, Lyubomirsky S. Achieving sustainable gains in happiness: Change your actions, not your circumstances. *J Happiness Stud.* 2006;7:55–86.
9. Smith J. Well-being and health from age 70 to 100: Findings from the Berlin Aging Study. *Eur Rev.* 2001;9:461–477.
10. George LK. Still happy after all these years: Research frontiers on subjective well-being in later life. *J Gerontol.* 2010;65:331–339.
11. George LK, Bearon LB. *Quality of Life in Older Persons: Meaning and Measurement.* New York: Human Sciences Press; 1980.
12. George LK, Landerman R. Health and subjective well-being: A replicated secondary data analysis. *Int J Aging Hum Dev.* 1984;19:133–156.
13. Bradburn NM. *The Structure of Psychological Well-Being.* Chicago: Aldine Publishing; 1969.
14. Neugarten BL, Havighurst RJ, Tobin SS. The measurement of life satisfaction. *J Gerontol.* 1961;16:135–143.
15. Lawton MP. The Philadelphia Geriatric Center Moral Scale: A revision. *J Gerontol.* 1975;15:85–89.
16. Saad L. (2003) A nation of happy people. Most are happy and satisfied with their lives. Gallup Poll News Services, January 4, 2004. Washington, DC: Gallup Organization. http://www.gallup.com/poll/10090/Nation-Happy-People.aspx.
17. Diener E, Suh EM, Lucas RE, Smith HE. Subjective well-being: Three decades of progress. *Psychol Bull.* 1999;125:276–302.
18. Okun MA, Stock WA. Correlates and components of subjective well-being among the elderly. *J Appl Gerontol.* 1987;6:95–112.
19. Okun MA, Stock WA, Haring MJ, Witter RA. Health and subjective well-being: a meta-analysis. *Int J Aging Hum Dev.* 1984;19:111–132.
20. Smith J, Borchelt M, Maier H, Jopp D. Health and well-being in the young old and oldest old. *J Soc Issues.* 2002;58:715–732.
21. Zautra A, Hempel A. Subjective well-being and physical health: A narrative literature review with suggestions for future research. *Int J Aging Hum Dev.* 1984;19:91–110.
22. Pressman SD, Cohen S. Does positive affect influence health? *Psychol Bull.* 2005;131:925–971.
23. Chida Y, Steptoe A. Positive psychological well-being and mortality: A quantitative review of prospective observational studies. *Psychosom Med.* 2008;70:741–756.
24. Howell RT, Kern ML, Lyubomirsky S. Health benefits: Meta-analytically determining the impact of well-being on objective health outcomes. *Health Psychol Rev.* 2007;1:83–136.
25. Snowdon DA. Healthy aging and dementia: Findings from the Nun Study. *Ann Internal Med.* 2003;139:450–454.
26. Danner DD, Snowdon DA, Friesen WV. Positive emotions in early life and longevity: Findings from the Nun Study. *J Pers Soc Psychol.* 2001;80:804–813.
27. Kaprio J, Sarna S, Koskenvuo M, Rantasalo I. The Finnish twin registry: Formation and compilation, questionnaire study, zygosity determination procedures, and research program. *Prog Clin Biol Res.* 1978;24:179–184.
28. Sarna S, Kaprio J, Sistonen P, Koskenvuo M. Diagnosis of twin zygosity by mailed questionnaire. *Hum Hered.* 1978;28:241–254.
29. Koivumaa-Honkanen H, Honkanen R, Viinamäki K, et al. Self-reported life satisfaction and 20-year mortality in healthy Finnish adults. *Am J Epidemiol.* 2000;152:983–991.
30. Koivumaa-Honkanen H, Honkanen R, Viinamäki K, et al. Life satisfaction and suicide: A 20-year follow-up study. *Am J Psychiatry.* 2001;158:433–439.
31. Haring MJ, Stock WA, Okun MA. A research synthesis of gender and social class as correlates of subjective well-being. *Hum Relat.* 1984;37:645–657.
32. Pinquart M, Sorensen S. Gender differences in self-concept and psychological well-being in old age: A meta-analysis. *J Gerontol.* 2001;56B:P195–P213.
33. Smith J, Baltes MM. The role of gender in very old age: Profiles of functioning and everyday life patterns. *Psychol Aging.* 1998;13:676–695.
34. Ehrlich BS, Isaacowitz DM. Does subjective well-being increase with age? *Perspect Psychol.* 2002;Spring:20–26.
35. Isaacowitz DM, Smith J. Positive and negative affect in very old age: Extending into later life. Unpublished manuscript. Berlin, Germany: Max Planck Institute for Human Development; 1999.
36. Diener E, Suh EM. Subjective well-being and age: An international analysis. *Annu Rev Gerontol Geriatrics.* 1998;17:304–324.
37. Mroczek DK, Kolarz CM. The effect of age on positive and negative affect: A developmental perspective on happiness. *J Pers Soc Psychol.* 1998;75:12333–12349.
38. Ryff CD. In the eye of the beholder: Views of psychological well-being among middle-aged and older adults. *Psychol Aging.* 1989;4:195–210.
39. Pinquart M. Age differences in perceived positive affect, negative affect, and affect balance in middle and old age. *J Happiness Stud.* 2001;2:375–405.
40. Charles ST, Reynolds CA, Gatz M. Age-related differences and change in positive and negative affect over 23 years. *J Pers Soc Psychol.* 2001;80:136–151.
41. Martin P, Poon LW, Johnson MA. Social and psychological resources in the oldest old. *Exp Aging Res.* 1996;22:121–139.
42. Gerstorf D, Ram N, Mayraz G, Hidajat M, Lindenberger U, Wagner GG, Schupp J. Late-life decline in well-being across adulthood in Germany, the United Kingdom, and the United States: Something is seriously wrong at the end of life. *Psychol Aging.* 2010;25:477–485.
43. Palgi YU, Shrira A, Ben-Ezra M, Spalter T, Dhmotkin D, Kavé G. Delineating terminal change in subjective well-being and subjective health. *J Gerontol.* 2010;65:61–64.
44. Bowling A, Windsor J. Towards the good life: A population survey of dimension of quality of life. *J Happiness Stud.* 2001;2:55–81.
45. Depner CE, Ingersoll-Dayton B. Supportive relationships in later life. *Psychol Aging.* 1988;3:348–357.
46. Pinquart M, Sorensen S. Influences of socioeconomic status, social network, and competence on psychological well–being in the elderly. *Psychol Aging.* 2000;15:187–224.
47. Moen P. The gendered life course. In: Binstock R, George LK, eds. *Handbook of Aging and the Social Sciences.* 4th ed. San Diego, CA: Academic Press; 2001:179–196.
48. Albert I, Labs K, Trommsdorff G. Are older adult German women satisfied with their lives? *GeroPsych.* 2010;23:39–49.
49. Heidrich SM, Ryff CD. Physical and mental health in later life: The self-system as mediator. *Psychol Aging.* 1993;8:327–338.
50. Gove WR, Hughes M, Style CB. Does marriage have positive effects on the psychological well-being of the individual? *J Health Soc Behav.* 1983;24:122–131.
51. Strawbridge WJ, Wallhagen MI. Chapter 1: Self-rated successful aging: Correlates and predictors. In: Poon LW, Gueldner SH, Sprouse BM, eds. *Successful Aging and Adaptation with Chronic Diseases.* New York: Springer Publishing Co.; 2003.
52. Farquhar M. Elderly people's definitions of quality of life. *Soc Sci Med.* 1995;41:1439–1446.
53. Bowling A. The most important things in life. Comparisons between older and younger population age groups by gender. Results from a national survey of The Public's Judgments. *Int J Health Sci.* 1996;6:169–175.
54. George LK. Sociological perspectives on life transitions. *Annu Rev Sociol.* 1993;19:353–373.
55. Pearlin LI. The life course and the stress process: Some conceptual comparisons. *J Gerontol* 2010;65:207–215.
56. Lee S, Shaw L. *From Work to Retirement: Tracking Changes in Women's Poverty Status.* Research Report. Washington, DC: AARP Public Policy Institute; 2008. http://www.aarp.org/money/low-income-assistance/info-02–2008/2008_03_poverty.html. Accessed September 8, 2010.
57. Moen P. Recasting careers: Changing reference groups, risks, and realities. *Generations.* 1998;22:40–45.
58. Aneshensel CS, Pearlin LI, Mullin JT, et al. *Profiles in Caregiving: The Unexpected Career.* New York: Academic Press; 1995.
59. Pearlin LI. The stress process revisited. In: Aneshensel CA, Phelan JC, eds. *Handbook of the Sociology of Mental Health.* New York, NY: Lower Academic/Plenum Publisher; 1999:395–415.
60. Brody EM. *Women in the Middle: Their Parent-Care Years.* New York: Springer; 1990.
61. Strawbridge WJ, Wallhagen MI, Shema SJ, Kaplan GA. New burdens or more of the same? Comparing grandparent, spouse and adult-child caregivers. *Gerontologist.* 1997;37:505–510.
62. Schulz R, Sherwood PR. Physical and mental health effects of family caregiving. *Am J Nurs.* 2008;109:23–27.
63. Pinquart M, Sorensen S. Differences between caregiving and non-caregiving in psychological health and physical health: A meta-analysis. *Psychol Aging.* 2003;18:250–267.
64. MetLife Mature Market Institute. *The MetLife Juggling Act Study: Balancing Caregiving with Work and the Costs Involved.* Westport, CT: Metropolitan Life Insurance Company; 1999. http://www.caregiving.org/data/jugglingstudy.pdf. Accessed September 8, 2010.

65. Raveis VH. The challenges and issues confronting family caregivers to elderly cancer patients. In: Carmel S, Morse CA, Torres-Gil FM, eds. *Lessons on Aging from Three Nations: Vol 2. The Art of Caring for Older Adults.* New York, NY: Baywood Press; 2007:85–97.

66. Kotkamp-Mothes N, Slawinsky D, Hindermann S, Strauss B. Coping and psychological well being in families of elderly cancer patients. *Crit Rev Oncol Hematol.* 2005;55:213–229.

67. Raveis VH, Karus D, Pretter S. Impact of cancer caregiving over the disease course: depressive distress in adult daughters. *Psychooncology.* 2004;13:S47.

68. Raveis VH. Facilitating older spouses' adjustment to widowhood: A preventive intervention program. *Soc Work Health Care.* 1999;29:13–32.

69. Raveis VH. Psychosocial impact of spousal caregiving at the end-of-life: Challenges and consequences. *Gerontologist.* 2004;44:191–120.

70. Osterweis M, Solomon F, Green M. *Bereavement: Reactions, Consequences, and Care: A Report of the Institute of Medicine, National Academy of Sciences.* Washington DC: National Academy Press; 1984.

71. Raveis VH. Bereavement. In Bruera E, Higginson I, Ripamonti C, von Gunten C, eds. *Textbook of Palliative Medicine.* London, UK: Hodder Arnold; 2006:1044–1050.

72. Baltes MM. *The Many Faces of Dependency in Old Age.* Cambridge: University Press; 1996.

73. Gignac AM, Cott C. A conceptual model of independence and dependence for adults with chronic physical illness and disability. *Soc Sci Med.* 1998;47:739–753.

74. Yang Y. Long and happy living: Trends and patterns of happy life expectancy in the U.S., 1970–2000. *Soc Sci Res.* 2008;37:1235–1252.

75. Baltes PB, Baltes MM. Psychological perspectives on successful aging: The model of selective optimization with compensation. In: Baltes PB, Baltes MM, eds. *Successful Aging: Perspectives from the Behavioral Sciences.* New York: Cambridge University Press; 1990:1–34.

76. Baltes MM, Carstensen LL. The process of successful ageing. *Ageing Soc.* 1996;16:397–422.

77. Kahana E, Kahana B. Conceptual and empirical advances in understanding aging well through proactive adaptation. In: Bengston VL, ed. *Adulthood and Aging: Research on Continuities and Discontinuities.* New York: Springer; 1996:18–40.

78. Rowe JW, Kahn RL. Successful Aging. New York, NY: Dell; 1998.

79. Ouwehand C, deRidder DTD, Bensing JM. A review of successful aging models: proposing proactive coping as an important additional strategy. *Clin Psychol Rev.* 2007;27:873–884.

80. Kahn RL. Chapter 3: Successful aging: Intended and unintended consequences of a concept. In: Poon LW, Gueldner SH, Sprouse BM, eds. *Successful Aging and Adaptation with Chronic Diseases.* New York: Springer; 2003.

81. Freund AM, Baltes PB. Selection, optimization, and compensation as strategies of life management: Correlations with subjective indicators of successful aging. *Psychol Aging.* 1998;13:531–543.

82. Baltes PB, Smith J. New frontiers in the future of aging: From successful aging of the young old to the dilemmas of the fourth age. *Gerontology.* 2003;49:123–135.

83. Freund AM, Baltes PB. Selection, optimization, and compensation as strategies of life management: Correction to Freud and Baltes. *Psychol Aging.* 1999;14:700–702.

The Impact of Falls and Fall Injuries on Older Women*

Judy A. Stevens, PhD, MPH; Grant T. Baldwin, PhD, MPH; Michael F. Ballesteros, PhD;
Rita K. Noonan, PhD; and David A. Sleet, PhD, FAAHB

Introduction

Falls and fall injuries among adults aged 65 years and older are a major public health concern. More than a third of older adults fall annually,[1,2] and those who fall are two to three times more likely to fall again within a year.[3] Between 20% and 30% of older adults who fall sustain moderate to severe injuries that reduce mobility and independence and increase the risk of premature death.[4,5] Women are disproportionately affected by falls in part because women outnumber men in the older age groups, but also because of they are more vulnerable to falling and sustaining fall-related injuries such as hip fractures.

This chapter describes the magnitude of this health issue and highlights how falls and fall injuries differentially affect women. It summarizes the epidemiology of older adult falls and describes our current knowledge about interventions that can reduce these injuries.

Background

Falls are the leading cause of both fatal and nonfatal injuries among people aged 65 and older (Figure 38-1).[6] In 2010 there were 41,300 unintentional injury deaths among older adults, of which 52% were caused by unintentional falls. Women accounted for slightly more than half (55%) of the fall-related deaths. But fatal falls represent only the "tip of the iceberg." In the same year, almost 2.4 *million* unintentional injuries among older adults were treated in emergency departments, of which 69% were nonfatal fall injuries; 69% of these fall injuries were sustained by women.

One of the most serious fall outcomes is hip fracture, an injury that often results in long-term functional impairment, nursing home admission and increased mortality.[7] More than 90% of hip fractures are caused by falls.[8] In 2007 there were 281,000 hospital admissions for hip fractures and women sustained 77.3% of these injuries.[9]

In addition to physical injuries, falls may have significant psychological and social consequences. Many people who fall, whether or not they sustain injuries, develop a fear of falling. Studies show that 12% to 39% of older adults report they are afraid of falling[10] and this fear can cause them to restrict their activities, which leads to reduced mobility, muscle weakness, and subsequent increased fall risk.[11] Fear of falling is more prevalent among women,[11] is strongly associated with future falls, and has been found to lead to deteriorating health, a decline in physical and social functioning, and nursing home admission.[12]

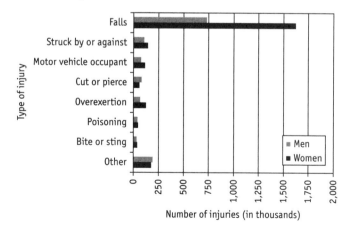

Figure 38-1 Leading Causes of unintentional non-fatal injuries among men and women aged ≥65, U.S., 2010.

Source: Reproduced from National Electronic Injury Surveillance System All Injury Program [NEISS-AIP] 2010. Centers for Disease Control and Prevention [CDC]. Web-based Injury Statistics Query and Reporting System (WISQARS). [database online]. www.cdc.gov/ncipc/wisqars.

Costs

The financial burden of falls is significant. In 2000, the direct medical costs of fall injuries among older adults totaled $1.79 million for fatal falls and $19 billion for nonfatal fall injuries.[28] This is equivalent to $26.3 billion in 2008 dollars. Although women comprised 58% of the American population over age 65, their medical expenditures were almost three times higher than the costs for men ($14 billion vs. $5 billion).

Community Settings

Approximately 96% of the 35 million adults aged 65 and older live independently (that is, not in assisted living or nursing homes), and many spend a large proportion of their time at home. Therefore it is not surprising that between one-half and two-thirds of all falls, and about half of fatal falls, happen in or around the home.[13,14] Studies show that most people fell from a standing height (e.g., by slipping or tripping while walking)[15] and most falls occurred on the same level rather than from heights (e.g., down stairs or off ladders).[16] Berg and colleagues found that the majority of falls (82%) occurred during the day, 14% in the evening, and only 4% at night.[13] People who experienced multiple falls were at greatly increased risk of sustaining serious injury.[17]

Nursing Homes

In 2004 approximately 1.3 million Americans aged 65 and older were living in nursing homes; half were 85 and older and three-quarters were women.[18] By 2030, the number of nursing home residents is projected to double.[19] In 2004, the median length of stay for nursing home residents was 511 days for women and 355 days for men. Nursing home residents are particularly vulnerable to falls and fall-related injuries. At least half of nursing home residents fall annually and the proportion is higher among certain at-risk populations such as people with dementia, where the incidence is 70–80%.[20] Compared to seniors living in the community, people in nursing homes are older, frailer, and have a higher prevalence of cognitive impairment. Nursing home residents also tend to have more, and more severe, chronic conditions, greater limitations in their basic activities of daily living, and a higher prevalence of gait problems,[21] all factors that are associated with falling.[22]

The fall rate among nursing home residents is two to three times the rate for seniors living in the community. The average incidence of falls is 1.5 falls per bed per year.[23] Each year, a typical 100-bed nursing home reports between 100 and 200 falls; this estimate is considered low as many falls are likely to be unreported.[24] Approximately 4% of falls result in fractures and another 12% cause severe injuries such as head trauma and severe lacerations. About 35% of fall-related injuries occur among nonambulatory residents.[25] Nursing home residents tend to fall repeatedly, which increases their chances of sustaining injuries.

Hospitals

Fall rates among hospital patients vary by patient population, type of hospital, and reasons for hospitalization. The highest rates are seen among the oldest patients. Within the geriatric population, the highest rates, from 8.9 to 17.1 falls per 1,000 patient-days, have been reported for departments of neuroscience, rehabilitation, and psychiatry.[26,27] Methods for calculating hospital fall rates differ. The most accurate approach is to report the number of falls per 1,000 patient bed-days. However, many studies calculate the fall rate as the number of falls per 100 hospital admissions. These differences make it difficult to compare fall rates among institutions.

Epidemiology

Fatal Falls

In 2010, 21,649 older adults (55% women) died from fall injuries, an average of one death every 25 minutes.[6] The higher proportion of women reflects the gender distribution in the over-65 population. In contrast, fall death rates are significantly higher for men in all age groups (Figure 38-2). In 2010, the age-adjusted fall death rate for men (61.3 per 100,000 population) was 40.5% higher than the rate for women (44.9 per 100,000).

For both men and women, fall death rates increase sharply with age; the greatest increase occurs after age 80 (Figure 38-2).[6] Fall death rates also differ by race. One study found that fall-related death rates for both men and women were highest among whites, and the rate for white women was approximately twice that for women of other races.[29] The cause of higher mortality from falls among men has not been fully explained. This disparity may be due to gender differences in underlying chronic conditions at similar ages, such as cardiovascular disease, or the differential may reflect more risk-taking behaviors, such as climbing on ladders.

National data indicate that fall death rates are increasing. From 2000 to 2010, age-adjusted rates increased 64% in men and 84% in women (Figure 38-3). Reasons for this increase are unclear. The number and rate of fatal fall injuries are calculated using vital records

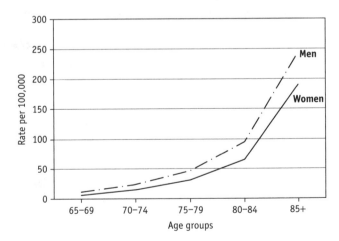

Figure 38-2 Fall death rates among men and women aged ≥65 by age group, U.S., 2010.

Data from National Center for Health Statistics. Vital Statistics, 2010. Centers for Disease Control and Prevention [CDC].

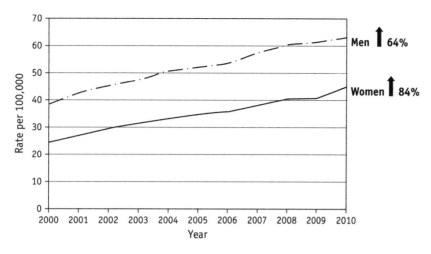

Figure 38-3 Trends in age-adjusted fall death rates for men and women aged ≥65, U.S., 2000-2010.

Data from National Electronic Injury Surveillance System all Injury Program [NEISS-AIP], 2000-2010 Centers for Disease Control and Prevention [CDC]. Web-based Injury Statistics Query and Reporting System (WISQARS). [database online]. www.cdc.gov/ncipc/wisqars.

data that are compiled by the National Center for Health Statistics. Although comprehensive, the quality of these data depends on the training and/or experience of the physician or medical examiner filling out the death certificate. The number of deaths attributable to falls may be undercounted if a fall did not occur close to the time of death.

Few studies have examined the specific causes of fall-related deaths although there is evidence that up to half are due to traumatic brain injuries (TBI). In an analysis of fall-related deaths in 2005 among people aged 65 and older, 50.3% were attributed to TBI.[30] Complications following fractures, especially hip fractures, also contribute significantly to fall deaths.[9,14]

Nonfatal Falls

In 2010, 2.4 million falls among people aged 65 and older were treated in hospital emergency departments and 68.9% of these injuries were to women.[6] The majority of fall injuries were mild to moderate; about three-quarters of patients were treated and released and one quarter were hospitalized. Nonfatal fall rates also have increased significantly. From 2001 to 2010, age-adjusted fall injury rates increased 23.5% for men and 25.8% for women.[6]

One out of five falls causes a serious nonfatal injury such as a fracture or head trauma, injuries that can limit mobility, reduce independence, and increase the risk of premature death.[5] In a population-based study, Stevens and Sogolow[31] found that fall-related injury rates for women were 40%–60% higher than for men of comparable age. Women also were more likely to sustain serious injuries such as fractures and head injuries that required hospitalization. In this study, the hospitalization rate for women was 1.8 times that for men, and women's hospital admission rates for fractures and lower trunk injuries were more than twice as high as men's rates. Similarly, in an analysis of Washington State hospital discharge data, researchers found that

the fall-related hospitalization rate for women was twice that for men.[32] About 46.7% of patients who were hospitalized for a fall injury were subsequently transferred to a skilled nursing facility.[32]

A recent analysis of the 2006 Current Medicare Beneficiary Survey (CMBS) data found that nearly seven million community-dwelling Medicare beneficiaries aged 65 and over reported having fallen in the past year; 61.1% of those who fell were women.[33] Over two million beneficiaries sought medical attention following a fall and women were significantly more likely than men to seek medical treatment for a fall (37.5% vs. 24.3%) and to talk with a healthcare provider about preventing future falls (31.2% vs. 24.3 %). This is consistent with other studies that have noted women's higher incidence of fall injuries.[31,34]

Women are disproportionately affected by nonfatal fall injuries (Figure 38-4). In 2010, after adjusting for age, the fall injury rate for women was 49% higher than for men.[6] One study found that the most prevalent nonfatal fall injuries were fractures, contusions or abrasions, and lacerations.[31] and compared to men, injury rates for women were 2.2 times higher for fractures, 70% higher for contusions or abrasions, and 10% higher for lacerations.[31]

Much of the gender disparity is due to women's greater susceptibility to hip fracture, an extremely serious fall injury that can result in disability, nursing home admission, and increased mortality.[35–37] Women sustain hip fractures at a significantly higher rate than men,[9] and white women are much more likely to sustain hip fractures than are African-American or Asian women.[15] Treatment typically includes surgery and hospitalization, frequently followed by admission to a nursing home and extensive rehabilitation.[38]

Falls are the strongest risk factor for hip fracture. However, a significant contributing factor is osteoporosis, a metabolic disease that affects postmenopausal women and elderly men. It is characterized by low bone mineral

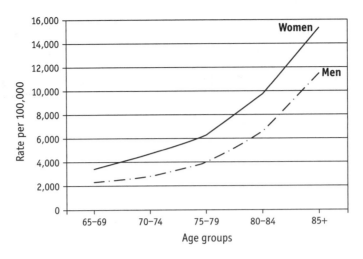

Figure 38-4 Nonfatal fall injury rates for men and women age ≥65 by age group, U.S., 2010.

Data from National Electronic Injury Surveillance System all Injury Program [NEISS-AIP], 2010. Centers for Disease Control and Prevention [CDC]. Web-based Injury Statistics Query and Reporting System (WISQARS). [database online]. www.cdc.gov/ncipc/wisqars.

density (BMD) and deterioration of bone structure making bones porous and susceptible to fracture. The National Osteoporosis Foundation estimates that more than 10 million people over age 50 in the United States have osteoporosis and 80% of those affected are women. An additional 34 million people have low BMD and are at risk for the disease.[39]

Bone mass for both men and women peaks around age 30 and then declines—about 0.5% per year for men and 1% per year for women.[40] In addition, women suffer rapid loss of bone mass during the first 5 years following menopause. A 1992 Rochester, Minnesota study found that 59% of 153 women over age 60 (and 84% of 50 women over age 80) had osteopenia, a preosteoporotic condition characterized by low bone mass two standard deviations below the mean for normal women under age 40.[41]

Although women's susceptibility to hip fracture is often attributed to reduced bone mass,[42,43] falling sideways onto the hip is usually necessary to cause a hip fracture.[44] Specialized hip protectors have been developed that assist reduce and deflect the force of impact on the hip joint when falls occur[45] and may prevent hip fractures among people at high risk.[46,47]

Fall Risk Factors

Epidemiologic studies have identified numerous fall risk factors and the prevalence of many of these increase with age. Risk factors frequently are classified as either intrinsic (i.e., originating within the body, such as age, female gender, leg weakness, balance disorders, and poor vision) or extrinsic (i.e., originating outside the body, such as environmental hazards). Some researchers have further expanded this classification to include behavioral and social/economic risk factors.[48] Table 38-1 lists major risk factors within each category.

Biological Factors

Some biological risk factors are important but cannot be modified, such as older age, being female and being cognitively impaired. Having certain chronic conditions also increases fall risk through various mechanisms. Some conditions, such as stroke and Parkinson's disease, adversely affect balance, gait, and muscular coordination;[50,51] diabetes can cause loss of vision and peripheral neuropathy leading to decreased sensation in the feet;[52] and arthritis affects flexibility[53] and may also cause chronic pain.[54]

However, a number of important risk factors are appropriate targets for prevention efforts because they can be modified. These include muscle weakness in the legs, gait and balance problems, and poor vision.[49] In addition, identifying and treating the symptoms of chronic conditions may reduce fall risk.[55]

Behavioral Factors

Behavioral factors are the focus of public health efforts because they are generally considered modifiable. Risky behaviors include climbing on ladders or chairs;[16] being inactive, which leads to poor physical conditioning and muscle weakness;[49] taking four or more medications; and taking medications that affect the central nervous system. Psychoactive medications such as tranquilizers, sedatives, and antidepressants have been most strongly associated with falls,[56] but diuretics, antihypertensive medications, and narcotic analgesics also increase fall risk.[57] Although all these factors are potentially modifiable through science-based interventions, it is well documented that human behavior is very difficult to change, especially for sustained periods of time. Changing older adults' behaviors to prevent falls is no exception.[58]

Environmental Factors

Some environmental factors, such as cold temperatures, uneven pavement, and poorly designed public spaces (e.g., street crossings and parking lots) are difficult or impossible to change. Fortunately, there are risk factors within the home that can be modified. Examples include clutter in walkways, tripping hazards, dim lighting, and lack of stair railings or grab bars in the bathroom.[59]

Table 38-1

Selected fall risk factors

Biological	Behavioral	Environmental	Social/Economic
Advanced age	Multiple medications	Lack of stair handrails	Low income
Previous falls	Psychoactive medications	Poor stair design	Lack of education
Female gender	Inactivity	Lack of bathroom grab bars	Poor living conditions
Muscle weakness	Risk-taking behaviors	Dim lighting or glare	Lack of social support
Poor balance & coordination	Fear of falling	Obstacles & tripping hazards	Living alone
Gait disorders	Improper or inappropriate use of mobility aids	Slippery or uneven surfaces	Illiteracy and/or language barriers
Chronic conditions: Arthritis, diabetes, stroke, Parkinson's, incontinence, dementia	Poor nutrition or hydration	Poor building design and/or maintenance	
Poor vision	Inappropriate footwear	Poorly designed or maintained public spaces	
Functional limitations	Alcohol use		
Acute illness			

Source: Adapted from Scott V. *Prevention of Falls and Injuries among the Elderly*. Vancouver, BC: British Columbia-Office of the Provincial Health Officer; 2004, and Rubenstein LZ, Josephson KR. Falls and their prevention in elderly people: what does the evidence show? *Med Clin North Am*. 2006;90:807–24.

Social and Economic Factors

Although evidence is limited, some research suggests that a number of risk and protective factors are related to social and economic conditions. For example, low income is highly associated with poor health status and disability that, in turn, are associated with increased fall risk.[60,61] Some psychosocial conditions such as depression also increase the risk of falls and fall-related injuries.[62–64] Conversely, social integration, as measured by the size and quality of family and friendship networks, has been shown to protect against falls[65] and fall-related fractures.[62] Fear of falling has been identified as a fall risk factor, particularly when it causes a reduction in physical activity, which may be protective.[66]

Risk Factor Interactions

Most falls result from interactions among multiple risk factors (Figure 38-5).[49] In an early study of community-dwelling older adults, Tinetti et al. found that the likelihood of falling increased with the number of risk factors present.[67] The proportion of people who fell increased from 27% for those with up to one risk factor to 78% for those with four or more risk factors.

Not all risk factors are equally important. Using meta-analysis, researchers have determined that a history of falling, muscle weakness, difficulties with gait and balance, use of psychoactive medications, functional limitations, visual impairment, arthritis, and depression

are the factors most strongly associated with falls.[49,68] Fall interventions have focused on these potentially modifiable fall risk factors.

Fall Interventions

The frequency of falls among older adults, combined with high susceptibility to injury due to age-related physiological changes (e.g., decreased muscle strength and endurance, delayed reaction times) and a high prevalence of chronic conditions, makes any fall potentially dangerous. Unfortunately, many older people are not aware of

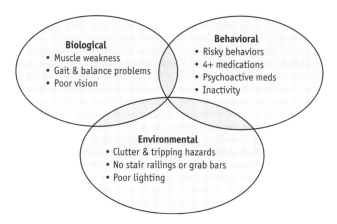

Figure 38-5 Risk factor interactions.

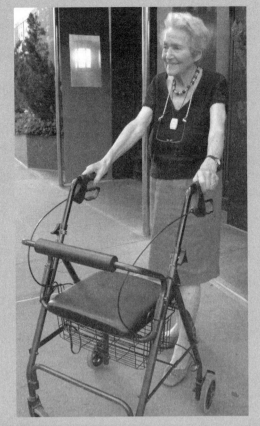

Figure 38-6 Inge Humbert 4/30/1918 –

In 1935 Ms. Humbert, who lived in Munich, Germany, was encouraged by her parents to leave her home country and join her uncle in New York. After immigrating, she held several jobs including that of a model, a secretary for a doctor, and a real estate saleswoman. While selling real estate, she met the man she married. She and her husband traveled a great deal, often spending summers in Italy. Although her husband died more than twenty years ago, Ms. Humbert has remained physically and socially active. Now age 94, Ms Humbert relies on her walker for mobility and on the assistance of a home health aide to remain independent. After experiencing a small stroke, she follows her doctors' orders to walk at least 30 minutes each day to avoid a recurrence.

their risk of falling or avoid discussing these issues with their healthcare providers.[58] Consequently, opportunities to implement prevention strategies are often missed.

Clinical Assessment and Risk Factor Reduction

In a meta-analysis of randomized controlled trials of fall interventions, Gillespie et al. concluded that the most effective fall intervention was a clinical assessment by a healthcare provider combined with individualized fall risk reduction, referral, and patient follow-up.[69]

The American Geriatrics Society (AGS) published clinical fall assessment guidelines in 2001[72] that were updated in 2010.[55] For high-risk patients, these guidelines recommend testing gait, balance, and neurological function; reviewing all medications; developing a tailored medical management approach; and making appropriate referrals.[72] However, primary care physicians have been slow to put these recommendations into clinical practice because many feel they do not have adequate knowledge about methods of risk assessment and/or fall prevention.[73–75]

Exercise

After clinical assessment with risk factor reduction, the most effective intervention is exercise, which can reduce fall risk on average by 24%.[76] However, recruiting participants and maintaining compliance with an exercise program can be problematic.

The Cochrane group conducted a meta-analysis of 43 randomized controlled trials of fall interventions that included exercise.[69] They concluded that multiple component exercise interventions were effective in reducing the rate and risk of falling. The evidence supported three different approaches: multiple component group exercise programs, individually prescribed multiple component exercise carried out at home, and tai chi as a group exercise.

In a randomized controlled trial (RCT) of a tai chi intervention, Li et al.[70] found the risk of falling was decreased 55% among participants in the tai chi group compared to the control group. In another RCT, Voukelatos et al.[71] studied the effectiveness of a community-based tai chi program and found that the fall rate in the tai chi group was 28% lower than in the control group after 16 weeks and 33% lower after 24 weeks.

Sherrington and colleagues carried out a meta-analysis of 44 fall intervention studies that devoted at least 25% of the time to exercise.[77] They found that including exercises that challenged balance, making exercises progressive, and having at least 50 hours of exercise were the key factors associated with program effectiveness. Including a walking program did not contribute to reducing fall rates, possibly because the time spent walking took the place of time spent improving balance.[77] However, walking programs have other health benefits including improved fitness, weight loss, and lowered blood pressure.[78] Research is needed to better understanding the effect of walking programs on fall risk.

Medication Management

Studies have clearly demonstrated that psychoactive medications, specifically benzodiazepines, antidepressants, and sedatives/hypnotics, increase fall risk.[56,79–81] Medication management involves a doctor or pharmacist first reviewing all prescription and the over-the-counter medications an older adult is taking and then reducing the number of medications, finding alternative drugs, and/or adjusting dosages so as to reduce side effects and interactions that may lead to falls.[56,79] A relatively small study by Campbell et al.[82] found that eliminating psychoactive medication use among community-dwelling seniors reduced fall rates by 66%. However, one month after the study ended, 47% of the participants had resumed taking their psychoactive medications.

Vision Enhancement

Impaired vision, which encompasses poor visual acuity, reduced contrast sensitivity and depth perception, and visual field loss, increases the risk of falling.[83,84] Eye examinations and vision correction can help reduce this risk. Many older adults use glasses with multifocal lenses that can reduce edge contrast and depth perception, creating a fall hazard;[85] single vision lenses may be a better choice for activities such as walking that require good depth perception. Evidence that cataract surgery reduces falls is inconclusive.[86] Some studies have found that removing cataracts in both eyes reduces falls whereas others have not.

Home Modification

More than half of falls in community-dwelling older adults occur in or around the home,[12,15] so the home environment is a natural setting for fall prevention efforts. Although it remains a popular fall prevention strategy, simply reducing environmental risks, such as by improving lighting and removing tripping hazards, has not been shown to reduce falls among older adults.[87,88] Day and colleagues conducted a factorial trial of three fall interventions: exercise, vision enhancement, and home hazard reduction.[59] Individually, only the exercise program was effective; this intervention reduced falls by 18%. However, when home hazard reduction was combined with the exercise program, falls were reduced by 24%, and when the intervention included all three components, falls were reduced by 33%.

Two home modification interventions have been shown in randomized controlled trials to effectively reduce falls. These individualized interventions involved home visits by occupational therapists who discussed behavioral changes with each client, tailored environmental changes to the client's specific needs, and facilitated recommended home modifications.[89,90]

Vitamin D

Vitamin D has a direct effect on muscle strength, calcium absorption, and bone growth. Calcium combined with vitamin D may help decrease the risks of falls and fractures in older adults.[91] Sources of vitamin D include food (such as fish, eggs, and fortified milk), sun exposure, and dietary supplements. After conducting a meta-analysis of eight randomized clinical trials, Bischoff-Ferrari and colleagues concluded that vitamin D supplementation in a dose of 700 to 1000 IU a day reduced the risk of falls among older adults by 19%,[92] and a Cochrane review reported that vitamin D supplements reduced falls in community-dwelling older adults with initially low 25-hydroxyvitamin D levels.[93] However, a systematic review by the Agency for Healthcare Research and Quality (AHRQ) concluded that the evidence regarding the benefit of vitamin D in reducing falls and fractures was inconclusive.[94] Vitamin D as a fall prevention strategy is appealing because it is inexpensive and would be acceptable to high-risk older adults.[95]

Multifactorial Interventions

Falls often are caused by a complex interaction between the individual and the environment. In 1994, Tinetti and colleagues published the results of a landmark fall intervention study that focused on a number of risk factors: balance, gait, impaired arm or leg strength or range of motion, use of sedatives, use of four or more prescription medications, postural hypotension, and ability to transfer safely (i.e., move from the bed to a chair).[96] This study demonstrated that an intervention that addressed multiple risk factors could significantly reduce falls among community-dwelling seniors. The majority of effective interventions include multiple components that address a variety of risk factors. These may incorporate risk factor screening and treatment or referrals to specialists to reduce fall risk; exercise programs or physical therapy to improve gait, balance and strength; medication management; environmental modification; and other elements such as education about fall risk factors and vision assessment and correction.[97–99]

Possible Reasons for Gender Differences

Studies have consistently shown that women have a higher risk of falling and of sustaining fall injuries than men.[30,32] The difference in fracture rates, particularly hip fractures, is especially striking. This disparity may be related to the amount of physical activity, lower body strength, bone mass, circumstances surrounding the fall, or willingness to seek medical attention. Because women are more likely to seek medical treatment,[100] the prevalence of falls among women may be somewhat inflated. However, reporting bias would not affect the gender differences observed for serious injuries such as fractures[30,101] and traumatic brain injuries, diagnoses that are based on medical records and diagnostic codes in the *International Classification of Diseases, 9th Revision, Clinical Modification*.[102]

Much of the gender disparity is probably attributable to differences in physical activity levels. Muscle weakness and loss of lower-body strength, often caused by inactivity, is a well-known risk factor for falling.[72] Data from the 1982–1984 National Health and Nutrition Examination Survey (NHANES 1) Follow-up Survey established that older women were less physically active than older men,[103] and a 1993–1995 study of 2,025 California residents found that men had greater lower body strength than women.[104]

Research Gaps

Research has identified effective interventions for community-dwelling older adults,[105] but fall interventions for nursing home residents and hospital patients are more limited. There is evidence that multifactorial interventions and supervised exercise reduce falls and fall risk in hospital patients, and vitamin D supplementation can reduce fall rates in nursing home residents.[106]

Further research is needed now to tailor interventions for subpopulations with differing characteristics and risk factors, such as those with chronic conditions or differing levels of functional impairment; to determine the underlying causes and/or circumstances of falls; and to understand how these factors differ for men and women. Clarifying these differences as well as collecting information about the location and events preceding a fall or fall-related injury is vital to identifying high-risk behaviors and situations and for developing and implementing targeted fall prevention strategies.

Summary

Falls and fall-related injuries are age-related problems and the U.S. population is aging rapidly. People over 85 are the fastest growing segment of the older population and have the highest fall injury rate. In 2010, there were 3.9 million women aged 85 and older and by 2040 this number will reach 8.7 million.[107] Because women live longer than men and typically marry men older than themselves, many more older women than men will be affected by fall-related injuries unless we take preventive action.

Much is known about effective fall prevention strategies.[55] We now need to refine these proven interventions to broaden their use across diverse populations, create an infrastructure to train implementers how to use proven strategies, disseminate effective fall prevention programs, and support widespread adoption at the local level. We also must enhance provider training to incorporate fall risk assessment and interventions into clinical settings. Such a multifaceted approach would support broad implementation of effective fall interventions and would reduce the personal and societal burden associated with older adult falls.

Discussion Questions

1. What are likely reasons for the increasing trend in fall death rates? How might these affect men and women differently?
2. List six important fall risk factors and discuss how you would design a community-based fall prevention program to address these factors.
3. Discuss why women are more likely than men to sustain nonfatal fall injuries.
4. What fall prevention interventions would be most helpful to women?

Fall Prevention Resources

Articles:
Self-Reported Falls and Fall-Related Injuries Among Persons Aged ≥ 65 Years—United States, 2006
http://www.cdc.gov/mmwr/preview/mmwrhtml/mm5709a1.htm

CDC Publications:
Preventing Falls: What Works—A CDC Compendium of Effective Community-Based Interventions
http://www.cdc.gov/HomeandRecreationalSafety/Falls/compendium.html
Preventing Falls: How to Develop Community-based Fall Prevention Programs
http://www.cdc.gov/HomeandRecreationalSafety/Falls/community_preventfalls.html

Fact sheets:
Falls Among Older Adults: An Overview
http://www.cdc.gov/HomeandRecreationalSafety/Falls/adultfalls.html
Costs of Falls among Older Adults
http://www.cdc.gov/HomeandRecreationalSafety/Falls/fallcost.html
Hip Fractures among Older Adults
http://www.cdc.gov/HomeandRecreationalSafety/Falls/adulthipfx.html
Falls in Nursing Homes
http://www.cdc.gov/HomeandRecreationalSafety/Falls/nursing.html

Podcasts:
Adult Falls—Date Released: June 8, 2007. Series: A Cup of Health with CDC.
http://www2c.cdc.gov/podcasts/player.asp?f=5812
Falls Among Older Adults—Date Released: March 13, 2008. Series: A Cup of Health with CDC.
http://www2c.cdc.gov/podcasts/player.asp?f=8521
Preventing Older Adult Falls and TBI—Date Released: March 7, 2008. Series: CDC Featured Podcasts.
http://www2c.cdc.gov/podcasts/player.asp?f=6052658

References

1. Hornbrook MC, Stevens VJ, Wingfield DJ, et al. Preventing falls among community-dwelling older persons: results from a randomized trial. *Gerontol.* 1994;34:16–23.
2. Hausdorff JM, Rios DA, Edelber HK. Gait variability and fall risk in community-living older adults: a 1-year prospective study. *Arch Phys Med & Rehabil.* 2001;82:1050–56.
3. Teno J, Kiel DP, Mor V. Multiple stumbles: a risk factor for falls in community-dwelling elderly. A prospective study. *J Am Geriatr Soc.* 1990;38:1321–1325.
4. Alexander BH, Rivara FP, Wolf ME. The cost and frequency of hospitalization for fall-related injuries in older adults. *Am J Pub Health.* 1992;82:1020–1023.
5. Sterling DA, O'Connor JA, Bonadies J. Geriatric falls: injury severity is high and disproportionate to mechanism. *J Trauma.* 2001;50:116–119.
6. Centers for Disease Control and Prevention (CDC). Web-based Injury Statistics Query and Reporting System (WISQARS). National Center for Injury Prevention and Control, Centers for Disease Control and Prevention. www.cdc.gov/ncipc/wisqars. Accessed December 1, 2009.
7. Stevens JA. Falls Among Older Adults—Risk Factors and Prevention Strategies. In: *Falls Free: Promoting a National Falls Prevention Action Plan: Research Review Papers.* Washington, DC: National Council on Aging, Center for Healthy Aging; 2005:3–18.
8. Nyberg L, Gustafson Y, Berggren D, et al. Falls leading to femoral neck fractures in lucid older people. *J Am Geriatr Soc.* 1996;44:156–60.
9. Centers for Disease Control and Prevention, National Center for Health Statistics. National Hospital Discharge Survey (NHDS). http://www.cdc.gov/nchs/nhds.htm. Accessed February 2, 2009.
10. Scheffer AC, Schuurmans MJ, Van Dijk N, Van Der Hoof T. Fear of falling: measurement strategy, prevalence, risk factors and consequences among older persons. *Age Ageing.* 2008;37:19–24.
11. Vellas BJ, Wayne SJ, Romero LJ, et al. Fear of falling and restriction of mobility in elderly fallers. *Age Ageing.* 1997;26:189–193.
12. Tinetti ME, Williams CS. The effect of falls and fall injuries on functioning in community-dwelling older persons. *J Gerontol A Biol Sci Med Sci.* 1998;53:M112–M119.

13. Berg WP, Alessio HM, Mills EM, et al. Circumstances and consequences of falls in independent community-dwelling older adults. *Age Ageing.* 1997;26:261–268.

14. Deprey SM. Descriptive analysis of fatal falls of older adults in a Midwestern counting in the year 2005. *J Geriatr Phys Ther.* 2009;32:23–28.

15. Ellis AA, Trent RB. Hospitalized fall injuries and race in California. *Inj Prev.* 2001;7:316–320.

16. Nachreiner NM, Findorff MJ, Wyman JF, et al. Circumstances and consequences of falls in community-dwelling older women. *J Women's Health.* 2007;16:1437–1446.

17. Nevitt MC, Cummings SR, Hudes ES. Risk factors for injurious falls: a prospective study. *J Gerontol.* 1991:46:M164–M170.

18. Jones Al, Dwyer LL, Bercovitz AR, Strahan GW. The National Nursing Home Survey: 2004 overview. National Center for Health Statistics. *Vital Health Stat.* 2009;13(167).

19. Sahyoun NR, Pratt LA, Lentzner H, et al. *The Changing Profile of Nursing Home Residents: 1985-1997.* Aging Trends; No. 4. Hyattsville, MD: National Center for Health Statistics; 2001.

20. Shaw FE. Prevention of falls in older people with dementia. *J Neural Transm.* 2007;114:1259–64.

21. Bedsine RW, Rubenstein LZ, Snyder L, eds. *Medical Care of the Nursing Home Resident.* Philadelphia, PA: American College of Physicians; 1996.

22. Ejaz FK, Jones JA, Rose MS. Falls among nursing home residents: an examination of incident reports before and after restraint reduction programs. *J Am Geriatr Soc.* 1994;42:960–964.

23. Rubenstein LZ, Josephson KR, Robbins AS. Falls in the nursing home. *Ann Intern Med.* 1994;121:442–451.

24. Rubenstein LZ. Preventing falls in the nursing home. *JAMA.* 1997;278:595–596.

25. Thapa PB, Brockman KG, Gideon P, et al. Injurious falls in nonambulatory nursing home residents: a comparative study of circumstances, incidence and risk factors. *J Am Geriatr Soc.* 1996;44:273–278.

26. Nyberg L, Gustafson Y, Janson A, et al. Incidence of falls in three different types of geriatric care. *Scand J Soc Med.* 1997;25:8–13.

27. Rhode JM, Myers AH, Vlahov D. Variation in risk for falls by clinical department: implications for prevention. *Infect Control Hosp Epidemiol.* 1990;11:521–524.

28. Stevens JA, Corso PS, Finkelstein EA, Miller TR. Cost of fatal and nonfatal falls among older adults. *Inj Prev.* 2006;12:290–295.

29. Stevens JA, Dellinger AM. Motor vehicle and fall related deaths among older Americans 1990–98: sex, race, and ethnic disparities. *Inj Prev.* 2002;8:272–275.

30. Thomas KE, Stevens JA, Sarmiento K, Wald MM. Fall-related traumatic brain injury deaths and hospitalizations among older adults—United States, 2005. *J Safety Res.* 2008;39:269–272.

31. Stevens JA, Sogolow ED. Gender differences for nonfatal unintentional fall-related injuries. *Inj Prev.* 2005;11:115–119.

32. Guse CE, Porinsky R. Risk factors associated with hospitalization for unintentional falls: Wisconsin hospital discharge data for patients aged 65 and over. *WMJ.* 2003;102:37–42.

33. Stevens JA, Ballesteros MF, Mack KA, Rudd RA, DeCaro E, Adler G. Gender differences in seeking care for falls in the aged Medicare population. *American Journal of Preventive Medicine.* 2012;43(1):59–62.

34. Tinetti ME, Doucette J, Claus E, Marottoli R. Risk factors for serious injury during falls by older persons in the community. *J Am Geriatr Soc.* 1995;43:1214–1221.

35. Wolinsky FD, Fitzgerald JF, Stump TE. The effect of hip fracture on mortality, hospitalization, and functional status: a prospective study. *Am J Pub Health.* 1997;87:398–403.

36. Hall SE, Williams, JA, Senior JA, et al. Hip fracture outcomes: quality of life and functional status in older adults living in the community. *Aust NZ J Med.* 2000;30:327–332.

37. Braithwaite RS, Co NF, Wong JB. Estimating hip fracture morbidity, mortality and costs. *J Am Geriatr Soc.* 2003;51:364–370.

38. Marks R, Allegrante JP, MacKenzie CR, et al. Hip fractures among the elderly: causes, consequences and control. *Ageing Res Rev.* 2003;2:57–93.

39. National Osteoporosis Foundation (NOF). *Clinician's Guide to Prevention and Treatment of Osteoporosis.* http://www.nof.org/professionals/clinical-guidelines. Accessed October 11, 2012.

40. Riggs BL, Wahner HW, Dunn WL, et al. Differential changes in bone mineral density of the appendicular and axial skeleton with aging. *J Clin Invest.* 1981;67:328–335.

41. Melton LJ, Chrischilles EA, Cooper C, et al. How many women have osteoporosis? *J Bone Miner Res.* 1992;7:1005–1010.

42. Birge SJ. Osteoporosis and hip fracture. *Clin Geriatr Med.* 1993;9:69–86.

43. Greenspan SL, Myers ER, Maitland LA, et al. Fall severity and bone mineral density as risk factors for hip fracture in ambulatory elderly. *JAMA.* 1994;271(2):128–133.

44. Hayes WC, Myers ER, Morris JN, et al. Impact near the hip dominates fracture risk in elderly nursing home residents who fall. *Calcif Tissue Int.* 1993;52:192–198.

45. Robinovitch SN, Hayes WC, McMahon TA. Energy-shunting hip padding system attenuates femoral impact force in a simulated fall. *J Biomech Eng.* 1995;117:409–413.

46. Parker MJ, Gillespie LD, Gillespie WJ. Hip protectors for preventing hip fractures in the elderly (Cochrane Review). In: *The Cochrane Library,* Issue 2. Oxford: Update Software; 2002.

47. Howland J, Peterson E, Kivell E. Hip protectors efficacy and barriers to adoption to prevent fall-related injuries in older adults: findings and recommendations from an international workgroup. *J Safety Res.* 2006;37:421–424.

48. Scott V. *Prevention of Falls and Injuries among the Elderly.* Vancouver, BC: British Columbia-Office of the Provincial Health Officer; 2004.

49. Rubenstein LZ, Josephson KR. Falls and their prevention in elderly people: what does the evidence show? *Med Clin North Am.* 2006;90:807–824.

50. Mackintosh SFH, Goldie P, Hill K. Falls incidence and factors associated with falling in older, community-dwelling, chronic stroke survivors (>1 year after stroke) and matched controls. *Aging Clin Exp Res.* 2005;17:74–81.

51. Gray P, Hildebrand K. Fall risk factors in Parkinson's disease. *J Neurosci Nurs.* 2000;32:222–229.

52. Patel S, Hyer S, Tweed K, et al. Risk factors for fractures and falls in older women with Type 2 diabetes mellitus. *Calcif Tissue Int.* 2008;82:87–91.

53. Lawlor DA, Patel R, Ebrahim S. Association between falls in elderly women and chronic diseases and drug use: cross sectional study. *BMJ.* 2003;327:1–6.

54. Leveille SG, Jones RN, Kiely DK, et al. Chronic musculoskeletal pain and the occurrence of falls in an older population. *JAMA.* 2009;302:2214–2227.

55. *AGS/BGS Clinical Practice Guideline: Prevention of Falls in Older Persons.* New York: American Geriatrics Society; 2010. http://www.americangeriatrics.org/health_care_professionals/clinical_practice/clinical_guidelines_recommendations/2010/. Accessed October 11, 2012.

56. Ray WA, Griffin MR. Prescribed medications and the risk of falling. *Top Geriatr Rehabil.* 1990;5:12–20.

57. Weiner DK, Hanlon JT, Studenski SA. Effects of central nervous system polypharmacy on falls liability in community-dwelling elderly. *Gerontology.* 1998;44:217–221.

58. Stevens JA, Noonan RK, Rubenstein LZ. Older adult fall prevention: perceptions, beliefs, and behaviors. *Am J Lifestyle Med.* 2010;4:16–20.

59. Day L, Fildes B, Gordon I, et al. Randomised factorial trial of falls prevention among older people living in their own homes. *BMJ.* 2002; 325:1–6.

60. Evans RG, Barer ML, Marmor TR, eds. *Why Are Some People Healthy and Others Are Not? The Determinants of Health of Populations.* New York: Aldine De Gruyter; 1994.

61. Gallagher EM, Hunter M, Scott VJ. The nature of falling among community dwelling seniors *Can J Aging.* 1999;18;348–362.

62. Peel NM, McClure RJ, Hendrikz JK. Psychosocial factors associated with fall-related hip-fractures. *Age Ageing.* 2007;36:145–151.

63. Forsen L, Meyer HE, Sogaard AJ, Naess S, Schei B, Edna TH. Mental distress and risk of hip fracture. Do broken hearts lead to broken bones? *J Epidemiol Community Healthi.* 1999;53:343–347.

64. Luukinen H, Koski K, Kivela S-L, Laippala P. Social status, life changes, housing conditions, health, functional abilities and life-style as risk factors for recurrent falls among the home-dwelling elderly. *Public Health.* 1996;110:115–118.

65. Faulkner KA, Cauley JA, Zmuda JM, Griffin JM, Nevitt MC. Is social integration associated with risk of falling in older community-dwelling women? *J Gerontology.* 2003;10:954–959.

66. Wijlhuizen GJ, de Jong R, Hopman-Rock M. Older persons afraid of falling reduce physical activity to prevent outdoor falls. *Prev Med.* 2007;44:260–264.

67. Tinetti ME, Williams TF, Mayewski R. Fall risk index for elderly patients based on number of chronic disabilities. *Am J Med.* 1986:80:429–434.

68. Rubenstein LZ, Josephson KR. The epidemiology of falls and syncope. *Clin Geriatric Med.* 2002;18:141–158.

69. Gillespie LD, Gillespie WJ, Robertson MC et al. Interventions for preventing falls in elderly people. *Cochrane Database Syst Rev.* 2003;4:CD000340.

70. Li, F, Marmer, P Fisher, J, et al. Tai chi and fall reductions in older adults: a randomized controlled trial. *J Gerontol. A Biol Sci Med Sci.* 2005;60A:187–194.

71. Voukelatos, A, Cumming RG, Lord SR, Rissel, C. A randomized controlled trial of tai chi for the prevention of falls: the central Sydney tai chi trial. *J Am Geriatr Soc.* 2007;55:1185–1191 2007.

72. American Geriatrics Society, British Geriatrics Society, and American Academy of Orthopaedic Surgeons Panel on Falls Prevention. A guideline for the prevention of falls in older persons. *J Am Geriatr Soc.* 2001;49(5):664–672.

73. Fortinsky RH, Iannuzzi-Sucich M, Baker DI, et al. Fall-risk assessment and management in clinical practice: views from healthcare providers. *J Am Geriatr Soc.* 2004;52:1522–1526.

74. Rubenstein LZ, Solomon DH, Roth CO, et al. Detection and management of falls and instability among vulnerable elders by community physicians. *J Am Geriatr Soc.* 2004;52:1527–1531.

75. Chou WC, Tinetti ME, King MB, et al. Perceptions of physicians on the barriers and facilitators to integrating fall risk evaluation and management into practice. *J Gen Intern Med.* 2006;21:117–122.

76. Chang JT, Morton SC, Rubenstein LZ, et al. Interventions for the prevention of falls in older adults: systematic review and meta-analysis of randomized clinical trials. *BMJ.* 2004;328;1–7.

77. Sherrington C, Whitney JC, Lord SR, et al. Effective exercise for the prevention of falls: a systematic review and meta-analysis. *J Am Geriatr Soc.* 2008;56:2234–2243.

78. Murphy MH, Nevill AM, Murtagh EM, Holder RL. The effect of walking on fitness, fatness and resting blood pressure: a meta-analysis of randomised, controlled trials. *Prev Med*. 2007;44:377–385.

79. Cumming RG. Epidemiology of medication-related falls and fractures in the elderly. *Drugs Aging*. 1998;12: 43–53.

80. Leipzig RM, Cumming RG, Tinetti ME. Drugs and falls in older people: a systematic review and meta-analysis: I. Psychotropic drugs. *J Am Geriatr Soc*. 1999;47:30–39.

81. Ensrud KE, Blackwell T, Mangione CM, et al. Central nervous system active medications and risk for fractures in older women. *Arch Intern Med*. 2003;163:949–957.

82. Campbell AJ, Robertson MC, Gardner MM, et al. Psychotropic medication withdrawal and a home-based exercise program to prevent falls: a randomized controlled trial. *J Am Geriatr Soc*. 1999;47:850–853.

83. Lord SR, Dayhew J. Visual risk factors for falls in older people. *J Am Geriatr Soc*. 2001;49:508–515.

84. De Boer MR, Pluijm SMF, Lips P, et al. Different aspects of visual impairment as risk factors for falls and fractures in older men and women. *J Bone Miner Res*. 2004;19:1539–1547.

85. Lord SR, Dayhew J, Howland A. Multifocal glasses impair edge-contrast sensitivity and depth perception and increase the risk of falls in older people. *J Am Geriatr Soc*. 2002;50:1760–1766.

86. Desapriya E, Subzwari S, Scime-Beltrano G. Vision improvement and reduction in falls after expedited cataract surgery. A systematic review and meta-analysis. *J Cataract Refract Surg*. 2010;36:13–19.

87. Lord SR, Menz HB, Sherrington C. Home environment risk factors for falls in older people and the efficacy of home modifications. *Age Ageing*. 2006; 35-S2:ii55–ii59.

88. Lyons RA, John A, Brophy S, et al. Modification of the home environment for the reduction of injuries. *Cochrane Database Syst Rev*. 2006;4:CD003600.

89. Cumming RG, Thomas M, Szonyi G, et al. Home visits by an occupational therapist for assessment and modification of environmental hazards: a randomized trial of falls prevention. *J Am Geriatr Soc*. 1999;47:1397–1402.

90. Nikolaus T, Bach M. Preventing falls in community-dwelling frail older people using a home intervention team (HIT): results from the randomized Falls-HIT trial. *J Am Geriatr Soc*. 2003;51:300–305.

91. Johnson MA, Kimlin MG, Porter KN. Vitamin D and injury prevention. *Am J Lifestyle Med*. 2010;1:21–24.

92. Bischoff-Ferrari HA, Dawson-Hughes B, Willett WC, et al. Effect of vitamin D on falls: a meta-analysis. *JAMA*. 2005;291:1999–2006.

93. Gillespie, LD, Robertson, MC, Gillespie, WH et al. Interventions for preventing falls in older people living in the community. *Cochrane Database Syst Rev*. 2009;(2):CD 007146.

94. Chung M, Balk EM, Brendel M, et al. *Vitamin D and Calcium: A Systematic Review of Health Outcomes*. Evidence Report No. 183. (Prepared by the Tufts Evidence-based Practice Center under Contract No. HHSA 290-2007-10055-I.) Rockville, MD: Agency for Healthcare Research and Quality; 2009. AHRQ Publication No. 09-E015.

95. McInnes E, Askie L. Evidence review on older people's views and experiences of falls prevention strategies. *Worldviews Evid Based Nurs*. 2004;1:20–37.

96. Tinetti ME, Baker DI, McAvay G, et al. A multifactorial intervention to reduce the risk of falling among elderly people living in the community. *N Engl J Med*. 1994;331:821–827.

97. Close, JCT. Prevention of falls–a time to translate evidence into practice. *Age Ageing*. 2005;34(2):98–100.

98. Clemson L, Cumming RG, Kendig H, et al. The effectiveness of a community-based program for reducing the incidence of falls in the elderly: a randomized trial. *J Am Geriatr Soc*. 2004;52:1487–1494.

99. Davidson J, Bond J, Dawson P, et al. Patients with recurrent falls attending Accident & Emergency benefit from multifactorial intervention—a randomized controlled trial. *Age Ageing*. 2005;43:162–168.

100. Macintyre S, Hunt K, Sweeting H. Gender differences in health: are things really as simple as they seem? *Soc Sci Med*. 1996;42:617–624.

101. Lane JM, Serota AC, Raphael B. Osteoporosis: differences and similarities in male and female patients. *Orthop Clin N Am*. 2006;37:601–609.

102. U.S. Department of Health and Human Services, National Center for Health Statistics. *The International Classification of Diseases, 9th revision, Clinical Modification: ICD-9-CM*. Atlanta, GA: Centers for Disease Control and Prevention; 2003. www.cdc.gov/nchs/icd.htm. Accessed April 14, 2010.

103. Davis MA, Neuhaus JM, Moritz DJ, et al. Health behaviors and survival among middle-aged and older men and women in the NHANES I Epidemiologic Follow-up Study. *Prev Med*. 1994;23:369–376.

104. Oman D, Reed D, Ferrara A. Do elderly women have more physical disability than men do? *Am J Epidemiol*. 1999;150:834–842.

105. Stevens JA, Sogolow ED. *Preventing Falls: What Works. A CDC Compendium of Effective Community-Based Interventions from Around the World*. Atlanta, GA: Centers for Disease Control and Prevention, National Center for Injury Prevention and Control; 2008. http://www.cdc.gov/HomeandRecreationalSafety/Falls/compendium.html. Accessed October 11, 2012.

106. Cameron ID, Murray GR, Gillespie LD, et al. Interventions for preventing falls in older people in nursing care facilities and hospitals. *Cochrane Database Syst Rev*. 2010;Issue 1. Art. No.:CD005465. DOI: 10.1002/14651858. CD005465.pub2.

107. Bureau of the Census. Population Projections—2008 National Population Projections, Summary Tables. www.census.gov/population/www/projections/summarytables.html. Accessed April 2, 2010.

Alzheimer's Disease in Women

Sarah C. Janicki, MD, MPH

Introduction

Cognitive health is an essential component of personal health that includes abilities with language, thought, memory, judgment, and the capacity to plan and carry out tasks. Changes in cognitive function occur over time among older adults due to aging and a combination of genetics, lifestyle, social and environmental factors as well as comorbid conditions. Risk factors, age at onset, and speed of deterioration vary considerably among people of the same chronological age.[1] Varying rates of diminished function among older adults may reflect differences in genetic susceptibility and timing of exposures over the life course.[2] Exposure to tobacco smoke, weight gain, hormone use, and onset of treatment for chronic conditions may influence brain function many years after initiation. Alzheimer's disease (AD), the most common type of dementia in elderly people, was first described in 1906 by the German psychiatrist Alois Alzheimer when he noted plaque between nerve cells in the brain of a patient with dementia. This chapter discusses the epidemiology of AD in women, with a focus on potential role of gender and hormones in disease. It also presents information regarding the genetics of AD, summarizes studies regarding diet and lifestyle factors in disease modification, and provides a synopsis of AD pathogenesis, clinical findings, and current treatments.

Incidence and Mortality

Alzheimer's disease currently affects 1 in 8 men and women over age 65. The prevalence of AD is expected to quadruple by the year 2047. If greater progress in prevention has not occurred by 2050, 11–16 million cases are anticipated given an estimated 10% of Americans will be age 65 or older by the middle of the 21st century.[3] The disorder is a growing public health concern with potentially devastating effect. There are no known cures or preventions for AD. Even delaying the onset by a few years would decrease its prevalence and burden on public health systems. In January 2011 a major congressional initiative, the National Alzheimer's Project Act (NAPA), was signed into law by the President (Public Law 111-375). NAPA calls for a national strategic plan to coordinate activities among federal agencies addressing the rapidly escalating incidence of Alzheimer's disease among Americans.[4] Among the planned activities provided by NAPA is the development of a population-based surveillance system with routinely timed follow-up to provide measures of the public health burden associated with cognitive decline. In addition to educating the public about risk and protective factors, the initiative calls for research including clinical trials to assess the role of physical activity in reducing cognitive decline and improving function.[4]

Pathogenesis

Diagnosis of AD requires both the presence of dementia and a characteristic pattern of brain changes, including atrophy, neuronal loss, the presence of extracellular plaques containing beta amyloid peptides, intracellular neurofibrillary tangles, and granulovacuolar cytoplasmic changes in the neocortical association areas, hippocampus, and other brain regions.

Gender Differences in Cognitive Decline and AD

The evidence for differences in cognitive decline and dementia of women compared with men is mixed. Four population-based studies of differences in dementia by gender published before 2000 reported a higher prevalence of AD in women; however, four others reported no difference. Inconsistencies may be due to earlier mortality and greater morbidity in men compared with women. Thus studies that look at the age-specific incidence of AD would best capture gender-specific differences. In the EURODEM Incidence Research Study, there was a higher incidence of AD in women compared with men (RR = 1.54, 95% CI = 1.21–1.96) in all age groups combined.[5] Likewise, a Swedish cohort demonstrated a higher incidence of AD in women than in men among all age groups, with the greatest difference seen in those over 90 years old.[6] In contrast, the MoVIES study,[7] the Rochester study,[8] the Framingham study,[9] the Baltimore Longitudinal Study of Aging,[10] the East Boston Study,[11] and the Adult Changes in Thought (ACT) cohort study[12] provided no support for a greater incidence of dementia or AD among women than men. To better understand potential gender differences in AD prevalence or incidence, a summary of the role of estrogen in neuroprotection is provided.

Estrogen in Neuroprotection and Risk for AD

Estrogens are a group of steroid compounds that function as primary female sex hormones. They are produced primarily by developing follicles in the ovaries as well as by the corpus luteum and the placenta. Some estrogens are also produced in smaller amounts by other tissues such as the liver, adrenal glands, and adipose tissue. These secondary sources of estrogen are important sources of endogenous estrogen in postmenopausal women. Estrogen interacts with different types of receptors including ER-α and ER-β. Both receptors are highly expressed in the brain, although ER-α receptors are present in higher concentrations in the hippocampus and ER-β receptors are present in higher concentrations in the basal forebrain and cerebral cortex.[13]

Several hundred published papers have established that estrogen has beneficial effects on brain tissue and physiology in cell culture and animal models, including nonhuman primates; however, the mechanisms underlying estrogen neuroprotection have not been completely elucidated. Estrogen promotes the growth and survival of cholinergic neurons,[14,15] increases cholinergic activity,[16] has antioxidant properties,[17] and promotes the nonamyloidogenic metabolism of the amyloid precursor protein.[18] Although significant neuroprotective actions of estrogen have been demonstrated in vitro and in animal studies, the evidence is less consistent in studies of aging women. Although individual study results are inconsistent, overall data from epidemiologic studies, observational studies, and clinical trials of hormone replacement therapy (HRT), studies of endogenous hormones and evaluations of genetic variants involved in estrogen biosynthesis and receptor activity indicate that estrogen plays an important role in the pathogenesis of cognitive decline and risk of AD in both men and women. Looking ahead, genetic studies may help to clarify some of the ambiguity in the existing data.

Observational Studies of Hormone Replacement Therapy

The hypothesis that hormone therapy might protect against cognitive aging arose from observational studies that demonstrated a lower risk of AD among women who had been treated with hormone therapy compared with those who had not. In many observational studies, postmenopausal women who used estrogen-only or estrogen combined with progestogen showed slower decline in cognitive function and decreased risk of AD,[19–24] but not all studies found beneficial effects. Some inconsistencies may be related to the timing of hormone use. The Cache County Study found evidence that prior use of hormones typically initiated early in the menopausal transition

protected against AD, whereas use at older ages did not protect against AD unless hormone use was initiated before age 63 on average.[24] The authors concluded that there was a limited window of time during which sustained hormone exposure appeared to lower risk of AD.[24] Several articles since have raised the possibility that there is a critical period in which hormones exert cognitive benefits, possibly early in the perimenopausal period or just after last menses.[25,26] In addition, prior hormone use has been associated with higher educational levels and better access to medical care, which could be the protective factors associated with lower risk of cognitive decline.

Clinical Trials of Hormone Replacement Therapy

Although clinical trials of hormone therapy can correct for selection bias and confounding inherent in observational studies, they have demonstrated limited benefit of hormone use in maintaining cognitive function, primarily assessed as verbal memory, or on lowering the risk for AD. Overall, these studies indicate no effect of estrogen alone and a detrimental effect of combined estrogen-progestogen treatment on verbal memory. It is helpful to group study results by population and hormone formulation in order to evaluate result trends.

Three randomized, placebo-controlled trials of unopposed estrogen therapy on episodic verbal memory in women younger than age 65 demonstrated improvement in test scores of verbal recall associated with estrogen-only supplementation.[27–29] Results were limited by sample sizes of 50 women or fewer and most or all of the women in these studies were surgically menopausal. Despite the small study samples and design limitations, the results of these studies support the hypothesis that estrogen alone either enhances or has no effect on verbal memory in younger women during short-term follow-up. Unopposed estrogen therapy among older women has demonstrated no influence on cognition.

Although unopposed estrogen therapy has demonstrated positive effects on cognitive outcomes in younger women and neutral effects in older women, the results from combination estrogen-progestogen treatment trials are less encouraging in both age groups. The Cognitive Complaints in Early Menopause Trial was the largest study of any form of hormone therapy on verbal memory in women younger than age 65,[30] which indicated conjugated equine estrogen/medroxyprogesterone acetate (CEE/MPA) was associated with a nonsignificant decline in both short- and long-delayed free recall compared with placebo ($P < 0.07$). A second study in younger women found that combined therapy of estrogen plus progestogen (dienogest) enhanced verbal memory compared with either placebo or estradiol.[31] The two studies suggest that specific forms of progestogens have different effects on cognitive function in younger women, with negative effects of MPA and positive effects of dienogest, a progestogen with antiandrogenic effects, on verbal memory.

A number of trials have evaluated combined estrogen/progestogen treatment in women over 65 years of age. Out of four randomized trials evaluating combined therapy on cognition in postmenopausal women, three showed either a negative effect of hormone therapy,[32,33] or a trend toward a negative effect ($P < 0.06$).[34] These findings suggest a consistent, detrimental effect of combined hormone therapy on verbal memory. The Women's Health Initiative Memory Study (WHIMS),[35] the largest trial to date, examined incidence of dementia in women age 65 or older associated with CEE in women with prior hysterectomy and the impact of CEE/MPA in naturally postmenopausal women. In the combined therapy arm, CEE/MPA doubled the risk for all-cause dementia (HR = 2.01; 95th % CI = 1.21–3.48).[36] In the estrogen-alone arm there was no evidence that CEE changed the risk of all-cause dementia (HR = 1.49; 95% CI = 0.83–2.66).[37] However, the negative effects of the WHIMS trials may be related to the timing of treatment, the specific formulation of HRT provided, and the dosage and schedule used. Interestingly, analysis of prior hormone use in the perimenopausal period in the WHIMS population was associated with a lower incidence of dementia regardless of the treatment arm. When AD was analyzed apart from other causes of dementia, prior hormone therapy was associated with a 64% reduction in incidence.[37] In sum, results of clinical trials vary depending on the type of therapy used and the age of initiation. The true effects of combined therapy on brain function are complicated by the varying effects of different types of progestogens. MPA, but not others, may antagonize the effects of estrogen on the hippocampus[38] providing motivation for exploring the impact of different estrogen/progestogen combinations and dosages on verbal memory.

Modes of hormone delivery also need to be evaluated. Transdermal applications enable hormone absorption directly into the bloodstream bypassing first-pass metabolism in the liver, which may have differing effects on cognitive outcome. In addition, the critical window hypothesis highlights the need to define the time period of effective intervention in order to optimize any beneficial effect of hormone therapy on cognition. Finally, studies need to determine optimum duration of hormone use for maximum benefit. The answer may be provided in part by the results of PREPARE (PREventing Post-menopausal Alzheimer's disease with Replacement Estrogens), a randomized trial of women age 65 or older with a family history of dementia in a first-degree relative. The study was designed to determine whether hormone use delays AD or memory loss in women at increased risk for cognitive change.[39] Although active study treatment was discontinued in response to the WHI Memory Study report, the study will continue to follow participants for a total of 5 years blinded to the original medication assignment. Future results will address whether there are lasting or delayed effects of estrogen or combined therapy on cognition after treatment is discontinued.

Two large clinical trials may provide important information on the effect of HRT on cognitive function in younger and older postmenopausal women. The Kronos Early Estrogen Prevention Study (KEEPS) is a 5-year, multicenter clinical trial that will enroll women who are within 36 months of their final menstrual period. Participants will be randomized to receive oral CEE plus progesterone, transdermal estradiol plus micronized progesterone, or placebo. The trial was designed to address the dual concerns associated with the WHI: the older mean age of participants may have affected response to HRT and the mode of HRT administration may have affected health outcome.[40] Although incidence and progression of atherosclerosis is the primary study outcome, cognitive changes will be assessed in a secondary analysis. Before enrollment women will complete the structured mental status test, Mini Mental State Exam (MMSE) and will be included only if their MMSE score is 23 or greater. The Early versus Late Intervention Trial with Estradiol (ELITE) at UCLA is a single study with 504 postmenopausal women enrolled who are less than 6 years postmenopausal (early) versus 10 years or more from menopause (late) randomized to either oral estradiol or placebo.[41] Both KEEPS and ELITE will examine verbal memory as a primary outcome and focus on naturally menopausal women.

Endogenous Estrogen and Cognition

The ability of current hormone therapy trials to address whether estrogen protects against AD is limited by different patterns of use and different formulations. Studies of endogenous estrogen could potentially address the role of estrogen in the pathogenesis of AD more directly; however, results of these studies have also been inconsistent. In the Study of Osteoporotic Fractures, women with the highest estrone levels had significantly poorer performance in some cognitive test scores over 5 years.[42] In contrast, a large cross-sectional study from the Netherlands found that women in the highest quintile of either estradiol or estrone were 40% less likely to be cognitively impaired than women in the lowest quintile.[43] Among postmenopausal women with Down Syndrome (DS), women with early onset of menopause at ages younger than 46 years had earlier onset and increased risk of dementia compared with women with onset of menopause after 46 years.[44] This suggests that lower lifetime endogenous estrogen exposure increases the risk of dementia in this population.

Additional data regarding endogenous estrogen exposure and cognition come from review of studies of women undergoing oophorectomy. Current evidence on the association between oophorectomy and cognitive performance was provided by observational studies and from small-scale clinical trials. In the Mayo Clinic Cohort Study of Oophorectomy and Aging, women who underwent bilateral oophorectomy before the onset of menopause had an increased risk of cognitive impairment or dementia compared with controls (HR 1.33; 95% CI = 0.98–1.81).[45] The risk increased with younger age at oophorectomy, and women under age 43 years had the greatest risk (HR 1.74; 95% CI = 0.97–3.14). Interestingly, the risk was restricted to women who underwent oophorectomy before age 49 years and were not treated with estrogen until at least age 50 years (HR 1.89; 95% CI = 1.27–2.83).[45] Another study performed an evaluation of neuropsychological tasks in 27 surgically menopausal women following hysterectomy with bilateral oophorectomy and 76 naturally menopausal women at a mean age of 52 years. Women who underwent oophorectomy scored significantly worse on recall from a word-list memory task. In addition, scores tended to be lower when oophorectomy occurred at younger ages.[46] In a longitudinal study from Egypt, 35 premenopausal women with a mean age of 41 years underwent neuropsychological testing before and after oophorectomy with hysterectomy, and results were compared with those of 18 premenopausal women matched for age, education, parity, weight, and height. Surgically menopausal women had significant decreases in global cognitive functioning scores and Wechsler Memory Scale subtests 6 months after oophorectomy, compared with the premenopausal women who experienced no decline.[47]

However, not all observational studies of women undergoing oophorectomy have found cognitive decline. In the Rancho Bernardo Study, which evaluated older postmenopausal women at a mean age of 74 years in a southern California community, women with prior bilateral oophorectomy with hysterectomy performed significantly poorer on certain memory tests (serial sevens and Trails B), but the difference was reported to be of limited clinical significance.[48] There were no differences in mean cognitive function scores between women in this cohort who underwent bilateral oophorectomy (n = 190) versus hysterectomy with ovarian preservation (n = 225), and no differences compared with women who were naturally menopausal (n = 470). Likewise, in a British cohort of 1,261 women with a mean age of 53 years, there were no significant differences in mean cognitive test scores between women who had undergone hysterectomy, bilateral oophorectomy, or natural menopause.[49]

Clinical trials evaluating the effects of oophorectomy and estrogen therapy on cognitive function have also reported contrasting results. Sherwin reported a greater decline in cognitive function tests in 40 premenopausal women who underwent hysterectomy with bilateral oophorectomy and were randomized to placebo compared with women randomized to estrogen or testosterone therapy for 3 months following surgery.[29] In a subsequent randomized controlled trial evaluating 19 premenopausal women before and after surgical menopause with a larger battery of neuropsychological tests, women were randomized to estradiol versus placebo. The women given estradiol following hysterectomy with oophorectomy performed significantly better on tests of verbal memory than women given placebo.[28] Four other randomized controlled trials reported no cognitive benefit of estrogen after surgical menopause, but the trials were not well controlled in that estrogen was not given immediately after surgery, and baseline testing before surgical menopause was not performed.[50–54]

In evaluating the impact of endogenous estrogen, it is important to assess bioavailable hormone levels, which may differ from total estrogen levels. An estimated 37% of estradiol in older women circulates bound to sex hormone binding globulin (SHBG) and only the non-SHBG bound fraction (e.g., bioavailable estradiol) is thought to cross the blood–brain barrier. Several observational studies have found an association between elevated SHBG and cognitive decline or AD.[23,44,55] In the Study of Osteoporotic Fractures, women with high concentrations of free and bioavailable estradiol (E2) were less like to develop cognitive impairment after 6 years than were women with low concentrations.[23] Among postmenopausal women with Down Syndrome, those with lower levels of bioavailable E2 at baseline were four times as likely to develop AD (HR = 4.1, 95% CI = 1.2–13.9).[56] These studies suggest that low bioavailable estrogen levels associated with high SHBG after menopause may accelerate the development of AD. Again, however, the literature is conflicting, as both the Rancho Bernardo Study[19] and the Rotterdam Study[57] either failed to identify consistent associations of total or bioavailable estradiol on cognitive test outcomes[19] or demonstrated that women with higher calculated bioavailable estradiol levels had significantly poorer results in delayed recall.[57] These inconsistencies may be related to variable hormone measurement procedures or may be due to the difficulty of measuring circulating estradiol in older women who have been postmenopausal for many years.

Genetics of the Estrogen Pathway

Genes involved in estrogen biosynthesis and estrogen receptor activity are also potential contributors to risk of AD. Variants of these genes could influence age at onset or risk of AD by affecting the neuroprotective activity of estrogen or by altering estrogen levels over long periods of time. In addition, examination of polymorphisms in estrogen genes may serve as a marker of hormone status in cohorts of elder women where measurement of hormone levels may not be informative. Five candidate genes *ESR1*, *ESR2*, *CYP17*, *CYP19*, and *HSD17B1* are likely to be contributors. Although variants in these genes have been associated with differences in estrogen levels and with increased risk for estrogen-related disorders such as osteoporosis, breast cancer, or endometrial cancer and some risk for AD, their contribution to risk of AD has not yet been systematically examined, with all genes assessed in the same population.

Two estrogen receptors, ER-α and ER-β, have been identified in the brain and have been found in regions affected by AD, including the hippocampus, basal forebrain and

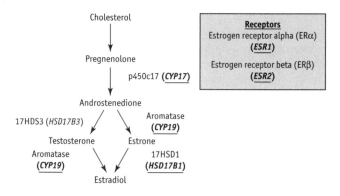

Figure 39-1 Estradiol biosynthetic pathway and receptors, with associated genes (in parentheses)

amygdala. Two closely linked restriction fragment length polymorphisms (RFLPs), *Pvu*II and *Xba*I, located in the first intron of *ESR1*, the gene for ER-α, have been reported to influence estrogen receptor expression and, in turn, may influence risk for AD. In several case-control studies, the XX or PP genotypes and the XXPP haplotype of the *ESR1* gene have been associated with increased risk for AD in Asian and European populations and in women with DS.[58–62] However, not all studies have found positive associations and risk alleles have been inconsistent across studies. In addition, the association between the XX and PP genotypes or the XXPP haplotype and risk for AD may vary by the presence of the *APOE* ε4 allele and by gender in some, but not all, studies. These findings, although not conclusive, suggest that *ESR1* genotype may influence risk for AD by affecting estrogen receptor expression. In addition, variants in *ESR2*, the gene for ER-β, have been associated with increased risk for AD in women.[63] The Health ABC study reported that two single nucleotide polymorphisms on *ESR2* were associated with development of cognitive impairment among both nondemented community dwelling men and women.[64]

Two key genes, *CYP17* and *CYP19*, are involved in the peripheral synthesis of estrogens. Polymorphisms in *CYP17* and *CYP19* have been repeatedly associated with variation in hormone levels, age at onset of menopause, and increased risk of estrogen-related diseases such as bone mass, fracture risk, breast cancer, and osteoporosis. Several studies have found associations between single nucleotide polymorphisms (SNPs) and haplotype blocks in *CYP19* and risk for AD in both men and women,[65,66] whereas others have found associations with AD primarily among women.[67,68] The *HSD17B1* gene encodes the enzyme 17β-hydroxysteroid dehydrogenase 1, which catalyzes the conversion of estrone to estradiol. The Ser312/Gly coding common variant of *HSD17B1*, SNP rs#605059 in Exon 6, is of particular interest as it has been associated with risk for breast cancer and endometriosis. Other common variants of *HSD17B1* are also candidate genetic susceptibility factors for AD, but no study to date has examined their relation to age at onset or risk of AD. Existing studies have examined only a few SNPs and several genes of interest have not been examined. Further study of polymorphisms in these genes and in other genes that are involved in estrogen pathways may clarify biological mechanisms relating variation in estrogen to risk of AD.

Other Genetic Influences in AD

AD is a genetically heterogeneous disorder. Four genes have been identified that are clinically available for genetic testing, and additional chromosomal regions and genes are being investigated. Three of the four genes are causative genes in which mutations result in autosomal dominant, early-onset AD (EOAD), typically defined as onset before 60 years of age. Mutations in these three genes, *PSEN1*, *PSEN2*, and *APP*, account for fewer than 5% of all cases of AD.[69] As a result, it is anticipated that there are additional genes involved in EOAD that have yet to be identified. The fourth gene, *APOE*, is a known susceptibility gene for AD

and is distinct among the causative genes because it alone is neither sufficient nor necessary to cause AD. *APOE* has three isoforms: ε2, ε3, and ε4. The ε4 variant of *APOE* is associated with an increased risk for AD. Risk figures associated with *APOE* ε4 vary between studies, suggesting a two- to threefold increased risk for ε4 heterozygotes and a two- to tenfold risk for ε4 homozygotes. Due to the disparity in these risk estimates, they are not clinically useful for individual risk assessment. Family history of AD may be just as useful as *APOE* genotype for risk assessment. First-degree relatives of an affected individual in sporadic or familial cases are estimated to have a two- to fourfold risk for AD compared to the general population.[69] Genetic testing for diagnostic and predictive purposes is available for EOAD; however, genetic counseling prior to and after testing is strongly recommended. For individuals who present with late-onset dementia, *APOE* genotyping may be part of the diagnostic workup but *APOE* genotyping without clinical evaluation is not warranted because it lacks sufficient sensitivity and specificity to make a diagnosis of AD by itself. Although predictive testing for both causative and susceptibility genes for AD is currently limited, family members of patients with AD may benefit from genetic counseling, which includes information about the genetic influences of AD, a risk assessment via pedigree analysis, and current information about ongoing genetic research studies.

Prevention

No specific environmental risk factor has been definitively identified as being associated with AD. Epidemiologic research has focused on genetic risks, comorbidity, and personal health behaviors that may be reduce the risk or delay onset of dementia and subsequent Alzheimer's. Healthy lifestyle including adequate exercise, weight control, moderate alcohol, and avoidance of tobacco should preserve blood circulation to the brain and lower onset of diminishing brain function. Maintaining social interaction with family and friends is also considered an essential health maintenance strategy.

Diet

There is evidence that oxidative stress, vitamins, fats, and alcohol have a role in the pathogenesis of AD. Few large epidemiological studies have explored the associations between nutrients and AD, and there has been only one trial of vitamin E in the prevention of AD. Some studies suggest that high intake of vitamins C, E, B6, B12, and folate; unsaturated fatty acids; and fish is related to a low risk of AD, but reports are inconsistent. Modest to moderate alcohol intake, particularly wine, may be related to a low risk of AD. Available data do not permit definitive conclusions regarding diet and AD or specific recommendations on diet modification for the prevention of AD. One of the main limitations of studies of diet in AD is potential error in the measurement of nutrients.[70] In addition, development of AD may be the consequence of lifelong exposures. The latency period of AD is unknown but may be as long as several decades although most studies of the association between diet and AD have been done in people over age 65. Individuals in this age group may be in an advanced stage in the latency period of AD. As a result, the capacity to change the course of disease with dietary interventions may be limited. Randomized clinical trials represent the ideal way to study diet and disease but the potentially long duration of preclinical AD limits the possibility of studying primary prevention through diet.

Antioxidants

Reactive oxygen species are associated with neuronal damage in AD.[71] The possibility that the production of reactive oxygen species is a cause in AD pathology has led to research exploring how antioxidants in foods and supplements can affect AD. These antioxidants include tocopherol (vitamin E), ascorbic acid (vitamin C), and carotenes. In vitro, vitamin E decreases Aβ-induced lipid peroxidation and oxidative stress[72] and suppresses inflammation-signaling cascades. Vitamin C blocks the creation of nitrosamines through the reduction of nitrites but may also affect catecholamine synthesis, whereas carotenes affect lipid peroxidation.[72,73] Evidence supports an association between intake of dietary antioxidants and low risk of stroke[74,75] and secondarily lower risk of AD.[76,77] Cerebrovascular disease may be another pathway linking antioxidant vitamins and AD.

Several studies have explored the relationship between plasma concentrations of antioxidants and cognition. Some of these studies have found low concentrations of antioxidants in the blood of people with cognitive impairment and AD.[78,79] Other studies have found conflicting results relating peripheral concentrations of antioxidants to cognitive function.[80] The interpretation of studies relating blood concentrations of antioxidants and cognition is complicated because antioxidants could be depleted owing to the oxidation that accompanies aging and AD progression.

Data from prospective studies relating intake of antioxidant vitamins and AD are conflicting.[81–87] Some studies report a low risk of AD in relation to vitamin E supplements,[83] whereas others report no decreased risk associated with supplements but a decreased risk associated with high dietary intake.[84,86] Only one trial assessed prevention of disease progression among patients with moderate AD by antioxidant vitamin supplementation. A total of 341 patients received the selective monoamine oxidase inhibitor selegiline (10 mg a day), alpha-tocopherol (vitamin E, 2000 IU a day), both selegiline and alpha-tocopherol, or placebo for 2 years. The study found that intake of vitamin E supplements was related to a longer time to institutionalization but was not related to cognitive outcomes.[88] A recent trial of vitamin E supplementation in persons with amnestic mild cognitive impairment (MCI), a transitional stage between normal cognition and AD, failed to show prevention of progression to AD.[89] The safety of antioxidant supplements has recently been questioned given results of a recent meta-analysis of vitamin

E supplementation for prevention of heart disease. That study found increased mortality among individuals randomized to the supplements.[90] Thus, the most conservative approach given current evidence is not to recommend antioxidant supplements for the prevention of AD. The data relating vitamins B12, B6, and folate to cognitive decline and AD are also inconsistent.[91–96] There are data from small nonrandomized trials in people with low concentrations of vitamin B12 that suggest that supplementation improves cognitive performance.[94] Participants with low concentrations of vitamin B12 and folate should be treated for reasons including the prevention of pernicious anemia, peripheral neuropathy, and other neuropsychiatric outcomes, but data from randomized trials are not available to support the use of these vitamins for the prevention of cognitive decline. There are no data with longer follow-up that include cognition, and there are no data on primary prevention.

Dietary Fats

Intake of unsaturated fats, low intake of hydrogenated and saturated fats, and high intake of n-3 polyunsaturated fatty acids (PUFA) from fish or vegetable sources can lower the risk of cardiovascular disease[97] and potentially lower the risk of AD through vascular mechanisms. Dietary fats may also influence AD through other mechanisms. Higher intake of hydrogenated and saturated fats is related to insulin resistance,[98] and high insulin concentrations may be related to a high risk of AD.[99] High intake of fats may also cause oxidation,[100] which can result in cardiovascular disease and in AD. Other observations provide compelling support for a role of fat intake in the pathogenesis of AD. High intake of dietary cholesterol increases the deposition of Aβ in animal brains,[101] and hypercholesterolemic rabbits have increased neuronal Aβ accumulation.[102]

Several prospective studies have found associations between intake of dietary fats and the risk of AD[103–109] but the mechanisms for these associations are unknown. Among 980 elderly people studied for 4 years, the risk of AD was highest in those in the highest quartiles of total fat and calorie intake who had the *APOE* ε4 allele.[103] Another study found that high intakes of saturated and polyunsaturated fatty acids were associated with a high risk of AD regardless of the *APOE* genotype and a high risk of cognitive decline.[108] This study also found that intake of fish and fish-related fats was related to a low risk of AD.[105] However, fat intake of any type was not related to dementia or AD in a study of more than 5,000 people age 55 years or older.[106]

In summary, there are few and inconsistent studies relating intake of different types of fats and the risk of AD. There are no trial data and recommendations cannot be made on the basis of these studies. However, a diet low in saturated and trans fatty acids and high in monounsaturated, polyunsaturated, and fish-related fats is associated with a low risk of vascular disease[97,110] and it may be reasonable to extend their benefits to the prevention of cognitive decline and AD.

Alcohol

Alcohol is a neurotoxin, and rat models show that different exposures to alcohol can result in oxidative brain damage.[110] Moderate alcohol consumption in human beings is related to greater brain atrophy, but also fewer silent brain infarcts, less white-matter disease, and a lower risk of clinical stroke.[111] Alcohol consumption increases concentrations of high-density lipoprotein, decreases platelet adhesiveness, and improves endothelial function,[112–114] which may help to explain the association between moderate alcohol intake and better cardiovascular outcomes. Wine in particular may contain antioxidants, such as flavonoids, not present in beer and spirits, which may have additional benefits to those of alcohol.[115] Thus, alcohol may have paradoxical and competing effects in the brain: on the one hand lowering the risk of cerebrovascular disease, but on the other hand acting as a neurotoxin.

There are several prospective studies that have explored the relation between alcoholic drinks and AD.[116–120] One nested case-control study in people age 65 years and older showed that consumption of one to six drinks of alcohol weekly, regardless of type, was related to a lower risk of AD than that in nondrinkers.[117] Another study showed that people who consumed up to three servings of alcohol a day had a low risk of AD compared with those who never drank alcohol; again there were no associations by beverage type.[116] A nested case-control study of individuals age 65 years and older found that monthly or weekly intake of wine, but not other alcoholic drinks, was associated with a low risk of dementia including AD.[118] Similarly, a cohort study of individuals age 65 and older indicated that intake of up to three servings of wine per day, but not other alcoholic beverages, was associated with a low risk of AD.[119] Most of these studies produced data suggesting that heavy alcohol intake (four or more servings daily) was related to a high risk of dementia, but the results were not statistically significant given the small number of elderly people who reported heavy alcohol intake. Alcohol, wine in particular, is related to better cardiovascular[121] and cognitive outcomes in observational studies. However, there are no available randomized trials of the effects of alcoholic drinks on these outcomes and no recommendations can be made.[121] In summary, those who drink should maintain moderation (less than three servings of wine a day) on the basis of the evidence reviewed. It also seems reasonable not to recommend alcohol intake to those who do not drink in light of the potential for abuse and addiction, and other potential adverse events, such as falls in elderly people.[122]

Diagnosis

Clinical Findings

AD is characterized by a gradual progressive decline in cognition associated with impairment in memory, judgment and problem solving, orientation, language skills, and visual spatial function. Potential psychiatric comorbidities may include changes in personality and mood including apathy and depression, agitation, aggression, paranoia and other delusions, and hallucinations and illusions.

Standardized rating instruments are available for the staging of AD, including the Clinical Dementia Rating Scale (CDR) and the Global Deterioration Scale (GDS). The CDR divides AD into broad categories of mild, moderate, and severe dementia based on review of the patient's capabilities in six categories, including memory, orientation, judgment and problem solving, community affairs, home and hobbies, and personal care.[123] Staging is useful in order to follow disease progression and may have value for family counseling and patient management.

Mild AD is categorized by impairment of work or social activities with ability to maintain independent living including appropriate judgment and hygiene. Patients may demonstrate forgetfulness, word-finding difficulties, and difficulty with more complex tasks such as following directions, managing finances, taking medications, planning meals, shopping, driving, maintaining hobbies, and problem solving. Behavioral changes in mild AD include apathy, withdrawal, and depression.

Moderate AD is distinguished by the need for supervision with impaired recent memory, orientation and insight. Patients require help with activities of daily living (ADLs) such as the sequencing and selection of clothing and dressing. Behavioral manifestations in this stage include wandering, agitation, and delusions. Sleep disturbance may become apparent.

Severe AD is characterized by significant impairment of ADLs resulting in the need for constant supervision and personal care. Patients have very limited language capabilities and are unable to manage their basic needs including eating, dressing, bathing, and toileting. Frequent incontinence results and weight loss is common. Patients may also require assistance with walking as the disease progresses. In the final stages of AD, patients may become bedridden with flexion deformities, mutism, and inability to swallow.

Diagnostic Criteria

In 1984, the National Institute of Communicative Disorders and Stroke and the Alzheimer's Disease and Related Disorders Association (NINCDS-ADRDA) proposed criteria to enable clinicians to have a range of certainty in diagnosing AD: probable, possible, and definite.[124] Through use of these criteria, it is estimated that the clinician can achieve 85% accuracy in the diagnosis of AD.[125]

Probable AD—Patients are 40 to 90 years old and have cognitive decline that can be documented by neuropsychological tests. Memory and at least one of the following higher brain functions must be defective: judgment, language, perception, or cognition. Patients also demonstrate decreased independence in ADLs. Systemic diseases or other brain disorders that might cause dementia or altered consciousness such as thyroid disease, pernicious anemia, tertiary syphilis or other chronic infections of the central nervous system, normal pressure hydrocephalus,

Creutzfeldt-Jakob disease (CJD), subdural hematoma, and brain tumors must be absent, and laboratory studies must be generally normal. Conditions that can cause cognitive impairment and mimic AD, such as Parkinson's disease, depression, vascular dementia, or drug intoxications also must be excluded.

Possible AD—This category is used when a second condition that might contribute to dementia is present but is not considered to be a causal factor. A diagnosis of possible AD may also be used if the presentation or clinical course is atypical.

Definite AD—This classification is reserved for patients who meet the clinical criteria and have autopsy or brain biopsy confirmation of diagnosis (including neurofibrillary tangles and senile plaques). As a result, this category of diagnosis is rare in living patients.

Imaging and Diagnostic Studies

In 2001, the Quality Standards Subcommittee of the American Academy of Neurology (AAN) revised the guidelines for the evaluation of dementia.[126] The evaluation usually consists of neurologic, neuropsychological, and psychiatric assessment and neuroimaging and blood evaluations. Although not all of these tests may be necessary in patients with clear histories and advanced symptoms, individuals with subtle complaints may require the full set of tests to discriminate the earliest symptoms of mild cognitive impairment from early AD.

Mental status assessment—One structured mental status test is the Mini Mental State Exam (MMSE), an 11-item test used to measure memory, language, attention, calculations, fund of knowledge, and orientation.[127] Scores may range from 0 to 30, with lower scores indicating increased impairment (mild dementia 20–26; moderate dementia 10–19; and severe dementia 0–9). This test may be administered serially to monitor disease progression.

Routine laboratory blood tests are performed to eliminate metabolic derangements of other conditions associated with cognitive impairment. The standard workup consists of blood count, electrolytes, blood urea nitrogen/creatinine, liver function tests, thyroid function tests, and serum vitamin B12 level. Optional tests include screening for syphilis, serum folate, erythrocyte sedimentation rate, and HIV, to rule out these conditions, which may also present with memory complaints.

Lumbar puncture is useful in patients with cancer, reactive serum syphilis serology, rapidly progressive dementia, immunosuppression, patients with connective tissue disease in whom central nervous system (CNS) vasculitis is suspected, or patients under age 55. In addition to ruling out other conditions that may cause cognitive complaints, cerebrospinal fluid (CSF) examination may be used to identify biochemical markers which are abnormal in AD. CSF phosphorylated tau levels are elevated and β-amyloid levels are reduced in patients with AD. Lumbar puncture can be a useful screening tool to ascertain the level of these biomarkers for diagnosis of AD in clinically questionable cases. Future utility may include prediction of AD in patients with mild cognitive impairment, but the sensitivity and specificity of CSF evaluation are currently being evaluated for this indication.

Structural neuroimaging studies are not diagnostic of AD but is recommended to rule out conditions such as brain tumors, hydrocephalus, or active CNS infection or inflammation which may contribute to the patient's cognitive complaints. Brain imaging with computed tomography (CT) demonstrates that individuals with AD have greater general brain atrophy; however, this finding is not specific to patients with AD, limiting its diagnostic utility.[128] Magnetic resonance imaging (MRI) has greater resolution than CT and generates coronal and sagittal views to better visualize the hippocampus. In addition, the atrophy rates of the medial temporal lobe and hippo-

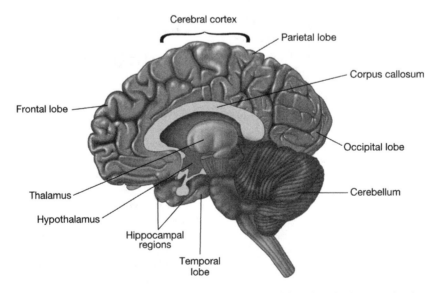

Figure 39-2 Midline image of the brain with hippocampus and frontal, parietal, temporal and occipital lobes

Source: © Jones & Bartlett Learning

campus as assessed by MRI are correlated with cognitive decline in individuals with AD.[129]

Molecular brain imaging, including positron emission testing (PET) and single-photon emission tomography (SPECT) has developed in parallel to structural imaging. PET enables imaging of biological activity and can be used to identify abnormal biological activity in AD. Regional differences in brain glucose metabolism using PET have been examined, and 18F 2-fluoro-2-deoxy-D-glucose (FDG-PET) has become the most widely investigated radioligand.[130] Glucose hypometabolism identified in FDG-PET is thought to represent local decreases in synaptic activity in neurons affected by Alzheimer pathologic changes as well as decreased synaptic activity in regions receiving projections from these disease neurons.[130] As a result, abnormalities in regional cerebral metabolism found in FDG-PET are thought to reflect the pattern of neuropathologic development of AD with early metabolic changes seen in the medial temporal cortex. These studies demonstrate that FDG-PET is a useful supplement to current neuroimaging techniques for AD diagnosis.

The presence of Aβ plaques in the brain of AD patients is currently being studied as a possible biomarker for AD. PET tracers have been developed for in vivo imaging of Alzheimer's disease pathology. Six amyloid PET ligands, including 18F-FDDNP, 11C-PIB, 11C-SB13, 11C-BF-227, 18F-BAY94-9172, and AZD2184, have been tested in PET studies in individuals with AD. The most comprehensively studied compounds have been 18F-FDDNP, developed in 2002 as the first amyloid ligand studied in patients, and 11C-Pittsburgh compound B (PiB). 11C-PiB was designed to measure the amount of amyloid plaque deposits. Individuals with AD show higher PiB retention in the frontal, temporal, parietal, and occipital cortices compared with healthy controls.[130]

Neuropsychological testing is considered optional. Tests that assess orientation, memory (including recall and recognition), language skills, constructional ability, attention, visual perception, and problem-solving skills are performed and can yield information about the pattern of impairment. Neuropsychological testing may be valuable in diagnosing early dementia and can be used to assess progression of disease. It may also be useful in distinguishing depression from dementia.

Mild Cognitive Impairment

Mild cognitive impairment (MCI) is a syndrome, not a disease, and is considered to be a transitional state between normal cognition and Alzheimer's disease. Although a diagnosis of MCI may be given for deficiencies in many cognitive domains, many clinicians and researchers focus on the amnestic subtype, which has been shown in longitudinal studies to exhibit a high conversion rate to AD (approximately 10–15% of individuals with this diagnosis per year will progress to a diagnosis of AD, compared to 1–2% of the general population).[131]

The criteria for diagnosis of MCI include memory complaints in the setting of normal capabilities in activities of daily living, coupled with abnormal memory for age

and education when compared with normally functioning individuals.[132] The current gold standard for diagnosis is behavioral neurological examination coupled with neuropsychological testing. Neurologic evaluation should eliminate comorbid psychiatric conditions such as depression or anxiety or potential medication side effect (particularly due to anticholinergic action) as potential contributing causes to the cognitive complaint. Neuropsychological testing for individuals with MCI demonstrates deficits in verbal memory and possibly category naming. Some studies have shown that deficits in delayed recall on neuropsychological testing were predictive of conversion to AD in nondemented subjects.[133]

Individuals with MCI typically demonstrate no clinically significant findings on structural brain imaging, including computed tomography (CT) or magnetic resonance imaging (MRI).[134] The utility of functional brain imaging, including 18F 2-fluoro-2-deoxy-D-glucose positron emission tomography (FDG-PET) as a prognostic indicator in individuals with MCI is still unclear. Although there are few existing longitudinal FDG-PET studies in MCI and progression to AD, there is some evidence that FDG-PET may predict subsequent decline and conversion to AD.[135] However, these studies have relatively small sample sizes and have not established strong evidence for longitudinal associations between cognitive measures and FDG-PET findings. Detection of amyloid deposition with 11C- Pittsburgh compound B (PIB) PET in individuals with MCI may provide useful prognostic information. PIB-positive individuals with MCI are significantly more likely to convert to AD than PIB-negative individuals.[135] There are no treatments approved by the Food and Drug Administration (FDA) for MCI. Studies of cyclooxygenase-2 inhibitors or cholinesterase inhibitors as prevention of conversion from MCI to AD failed to demonstrated efficacy.[136,137] Regular exercise, adherence to a low cholesterol high fiber diet, and routine cognitive stimulation may have long-term beneficial effects.[138,139]

Treatment in AD

Early degenerative changes in the basal forebrain that lower the concentration of acetylcholine have been related to the memory symptoms of Alzheimer's disease. The decrease in acetylcholine is the target of symptomatic treatment with cholinesterase inhibitors.[144] Cholinesterase inhibitors are used to enhance cholinergic function by blocking the breakdown of acetylcholine. Four cholinesterase inhibitors have been approved by the FDA for the treatment of mild-to-moderate AD; three of these agents (donepezil, rivastigmine, and galantamine) are commonly used to treat AD. In a double-blind placebo-controlled trial, donepezil demonstrated a significant benefit over placebo in terms of rate of change in cognitive measures and clinical global scales.[140] The most frequent side effects are nausea, diarrhea, abdominal discomfort, headache, insomnia, fatigue, and nightmares. The medication can be administered in the morning or at bedtime. If gastrointestinal side effects occur, they may be minimized by taking medication during or immediately after a meal or in the evening before bed. Sleep disturbance side effects may be lessened by morning administration. All three of the commonly used agents are available in pill form; in addition, rivastigmine is available in a transdermal patch formulation, which has been demonstrated to cause fewer gastrointestinal side effects. Galantamine is also available as an extended-release oral formulation designed to reduce gastrointestinal side effects.

The N-methyl-D-aspartate (NMDA) receptor is a glutamate receptor that may be relevant in the production of pathologic changes in AD. Glutamate receptor blockade may protect against excitatory amino acid-mediated toxicity, which has been found to lead to cell death. Memantine is a noncompetitive, low-to-moderate affinity NMDA-receptor antagonist that may selectively block the excitotoxic effects associated with abnormal transmission of glutamate while allowing for the physiologic transmission associated with normal cell functioning. Memantine has been approved by the FDA for the treatment of moderate-to-severe AD. In double-blind, placebo-controlled trials in patients with moderate-to-severe AD, treatment slowed the rate of cognitive and functional decline.[140] A similarly designed trial demonstrated benefit of memantine/donepezil combination therapy compared with donepezil alone in patients with moderate AD.[140] The most frequent side effects of memantine include dizziness, headache, constipation, and confusion.

Prognosis

Although the disease duration in AD may range from 3 to 20 years, the usual duration is 7 to 10 years with slow progression.[141] Longitudinal studies suggest that patients remain in the early stage for 1–2 years, the middle stage for 2–12 years, and the late stage for 1–2 years depending on the type of care that they receive.[142] Studies suggest that rigidity and psychosis, including the presence of hallucinations and delusions, predict more rapid cognitive and functional decline.[143] Patients with AD are susceptible to unintentional injuries and infections, and death is most likely to occur from pneumonia, malnutrition, dehydration, and sepsis resulting from pressure ulcers or urinary tract infections.

Summary

Alzheimer's disease is a growing public health concern with potentially devastating effect. There are no known cures or preventions for AD, however even delaying the onset by a few years would decrease its prevalence and burden on public health systems. Evidence for sex differences in cognitive decline and dementia is mixed. The variable effects of endogenous hormones and hormone supplementation on risk for AD demonstrated in observational studies and clinical trials may be related to the timing of hormone exposure or treatment, the specific formulation of HRT provided, and schedule used. Looking ahead, genetic studies may help to clarify some of the ambiguity in the existing data. Data regarding diet in prevention of AD is also

conflicting. In summary, there are few and inconsistent studies relating intake of different types of fats, antioxidants, and alcohol and the risk of AD. However, a diet low in saturated and trans fatty acids and high in monounsaturated, polyunsaturated, and fish-related fats is associated with a low risk of vascular disease, and it may be reasonable to extend their benefits to the prevention of cognitive decline and AD. Finally, accurate diagnosis of AD has been guided by the establishment of comprehensive clinical criteria and neuroimaging techniques, which continue to develop. As new treatments for AD hopefully develop in the near future, early and accurate diagnosis will be critical to providing early intervention to those at highest risk.

Discussion Questions

1. Describe the incidence and mortality patterns of Alzheimer's disease in the United States.
2. Compare and contrast the association between risk of Alzheimer's disease and use of estrogen versus estrogen-protestogen supplementation. How do the findings vary by age of supplementation?
3. Summarize data regarding use of antioxidant supplements, dietary fats, and alcohol in prevention of Alzheimer's disease.
4. Discuss different imaging modalities that can be used for patients with Alzheimer's disease and the reasons for their use.
5. Summarize current treatments available for patients with Alzheimer's disease.

References

1. Satariano W. *Epidemiology of Aging: An Ecological Approach.* Sudbury, MA: Jones and Bartlett Publishers, 2006.
2. Lang JE, Anderson L, LoGerfo J, et al. The Prevention Research Centers Healthy Aging Research Network. *Prev Chronic Dis.* 2006;3:A17.
3. Steenland K, MacNeil J, Vega I, Levey A. Recent trends in Alzheimer disease mortality in the United States, 1999 to 2004. *Alzheimer Dis Asso Disord.* 2009;23:165–170.
4. Prevention CDC. The CDC Healthy Brain Initiative: Progress 2006–2011. http://www.cdc.gov/aging. Accessed January 27, 2012.
5. Andersen K, Launer LJ, Dewey ME, et al. Gender differences in the incidence of AD and vascular dementia: The EURODEM Studies. EURODEM Incidence Research Group. *Neurology.* 1999;53:1992–1997.
6. Fratiglioni L, Viitanen M, von Strauss E, et al. Very old women at highest risk of dementia and Alzheimer's disease: incidence data from the Kungsholmen Project, Stockholm. *Neurology.* 1997;48:132–138.
7. Ganguli M, Dodge HH, Chen P, et al. Ten-year incidence of dementia in a rural elderly US community population: the MoVIES Project. *Neurology.* 2000;54:1109–1116.
8. Rocca WA, Cha RH, Waring SC, Kokmen E. Incidence of dementia and Alzheimer's disease: a reanalysis of data from Rochester, Minnesota, 1975–1984. *Am J Epidemiol.* 1998;148:51–62.
9. Bachman DL, Wolf PA, Linn RT, et al. Incidence of dementia and probable Alzheimer's disease in a general population: the Framingham Study. *Neurology.* 1993;43:515–519.
10. Kawas C, Gray S, Brookmeyer R, Fozard J, Zonderman A. Age-specific incidence rates of Alzheimer's disease: the Baltimore Longitudinal Study of Aging. *Neurology.* 2000;54:2072–2077.
11. Hebert LE, Scherr PA, Beckett LA, et al. Age-specific incidence of Alzheimer's disease in a community population. *JAMA.* 1995;273:1354–1359.
12. Kukull WA, Higdon R, Bowen JD, et al. Dementia and Alzheimer disease incidence: a prospective cohort study. *Arch Neurol.* 2002;59:1737–1746.
13. McEwen BS. Invited review: Estrogens effects on the brain: multiple sites and molecular mechanisms. *J Appl Physiol.* 2001;91:2785–2801.
14. Goodman Y, Bruce AJ, Cheng B, Mattson MP. Estrogens attenuate and corticosterone exacerbates excitotoxicity, oxidative injury, and amyloid beta-peptide toxicity in hippocampal neurons. *J Neurochem.* 1996;66:1836–1844.
15. Toran-Allerand CD, Miranda RC, Bentham WD, et al. Estrogen receptors colocalize with low-affinity nerve growth factor receptors in cholinergic neurons of the basal forebrain. *Proc Natl Acad Sci.* 1992;89:4668–4672.

16. Luine VN. Estradiol increases choline acetyltransferase activity in specific basal forebrain nuclei and projection areas of female rats. *Exp Neurol.* 1985;89:484–490.

17. Behl C, Widmann M, Trapp T, Holsboer F. 17-beta estradiol protects neurons from oxidative stress-induced cell death in vitro. *Biochem Biophys Res Commun.* 1995;216:473–482.

18. Jaffe AB, Toran-Allerand CD, Greengard P, Gandy SE. Estrogen regulates metabolism of Alzheimer amyloid beta precursor protein. *J Biol Chem.* 1994;269:13065–13068.

19. Barrett-Connor E, von Muhlen D, Laughlin GA, Kripke A. Endogenous levels of dehydroepiandrosterone sulfate, but not other sex hormones, are associated with depressed mood in older women: the Rancho Bernardo Study. *J Am Geriatr Soc.* 1999;47:685–691.

20. Jacobs DM, Tang MX, Stern Y, et al. Cognitive function in nondemented older women who took estrogen after menopause. *Neurology.* 1998;50:368–373.

21. Paganini-Hill A, Henderson VW. Estrogen deficiency and risk of Alzheimer's disease in women. *Am J Epidemiol.* 1994;140:256–261.

22. Tang MX, Jacobs D, Stern Y, et al. Effect of oestrogen during menopause on risk and age at onset of Alzheimer's disease. *Lancet.* 1996;348:429–432.

23. Yaffe K, Lui LY, Grady D, et al. Cognitive decline in women in relation to non-protein-bound oestradiol concentrations. *Lancet.* 2000;356:708–712.

24. Zandi PP, Carlson MC, Plassman BL, et al. Hormone replacement therapy and incidence of Alzheimer disease in older women: the Cache County Study. *JAMA.* 2002;288:2123–2129.

25. Henderson VW. Aging, estrogens, and episodic memory in women. *Cogn Behav Neurol.* 2009;22:205–214.

26. Resnick SM, Henderson VW. Hormone therapy and risk of Alzheimer disease: a critical time. *JAMA* 2002;288:2170–2172.

27. Joffe H, Hall JE, Gruber S, et al. Estrogen therapy selectively enhances prefrontal cognitive processes: a randomized, double-blind, placebo-controlled study with functional magnetic resonance imaging in perimenopausal and recently postmenopausal women. *Menopause.* 2006;13:411–422.

28. Phillips SM, Sherwin BB. Effects of estrogen on memory function in surgically menopausal women. *Psychoneuroendocrinology.* 1992;17:485–495.

29. Sherwin BB. Estrogen and/or androgen replacement therapy and cognitive functioning in surgically menopausal women. *Psychoneuroendocrinology.* 1988;13:345–357.

30. Maki PM, Gast MJ, Vieweg AJ, Burriss SW, Yaffe K. Hormone therapy in menopausal women with cognitive complaints: a randomized, double-blind trial. *Neurology.* 2007;69:1322–1330.

31. Linzmayer L, Semlitsch HV, Saletu B, et al. Double-blind, placebo-controlled psychometric studies on the effects of a combined estrogen-progestin regimen versus estrogen alone on performance, mood and personality of menopausal syndrome patients. *Arzneimittelforschung.* 2001;51:238–245.

32. Pefanco MA, Kenny AM, Kaplan RF, et al. The effect of 3-year treatment with 0.25 mg/day of micronized 17beta-estradiol on cognitive function in older postmenopausal women. *J Am Geriatr Soc.* 2007;55:426–431.

33. Resnick SM, Maki PM, Rapp SR, et al. Effects of combination estrogen plus progestin hormone treatment on cognition and affect. *J Clin Endocrinol Metab.* 2006;91:1802–1810.

34. Grady D, Yaffe K, Kristof M, Lin F, Richards C, Barrett-Connor E. Effect of postmenopausal hormone therapy on cognitive function: the Heart and Estrogen/progestin Replacement Study. *Am J Med.* 2002;113:543–548.

35. Shumaker SA, Reboussin BA, Espeland MA, et al. The Women's Health Initiative Memory Study (WHIMS): a trial of the effect of estrogen therapy in preventing and slowing the progression of dementia. *Control Clin Trials.* 1998;19:604–621.

36. Shumaker SA, Legault C, Rapp SR, et al. Estrogen plus progestin and the incidence of dementia and mild cognitive impairment in postmenopausal women: the Women's Health Initiative Memory Study: a randomized controlled trial. *JAMA.* 2003;289:2651–2662.

37. Shumaker SA, Legault C, Kuller L, et al. Conjugated equine estrogens and incidence of probable dementia and mild cognitive impairment in postmenopausal women: Women's Health Initiative Memory Study. *JAMA.* 2004;291:2947–2958.

38. Nilsen J, Brinton RD. Divergent impact of progesterone and medroxyprogesterone acetate (Provera) on nuclear mitogen-activated protein kinase signaling. *Proc Natl Acad Sci U S A.* 2003;100:10506–10511.

39. Sano M, Jacobs D, Andrews H, et al. A multi-center, randomized, double blind placebo-controlled trial of estrogens to prevent Alzheimer's disease and loss of memory in women: design and baseline characteristics. *Clin Trials.* 2008;5:523–533.

40. Miller VM, Black DM, Brinton EA, et al. Using basic science to design a clinical trial: baseline characteristics of women enrolled in the Kronos Early Estrogen Prevention Study (KEEPS). *J Cardiovasc Transl Res.* 2009;2:228–239.

41. Clinicaltrials.gov. ELITE: Early vs Late Intervention Trial with Estradiol. http://clinicaltrials.gov/ct2/show/NCT00114517. Accessed January 27, 2012.

42. Yaffe K, Grady D, Pressman A, Cummings S. Serum estrogen levels, cognitive performance, and risk of cognitive decline in older community women. *J Am Geriatrics Soc.* 1998;46:816–821.

43. Lebrun CE, van der Schouw YT, de Jong FH, Pols HA, Grobbee DE, Lamberts SW. Endogenous oestrogens are related to cognition in healthy elderly women. *Clin Endocrinol (Oxf).* 2005;63:50–55.

44. Schupf N, Pang D, Patel BN, et al. Onset of dementia is associated with age at menopause in women with Down's syndrome. *Ann Neurol.* 2003;54:433–438.

45. Rocca WA, Bower JH, Maraganore DM, et al. Increased risk of cognitive impairment or dementia in women who underwent oophorectomy before menopause. *Neurology.* 2007;69:1074–1083.

46. Nappi RE, Sinforiani E, Mauri M, et al. Memory functioning at menopause: impact of age in ovariectomized women. *Gynecol Obstet Invest.* 1999;47:29–36.

47. Farrag AK, Khedr EM, Abdel-Aleem H, Rageh TA. Effect of surgical menopause on cognitive functions. *Dement Geriatric Cogn Disord.* 2002;13:193–198.

48. Kritz-Silverstein D, Barrett-Connor E. Hysterectomy, oophorectomy, and cognitive function in older women. *J Am Geriat Soc.* 2002;50:55–61.

49. Kok HS, Kuh D, Cooper R, et al. Cognitive function across the life course and the menopausal transition in a British birth cohort. *Menopause.* 2006;13:19–27.

50. Polo-Kantola P, Portin R, Polo O, et al. The effect of short-term estrogen replacement therapy on cognition: a randomized, double-blind, cross-over trial in postmenopausal women. *Obstet Gynecol.* 1998;91:459–466.

51. Schiff R, Bulpitt CJ, Wesnes KA, Rajkumar C. Short-term transdermal estradiol therapy, cognition and depressive symptoms in healthy older women. A randomised placebo controlled pilot cross-over study. *Psychoneuroendocrinology.* 2005;30:309–315.

52. Almeida OP, Lautenschlager NT, Vasikaran S, et al. A 20-week randomized controlled trial of estradiol replacement therapy for women aged 70 years and older: effect on mood, cognition and quality of life. *Neurobiol Aging.* 2006;27:141–149.

53. Espeland MA, Rapp SR, Shumaker SA, et al. Conjugated equine estrogens and global cognitive function in postmenopausal women: Women's Health Initiative Memory Study. *JAMA.* 2004;291:2959–2968.

54. Henderson VW, Sherwin BB. Surgical versus natural menopause: cognitive issues. *Menopause* 2007;14:572–579.

55. Hoskin EK, Tang MX, Manly JJ, Mayeux R. Elevated sex-hormone binding globulin in elderly women with Alzheimer's disease. *Neurobiol Aging.* 2004;25:141–147.

56. Schupf N, Winsten S, Patel B, et al. Bioavailable estradiol and age at onset of Alzheimer's disease in postmenopausal women with Down syndrome. *Neurosci Lett.* 2006;406:298–302.

57. Geerlings MI, Launer LJ, de Jong FH, et al. Endogenous estradiol and risk of dementia in women and men: the Rotterdam Study. *Ann Neurol.* 2003;53:607–615.

58. Brandi ML, Becherini L, Gennari L, et al. Association of the estrogen receptor alpha gene polymorphisms with sporadic Alzheimer's disease. *Biochem Biophys Res Commun.* 1999;265:335–338.

59. Corbo RM, Gambina G, Ruggeri M, Scacchi R. Association of estrogen receptor alpha (ESR1) PvuII and XbaI polymorphisms with sporadic Alzheimer's disease and their effect on apolipoprotein E concentrations. *Dement Geriatr Cogn Disord.* 2006;22:67–72.

60. Isoe-Wada K, Maeda M, Yong J, et al. Positive association between an estrogen receptor gene polymorphism and Parkinson's disease with dementia. *Eur J Neurol.* 1999;6:431–435.

61. Ji Y, Urakami K, Wada-Isoe K, Adachi Y, Nakashima K. Estrogen receptor gene polymorphisms in patients with Alzheimer's disease, vascular dementia and alcohol-associated dementia. *Dement Geriatr Cogn Disord.* 2000;11:119–122.

62. Schupf N, Lee JH, Wei M, et al. Estrogen receptor-alpha variants increase risk of Alzheimer's disease in women with Down syndrome. *Dement Geriatr Cogn Disord.* 2008;25:476–482.

63. Pirskanen M, Hiltunen M, Mannermaa A, et al. Estrogen receptor beta gene variants are associated with increased risk of Alzheimer's disease in women. *Eur J Hum Genet.* 2005;13:1000–1006.

64. Yaffe K, Lindquist K, Sen S, et al. Estrogen receptor genotype and risk of cognitive impairment in elders: findings from the Health ABC study. *Neurobiol Aging.* 2009;30:607–614.

65. Huang R, Poduslo SE. CYP19 haplotypes increase risk for Alzheimer's disease. *J Med Genet.* 2006;43:e42.

66. Iivonen S, Corder E, Lehtovirta M, et al. Polymorphisms in the CYP19 gene confer increased risk for Alzheimer disease. *Neurology.* 2004;62:1170–1176.

67. Butler HT, Warden DR, Hogervorst E, Ragoussis J, Smith AD, Lehmann DJ. Association of the aromatase gene with Alzheimer's disease in women. *Neurosci Lett.* 2010;468:202–206.

68. Corbo RM, Gambina G, Ulizzi L, Moretto G, Scacchi R. Genetic variation of CYP19 (aromatase) gene influences age at onset of Alzheimer's disease in women. *Dement Geriatr Cogn Disord.* 2009;27:513–518.

69. Rocchi A, Pellegrini S, Siciliano G, Murri L. Causative and susceptibility genes for Alzheimer's disease: a review. *Brain Res Bull.* 2003;61:1–24.

70. Thiebaut AC, Freedman LS, Carroll RJ, Kipnis V. Is it necessary to correct for measurement error in nutritional epidemiology? *Ann Intern Med.* 2007;146:65–67.

71. Markesbery WR. Oxidative stress hypothesis in Alzheimer's disease. *Free Radic Biol Med.* 1997;23:134–147.

72. Butterfield DA, Castegna A, Drake J, Scapagnini G, Calabrese V. Vitamin E and neurodegenerative disorders associated with oxidative stress. *Nutr Neurosci.* 2002;5:229–239.

73. Pitchumoni SS, Doraiswamy PM. Current status of antioxidant therapy for Alzheimer's Disease. *J Am Geriatr Soc.* 1998;46:1566–1572.

74. Ascherio A. Antioxidants and stroke. *Am J Clin Nutr.* 2000;72:337–338.

75. Hirvonen T, Virtamo J, Korhonen P, Albanes D, Pietinen P. Intake of flavonoids, carotenoids, vitamins C and E, and risk of stroke in male smokers. *Stroke.* 2000;31:2301–2306.

76. Honig LS, Tang MX, Albert S, et al. Stroke and the risk of Alzheimer disease. *Arch Neurol.* 2003;60:1707–1712.

77. Vermeer SE, Prins ND, den Heijer T, Hofman A, Koudstaal PJ, Breteler MM. Silent brain infarcts and the risk of dementia and cognitive decline. *N Engl J Med.* 2003;348:1215–1222.

78. Berr C, Richard MJ, Roussel AM, Bonithon-Kopp C. Systemic oxidative stress and cognitive performance in the population-based EVA study. Etude du Vieillissement Arteriel. *Free Radic Biol Med.* 1998;24:1202–1208.

79. Rinaldi P, Polidori MC, Metastasio A, et al. Plasma antioxidants are similarly depleted in mild cognitive impairment and in Alzheimer's disease. *Neurobiol Aging.* 2003;24:915–919.

80. Launer LJ. Is there epidemiologic evidence that anti-oxidants protect against disorders in cognitive function? *J Nutr Health Aging.* 2000;4:197–201.

81. Masaki KH, Losonczy KG, Izmirlian G, et al. Association of vitamin E and C supplement use with cognitive function and dementia in elderly men. *Neurology.* 2000;54:1265–1272.

82. Grodstein F, Chen J, Willett WC. High-dose antioxidant supplements and cognitive function in community-dwelling elderly women. *Am J Clin Nutr.* 2003;77:975–984.

83. Zandi PP, Anthony JC, Khachaturian AS, et al. Reduced risk of Alzheimer disease in users of antioxidant vitamin supplements: the Cache County Study. *Arch Neurol.* 2004;61:82–88.

84. Engelhart MJ, Geerlings MI, Ruitenberg A, et al. Dietary intake of antioxidants and risk of Alzheimer disease. *JAMA.* 2002;287:3223–3229.

85. Morris MC, Evans DA, Bienias JL, Tangney CC, Wilson RS. Vitamin E and cognitive decline in older persons. *Arch Neurol.* 2002;59:1125–1132.

86. Morris MC, Evans DA, Bienias JL, et al. Dietary intake of antioxidant nutrients and the risk of incident Alzheimer disease in a biracial community study. *JAMA.* 2002;287:3230–3237.

87. Luchsinger JA, Tang MX, Shea S, Mayeux R. Antioxidant vitamin intake and risk of Alzheimer disease. *Arch Neurol.* 2003;60:203–208.

88. Sano M, Ernesto C, Thomas RG, et al. A controlled trial of selegiline, alpha-tocopherol, or both as treatment for Alzheimer's disease. The Alzheimer's Disease Cooperative Study. *N Engl J Med.* 1997;336:1216–1222.

89. Petersen RC, Thomas RG, Grundman M, et al. Vitamin E and donepezil for the treatment of mild cognitive impairment. *N Engl J Med.* 2005;352:2379–2388.

90. Miller ER, 3rd, Pastor-Barriuso R, Dalal D, Riemersma RA, Appel LJ, Guallar E. Meta-analysis: high-dosage vitamin E supplementation may increase all-cause mortality. *Ann Intern Med.*2005;142:37–46.

91. Clarke R, Smith AD, Jobst KA, Refsum H, Sutton L, Ueland PM. Folate, vitamin B12, and serum total homocysteine levels in confirmed Alzheimer disease. *Arch Neurol.* 1998;55:1449–1455.

92. Kwok T, Tang C, Woo J, Lai WK, Law LK, Pang CP. Randomized trial of the effect of supplementation on the cognitive function of older people with subnormal cobalamin levels. *Int J Geriatr Psychiatry.* 1998;13:611–616.

93. Eastley R, Wilcock GK, Bucks RS. Vitamin B12 deficiency in dementia and cognitive impairment: the effects of treatment on neuropsychological function. *Int J Geriatr Psychiatry.* 2000;15:226–233.

94. Nilsson K, Gustafson L, Hultberg B. Improvement of cognitive functions after cobalamin/folate supplementation in elderly patients with dementia and elevated plasma homocysteine. *Int J Geriatr Psychiatry.* 2001;16:609–614.

95. Crystal HA, Ortof E, Frishman WH, Gruber A, Hershman D, Aronson M. Serum vitamin B12 levels and incidence of dementia in a healthy elderly population: a report from the Bronx Longitudinal Aging Study. *J Am Geriatr Soc.* 1994;42:933–936.

96. Wang HX, Wahlin A, Basun H, Fastbom J, Winblad B, Fratiglioni L. Vitamin B(12) and folate in relation to the development of Alzheimer's disease. *Neurology.* 2001;56:1188–1194.

97. Hu FB, Willett WC. Optimal diets for prevention of coronary heart disease. *JAMA.* 2002;288:2569–2578.

98. Bray GA, Lovejoy JC, Smith SR, et al. The influence of different fats and fatty acids on obesity, insulin resistance and inflammation. *J Nutr.* 2002;132:2488–2491.

99. Luchsinger JA, Tang MX, Shea S, Mayeux R. Hyperinsulinemia and risk of Alzheimer disease. *Neurology.* 2004;63:1187–1192.

100. Cohn JS. Oxidized fat in the diet, postprandial lipaemia and cardiovascular disease. *Curr Opin Lipidol.* 2002;13:19–24.

101. Hardy JA, Higgins GA. Alzheimer's disease: the amyloid cascade hypothesis. *Science.* 1992;256:184–185.

102. Sparks DL, Martins R, Martin T. Cholesterol and cognition: rationale for the AD cholesterol-lowering treatment trial and sex-related Differences in beta-amyloid accumulation in the brains of spontaneously hypercholesterolemic Watanabe rabbits. *Ann N Y Acad Sci.* 2002;977:356–366.

103. Luchsinger JA, Tang MX, Shea S, Mayeux R. Caloric intake and the risk of Alzheimer disease. *Arch Neurol.* 2002;59:1258–1263.

104. Morris MC, Evans DA, Bienias JL, et al. Dietary fats and the risk of incident Alzheimer disease. *Arch Neurol.* 2003;60:194–200.

105. Morris MC, Evans DA, Bienias JL, et al. Consumption of fish and n-3 fatty acids and risk of incident Alzheimer disease. *Arch Neurol.* 2003;60:940–946.

106. Engelhart MJ, Geerlings MI, Ruitenberg A, et al. Diet and risk of dementia: Does fat matter?: The Rotterdam Study. *Neurology.* 2002;59:1915–1921.

107. Barberger-Gateau P, Letenneur L, Deschamps V, Peres K, Dartigues JF, Renaud S. Fish, meat, and risk of dementia: cohort study. *BMJ.* 2002;325:932–933.

108. Morris MC, Evans DA, Bienias JL, Tangney CC, Wilson RS. Dietary fat intake and 6-year cognitive change in an older biracial community population. *Neurology.* 2004;62:1573–1579.

109. Kris-Etherton P, Daniels SR, Eckel RH, et al. Summary of the scientific conference on dietary fatty acids and cardiovascular health: conference summary from the nutrition committee of the American Heart Association. *Circulation.* 2001;103:1034–1039.

110. Agar E, Demir S, Amanvermez R, Bosnak M, Ayyildiz M, Celik C. The effects of ethanol consumption on the lipid peroxidation and glutathione levels in the right and left brains of rats. *Int J Neurosci.* 2003;113:1643–1652.

111. Sacco RL, Elkind M, Boden-Albala B, et al. The protective effect of moderate alcohol consumption on ischemic stroke. *JAMA.* 1999;281:53–60.

112. Howard A, Chopra M, Thurnham D, Strain J, Fuhrman B, Aviram M. Red wine consumption and inhibition of LDL oxidation: what are the important components? *Med Hypotheses.* 2002;59:101–104.

113. Bertelli AA, Migliori M, Panichi V, et al. Oxidative stress and inflammatory reaction modulation by white wine. *Ann N Y Acad Sci.* 2002;957:295–301.

114. Belleville J. The French paradox: possible involvement of ethanol in the protective effect against cardiovascular diseases. *Nutrition* 2002;18:173–177.

115. Heinonen IM, Lehtonen PJ, Hopia AI. Antioxidant activity of berry and fruit wines and liquors. *J Agric Food Chem.* 1998;46:25–31.

116. Ruitenberg A, van Swieten JC, Witteman JC, et al. Alcohol consumption and risk of dementia: the Rotterdam Study. *Lancet.* 2002;359:281–286.

117. Mukamal KJ, Kuller LH, Fitzpatrick AL, Longstreth WT, Jr., Mittleman MA, Siscovick DS. Prospective study of alcohol consumption and risk of dementia in older adults. *JAMA.* 2003;289:1405–1413.

118. Galanis DJ, Joseph C, Masaki KH, Petrovitch H, Ross GW, White L. A longitudinal study of drinking and cognitive performance in elderly Japanese American men: the Honolulu-Asia Aging Study. *Am J Public Health.* 2000;90:1254–1259.

119. Luchsinger JA, Tang MX, Siddiqui M, Shea S, Mayeux R. Alcohol intake and risk of dementia. *J Am Geriatr Soc.* 2004;52:540–546.

120. Truelsen T, Thudium D, Gronbaek M. Amount and type of alcohol and risk of dementia: the Copenhagen City Heart Study. *Neurology.* 2002; 59:1313–1319.

121. Goldberg IJ, Mosca L, Piano MR, Fisher EA. AHA Science Advisory: Wine and your heart: a science advisory for healthcare professionals from the Nutrition Committee, Council on Epidemiology and Prevention, and Council on Cardiovascular Nursing of the American Heart Association. *Circulation.* 2001;103:472–475.

122. Resnick B, Junlapeeya P. Falls in a community of older adults: findings and implications for practice. *Appl Nurs Res.* 2004;17:81–91.

123. Morris JC. The Clinical Dementia Rating (CDR): current version and scoring rules. *Neurology.* 1993;43:2412–2414.

124. McKhann G, Drachman D, Folstein M, Katzman R, Price D, Stadlan EM. Clinical diagnosis of Alzheimer's disease: report of the NINCDS-ADRDA Work Group under the auspices of Department of Health and Human Services Task Force on Alzheimer's Disease. *Neurology.* 1984;34:939–944.

125. Blacker D, Albert MS, Bassett SS, Go RC, Harrell LE, Folstein MF. Reliability and validity of NINCDS-ADRDA criteria for Alzheimer's disease. The National Institute of Mental Health Genetics Initiative. *Arch Neurol.* 1994;51:1198–1204.

126. Doody RS, Stevens JC, Beck C, et al. Practice parameter: management of dementia (an evidence-based review). Report of the Quality Standards Subcommittee of the American Academy of Neurology. *Neurology.* 2001;56:1154–1166.

127. Folstein MF, Folstein SE, McHugh PR. "Mini-mental state." A practical method for grading the cognitive state of patients for the clinician. *J Psych Res.* 1975;12:189–198.

128. Bloudek LM, Spackman DE, Blankenburg M, Sullivan SD. Review and meta-analysis of biomarkers and diagnostic imaging in Alzheimer's disease. *J Alzheimer Dis.* 2011;26:627–645.

129. McDonald CR, McEvoy LK, Gharapetian L, et al. Regional rates of neocortical atrophy from normal aging to early Alzheimer disease. *Neurology.* 2009;73:457–465.

130. Quigley H, Colloby SJ, O'Brien JT. PET imaging of brain amyloid in dementia: a review. *Int J Geriat Psych.* 2011;26:991–999.

131. Petersen RC. Early diagnosis of Alzheimer's disease: is MCI too late? *Curr Alzheimer Res.* 2009;6:324–330.

132. Petersen RC, Doody R, Kurz A, et al. Current concepts in mild cognitive impairment. *Arch Neurol.* 2001;58:1985–1992.

133. Petersen RC, Roberts RO, Knopman DS, et al. Mild cognitive impairment: ten years later. *Arch Neurol.* 2009;66:1447–1455.

134. Petersen RC, Jack CR, Jr. Imaging and biomarkers in early Alzheimer's disease and mild cognitive impairment. *Clin Pharm Therapeut.* 2009;86:438–441.

135. Weiner MW, Aisen PS, Jack CR, Jr., et al. The Alzheimer's disease neuroimaging initiative: progress report and future plans. *Alzheimer Dement.* 2010;6:202–211 e207.

136. Raschetti R, Albanese E, Vanacore N, Maggini M. Cholinesterase inhibitors in mild cognitive impairment: a systematic review of randomised trials. *PLoS Med.* 2007;4:e338.

137. Thal LJ, Ferris SH, Kirby L, et al. A randomized, double-blind, study of rofecoxib in patients with mild cognitive impairment. *Neuropsychopharmacology.* 2005;30:1204–1215.

138. Baker LD, Frank LL, Foster-Schubert K, et al. Effects of aerobic exercise on mild cognitive impairment: a controlled trial. *Arch Neurol.* 2010;67:71–79.

139. Solfrizzi V, Panza F, Frisardi V, et al. Diet and Alzheimer's disease risk factors or prevention: the current evidence. *Expert Rev Neurotherapeutics.* 2011;11:677–708.

140. Cummings JL. Treatment of Alzheimer's disease: current and future therapeutic approaches. *Reviews Neurol Dis.* 2004;1:60–69.

141. Brookmeyer R, Corrada MM, Curriero FC, Kawas C. Survival following a diagnosis of Alzheimer disease. *Arch Neurol.* 2002;59:1764–1767.

142. Larson EB, Shadlen MF, Wang L, et al. Survival after initial diagnosis of Alzheimer disease. *Ann Int Med.* 2004;140:501–509.

143. Stern Y, Tang MX, Albert MS, et al. Predicting time to nursing home care and death in individuals with Alzheimer disease. *JAMA.* 1997;277:806–812.

144. Mayeux R, Sano M. Treatment of Alzheimer's disease. *N Engl J Med.* 1999;341:1670–1679.

39-1

One Caregiver's Perspective

Marilyn Hillman

I'm huddled over a book at my neighborhood diner, but I can't focus. All I can think about is my new status as my husband's primary caregiver, a job I never signed on for, never gave any thought to during the past thirty-odd years of our marriage, and certainly never wanted.

My husband—a once-formidable marketing strategist and executive vice president of a global advertising firm—is denying the dementia that is steadily fogging his brain, and I am trying to pick up the pieces of his life, while his brain staggers under the burden of unwanted amyloid deposits and tau tangles.

While I ponder Murray's dementia, his geriatric psychiatrist slides into the seat opposite me. Dr. White has generously consented to meet me in a neutral place to discuss my anxieties about caregiving. In my life I've been good at some things, superb at nothing. Chances are I won't excel in this new role either. Frankly, I think I do not wish to become an ace caregiver. That would imply many years ahead in which to polish my skills while losing my life.

I detail my fears while Dr. White listens patiently. He then enumerates the problems I'll be facing as my husband's vascular dementia progresses. I'm dumbfounded as I try to absorb all the bad news at once. Swallowing problems. Oh yes, Murray already has that, but who knew that swallowing skills could be compromised by a deteriorating brain? Dr. White advises me to put my husband's pills in applesauce or mashed potatoes to make the swallowing easier.

Then there's the twenty-four-hour care my husband will require when he becomes oblivious to me and the rest of the world. Dr. White counsels me that a nursing home is not the only solution if I choose to keep him at home. Many families manage this, the psychiatrist tells me, despite the incontinence and possible aggressive behavior that can accompany severe dementia. Am I kidding myself? Can I really handle incontinence and aggression? Can anyone?

Dr. White is like the TV weather guy you trust but refuse to believe as he describes the approaching perfect storm. He's direct, so direct that I think I need a flak jacket to ward off the bulletins of bad news he shoots my way. And he makes house calls. House calls? Yes, this dedicated and insightful physician actually visits us in our apartment a few times a month. Kill me now, I think. Life doesn't get much better than this.

I listen to myself—thrilled about psychiatric house calls instead of an upcoming trip to Rome. How pathetic is that? Equally pathetic—I've memorized the phone numbers of Murray's cardiologist and our local pharmacy. And I have more than a nodding acquaintance with Head Nurse Christine on the cardiology floor at the hospital. My husband has had three go-rounds of heart failure in the past two years—more than enough time for me to be on "hi-how've-you-been" terms with Four North's cardiology staff.

This is my life? Well it doesn't have to be your life, my friends tell me as they pile on the advice. Get help. Get a life. Have an affair. *An affair*? Who has the time or energy for that? Take classes. Write. *Write*? Assemble a coherent narrative out of the chaos of my life? This will keep me sane?

Decathect. *Decathect*? That's the stopper my friend the social work professor throws out one day at lunch. My online dictionary tells me that to decathect is to stop investing emotional energy in a person. I consider this advice. Is she kidding? Just coldly stop caring about my husband of thirty-four years? How do I do that? Another friend—a psychiatrist—advises me to accept my losses. Grieve. Mourn. And move on. Excuse me? Mourn my husband while I'm making his breakfast?

And here's the advice that makes me the craziest—join a support group. Do what? Spend my precious outside time trading tips on caring for a spouse with cognitive impairment? I'd rather join a writers' group and trade tips on getting published.

So here's one of my favorite things about Dr. White. He hasn't raised the dreaded support group thing, hasn't even dropped the most casual hint. Maybe in his extensive experience he's learned that support groups don't suit everyone—that they might even do more harm than good, as beginners like me hear our darkest fears spelled out by caregivers handling worse cases. Or maybe Dr. White figures I've already got a handle on staying afloat on a boat about to be sucked up in a dementia tsunami. Well that makes one of us, I think.

I read a book on geriatric mental health care for primary caregivers. I assume the author means me, but after reading the introduction to the book, I realize that primary caregivers are family physicians. I read the book anyway, finding it accessible and helpful, particularly on the delineation and progression of the different dementias.

The author writes in a straight-talking style, and while I have to look up aphasia, apraxia, and agnosia—I think of them as the three A's of dementia—I finish the book, skipping the scariest nursing home stuff.

Armed with the new words in my vocabulary, I imagine myself as a contestant on *Jeopardy*. Alex Trebek announces, "The answer is—partial or total loss of the ability to articulate ideas or comprehend spoken or written language resulting from damage to the brain caused by injury or disease." Quick. I've got it. "What is aphasia?" I belt out with confidence.

I learn that Murray's vascular dementia is proceeding in stepwise fashion, with occasional plateaus where he can hang on to whatever he still has in the cognition department before the next drop-off, unlike an Alzheimer's patient whose progression is a steep slope downward without benefit of rest stops.

The more I learn about my husband's cognitive impairment including the obliteration of his executive function skills—those skills which once allowed him to plan his day, not to mention his life—the more I wonder if I can cope. I don't know. What I do know is that some days I'm in way over my head, slogging through the responsibilities and hassles of daily caregiving. Look at that, I think. I'm shameless, tossing caregiving and hassles into the same sentence like it's some kind of chopped salad. Then instead of oil and vinegar, I throw in a pinch of anger. And a teaspoon of disappointment.

Yes, I admit it. I am not a saint. And there are days when my patience wears thin. Very thin. I worry about my own sanity. I read several books on dementia and the burden it places on family caregivers who face an elevated risk of depression, a loss of social ties, and poorer physical health than noncaregivers. I am particularly shocked to learn that 20 to 60% of family caregivers, most of whom are women, end up clinically depressed, some requiring medication. I do not want to go down that dark road.

Yes, I understand my risks, but what about Murray? We skirt around the subject of his cognitive deterioration, and I can see that he feels like he's caught in a riptide pulling him further and further away from the safety of the beach. No lifeguards in sight. Just me, Dr. White, and an assortment of other medical professionals cheering my husband on and throwing him a life raft during an occasional crisis.

One day Murray tells Dr. White, "My mind was my weapon. I used it with precision, and it always served me well. And now it's gone. I've got holes where ideas used to be." This is the first time he's named his losses, and I'm suddenly flooded with compassion for my husband. I tell him he's brave. And sweet. And I wish I could fix the problem for him. But I'm also thinking, Please God, do not let this happen to me.

Then a hotshot author on PBS scares me with the fact that alcohol—even the smallest amount of wine—shrinks brain cells. Oh no, not that. So I give up my glass of wine with dinner. Because no way do I want to be dealing with my own dementia down the road. Then I read another expert's research stating that moderate wine drinkers lose two per cent of their brain cells every ten years. I imagine a tiny fragment of my brain breaking loose and waving goodbye. I wave back, regretting all those lovely French Bordeaux wines I've indulged in for years. Adieu, my vanishing thought cells.

Hoping to prevent any further cognitive losses, I engage in mental gymnastics, like counting back from 100 by sevens. Or trying to recall as many words as I can, starting with the letter F. Or S. Or any other letter I can still remember. While I swim laps, I match up alphabetic sequences with consecutive numbers, starting backwards from Z-26 to A-1.

But sometimes, depending on how much I let my fears shape my thoughts, I skip the mental judo and just let anxiety take me over, as I teeter on the edge of the abyss. Don't look down, I think. You don't want to know.

I wish I could make this part of my life disappear—make my husband whole again. And while I'm at it, I wish I could write an upbeat ending to this narrative. But this story will not end well. And it will be endless until it ends. Meanwhile, Murray and I are just trying to put one foot in front of the other and keep moving. In my husband's case, this will become increasingly difficult—and finally impossible.

Five years later I've pretty much been seen it all, from Murray's incontinence, to occasional wandering, and sadly, to outbursts of rage when he feels totally helpless. Dr. White has become indispensable to my sanity as he helps me navigate from one crisis to the next. Without his expertise and deep understanding of the problems I face, I might not survive mentally or physically intact.

I speak on caregiving at some dementia symposiums, detailing my personal tools for survival, first and foremost my quirky sense of humor. Without an ability to laugh at the absurd facets of life with a demented husband, I would have either fled the premises by now, or been put on serious meds.

After five years of battling his cognitive demons, Murray survives hip fracture surgery and two bouts of pneumonia. Even with constant physical therapy, he eventually becomes weaker and more frail.

We visit his cardiologist and internist. Neither physician can find a reason for his physical deterioration. Then his speech becomes garbled. It is Dr. White who tells me that Murray's motor system is shutting down. "This is global, Marilyn. It will involve all of his organs. He will die within weeks."

Laying aside his white coat of immunity for the moment, Dr. White tells me how sad it makes him to see Murray in this condition. I sense that we're *both* devastated by the fact of Murray's approaching death. And I am struck by the physician's compassion and innate humanity.

As for Murray, my determined husband has waged a gallant struggle against an implacable disease, but it's a battle he finally loses.

Impact of Research: Lessons from the Past, Challenges of the Future

An Overview of Breast Screening

Cornelia J. Baines, MD, MSc, FACE

Introduction

One can read on a U.S. government information website the following:

> Many women are fearful of breast cancer. One reason is that breast cancer is personal. Breast cancer affects one in eight women during their lives and many of us know someone who has had it. Another reason is that breast cancer is a real threat to women. It is the second-leading cancer killer of women in the United States…Thanks to screening, breast cancer can often be found early, when the chance of successful treatment is best. In fact many women are even cured of their disease.[1]

What the text states will not be disputed, except for the "one in eight" statement, which would be better presented as a woman having a one in eight chance of getting breast cancer by the time she is 80 years old, not before. Other than this readily misinterpreted statement, the quote leads directly into the topic of breast screening to potentially detect breast cancer early, change its "natural history," and prevent death from breast cancer. Early detection is primarily achieved by screening mammography, although historically clinical breast examination and breast self-examination were also recommended as early detection modalities.

Distinguishing between screening mammography and diagnostic mammography is essential. The former screens presumably healthy women for early disease on a recommended schedule influenced by age. The latter evaluates abnormalities in symptomatic women of any age. Women should be advised that the early detection achievable with mammography may not be early enough to prevent death from breast cancer in *all* women with screen-detected breast cancer, as some tumors are very aggressive and may rapidly metastasize to other organs.

At best, one mammography trial provided a 30% reduction in breast cancer mortality. If this were generally achieved, it means that for every 10 women destined to die of breast cancer if not screened, 7 will still die even with breast screening. Furthermore screening unavoidably increases the incidence of breast cancer.[2] By detecting cancers earlier, more tumors will be detected at an earlier point in time than would have occurred otherwise clinically. The interval between screen detection and clinical detection of a cancer is called *lead time*. Lead time bias lengthens survival time without necessarily reducing the risk of dying from breast cancer. Therefore, the stage-specific survival comparisons presented in a 2010 *Morbidity and Mortality Weekly Report* from the Centers for Disease Control and Prevention stating that "the 5-year survival rate for women who receive a diagnosis of localized breast cancer is 98% compared with 84% for regional stage and 23% for distant stage" constitutes an erroneous argument encouraging screening.[1]

When early screening trials were first initiated, the researchers assumed that the early increase in breast cancer incidence detected by yearly mammography would eventually be matched by cancers diagnosed later in the comparison group. Eventually the numbers of cases would equalize in the study and control groups. Unfortunately, we now know that the number of cases in screened populations always remains greater than the number in the control group, leading to the inevitable conclusion that some screen-detected cancers are "overdiagnosed." This phenomenon is described later in the chapter. Fortunately, U.S. incidence and mortality data indicate that the majority of women diagnosed with breast cancer do not die of the disease. Figure 40-1 shows that the mortality rate from breast cancer has been declining during the past 10 years or more.

Randomized Controlled Trials

Large randomized controlled screening trials conducted over the past 50 years have been carefully evaluated by the scientific committee charged with revising screening recommendations issued by the United States Preventive Services Task Force (USPSTF). This section reviews the contributions of randomized controlled trials (RCT), the "gold standard" for testing efficacy of procedures, to the current body of scientific knowledge used in developing clinical guidelines.

Current standards require ethical approval of proposed trials by an institutional review board. Participants must sign an informed consent document that describes

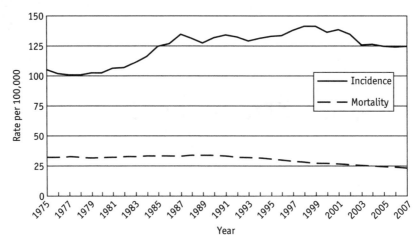

Figure 40-1 Breast cancer incidence and mortality rates per 100,000 by year.

Source: Data from SEER Cancer Statistics Review, 1975–2007, National Cancer Institute http://seer.cancer.gov/csr/1975_2007/. US Mortality Files, National Center for Health Statistics, Centers for Disease Control and Prevention. Rates are per 100,000 and are age-adjusted to the 2000 US Standard Population.

benefits and risks to participants, obligations of participants including routine follow-up, the purpose of the trial, sources of funding, names and affiliations of the research team, and how to reach them if necessary. Women meeting entry criteria and agreeing to participate must be randomly assigned to intervention or control status. Exclusion criteria must be specifically defined. Randomization minimizes imbalance of both known and unknown demographic and behavioral variables in order to ensure that the two study groups will be as similar as possible; the single difference should be that the intervention is offered to only one group. In screening trials, women receiving one intervention (in this case mammography) should be similar (with respect to age, marital status, age at menarche, age at first birth, etc.) to those randomized as controls (no mammography). The intervention should be subjected to quality control measures. Compliance with assignment must be carefully monitored. And outcome assessment should be assessed by an external monitoring committee.

An Overview of Screening Trials

New York Health Insurance Plan—1960s

A complete overview of breast cancer screening trials is provided at the National Cancer Institute (NCI) website.[3] Screening mammography was first evaluated in the New York Health Insurance Plan Study (HIP). In 1963 HIP randomized women ages 40 to 64 to receive annual two-view mammography and clinical breast examination for three annual screens or to receive "usual" clinical care as provided by the medical program. In all, 30,000 women were randomly assigned to each arm of the study. Although 35% of the intervention group did not attend the first screening, they were included in an intention-to-treat analysis. Mammography quality at that time did not match the excellence of current standards. The HIP study's 15-year follow-up revealed an overall statistically significant reduction in breast cancer mortality of 23% but no benefit was seen from screening women ages 40–49.[4] An unexpected

transient and paradoxical increase in breast cancer mortality was observed in women ages 40–49 who received screening compared to no screening. This paradox would be observed in subsequent screening studies.[5]

Randomized Trials Conducted in Sweden—1970s

In 1976 another study was initiated in Malmö, Sweden for those aged 45–69 years, with about 21,000 women in the study group and another 21,000 in the control group. After 12 years a statistically nonsignificant breast cancer mortality reduction of 20% was observed.[6] The Swedish Two-County trial initiated in 1977 had two components, each of which involved women ages 40 to 74 who were randomized by geographic clustering rather than by individual assignment.[7,8]

The Östergötland trial recruited approximately 39,000 in the study group and 37,500 in the control group. The intervention was single-view mammography every 2 years for women less than 50 years of age and every 33 months for women 50 and over. At 12-year follow-up the breast cancer mortality reduction encompassing all ages was 18%, again not statistically significant.

The Kopparberg trial included approximately 38,800 women in the study group and 18,600 in the control group although the sample size varied over publications. The intervention was the same as for the Östergötland trial. At 12-year follow-up a statistically significant reduction in mortality of 32% was observed, although at 14-year follow-up no significant breast cancer mortality reduction was observed among women ages 40–49 in either county.

Randomized Trial in United Kingdom (UK)—1970s

The Edinburgh (UK) trial was initiated in 1978 recruiting women aged 45–64 years with 23,226 in the study group and 21,904 in the control group.[9] The method used to randomize general practice units (rather than individual women) was never described although reports indicated that participants from practices "randomized" to receive screening were of much higher socioeconomic status than those in the control practices. This serious discrepancy in socioeconomic status accounted for the higher all-cause mortality seen in the control group. The lack of appropriate randomization may also have exaggerated any observed benefit of screening voiding any contribution of the results to an understanding of screening efficacy.

Changing Mammography Screening Trial Designs

In the early 1970s, the Breast Cancer Demonstration Project (BCDDP) funded by the National Cancer Institute (NCI) and the American Cancer Society (ACS) was launched. Mammography screening and clinical breast examination were provided at no cost to self-selected women who were concerned about breast cancer.[10] This was not a "gold standard" randomized controlled trial. By 1979, researchers interested in screening in North America had concluded that the HIP study had lacked adequate power to demonstrate a screening benefit for women ages 40–49 because breast cancer incidence is so much lower in younger women. The BCDDP could not answer this question either. Clearly, a larger study population of women ages 40–49 was needed in the context of a randomized controlled trial. The HIP study had also raised the question of the incremental benefit of mammography over and above clinical examination of the breasts.

A working group was therefore convened by the funding organizations to evaluate available data from the BCDDP on breast cancer screening.[11] Two recommendations emerged. The first was that a larger study was needed to determine whether screening was effective in women aged 40–49; the screening intervention should be both mammography and clinical breast examination, and the comparison should be combined screening versus no screening. The second recommendation was that the incremental effect of mammography over and above clinical breast examination (in reducing breast cancer mortality) needed to be studied in women ages 50–59. This required women receiving both mammography and clinical breast examination to be compared with women receiving only clinical breast examination (CBE).

These two recommendations determined the design of the Canadian National Breast Screening Study (CNBSS), which commenced recruitment in 1980 at 15 collaborating medical centers across Canada from Halifax to Vancouver. Radiation exposure from mammography had been raised as a hazard before the CNBSS was launched but these fears were addressed by the research team.[12] CNBSS-1 recruited women aged 40 to 49 years: 25,214 in the study group and 25,216 in the control group. The intervention was four or five annual two-view mammograms accompanied by CBE performed by carefully trained nurses in all centers except those in Quebec where physicians were the examiners. Controls received one CBE on entry as required for informed consent and subsequently received usual care in the community. Annual questionnaires provided

information on the health status of controls. After CBE was performed by a nurse-practitioner, women were individually randomized by the center coordinators, who were blind to the CBE results. All women entering the screening trial were retained in the arm to which they were randomized regardless of any clinical findings. At 13-year follow-up, mortality reduction was a statistically nonsignificant 3% among women in the intervention group.[13]

CNBSS-2 recruited women aged 50 to 59 years with individual randomization assigning 19,711 to the study group and 19,694 to the control group. The study group received four to five annual two-view mammograms and CBEs; the controls received four to five annual CBEs. The relative risk of death comparing screened women to controls was 1.02 (95% CI = 0.62–1.52) clearly no benefit was gained from mammography screening over CBE.[14] Both components of CNBSS included instruction in breast self examination (BSE).[15,16]

Additional European Screening Trials—1980s

Other trials comparing mammography screening to no screening were being conducted in Europe. In 1981 the Stockholm, Sweden trial started recruiting women aged 40 to 64 years. Cluster randomization by birth date was employed and the numbers in the study and control groups changed between published reports. The intervention was single-view mammography done twice with an interval of 28 months. No mortality reduction was reported in women aged 40–49 after 11.4-year follow-up.[17]

In 1982 the Göteborg, Sweden trial started recruiting women aged 39 to 59 years, 21,650 in the study group and 29,961 in the control group. A complex form of cluster randomization was employed. At 12- to 14-year follow-up no statistically significant mortality reduction was observed for women 39–59 and for women 50–54 no reduction significant or otherwise was observed as noted on the NCI website.[3] In marked contrast, for women 45–49 others have claimed a 48% significant reduction.[2]

Similar to the BCDDP providing mammography to American women, the Forrest Report[18] in 1986 recommended the introduction of a National Health Service Breast Screening Program in the United Kingdom offering mammography once every 3 years to women aged 50 to 64. The English program established in 1988 invited 110,700 women between the ages of 50 and 64 for screening. This program, lacking a comparison group like the BCDDP, was not a "gold standard" randomized controlled trial.

Recent Mammography Screening Trials

The most recent study conducted between 1991 and 1997, the UK Age trial, was designed to assess screening among women ages 40–49.[19] All other trials displayed "age creep" in that women recruited in their late 40s entered their 50s within a few years although analyses were based on age group at entry. Women 49 and younger are more likely to be premenopausal when breast tissue density adversely affects the sensitivity of mammography compared to women ages 50 and older when menopause accompanied by reduced hormonal stimulation is associated with a reduction in density and an increase in mammography sensitivity. By recruiting 160,291 women aged 39–41 and randomizing them in a ratio of 1:2 to screening or a control group, the UK researchers were able to recruit a study population that remained in their 40s at 10-year follow-up. Although a 17% breast cancer mortality reduction was observed at a mean follow-up of 10.7 years, it was not statistically significant. Unfortunately, the UK researchers have not revealed annual cumulative breast cancer mortality as provided by others, limiting our ability to compare results across clinical trials.[5]

Table 40-1 reveals the diversity of the trials. Compliance in attendance at first screen varied from 61% to 100% across trials. In some trials, single-view mammography was used; in others two-view mammography. The interval between screens varied from 12 to 33 months; between 2 and 10 screens were performed. Ages at entry ranged from 39 to 75. Differing methods of randomization were used: cluster (geographic region, birth date, or medical practice) or individual, the gold standard. Clinical examination of the breast was included in some trials but not others.

Table 40-2 shows data for breast cancer mortality reduction at 13-year follow-up, including all ages. Only three trials presented substantial breast cancer mortality reductions: the HIP Study, Göteborg, and the Swedish Two-County trial. The HIP Study is really borderline given the confidence interval includes 1.0.

Translating Mammography Research to Clinical Practice

After years of follow-up, combined data from the trials demonstrate a 15 to 16% reduction in overall breast cancer mortality.[20,21] Looking specifically at the benefit from screening women ages 40–49, the Swedish Overview[22] revealed a 9% reduction, which was not statistically significant, the UK trial a 17% reduction, not significant,[19] and the review by the USPSTF[21] indicated a nonsignificant 15% reduction. When the estimated reduction is translated into the absolute benefit, one death is prevented per 2,000 women screened annually for 10 years. More specifically, Moss et al. reported that more than 2,500 women aged 40–49 would need to be screening annually for 7 to 9 years to prevent one death from breast cancer.[19] That small opportunity for benefit must be balanced against the 25% of screen-detected cancers that are overdiagnosed[23] and radiation exposure among premenopausal women.

Table 40-1							
Basic features of randomized controlled trials of breast screening[2,19]							
Study & Year	Age on Entry (years)	# Women	Random- ization	Screen Modality	Interval (months)	# Rounds	Compliance First Screen
HIP Study 1963–66	40–64	60,995	Individual	2-view MA+CBE	12	4	67%
Malmö 1976–90	43–70	60,076	Individual	2-view MA	18–24	1–7	75–80%
2-County 1977–81	40–75	133,065	Cluster	1-view MA	24, 33	2–4	89%
Edinburgh 1979–86	45–64	44,268	Cluster	2-view MA+CBE	24	2–4	61%
CNBSS-1 1980–85	40–49	50,430	Individual	2-view MA+CBE	12	4, 5	100%
CNBSS-2 1980–85	50–59	39,405	Individual	2-view MA+CBE	12	4, 5	100%
Stockholm, 1981–83	40–64	60,117	Cluster	1-view MA	28	2	81%
Göteborg 1982–84	39–49	51,611	Cluster	2-view MA	18	4–5	84%
UK Age Trial 1991–97	39–41	160,291	Individual	First screen 2-view MA; then 1-view	12	7–9	68%

HIP: New York Health Insurance Plan Study; MA: mammography; CBE: clinical breast examination; CNBSS: Canadian National Breast Screening Study

Table 40-2

Study	Risk Ratio	CI	% Reduction
HIP	0.83	0.70–1.00	17
Malmö	0.81	0.61–1.07	19
Kopparberg	0.58	0.45–0.76	42
Östergötland	0.76	0.61–0.95	24
CNBSS-1	0.97	0.74–1.29	3
CNBSS-2	1.02	0.78–1.33	-
Stockholm	0.73	0.50–1.06	27
Göteborg	0.75	0.58–0.97	25
UK Age Trial	0.83	0.66–1.04	17

Breast cancer mortality reduction at 13 years follow-up[20]

Source: Data from Gøtzsche PC, Nielsen M. Screening for breast cancer with mammography. *Cochrane Database Syst Rev*. 2011;1:CD001877.

Other Screening Modalities

Clinical Examination of the Breasts (CBE)

Only the CNBSS trial provided data on the efficacy of CBE. The structured protocol required a visual examination of the breasts with arms akimbo, arms elevated, bending at the waist, and torsion at the waist. Palpation followed a grid pattern, included examination of the axillae and the supraclavicular region. The physician and nurse-examiners were observed at regular intervals. In short, CBE in the CNBSS began with a structured protocol, followed by intensive training and routine monitoring. Furthermore, CBE duration could be as little as 5 minutes but when women had large or tender breasts, were nervous, or had many questions much longer examinations were required.

As to the efficacy of CBE it is interesting that in CNBSS-2, women aged 50–59 receiving both mammography and CBE had smaller tumors and higher cancer detection rates than those who received only CBE. However, no reduction in breast cancer mortality was achieved by mammography at 13-year follow-up compared with CBE.[14]

Breast Self-Examination (BSE)

Based on results from a large trial conducted in China, the current consensus is that breast self-examination should not be recommended. Chinese factories were randomized; their female employees age 30 and older either received BSE training or were considered controls. The results were not hugely compelling.[24] Questions have been raised about the selection of the targeted age group and the country. The breast cancer incidence rate among Chinese women is among the lowest internationally. Furthermore, women did move from one factory to another, complicating assessment by factory assignment. Another trial was initiated in Russia, again with no positive results.[25] During a site visit the quality of BSE instruction in Russia was judged as inadequate and the BSE performance level did not meet high standards.

A major contrast in BSE findings was afforded by the CNBSS. Women were given BSE training by the physician and nurse-examiners who followed a structured protocol. At every scheduled visit their BSE performance was evaluated in a structured fashion; BSE scores were tabulated from the second to the final screening visit. On the basis of this information, a nested case-control study was implemented; participants with higher scores 2 years prior to their breast cancer diagnosis had lower odds ratios for risk of breast cancer death.[16] At a pragmatic level it must be recognized that training and monitoring BSE performance is not undertaken lightly and the infrastructure for doing so does not exist. However, the visual examination was found to be the most important component of BSE indicating that subtle asymmetries of contour should not be ignored.

Screening Policy

In spite of being based on common data sources, by the early 1990s, screening recommendations varied enormously both within the United States, between the United States and Canada, and between the United States and some European countries. In a 1993 publication, a table listing organizations that endorsed or did not endorse screening under the age of 50 was published.[26] Those in favor included the American Academy of Family Physicians, the American Association of Women Radiologists, the American Cancer Society, the American College of Radiology, the American Medical Association, the American Society of Internal Medicine, the American Society for Therapeutic Radiology and Oncology, the College of American Pathologists, the U.S. National Cancer Institute, the U.S. National Medical Association, the American Osteopathic College of Radiology, and the British Columbia Ministry of Health.

Those not endorsing screening for women under 50 included the Canadian Task Force on Periodic Health Examination, the Canadian Workshop Group (Canadian

Cancer Society, Department of National Health and Welfare and the National Cancer Institute of Canada), the U.S. Preventive Services Task Force, the American College of Physicians, the UK Forrest Report, the International Union Against Cancer, the European Group for Breast Cancer Screening, the New Zealand Cancer Society, the British Medical Association, and national policies in Finland, Denmark, and Holland.

Positions have changed in the ensuing years, sometimes due to political interference as in 1997 when the conclusions of the National Institutes of Health consensus conference were overturned,[27] but the underlying scientific evidence has not changed. However, association recommendations and national policy have limited influence on screening behaviors in North America. Most physicians and most women believe that screening is beneficial and even an inalienable right. This was illustrated vividly in the outcry against USPSTF 2009 guidelines[28] that concluded 1,904 women aged 39 to 49 had to receive 10 annual mammography screenings to prevent one breast cancer death, resulting in potential overdiagnosis and radiation exposure among the remaining 1,903 women. Corresponding figures for women aged 50–59 and 60–69 were 1,339 and 377 respectively. USPSTF recommendations were as follows:[28]

- Because the additional benefit achieved by commencing screening at age 40 is small, and because harms are indisputable, routine screening of women in their 40s was not recommended.
- Consideration can be given to initiating biennial screening mammography in the 40s given particular patient values.
- Biennial screening for women 50 to 74 years of age is recommended.
- Current evidence is insufficient to assess benefits from screening women 75 and over.
- Teaching breast self-examination is not recommended and there is insufficient evidence to determine whether clinical breast examination is beneficial.
- Biennial screening achieves most of the benefit of annual screening with less harm.

Response to the USPSTF 2009 Guidelines

In response to the USPSTF guidelines the American College of Radiology declared that "two decades of decline in breast cancer mortality could be reversed and countless American women may die needlessly from breast cancer each year."[30] This statement conveniently ignored the evidence that breast cancer mortality has declined even in the absence of screening due to improved therapy.[31–33] The college additionally claimed that the USPSTF guidelines were "flawed, shocking and unconscionable." A radiologist and screening advocate stated that the USPSTF was telling women to wait until their breast cancers were so large they could no longer be ignored. Interestingly, the American College of Radiology has received donations of at least $1 million each from GE Healthcare and Siemens

AG. Both companies make mammography equipment and magnetic resonance imaging (MRI) scanners. The lobbying group that led the charge in Washington against the new USPSTF guidelines included GE Healthcare, Siemens, and the American College of Radiology, all of whom financially benefit from screening.[30] Although some radiologists were vehemently opposed to the revised screening recommendations, others had more reasonable responses to the USPSTF guidelines. Two radiologists concluded that the credentials of the task force were impeccable and that the response by the radiologic community was needlessly confrontational and not in the best interest of women seeking guidance for frequency of screening for breast cancer.[30]

Dr. Robert Aronowitz pointed out that those who most strongly advocate screening fail to acknowledge that the very small numbers of lives potentially saved by screening younger women are outweighed by the health risks, psychological stress, and financial costs of overdiagnosis. He concluded Americans are addicted to mammograms.[34] A news article in the *Journal of the National Cancer Institute* noted that the USPSTF 2009 conclusions were remarkably similar to those reached at a U.S. National Institutes of Health Consensus Development Conference in 1997. Then as now, the recommendations were repudiated.[35] A blunt warning was recently issued to the effect that obvious conflicts of interest should not be ignored in the "mammography wars" and that "vested interests" should not have the loudest voices.[36] Impartial multidisciplinary bodies such as the USPSTF and the Cochrane Collaboration offer the most objective evaluations of evidence.

Anomalies in Critiquing Trials

First let us consider two trials, Trial A and Trial B.

- Trial A has informed consent and individual randomization. Trial B has no informed consent and uses cluster randomization.
- Trial A maintains consistent numbers of participants and deaths over years of follow-up. Trial B does not.[20]
- Trial A has 100% compliance at first screen; not so for Trial B.
- Trial A used two-view mammography, Trial B single-view mammography.
- Trial A screens women every 12 months. Trial B screens every 33 months.
- Trial A has an external audit of mammography based on stratified sampling. Trial B does not.
- Trial A has a higher cancer detection rate with smaller tumor size at first screen than Trial B.[37]
- Trial A has external pathology reviews to confirm all biopsies performed. Trial B does not.
- Trial A has an external review panel to determine cause of death of each case known to have been diagnosed with breast cancer during the trial or suspected of having breast cancer after linkage with a national data base. Trial B did not.

Rationally one would expect that Trial A to be deemed superior to Trial B; however, such is not the case. Recently Trial B was described as flawless and meticulously conducted by a screening advocate. Trial A is the CNBSS and Trial B is the Two-County trial of Sweden, the two trials representing the two extremes of the screening controversy. The CNBSS showed a null effect of screening and the Two-County trial—even with only single-view mammography and a frequency of 33 months—showed the largest benefit of any trial. There were flaws in both trials; balanced criticism has been absent. Criticisms of the CNBSS continue even in 2010[38] with detailed counter-responses.[39]

Understanding how socioscientific controversy arises is important, not only in the case of breast screening but also for other issues such as whether there is or is not global climate change, or decades ago, whether smoking was related to lung cancer. Always there are two opposing views; some strongly advocate breast screening and others are more cautious. In this review I have shown first that a careful comparison of the CNBSS and the Swedish Two-County trial reveals how so-called flaws are differentially reported and second that a combined analysis of all screening studies by an impartial panel with diverse expertise shows only a small benefit for women in their 40s and a modest benefit for women 50 and older. But it is indisputable that this information is unwelcome or unknown to most of the public and to most physicians. And even when it is known, women regard the one chance in 2,000 of avoiding breast cancer death as very persuasive—much better than the usual odds in a lottery.

Are There Downsides of Mammography Screening?

Many are familiar with at least some of the downsides:

- False-positives, which can affect up to 30% of women who are screened multiple times in their 40s leading to unnecessary biopsies[40]
- False-negatives when a cancer diagnosis is delayed and the woman is falsely reassured (Mammography is never 100% accurate but is known to miss approximately 20% of invasive tumors.[41])
- Anxiety either before screening is scheduled or when a positive call is made on a mammogram

However, there are other downsides that have been more recently recognized:

- Overdiagnosis, represented by ductal carcinoma in situ, and constituting 25% and more of all screen-detected cancers leads to unnecessary treatment for breast cancer[23,40,42]
- An increase in mastectomies in screened women even though it was expected that screening would be followed by fewer mastectomies[20,43]
- The mortality paradox where more screened women aged 40–49 die of breast cancer in the first few years after screening is initiated, compared to controls although this excess is not statistically significant[5]

Overdiagnosis

Overdiagnosis of breast cancer occurs when the tumor is so indolent that it would never progress to cause problems. It is not misdiagnosis.[40,42] Recently it has been estimated that at least 25% of screen-detected breast cancers are overdiagnosed. In contrast to the disadvantages of false-positive screens, which are transitory, the downside of overdiagnosis is the lifelong adverse effects of treatment as well as the psychological burden affecting quality of life.[23]

The estimated proportion of cases overdiagnosed varies considerably. How did the concept of overdiagnosis arise? When the trials were being planned, it was predicted that in the screened group there would be an initial increased incidence of early stage breast cancer and that later there would be a corresponding decline in invasive cancer. In fact, U.S. Surveillance, Epidemiology and End Results data reveal that the expected correlation between an initial increase in early cancers and later decline in invasive cancers did not occur in the period 1983–2005. The early increase occurred, but there was no subsequent decline in advanced cancers.[40] Similar observations have been made in Europe.[20,42]

It would be helpful if the increased incidence of early cancer associated with screening explained declining mortality rates, but this does not appear to be the case. A Danish study compared breast cancer death rates in 20% of the Danish population who lived in counties where breast screening was offered to death rates in the 80% of the population who lived in counties where none was offered.[31] The authors examined data over the period 1971 to 2005.

Surprisingly, breast cancer deaths in the Danish population decreased in both screened and unscreened populations up to the age of 74. No decline was observed in women over 74. More surprising was that breast cancer deaths declined even in younger women who were ineligible for screening and who were not screened. Also of interest, breast cancer deaths were declining in the 10 years prior to initiation of screening. In fact a decline in breast cancer mortality rates in women too young to be screened has been observed in other jurisdictions.[32,33] Improved therapy and increased awareness account for these findings.

Excess Mastectomies

A review of eight screening trials concluded that screened women had a 20 to 30% significantly elevated risk of having a mastectomy compared to control women.[20] In light of the expectation that early detection would result in more conservative surgery, this is to some shocking. Others have reported similar observations.[43]

Mortality Paradox

More distressing than the null results observed in some screening trials for women aged 40–49 is the observation that for 10 or more years after screening begins, more breast cancer deaths occur in women who receive mammography screening than in the controls.[5,44] At 10-year follow-up, CNBSS results revealed a 14% statistically nonsignificant (but clearly paradoxical) excess of breast cancer deaths in screened women aged 40–49.[44] The Swedish Two-County trial when first reported in 1985 revealed a 26% excess breast cancer mortality in women ages 40 to 49 who were screened and an excess persisted until 10 years of follow-up were completed.[7] The paradoxical mortality excess in screened women is a generally observed and early phenomenon in screening trials[5] but it is rarely acknowledged. Surgical removal of a primary breast tumor from premenopausal women with involved lymph nodes may trigger the growth of temporarily dormant micrometastases in 20% of patients.[44,46] In this group of women, growth factors promoting wound healing after surgery could reasonably promote residual tumor growth.

Women may ask:

- How much does fear play into the screening controversy? Are the fears valid?
- Because breast cancer is a terrible disease, afflicting too many women including this author, is any effort to remediate it, no matter how limited, better than none?
- How much is screening advocacy by professionals associated with financial conflict of interest?

So What Should Women Do?

Women could remember that the major lesson to be learned from the breast screening controversy is the huge importance of critically appraising information. Les Irwig in his book *Smart Health Choices*[47] has suggested that women thinking about health choices should consider five factors:

1. What will happen if I wait and watch?
2. What are my test or treatment options?
3. What are the benefits and harms of these options?
4. How do the benefits and harms added up for me?
5. Do I have enough information to make a choice?

A very informative pamphlet for women who are considering mammography screening is now available in multiple languages.[48]

Finally, Peter Gøtzsche, Director of the Nordic Cochrane Center (personal communication), has wisely said: "It may be reasonable to attend for breast cancer screening with mammography, but it may also be reasonable not to attend as screening has both benefits and harms."

Discussion Questions

1. Why are clinical trials more appropriate than observational studies for evaluating the contribution of screening modalities to reduce breast cancer deaths?
2. Screening is often called "prevention." Is this accurate? How do you define cancer prevention?
3. How may age influence the contribution of mammographic screening to breast tumor detection?
4. Screening is scheduled at different frequencies in countries promoting mammography. What might explain these differing recommendations?

References

1. Henley SJ, King JB, German RR, et al. *MMWR Surveillance Summaries.* 2010:59:1–25.
2. Vainio H, Bianchini F. *Breast Cancer Screening.* Lyon, France: IARC Press; 2002. IARC Handbooks of Cancer Prevention; vol 7.
3. National Cancer Institute. Breast cancer screening (PDQ®). Harms of screening. www.cancer.gov/cancertopics/pdq/screening/breast/healthprofessional/Page6
4. Shapiro S. Evidence on screening for breast cancer from a randomized trial. *Cancer.* 1977;39:2772–2782.
5. Cox B. Variation in the effectiveness of breast screening by year of follow-up. *J Natl Cancer Inst Monogr.* 1997;22:69–72.
6. Andersson I, Aspegren K, Janzon L et al. Mammographic screening and mortality from breast cancer: the Malmö mammographic screening trial. *BMJ.* 1988;297:943–948.
7. Tabár L, Fagerberg G, Duffy SW et al. Update of the Swedish two county program of mammographic screening for breast cancer. *Radiol Clin North Am.* 1992;30:187–210.
8. Tabár L, Chen H-H, Fagerberg G, et al. Recent results from the Swedish two-county trial: the effects of age, histologic type and mode of detection on the efficacy of breast cancer screening. *J Natl Cancer Inst Monogr.* 1997;22:43–47.
9. Roberts MM, Alexander FE, Anderson TJ et al. Edinburgh trial of screening for breast cancer: mortality at seven years. *Lancet.* 1990;335:241–246.
10. Cunningham MP. The Breast Cancer Detection Project 25 years later. *CA Cancer J Physicians.* 1997;47(3):131–133.
11. Working Group. Report of the Working Group to Review the National Cancer Institute-American Cancer Society Breast Cancer Detection Demonstration Projects. *J Natl Cancer Inst.* 1979;62:639–709.
12. Baines CJ. Impediments to recruitment in the Canadian National Breast Screening Study: response and resolution. *Control Clin Trials.* 1984;5:129–140.
13. Miller AB, To T, Baines CJ, Wall C. The Canadian National Breast Screening Study-1:breast cancer mortality after 11–16 years of follow-up. A randomized screening trial of mammography in women age 40–49 years. *Ann Int Med.* 2002;137:305–312.
14. Miller AB, Baines CJ, To T, Wall C. The Canadian National Breast Screening Study-2. 13-year results of a randomized trial in women aged 50–59 years. *J Natl Cancer Inst.* 2000;92:1490–1499.
15. Baines CJ, To T. Changes in breast self-examination behaviour achieved by 89,835 participants in the Canadian National Breast Screening Study. *Cancer* 1990;66:295–298.
16. Harvey BJ, Miller AB, Baines CJ, Corey PN. Effect of breast self-examination techniques on the risk of death from breast cancer. *CMAJ.* 1997;157:1205–1212.
17. Frisell J, Eklund G, Hellstrom L, et al. Randomized study of mammographic screening—preliminary report in the Stockholm trial. *Breast Cancer Res Treat.* 1991;18:49–56.
18. Forrest, A.P., *Breast Cancer Screening: Report to the Health Minister of England, Wales, Scotland and Northern Ireland.* London, HMSO; 1986.
19. Moss SM, Cuckle H, Evans A et al. Effect of mammographic screening from age 40 years on breast cancer mortality at 10 years' follow-up: a randomized controlled trial. *Lancet.* 2006;368:2053–2060.
20. Gøtzsche PC, Nielsen M. Screening for breast cancer with mammography. *Cochrane Database Syst Rev.* 2011;1:CD001877.
21. Humphrey LL, Helfand M, Chan BK, Woolf SH. Breast cancer screening: a summary of the evidence for the U.S. Preventive Services Task Force. *Ann Intern Med.* 2002;137:347–369.
22. Nyström L, Andersson I, Bjurstam N, et al. Long-term effects of mammography screening: updated overview of the Swedish randomized trials. *Lancet.* 2002;359:909–919.
23. Welch GH, Black WC. Over-diagnosis in cancer. *J Natl Cancer Inst.* 2010;102:605–613.
24. Thomas DB, Gao DL, Self SG et al. Randomized trial of breast self-examination in Shanghai: methodology and preliminary results. *J Natl Cancer Inst.* 1997;89:355–365.
25. Semiglazov VF, Sagaidak VN, Moisyenko VM, Mikhailov EA. Study of the role of breast self-examination in the reduction of mortality from breast cancer: the Russian Federation/World Health Organization Study. *Eur J Cancer.* 1993;29A:2039–2046.
26. Baines CJ. Searching for the truth about breast cancer screening. *Can J Diagnosis.* 1993:95–103.
27. Fletcher SW. Whither scientific deliberation in health policy recommendations? Alice in the Wonderland of breast cancer screening. *N Engl J Med.* 1997;336:1180–1183.
28. US Preventive Services Task Force. Screening for breast cancer: US Preventive Services Task Force Recommendation Statement. *Ann Intern Med.* 2009;151:716–726.
29. Mandelblatt JS, Cronin KA, Bailey S et al. Effects of mammography screening under different screening schedules: model estimates of potential benefits and harms. *Ann Intern Med.* 2009;151:738–747.
30. Berlin L, Hall FM. More mammography muddle: emotions, politics, science, costs and polarization. *Radiology.* 2010;255:311–316.
31. Jørgensen KJ, Zahl P-H, Gøtzsche PC. Breast cancer mortality in organized mammography screening in Denmark: comparative study. *BMJ.* 2010;340:c1241 doi:10.1136/bmj.c1241.

32. Levi F, Bosetti C, Lucchini F, Negri E, Vecchia CL. Monitoring the decrease in breast cancer mortality in Europe. *Eur J Cancer Prev*. 2005;14:487–502.

33. Autier P, Boniol M, LaVecchia C et al. Disparities in breast cancer mortality trends between 30 European countries: retrospective trend analysis of WHO mortality database. *BMJ*. 2010;341:c3620 doi:10.aa36/bmj.c3620.

34. Aronowitz R. Addicted to mammograms. *The New York Times*, November 20, 2009.

35. Peres J. Mammography screenings: after the storm, calls for more personalized approaches. *J Natl Cancer Inst*. 2010;102:9–11.

36. Quanstrum KH, Hayward RA. Sounding board: lessons from the mammography wars. *N Engl J Med*. 2010;363:1076–1079.

37. Narod SA. On being the right size: a reappraisal of mammography trials in Canada and Sweden. *Lancet*. 1997;349:1869.

38. Kopans DB. Why the critics of screening mammography are wrong: they distort data, rely on weak science, but refuse to defend when challenged. *Diagnostic Imaging*. 2009;31:18–24.

39. Baines CJ. Rational and irrational issues in breast cancer screening. *Cancers* 2011;3(1):252–266. doi:10.3390/cancers3010252

40. Croswell JM, Ransohoff DF, Kramer BS. Principles of cancer screening: lessons from history and study design issues. *Sem Oncology*. 2010;37:202–215.

41. Kopans DB. Detecting breast cancer not visible by mammography (Editorial) *J Natl Cancer Inst*. 1992;84:745–747.

42. Jorgensen KJ, Gøtzsche PC. Overdiagnosis in publicly organised mammography screening programmes: systematic review of incidence trends. *BMJ*. 2009;339:b2587.

43. Dixon JM. Breast screening has increased the number of mastectomies. *Breast Cancer Res*. 2009;11(suppl 3):S19.

44. Baines CJ. Mammography screening: are women really giving informed consent? *J Natl Cancer Inst*. 2003;95:1508–1511.

45. Miller AB, To T, Baines CJ, Wall C. The Canadian Breast Screening Study: update on breast cancer mortality. *J Natl Cancer Inst Monogr*. 1997;22:37–41.

46. Retsky M, Demicheli R, Hrushesky W. Premenopausal status accelerates relapse in node positive breast cancer: hypothesis links angiogenesis, screening controversy. *Breast Cancer Res Treat*. 2001;65:217–224.

47. Irwig L, Irwig J, Trevena L, Sweet M. *Smart Health Choices: Making Sense of Health Advice*. London: Hammersmith Press; 2007. http://sydney.edu.au/medicine/public-health/shdg/resources/smart_health_choices.php

48. Screening for breast cancer with mammography published by The Nordic Cochrane Centre 2012. Available at: http://www.cochrane.dk/screening/mammography-leaflet.pdf

The Future Role of Genetics in Women's Health Research and Clinical Care

Wendy Chung, MD, PhD

Introduction

In the over 50 years since the structure of DNA was described by Watson and Crick, there have been remarkable advances in our understanding of the genetic basis for human variation and disease. As of 2007, research had defined the genetic basis for more than 2,600 monogenic human disorders, and clinical genetic tests were available for over 1,500 conditions.[1] Despite the remarkable advances in our scientific understanding of genetics, the impact of such information on medical care for common clinical conditions has been modest. With the complete sequence of the human genome and many other model organisms, as well as detailed characterization of the human haplotype structure, which has stimulated large-scale genomewide association studies for virtually all diseases with any heritable component, scientists are beginning to understand the complex genetic basis for common diseases such as macular degeneration,[2–8] obesity,[9] hypertension,[10] coronary artery disease,[11] inflammatory bowel disease,[12,13] breast cancer,[14] and Alzheimer's disease.[15] As these scientific discoveries unfold, physicians are being challenged on how to clinically integrate this new information into routine patient care to improve health and quality of life in a cost-effective, socially acceptable manner. Early adopters of this new genetic information are providing invaluable experience to guide future implementation strategies.

This chapter reviews the current and projected future use of genetics and genomics in clinical medicine to (1) refine treatment for diagnosed conditions; (2) prevent disease, based on both family history and population-based genetic testing; and (3) define the steps to overcome patient, healthcare provider, and third-party payer hurdles to allow successful integration of genetic medicine to improve the quality of health care. Limitations based on our current scientific understanding and realistic expectations are also explored.

Genetic Stratification that Enables Personalized Medical Care after Diagnosis

In what way will germline genomic variation (present in all cells of the body and transmitted to future generations) be clinically used? There are emerging data suggesting that genetic stratification of phenotypically similar diseases has important therapeutic implications. Genetic characterization after an initial diagnosis may clarify prognosis and response to therapy. The following four examples illustrate this point.

Hereditary Breast/Ovarian Cancer (HBOC)

Hereditary breast/ovarian cancer syndrome has variable expression and can present in families with breast cancer only, ovarian cancer only, or with both breast and ovarian cancers. HBOC should be considered when two or more first-degree relatives have breast and/or ovarian cancer, especially if diagnosis occurred before age 40, if cancer is multifocal or bilateral, if breast and ovarian cancer occur in the same individual, and if a male in the family is diagnosed with breast cancer. In addition, Ashkenazi Jewish ancestry is associated with a higher prevalence of breast and ovarian cancers resulting from HBOC.

The two major HBOC cancer susceptibility genes identified, *BRCA1* and *BRCA2*, are tumor suppressor genes that are autosomal dominantly inherited. Mutations in *BRCA1* and *BRCA2* are characterized by high lifetime risks for development of breast cancer (55 to 85%) and ovarian cancer (20 to 44%)[16] (Figure 41-1), as well as more limited increased risks of prostate cancer, colon cancer, pancreatic cancer, melanoma, male breast cancer, and other cancers.[17,18] More than 2,000 distinct pathogenic mutations have been identified in these two genes. There are founder mutations in certain populations, such as the Ashkenazim,[19,20] Dutch,[21,22] Icelandics,[23] and French Canadians.[23] Importantly, among Ashkenazi Jewish individuals one of the three founder mutations, 185delAG and 5382insC in *BRCA1* and 6174delT in *BRCA2*, accounts for 20 to 35% of early-onset breast cancer and ovarian cancer at any age in Ashkenazi women.[18] In other populations found to carry germline *BRCA1* and *BRCA2* mutations, these susceptibility genes account for only 5 to 10% of young patients with breast cancer or ovarian cancer.[24,25]

DNA-based testing for *BRCA1* and *BRCA2* cancer-predisposing mutations is available on a clinical basis for individuals identified by personal or family history to be at increased risk for having a germline *BRCA1/BRCA2* mutation and for at-risk relatives of an individual with an

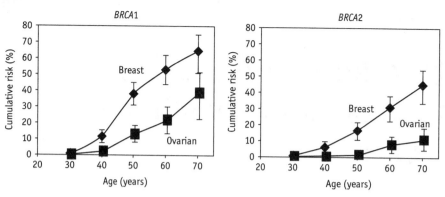

Figure 41-1 Cumulative BRCA-related risk of breast and ovarian cancer.

Source: Reproduced from Antoniou A, Pharoah PDP, Narod S, et al. Average risks of breast and ovarian cancers associated with BRCA1 or BRCA2 mutations detected in case series unselected for family history: a combined analysis of 22 studies. *Am J Human Genetics.* 2003;72:1117–1130, with permission from Elsevier.

identified *BRCA1/BRCA2* mutation. At present, the available clinical testing includes direct sequence analysis of all coding exons and splice sites and analysis of common deletions. More extensive assessment for deletions, duplications, and complex rearrangements in *BRCA1* and *BRCA2* called BART testing (*BRCA* Analysis Rearrangement Test) became available in 2007, but is only performed by request or reflexively for patients with normal *BRCA1/BRCA2* sequence and a high pretest probability of carrying a mutation, such as families with breast and ovarian cancer or three or more relatives with premenopausal breast cancer. Current clinical testing is estimated to have an analytical sensitivity of at least 90%. There can be false negatives due to limitations of testing methodology or parts of genes such as regulatory regions and introns that are not analyzed. False positives rarely occur and would be the result of a sample switch.

Given the substantially increased risk of breast, ovarian, and other cancers in HBOC, the management of individuals with *BRCA1/BRCA2* cancer-predisposing mutations includes discussion of enhanced cancer screening protocols, chemoprevention strategies, and options for prophylactic mastectomy and/or salpingo-oophorectomy. None of these strategies has been assessed by randomized clinical trials or case-control studies in high-risk women, and current recommendations are made on the basis retrospective studies and expert clinical opinion.

Recommendations of the National Comprehensive Cancer Network[26] for breast and ovarian cancer screening specifically for women with a *BRCA1/BRCA2* mutation are listed in Table 41-1.

Chemoprevention strategies should be discussed with *BRCA1/BRCA2* mutation carriers. The efficacy of tamoxifen for breast cancer risk reduction in women with *BRCA1* and *BRCA2* mutations is controversial. Although a randomized clinical trial of treatment with tamoxifen in women identified by the Gail breast cancer risk model indicated a 49% reduction in breast cancer among treated women,[27] tamoxifen was found to reduce the incidence of breast cancers that were estrogen-receptor positive but not estrogen-receptor negative. Because breast cancers occurring in women with *BRCA1* mutations are more likely to be estrogen-receptor negative, it is difficult to estimate the benefit of tamoxifen prophylaxis in *BRCA1* carriers, although there does appear to be some benefit. It is possible that premalignant lesions in *BRCA1* carrier are estrogen responsive and amenable to tamoxifen prophylaxis at least at some point during the premalignant phase. Oral contraceptives reduce the risk of ovarian cancer in women with *BRCA1* or *BRCA2* mutations who used contraceptive pills for more than 3 years.[28]

Because early detection does not prevent cancer, it is necessary to discuss the options of risk-reducing surgery including prophylactic mastectomy and prophylactic

---

Table 41-1

Recommendations of the National Comprehensive Cancer Network for cancer screening of individuals with a BRCA1/BRCA2 mutation

Breast Cancer Screening

- Breast self-exam training and education starting at age 18 years.
- Clinical breast exam, every 6-12 months, starting at age 25 years.
- Annual mammogram and breast MRI screening starting at age 25 years, or individualized based on earliest age of onset in family.

Ovarian Cancer Screening

- Consider concurrent transvaginal ultrasound (preferably day 1–10 of menstrual cycle in premenopausal women) + CA-125 (preferably after day 5 of menstrual cycle in premenopausal women) every 6 months starting at age 30 years or 5–10 years before the earliest age of first diagnosis of ovarian cancer in the family.

---

salpingo-oophorectomy. Tissue removed prophylactically should be carefully examined for malignancy, a finding that could alter medical management. At the time of prophylactic oophorectomy, ovarian or fallopian tube cancer is detected in 2–5% of cases. Theoretical modeling and epidemiologic studies suggest that prophylactic surgeries do significantly decrease the risk of developing these cancers by greater than 90% but do not completely eliminate all cancer risk. Prophylactic mastectomy can be effectively performed with skin-sparing procedures enabling breast reconstruction. Prophylactic mastectomy can also be performed with nipple preservation although this procedure has a higher residual risk of breast cancer.

Prophylactic oophorectomy decreases the risk of breast cancer by up to 50% if performed before age of 40 and not followed by hormone replacement. However, hormone replacement after bilateral oophorectomy for a short period of time is acceptable in women without a history of breast cancer and should not significantly increase the risk of breast cancer above the baseline in *BRCA1* and *BRCA2* mutation carriers. Another treatment options for consideration is total abdominal hysterectomy to either decrease the risk of endometrial cancer if tamoxifen is considered or to use unopposed estrogens for hormone replacement, which may be associated with less breast cancer risk than estrogen combined with progesterone. Even after prophylactic oophorectomy and removal of unaffected ovaries, a small residual risk of primary peritoneal cancer remains.

Many women with diagnosed breast or ovarian cancer are appropriate candidates for genetic testing to guide medical and surgical decisions. Women with breast cancer due to mutations in *BRCA1/BRCA2* have an increased risk for a second primary malignancy, usually in the opposite breast or ovaries, for which increased surveillance, chemoprevention, or prophylactic surgery are recommended.[29]

Women with a mutation may choose more aggressive surgical options, including mastectomy rather than lumpectomy or contralateral prophylactic mastectomy.

Genetic status may also be used in making decisions about chemotherapy (Figure 41-2). Women with a *BRCA1* mutation are likely to derive relatively more benefit from chemotherapy and may decrease the relative risk of cancer related death by 50% compared to mutation negative women with breast cancer.[30] In addition, new molecularly based therapies of poly ADR ribose polymerase (PARP) inhibitors are in phase II clinical trials[31] and are being specifically targeted for *BRCA1/2* mutation carriers, taking advantage of the cancer cells' inherent susceptibility to cell death due to defective double-stranded break repair.

Hereditary Nonpolyposis Colon Cancer

Hereditary nonpolyposis colon cancer (HNPCC) or Lynch syndrome is an autosomal dominantly inherited predisposition to colon carcinoma that is not associated with polyposis, or the finding of hundreds of polyps. Several other types of cancer can also be associated with HNPCC including endometrial, small intestinal, ovarian, stomach, urinary tract, and brain cancer[32-34] HNPCC is genetically heterogeneous and involves inactivating mutations in one of several mismatch repair genes including *MHS2*, *MLH1*, *MSH6*, *PMSl*, and *PMS2*. Mutations in *MSH2* and *MLH1* account for 31% and 33% of families with HNPCC.[35]

Identification of the underlying genetic basis for HNPCC revealed a new mechanism of cancer progression with hypermutability leading to accumulation of changes in the DNA that ultimately lead to uncontrolled cell growth and division. This hypermutability can be detected in colonic polyps as acquired microsatellite instability (MSI), resulting from mutations of simple repetitive elements (usually dinucleotide repeats) called microsatellites. This

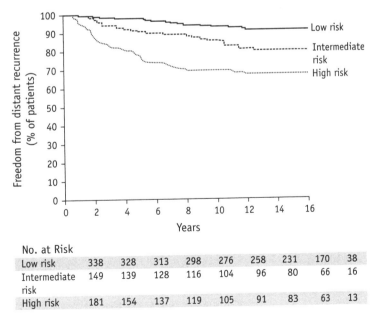

No. at Risk									
Low risk	338	328	313	298	276	258	231	170	38
Intermediate risk	149	139	128	116	104	96	80	66	16
High risk	181	154	137	119	105	91	83	63	13

Figure 41-2 Predicting breast cancer recurrence.

Source: Reproduced from Paik S, Shak S, Tang G, et al. A multigene assay to predict recurrence of tamoxifen-treated, node-negative breast cancer. *N Engl J Med.* 2004;351:2817–2826. © 2004 Massachusetts Medical Society. All rights reserved.

hypermutability leaves cells susceptible to the accumulation of pathogenic mutations that ultimately lead to neoplasia. Clinical criteria, called the Amsterdam criteria,[36] define the components required for diagnosis of Lynch syndrome. These are more liberal than Bethesda criteria as they emphasize that women with an early age of diagnosis (age younger than 45), with multiple synchronous or metachronous HNPCC-related cancers, multiple close family members with HNPCC-related cancers, right-sided colon cancers, and colon cancer with specific pathological features including signet ring morphology, lymphocytic infiltrate, and mucinous features are more likely to have HNPCC. Once a clinical diagnosis has been made, genetic testing can be used for risk assessment of unaffected members of the family, and the utility of genetic testing has been validated by Evaluation of Genomic Applications in Practice and Prevention (EGAPP).[37] Screening for HNPCC can also be directly performed on the tumor by testing the tissue for MSI or lack of immunohistochemistry (IHC) for *MHS2*, *MLH1*, and *MSH6*. The most sensitive and efficient method to identify symptomatic HNPCC mutation carriers has not yet been rigorously validated[37] Some IHC tumors will be negative due to epigenetic changes rather than germline mutations, so IHC should be considered only a screening test and may be followed by germline testing or other molecular tests on the tumor for the *BRAF* somatic mutation V600E that is almost never present in HNPCC carriers.[38]

The clinical manifestations of HNPCC are sex dependent. Men with HNPCC mutations are most likely to develop colon cancer, whereas women with HNPCC mutations are most likely to develop endometrial cancer. The lifetime risk of endometrial cancer has been estimated at 61% and 42% for *MSH2* and *MLH1* mutations, respectively[39] compared with the population risk of 3%. The median age of endometrial cancer diagnosis is 46 years.[33] The relative risk for other extracolonic HNPCC associated cancers is 4.1 to 4.4 for stomach, 6.4 to 8.0 for ovarian, 103 to 292 for small intestinal, and 75.3 for renal and ureteral.[39] The relative risk varies somewhat depending on the specific gene implicated. Identification of patients with

HNPCC is important because of the high probability of a metachronous cancer after successful treatment of the first neoplasm. Prognosis of colon cancer is however no worse and may be somewhat better with HNPCC-associated colon cancer. Presymptomatic mutation carriers should follow a cancer surveillance protocol consisting of colorectal cancer surveillance and endometrial carcinoma screening starting at the age of 25 to 35. There is no consensus about the optimal method of endometrial carcinoma screening, but ultrasound and endometrial biopsy are usually done on an annual basis. Ovarian cancer screening consists of annual CA-125 and transvaginal ultrasound, but it is not associated with decreased mortality. Therefore, mutation carriers may consider prophylactic total hysterectomy to maximally reduce their cancer risk once childbearing is complete. Screening methods and frequency for other HNPCC-associated cancers has not yet been standardized but is dependent upon whether or not there is a family history of those other related cancers.

Long QT Syndrome: Genetic Testing Can Guide Therapy and Risk Stratification

Long QT syndrome (LQTS) is an autosomal dominantly inherited predisposition to cardiac arrhythmias, characterized by a prolonged QT interval on an electrocardiogram, that are associated with syncope and sudden cardiac death. Currently, there are 12 different genetically identified causes of LQTS, all affecting cardiac ion channel conductance, that are clinically difficult to distinguish. The three most common forms of LQTS (LQT1, LQT2, and LQT3) have specific triggers for arrhythmias that can be avoided, such as exercise-induced tachycardia in LQT1 and auditory stimuli during sleep in LQT2 (Figure 41-3).[40] Specific molecular-based pharmacologic intervention is also now available. Patients with LQT3, caused by mutations in the cardiac sodium channel gene *SCN5A* that inappropriately activate and open the sodium channel, respond to sodium channel blockers such as flecainide.[41] LQT3 patients are more likely to have arrhythmias at times of bradycardia. However, β-blockers have historically been routinely prescribed for all patients with LQTS and are effective for

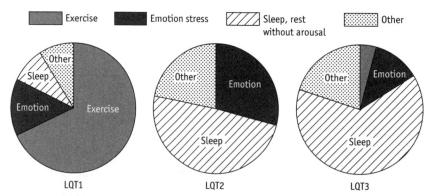

This study identified patients of a known genotype who experienced significant cardiac events. The pattern of triggers differed by genotype.

Figure 41-3 Gene-specific triggers for Long QT cardiac events.

Source: Adapted from Schwartz PJ, Priori SG, Spazzolini C, et al. Genotype-phenotype correlation in the Long-QT syndrome. *Circulation*. 2001;103:89–95.

LQTS1, but may by counterproductive for LQT3 because they induce bradycardia. Therefore, identifying the molecular subtype of LQTS allows for the selection of the most appropriate medication, avoidance of specific triggers. Risk of sudden cardiac death can be stratified by type of long QT, age, gender, maximal QT interval, and number of episodes of syncope or cardiac arrest within the prior 2 years.[42] Women with LQT2 are generally at higher risk than men, and the postpartum period is a time of particular vulnerability.[43] The level of risk may be used clinically to guide placement of Automatic Implantable Cardiac Defibrillators (AICDs) in appropriate candidates for either primary or secondary prevention.

Maturity Onset Diabetes of the Young: Prognostic Information obtained from Genetic Testing May Guide Management

A rare autosomal dominantly inherited form of diabetes termed maturity onset diabetes of the young (MODY) is genetically heterogeneous and caused by mutations in eight different genes. Women with MODY often are diagnosed by an oral glucose tolerance test during pregnancy and are thought to have gestational diabetes, but without resolution after delivery. Prognosis, including diabetic complications, for patients with mutations in glucokinase (MODY2) is more optimistic than for other forms of MODY. Molecular diagnosis can now provide reassurance that tight glycemic control is unnecessary to prevent diabetic complications specifically in MODY2 patients, who will remain only mildly hyperglycemic.[44] In addition, patients with mutations in hepatocyte nuclear transcription factor 1α (MODY3) are extremely sensitive to sulfonylureas, and this information may assist with pharmacologic management.[45] Identification of the mutation within a family can be used to identify relatives at increased risk and to provide guidance for medical management of the index patient.

Population-Based Germline Genomic Screening

Rather than waiting until a diagnosis is made, genetic variation can be used to prevent disease. Population-based genetic screening could provide the opportunity to improve health outcomes by disease prevention and increased surveillance to facilitate early diagnosis. It would allow population stratification to identify individuals at increased risk who are most likely to benefit from preventative medications or interventions for which population-based therapy would not be appropriate because of potential adverse effects of treatment and cost. Data to support an individual's susceptibility to disease may provide the necessary motivation to increase compliance with recommended health behaviors, such as routine exercise and weight control for individuals at increased risk for diabetes and smoking cessation for those at risk of emphysema due to alpha 1 antitrypsin deficiency. Screening those at risk for adverse effects from specific environmental exposures would allow susceptible individuals to modify their work or home environment to minimize exposure. Screening individuals for adverse pharmacologic reactions would provide a rational basis for drug selection and avoid harmful adverse effects. Such a strategy would ultimately increase the total number of drugs available for clinical use and decrease the cost of drug development by identifying and eliminating drug exposure in the small number of patients who would have adversely responded to the medication.

The genetic basis for most common diseases is, however, complex, involving multiple genetic variants and interactions with the environment. Researchers are only beginning to catalog the genetic variants that predispose humans to common diseases, many of which have modest individual effects on disease risk. A flurry of recent publications on genomewide associations are now providing replicated data identifying common variants for common diseases such as type 2 diabetes mellitus (DM),[5,6,8] obesity,[9] and breast cancer.[14] These studies include as many as 40,000 subjects and multiple replication sets and highlight the need for large numbers of subjects to identify and confirm genetic susceptibility to common diseases. The genetic variants identified in these studies confer a modest relative risk of disease less than RR = 2. A composite panel may be necessary to identify multiple susceptibility/protective alleles linked with individual patient characteristics such as gender, weight, and biomarker data—to accurately predict risk for common diseases. Although a future goal of genomic medicine is to provide accurate population-based risk stratification for most common variants of common diseases, in fact, studies using common genetic variants of modest risk have failed to predict risk of diabetes any better than routine clinical risk factors currently in practice.[46] Nevertheless, several companies such as 23andMe (https://www.23andme.com/), Navigenics (http://www.navigenics.com/), and deCODEme (http://www.decodeme.com/) have launched direct-to-consumer tests designed to identify future risk for common diseases including cancers, diabetes, and Alzheimer's disease.

Population-based screening holds great promise, but it is important to ensure that both natural history and clinical utility have been adequately defined before these procedures are introduced into clinical care. For example, consider the case of hereditary hemochromatosis (HH). This condition is autosomal recessively inherited and therefore runs in families and can produce common symptoms including diabetes, depression, and heart failure. Two common mutations in a single gene, *HFE*, account for most of the autosomal recessively inherited HH in Europeans.[47] Furthermore, because the complications of HH are completely preventable by reducing iron stores through phlebotomy (which is inexpensive), presymptomatic screening for HH could be clinically useful. With a frequency of 1 in 400 white individuals carrying one or both of the two common mutations in *HFE*, large-scale population-based screening is technically feasible. When many experts considered introducing HH screening on a population-wide basis, it became increasingly apparent that the natural history of mutation carriers was incompletely understood, and that the disease penetrance was less than 1%[48] and was reduced in women compared with men, owing to menstrual blood losses. Although population-based screening for HH may still have clinical utility when coupled with iron studies, the frequency of clinical manifestation with a positive genetic test is lower than had once been anticipated, dramatically altering the cost-to-benefit ratio, especially for women.

Population based genetic screening is being used for reproductive purposes for women. All women trying to conceive or currently pregnant are offered carrier testing for the autosomal recessive condition cystic fibrosis and are screened for hemoglobinopathies. In addition, women of Ashkenazi Jewish descent are screened for Tay-Sachs disease and as many as 14 other recessive conditions of increased prevalence in the Ashkenazim. This list has frequently expanded as additional founder mutations for recessive conditions are identified and are easily added to the screening panel.

Pharmacogenomics

Screening for variation in drug metabolism and adverse effects, termed *pharmacogenomics*, may permit safer and more efficacious use of drugs. There is heritable variation in drug metabolism that alters the levels of active drugs and metabolites, thereby producing differential therapeutic effect and toxicity in different patients receiving the same dose of medication, due to differences in drug levels. There are also genetic differences in drug targets that may differentiate responders from nonresponders. Pharmacogenomic variation is common within the population and affects the majority of patients taking medications.[49] Approximately 20% to 40% of patients do not respond to medications commonly prescribed for hypertension, depression, and diabetes.[49] With genetic characterization of the genes involved in drug metabolism and drug action, it should be possible to more accurately predict the dosage of medication required to remain in the therapeutic window and circumvent the current practice of trial and error that results in harmful adverse effects and delayed time to effective treatment. Pharmacogenetics can be used to accurately define patients at high risk of adverse outcomes, such as hypersensitivity to abacavir for treatment of HIV in HLA-B*5701 carriers, and allowed resurrection of this nucleoside inhibitor that otherwise would not have been approved by the Food and Drug Administration due to the serious adverse consequences.[50] There are now clinically available diagnostic panels for some drugs. For some medications (e.g., warfarin and irinotecan), package inserts now contain dosing information specific to the predicted metabolizing phenotype.

Anticoagulation therapy is common, with 31 million outpatients treated in 2004,[51] and can prove difficult. Empiric dose determination is required to determine the correct dose of warfarin to simultaneously prevent thrombophilia and bleeding. Unfortunately, while the dose of warfarin is being adjusted, ~29,000 patients will have bleeding complications requiring emergency room visits. Pharmacogenomic assays for the both the warfarin-metabolizing gene *CYP2C9* and the target vitamin K receptor *VKORC1* are now available clinically and may be useful, in conjunc-

tion with other known variables affecting warfarin dosing (age, sex, weight, ethnicity, diabetes, smoker status), to select an initial dose and minimize the length of time to achieve the therapeutic target.[52,53] To determine the efficacy of including the *CYP2C9* and *VKORC1* genotypes in dosing, prospective randomized controlled clinical trials[54,55] are now ongoing for patients beginning chronic warfarin therapy for atrial fibrillation, deep vein thrombosis, or postorthopedic surgery prophylaxis. These studies will provide the data necessary to determine the efficacy of using patients' genotypes to more efficiently dose warfarin within its narrow therapeutic window.

Within the field of oncology, several widely used medications are known to have common polymorphisms in genes that metabolize the drugs that can produce toxic adverse effects. Irinotecan, 5-fluorouracil, 6-mercaptopurine, and methotrexate have common mutations/polymorphisms in the drug-metabolizing genes dihydropyrimidine dehydrogenase,[56] UDP-glycosyltransferase I,[57] thiopurine methyltransferase,[58] and 5,10-methylenetetrahydrofolate reductase,[59] respectively. Mutations in these genes are associated with toxicity that can be easily screened at any time before administration of the medication. Genetic variation in *CYP2D6* and *SULT1A1* determines in part the levels of the active metabolite of tamoxifen and may in the future be used to determine dose of tamoxifen or which patients should receive an aromatase inhibitor rather than tamoxifen for breast cancer.[60] In the future, each patient may have a unique pharmacogenetic profile for drug-metabolizing genes in their electronic medical record that will automatically either warn prescribers against or for prescribing certain medications or suggest altered dosing.

Using pharmacogenomics to rationally select the appropriate medication at the correct dose to prevent and treat disease should be economically efficient, with less money spent on ineffective drugs or drug doses, fewer adverse outcomes and complications, and an increased number of medications that may safely be prescribed to properly screened patients. However, before pharmacogenomic testing can be effectively used clinically, more data are necessary from randomized controlled clinical trials to determine the efficacy, utility, and algorithms for using genotypes in combination with standard clinical parameters for appropriate selection and dosing of medications.

Somatic Genomic Variation

In addition to testing for heritable germline genetic characteristics, characterizing somatic variation in tumor specimens is now common practice. Cancer treatment is likely to be rapidly redefined with genomic characterization of tumors, using a combination of comparative genomic hybridization, quantification of gene amplifications/deletions, identification of acquired genetic mutations, and gene expression profiling. Targeted medications with fewer adverse effects will be more forthcoming as we rationally develop drugs based on specific molecular targets. Examples already include the tyrosine kinase inhibitor imatinib mesylate for chronic myelogenous leukemia and gastrointestinal stromal tumors that overexpress the tyrosine kinases, trastuzumab for HER2 overexpressing breast cancer, and gefitinib for activating mutations in epidermal growth factor receptor for non-small cell lung cancer.[61] These medications offer the possibility of increased efficacy, and their use critically relies on accurate molecular tumor characterization to identify the subset of patients who will likely respond to these expensive therapies. Another form of genomic tumor characterization is also available: a limited expression profiling array of genes for estrogen-receptor positive, node-negative, stage 1 or 2 breast cancer (Oncotype Dx, Genomic Health, Inc., Redwood City, California and MammaPrint, Agendia, Huntington Beach, California). The expression profiles quantify the likelihood of breast cancer recurrence in women with newly diagnosed, early-stage breast cancer and assesses the benefit of chemotherapy with a numerical scoring system (Figure 41-2).[62] The ability to simply numerically quantify and integrate complex genomic information facilitates physician and patient communication and understanding, and enables them to make more rational decisions about therapy. Multiple oncology clinical trials are currently in progress to determine both the precise algorithms by which expression profiles will be weighted and analyzed and the clinical utility for prognosis and treatment efficacy.[63] It is likely that more clinically relevant diagnostic tools to assist with oncologic management will be available for multiple tumor types.

Novel Sources of Genomic Variation

In addition to the nuclear germline and somatic mutations resulting from alteration in one or a small number of nucleotides, there are additional sources of genomic variation the clinical significance of which is not yet fully appreciated. Human genomic architecture and variation are now being characterized.[64] Previously undetected variation in the copy number of genes will underlie a significant fraction of birth defects, mental retardation, and autism.[65,67] Oligonucleotide microarrays are now offered prenatally to provide greater resolution than is available using standard methods for karyotyping. It is likely that chromosome microarrays will soon supplant the karyotype for invasive prenatal testing for chromosomal disorders. However, we still have much to learn about the normal genomic architecture and the range of phenotypes associated with these genetic copy number variants. It is also possible that copy number variation increases susceptibility to common psychiatric, neurological, and medical conditions.[68] Clinical trials are currently underway evaluating chromosome microarrays in the prenatal setting and will provide the foundation of experience for future clinical implementation.

Genetic Information Nondiscrimination Act

Some patients have concerns about the misuse of their genetic information. The Genetic Information Nondiscrimination Act passed by Congress in 2008 and in effect in 2009, provided Americans with protection against discrimination in employment and health insurance underwriting of group and individual health care policies.[69] However, the law does not protect individuals against discrimination in life insurance, long-term disability, or long-term care insurance. To date, there have been no documented legal cases of health insurance discrimination on the basis of genetic predisposition that have not been settled in the patient's interest.

Summary

We will increasingly be able to determine our susceptibility to disease and the susceptibility of our future children. Steps have become available to effectively intervene in disease prevention, with lifestyle changes, pharmacologic interventions, and increased surveillance to improve health outcomes and decrease adverse effects. However, realistic expectations require adequate time to complete research before implementing these improvements in genetic medicine. Clinical validation and utility take time but should be rigorously demonstrated through clinical trials and evidence-based revised by working groups such as Evaluation of Genomic Applications in Practice and Prevention (EGAPP) before clinical implementation. This will not happen as quickly as some might expect, and fostering unrealistic public expectations will surely lead to disappointment. Improvements in technologies to characterize our genes will drive down the cost of genetic characterization to the ultimate goal of the $1,000 genome, leading to a bottleneck of insufficient numbers of clinically well-characterized patients to robustly demonstrate the associations between genetic variants and health and disease and demonstrate clinical utility. However, investing now in collection of DNA specimens on clinically well-characterized cohorts will provide an unprecedented opportunity to improve the future of individualized medical care.

Discussion Questions

1. Name several common conditions for which genetic analyses have already contributed to clinical care. How has knowing mutation status affected treatment?
2. How may individual patients benefit from personal knowledge of their family history of diseases? What may be recommended for affected and unaffected relatives?
3. Given the future role of genetics in the health of women and the many chronic conditions discussed in this textbook, can you anticipate population-based benefits from the genomic era?

Acknowledgment

Josue Martinez provided assistance with manuscript preparation.

References

1. University of Washington. GeneTests. 2007. http://www.genetests.org/. Accessed August 28, 2007.
2. Edwards AO, Ritter R, 3rd, Abel KJ, Manning A, Panhuysen C, Farrer LA. Complement factor H polymorphism and age-related macular degeneration. *Science*. 2005;308:421–424.

3. Haines JL, Hauser MA, Schmidt S, et al. Complement factor H variant increases the risk of age-related macular degeneration. *Science*. 2005; 308:419–421.

4. Klein RJ, Zeiss C, Chew EY, et al. Complement factor H polymorphism in age-related macular degeneration. *Science*. 2005;308:385–389.

5. Saxena R, Voight BF, Lyssenko V, et al. Genome-wide association analysis identifies loci for type 2 diabetes and triglyceride levels. *Science*. 2007;316:1331–1336.

6. Scott LJ, Mohlke KL, Bonnycastle LL, et al. A genome-wide association study of type 2 diabetes in Finns detects multiple susceptibility variants. *Science*. 2007;316:1341–1345.

7. Yates JR, Sepp T, Matharu BK, et al. Complement C3 variant and the risk of age-related macular degeneration. *N Engl J Med*. 2007;357:553–561.

8. Zeggini E, Weedon MN, Lindgren CM, et al. Replication of genome-wide association signals in UK samples reveals risk loci for type 2 diabetes. *Science*. 2007;316:1336–1341.

9. Frayling TM, Timpson NJ, Weedon MN, et al. A common variant in the FTO gene is associated with body mass index and predisposes to childhood and adult obesity. *Science*. 2007;316:889–894.

10. Hamet P, Seda O. Current status of genome-wide scanning for hypertension. *Curr Opin Cardiol*. 2007;22:292–297.

11. McPherson R, Pertsemlidis A, Kavaslar N, et al. A common allele on chromosome 9 associated with coronary heart disease. *Science*. 2007;316:1488–1491.

12. Duerr RH, Taylor KD, Brant SR, et al. A genome-wide association study identifies IL23R as an inflammatory bowel disease gene. *Science*. 2006;314:1461–1463.

13. Hampe J, Franke A, Rosenstiel P, et al. A genome-wide association scan of nonsynonymous SNPs identifies a susceptibility variant for Crohn disease in ATG16L1. *Nature Genetics*. 2007;39:207–211.

14. Easton DF, Pooley KA, Dunning AM, et al. Genome-wide association study identifies novel breast cancer susceptibility loci. *Nature*. 2007;447:1087–1093.

15. Coon KD, Myers AJ, Craig DW, et al. A high-density whole-genome association study reveals that APOE is the major susceptibility gene for sporadic late-onset Alzheimer's disease. *J Clin Psychiatry*. 2007;68:613–618.

16. Antoniou A, Pharoah PD, Narod S, et al. Average risks of breast and ovarian cancer associated with BRCA1 or BRCA2 mutations detected in case Series unselected for family history: a combined analysis of 22 studies. *Am J Hum Genet*. 2003;72:1117–1130.

17. Ford D, Easton DF, Bishop DT, Narod SA, Goldgar DE. Risks of cancer in BRCA1-mutation carriers. Breast Cancer Linkage Consortium. *Lancet*. 1994;343:692–695.

18. Struewing JP, Hartge P, Wacholder S, et al. The risk of cancer associated with specific mutations of BRCA1 and BRCA2 among Ashkenazi Jews. *N Engl J Med*. 1997;336:1401–1408.

19. Oddoux C, Struewing JP, Clayton CM, et al. The carrier frequency of the BRCA2 6174delT mutation among Ashkenazi Jewish individuals is approximately 1%. *Nat Genet*. 1996;14:188–190.

20. Roa BB, Boyd AA, Volcik K, Richards CS. Ashkenazi Jewish population frequencies for common mutations in BRCA1 and BRCA2. *Nat Genet*. 1996;14:185–187.

21. Petrij-Bosch A, Peelen T, van Vliet M, et al. BRCA1 genomic deletions are major founder mutations in Dutch breast cancer patients. *Nat Genet*. 1997;17:341–345.

22. Verhoog LC, Berns EM, Brekelmans CT, Seynaeve C, Meijers-Heijboer EJ, Klijn JG. Prognostic significance of germline BRCA2 mutations in hereditary breast cancer patients. *J Clin Oncol*. 2000;18:119S-124S.

23. Thorlacius S, Olafsdottir G, Tryggvadottir L, et al. A single BRCA2 mutation in male and female breast cancer families from Iceland with varied cancer phenotypes. *Nat Genet*. 1996;13:117–119.

24. Couch FJ, DeShano ML, Blackwood MA, et al. BRCA1 mutations in women attending clinics that evaluate the risk of breast cancer. *N Engl J Med*. 1997;336:1409–1415.

25. FitzGerald MG, MacDonald DJ, Krainer M, et al. Germ-line BRCA1 mutations in Jewish and non-Jewish women with early-onset breast cancer. *N Engl J Med*. 1996;334:143–149.

26. National Comprehensive Cancer Network. Clinical practice guidelines in oncology: genetic/familial high-risk assessment: breast and ovarian. Version 1.2008. In: NCCN Guidelines for Detection, Prevention, & Risk Reduction. Fort Washington, PA: Author; 2008. http://www.nccn.org/professionals/physician_gls/PDF/genetics_screening.pdf.

27. Fisher B, Costantino JP, Wickerham DL, et al. Tamoxifen for prevention of breast cancer: report of the National Surgical Adjuvant Breast and Bowel Project P-1 Study. *J Natl Cancer Inst*. 1998;90:1371–1388.

28. Narod SA, Risch H, Moslehi R, et al. Oral contraceptives and the risk of hereditary ovarian cancer. Hereditary Ovarian Cancer Clinical Study Group. *N Engl J Med*. 1998;339:424–428.

29. Verhoog LC, Brekelmans CT, Seynaeve C, et al. Survival and tumour characteristics of breast-cancer patients with germline mutations of BRCA1. *Lancet*. 1998;351:316–321.

30. Rennert G, Bisland-Naggan S, Barnett-Griness O, et al. Clinical outcomes of breast cancer in carriers of BRCA1 and BRCA2 mutations. *N Engl J Med*. 2007;357:115–123.

31. Fong PC, Boss DS, Yap TA, et al. Inhibition of poly(ADP-ribose) polymerase in tumors from BRCA mutation carriers. *N Engl J Med* 2009;361:123–134.

32. Lynch HT, Ens J, Lynch JF, Watson P. Tumor variation in three extended Lynch syndrome II kindreds. *Am J Gastroenterol*. 1988;83:741–747.

33. Lynch HT, Lanspa S, Smyrk T, Boman B, Watson P, Lynch J. Hereditary non-polyposis colorectal cancer (Lynch syndromes I & II). Genetics, pathology, natural history, and cancer control, Part I. *Cancer Genet Cytogenet*. 1991;53:143–160.

34. Vasen HF, Offerhaus GJ, den Hartog Jager FC, et al. The tumour spectrum in hereditary non-polyposis colorectal cancer: a study of 24 kindreds in the Netherlands. *Int J Cancer*. 1990;46:31–34.

35. Leach FS, Nicolaides NC, Papadopoulos N, et al. Mutations of a mutS homolog in hereditary nonpolyposis colorectal cancer. *Cell*. 1993;75:1215–1225.

36. Vasen HF, Mecklin JP, Khan PM, Lynch HT. The International Collaborative Group on Hereditary Non-Polyposis Colorectal Cancer (ICG-HNPCC). *Dis Colon Rectum* 1991;34:424–425.

37. Recommendations from the EGAPP Working Group: genetic testing strategies in newly diagnosed individuals with colorectal cancer aimed at reducing morbidity and mortality from Lynch syndrome in relatives. *Genet Med*. 2009;11:35–41.

38. Palomaki GE, McClain MR, Melillo S, Hampel HL, Thibodeau SN. EGAPP supplementary evidence review: DNA testing strategies aimed at reducing morbidity and mortality from Lynch syndrome. *Genet Med*. 2009;11:42–65.

39. Vasen HF, Wijnen JT, Menko FH, et al. Cancer risk in families with hereditary nonpolyposis colorectal cancer diagnosed by mutation analysis. *Gastroenterology*. 1996;110:1020–1027.

40. Schwartz PJ, Priori SG, Spazzolini C, et al. Genotype-phenotype correlation in the long-QT syndrome: gene-specific triggers for life-threatening arrhythmias. *Circulation*. 2001;103:89–95.

41. Moss AJ, Windle JR, Hall WJ, et al. Safety and efficacy of flecainide in subjects with Long QT-3 syndrome (DeltaKPQ mutation): a randomized, double-blind, placebo-controlled clinical trial. *Ann Noninvasive Electrocardiol*. 2005;10:59–66.

42. Priori SG, Schwartz PJ, Napolitano C, et al. Risk stratification in the long-QT syndrome. *N Engl J Med*. 2003;348:1866–1874.

43. Seth R, Moss AJ, McNitt S, et al. Long QT syndrome and pregnancy. *Ann Noninvasive Electrocardiol*. 2007;49:1092–1098.

44. Codner E, Deng L, Perez-Bravo F, et al. Glucokinase mutations in young children with hyperglycemia. *Diabetes Metab Res Rev*. 2006;22:348–355.

45. Pearson ER, Starkey BJ, Powell RJ, Gribble FM, Clark PM, Hattersley AT. Genetic cause of hyperglycaemia and response to treatment in diabetes. *Lancet*. 2003;362:1275–1281.

46. Meigs JB, Shrader P, Sullivan LM, et al. Genotype score in addition to common risk factors for prediction of type 2 diabetes. *N Engl J Med*. 2008;359:2208–2219.

47. Jazwinska EC, Cullen LM, Busfield F, et al. Haemochromatosis and HLA-H. *Nature Genetics*. 1996;14:249–251.

48. Beutler E, Felitti VJ, Koziol JA, Ho NJ, Gelbart T. Penetrance of 845G→A (C282Y) HFE hereditary haemochromatosis mutation in the USA. *Lancet*. 2002;359:211–218.

49. Haga SB, Burke W. Using pharmacogenetics to improve drug safety and efficacy. *JAMA*. 2004;291:2869–2871.

50. Mallal S, Phillips E, Carosi G, et al. HLA-B*5701 screening for hypersensitivity to abacavir. *N Engl J Med*. 2008;358:568–579.

51. Wysowski DK, Nourjah P, Swartz L. Bleeding complications with warfarin use: a prevalent adverse effect resulting in regulatory action. *Arch Intern Med*. 2007;167:1414–1419.

52. Aquilante CL, Langaee TY, Lopez LM, et al. Influence of coagulation factor, vitamin K epoxide reductase complex subunit 1, and cytochrome P450 2C9 gene polymorphisms on warfarin dose requirements. *Clin Pharmacol Ther*. 2006;79:291–302.

53. Carlquist JF, Horne BD, Muhlestein JB, et al. Genotypes of the cytochrome p450 isoform, CYP2C9, and the vitamin K epoxide reductase complex subunit 1 conjointly determine stable warfarin dose: a prospective study. *J Thromb Thrombolysis*. 2006;22:191–197.

54. A pharmacogenetic study of warfarin dosing, "the COUMA-GEN study." ClinicalTrials.gov, 2006. http://clinicaltrial.gov/ct/show/NCT00334464?order=1. Accessed August 28, 2007.

55. Modeling genotype and other factors to enhance the safety of coumadin prescribing. ClinicalTrials.gov, 2007. http://clinicaltrial.gov/ct/show/NCT00484640?order="1. Accessed August 28, 2007

56. Gonzalez FJ, Fernandez-Salguero P. Diagnostic analysis, clinical importance and molecular basis of dihydropyrimidine dehydrogenase deficiency. *Trends Pharmacol Sci*. 1995;16:325–327.

57. Iyer L, King CD, Whitington PF, et al. Genetic predisposition to the metabolism of irinotecan (CPT-11). Role of uridine diphosphate glucuronosyltransferase isoform 1A1 in the glucuronidation of its active metabolite (SN-38) in human liver microsomes. *J Clin Invest*. 1998;101:847–854.

58. Tai HL, Krynetski EY, Yates CR, et al. Thiopurine S-methyltransferase deficiency: two nucleotide transitions define the most prevalent mutant allele associated with loss of catalytic activity in Caucasians. *Am J Hum Genet*. 1996;58:694–702.

59. Ulrich CM, Yasui Y, Storb R, et al. Pharmacogenetics of methotrexate: toxicity among marrow transplantation patients varies with the methylenetetrahydrofolate reductase C677T polymorphism. *Blood*. 2001;98:231–234.

60. Goetz MP, Knox SK, Suman VJ, et al. The impact of cytochrome P450 2D6 metabolism in women receiving adjuvant tamoxifen. *Breast Cancer Res Treat*. 2007;101:113–121.

61. Lynch TJ, Bell DW, Sordella R, et al. Activating mutations in the epidermal growth factor receptor underlying responsiveness of non-small-cell lung cancer to gefitinib. *N Engl J Med.* 2004;350:2129–2139.

62. Paik S, Shak S, Tang G, et al. A multigene assay to predict recurrence of tamoxifen-treated, node-negative breast cancer. *N Engl J Med.* 2004;351:2817–26.

63. Buckhaults P. Gene expression determinants of clinical outcome. *Curr Opin Oncol.* 2006;18:57–61.

64. Redon R, Ishikawa S, Fitch KR, et al. Global variation in copy number in the human genome. *Nature.* 2006;444:444–454.

65. de Vries BB, Pfundt R, Leisink M, et al. Diagnostic genome profiling in mental retardation. *Am J Hum Genet.* 2005;77:606–616.

66. Schoumans J, Ruivenkamp C, Holmberg E, et al. Detection of chromosomal imbalances in children with idiopathic mental retardation by array based comparative genomic hybridisation (array-CGH). *J Med Genetics.* 2005;42:699–705.

67. Sebat J, Lakshmi B, Malhotra D, et al. Strong association of de novo copy number mutations with autism. *Science.* 2007;316:445–449.

68. Sebat J, Lakshmi B, Troge J, et al. Large-scale copy number polymorphism in the human genome. *Science.* 2004;305:525–528.

69. Korobkin R, Rajkumar R. The Genetic Information Nondiscrimination Act—a half-step toward risk sharing. *N Engl J Med.* 2008;359:335–337.

ACA: Patient Protection and Affordable Care Act
ACOG: American Congress of Obstetricians and Gynecologists
ACS: American Cancer Society
ACTH: Adrenocorticotrophic hormone
AIDS: Acquired immune deficiency syndrome
AMD: Age-related macular degeneration causing visual impairment
APS: Antiphospholipid antibody syndrome
AREDS: Age-Related Eye Disease Study
ART: Assisted reproductive technology
BCDDP: Breast Cancer Detection Demonstration Project
BMD: Bone mineral density
BMI: Body-Mass Index (kg/m²)
BOT: Borderline ovarian tumor
BP: Bipolar Disorder
BRCA1: A tumor suppressor gene
BRCA2: A tumor suppressor gene
BRFSS: Behavioral Risk Factor Surveillance Survey
CASH: Cancer and Steroid Hormone Study
CDC: Centers for Disease Control and Prevention
CEE: Conjugated equine estrogen
CHD: Coronary heart disease
CI: Confidence interval
CT: Computed tomography
CVD: Cardiovascular disease
DES: Diethylstilbestrol
DNA: Deoxyribonucleic acid
DSM: Diagnostic and Statistical Manual of Mental Disorders
EDC: Estrogen disruptor chemical
EOC: Epithelial ovarian cancer
ERT: Estrogen replacement therapy
FDA: U.S. Food and Drug Administration
FFQ: Food frequency questionnaire
FSH: Follicle-stimulating hormone
HCG: Human chorionic gonadotropin
HDL: High-density lipoprotein cholesterol
HIP: Health Insurance Plan [of New York]
HIV: Human immunodeficiency virus
HMG: Human menopausal gonadotropin
HPV: Human papilloma virus
HR: Hazard ratio; risk of disease or death
HRQOL: Health-related quality of life
HRT: Hormone replacement therapy
ICD: International Classification of Diseases
ICSI: Intracellular sperm injection
IOM: Institute of Medicine
IPV: Intimate partner violence
IUD: Intrauterine device

IVF: In vitro fertilization
LBW: Low birth weight
LDL: Low-density lipoprotein cholesterol
LH: Luteinizing hormone
LMP: Last menstrual period
MCI: Mild cognitive impairment
MDD: Major Depressive Disorder
MPA: Medroxyprogesterone acetate
MRI: Magnetic resonance imaging
NCEA: National Center for Elder Abuse
NCHS: National Center for Health Statistics
NCI: National Cancer Institute
NEISS-AIP: National Electronic Injury Surveillance System All Injury Program
NHANES: National Health and Nutrition Examination Survey
NHDS: National Hospital Discharge Survey
NHIS: National Health Interview Survey
NHS: Nurses' Health Study
NIH: National Institutes of Health
NSABP: National Surgical Adjuvant Breast Prevention
NSAIDs: Nonsteroidal anti-inflammatory drugs
NSFG: National Survey of Family Growth
OC: Oral contraceptive
OR: Odds ratio
PAF: Population attributable fraction
PCOS: Polycystic ovarian syndrome
PET: Positron emission testing
PGD: Preimplantation genetic diagnosis
PID: Pelvic inflammatory disease
PPV: Positive predictive value
PRAMS: Pregnancy Risk Assessment Monitoring System
RR: Relative risk
SEER: Surveillance Epidemiology and End Results
SERM: Selective estrogen modulator
SIDS: Sudden infant death syndrome
SIR: Standardized incidence ratio
SMR: Standardized mortality rate
STRIDE: Study titled: Do stage transitions result in detectable effects?
SWAN: Study of Women's Health Across the Nation
USPSTF: United States Preventive Services Task Force
UTI: Urinary tract infection
WHI: Women's Health Initiative
WHO: World Health Organization
WISQARS: Centers for Disease Control and Prevention's web-based injury statistics query and reporting system
WREI: Women's Research & Education Institute

"ABC": Avonex-Betaseron-Copaxone, approved drugs for multiple sclerosis treatment

Absolute risk: Risk of developing a disease over a set time interval

Acinetobacter: Bacterium infecting the upper respiratory tract possibly associated with multiple sclerosis

ACTH: Adrenocorticotrophic hormone produced in the brain and stored in the pituitary gland

A1C: Test that assesses blood glucose levels during past 2 to 3 months indicating the amount of glucose adhering to red blood cells

Adipose tissue: Specialized connective tissue composed of adipocytes (fat cells)

Adult-onset diabetes: Former term for type 2 diabetes

Allele: One of two or more versions of a genetic sequence at a particular location in the genome

Amenorrhea: Absence of menses after menarche lasting 3 months or longer

Amniotic fluid: Fluid surrounding an unborn fetus containing fetal cells available for genetic testing

Amyloid: Abnormal insoluble fibrous extracellular substances deposited between cells

Androgen: A sex hormone responsible for the development and maintenance of male sex characteristics

Androstenedione: An androgenic steroid secreted by the ovaries and adrenal cortex

Aneuploidy: Having too few or too many chromosomes, the cause of approximately 50% of clinical miscarriages, 5% of stillbirths, and (rarely) live births of infants with birth defects

Antepartum: During pregnancy, before the onset of labor

Antibody: Protein produced by B-cells of the immune system defending against infectious agents or stimulated by an antigen. An antibody may be directed against one's own tissues resulting in autoimmune disease

Antigen: Any substance (bacterium, virus, or single molecule) that stimulates an immune response, resulting in production of antibodies or a cellular reaction

Antigen-antibody complex: Immune complex formed by the binding of an antibody to an antigen in the blood

Antiphospholipid antibody syndrome [APS]: An autoimmune condition causing antibody production against normal components of blood and cell membranes

Apgar score: Assessment of health status of newborn at 1 minute and 5 minutes after birth, based on the infant's heart rate, respiratory effort, muscle tone, reflex irritability, and skin tone with each given a score of zero to 2

Apoptosis: Naturally occurring programmed cell death required for maintenance of healthy tissue

Aromatase: An enzyme that catalyzes the conversion of testosterone to estradiol

Artificial insemination: Pregnancy by artificial means; commonly donor semen is injected mechanically into the woman's vagina

Ascites: Fluid collection within the abdominal cavity

Assisted reproductive technology (ART): Procedures assisting couples to achieve pregnancy

Asthma: Chronic respiratory disease characterized by constriction of the alveoli causing wheezing, coughing and difficulty breathing

Asymptomatic: Without observable signs or reportable symptoms of illness

Atherosclerosis: Inflammatory process occurring in arteries; clogging, narrowing, and hardening of large arteries, impeding circulation

Attributable risk: Risk difference among exposed individuals compared to the unexposed; the calculation is used to estimate the percentage of risk attributable to a specific exposure

Autoimmunity: Activated immune system resulting in antibody production targeting the body's own tissue

Avascular necrosis: Death of bone cells due to treatment of lupus with steroids

Benign: Noncancerous growth confined to an organ without any evidence of invading adjacent tissue

Biofeedback: A training technique that enabling voluntary control over autonomic function

Biomarker: Biochemical measure of genetic, cellular or molecular alterations, potential indicator of a biological process predictive of a disease

Birth defect: Abnormal condition occurring during prenatal development or at birth

Birth interval: Months or years between deliveries

Blastocyst: Early stage post conception of embryo development when implantation occurs

Body Mass Index [BMI]: Adiposity calculated from an individual's weight and height (kg/m^2)

BRCA1/BRCA2: Human tumor suppressor genes linked to hereditary breast and ovarian cancers

Cardiac arrest: Cessation of normal heart functioning, disrupting circulation

Carrier status: Knowledge of disease-causing mutation status determined by genetic testing

Cellular casts: Blood cells excreted in urine indicative of kidney damage

Cesarean delivery: Extraction of the infant, placenta, and membranes through an incision in the maternal abdominal and uterine walls

Chemotherapy: Treatment of cancer and other conditions with medications

Chemoprevention: Medications prescribed to prevent cancer in healthy women and men

Chromosomes: Structures within the cell that store and transmit genetic information; there are a total of 22 pairs of nonsex and 2 sex chromosomes

Conception: Fertilization of an ovum by a sperm

Congenital anomaly: Structural or functional abnormality of fetus

Damage index: A summation of clinical features or characteristics of lupus used to estimate irreversible tissue damage caused by underlying disease, side effects of therapy, and/or comorbid conditions

Death rate: Total number of deaths per 100,000 population for a specific time interval

Diagnostic testing: Test or procedure required to confirm the presence or absence of a specific disease or condition following detection of an abnormality during a screening procedure

DNA banking: Process of preserving and storing a DNA sample

Dysmenorrhea: Painful menstruation

Ectopic pregnancy: Implantation of blastocyst outside the uterus, usually in an oviduct

Embolization: Treatment of uterine fibroids by blocking blood supply and impairing continued growth

Endogenous estrogens: Naturally circulating hormones produced by ovaries and other organs

Endometrium: Lining of the uterus which prepares for implantation with each menstrual cycle; in the absence of conception, the lining is shed resulting in menstruation

Epidemiology transition: Shift during 20th century in primary causes of death from infectious to chronic conditions

Epigenetic changes: Alterations to genetic material caused by mechanisms other than changes in DNA

Estrogen disruptor chemicals (EDCs): Chemicals that alter the normal production and function of endogenous estrogens

Family relationships: First degree: direct relatives, e.g., parents and children, or siblings
Second degree: grandparents, maternal and paternal aunts and uncles
Third degree: maternal and paternal cousins

Fecundity: Capacity to conceive and deliver a baby; repeated fertilization

Fertility: The capacity to achieve pregnancy and deliver a baby

Fertilization: Joining of genetic material of an ovum and sperm

Fetus: Stage of development beginning 8 weeks after conception following the embryonic stage

Follicular phase: First phase of the menstrual cycle from onset of menses to ovulation, duration is person-specific ranging from 10 to 50 days

Gail model: A statistical model developed by the NCI to guide patients and clinicians in estimating an individual woman's risk of developing breast cancer

Genitourinary: Affecting reproductive and urinary organs

Gestation: Status of being pregnant (gravid)

Gestational diabetes mellitus: Onset of carbohydrate intolerance first recognized during pregnancy

Gravidity: Number of pregnancies including miscarriages as opposed to number of births

Hassles index: A tally of small, irritating, frustrating, distressing day-to-day demands

Hormone: Secretion from an endocrine organ including adrenal glands and ovary

Hereditary germline mutation: Change in DNA of an egg or sperm passed from parent to offspring

Hyperglycemia: Postprandial blood glucose above normal level 1 to 2 hours after a person has eaten

Hypoglycemia: Blood glucose lower than normal, less than 70 mg/dL; associated with hunger, nervousness, shakiness, perspiration, dizziness or light-headedness, sleepiness, and confusion

Hysterectomy: Surgical removal of the uterus with or without bilateral oophorectomy, removal of ovaries

Impaired fasting glucose: Blood test meeting the criteria of pre-diabetes, higher than normal glucose levels after an 8- and 12-hour fast

Implantation: Attachment of the blastocyst to the uterine lining occurring 6 to 12 days after conception

Induced abortion: Interruption of a pregnancy by medical or surgical intervention

Infant mortality: Death during the first year of life

Infant mortality rate: Number of infant deaths per 1,000 live births

Infertility: Inability of couple to achieve pregnancy during 12 months of unprotected sexual intercourse

Inflammation: Accumulation of fluid, plasma proteins, and white blood cells resulting from injury, infection, or local immune response

Insulin: A hormone secreted by the beta cells of the pancreas enabling the body to use glucose for energy

Insulin resistance: Prediabetes condition associated with increased risk of type 2 diabetes

Intrapartum: Events occurring during labor but before delivery

In vitro fertilization (IVF): Fertilization by clinical intervention outside the body; fertilization occurs in a petri dish

Kappa agreement: The measure of agreement between two independent evaluations to assess the level of observed agreement after accounting for chance. The higher the magnitude of the kappa value indicates greater reliability of the independent measures

Lactation: Breastfeeding to provide nourishment to newborn baby

Lesbian: A woman who engages in sexual behavior with a woman or has sexual attraction to women

Li-Fraumeni syndrome: A rare hereditary cancer susceptibility condition associated with development of multiple sites of malignancy resulting from inherited mutations of the *p53* tumor suppressor gene

Low birthweight: Infant weighing less than 2,500 grams at birth

Luteal phase: The second phase of the menstrual cycle after ovulation, approximately 13 days before the next menses

Luteinizing hormones: A hormone produced by the pituitary that triggers ovulation in response to ovarian estrogen stimulation

Macrosomia: Abnormally large infant often associated with gestational diabetes

Maternal mortality: Death of a woman due to pregnancy or within 40 days of childbirth

Menarche: First menstrual cycle indicating female sexual maturation

Menopause: Permanent cessation of menstrual cycles

Menorrhagia: Excessive menstrual discharge

Menstrual cycle: Pattern of monthly menstrual bleeding stimulated by ovarian hormones

Metabolic Syndrome: Obesity and associated abdominal fat elevating risk of hypertension, high cholesterol levels, and heart disease

Miscarriage: Spontaneous termination of pregnancy usually within 20 weeks of conception

Mutation: Alteration in the structure of DNA influencing the normal function of a gene

Myomectomy: Surgical removal of uterine leiomyoma (fibroid tumor)

National Health and Nutrition Examination Survey (NHANES): Physical examinations and data collection surveys conducted by the National Center for Health Statistics, Centers for Disease Control and Prevention

National Hospital Discharge Survey: Annual sampling of inpatient discharges from nonfederal, short-stay hospitals

Neonatal mortality: Death of a newborn child within 28 days of birth

Nulliparity: Never having given birth

Obesity: Body mass index of 30 or greater characterized by excessive body fat

Oligomenorrhea: Absence of menses for intervals of 1 to 2 months or unevenly spaced menstrual cycles ranging from 35 to 90 days

Oral glucose tolerance test (OGTT): Blood test to diagnose prediabetes; after an overnight fast and consumption of a high-glucose beverage; blood samples are drawn for 2 to 3 hours to assess rate of glucose level

Organogenesis: the formation of organs in a developing fetus occurring during the first trimester of pregnancy (prior to 16 weeks gestation)

Parity: Number of live or stillborn births

Passive smoking: Inhalation of environmental tobacco smoke

Penetrance: Probability that a mutation carrier will develop the genetically related condition

Perimenopause: An interval before menopause when ovarian hormone production becomes less regular resulting in less predicable frequency and duration of menses

Polydipsia: Excessive thirst, potential indicator of diabetes

Postterm delivery: Birth following 42 weeks or more gestation

Pre-diabetes: Blood glucose levels higher than normal although not reaching diagnostic criteria of diabetes

Premature menopause: Natural cessation of ovarian function before age 40

Premature mortality: Death before age 65

Preterm delivery: Birth before 37 weeks gestation

Primary amenorrhea: Lack of a menstrual cycle by age 16

Prophylactic surgery: Removal of healthy tissue to prevent disease

Puberty: Growth during childhood culminating in sexual maturity

Replacement fertility rate: The birth rate of a given generation to exactly replace itself, generally considered to be 2,100 births per 1,000 women

Salpingo-oophorectomy: Surgical removal of fallopian tubes and ovaries

Sarcopenia: Degenerative loss of muscle mass and strength associated with aging and frailty syndrome

Serositis: Inflammation of the lining of organs such as lungs, heart or the inner lining of the abdomen

Single nucleotide polymorphisms (SNPs): Gene alterations that may be associated with specific diseases

Sjogren's Syndrome: An autoimmune disease that selectively attacks salivary and tear glands causing inflammation and tissue damage

Stillbirth: Birth of an infact at a gestational age of viability with no evidence of life at delivery

Sterility: Complete inability of a couple to conceive due to reproductive health problems in either the woman or man

Sudden Infant Death Syndrome (SIDS): Unexpected and unexplained death of an infant between 3 weeks and 9 months of age

Synchronous: Multiple tumors occurring at the same time

Telomeres: Ends of chromosomes, DNA sequences that protect chromosomes from damage during mitosis

Telomerase: An enzyme that repairs telomeres after mitosis

Teratogen: A drug or other agent that disrupts normal embryonic or fetal development

Term pregnancy: Delivery between 37 and 41 weeks of gestation

Trimester: A period of 3 months, one-third of the gestational interval between LMP and delivery

Twins, Dizygous/Fraternal: Two infants in same pregnancy conceived from two separately fertilized ova

Twins, Monozygous/Identical: Two infants in same pregnancy conceived from a single fertilized ovum

Type 1 diabetes: Lack of insulin resulting from the immune system attacking insulin-producing cells of the pancreas

Type 2 diabetes: High blood glucose levels caused either by lack of insulin or the body's inability to use insulin efficiently occurring most frequently among middle and older aged adults

Unplanned pregnancy: Unwanted, unintended, or poorly timed pregnancy

Uterine atony: Failure of the uterus to contract following delivery increasing the risk of postpartum hemorrhage

Very preterm birth: Birth before 32 weeks of gestation

Note: Italicized page locators indicate figures/illustrations; tables are noted with *t*.

Hygiene hypothesis, asthma and, 274, 275–276
Hyperemesis gravidarum
  migraine and, 431, 432
  obesity and, 432
Hyperglycemia, 299
Hypertension, 26, 125, 481, 535
  Bipolar Disorder and, 230
  cardiovascular disease and, 414, 417
  defined, 417
  diet and, 74
  endometrial cancer and, 378
  fibroids and, 131
  gestational, 68
  older women and, 476–477
  placental abruption and, 145
  preventing or controlling, 58
Hypertriglyceridemia, HIV and, 188
Hypomania, 226, 227, 228, 229t
Hypothalamic-pituitary-adrenal axis, posttraumatic stress disorder and, 243
Hypothalamic-pituitary-gonadal axis, Bipolar Disorder and, 233, 234
Hysterectomy, 161, 376, 389, 421, 422, 478, 537
  with bilateral oophorectomy
    breast cancer risk and, 339
    cognitive impairment and age at time of, 509–510
    migraine and, 432
    percentage of, by age group, U.S. (1994–1999), 157
  fibroid treatment and, 130–131
  ovarian cancer and, 363–364, 365, 367
  race, ovarian cancer risk and, 367
  rates of, by age group, U.S. (1994–1999), 156
  rates of, by geographic region, U.S., 156
  surgical menopause and, 156–157

I

IARC. *See* International Agency for Research on Cancer
Ibandronate, osteoporosis prevention and, 461t, 462
IgE, asthma and, 273
Illicit drug use, 249
Immigration status
  asthma and, 274
  intimate partner violence and, 261
Immunizations, diabetes and, 306
Immunotherapy, for asthma, 276, 277
Implanon, 118t, 119
Implantation, conception and, 128–129
Implants, contraceptive, 119
Incarceration, Bipolar Disorder and, 227
Incessant ovulation hypothesis, ovarian cancer and, 360
Incidence of disease, 17
Inclusion cysts, in ovaries, 357
Indoor air pollution

asthma and, 274
lung cancer and, 317
Infant mortality rate, 145–146
  maternal contributors to, 146
  prenatal care and, 136–137
  reduction in, 125
  U.S. (1940–2006), 146
Infection, lung cancer and, 318
Infectious diseases
  American women and epidemics of, 5
  reporting, 22
  trends in mortality, 5
Infertility
  breast cancer and, 338
  conditions contributing to
    endometriosis, 131
    maternal age, 129
    polycystic ovary syndrome, 130
    premenstrual syndrome, 129–130
    sexually transmitted infections, 130
    uterine leiomyomata, 130–131
  DES and, 132t
  eating disorders and, 132
  endometrial cancer and, 377
  following cancer treatment, 131
  ovarian cancer and, 363
  prenatal exposure to DES and, 132
  treatment of—assisted reproduction technology
    donor oocytes or embryos, 134
    gestational carriers, 134–135
    in-vitro fertilization, 133–134
    multiple births, 135–136
    ovarian stimulation, 132
    preimplantation genetic diagnosis, 135
Inflammation
  cardiovascular disease and, 418
  endometrial cancer and, 378
  periodontal disease, heart disease and, 86
Inflammatory bowel disease, 535
Influenza
  during pregnancy, 137
  vaccine, 54
Informed consent, population-based recruitment and, 22
Inhaled corticosteroids, for asthma, 276
Inhibin B, menopausal transition and, 153, 154
Injectable hormones, prevention of HIV/AIDS and, 204
Injection drug users, 196
  community-wide approach to, 201
  HIV/AIDS and, 189
Injury deaths, women's experience across the life span and, 35–36
Injury(ies)
  adverse effects of medical care and drugs, 45
  age- and race-specific mortality due to, among women, 39
  drowning and environmental and human-caused disasters, 45

estimated cost of all causes of, from ED visits, hospitalizations and deaths (2005), 39t
  firearm, all intents, 44
  home and homelessness-related, 46
  magnitude of, relative to total disease burden in U.S., 37–39
    healthcare costs, 38–39
    morbidity, 38
    years of potential life lost, 38
  occupational, 46
  percent of deaths due to, among females, U.S. (2007), 37t
  recreational and sports-related, 45–46
  relation of, to age and gender structure of U.S. population, 36, 36–37
  relative rank of, in females by YPLL before age 65, cause of death, hospitalization, and ED visits, 38t
  unintentional, 41–44, 47
Insoluble fiber, 74
Insomnia, older women and, 478
Institute of Medicine, 4, 5, 126, 148, 394
  dietary reference nutrients of, 71t
  on effective preventive services for women, 52
  on IPV and health professionals role, 262
  on sodium limits, 5858
  weight gain during pregnancy guidelines, 137–138
Insulin-dependent diabetes (type 1 diabetes), onset of, 299
Integrative medicine, 92
Intelligence quotient, PTSD incidence patterns and, 244
Intentional injury mechanisms, 39–41
  homicide, 40
  suicide, 41
Interaction (or effect) modification, 28
Intercourse, after menopause, 159–160
INTERHEART study, 415, 417, 418
International Agency for Research on Cancer, 316, 317, 404
International Classification of Diseases, 9th Revision, Clinical Modification, 504
International Committee for Research on Women, 196
International Headache Society, 427, 430
International Lung Cancer Consortium, 317
International Study of Asthma and Allergies in Childhood, 274
International Survey on Drug Utilization in Pregnancy (WHO), 432
International Union Against Cancer, 529
Internet, population-based recruitment via, 22
Interpersonal therapy, for Bipolar Disorder, 232, 234
Intimate partner violence, 10, 257–265
  asthma and, 272, 275
  costs to individuals and society, 257
  data sources on, 259–260

Modeling, bone, 455, *456*

MODY. *See* Maturity onset diabetes of the young

Molecular brain imaging, 515

Molecular markers, 25

Molecular mimicry, 283

Monosaturated fatty acids, 73

Monozygous twins, 128

Mons pubis, 116, *116*

Montagnier, Luc, 181, *182t*

Montelukast, for asthma, 276

Mood disorders, 146, 225

Mood stabilizers, 231, 232, 233–234

Morbidity

    injury-related, 38

    prevention, 8–9

    recreational and sports injuries, 45–46

Morbidity and Mortality Weekly Report, 177, 393

Morphine, 58

Mortality

    age-adjusted rates, life expectancy and, 468

    all-cause, early menarche and, 109

    marriage and, 114

    obesity and, 8

    percent decline in, by age group over 75 years between 1935 and 2010 in U.S., *50*

Morula, *117*

Mother Teresa, 493

Motor vehicle traffic deaths, 41–42

    among females per 100,000 by age group and race, *42*

    leading cause of injury death, and YPLL in women, 37, *38t*

    occupant injury deaths, race, gender, and age, 41–42

    rates of, U.S. (1980–2008), *60*

Movement therapies, 92

Movies, smoking in, young audiences and, 57

Movies Study, 507

MRI. *See* Magnetic resonance imaging

MRSA. *See* Methycillin resistant *Staphylococcus aureus*

MS. *See* Multiple sclerosis

MSH6, 537, 538

Mucinous ovarian cancer, 367

Multiethnic Cohort Study, 155, 156

Multi-Ethnic Study of Atherosclerosis, 422

Multifactorial research, 28

Multiple births, 135–136, 363

Multiple sclerosis, 10, 281–288

    chromosome 6 and, 282, *283*

    clinical course of, *282*

    clinical manifestations of, *281*, 281–282

    detection methods and screening patterns for, 284–285

    diagnosis of, 285

    environmental risks related to, 285–286

    genetic research and, 282–283

    genetic risk for, 285

    geographic distribution of, 283

    immunopathogenesis of, *281*

    incidence and prevalence rates for, 283

    management of acute relapses with, 287

    mean ages at diagnosis and changes over time, 283–284

        emotional stress, 284

        pregnancy, 284

    morbidity and mortality, 284

    oral bacteria and, 85

    pregnancy and, 286

    prevention, control, and adherence patterns, 287–288

        relapse prevention, 288

        smoking, 288

        vitamin D deficiency, 287

    reducing risk of relapses and neurologic disability, 287

    secondary progressive, 282

    sources of data on, 282

    symptomatic treatment of, 286–287

    vitamin D deficiency and risk of, 286

Multivitamins, pregnancy and, 68

Murders, intimate partner, 263

Muscatine Study, 419

Musculoskeletal pain, nonmalignant, 435

Mutual violent control, 258

Mycophenolate mofetil, 293, 296

Myocardial infarction, acute, 413

Myomectomy, 131

Myriad Genetics, 333, 349, 361

N

N-Acetyltransferase 2, 341

Nadolol, for migraine, 429

NAEPP. *See* National Asthma Education and Prevention Program

Naltrexone, 253t

NAPA. *See* National Alzheimer's Project Act

Natalizumab, for multiple sclerosis, 287

National Alzheimer's Project Act, 507

National Arthritis Data Workgroup, 444

National Asthma Education and Prevention Program, 276

National Birth Defects Prevention Study, 138, 140

National Breast and Cervical Cancer Early Detection Program, 328, 347

National Cancer Act, 11

National Cancer Act Amendments, 389

National Cancer Institute, 11, 323, 357, 358, 400, 526, 529

National Cancer Institute Combined Cohort Study, 155

National Center for Complementary and Alternative Medicine, 92, 448

National Center for Health Statistics, 22, 127, 190, 477, 499

National Center for Injury Prevention and Control, 259

National Center on Addiction and Substance Abuse, 249

National Center on Elder Abuse, 485

National Colonoscopy Study, 404

National Comorbidity Study Replication, 226

National Comorbidity Survey, 226

National Comorbidity Survey Replication, 218, 219–220

National Comprehensive Cancer Network, BRCA1/BRCA2 mutations and screening recommendations of, 536t

National Crime Victimization Survey, 259

National Electronic Injury Surveillance System, 259

National Guidelines Task Force, sexuality guidelines, 112

National Health and Nutrition Examination Survey I, 22, 70, 155, 177, 341, 343, 385, 414, 469, 504

    on chlamydia prevalence, 172

    on heart disease, 54

National Health and Nutrition Examination Survey III, 444, 444t

    on age at menarche, 105

    on dental care during pregnancy, 141

    on periodontal disease and cognitive skills, 86

    on tooth loss and pregnancy, 84

National Health and Social Life Survey, 113

National Health Examination Study, on obesity, 7, *7*

National Health Interview Survey, 12, 81, 93, 154, 272, 328, 389, 402, 443, 480

    on CAM, 91

    on HIV testing, 190

National Health Service Breast Screening Program (UK), 527

National Heart Lung Blood Institute, 423

    diagnostic criteria for metabolic syndrome, 74t

National Growth and Health Study, 107

National HIV/AIDS Strategy, 195, 200, 201, 204

National Hospital Ambulatory Medical Care Survey, 259

National Hospital Discharge Survey, 156

National Institute of Aging, 467, 469

National Institute of Arthritis and Musculoskeletal and Skin Diseases, 448

National Institute of Child Health and Human Development, Maternal-Fetal Medicine Units Network, 143

National Institute of Communicative Disorders and Stroke, 513

National Institute of Justice, 259, 265

National Institute of Mental Health, 232

National Institutes of Health, 49, 161, 265, 529

    first female director of, 4

    Office of AIDS Research, 195

National Longitudinal Study of Adolescent Health, 177

National Long-Term Care Surveys, 480

Nationally Notifiable Infectious Conditions, 176

R

RA. *See* Rheumatoid arthritis
Race/ethnicity, 18
 age at menarche and, 105, 106, 109
 arthritis and, 443
 asthma and, 274
 Binge Eating Disorder and, 211
 birth rates per 1,000 females aged 15–19
  by (2000–2010), *121*
 breast cancer, prognostic factors and,
  347
 breast cancer risk and, 331
 breast development and, 106
 CAM use and, 93
 cardiovascular disease and, 413
 cervical cancer and, *384*
 colorectal cancer and, 398, 399*t*,
  403–404
 colorectal screening disparities and, 402
 coronary heart disease and, *414*
 CVD knowledge and, 423
 deaths of adults and adolescent females
  with diagnosis of HIV by (2009), *186*
 diabetes and, 300–301
  in older years, 306
  in youth, 302–303, *303*, 304*t*
 drowning and, 45
 ectopic pregnancy, mortality rate due to
  and, 128
 endometrial cancer and, 374, *374*
 fatal falls and, 50
 fire and burn deaths and, *43*, 43–44
 firearm injuries and deaths and, 44, *45*
 HAART use and, 191
 happy life expectations and, 493
 health status at various life stages and, 63
 heart disease and, 416, *416*, 420
 HIV/AIDS rates and, 184
 HIV diagnoses among adult and
  adolescent females by (2010), 185*t*
 homicide rate and, 40, *40*, 41
 infant mortality and, 146
 intimate partner violence and, 260–261
 life expectancy and, 468
 lupus and, 291
 mammography among women ages 40
  and older, U.S. (2008), 329*t*
 maternal age and, 129
 maternal mortality and, 145–146
 menopausal symptoms, CAM use and, 94
 motor vehicle traffic deaths by, *42*
 multiple sclerosis and, 283
 nutrition, body size, puberty and, 107
 oral health in older years and, 475
 osteoarthritis and, 446
 osteoporosis and, 457
 ovarian cancer and, 357, 367
 periodontal disease, diabetes and, 86
 prenatal care and, 136–137
  for mothers with live births by (1970–
   2001), *137*
 preterm and low birth weight and,
  144–145

prevalence of substance use disorders
 among girls and women by, *250*
pubic hair development and, 105, 106
recession of 2008, declining fertility rate
 and, 127
sexually transmitted infections and, 188
spina bifida and, 141
stillbirths and, 145
suicide rate and, 41, *41*
systemic lupus erythematosus and, 295
unintentional injuries and, 41
unintentional poisoning and, 42–43, *43*
uterine fibroids and, 130–131
Race-specific injury mortality, among
 women, 39, *40*
Racial discrimination, health status
 adversely impacted by, 52
Radiation
 breast cancer and, 340–34
 ovarian cancer and, 366
 preventing excess exposure to, 61–62
Radiation therapy
 breast cancer and, 346
 endometrial cancer and, 379
 rectal cancer and, 407
Radon, lung cancer risk and indoor
 exposure to, 317, 320
Raloxifene, 346, 349
 endometrial cancer risk and, 376
 osteoporosis prevention and, 461–462,
  461*t*
Rancho Bernardo Study, 510
Randomized controlled trials, 21, 25
RAND-36 questionnaire, 160
Rape, 147, 257
Rapid eye movement (REM) sleep, 478
RCTs. *See* Randomized controlled trials
Rebif, for multiple sclerosis, 287, 288
Recall bias, avoiding, 24
Recession of 2008, declining fertility rate
 and, 127
Reconstruction, breast, 346–347
Recreational injury morbidity, 45–46
Rectal cancer, 404, 406, 407
Reiki, 92, 96
Relative risk, 26, 27, 27*t*–28*t*
Renal failure, Bipolar Disorder comorbid
 with, 230
Repetitive movement
 osteoarthritis and, 446
  avoidance of, 448
"Replacement" fertility rate, 127
Replens, 159
Replication studies, 26–27
Reproduction technology. *See* Assisted
 reproduction technology
Reproductive anatomy, female, 116, *116*
Reproductive health
 conception and implantation, 128–129
 contraception, 126–127
 epidemiology of, 125–148
 exposures complicating pregnancy and
  birth outcomes, 137–142
 infertility

assisted reproduction technology,
 132–136
 conditions contributing to, 129–132
 preconception and prenatal care,
  136–137
 progress and challenges in, 125
 reproductive outcomes, 142–148
 reproductive potential, 127–128
Reproductive history, breast cancer risk
 and, 335–337
Reproductive outcomes, 142–148
 birth defects, 144
 breastfeeding, 147
 Cesarean delivery, 142–143
 maternal and infant mortality, 145–146
 miscarriage and stillbirth, 145
 placental abruption and placenta previa,
  145
 postpartum depression, 146
 preterm and low birth weight, 144
 vaginal birth, 142
Reproductive potential, 127–128
Reproductive years, oral health and,
 84–85
Rescue medications, for asthma, 276
Research, 13. *See also* Epidemiologic
 research
Residential care facilities, 480
Respiratory disease, oral health and, 81, 88
Respiratory infections, asthma and, 274
Restless leg syndrome, 478
Restriction fragment length
 polymorphisms, 511
Retirement, phased, 470
Retrospective cohort studies, 20–21
Retrospective data collection, prospective
 data collection vs., 24
RFLPs. *See* Restriction fragment length
 polymorphisms
Rheumatoid arthritis, 437, 443, 448–452
 age and, 449
 clinical manifestation with, 450
 complementary/alternative therapy for,
  451–452
 diagnosis of, 450
 drugs for, 450–451
 fetal origin and, 449
 gender and, 449
 genetic susceptibility and, 449
 geographic residence and, 450
 infectious agents and, 450
 nonpharmacologic therapy for, 451
 nutrition and, 451, 452
 oral contraceptives and, 449
 oral health and, 88
 parity and, 449
 pathophysiology of, 450
 periodontitis and, 85
 prevalence of, 448
 prevention of, 452
 smoking and, 449–450
 surgery for, 451
Rheumatoid factor (RF), detection of, 450
Rimonabant, 253*t*

Risedronate, osteoporosis prevention and, 461t, 462
Rituximab, for systemic lupus erythematosus, 293, 296
Rivastigmine, for Alzheimer's disease, 515
Rochester study, 507
Rockefeller, Margaretta (Happy), 330
Rosenberg Self-Esteem Scale, 489
Rotterdam Study, 510
RR. *See* Relative risk
RU486, 131
Rubella, 176
Rubinstein, Arthur, 494
Russia, breast self-examination in, 529
RV144 Prime-Boost HIV Vaccine Clinical Trial, 189

S

Sadness, depression vs., 217
Safe Mobile Care (UK), 485
Saliva, biomarkers in, 83
Salivary flow rate, estrogen and, 85
Salmeterol, for asthma, 276
Salpingo-oophorectomy, prophylactic, 536–537
Salt restriction, 58
   projected annual reductions in cardiovascular events associated with, 58, 59
"Sandwich generation," 492
Saquinavir, 181, 183t
Sarcopenia, preventing, 75
SARS. *See* Severe Acute Respiratory Syndrome
Saturated fats, dietary, 73
Saving Lives Now, 197
SC. *See* Small cell carcinoma
Scabies (*Sarcoptes scabei*), sexually transmitted, 169
Scans, during pregnancy, 141–142
SCC. *See* Squamous cell carcinoma
Scheinberg, Peritz, 283
Schizoaffective disorder, 217
Schizophrenia, 225, 251
Schumacher criteria, for multiple sclerosis, 285
SCLC. *See* Small cell lung cancer
Scleroderma, 85, 291
SCN5A, 538
SCORE trial, 400
Screening
   for breast cancer, 327–330
   for cancer, 13
   for cervical cancer, 389–392, 394
      current recommendations, 390–392
      reliability of Pap tests, 390
   for colorectal cancer, 397
   HIV, 190–191
   for intimate partner violence, 258–259
   for lung cancer, 319–320
   for multiple sclerosis, 284–285
   for older women, 475
   for ovarian cancer, 358–360

population-based, 539–540
   potentially adverse effects of, 19
   for substance use, 252
   for systemic lupus erythematosus, 293
Screening methods, statistical assessment of, 25–26
SEARCH for Diabetes in Youth Study, 302, 303, *303*, 308
Seat belts, 60
Secondary prevention, 18–19, 50
Secondary progressive multiple sclerosis, 282
Secondhand smoke, 6, 56
Sedentary lifestyle, obesity and, 60
SEER program. *See* Surveillance, Epidemiology, and End Results (SEER) program
Selective estrogen receptor modulators, 346, 376
Selective Optimization and Compensation (SOC) Model, successful aging and, 494
Selective reduction, 133
Self-concept deficits, risk factors for, 211, 212
Self-neglect syndrome, older population and, 484–485
Self-reported data, reliability of, 23
Semmelweiss, Ignac, 17
Senior Citizens Freedom to Work Act of 2000, 470
Senior Risk Reduction Demonstration (SRRD), 472
Seniors. *See* Aging population; Older women
Sensitivity, screening tests and, 25
Sentinel lymph node biopsy, 346
September 11, 2001 terrorist attacks, asthma and occupational exposure during, 271
SERMs. *See* Selective estrogen receptor modulators
Seropositive people, interventions among, 203
Serositis, systemic lupus erythematosus and, 292t
Serotonin, eating disorders and levels of, 212
Serous ovarian cancer, 367
Serrated polyp pathway, colorectal cancer and, 397
SES. *See* Socioeconomic status
Seventh-Day Adventists cohort, life expectancy, menopause and, 157
Severe Acute Respiratory Syndrome, 178
Sex hormone-binding globulin, 129
Sex hormones, asthma and, 275
Sexual abuse, 257
   dental anxiety and, 84
   eating disorders and, 212
   health consequences of, 263
   homelessness and history of, 261
   intimate partner violence and, 264
   of older persons, 485

PTSD in women and, 241
   STIs in prepubertal children and, 177
Sexual behavior, cervical cancer and, 386–387
Sexual debut, deferring, prevention of HIV/AIDS and, 197, 200
Sexual dysfunction, in men and women, 115
Sexual health
   across the life span, 9
   of older women, 479
Sexual identity, adolescents and, 113
Sexual intercourse, first, age of, 113
Sexuality, 122
   adolescent sexual development, 113
   adult sexual behavior, 113–114
   body image, 112–113
   defined, 111
   human sexual response cycle, 114–115
   interacting circles of, *111*
   learning about, 112
   life course and, 112
   marriage, 114
   masturbation, 113
   menopause and, 159–160
   sexual dysfunction, 115
   views of and communication about, 176
Sexually transmitted diseases, 112, 125, 169
   CAM used by women with, 94–95
   condom use and reducing risk of, 119
   substance use disorders and, 252
Sexually Transmitted Disease Surveillance (CDC), 177
Sexually transmitted infections, 9–10, 159, 169–179, 196
   chlamydia, 172–173
   common, 170t–171t
   emerging, 178
   epidemiology of, 176–178
      ascertainment and data sources, 176–177
      contact tracing and case investigation, 177
      risk factors and disparities in, 177–178
   fibroids and, 131
   gonorrhea, 171
   herpes simplex type 2, 173–174
   HIV and, 188–189
   human papillomaviruses, 174–175
   infertility and, 130–131
   intimate partner violence and, 264
   overview of, 169
   pelvic inflammatory disease, 175–176
   prospects for future, 178
   syphilis, 171–172
Sexual maturation, puberty and, 103
Sexual orientation, 112, 122, 479
   adolescence and, 113
   cervical cancer screening relative to, 392
Sexual relationships, 114
Sexual violence, 258
SFR. *See* Salivary flow rate

SGA. *See* Small for gestational age
SHBG. *See* Sex hormone-binding globulin
Shingles, 54, 173
Sidestream smoke, lung cancer and, 317
SIDS. *See* Sudden infant death syndrome
Siemens, 530
Sigmoidoscopy
    advantages/disadvantages of, 400*t*
    screening rates and adherence patterns, 402
Single nucleotide polymorphisms, 335, 362, 475, 511
SISTA project, 202
Situational couple violence, 258
6-mercaptopurine, 540
Sjögren's syndrome, 82, 85, 291
SLE. *See* Systemic lupus erythematosus
Sleep disorders, older women and, 478
Sleep position, reducing suffocation in young children and, 44
Small cell carcinoma, 315
Small cell lung cancer, 315, 317
Small for gestational age, age at menarche and, 108
Smallpox, 9
Smoking
    age at puberty and prenatal exposure to, 108
    asthma and, 274, 277
    average years of, before age 40 among women and men by birth cohort, 56
    avoiding, 18
        prevention by, 55–57
    breast cancer and, 341–342, 347
    cancer and, 251–252
    cardiovascular disease, stroke and, 417
    cervical cancer and, 388–389
    colorectal cancer and, 404
    dental disease and, 86
    endometrial cancer and, 378
    fibroids and, 131
    fire and burn fatalities and, 44
    gender and, 250
    health events and, U.S. (1900–1998), *6*
    identifying as leading cause of death, 49
    life span and residual effects of, 472
    lung cancer and, 17, 55–56, 316–317
    lung disease and, 50
    maternal, asthma and, 275
    menopause and, 154, 155
    multiple sclerosis and, 286, 288
    obesity and, trends in, U.S. (1960–2010), 7
    oral cancer and, 87
    osteoporosis and, 459
    ovarian cancer and, 366
    PAR for lung cancer associated with, 26
    percent of smokers engaging in before age 20 by year of birth, *56*
    periodontal disease in teens and, 83
    placental abruption and, 145
    pregnancy and, 140
    premenstrual dysphoric disorder and, 222
    reduced life expectancy and, 53

    reducing, mass media campaigns and, 62–63
    rheumatoid arthritis and, 449–450
    risk of death within 10 years per 1000 men and women by 5 year age groups, *472*
    stillbirths and, 145
    Surgeon General's reports on, 24, 55
    women's health and impact of, 5–7
Smoking cessation programs, 136, 253*t*
    ACA and cost of, 55
    older women and, 472–473, 479
Snow, John, London cholera outbreak and, 17
SNPs. *See* Single nucleotide polymorphisms
Social integration, gender and, 491, 494
Social network, CVD morbidity and mortality and, 419
Social phobias, migraine and, 427
Social roles, posttraumatic stress disorder and, 242
Social Security, 470
Social support
    older women and, 471–472
    systemic lupus erythematosus and, 295
Socioeconomic status
    age at menarche and, 106–107, 109
    asthma and, 274
    colorectal cancer and, 404
    falls and, 501
    heart disease and, 419–421
    older women and, 479
Sodium intake, reducing, blood pressure and, 74
Soluble fiber, 74
Somatic genomic variation, 540–541
Someday Melissa, Inc., 209
Sonograms, breast tumor detection and, 330
South Africa, estimated increase in HIV/AIDS-related deaths in (1994–1999), *196*
Soviet Union, dissolution of, increased adult mortality and, 63
Soy
    public health perspective on use of, 97
    review of therapeutic role of, in menopause, 164
Special Supplemental Nutrition Program for Women, Infants, and Children (WIC), 85
Specificity, 24–25, 26
Spermatogenesis, 116
Spermicides, 118*t*, 120
Spina bifida, 141, 233
Spinal manipulation, 92
Spine fractures, 457, 458
Spine pain, 437–438
    epidemiology of
        low back pain, 437–438
        neck pain, 438
    risk factors for, 438
Sponges, contraceptive, 120
Sports injury morbidity, 45–46
Spousal assault, 257

Squamous cell carcinoma, 315, 316, 385
Stalking, 257, 258
STAR. *See* Study of Tamoxifen and Raloxifene
STAT3, 318
Statins, colorectal cancer and, 406
Statistical power, 29
STDs. *See* Sexually transmitted diseases
STD Surveillance System, 177
Stem cell research, 134
Sterilization, 117, 121, 148
Steroids
    multiple sclerosis and, 287
    systemic lupus erythematosus and, 291, 293
Stillbirths, 145
    DES and, 132*t*
    substance use disorders and, 251
STIs. *See* Sexually transmitted infections
Stockholm Female Coronary Risk Study, 419
Stomach cancer, 11, 28
Stool-based tests, 398
    genetic stool tests, 402
    stool blood tests, 401–402
Stool blood tests, 401–402
    FIT, 402
    gFOBT, 401–402
Strength of the association, 24
Strep mutans, 82
Stress
    age at menarche and, 107
    asthma and, 275
    cardiovascular disease and, 418–419
    depression and, 221
    multiple sclerosis and, 284
    social origins of, 492
Stress buffering model, 489
Stress incontinence, 158, 159, 478
STRIDE study, 160
Stroke, 49
    age-adjusted death rate for, by state, U.S. (2005–2007), *420*
    age-adjusted death rates for, by race/ethnicity and sex, U.S. (1999–2008), *415*
    age-adjusted death rates for, U.S. (1960–2007), *11*
    defined, 414
    dietary salt reduction and projected annual reduction in, 58, *59*
    falls and, 500
    history of, 416
    hypertension and, 58
    ischemic *vs.* hemorrhagic, 413
    migraine and, 431
    older population and, 481
    oral health and, 87
    periodontal disease and, 81, 86
    reducing, diet and, 73
    risk factors for, 415–418
    Women's Health Initiative RCTs, risk of, among women randomized to hormones compared with placebo, 162*t*